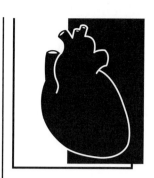

5TH Edition

The Clinical Recognition of Congenital Heart Disease

Joseph K. Perloff, MD

Streisand/American Heart Association Professor of Medicine and Pediatrics,
   Emeritus
Founding Director, Ahmanson/UCLA Adult Congenital Heart Disease Center
UCLA School of Medicine
Los Angeles, California

SAUNDERS

An Imprint of Elsevier

SAUNDERS
An Imprint of Elsevier
The Curtis Center
Independence Square West
Philadelphia, PA 19106

Library of Congress Cataloging-in-Publication Data

The clinical recognition of congenital heart disease / Joseph K. Perloff—5th ed.
   p. ; cm.
Includes bibliographical references and index.
ISBN 0-7216 9730-5
   1. Congenital heart disease—Diagnosis. I. Title.
   [DNLM: 1. Heart Defects, Congenital-diagnosis. WG 220 P451c.2003]
RC6B7.P38 2003
616.12043—dc21   2003042441

Publisher: Anne Lenehan
Publishing Services Manager: Frank Polizzano
Book Designer: Karen O'Keefe Owens

Printed in the United States of America

Last digit is the print number: 9 8 7 6 5 4 3

In memory of my parents,
Rose and Richard,
And with high hopes for
Alexandra, Benjamin and Nicholas

Preface

Because of the advances in knowledge of congenital heart disease since the fourth edition in 1994, each chapter in the fifth edition has undergone significant, if not major revision. There is a new chapter on Congenital Abnormalities of the Pericardium, a topic not formally addressed in other textbooks of congenital heart disease. The historical background of each malformation has been elaborated, and the sections on genetics and developmental biology have been expanded. The original of every figure reprinted from previous editions has been retrieved and digitized to create fifth edition figures that look new. Phonocardiograms have increased in number and quality and represent a unique resource that cannot be duplicated.

Contemporary imaging techniques illustrate anatomic details of both simple and complex malformations. References are up-to-date, but key references to original or important early publications have been retained, increasing the richness of the bibliographies.

Despite high technology diagnostic methods, the *clinical* recognition of congenital heart disease remains an exciting discipline in logical thinking, a stimulating challenge, and a gratifying source of self-education. Therein lies the essence of my book.

JOSEPH K. PERLOFF
LOS ANGELES, CALIFORNIA

Acknowledgments

As in the 4th edition, I begin by recognizing the Streisand Foundation and the American Heart Association that provided me with the resources of an Endowed Chair. I now wish to recognize a second endowment, this one from the Ahmanson Foundation whose largess provided pivotal support for the UCLA Adult Congenital Heart Disease Center. I also acknowledge Judah Hertz and the Hertz Group for generous support of the Center.

Special thanks to special colleagues: Dr John S. Child, Director of the Ahmanson/UCLA Adult Congenital Heart Disease Center; Pamela D. Miner, Nurse Practioner of the Center; Dr Hillel Laks, Chief, Division of Cardiothoracic Surgery; Dr Thomas Klitzner, Chief, Division of Pediatric Cardiology; and to my pediatric cardiology colleagues for fostering an atmosphere of collaboration that made it possible for congenital heart disease to be looked upon as a continuum from birth to adulthood.

As I did in the past editions, I acknowledge Marjorie Gabrielle Perloff who has served as a model of scholarly integrity and academic achievement, who has determined my standards, and who remains my most effective critic. Her tolerance of my many idiosyncrasies was not the least of her many virtues.

JOSEPH K. PERLOFF
LOS ANGELES, CALIFORNIA

Contents

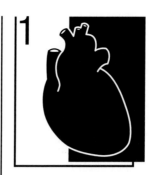

Introduction: Formulation of the Problem

The disaster that Hesiod sees threatening a community that disregards justice . . . is not an eternity of damnation but the failure of nature to work—of crops to grow, of herds to bear, of women to produce normal children.[6]

Congenital heart disease has been defined as "present at birth" (*con*, "together"; *genitus*, "born"). However, the implication that *congenital* simply refers to a gross structural abnormality of the heart, great arteries, or great veins that is "present at birth" requires qualification and elaboration. The heart is the first organ to form in vertebrate embryos[8,12] and has been characterized as the "youngest, most diverse, most fluid, most changeable, most versatile part of creation" (Goethe).[15] Beginning about embryonic day 20 in the human fetus, progenitor cells within the lateral plate mesoderm become committed to a cardiogenic fate.[12] The timing and location of cardiogenic lineage specification and determination in vertebrate embryos occurs at gastrulation, if not earlier.[8]

The majority of congenital cardiac malformations compatible with 6 months of intrauterine life permit live offspring at term. A given malformation may exist in relative harmony with the fetal circulation, only to be modified considerably, at least physiologically, by the dramatic circulatory adjustments at birth.[11] Weeks, months, or years may elapse before the anomaly reveals itself as "typical." Physiologic and structural changes may continue (a congenitally bicuspid aortic valve that is functionally normal at birth may take decades to fibrose, calcify, and present as overt aortic stenosis), or conversely, the malformation may "vanish" (spontaneous closure of a ventricular septal defect, or delayed closure of a patent ductus in premature infants). Thus, congenital heart diseases are not fixed anatomic defects that appear at birth but instead are dynamic anomalies that originate in the early embryo, evolve during gestation, and change considerably during the course of extrauterine life. Certain defects that are actually or potentially of functional significance are not gross structural malformations. Examples include major congenital electrophysiologic abnormalities, such as complete heart block, either isolated (see Chapter 4) or with congenitally corrected transposition of the great arteries (see Chapter 6) or left isomerism (see Chapter 3); Wolff-Parkinson-White preexcitation either isolated or complicated (see Chapter 13); absence of a sinus node and hence absence of sinus rhythm, as with superior vena cava sinus venosus atrial septal defect (see Chapter 15) or left isomerism (see Chapter 3); and ventricular tachycardia as with the long QT syndromes,[3] or arrhythmogenic right ventricular dysplasia (see Chapter 13). Still other abnormalities, such as Marfan syndrome which results from mutations in the FBN1 gene that encodes fibrillin-1, are actually or potentially of functional significance but may not be manifest at birth as a gross structural malformation and, as a matter of convention, are generally not classified as congenital heart disease.[10] Finally, there are a handful of odd defects that tend to escape inclusion, such as congenital kinking of the internal carotid artery.[7]

In light of the intimate interplay between congenital malformations of the heart and the fetal circulation, let us now turn to the fetal circulation per se, and the remarkable circulatory changes that occur at birth.[9,11] In utero patterns of blood flow have been determined in fetal lambs after insertion of catheters into limb vessels,[11] and in utero left and right ventricular outputs and flow distributions through the foramen ovale, ductus arteriosus, and pulmonary bed have been determined in human fetuses with high-resolution color Doppler ultrasonography.[1,9] In the fetus, the right and left ventricles do not function in series as they do in the normal extrauterine circulation. Gas exchange occurs in the placenta, not in the lungs. About two thirds of the right ventricular output is diverted away from the lungs through the widely patent ductus arteriosus into the descending thoracic aorta, from which a large portion enters the umbilical circulation for oxygenation in the placenta. Pulmonary blood flow is low but meets nutritional requirements for growth of the lungs. Inferior vena cava blood, which is a composite from the umbilical vein, the left and right hepatic veins, the ductus venosus, and the distal inferior vena cava, streams in the direction of the foramen ovale, assisted by the eustachian valve, and enters the left atrium and then the left ventricle. About 60% of umbilical venous return that is oxygenated in the placenta bypasses the liver through the ductus venosus and enters the inferior vena cava and right atrium. Blood from the superior vena cava is deflected within the right atrium toward the tricuspid valve, across which it enters the right ventricle. About 70% of the relatively oxygen-rich blood ejected from the left ventricle is distributed to the coronary circulation (and thus the myocardium), the head and neck (and thus the brain), and the forelimbs. Almost 90% of the relatively oxygen-poor blood ejected by the right ventricle passes through the ductus arteriosus into the descending aorta to be oxygenated in the placenta. Accordingly, the fetal circulation is designed so that blood with higher oxygen saturation preferentially reaches the myocardium and brain, and less saturated blood preferentially reaches the placenta.

Remarkable circulatory changes occur at birth. The umbilical/placental circulation is eliminated, the lungs expand, rhythmic ventilation commences, oxygen tension rises as alveolar fluid is eliminated and ambient air is breathed, pulmonary vascular resistance falls, and pulmonary blood flow increases 8- to 10-fold, thus increasing venous return to the left atrium. Left atrial pressure rises, the valve of the foramen ovale closes, and the ductus arteriosus functionally closes (constricts) within hours after birth, effectively separating the pulmonary and systemic circulations.[11] These profound birth-related changes occur almost simultaneously.

A number of important delayed events complete the transition from the fetal circulation to the maturing circulation after birth. During the course of gestation, pulmonary vascular resistance falls progressively as new resistant arterioles develop. Regulation of the perinatal pulmonary circulation reflects a complex interplay between vasoconstrictor and vasodilator factors, but the net effect is the dramatic increase in pulmonary blood flow initiated by expansion of the lungs and rhythmic ventilation at birth that reflects a shift from active pulmonary vasoconstriction in the fetus to active vasodilatation in the neonate.[11] Failure of this shift to occur results in persistent fetal circulation (pulmonary hypertension) of the newborn (see Chapter 14). The thick-walled fetal pulmonary arterioles are designed to meet the full force of systemic right ventricular pressure the instant the lungs expand. As respiration is established, there is a marked increase in alveolar and systemic arterial oxygen tensions, to which pulmonary arterioles are exquisitely sensitive, setting the stage for dilatation and involution of the fetal arterioles. The large pulmonary arteries also play a role, although a much lesser one, in determining the total drop in pressure across the lungs.

Maturational changes have an impact on the neonatal disparity in size between the main and branch pulmonary arteries, as well as on the angulation at the origins of the right and left branches (see Chapter 11). Both of these factors are responsible for a physiologic drop in pressure distal to the pulmonary trunk. Another important delayed change relates to the fetal right ventricle, which slowly loses its relative thickness. With the stimulus of afterload eliminated, there is a gradual reduction in right ventricular wall thickness relative to the ventricular septum and left ventricle. The neonatal right ventricle does not undergo regression but instead does not increase its mass as rapidly as the left ventricle in the growing infant. Normal physiologic adaptations at birth are remarkable in their own right. It is therefore not surprising that congenital malformations of the heart or circulation will, to varying degrees, interact with or be modified by extrauterine life.

The principle to be extracted is clear. The anatomy and physiology of the heart and circulation in the presence of congenital heart disease change with the passage of time from the fetus to the neonate to the infant, child, adolescent, and adult. Some of these changes result in neonatal death, whereas others express themselves gradually over weeks, months, years, or even decades. A realistic comprehension of the clinical manifestations—and therefore the *clinical recognition*—of congenital heart disease requires that these various patterns be taken into account.

The clinical diagnosis of congenital malformations of the heart and circulation represents the epitome of applied logic. When correct inferences are drawn from accurate observations, diagnoses emerge with gratifying frequency. "One of the most wondrous features of animate nature must surely be the perfect harmony existing between structure and function."[14] No mammalian organ system better exemplifies this principle than the heart and circulation. In this book, the clinical expressions of congenital heart disease are dealt with in terms of the anatomic and physiologic mechanisms responsible for their production. Logical thought is encouraged and memorization minimized. In each chapter, the gross morphology is first established in order to shed light on the physiologic derangements. The question is then asked: What clinical manifestations might result from these anatomic and physiologic derangements? The stage is then set for *clinical recognition* (diagnosis)—the thesis of this book—which depends on a synthesis of information from the history, the physical signs, the electrocardiogram, and the chest x-ray.

The *history*, which is really an *interview*, is designed to extract important information and benefits from studying the techniques used by professional interviewers on television.

Physical diagnosis consists of a synthesis of information from five sources: physical appearance, the arterial pulse, the jugular venous pulse, precordial percussion, movement and palpation, and auscultation.[13] It is relevant that the stethoscope is the oldest cardiovascular diagnostic instrument in continuous clinical use.

The *electrocardiogram* (developed in 1903 by Willem Einthoven), when read carefully and interpreted in clinical context, provides gratifying diagnostic insights, even in cases of complex congenital heart disease. Meticulous sequential attention must be devoted to the P wave, the P duration, the PR interval, the QRS, the QT interval, and the T wave. The names of the waves in the electrocardiogram have been attributed to Rene Descartes, 18th century French philosopher and scientist[5] who was surely known to Einthoven.

The *chest x-ray* (developed in 1895 by Wilhelm Conrad Roentgen) must also be read meticulously, both posteroanterior and lateral views, according to a planned sequence that minimizes inadvertent oversight: technique (penetration, rotation, degree of inhalation), age and sex of the patient, right/left orientation, thoracic and abdominal situs positions and malpositions (above and below the diaphragm), the bones, the extrapulmonary soft tissue densities, the intrapulmonary soft tissue densities (vascular and parenchymal), the great arteries and great veins, the atria, and the ventricles. There is much to be said for learning radiologic interpretation by reading x-rays with professional chest radiologists. As with the electrocardiogram, so too with the chest x-ray: the amount of diagnostic information that can be extracted is gratifying.

It is axiomatic that emphasis should be placed on the relationship of *the parts to the whole*, a relationship that ideally results in a harmonious picture devoid of contradictions, rather than a collection of loosely related observations. Maximum information should be extracted from each clinical source while relating information from one source to that of another. A simple principle emerges: on the one hand, depth and refinement, on the other hand, synthesis. Each step should advance our thinking and narrow the diagnostic possibilities. By the end of the clinical assessment, untenable considerations should have been discarded, the possibilities retained for further consideration, and the probabilities brought into focus. This process reflects Herophilus' adage that the best physician is one who is able to distinguish between the possible and the impossible.

Once a diagnostic consideration is reached from an analysis of the initial step in the clinical assessment, that impression necessarily influences the objectivity with which subsequent steps are appraised. Thus, if the same sequence of evaluation is always employed, the later steps cannot be objectively evaluated. It is therefore useful to vary the sequence with which information is assembled. Begin, for example, by reading the chest x-ray or electrocardiogram; or, with infants, it is often practical to take advantage of temporary periods of calm and start with the physical examination, which shortly may be difficult or impossible to perform. It is not the sequence that matters but rather the depth and synthesis of analysis. Irrespective

of how the order of information access is arranged, two questions must always be asked: How does one step relate to the next? How do the parts relate to the whole?

Diagnostic thinking benefits from employing the devices of *anticipation* and *supposition*. Anticipate what the next step might reveal. After drawing tentative conclusions from the history, it is useful to pause and ask: If these assumptions are correct, what can I expect from the physical examination, or what specific points might I anticipate in the electrocardiogram or x-ray to support or refute the initial impressions? The device of anticipation not only helps achieve synthesis of a given step with the next but also heightens interest as the clinical assessment progresses. As a result, confirmation comes as a source of satisfaction, and errors stand out in bold relief. Nor should we be afraid of mistakes. The truth emerges sooner from error than from confusion.

The anatomic and physiologic basis and the clinical manifestations of congenital heart disease are best understood when information is handled within the framework of an orderly classification. The classification system given in Table 1–1 and in Figure 1–1 and Figure 1–2 is employed because it is practical, clinically accurate, and applicable irrespective of which source of information one is dealing

Table 1–1	Clinical Classification of Congenital Heart Disease

General

Innocent or normal murmurs

Cardiac malpositions

Ventricular inversion (congenitally corrected transposition of the great arteries)

Complete heart block

Acyanotic without a shunt (normal or decreased pulmonary arterial blood flow)

Malformations originating in the right side of the heart (from most proximal to most distal)

Malformations originating in the left side of the heart (from most proximal to most distal)

Acyanotic with a shunt (left to right, increased pulmonary arterial blood flow)

Shunt at atrial level

Shunt at ventricular level

Shunt between aortic root and right side of heart

Shunt at aortopulmonary level

Shunts at more than one level

Cyanotic

Increased pulmonary arterial blood flow

Normal or decreased pulmonary arterial blood flow

Dominant left ventricle

Dominant right ventricle

With pulmonary hypertension

Without pulmonary hypertension

Normal or nearly normal ventricles

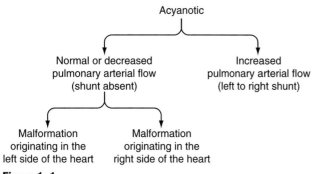

Figure 1–1
Algorithm for diagnosis in acyanotic patients.

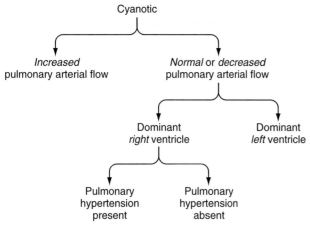

Figure 1–2
Algorithm for diagnosis in cyanotic patients.

with. There are shortcomings in any classification system, but shortcomings should not obscure the value of a practical, orderly approach. The fact that a number of defects are listed in more than one category emphasizes the variability of their clinical expressions. A similar classification was proposed by Paul Wood decades ago and is based essentially on answers to five questions (Table 1–2). It is not necessary to ask all five questions in each case, although the first two questions are obligatory. When approached according to the principles espoused, the clinical recognition of congenital heart disease is at once a stimulating challenge, a satisfying discipline in logical thinking, and a constant source of self-education. The intensity of inquiry and the analytical standards employed at the bedside should be the same as in the diagnostic or research laboratory.

Table 1–2	Five Basic Questions

1. Is the patient acyanotic or cyanotic?
2. Is pulmonary arterial blood flow increased or not?
3. Does the malformation originate in the left or right side of the heart?
4. Which is the dominant ventricle?
5. Is pulmonary hypertension present or not?

The Preface to the first edition contained the statement, "I hope to stimulate clinicians to use the tools at their disposal (the history, physical examination, electrocardiogram, and chest x-ray) and to feel that many insights can be gained apart from the laboratory." The Preface to the third edition contained the statement, "Two-dimensional echocardiography was in its infancy when the second edition appeared but is now a routine laboratory procedure along with the electrocardiogram and chest x-ray." Cardiac catheterization and angiography were the first major diagnostic steps forward, followed by transthoracic and transesophageal echocardiography. Now cine magnetic resonance imaging (MRI), three-dimensional reconstruction of gadolinium-enhanced magnetic resonance angiography, and three-dimensional computed tomographic angiography provide exquisite anatomic detail and refined physiologic information.

In light of these advances in imaging techniques, and with the prospect of even more advanced methods in the offing, does my emphasis on the history, physical examination, electrocardiogram, chest x-ray, and transthoracic echocardiogram remain acceptable? "Intelligent selection of investigative procedures from the ever-increasing array of tests now available requires far more sophisticated decision-making than was necessary when the choices were limited to electrocardiography and chest roentgenography. The clinical examination provides the critical information necessary for most of these decisions. With the increasing emphasis on the cost of medical care, it is likely that there will be a resurgence of interest in the relatively inexpensive and absolutely safe clinical examination."[2]

Several additional points need to be made. First, the term *natural history* is not used. The *Oxford Dictionary of Natural History* defines the term *natural* as "a community that would develop if human influences were removed completely and permanently." More relevant is Julien Hoffman's definition: "The natural history of any disease is a description of what happens to people with the disease who do not receive treatment for it."[4] Accordingly, *natural history* is not synonymous with "unoperated," and *unnatural history* is not synonymous with "postoperative." Longevity patterns based on the benefits of nonsurgical therapeutic armamentariums that include pharmacologic resources, pacemakers, defibrillators, and interventional catheterization can hardly be considered natural. Second, traditional considerations of *differential diagnoses* are not employed. Instead, each chapter ends with a concise summary of the principal manifestations that permit clinical recognition of the congenital anomaly covered in the text. These summaries bring together highlights of the clinical features of each malformation and serve as reminders for the reader's convenience. Finally, a comment on *terminology*, which is always a contentious topic. The terms used to describe congenital malformations of the heart and circulation include the older latinized terminology and the more recent anglicized terminology. Attempts to "purify" either latinized or anglicized versions by excluding the other have not succeeded. The vocabulary of congenital heart disease is replete with abbreviations understood only by the initiated. Accordingly, when abbreviations find their way into the text, they will first be defined for the reader's enlightenment, but full terms will then be used. New terms are not used when old terms suffice, which is usually the case. Acronyms, which are generally self-serving, are avoided. Importantly, the Third World Congress of Pediatric Cardiology and Cardiac Surgery in Toronto hosted an International Summit on Nomenclature for Congenital Heart Disease that may help us all.

I have tried to ensure that the material in this book is understood by a relatively broad audience. The words that I have chosen—terminology or nomenclature—were as assiduously addressed as grammar and syntax and were based on decades of personal experience. My principal objectives have always been to excite interest and to be understood.

REFERENCES

1. Alcazar JL, Rovira J, Ruiz-Perez ML, Lopez-Garcia G: Transvaginal color Doppler assessment of fetal circulation in normal early pregnancy. Fetal Diagn Ther 12:178, 1997.

2. Braunwald E: Foreword. In Perloff JK (ed): Physical Examination of the Heart and Circulation. Philadelphia, WB Saunders, 2000.

3. Chiang C, Roden DM: The long QT syndromes: Genetic basis and clinical implications. J Am Coll Cardiol 36:1, 2000.

4. Hoffman JIE: Reflections on the past, present and future of pediatric cardiology. Cardiol Young 4:208, 1994.

5. Hurst JW: Naming of the waves in the ECG, with a brief account of their genesis. Circulation 98:1937, 1998.

6. Jameson MH: A Greek countryside. Report from the Argolid exploration project. Expedition—The Magazine of Archeology/Anthropology 19:2, 1976.

7. Le Bret E, Pineau E, Folliguet T, et al: Congenital kinking of the internal carotid artery in twin brothers. Circulation 102:173, 2000.

8. Lyons GE: Vertebrate heart development. Curr Opin Genet Dev 6:454, 1996.

9. Mielke G, Benda N: Cardiac output and central distribution of blood flow in the human fetus. Circulation 103:1662, 2001.

10. Milewicz DM: Molecular genetics of Marfan syndrome and Ehlers-Danlos type IV. Curr Opin Cardiol 13:198, 1998.

11. Moller JH, Hoffman JE (eds): Pediatric Cardiovascular Medicine. New York, Churchill Livingstone, 2000.

12. Olson EN, Srivastava D: Molecular pathways controlling heart development. Science 272:671, 1996.

13. Perloff JK: The Physical Examination of the Heart and Circulation. Philadelphia, WB Saunders, 2000.

14. Qvist G: John Hunter 1728–1793. London, William Heinemann Medical Books, 1981.

15. Williams JR: The Life of Goethe. Oxford, Blackwell Publishers, 1998.

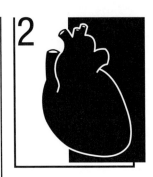

2

Normal or Innocent Murmurs

Murmurs that occur in the absence of either morphologic or physiologic abnormalities of the heart or circulation have been called *normal, innocent, functional, physiologic,* or *benign. Normal* is perhaps the best term because it is unambiguous.[25] Normal murmurs are common, are virtually ubiquitous in children, and can with few exceptions be diagnosed by the physical examination alone. The index of suspicion is the murmur itself. Auscultation is otherwise normal, and the history, physical appearance, arterial pulse, jugular venous pulse, precordial palpation, electrocardiogram, chest x-ray, and echocardiogram are normal.[17]

There are seven types of normal systolic murmurs and three types of normal continuous murmurs (Table 2–1). Normal systolic murmurs include the vibratory murmur, the main pulmonary artery murmur, the branch pulmonary artery murmur of the neonate, the supraclavicular systolic murmur, the systolic mammary souffle, the aortic systolic murmur of older adults, and the cardiorespiratory systolic murmur. All normal systolic murmurs except the mammary souffle are midsystolic and are not loudest at the right base.[52] Normal continuous murmurs include the venous hum, the continuous mammary souffle, and the continuous cephalic (cranial) murmur (see Table 2–1).

Normal murmurs are not solely diastolic, with one exception—the transient left basal holodiastolic or mid-diastolic ductus arteriosus murmur sometimes heard during the first 3 or 4 days of life.[48] A valvelike structure at the pulmonary artery end of the ductus (see Chapter 20) is held responsible for selective diastolic flow.[35,48]

Normal Systolic Murmurs

THE VIBRATORY SYSTOLIC MURMUR

The vibratory midsystolic murmur was described by George F. Still in 1909 (Fig. 2–1 and Fig. 2–2).[66] Still wrote, "It is heard usually just below the level of the nipple, and about halfway between the left margin of the sternum and the vertical nipple line. . . .Its characteristic feature is a twanging sound very like that made by twanging a piece of tense string. . . .Whatever may be its origin, I think it is clearly functional, that is to say, not due to any organic disease either congenital or acquired."

Still's murmur is seldom heard in infants[4] but is prevalent after the age of 3 years, with diminishing frequency toward adolescence.[15,18,30] The murmur ranges from grade 1 to 3 of 6 and is loudest between the apex and lower left sternal edge in the supine position.[8,18,38,59,69] During exercise, excitement, or fever, the murmur intensifies (see Fig. 2–1).[18] The quality is distinctive[18,23]: vibratory or buzzing with a uniform, medium, pure frequency (70 to 130 cycles per second)[27] requiring the stethoscopic bell for best assessment.[8,52] The closest acoustic analogy is Still's twanging of a taut rubber band or string. The murmur begins shortly after the first heart sound and is typically confined to the first half of systole with a relatively long gap between the end of the murmur and the second heart sound (see Figs. 2–1 and 2–2).

The mechanism of Still's murmur remains to be established, but theories must take into account the distinctive frequency composition and configuration, location on the chest wall, and the incidence according to age. The pure

Table 2–1	Normal Murmurs

Systolic

    The vibratory systolic murmur of Still

    The pulmonary artery systolic murmur

    The branch pulmonary artery systolic murmur

    The supraclavicular systolic murmur

    The systolic mammary souffle

    The aortic sclerotic systolic murmur

    The cardiorespiratory systolic murmur

Continuous

    The venous hum

    The continuous mammary souffle

    The cephalic continuous murmur

medium frequency implies that a cardiac structure is set into periodic vibration during ventricular systole. Origin in the right side of the heart has been assigned to the pulmonary valve itself when "trigonoidation" of the leaflets results in periodic vibrations of the base of the cusps.[30,42] A catheter across the pulmonary valve can tense the cusps and generate a transient pure-frequency midsystolic murmur (Fig. 2–3B). The relatively low right ventricular ejection pressure and velocity are believed to cause the attachments of the pulmonary cusps to vibrate at a low to medium frequency. A murmur produced by a vibrating semilunar valve at its arterial attachment tends to be trans-

mitted into the cavity of the concordant ventricle,[20,51,52,57] which could account for the thoracic location of Still's murmur between the apex and lower left sternal edge— that is, topographically over the right ventricle. In children with Still's murmur, Doppler echocardiography has identified systolic vibrations in the aortic valve and higher maximum acceleration of flow in the left ventricular outflow tract.[36,61,69] However, a murmur originating in a vibrating aortic valve would be transmitted into the left ventricular cavity and heard best over the left ventricular impulse. Midsystolic murmurs in adults have been ascribed to high intraventricular velocities generated by vigorous left ventricular contraction associated with an increase in left ventricular mass.[63]

The origin of Still's murmur has also been assigned to the left ventricular cavity, a location that is in accord with delayed response to the Valsalva maneuver.[2] Left ventricular bands or false tendons (Fig. 2–3A) are believed to vibrate periodically during ventricular systole and transmit their vibrations to the chest wall.[13,40,53] A high percentage of patients with Still's murmur reportedly have left ventricular bands, especially in the outflow tract.[13,22,40,53] However, the prevalence of Still's murmur declines from childhood to adolescence,[18,30] whereas the prevalence of left ventricular bands is the same in children, adolescents, and adults.[13,21,40] The incidence of Still's murmur is believed to exceed the incidence of left ventricular bands,[69] although the incidence depends largely on the avidity with which bands are sought with echocardiography.

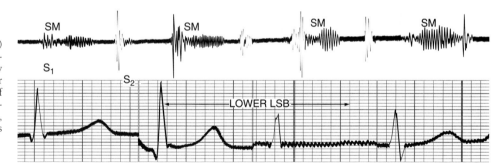

Figure 2–1

Vibratory midsystolic murmurs (SM) from four normal children. The murmurs are pure frequency, relatively brief, and maximal along the lower left sternal border (LSB). The last of the four murmurs was from a 5-year-old febrile girl. After defervescence, the murmur decreased in loudness and duration.

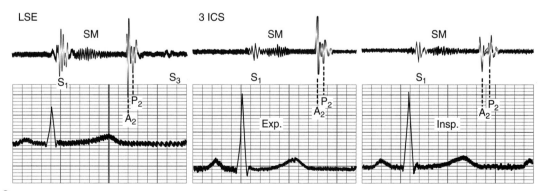

Figure 2–2

A vibratory midsystolic murmur (SM) from a normal 7-year-old boy. The murmur is maximal along the lower left sternal edge (LSE) and is accompanied by a physiologic third heart sound (S_3) and normal respiratory splitting of the second heart sound. A_2/P_2, aortic and pulmonary components; 3ICS, third intercostal space.

THE PULMONARY ARTERY SYSTOLIC MURMUR

The normal systolic murmur in the main pulmonary artery is most prevalent in children, adolescents, and young adults.[8,18,52] The murmur is midsystolic, with maximum intensity in the second left intercostal space next to the sternum (Fig. 2–4), and ranges from bare audibility to grade 3/6 in response to exercise, fever, or excitement. The frequency composition is medium-pitched and impure, best heard in the supine position with the stethoscopic diaphragm or moderate pressure of the bell during full held exhalation.[8,18,59] The murmur represents normal ejection vibrations that reach the threshold of audibility from within the main pulmonary

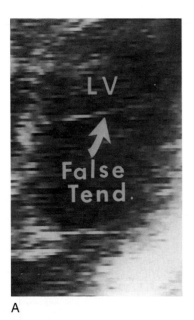

A

artery during right ventricular systole. The chest wall location is appropriate for origin in the pulmonary trunk, and intracardiac phonocardiograms record midsystolic murmurs within the pulmonary trunk in normal young subjects.[39]

These murmurs are commonly heard during pregnancy and in subjects with anemia or hyperthyroidism. Loss of thoracic kyphosis increases the proximity of the pulmonary trunk to the chest wall and increases the incidence of pulmonary systolic murmurs in the second left interspace.[14]

THE BRANCH PULMONARY ARTERY SYSTOLIC MURMUR

Branch pulmonary artery systolic murmurs are occasionally heard in normal neonates, especially premature neonates.[3,12,58] These murmurs are typically grade 1 to 2/6 and are medium-pitched and impure but, most importantly, are distributed to the left and right anterior chest, axillae, and back. The similarity of frequency composition to breath sounds, the rapid respiratory rate of infants, and the nonprecordial locations of pulmonary artery systolic murmurs cause oversight. Audibility is improved if respiration is momentarily arrested by pinching the nostrils while the infant sucks a pacifier. Auscultation is best carried out by examining the infant in both the supine and prone positions and by using the stethoscopic diaphragm applied to the right and left anterior chest, back, and axillae. The murmurs are typically confined to neonates, are usually absent at the first well-baby examination, and seldom persist beyond 3 to 6 months of age.[1,58,59]

The transient branch pulmonary artery systolic murmur in normal neonates is indistinguishable from the peripheral murmur of fixed stenosis of the pulmonary

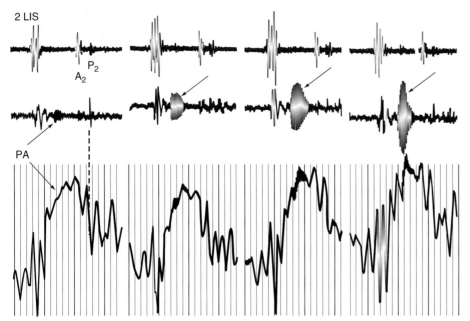

B

Figure 2–3

A, Echocardiogram (apical view) from a 12-year-old boy with a left ventricular (LV) false tendon that was an incidental finding. The boy did *not* have Still's murmur. *B*, Phonocardiogram recorded from within the main pulmonary artery (PT) distal to a normal pulmonary valve. The catheter transiently tensed the pulmonary cusps, setting them into pure-frequency periodic vibration (*arrows*).

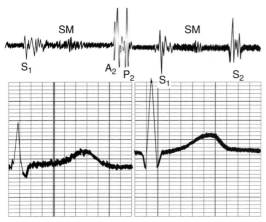

Figure 2–4

Pulmonary artery systolic murmurs (SM) recorded from the second left intercostal space of two normal children aged 8 and 11 years. The murmurs are brief, midsystolic, and mixed frequency.

artery and its branches (see Chapter 11). The analogy sheds light on the mechanism of production.[3,12,58] The pulmonary trunk in the fetus is a relatively dilated domed structure because it receives the output of the high-pressure right ventricle. Proximal right and left pulmonary arteries arise from the pulmonary trunk as comparatively small lateral branches that receive a paucity of intrauterine blood flow. When the lungs expand at birth, the difference in size between the pulmonary trunk and its right and left branches transiently persists, especially in premature infants (Fig. 2–5).[1] In addition to the disparity in size, the branches arise at relatively sharp angles from the inferior and posterior walls of the pulmonary trunk. These anatomic arrangements account for both the turbulence and the physiologic drop in systolic pressure from pulmonary trunk to proximal branches and for generation of the branch pulmonary artery systolic murmur.[12,58]

THE SUPRACLAVICULAR SYSTOLIC MURMUR

Normal supraclavicular systolic arterial murmurs are typically heard in children and young adults, are always maximal above the clavicles, are generally bilateral but tend to be louder on the right, and are prominent in the suprasternal notch (Fig. 2–6).[52,64] The weight of evidence assigns supraclavicular systolic murmurs to the aortic origins of major brachiocephalic arteries, especially the subclavians.[19,52] Intensity can reach grade 4/6,

Figure 2–5

Casts from the pulmonary arteries of two lambs at 12 hours and 4 months of age. There is a decrease in the ratio of the size of the pulmonary trunk to its branches and a loss of acute angulation of the branches. (From Danilowicz DA, Rudolf AM, Hoffman JIE, Heymann M: Physiologic pressure differences between the main and branch pulmonary arteries in infants. Circulation 45:410, 1972; by permission of the American Heart Association, Inc.)

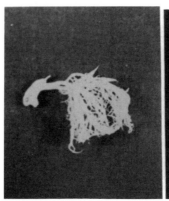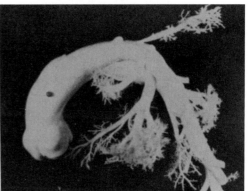

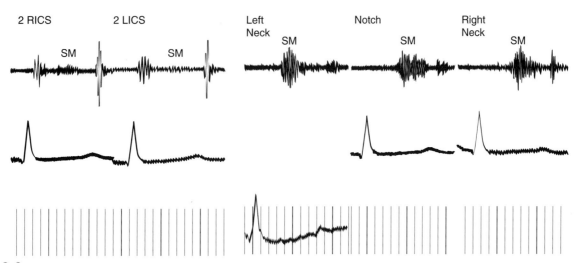

Figure 2–6

A supraclavicular systolic murmur (SM) in a normal 8-year-old girl. Maximal intensity is above the clavicles (left neck, right neck). Onset is abrupt, duration is brief, and timing is maximal in the first half of systole. The murmur is well recorded in the suprasternal notch. There is radiation to the second right and left intercostal spaces (2 RICS, 2 LICS) but with considerable attenuation.

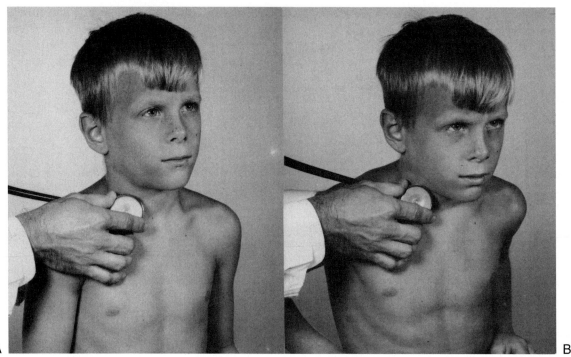

A   B

Figure 2–7

A, Shoulder maneuvers for assessing normal supraclavicular systolic murmurs. Auscultation is initially performed while the patient sits with shoulders relaxed and arms in front of the chest. *B,* When the elbows are brought well behind the back, hyperextending the shoulders, the supraclavicular murmur diminishes or disappears.

may generate a thrill, and may be sufficient for radiation below the clavicles but with distinct attenuation (see Fig. 2–6). The configuration of the supraclavicular systolic murmur is crescendo-decrescendo, the onset is abrupt, the duration is brief, and the timing is maximal in the first half or two thirds of systole (see Fig. 2–6). The frequency composition is uneven, but the murmur is seldom noisy even when loud. Partial compression of the subclavian artery intensifies the murmur, whereas compression sufficient to obliterate the ipsilateral radial pulse has the opposite effect.

Auscultation is most effectively carried out when the patient is sitting upright and looking straight ahead with shoulders relaxed and forearms and hands on the lap (Fig. 2–7A).[44,52] The stethoscopic bell is applied above the medial aspect of the right clavicle. The shoulders are then hyperextended with the elbows brought sharply behind the back until the shoulder girdle muscles are taut (Fig. 2–7B). When this maneuver is done smoothly but rapidly, the supraclavicular murmur diminishes considerably or disappears altogether.[44]

THE SYSTOLIC MAMMARY SOUFFLE

The souffle is either confined to systole or is louder in systole even when continuous (see later). As the name implies, the murmur is heard over the breasts late in pregnancy but especially postpartum in lactating women (Fig. 2–8). The systolic component was recognized by van den Bergh in 1908.[68] The murmur begins distinctly after the first heart sound because sufficient time must elapse from left ventricular ejection to arrival at the artery of origin.

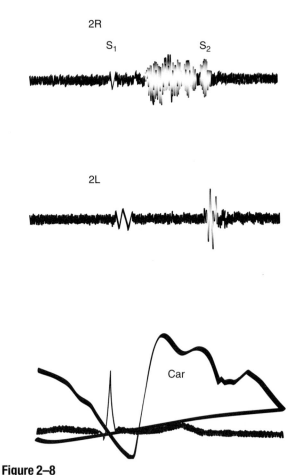

Figure 2–8

Systolic mammary souffle in the second right intercostal space (2R) of a normal 24-year-old lactating woman. The murmur begins at a distinct interval after the first heart sound (S_1), is crescendo-decrescendo, and fades toward the second heart sound (S_2). 2L, second left intercostal space; Car, carotid.

The length of the murmur ranges from short (midsystolic), to long (up to the second heart sound), to beyond the second heart sound into diastole (continuous; see later).

THE AORTIC SYSTOLIC MURMUR IN OLDER ADULTS

The most common form of normal midsystolic murmur in older adults is caused by fibrous or fibrocalcific thickening of the bases of inherently normal aortic cusps as they insert into the sinuses of Valsalva (Fig. 2–9B).[5,16,54] As long as the fibrous or fibrocalcific thickening is confined to the base of the leaflets, the cusps move well, so there is no functional deficit. These structural alterations of inherently normal trileaflet aortic valves affect 20% to 25% of adults older than 65 years.[5,29,47,50,52,54,65] The fibrous, ridgelike thickenings that are initially confined to the base of the aortic cusps may subsequently extend to the free edges as fibrocalcific changes without commissural fusion. Because the initial morphologic alterations do not impair cusp mobility and therefore do not cause obstruction, the accompanying murmur has been called the functionally normal aortic sclerotic systolic murmur of older age. Intra-arterial phonocardiography has identified midsystolic murmurs above the aortic valve before there is audibility on the chest wall in clinically normal adults older than 40 years.[65]

The fully developed aortic sclerotic murmur has two mechanisms and represents a combination of two murmurs. The murmur in the second right intercostal space is midsystolic, impure, and grade 2 or 3/6 and originates within the aortic root (mixed-frequency ejection vibrations of nonlaminar flow). The murmur heard over the left ventricular impulse is midsystolic, pure high-frequency musical, and grade 2 to 3/6 and originates from periodic vibrations of the bases of aortic cusps and their stiffened sinus of Valsalva attachments (Fig. 2–9).[5,51,52,57] These periodic vibrations have been recorded from aortic valve leaflets with M-mode echocardiography.[52] Intracardiac phonocardiography detects the musical high-frequency murmur within the left ventricular cavity and detects the harsh, impure, right basal murmur within the aortic root (Gallavardin dissociation) (see Fig. 2–9A).[20,52] What begins as a functionally benign aortic sclerotic murmur can culminate in severe calcific aortic stenosis. In adults with increased anteroposterior chest dimensions, the precordial murmur of calcific aortic stenosis can be deceptively soft and is best heard in the suprasternal notch.[52]

There is reason to believe that the essential morphologic substrate for the development of aortic sclerosis on an inherently normal trileaflet aortic valve is cuspal inequality, a congenital variation of normal, as originally proposed by Roberts.[56] The ideal aortic valve is equipped with cusps of identical size so that closing forces are equally distributed on the aortic surfaces of the three leaflets. Congenital variations in aortic leaflet size—cuspal inequality—is the rule rather than the exception and results in unequal distribution of tension during valve closure, the long-term effects of which are believed to culminate in the morphologic changes of aortic sclero-

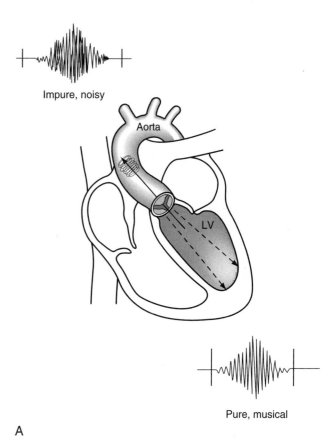

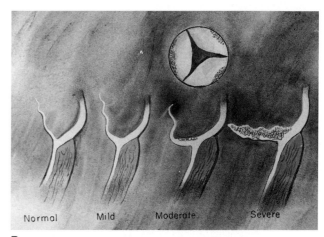

Figure 2–9

A, Illustration of Gallavardin dissociation of the two murmurs associated with fibrocalcific aortic stenosis of an inherently normal trileaflet aortic valve. The impure midsystolic murmur at the right base originates within the aortic root because of turbulence caused by the high-velocity jet. The pure musical midsystolic murmur at the apex originates from periodic high-frequency vibrations of the fibrocalcific aortic leaflets and radiates into the left ventricular cavity (LV). *B*, Schematic illustrations that begin with the normal attachment of an aortic cusp to its sinus of Valsalva (*left*). The initial alteration is a ridge-like fibrous thickening at the base of the aortic cusp as it inserts into its sinus. Calcium is subsequently deposited on the aortic surface of the leaflet (*severe*), converting an inherently normal trileaflet valve into calcific aortic stenosis.

sis/stenosis.[70] At its inception, the process is functionally benign, although there is a reported association between aortic valve sclerosis and cardiovascular mortality and morbidity.[47]

Echocardiography can detect focal areas of increased echogenicity and thickening at aortic cusp attachments to the sinuses of Valsalva without restriction of leaflet motion.[47] The auscultatory diagnosis of aortic sclerosis (see earlier) requires nothing more than proper use of a stethoscope.

THE FUNCTIONALLY NORMAL BICUSPID AORTIC VALVE

More than 400 years ago, Leonardo da Vinci sketched and described the bicuspid aortic valve.[45] He wrote, "Diagrams to illustrate . . . the triangular shape of the aortic aperture. In fig. 2 the customary three cusps are illustrated. In fig. 3 only two cusps fill the orifice."[45] *Functionally normal* refers to a bicuspid aortic valve that has the trivial gradient and the trivial regurgitation inherent in a mechanism equipped with two rather than three leaflets. A bicuspid aortic valve at birth is either functionally normal, intrinsically stenotic, can become "thick and unyielding," or conversely can become incompetent so that "blood which has entered the aorta is allowed to regurgitate into the ventricle," as Thomas Peacock observed in 1858.[49] William Osler in 1866 called attention to the susceptibility of bicuspid aortic valves to infective endocarditis.[46]

Because of potential hazards, it is important to distinguish the murmur of a functionally normal congenitally bicuspid aortic valve from normal systolic murmurs that prevail in the same age group. Normal systolic murmurs in young persons, with the exception of a systolic mammary souffle, are not heard maximally at the right base.[52] A midsystolic murmur that is most prominent in the second right intercostal space in children or young adults arouses suspicion of a functionally normal bicuspid aortic valve, especially in males (relative male prevalence is 70% to 75%).[56] Auscultation should then seek the confirmatory evidence of an aortic ejection sound that is most prominent at the apex, where it is readily mistaken for the second component of a split first heart sound.[37,52] The initial component of a normally split first heart sound is louder at the apex, and the second component is louder at the lower left sternal border.[52] Additional evidence of a functionally normal bicuspid aortic valve is the soft high-frequency early diastolic murmur of bicuspid aortic regurgitation that adds materially to the diagnosis. The murmur is heard best when firm pressure of the stethoscopic diaphragm is applied at the midleft sternal edge during held exhalation as the patient sits and leans forward. Isometric exercise (clenched fists) or squatting improves audibility.[52]

The combination of a midsystolic murmur at the right base, an aortic ejection sound at the apex, and a soft high-frequency early diastolic murmur at the left sternal border in a young male patient establishes the diagnosis of bicuspid aortic valve. When the ejection sound is equivocal and the aortic regurgitation murmur is absent, clinical suspicion rests on the right basal midsystolic murmur alone. The echocardiogram then plays a pivotal role. The normal trileaflet aortic valve in the short axis resembles the letter Y during diastole (Fig. 2–10A) and resembles an inverted triangle during systole.[10] A congenitally bicus-

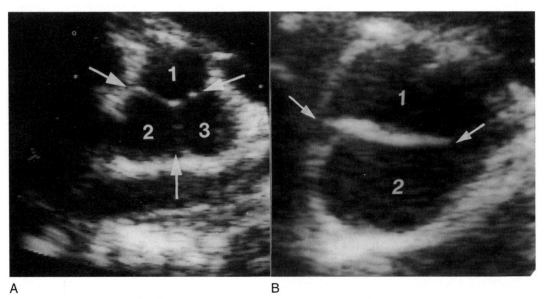

A   B

Figure 2–10
Echocardiogram (short-axis) of a normal trileaflet aortic valve in diastole (*A*), and a functionally normal congenitally bicuspid aortic valve in diastole (*B*). The diastolic configuration of the trileaflet valve resembles the letter Y (*arrows*). The bicuspid valve is characterized in diastole by a single linear band (*arrows*).

pid aortic valve appears as a single linear band in diastole (Fig. 2–10B) and appears as a fish mouth in systole.[10] Color flow imaging detects mild inaudible aortic regurgitation.

THE CARDIORESPIRATORY MURMUR

In 1915, Richard Cabot wrote,[6] "Such murmurs may be heard under the left clavicle or below the angle of the left scapula, as well as near the apex of the heart—less often in other parts of the chest . . . Cardiorespiratory murmurs may be either systolic or diastolic, but in the vast majority of cases are systolic. The area over which they are audible is usually a very limited one. They are generally affected by a position and by respiration, and are heard most distinctly if not exclusively during inspiration, especially at the end of that act."

Cardiorespiratory murmurs were known to Laënnec, but James Hope's description is the most colorful.[28] Hope described his examination of two university students: "Both wore very tight waistcoats, preventing the expansion of the lower ribs. During this state of breathing, a bellows murmur . . . existed in both. In both, the murmur ceased entirely when, unbuttoning their waistcoats and waistbands of their trousers, they breathed with the lungs naturally inflated. By altering the circumstances, the murmur could be created or removed at pleasure. I presume therefore that it proceeded from a cause exterior to the heart."

The mechanism responsible for the cardiorespiratory murmur is unclear, but its benign nature as well as its location, timing, and relation to respiration remain as Cabot originally described.[6]

Normal Continuous Murmurs

THE VENOUS HUM

The venous hum was described by Potain in 1867[55] and is the most common type of normal continuous murmur. It is universal in children and occurs in normal young adults[26,33] even in the absence of thyrotoxicosis, anemia, or pregnancy.[52] Maximal intensity is in the supraclavicular fossa just lateral to the sternocleidomastoid muscle. The

hum may radiate widely and is often bilateral but is usually more prominent on the right (Fig. 2–11). A loud venous hum, especially in children, may radiate below the clavicles and may be mistaken for a patent ductus arteriosus.[41] Abolition of the hum by digital compression prevents this error (Figs. 2–11 and 2–12). Intensity varies from faint to grade 6/6, and occasional patients are subjectively and unpleasantly aware of a loud hum, which is sensed as audible pulsatile tinnitus.[7,9,43,60]

A venous hum is best elicited with the patient sitting upright. The stethoscope is held in the right hand of the examiner, and the bell is applied to the medial aspect of the supraclavicular fossa while the examiner's left hand grasps the patient's chin from behind and pulls it tautly to the left and upward (see Fig. 2–12A).[52] Occasionally, the hum develops or increases when the chin is simply tilted upward, and a prominent hum is sometimes audible without neck maneuvers and irrespective of position. In a child who is either sitting or supine, a venous hum may appear when the patient's head is voluntarily turned to the left or tilted upward. The hum may appear when the child looks up at the examiner and may disappear when the child looks down at the stethoscope. The hum is reduced or abolished by digital compression of the ipsilateral internal jugular vein (see Fig. 2–12B), by removing the stretch on the neck as the head is returned to a neutral position, by the Valsalva maneuver, or by recumbency. The simplest procedure for abolishing the hum is compression of the deep jugular vein with the thumb of the free hand (see Fig. 2–12B). Compression causes instantaneous obliteration of the hum (see Fig. 2–11), which suddenly and transiently intensifies as pressure is released.[33,52]

The term *hum* does not necessarily characterize the quality of these cervical venous murmurs, which can be rough and noisy and are occasionally accompanied by a high-pitched whine.[33] The hum is truly continuous (see Fig. 2–11), although typically louder in diastole, as is the case with venous continuous murmurs in general (Fig. 2–13). The mechanism responsible for the venous hum is unsettled. Laminar flow in the internal jugular vein may be disturbed by deformation at the level of the transverse process of the atlas during head rotation.[11]

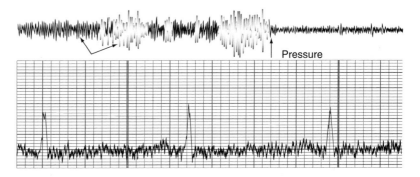

Figure 2–11

Continuous venous hum in a normal 24-year-old woman. The diastolic component of the hum is louder (*paired arrows*). Digital pressure on the right internal jugular vein (*vertical arrow*) abolished the murmur.

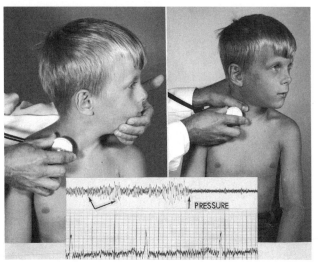

Figure 2–12

Maneuvers for eliciting or abolishing a venous hum. *A,* The bell of the stethoscope is applied to the medial aspect of the right supraclavicular fossa. The left hand grasps the patient's chin from behind and pulls it tautly to the left and upward. *B,* Digital compression of the right internal jugular vein obliterates the hum. The head has returned to a more neutral position.

THE CONTINUOUS MAMMARY SOUFFLE

A second but far less common benign continuous murmur occurs during late pregnancy and early postpartum in normal lactating women. A consensus supports the view that the mammary souffle is arterial in origin,[24,41,62,67] an opinion originally held by both van den Bergh[68] and Morgan-Jones.[32] Origin in the superficial veins of the breast has less credibility.[31] The delay in onset, the accentuation in systole, the relatively high frequency, and the persistence during the Valsalva maneuver are in accord with an arterial origin.[52]

The continuous mammary souffle was included in Morgan-Jones' 1951 book on heart disease in pregnancy.[32] *Souffle* is French, meaning "puff." *Soufflare* is Latin, meaning "to blow." The location of maximal intensity of the souffle can be anywhere over either breast, but there is a tendency for it to be louder in the second or third right or left intercostal space, and occasionally the souffle is bilateral.[67] A distinct gap between the first heart sound and the onset of the murmur represents the interval between ejection of blood from the left ventricle and arrival of blood at the artery that gives rise to the souffle.[24,62,67] The murmur is typically louder in systole, as is usually the case with continuous murmurs of arterial origin, with the diastolic portion often fading completely before the subsequent first heart sound (Figs. 2–13 and 2–14). The pitch may be relatively high, but the murmur is not musical.[67] Audibility is best with the patient supine, and the murmur may vanish in the upright position.[67] Light pressure with the stethoscope tends to augment the murmur and bring out its continuous features.[62] Firm pressure with the stethoscope or digital pressure adjacent to the site of auscultation can abolish the murmur completely.[31,62,67] Intensity may vary from beat to beat, from hour to hour, or from day to day.[67] The Valsalva maneuver does not affect the intensity.[62]

The location of a continuous mammary souffle may arouse suspicion of patent ductus arteriosus or of an arteriovenous fistula. However, the typical ductus murmur peaks before and after the second heart sound, whereas the mammary souffle peaks much earlier (see Fig. 2–14), and obliteration by local compression excludes patent ductus. An arteriovenous fistula may generate a continuous murmur that is maximal in systole and that attenuates with pressure, but the cycle-to-cycle or day-to-day variation of the mammary souffle and its invariable disappearance after termination of lactation resolve the problem.

THE CEPHALIC (CRANIAL) CONTINUOUS MURMUR

Low-intensity cephalic murmurs that are usually continuous and less often systolic are occasionally detected over the cranium of normal children younger than 4 years of age, especially in association with a febrile illness.[59] These murmurs tend to be most prominent over the anterior fontanel, the temporal regions, or the orbits and are best heard with the diaphragm of the stethoscope. Because auscultation is not routinely applied to the head, cephalic murmurs are overlooked. Their mechanism is unknown.

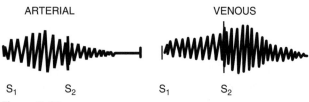

Figure 2–13

Schematic illustration of arterial and venous continuous murmurs. The arterial continuous murmur is louder in systole and the venous continuous murmur is louder in diastole.

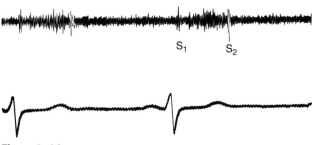

Figure 2–14

Continuous mammary souffle recorded at the upper left chest in a normal 26-year-old lactating woman. The murmur is continuous but is louder in systole and does not peak around the second heart sound (S_2). S_1, first heart sound.

REFERENCES

1. Arlettaz R, Archer N, Wilkinson AR: Natural history of innocent heart murmurs in newborn babies: Controlled echocardiographic study. Arch Dis Childh 18:F166, 1998.
2. Barlow JB, Bosman CK: The origin of the innocent vibratory systolic murmur. S Afr J Med Sci 30:96, 1965.
3. Barrillon A, Havy G, Scebat L, et al: Congenital pressure gradients between main pulmonary artery and its branches. Br Heart J 36:669, 1974.
4. Braudo M, Rowe RD: Auscultation of the heart: Early neonatal period. Am J Dis Child 101:575, 1961.
5. Bruns DL, van der Hauwaert LG: The aortic systolic murmur developing with increasing age. Br Heart J 20:370, 1958.
6. Cabot RC: Physical Diagnosis. New York, William Wood and Company, 1915.
7. Cary FH: Symptomatic venous hum. N Engl J Med 264:869, 1961.
8. Castle RF, Craige E: Auscultation of the heart in infants and children. Pediatrics 26:511, 1960.
9. Chandler JR: Diagnosis and cure of venous hum tinnitus. Laryngoscope 93:892, 1983.
10. Child JS: Transthoracic and transesophageal echocardiographic imaging: Anatomic and hemodynamic assessment. In Perloff JK, Child JS (eds): Congenital Heart Disease in Adults. Philadelphia, WB Saunders, 1998.
11. Cutforth R, Wiseman J, Sutherland RD: The genesis of the cervical venous hum. Am Heart J 80:488, 1970.
12. Danilowicz DA, Rudolph AM, Hoffman JIE, Heyman M: Physiologic pressure differences between the main and branch pulmonary arteries in infants. Circulation 45:410, 1972.
13. Darazs B, Hesdorffer CS, Butterworth AM, Ziady F: The possible etiology of the vibratory systolic murmur. Clin Cardiol 10:341, 1987.
14. DeLeon AC Jr, Perloff JK, Twigg H, Majd M: The straight back syndrome. Circulation 32:193, 1965.
15. deMonchy C, van der Hoeven GMA, Beneken JEW: Studies on innocent precordial vibratory murmurs in children. Br Heart J 35:685, 1973.
16. Edwards JE: An Atlas of Acquired Diseases of the Heart and Great Vessels. Philadelphia, WB Saunders, 1961.
17. Engle MA: Insurability and employability: Congenital heart disease and innocent murmurs. Circulation 56:143, 1977.
18. Fogel DH: The innocent systolic murmur in children: A clinical study of its incidence and characteristics. Am Heart J 59:844, 1960.
19. Fowler NO, Marshall WJ: Supraclavicular arterial bruit. Am Heart J 68:410, 1965.
20. Gallavardin L, Ravault P: Le souffle de retrecissement aortique peut changer de timbre et devenir musical dans sa propagation apexiene. Lyon Méd 135:523, 1925.
21. Gardiner HM, Joffe HS: Genesis of Still's murmurs: A controlled Doppler echocardiographic study. Br Heart J 66:217, 1991.
22. Gerlis LM, Wright HM, Wilson EF, Dickinson DF: Left ventricular bands: A normal anatomical feature. Br Heart J 52:641, 1984.
23. Goldblatt E: Innocent systolic murmurs in childhood. Br Med J 2:95, 1966.
24. Grant RP: A precordial systolic murmur of extracardiac origin during pregnancy. Am Heart J 52:944, 1965.
25. Groom D, Chapman W, Francis WW, et al: The normal systolic murmur. Ann Intern Med 52:134, 1960.
26. Hardison JE: Cervical venous hum. N Engl J Med 278:587, 1968.
27. Harris TN, Saltzman HA, Needleman HL, Lisker L: Spectrographic comparison of ranges of vibration frequency among some innocent cardiac murmurs in childhood and some murmurs of valvular insufficiency. Pediatrics 19:57, 1957.
28. Hope J: A Treatise on the Diseases of the Heart and Great Vessels. London, William Kidd, 1839.
29. Howard TH: Cardiac murmurs in old age: A clinico-pathological study. J Am Geriatr Soc 15:509, 1967.
30. Humphries JO, McKusick VA: Differentiation of organic and innocent systolic murmurs. Prog Cardiovasc Dis 5:152, 1962.
31. Hurst JW, Staton J, Hubbard D: Precordial murmur during pregnancy and lactation. N Engl J Med 259:515, 1958.
32. Jones AM: Heart Disease in Pregnancy. London, Harvey & Blythe, 1951.
33. Jones FL: Frequency, characteristics, and importance of the cervical venous hum in adults. N Engl J Med 267:658, 1962.
34. Kawabori I, Stevenson JG, Dooley TK, et al: The significance of carotid bruits in children. Am Heart J 98:160, 1979.
35. Keith TR, Sagarminaga J: Spontaneously disappearing murmur of patent ductus arteriosus. Circulation 24:1235, 1961.
36. Klewer SE, Donnerstein RL, Goldberg SJ: Still's-like innocent murmur can be produced by increasing aortic velocity to the threshold value. Am J Cardiol 68:810, 1991.
37. Leech G, Mills P, Leatham A: The diagnosis of a nonstenotic bicuspid aortic valve. Br Heart J 40:941, 1978.
38. Lessof M, Bridgen W: Systolic murmurs in healthy children and in children with rheumatic fever. Lancet 2:673, 1957.
39. Lewis DH, Ertugrul A, Deitz GW, et al: Intracardiac phonocardiography in the diagnosis of congenital heart disease. Pediatrics 23:837, 1959.
40. Malouf J, Gharzuddine W, Kutayli F: A reappraisal of the prevalence and clinical importance of left ventricular false tendons in children and adults. Br Heart J 55:587, 1986.
41. McKusick VA: Cardiovascular Sound in Health and Disease. Baltimore, Williams & Wilkins, 1958.
42. McKusick VA: Spectral phonocardiography. Am J Cardiol 4:200, 1959.
43. Nehru VI, Khaboori MJ, Kishore K: Ligation of the internal jugular vein in venous hum tinnitus. J Laryngol Otol 107:1037, 1993.
44. Nelson WP, Hall RJ: The innocent supraclavicular arterial bruit—utility of shoulder maneuvers in its recognition. N Engl J Med 278:778, 1968.
45. O'Malley CD, Saunders JB: Leonardo on the Human Body. New York, Dover Publications, 1983.
46. Osler W: The bicuspid condition of the aortic valve. Trans Assoc Am Physicians 2:185, 1886.
47. Otto CM, Lind BK, Kitzman DW, et al: Association of aortic valve sclerosis with cardiovascular mortality and mortality in the elderly. N Engl J Med 441:142, 1999.
48. Papadopoulos GS, Folger GM: Transient solitary diastolic murmurs in the newborn. Clin Pediatrics 22:548, 1983.
49. Peacock TB: On Malformations of the Human Heart. London, John Churchill, 1858.
50. Perez GL, Jacob M, Bhat PK, et al: Incidence of murmurs in the aging heart. J Am Geriatr Soc 24:29, 1976.
51. Perloff JK: Clinical recognition of aortic stenosis. Prog Cardiovasc Dis 10:323, 1968.
52. Perloff JK (ed): Physical Examination of the Heart and Circulation, 3rd ed. Philadelphia, WB Saunders, 2000.
53. Perry LW, Ruckman RN, Shapiro SR, et al: Left ventricular false tendons in children: Prevalence as detected by 2-dimensional echocardiography and clinical significance. Am J Cardiol 52:1264, 1983.
54. Pomerance A: Cardiac pathology and systolic murmurs in the elderly. Br Heart J 30:687, 1968.
55. Potain SC: Des mouvements et des bruits qui se passent dans les veines jugulaires. Bull Mém Soc Méd Hôp Paris 4:3, 1867.
56. Roberts WC: The congenitally bicuspid aortic valve. Am J Cardiol 26:72, 1970.
57. Roberts WC, Perloff JK, Costantino T: Severe valvular aortic stenosis in patients over 65 years of age. Am J Cardiol 27:497, 1971.
58. Rodriguez RJ, Riggs TW: Physiologic peripheral pulmonic stenosis in infancy. Am J Cardiol 66:1478, 1990.
59. Rosenthal A: How to distinguish between innocent and pathologic murmurs in childhood. Pediatr Clin North Am 31:1229, 1984.
60. Rothstein J, Hilger PA, Boies LR: Venous hum as a cause of reversible factitious sensorineural hearing loss. Ann Otol Rhinol Laryngol 94:267, 1985.
61. Schwartz ML, Goldberg SJ, Wilson N, et al: Relation of Still's murmur, small aortic diameter and high aortic velocity. Am J Cardiol 57:1344, 1986.
62. Scott JT, Murphy EA: Mammary souffle: Report of two cases simulating patent ductus arteriosus. Circulation 18:1038, 1958.
63. Spooner PH, Perry MP, Bradenberg RO, Pennock GD: Increased intraventricular velocities: An unrecognized cause of systolic murmur in adults. J Am Coll Cardiol 32:1589, 1998.
64. Stapleton JF, El-Hajj MM: Heart murmurs simulated by arterial bruits in the neck. Am Heart J 61:178, 1961.
65. Stein PD, Sabbah HN: Aortic origin of innocent murmurs. Am J Cardiol 39:665, 1977.

66. Still GF: Common Disorders and Diseases of Childhood. London, Frowde, Hodder & Stoughton, 1909.

67. Tabatznik B, Randall TW, Hersch C: The mammary souffle of pregnancy and lactation. Circulation 22:1069, 1960.

68. van den Bergh AAH: Een Schijnbaar Hartgeruisch. Nederl Tijdschr Geneesk 52:1104, 1908.

69. Van Oort A, Hopman J, Van Der Werf T, et al: The vibratory innocent heart murmur in schoolchildren: A case-controlled Doppler echocardiographic study. Pediatr Cardiol 15:275, 1994.

70. Vollebergh FE, Becker AE: Minor congenital variations of cusp size in tricuspid aortic valves: Possible link with isolated aortic stenosis. Br Heart J 39:1006, 1977.

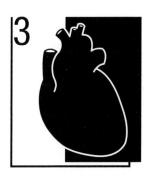

The Cardiac Malpositions

The heart may be congenitally misplaced in various ways, occupying either an unusual position within the thorax, or being situated external to that cavity.
Thomas B. Peacock, 1858

Dextrocardia in situs inversus was known to the anatomist-surgeon Marco Aurelio Severino in 1643, and was one of the first recognized congenital malformations of the heart.[22] Nearly a century and a half elapsed before Matthew Baillie's account of "complete transposition in the human subject, of the thoracic and abdominal viscera, to the opposite side from what is natural."[14]

Cardiac malpositions, which have a prevalence of 0.10 per 1000 live births,[43] refer to hearts that are located abnormally *within* the thoracic cavity, or that are located *outside* the thoracic cavity—*ectopia cordis*. In 1901, Paltauf published remarkable illustrations that distinguished the various types of dextrocardia,[97] and in 1928 the first useful classification of cardiac malpositions was proposed.[84] Subsequent observations by Lichtman[79] and by de la Cruz[34] shed light on the embryologic bases of the malpositions, and the landmark observations of van Praagh confirmed the validity of those assumptions.[142] Campbell's diagrams in the 1950s and 1960s,[24–26] and Elliott's radiologic classification in 1966,[42] set the stage for the *clinical recognition* of cardiac malpositions.

The genetics of cardiac midline and laterality defects occurs along three geometric axes: anteroposterior, dorsalventral, and left-right.[158] Genes expressed in dorsal midline cells coordinate the development of the three embryonic axes, driving the cardiac tube to loop in the appropriate direction relative to body axes. The left-right axis is established at approximately the 18th day after fertilization.[158] Both bilateral left-sidedness and bilateral right-sidedness have been reported in members of the same family, implying that the two conditions are different manifestations of a primary defect in lateralization.[28]

The first section of this chapter deals with the *three basic cardiac malpositions* in the presence of bilateral *asymmetry*.

The second section of the chapter deals with cardiac malpositions in the presence of bilateral *symmetry* (bilateral left-sidedness or bilateral right-sidedness). Certain organs or structures are in fact symmetric (the bronchi and lungs). Certain essentially unilateral organs, such as the liver, are transverse. Parts of certain structures, such as the atrial appendages, are symmetric, whereas the remainder of the atria are morphologically different.

The literature on cardiac malpositions is replete with an arcane vocabulary that often confounds rather than clarifies. Terms have been fully abbreviated, minimally abbreviated, or unabbreviated. In this chapter, unabbreviated terms will be used because they are accessible to the widest audience.[140]

Definitions and Terminology[11,140,143]

Cardiac position: Refers to the intrathoracic location of the heart as left-sided (levocardia), right-sided (dextrocardia), or midline (mesocardia).

Cardiac malposition: An abnormal intrathoracic location of the heart, or a location that is abnormal (inappropriate) relative to the position (situs) of the abdominal viscera.

Situs: Site or position.

Solitus: Usual or normal.

Situs solitus: Normal position (Fig. 3–1).

Inversus: Reverse or opposite.

Situs inversus: Opposite or reverse of normal (Fig. 3–2).

Ambiguus: Uncertain, indeterminant.

Situs ambiguus: Uncertain, indeterminant or ambiguous position.

17

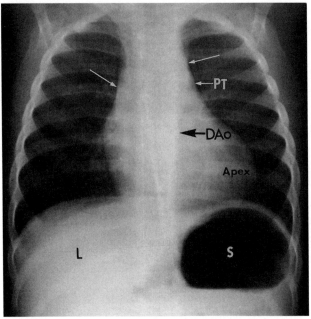

Figure 3–1
Normal heart and viscera in *situs solitus*. The stomach bubble (S) is on the left, the liver (L) is on the right, and the heart is left-sided with its base to apex axis pointing to the left. Despite a large stomach bubble (S), the left hemidiaphragm is lower than the right hemidiaphragm because the cardiac apex is on the left. The ascending aorta, the aortic knuckle (*unmarked white arrows*) and the pulmonary trunk (PT) are in normal positions. The descending aorta (DAo) is concordant on the left.

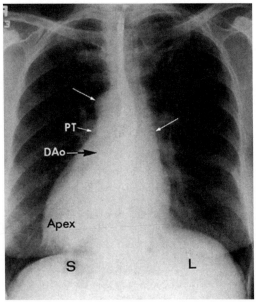

Figure 3–2
Chest x-ray from a 65-year-old female with complete *situs inversus*. The stomach bubble (S) is on the right, the liver (L) is on the left, the heart (apex) is on the right (dextrocardia), and the hemidiaphragm is lower on the side of the cardiac apex (right). The ascending aorta, the aortic knuckle (*unmarked white arrows*) and the pulmonary trunk (PT) are in their mirror image positions. The descending aorta (DAo) is concordant on the right,

Cardiac displacement: A *secondary* shift in intrathoracic cardiac position in response to eventration of a hemidiaphragm (Fig. 3–3B), agenesis of a lung (see Fig. 3–3A, C), or congenital complete absence of the pericardium (see Chapter 5).

Ectopia cordis: (Gr) *ektopos* = displaced. *Extrathoracic* location of the heart[71,75] (Fig. 3–4).

Chamber designations: Right and left refer to morphology rather than position, as right or left atrium, right or left ventricle.

Great arterial designations: Ascending aorta and pulmonary trunk are defined in terms of their ventricular alignments or their spatial relations to each other.

Heterotaxy: (Gr) *heteros* = other, different; *taxis* = arrangement.

Isomerism: (Gr) *isos* = equal; *meros* = part. Refers to the morphologic similarity of bilateral structures that are normally dissimilar such as right and left atrial appendages, right and left bronchi, right and left lungs.

Right isomerism: Refers to bilateral structures both of which have morphologic *right* characteristics, such as morphologic right atrial appendages, morphologic right bronchi, and bilateral trilobed lungs.

Left isomerism: Refers to bilateral structures both of which have morphologic *left* characteristics, such as morphologic left atrial appendages, morphologic left bronchi, and bilateral bilobed lungs.

Asplenia: Congenital absence of the spleen. Splenic tissue is either entirely absent or is rudimentary and nonfunctional.

Polysplenia: *Many spleens*, each of which is appreciably smaller than one normal-sized spleen. Multiple spleens of *polysplenia* differ from *accessory spleens* (splenules) that accompany one normal-sized spleen.

Ventricular loop: The right or left bend (loop) that forms in the straight heart tube of the embryo.

d-Loop: The normal *rightward* (dextro = d) bend in the embryonic heart tube. The d-loop designation as applied to the developed heart indicates that the sinus or inflow portion of the morphologic right ventricle lies to the right of the morphologic left ventricle.

l-Loop: A *leftward* (levo = l) bend in the embryonic heart tube. The l-loop designation as applied to the developed heart indicates that the sinus or inflow portion of the morphologic right ventricle lies to the left of the morphologic left ventricle.

Concordant: (L) *concordare* = to agree, i.e., agreeing or appropriate.

Concordant loop: Refers to a ventricular loop that agrees with (is appropriate for) the visceroatrial situs, i.e., d-loop in situs solitus, l-loop in situs inversus.

Atrioventricular concordance: Refers to appropriate (concordant) connection of a morphologic *right* atrium to a morphologic *right* ventricle via a morphologic *tricuspid* valve, and appropriate (concordant) connection of a morphologic *left* atrium to a morphologic *left* ventricle via a morphologic *mitral* valve. Each atrioventricular valve is normally *concordant* with the morphologic ventricle to which it is attached.

Infundibulum (conus): The ventriculo/great arterial segment that is normally subpulmonary.

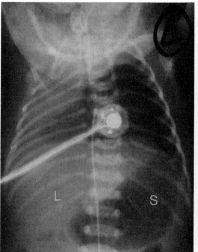
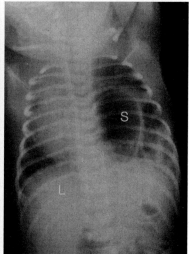

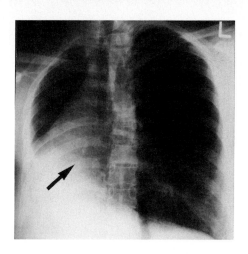

Figure 3–3

A, X-ray from a neonate in *situs solitus*. The stomach bubble (S) is on the left and the liver (L) is on the right, but the heart is in the right thoracic cavity because of displacement caused by congenital agenesis of the right lung. The proximity of the posterior ribs reflects the reduced size of the right hemithorax. *B*, X-ray from a neonate in *situs solitus*. The heart is displaced into the right hemithorax because of congenital eventration of the left hemidiaphragm through which the stomach (S) has entered the left thoracic cavity. The liver (L) is in its normal position on the right. *C*, Chest x-ray from a 29-year-old female in *situs solitus*. The heart is displaced into the right thoracic cavity because of congenital agenesis of the right lung. The right posterior ribs are in close proximity, and the right hemidiaphragm is elevated because the right hemithorax is reduced in size.

Ventriculoarterial concordance: Refers to appropriate (concordant) connection of a morphologic *right* ventricle to a *pulmonary trunk*, and appropriate (concordant) connection of a morphologic *left* ventricle to an aorta.

Discordant: Not agreeing, inappropriate.

Transposition of the great arteries: Each great artery is connected to a morphologically discordant ventricle (ventriculoarterial *discordance*). The *aorta* arises from a morphologic *right* ventricle, and the *pulmonary trunk* arises from a morphologic *left* ventricle.

Malposition of the great arteries: Refers to abnormal *spatial* relationships of the aorta and the pulmonary trunk to each other. Malpositions can be in either the lateral or the anteroposterior plane. The great arteries are *malposed* but not *transposed* because ventricular–great arterial concordance is maintained.

Inversion: Refers to *right/left* reversal with no change in anteroposterior or superoinferior relationships.

Atrioventricular discordance with ventriculoarterial discordance: *Atrioventricular* discordance applies when a morphologic *right* atrium connects to a morphologic *left* ventricle via a morphologic *mitral* valve, and when a morphologic *left* atrium connects to a morphologic

right ventricle via a morphologic *tricuspid* valve. *Ventriculoarterial* discordance applies when a morphologic *right* ventricle gives rise to the *aorta*, and a morphologic *left* ventricle gives rise to the *pulmonary trunk*. *Congenitally corrected transposition* applies when a *double* discordance (atrioventricular and ventriculoarterial) results in *physiologic correction*, so right atrial blood reaches the pulmonary artery through a morphologic left ventricle, and left atrial blood reaches the aorta through a morphologic right ventricle.

A systematic approach: Refers to sequential attention to the atria, the atrioventricular valves, the atrioventricular connections, the ventricles, the ventriculoarterial connections, the great arteries, and the positions or malpositions of the heart and abdominal viscera.[11,140,143] Let us first focus on *normal* cardiac and *normal* abdominal visceral positions (*situs solitus*), and then on the three major cardiac *malpositions* in the presence of right/left *asymmetry*.

Situs solitus (see Fig. 3–1): Because *atrial situs* and *abdominal situs* are usually concordant, *atrial situs solitus* can be inferred at the bedside by percussing a left-sided stomach, a right-sided liver, and a left-sided heart. The chest x-ray confirms the positions of the stomach, liver, and heart (see Fig. 3–1) and discloses bronchial

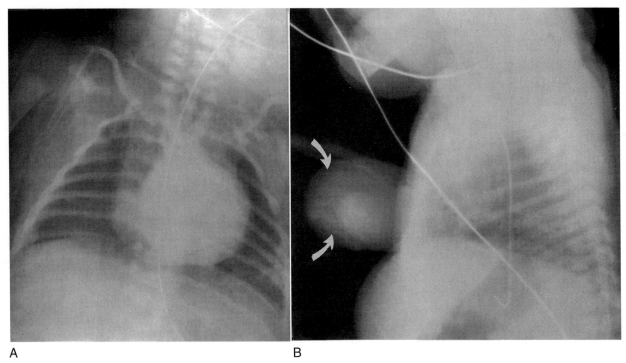

A   B

Figure 3–4
X-rays from a 2-day-old male with *ectopia cordis*. *A,* The external position of the heart cannot be inferred from the frontal projection, but is obvious (*arrows*) in the lateral projection (*B*).

morphology, which is a reliable predictor of atrial situs.[77,99,138,143] A morphologic *right* bronchus is relatively short and straight, whereas a morphologic *left* bronchus is relatively long and curved (Fig. 3–5).

A morphologic *right* bronchus is concordant with a *trilobed* morphologic *right* lung, and a morphologic *left* bronchus is concordant with a *bilobed* morphologic *left* lung. The chest x-ray establishes the direction of

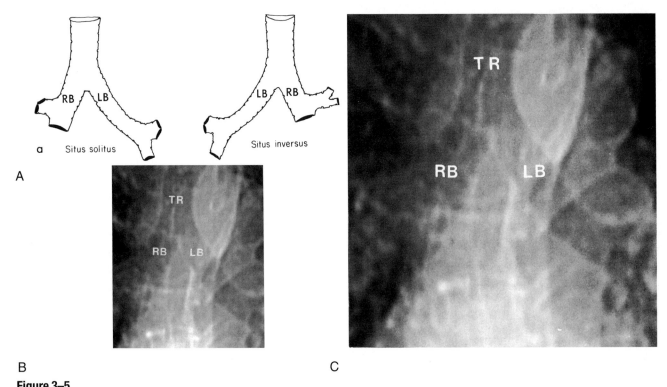

A

B   C

Figure 3–5
A, In *situs solitus,* the morphologic right bronchus (RB) is short, wide, relatively straight, and is right-sided. The morphologic left bronchus (LB) is long, thin, curved, and is left-sided. In *situs inversus* (mirror image), the morphologic right bronchus is left-sided and the morphologic left bronchus is right-sided. *B* and *C,* Tomograms showing the morphologic right bronchus (RB) and morphologic left bronchus (LB) in *situs solitus.* TR, trachea.

the base to apex axis which points to the left because the straight heart tube of the embryo initially bends to the right (d-loop) and then pivots to the left until the ventricular portion comes to occupy its normal left thoracic position[128,142,143] (see Fig. 3–1). The relative levels of the two hemidiaphragms are determined by the location of the cardiac apex, not by the location of the liver, so the left hemidiaphragm is normally lower than the right hemidiaphragm.[107] Thoracoabdominal *discordance* is represented by *thoracic situs solitus*, a *left* thoracic heart, and *abdominal situs inversus*[30,56,58,117,147] (Fig. 3–6), or by *thoracic situs inversus*, a *right* thoracic heart (dextrocardia), and *abdominal situs solitus*.[53]

The next step in the systematic analysis concerns the *great arteries*. The chest x-ray provides information on the spatial relationships of aorta and pulmonary trunk and on ventriculoarterial alignments. In *situs solitus* with atrioventricular and ventriculo/great arterial concordance, the ascending aorta forms a convex shadow at the right basal aspect of the cardiac silhouette, the aortic arch forms a left basal knuckle below which lies the slightly convex main pulmonary artery segment, and the descending thoracic aorta runs parallel to the left border of the vertebral column (see Fig. 3–1).

The Malpositions

Three major cardiac malpositions occur in the presence of right/left asymmetry (Figs. 3–7 and 3–8): 1) visceroatrial *situs inversus* with dextrocardia, 2) visceroatrial *situs solitus* with dextrocardia, and 3) visceroatrial *situs inversus* with levocardia. *Mesocardia*—a midline heart—is sometimes regarded as a fourth malposition. A midline heart in *situs solitus* with a d-bulboventricular loop is a variation of normal, but a midline heart with visceroatrial *situs inversus* and an l-bulboventricular loop occurs with major congenital malformations.[143]

Situs Inversus with Dextrocardia (see Fig. 3–2). Incidence in the general population is estimated at 1/8000.[39] The heart and the thoracic and abdominal viscera are mirror images of normal (see Fig. 3–2). The bronchi are inverted (see Fig. 3–5A), with the morphologic *right bronchus* concordant with the morphologic *right atrium* and the *trilobed lung*, and the morphologic *left bronchus* concordant with the morphologic *left atrium* and the *bilobed lung* (see Fig. 3–5). The heart is right-sided, and the right hemidiaphragm is lower than the left hemidiaphragm (see Fig. 3–2). The descending aorta is on the right, the ascending aorta, aortic knuckle, and pulmonary trunk are in their mirror image positions, and the anatomic right ventricle lies to the left of the anatomic left ventricle (l-bulboventricular loop), which is normal for *situs inversus* just as a d-bulboventricular loop is normal for *situs solitus*.

Situs Solitus with Dextrocardia. The lungs and abdominal viscera are *situs solitus*, but the heart is right thoracic (dextrocardia) (Figs. 3–7 through 3–10). The ascending aorta and aortic knuckle occupy their normal positions and the descending aorta runs its normal course along the left vertebral border (see Fig. 3–9), but the major cardiac shadow lies to the *right* of midline (dextrocardia), the base to apex axis points to the *right*, and the *right* hemidiaphragm is lower than the left hemidiaphragm (see Fig. 3–9). In the type of *situs solitus* with dextrocardia shown in Figure 3–9, the anatomic right ventricle lies to the right of the anatomic left ventricle (d-loop) because the straight heart tube of the embryo initially bent in a rightward direction (d-loop), but then failed to pivot into the left chest. Varying degrees of incomplete pivoting determine the degree to which the ventricular portion of the heart lies to the right of midline (see Fig. 3–10).

Situs Inversus with Levocardia. The defining characteristics of this malposition are *situs inversus* of thoracic and abdominal viscera in the presence of a left thoracic heart (levocardia) (Figs. 3–7 and 3–11). The left hemidiaphragm is lower than the right hemidiaphragm because the apex is on the left (see Fig. 3–11). Inversion of the bronchi (see Fig. 3–5A) coincides with inversion of the atria and lungs. The stomach is on the right and the liver is on the left (abdominal *situs inversus*) (see Fig. 3–11). The major cardiac mass lies in the left chest for one of two morphogenetic reasons. First, an embryonic l-loop which is *concordant* for *situs inversus*, fails to pivot into the right side of the chest. Second, an embryonic d-loop which is *discordant* for *situs inversus*, fails to pivot into the left side of the chest. When a d-loop in *situs inversus* is associated with congenitally corrected transposition of the great

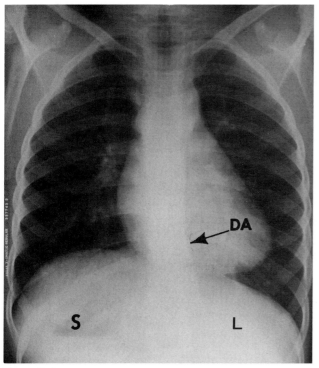

Figure 3–6
X-ray from an 8-year-old female with *thoracoabdominal discordance* represented by abdominal *situs inversus* but thoracic *situs solitus* with a left-sided heart. The stomach (S) lies in the right upper quadrant, and the liver (L) lies in the left upper quadrant. DA, descending aorta.

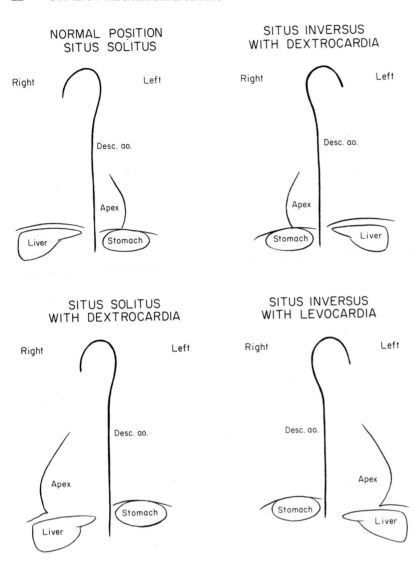

NORMAL POSITION
SITUS SOLITUS

SITUS INVERSUS
WITH DEXTROCARDIA

SITUS SOLITUS
WITH DEXTROCARDIA

SITUS INVERSUS
WITH LEVOCARDIA

Figure 3–7
Schematic illustrations of the four basic cardiac positions (normal and three malpositions) and the relationships of descending aorta, cardiac apex, stomach, and liver. The drawings are shown as projected from the frontal view of a chest x-ray. In *situs solitus*, the descending aorta, cardiac apex, and stomach are all on the *left*. In *situs inversus* with *dextrocardia*, the descending aorta, cardiac apex, and stomach are all on the *right*. In *situs solitus* with *dextrocardia*, the descending aorta and stomach are on the *left* (normal), but the cardiac apex is on the *right*. In *situs inversus* with *levocardia*, the descending aorta and stomach are on the *right* (situs inversus), but the cardiac apex is on the *left*.

arteries (ventricular inversion), the ascending aorta forms a smooth shadow at the left basal aspect of the heart (see Fig. 3–11).

Midline Heart (Mesocardia). The example shown in Figure 3–12 is a midline cardiac position in the presence of thoracic and abdominal *situs solitus*. The cardiac silhouette extends equally to the right and left of midline (see Fig. 3–12A). A d-bulboventricular loop stopped in the midline as it pivoted to the left[78,143] (see Fig. 3–12B). Much less commonly, mesocardia is associated with *situs inversus* and an l-loop that stops in the midline as it incompletely pivots to the *right*.[78,143]

In brief, there are two varieties of *right-thoracic hearts* (see Figs. 3–7 and 3–8), namely, *situs inversus* with dextrocardia and *situs solitus* with dextrocardia. There are two varieties of *left-thoracic hearts*, namely, *situs solitus* with levocardia (normal) and *situs inversus* with levocardia. A midline heart (mesocardia) is exceptional, but occurs either in *situs solitus* or rarely in *situs inversus*. Once the cardiac malposition has been defined, clinical assessment turns to the presence and type of associated congenital heart disease.

Situs inversus with *dextrocardia* (complete *situs inversus*, mirror image dextrocardia) (see Fig. 3–2) usually occurs without coexisting congenital heart disease.[86] Isolated atrial inversion is rare.[118] *Situs solitus* with *dextrocardia* is only occasionally associated with a structurally normal heart (see Figs. 3–9 and 3–10); left-to-right shunts at atrial level or ventricular level usually coexist. When *situs solitus* with *dextrocardia* occurs with a bulboventricular loop that initially bends to the *left* and then pivots to the *right* (where an l-loop *belongs*),[143] ventricular inversion, ventricular septal defect, and obstruction to venous ventricular outflow usually coexist.[42,120,143]

Situs inversus with *levocardia* is consistently associated with coexisting congenital heart disease[143] (see Fig. 3–11), whether the left thoracic heart results from a discordant d-loop that pivots into the left hemithorax or from a concordant l-loop that fails to pivot into the right hemithorax. A discordant d-loop in *situs inversus* results in ventricular inversion, as does a discordant l-loop in *situs solitus*.[143] Coexisting congenital heart disease is invariable and complex, but occurs without prevailing patterns.[42,114,143]

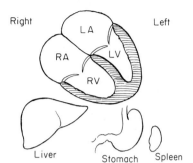

NORMAL POSITION
SITUS SOLITUS

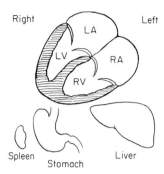

SITUS INVERSUS
WITH DEXTROCARDIA

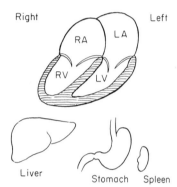

SITUS SOLITUS
WITH DEXTROCARDIA

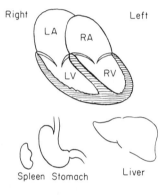

SITUS INVERSUS
WITH LEVOCARDIA

Figure 3–8
Schematic illustrations of the anatomic relationships of the descending aorta, left atrium, cardiac apex, and stomach in the four basic cardiac positions (normal and three malpositions). In *situs solitus*, the descending aorta, left atrium, cardiac apex, and stomach are all on the *left*. In *situs inversus* with *dextrocardia*, the descending aorta, left atrium, cardiac apex, and stomach are all on the *right*. In *situs solitus* with *dextrocardia*, the descending aorta, left atrium, and stomach are on the *left* (normal), but the cardiac apex is on the *right*. In *situs inversus with levocardia*, the descending aorta, left atrium, and stomach are on the *right* (situs inversus), but the cardiac apex is on the *left*. RA, right atrium; LA, left atrium; RV, right ventricle; LV, left ventricle; spleen as shown.

A *midline cardiac position* (mesocardia) occurs in *situs solitus* (see Fig. 3–12) or in *situs inversus*.[78,143] If the bulboventricular loop is discordant, ventricular inversion coexists.

The History

Situs inversus with *dextrocardia* and a structurally normal heart is usually discovered by chance in a chest x-ray which is often considered normal because the film is inadvertently reversed when first read. There is a reported tendency for left handedness in complete *situs inversus*,[22] but Matthew Baillie wrote: "The person seems to have used his right hand in preference to his left . . . which was readily discovered by the greater bulk and hardness of that hand as well as the greater fleshiness of the arm."[14] Baillie's conclusion has been confirmed.[74,131]

Important are investigations of the human brain which is midline but asymmetric in both structure and function.[74,131] The developmental factors that determine *functional* asymmetry of the brain independently recognize laterality (asymmetry) in visceral situs.[131] Developmental factors that determine *anatomic* asymmetry of the brain are distinct from those that determine visceral asymmetry and lateralization of language.[74]

Situs inversus with dextrocardia is the malposition most likely to occur with an otherwise structurally normal heart and with normal longevity. Symptoms caused by coexisting acquired cardiac or noncardiac disease may lead to the discovery of hitherto unsuspected *situs inversus*.[19,39,66,68,69,76] The pain of ischemic heart disease is located in the *right* anterior chest with radiation to the *right* shoulder and *right* arm.[66,68,76] The pain of appendicitis is referred to the *left* lower quadrant,[93] and the pain of biliary colic presents in the *left* upper quadrant (Fig. 3–13).

In 1933, Kartagener called attention to the association of sinusitis, bronchiectasis and *situs inversus*,[72] a combination subsequently called Kartagener syndrome or triad.[16,51,73,80,92,132] In the first English language publication of the syndrome (1937), as many as one fifth of patients with *situs inversus* had bronchiectasis, underscoring that the association was not fortuitous.[5] In 1986, a blinded controlled study of cilia ultrastructure in Kartagener syndrome found a widespread inherited ciliary disorder[40,95,98,133] that included the upper and lower respiratory tracts[54,73,133] (bronchitis, bronchiectasis, sinusitis) and the testis[4,6,7,49,103] (immobile sperm, male infertility). *Situs inversus* is common in infertile men, an observation that contributed to the identification of a generalized disorder of ciliary motility.[6,49] Respiratory symptoms are a significant part of the history and may lead to the discovery of *situs inversus*. The connection between abnormal cilia and laterality remains enigmatic.[7] Familial *situs inversus* has been reported,[23,135,159] and Kartagener syndrome is sometimes familial.[40,95,133] One family of six siblings included two cases of Kartagener syndrome and two cases of isolated bronchiectasis.[16]

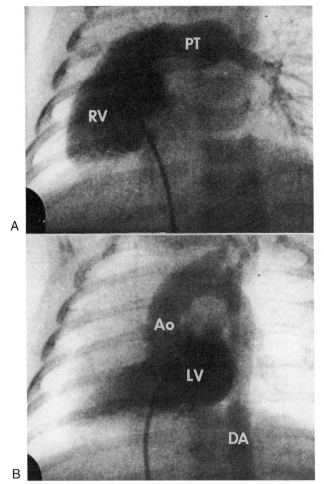

Figure 3–9

A, Right ventriculogram (anteroposterior) in a two-month-old female in *situs solitus* with dextrocardia and no associated congenital heart disease. The morphologic right ventricle (RV) occupies the apex on the right and gives rise to the pulmonary trunk (PT). The hemidiaphragm is lower on the side of the apex. *B*, The morphologic left ventricle (LV) is in a medial position, and gives rise to a normally positioned ascending aorta (Ao) and a left-sided descending aorta (DA).

Situs solitus with *dextrocardia* occasionally occurs without coexisting congenital heart disease and escapes recognition. A routine chest x-ray may provide the first evidence (see Fig. 3–10). As a rule, accompanying congenital cardiac malformations bring the patient to medical attention. *Situs inversus* with *levocardia* (see Fig. 3–11) invariably occurs with coexisting congenital heart disease that leads to the discovery of the cardiac malposition.

Physical Appearance, the Arterial Pulse, and the Jugular Venous Pulse

These features are determined by coexisting congenital heart disease rather than the cardiac malposition. The left testicle in the normal upright male is lower than the right testicle, whereas the opposite is the case in *situs inversus*.

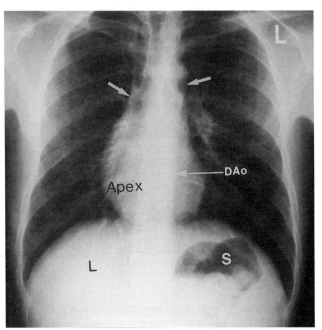

Figure 3–10

Chest x-ray from a 20-year-old male in *situs solitus* with dextrocardia and no associated congenital heart disease. The stomach (S) is on the left and the liver (L) is on the right. The base to apex axis points to the *right*, the cardiac shadow is chiefly to the right of midline, but the hemidiaphragms are at the same level. The ascending aorta and aortic knuckle (*unmarked white arrows*) are in their normal positions, and the descending thoracic aorta (DAo) is normally positioned along the left border of the vertebral column.

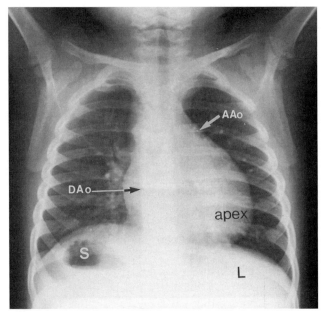

Figure 3–11

X-ray from a 2-year-old female in *situs inversus* with levocardia. The stomach (S) is on the right and the liver (L) is on the left, but the heart (apex) is to the left of midline. The left hemidiaphragm is lower than the right hemidiaphragm because the cardiac apex is on the left. The descending thoracic aorta (DAo) is on the right (concordant for *situs inversus*), but the position of the ascending aorta (AAo) indicates a discordant d-bulboventricular loop.

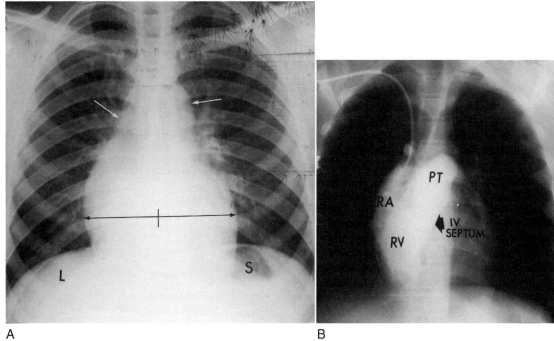

A   B

Figure 3–12

A, X-ray from a 16-year-old male in *situs solitus* with a midline heart (mesocardia) and no associated congenital heart disease. The stomach (S) is on the left, and the liver (L) is on the right. There is identical extension of the heart to the right and left of center (*equal black arrows*). The ascending aorta and aortic knuckle (*unmarked white arrows*) are in their normal positions. The cardiac silhouette is hump-shaped because the right atrium (RA) and right ventricle (RV) are super-imposed (see angiogram, *B*). The right hemidiaphragm is lower than the left hemidiaphragm because the base to apex axis points to the right. *B,* The position of the right ventricle (RV) and the interventricular septal plane (IV septum) indicate that mesocardia resulted from a d-bulboventricular loop in which leftward pivoting stopped at the midline. RA, right atrium; PT, pulmonary trunk.

Poland syndrome, which is characterized by absence of a pectoralis major muscle (usually right-sided), ipsilateral syndactyly, brachydactyly, and hypoplasia of a hand, has been reported with *situs solitus* and dextrocardia[46] (see Fig. 18–17), and the Goldenhar syndrome (oculoauricular vertebral dysplasia, hemifacial microsomia) has been reported with complete *situs inversus.*[52]

Percussion and Palpation

A *right* anterior chest bulge with asymmetry arouses suspicion of dextrocardia. Percussion and palpation are useful in the clinical recognition of cardiac malpositions because these physical signs are influenced by the malposition *per se,* and establish the right or left thoracic location of the heart and the abdominal location of hepatic dullness and gastric tympany. If the stomach is not sufficiently air-filled to generate a tympanitic percussion note, a carbonated beverage or deliberate aerophagia (an infant can suck an empty bottle) solves the problem. Percussion begins over the sternum and then compares left and right parasternal sites. The side of major cardiac dullness is more accurately established by percussing with the patient turned moderately to the left and then moderately to the right. The heart tends to fall to the side towards which the base to apex axis points. *Situs inversus* with *dextrocardia* is characterized by

gastric tympany on the right, hepatic dullness on the left and cardiac dullness on the right (see Figs. 3–2 and 3–7). *Situs solitus* with *dextrocardia* is characterized by normal locations of gastric tympany and hepatic dullness and by cardiac dullness on the right (see Figs. 3–7 and 3–10). *Situs inversus* with *levocardia* is the converse of *situs solitus* with *dextrocardia* (see Figs. 3–7 and 3–11).

Palpation is undertaken with the patient supine and then in both left and right lateral decubitus positions. The normal *situs solitus* heart (see Fig. 3–1) is represented by a morphologic left ventricle that occupies the apex in the left hemithorax and a morphologic right ventricle that underlies the lower left sternal border.[102] *Situs inversus* with *dextrocardia* (see Fig. 3–2) is represented by a morphologic left ventricle that occupies the apex in the *right* hemithorax and a morphologic right ventricle that underlies the lower *right* sternal border. *Situs solitus* with *dextrocardia* is represented by a right thoracic apical low-pressure morphologic *right* ventricle that retracts, and a high-pressure systemic morphologic *left* ventricle that generates outward systolic movement adjacent to the lower right sternal border (see Figs. 3–9 and 3–10). *Situs inversus* with *levocardia* and l-bulboventricular loop is represented by a left thoracic apical low-pressure morphologic right ventricle that retracts, and a high-pressure systemic morphologic left ventricle that generates outward systolic movement adjacent to the lower left sternal border (see Fig. 3–11).

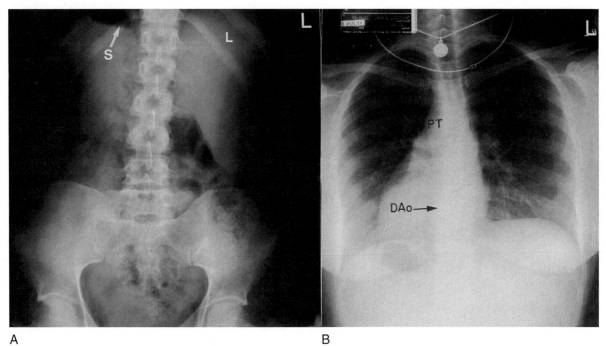

A   B

Figure 3–13
X-rays from a 28-year-old female who presented with acute *left* upper quadrant colic. *A,* The abdominal x-ray disclosed the stomach bubble (S) on the right and the liver (L) on the left, establishing the diagnosis of abdominal *situs inversus* which was appropriate for biliary colic referred to the *left* upper quadrant. *B,* The chest x-ray disclosed thoracic *situs inversus* with dextrocardia and abdominal situs inversus with stomach (S) on the right and liver (L) on the left. The pulmonary trunk (PT) is in its mirror image position, and the descending aorta (DAo) is along the right side of the vertebral column.

Auscultation

The relative prominence of auscultatory events should be compared in the left and right anterior hemithorax, more specifically along the left and right sternal borders and at the apices (Fig. 3–14). The stethoscope should alternate from one side to the other to compare analogous right and left thoracic sites. With dextrocardia, the first and second heart sounds are louder in the right anterior chest (see Fig. 3–14); splitting of the second sound in the second *right* intercostal space is a feature of dextrocardia just as splitting of the second heart sound in the second *left* interspace is a feature of a left thoracic heart. In *situs solitus* with dextrocardia and a d-bulboventricular loop (see Figs. 3–9 and 3–10), the position of the pulmonary valve results in splitting of the second sound in the second *right* interspace, and the anterior position of the aorta results in amplification of the aortic component (Fig. 3–15). In *situs inversus* with levocardia, splitting of the second sound is more prominent in the second *left* interspace.

The location and radiation of murmurs are governed by the type of cardiac malposition. In *situs inversus* with dextrocardia, murmur sites are the mirror images of normal. In *situs solitus* with dextrocardia, a pulmonary stenotic murmur is louder to the *right* of the sternum (Fig. 3–16) and radiates upward and to the *left* because of the direction taken by the pulmonary trunk (see Fig. 3–9A).

The Electrocardiogram

As early as 1889, well before the advent of electrocardiography, it was postulated that ventricular potentials in *complete situs inversus* should be diametrically opposite the ventricular potentials of the normal heart.[149] In *situs inversus* with dextrocardia, a mirror image sinus node lies at the junction of a *left* superior vena cava and the mirror image *left-sided* morphologic right atrium. The right and left bundle branches supply their corresponding mirror image right and left ventricles.[17] It is essential to be certain that the limb leads are properly attached before proceeding with interpretation of the 12-lead electrocardiogram.[1,41] Interpretation in mirror image dextrocardia is easier when the arm leads are *intentionally* reversed and when *right* precordial leads are *intentionally* recorded from locations that are the exact opposites of standard left precordial lead positions[25,66,68,76] (Fig. 3–17). In *situs solitus* with *dextrocardia,* the limb leads are best left unchanged, while the precordial leads are recorded from the right anterior chest (Fig. 3–18). This recommendation is appropriate because atrial situs is normal (sinus node is at the junction of the right superior vena cava and morphologic right atrium on the right),[17] and because the base to apex axis points to the right whether the bundle branches supply their corresponding ventricles as d-loop or l-loop.[17] In *situs inversus* with *levocardia,* standard limb lead and left precordial lead positions suffice (Fig. 3–19).

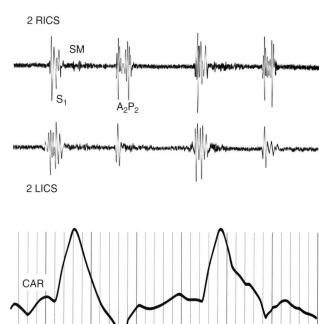

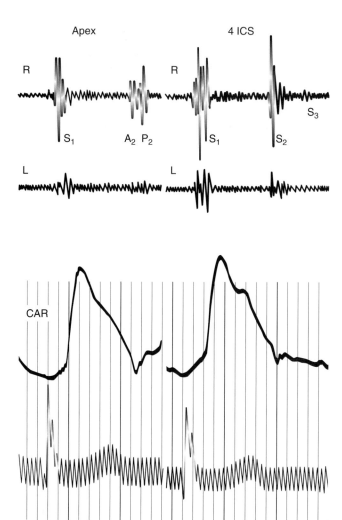

Figure 3–14

Phonocardiograms from a 7-year-old male in *situs solitus* with dextrocardia and an ostium secundum atrial septal defect. Heart sounds are louder on the right (R). L, left; 4 ICS, fourth intercostal space. The pulmonary component of the second sound (P_2) was recorded at the right cardiac apex because the apex was occupied by the right ventricle. CAR, carotid pulse.

Figure 3–15

Phonocardiograms from the 7-year-old male referred to in Figure 3–14. A short soft pulmonary midsystolic murmur was recorded in the second right interspace (2 RICS) together with persistent splitting of the second heart sound. A_2, aortic component; P_2, pulmonary component; CAR, carotid pulse; 2 LICS, second left intercostal space.

Analysis of the electrocardiogram commences with the P wave direction which is determined by atrial situs unless the atrial pacemaker is ectopic.[15,20,90,105,106] In *situs solitus* with either levocardia or dextrocardia, atrial depolarization proceeds from a normally positioned right sinus node, so upright P waves appear in leads 1 and aVL and an inverted P wave appears in lead aVR[25,26,88,90] (Fig. 3–20). Conversely, in *situs inversus* with either dextrocardia or levocardia, atrial depolarization proceeds from a *left* sinus node, so *inverted* P waves appear in leads 1 and aVL and an *upright* P wave appears in lead aVR[26,114] (Figs. 3–17 and 3–19). In the presence of a right sinus node, the direction of the P wave can be altered by a left atrial ectopic focus.[15,26,45,88,89,105] The Valsalva maneuver, ocular pressure, or exercise may transiently shift the ectopic focus to the right sinus node.[89] Left atrial ectopic rhythm is manifested by a negative P wave in lead 1 and isoelectric or negative P waves in left precordial leads (see Fig. 3–18). A less common but more distinctive configuration is the *dome*

and dart P wave in lead V_1[89] (Fig. 3–21). A negative P wave in lead 1 or lead V_1 does not distinguish *situs solitus* with a left atrial ectopic rhythm from *situs inversus*, but a dome and dart P wave in lead V_1 or V_2 confirms a left atrial ectopic focus irrespective of atrial situs.[45,55,85,89]

In *situs inversus* with *dextrocardia*, ventricular activation and repolarization are the reverse of normal as predicted in 1889[87,100,149] (see Fig. 3–17). In lead 1, the major QRS deflection is negative and the T wave is inverted; lead aVR resembles lead aVL and vice versa, and right precordial leads resemble leads from corresponding left precordial sites (see Fig. 3–17). Septal Q waves appear in *right* lateral precordial leads rather than in left lateral precordial leads because septal depolarization proceeds from right to left (see Fig. 3–17). The electrocardiogram can be "corrected" when limb leads are reversed and chest leads are recorded from right precordial sites (see earlier).

In *situs solitus* with *dextrocardia* and a d-loop, the left ventricle is relatively anterior and the right ventricle lies to the right (see Fig. 3–9); left ventricular electrical activity is directed anteriorly and right ventricular activity is directed to the right. Depolarization in the frontal plane is

2 RICS   2 LICS

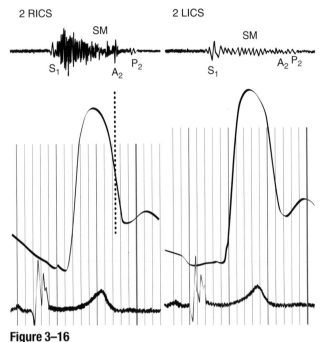

Figure 3–16

Phonocardiograms, carotid pulse, and electrocardiogram from a 15-year-old male in *situs solitus* with dextrocardia. There was pulmonary stenosis with a right-to-left shunt through a ventricular septal defect. The pulmonary stenotic murmur (SM) was appreciably louder in the second right intercostal space (2 RICS) compared to the second left intercostal space (2 LICS). A soft, delayed pulmonary component of the second (P_2) was more apparent on the right.

counterclockwise, so Q waves appear in leads 1 and aVL (see Figs. 3–18 and 3–20). Precordial leads display relatively prominent R waves in leads V_1 and V_2 (anterior left ventricular forces) and display prominent RS complexes in most of the remaining right precordial leads (see Fig. 3–18). Normal left to right septal depolarization (d- loop) results in Q waves in standard *left* precordial locations (see Figs. 3–18 and 3–20). The converse is the case for an l-loop with which Q

waves are *absent* in *left* precordial leads and are present in *right* precordial leads, indicating right-to-left septal depolarization (Fig. 3–22). *Left* ventricular hypertrophy is manifested by tall R waves in leads V_1 and V_2 while *right* ventricular hypertrophy is manifested by tall R waves in leads V_5R and V_6R and deep Q waves in lead 1 (see Figs. 3–18 and 3–20). In *situs inversus* with *levocardia* and l-loop, septal depolarization is right-to-left, so precordial Q waves are present at right thoracic sites and are absent on the left.[114]

The X-Ray

The x-ray permits confident recognition of cardiac malpositions.[42,138,143] The first necessity is to identify the orienting letters L and R or analogous symbols that designate left and right. From the radiologic point of view, this is all that is required to diagnose *situs inversus* with dextrocardia (see Fig. 3–2). The aorta is in its inverted position with the arch deviating the trachea toward the *left*, the descending thoracic aorta appears as a fine line along the right vertebral border, and the major cardiac shadow to the right of midline (see Fig. 3–2 and Fig. 3–23A). *Situs inversus* is missed if the film is inadvertently read in a reversed position, because it then appears *correct* except for the L and R designations that are on the wrong sides (see Fig. 3–23B). Complete *situs inversus* implies atrial situs inversus (visceroatrial concordance) (see Figs. 3–8 and 3–23) which is established by identifying the inverted morphologic right and left bronchi[99,138] (see Fig. 3–5).

Situs solitus with *dextrocardia* (see Figs. 3–9, 3–10, and 3–24) is represented by normal positions of the stomach, liver, descending thoracic aorta, and right and left bronchi, by the major cardiac shadow to the right of midline, and by the right hemidiaphragm lower than the left hemidiaphragm because the cardiac apex is on the right.[81,107,123,124,153] The position of the ascending aorta permits identification of

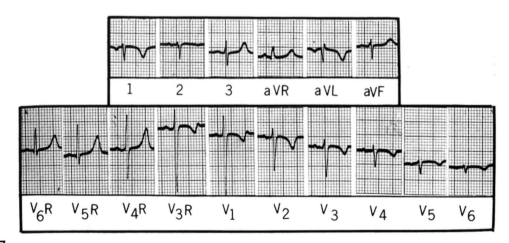

Figure 3–17

Electrocardiogram from an 11-year-old female in *situs inversus* with dextrocardia and no coexisting congenital heart disease. The P wave and T wave are inverted in lead 1, and the major QRS deflections are negative. Lead aVR and lead aVL are mirror images of normal. Precordial leads V_2 through V_6R resemble normal *left* precordial leads (mirror image).

Figure 3–18

Electrocardiogram from the 7-year-old male in *situs solitus* with dextrocardia referred to in Figure 3–14. The direction of the P wave is abnormal because of a left atrial ectopic focus. The frontal QRS axis is vertical. The deep Q wave in lead 1 is a sign of right ventricular hypertrophy. Septal depolarization proceeds from left to right as in normally positioned hearts. *Septal Q waves* in left precordial leads indicate that ventricular inversion does not coexist. The dominant R wave in V_6R is evidence of right ventricular hypertrophy because the right-sided right ventricle occupies the apex.

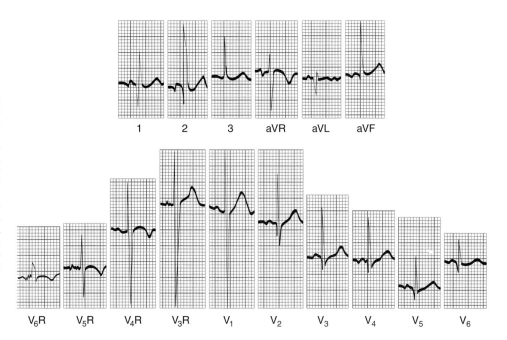

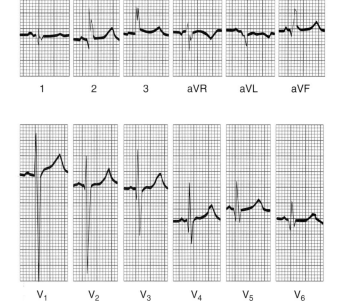

a d-bulboventricular loop (Fig. 3–24A) l-bulboventricular loop (Fig. 3-24B).

Situs inversus with *levocardia* is represented by inverted positions of the stomach, liver, descending aorta, and bronchi, while the major cardiac shadow is to the *left* of midline and the *left* hemidiaphragm is lower than the right hemidiaphragm because the cardiac apex is on the *left* (see Figs. 3–11, 3–25, and 3–26). When the bulboventricular loop is discordant for *situs inversus* (d- loop), the ascending aorta forms a smooth contour at the left basal aspect of the heart (see Fig. 3–25).

A *midline cardiac position*—mesocardia—is uncommon and is usually represented by *situs solitus* with a d-bulboventricular loop that stops at midline as it pivots from right to left (see Fig. 3–12). A hump-shaped contour of the right cardiac border is due to superimposition of right ventricular and right atrial shadows (see Fig. 3–12B).

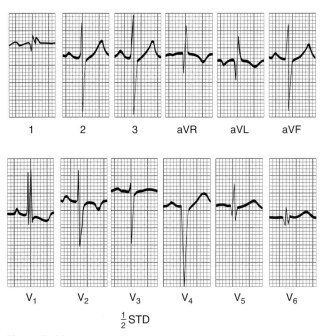

Figure 3–19

Electrocardiogram from an 11-year-old male in *situs inversus* with levocardia, severe pulmonary stenosis, ventricular septal defect, ventricular inversion, and a Blalock-Taussig shunt. Negative P waves in leads 1 and aVL indicate atrial situs inversus. Q waves in left precordial leads identify left to right septal depolarization of ventricular inversion.

Figure 3–20

Electrocardiogram from a 15- year-old male in *situs solitus* with dextrocardia, pulmonary stenosis, and a ventricular septal defect. The upright P wave in lead 1 indicates normal atrial situs. Right ventricular hypertrophy is responsible for a vertical QRS axis with a prominent Q wave and a small r wave in lead 1. Septal depolarization proceeds from left to right as in the normal heart, so septal Q waves appear in left precordial leads.

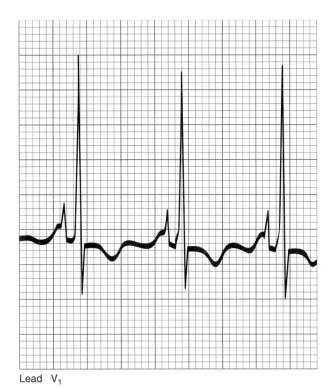

Lead V$_1$

Figure 3–21
Lead V$_1$ from a 5-year-old male in *situs solitus* with dextrocardia. The dome and dart P wave is characteristic of a left atrial ectopic rhythm.

The Echocardiogram

Echocardiography with color flow imaging lends itself to systematic segmental analysis of visceroatrial situs, atrioventricular connections, ventricular locations, and the spatial relationships and ventricular alignments of the great arteries.[11,64,65,127] Atrial morphology and atrial situs are established by identifying the right atrial appendage with its broad junction, and the left atrial appendage with its narrow junction. However, it is easier to infer atrial morphology and situs from the abdominal echocardiogram. The normal *situs solitus with left thoracic heart* is represented by an aorta on the *left* side of the spinal column and an inferior cava on the *right* side of the spinal column (Fig.

3–27). The morphologic right atrium resides on the same side as the inferior vena cava (atrial situs solitus). The inferior vena cava and aorta are distinguished from each other by color flow imaging and by systolic pulsations of the aorta. The liver is on the right and the stomach on the left—normal positions (see Fig. 3–27). Hepatic venous connections to the inferior vena cava can be identified as well as the course of the inferior vena cava to the right-sided morphologic right atrium.

Situs inversus with *dextrocardia* is the reverse—mirror image—of the normal arrangements.[64,65,127] The short-axis view recognizes the left atrial appendage with its narrow junction to the right of the aorta, and recognizes the right atrial appendage with its broad junction to the left of the aorta.[127] The abdominal echocardiogram identifies the aorta to the right of the spinal column and identifies the inferior vena cava to the left of the spinal column (Fig. 3–28*A*). Color flow imaging refines identification of the aorta and inferior vena cava (see Fig. 3–28*B*,*C*). The echocardiogram then determines hepatic venous connections to the inferior vena cava and determines the course of the left-sided inferior vena cava to the left-sided morphologic right atrium.[65] *Situs solitus* with *dextrocardia* has echocardiographic features of normal atrial situs. *Situs inversus* with *levocardia* has the echocardiographic features of atrial situs inversus. Once atrial situs is established, echocardiography focuses on the atrioventricular junction, ventricular morphology, ventricular location, and ventricular/great arterial connections.

Summary

The three basic cardiac malpositions in the presence of right/left asymmetry are *situs inversus* with *dextrocardia*, *situs solitus* with *dextrocardia*, and *situs inversus* with *levocardia*. *Situs inversus* with *dextrocardia* is characterized by a right thoracic heart, a right-sided stomach, a left-sided liver, a left-sided morphologic right bronchus and trilobed lung, a right-sided morphologic left bronchus and bilobed lung, and inverted positions of the atria. *Situs inversus* with *dextrocardia* (mirror image) is likely to be discovered inci-

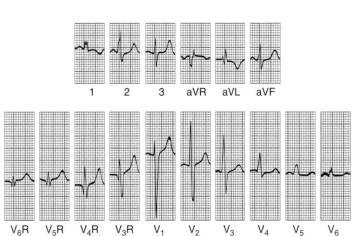

1   2   3   aVR   aVL   aVF

V$_6$R   V$_5$R   V$_4$R   V$_3$R   V$_1$ V$_2$ V$_3$ V$_4$ V$_5$ V$_6$

Figure 3–22
Electrocardiogram from a 26-year-old female in *situs solitus* with dextrocardia, ventricular inversion, pulmonary stenosis, and a ventricular septal defect. The upright P wave in lead 1 indicates normal atrial situs. Q waves in *right* precordial leads and *absent* Q waves in *left* precordial leads indicate the reversed septal depolarization of ventricular inversion.

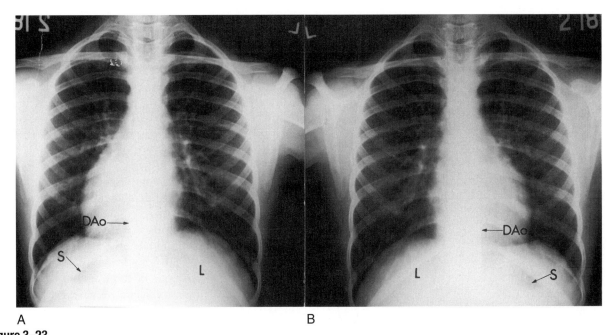

Figure 3–23
X-rays from an 11-year-old female in *situs inversus* with dextrocardia and no associated congenital heart disease (see Fig. 3–17). *A*, The L in the upper right corner of the film indicates that the x-ray is viewed properly. The stomach (S) and liver (L) are inverted. *B*, When the x-ray is reversed, it normalizes except for the L designation. DAo, descending aorta.

dentally on a routine chest x-ray, especially when the heart is structurally normal, which is usually the case. On physical examination, gastric tympany and cardiac dullness are on the right, hepatic dullness is on the left, and heart sounds are louder on the right side of the chest. The x-ray confirms the stomach bubble on the right, the liver on the left, and the cardiac silhouette to the right of midline. The electrocardiogram shows an inverted P wave, negative QRS complex and inverted T wave in lead 1, reversal of the QRS pattern in lead aVR and lead aVL, and reversal of corresponding right and left precordial leads. Echocardiography visualizes the inferior vena cava and the liver to the left of

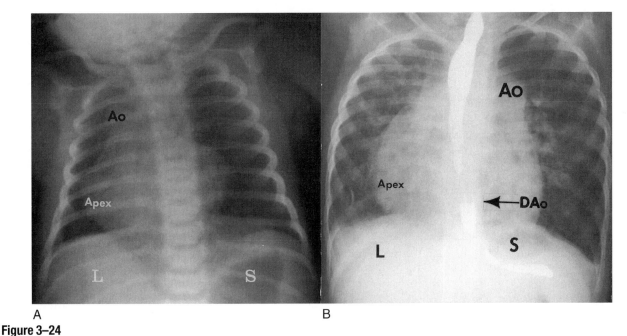

Figure 3–24
A, X-ray from a 3-week-old female in *situs solitus* with dextrocardia, d- bulboventricular loop, and a ventricular septal defect with pulmonary atresia. The liver (L) and stomach (S) are in normal positions, but the heart (apex) is on the right, so the right hemidiaphragm is lower than the left hemidiaphragm. The ascending aorta (Ao) is concordant with a d-bulboventricular loop and is relatively prominent because of pulmonary atresia. *B*, X-ray from a 4-year-old acyanotic male in *situs solitus* with dextrocardia, an l-bulboventricular loop and ventricular and atrial septal defects. The liver, stomach, and descending aorta (DAo) are in normal positions, but the base to apex axis points to the right, and the ascending aorta (Ao) forms a prominent leftward shadow appropriate for an l-loop.

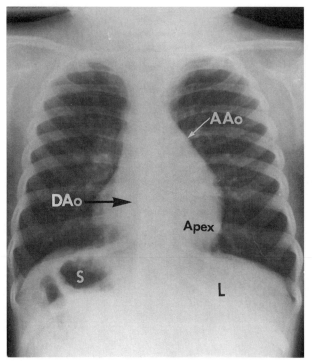

Figure 3–25

X-ray from a 4-year-old male in *situs inversus* with a left thoracic heart and discordant d-bulboventricular loop. The stomach (S), liver (L), and descending aorta (DAo) are in inverted positions, but the major cardiac shadow is to the left of midline. The smooth leftward silhouette of the *ascending* aorta (AAo) indicates a d-bulboventricular loop in *situs inversus* (ventricular inversion).

the spine, and the stomach and descending aorta to the right of the spine.

Situs solitus with *dextrocardia* is characterized by a right thoracic heart with normal locations of the stomach, liver, bronchi, lungs, and atria. The malposition usually comes to light because of coexisting congenital heart disease. Gastric tympany is on the left and hepatic dullness is on the right (normal), but cardiac dullness is on the *right* and heart sounds are louder in the right anterior chest (dextrocardia). The x-ray confirms normal positions of the stomach and liver, with the cardiac silhouette to the right of midline and the right hemidiaphragm lower than the left hemidiaphragm. The electrocardiogram shows an upright P wave in lead 1 with normal P wave patterns in leads aVR and aVL (atrial situs solitus), but the major precordial QRS voltage lies in the right hemithorax. Echocardiography visualizes normal positions of the liver and inferior vena cava to the right of the spine and normal positions of the stomach and aorta to the left of the spine.

Situs inversus with *levocardia* is characterized by reversed locations of the stomach, liver, bronchi, lungs, and atria, while the heart lies to the left of midline. The malposition comes to attention because of invariably coexisting congenital heart disease. Gastric tympany is on the right, hepatic and cardiac dullness are on the left, and heart sounds are louder in the left hemithorax. The x-ray confirms the heart to the left of midline, the stomach on the right, the liver on the left and the left hemidiaphragm lower than the right hemidiaphragm. The electrocardio-

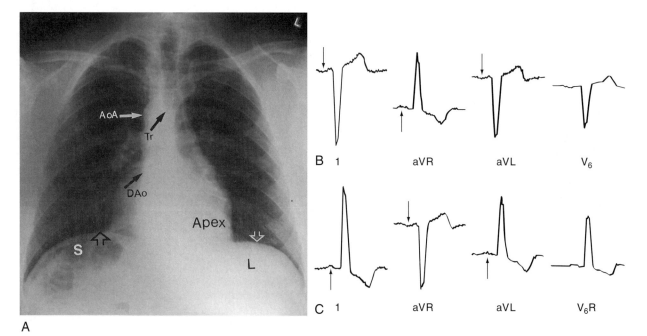

A

Figure 3–26

A, X-ray from a 35-year-old male in *situs inversus* with a left thoracic heart and ventricular inversion. The stomach (S) is on the right, the liver (L) is on the left, a right aortic arch (AoA) indents the right side of the trachea (Tr), and the aorta descends on the right. DAo, descending aorta; appropriate positions for *situs inversus*. The hemidiaphragm is lower on the side of the cardiac apex (left). B, Limb leads and precordial lead V_6. The P wave is inverted in leads 1 and aVL and upright in lead aVR, appropriate for atrial *situs inversus*. C, Reversed limb leads together with precordial lead V_6R. The P wave is now upright in leads 1 and aVL and inverted in lead aVR. The Q wave in lead V_6 (B) and the absent Q wave in lead V_6R (C) indicate the reversed septal depolarization of ventricular inversion.

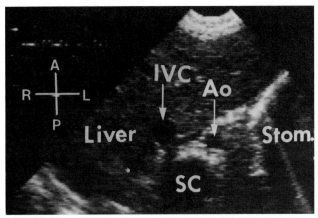

Figure 3–27

Abdominal echocardiogram from a normal 5-year-old male in *situs solitus*. The liver and inferior vena cava (IVC) are on the right, and the stomach (Stom) and descending aorta (Ao) are on the left. SC, spinal column; A, anterior; L, left; P, posterior; R, right.

Visceral Heterotaxy

Asplenia and *polysplenia* have been called into question as appropriate terms in patients with *bilateral symmetry*.[10,11,67,70,82,83,125,140,141,143,157] *Heterotaxy* is an alternative term that is derived from the Greek *heteros* = other + *taxis* = arrangement. *Isomerism* is a term that is derived from the Greek *isos* = equal + *meros* = part, and is used to designate bilateral similarity if not equivalence of structure. Visceral heterotaxy occurs in 0.8% of cases of congenital heart disease.[43] Isolated congenital asplenia in otherwise normal individuals is rare.[126]

Right and left bronchi are normally asymmetric (Figs. 3–29A and 3-30A); the right lung is trilobed, the left lung is bilobed, and the right and left atrial appendages are morphologically distinctive. The spleen is the only organ that is normally left-sided from its inception because it develops in the left side of the dorsal mesogastrium.[139] Unpaired structures such as the liver, spleen and stomach are normally confined to either the right or left upper quadrant of the abdomen.

The two bronchi can be morphologically right or morphologically left (see Figs. 3–29 and 3–30B), the two lungs can be bilaterally trilobed or bilaterally bilobed (see Fig. 3–29B), and the two atrial appendages can exhibit right or left morphologic features. A relationship exists,

gram shows inverted P waves in lead 1 and lead aVL and an upright P wave in lead aVR (atrial situs inversus). The major precordial QRS voltage resides to the left of midline. Echocardiography identifies the liver and inferior vena cava to the left of the spine and the stomach and descending aorta to the right of the spine (inverted).

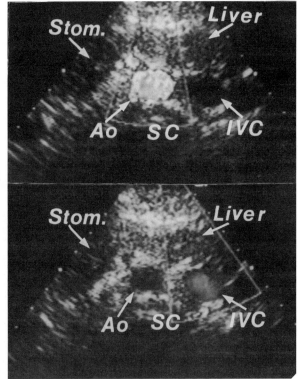

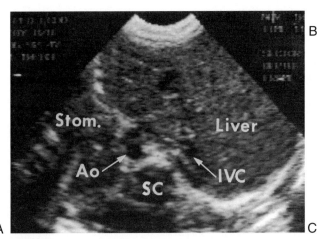

Figure 3–28

A, Abdominal echocardiogram from a 4-year-old male in *situs inversus*. The stomach (Stom) and descending aorta (Ao) are on the right, and the liver and inferior vena cava (IVC) are on the left. SC, spinal column. *B, C*, Abdominal echocardiogram with black and white print of a color flow image from a 12-year-old male in *situs inversus* with dextrocardia. The liver is on the left and the stomach is on the right. The abdominal aorta (Ao) lies on the right side of the spinal column (SC), and the inferior vena cava (IVC) lies on the left side of the left spinal column.

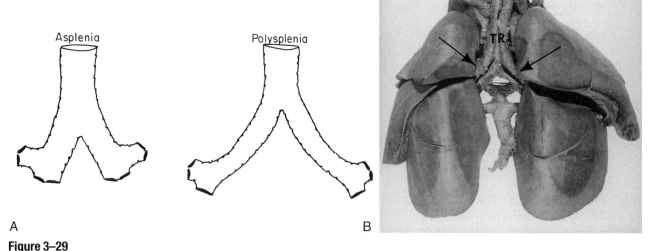

Figure 3–29

A, Schematic illustrations of bilateral morphologic *right* bronchi that are features of right isomerism, and bilateral morphologic *left* bronchi that are features of left isomerism. *B*, Gross specimen from an asplenic male neonate with bilateral morphologic right bronchi (*arrows*) and right isomerism. TR, trachea.

albeit imperfect, between *right isomerism* and *asplenia* and *left isomerism* and *polysplenia*.[134] In right isomerism (asplenia) and left isomerism (polysplenia), the liver is typically transverse (bilaterally symmetric) (Figs. 3–31 and 3–32*A*), and the superior vena cavae are typically bilateral (Figs. 3–33 and 3–34). There is strong but not invariable concordance between a morphologic *right* bronchus (see Fig. 3–30*A*), a morphologic *right* atrial appendage, and a trilobed morphologic *right* lung[134] (see Fig. 3–29*B*). There is similar strong but not invariable concordance between a morphologic *left* bronchus (see Fig. 3–30*A*), a morphologic *left* lung, and a bilobed morphologic *left* atrial appendage.[134] Accordingly, and with few exceptions,[134] *bilaterally symmetric* morphologic *right* bronchi (see Figs. 3–29 and 3–30*B*) are coupled with bilateral morphologic right atrial appendages and with bilateral trilobed right lungs (see Fig. 3–29*B*), and *bilaterally symmetric* morpho-

logic *left* bronchi (see Fig. 3–29*A*) are coupled with bilateral morphologic left atrial appendages and with bilateral bilobed left lungs. In about 15% of cases, splenic tissue does not coincide with the type of isomerism, and in about 5% of necropsy cases a normal-sized spleen is located in the *right* upper quadrant. Rarely, bronchial morphology is not concordant with atrial appendage morphology.[10,125,134]

Asplenia can be diagnosed by ultrasound or by computed tomography, and has been diagnosed with fetal ultrasound.[31] A simple and readily accessible method for identifying asplenia is the presence of Howell-Jolly bodies in peripheral blood smears[32,126] (Fig. 3–35), although Howell-Jolly bodies are occasionally found in normal infants during the first week of life.[18,106,113,126] *Pitted* red cells are also evidence of asplenia, but visualization of the pits requires examination of wet preparations with a

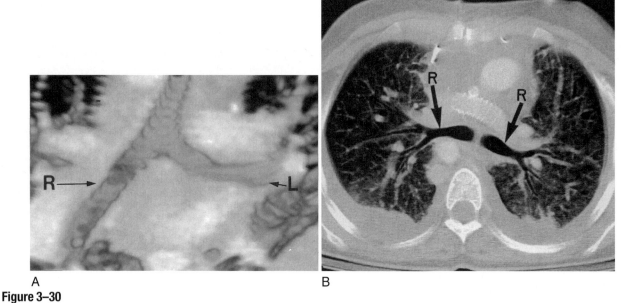

Figure 3–30

A, Thoracic computerized tomography from an 18-year-old male illustrating typical normal asymmetric morphologic right (R) and left (L) bronchi. *B*, Magnetic resonance image illustrating symmetric morphologic right bronchi (R and R) in a 4-year-old female with right isomerism.

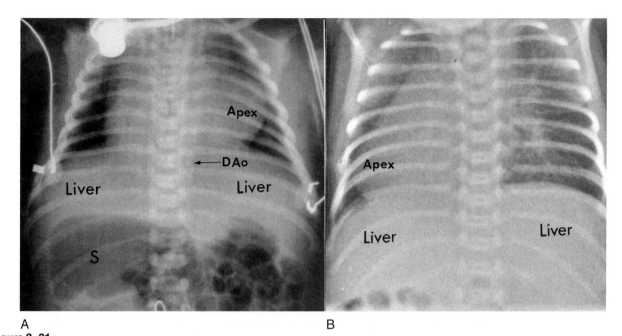

Figure 3–31

A, X-ray from an asplenic male neonate with right isomerism. The liver is transverse, the stomach (S) is on the right and the heart is midline, but the base to apex axis points to the left. *B*, X-ray from an asplenic male neonate with right isomerism. The liver is transverse, the base to apex axis points to the right, and the heart is to the right of midline. The ground glass appearance of the lungs was caused by total anomalous pulmonary venous connection with obstruction.

special optical system.[126] A *wandering spleen* is highly mobile, and may be located anywhere in the abdomen or pelvis. Failure to recognize a wandering spleen has resulted in the mistaken diagnosis of asplenia.[2,8,10] What is important in a *clinical* setting is not the presence, absence, or multiplicity of the spleen, but the relatively consistent relationships that exist between the type of isomerism and the type of congenital heart disease.[10,61] It is this relationship that forms the basis of the following sections.

Visceral Heterotaxy with Right Isomerism

Right isomerism as characterized in Table 3–1 is accompanied by the congenital cardiovascular malformations listed in Table 3–2. The heart is likely to reside to the left of midline.[57,119] The liver is transverse (see Figs. 3–31 and 3–34). The superior vena cavae are bilateral,[116] hence the tendency for bilateral sinus nodes.[17,36,82] Exceptionally, one vena cava is partially or completely atretic.[116] Bilateral morphologic right bronchi (see Figs. 3–29 and 3–30) are

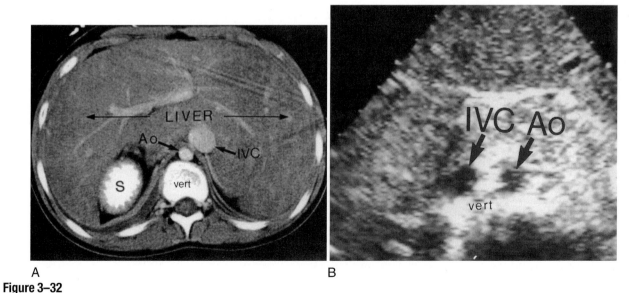

Figure 3–32

A, Abdominal magnetic resonance image from a 5-year-old male with left isomerism. The liver is transverse. The aorta (Ao) lies directly anterior to the vertebral column (vert), the inferior vena cava (IVC) is leftward, and the stomach (S) is on the right. *B*, Abdominal echocardiogram from an asplenic female neonate with right isomerism. The inferior vena cava (IVC) and aorta (Ao) are both anterior to the vertebral column (vert).

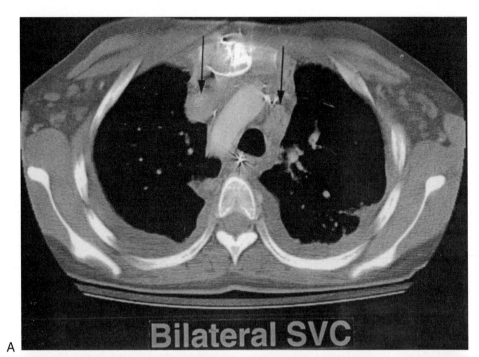

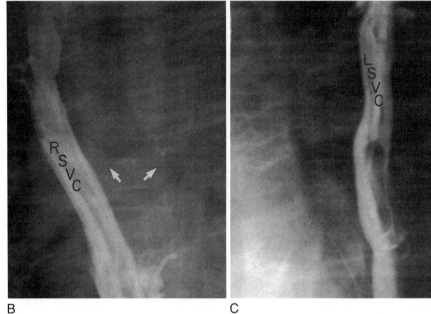

Figure 3–33

A, Magnetic resonance image from a 4-month-old female with left isomerism and bilateral superior vena cavae (*vertical arrows*). *B*, Angiographic visualization of the right superior vena cava (RSVC) and (*C*) of the left superior vena cava (LSVC). Paired *arrows* in *B* point to bilaterally symmetric morphologic left bronchi.

closely coupled with bilateral morphologic right atrial appendages and bilateral trilobed lungs[10,27,125,130,137] (see Fig. 3–29B). Ventricular/great arterial connections are usually discordant.[57] Total anomalous pulmonary venous connection is a common arrangement.[10,82,113,116,139] The ductus arteriosus may be bilateral.[44] Intracardiac malformations approximate a bilocular heart (see Fig. 3–34), namely, common atrium, common atrioventricular valve, functionally single ventricle (hypoplastic right or left ventricle) or anatomically single ventricle, and severe pulmonary stenosis or atresia.[10,57,82,113]

Extracardiac abnormalities have focused chiefly on the spleen, the largest lymphoid organ in the body.[108] Because of the spleen's manifold immunologic functions, *asplenia* is accompanied by recurrent, serious, and even life-threaten-ing infections.[126,150] Gastrointestinal abnormalities are the rule. Biliary atresia[60,94,145] and midline defects such as tracheoesophageal fistula are prevalent,[134] but the commonest gastrointestinal disorder is intestinal malrota-tion that predisposes to volvulus.[37,57,134] Midline defects also include the central nervous system (meningomyelo-cele, cerebellar agenesis, encephalocele), craniofacial (cleft lip and palate), genitourinary (horseshoe kidney), and musculoskeletal (kyphoscoliosis, pectus deformity).[57,134]

THE HISTORY

The sex distribution of visceral heterotaxy with right iso-merism is approximately equal[119] or with male predomi-nance.[113,139,134] Asplenia has been reported in siblings and in

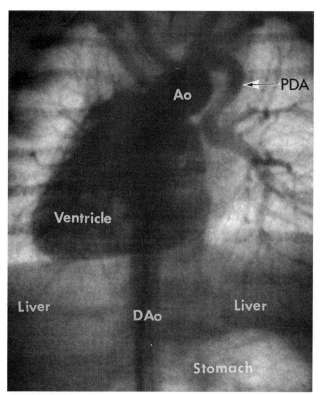

Figure 3–34
Angiocardiogram from an asplenic male neonate with right isomerism. The liver is transverse and the stomach and descending aorta (DAo) are on the same side. The heart was right-sided with single ventricle and pulmonary atresia. Ao, dilated aorta.

families.[113] Cyanosis is often evident in the first 24 hours.[57] Survival is determined chiefly by coexisting congenital heart disease (see Table 3–2), but extracardiac anomalies (see earlier) weigh heavily in determining morbidity and mortality. The majority of deaths are within the first few months of life with only sporadic survivals after the first year[113,129,139] and a single remarkable survival to age 21 years.[154] Because asplenia increases the risk of bacterial infection and septicemia,[18,126,143,148,150] the clinical presentation may be characterized by high fever, vomiting, hypotension, coma, and death shortly after the onset of symptoms.[126]

Table 3–1	**Characteristics of Right Isomerism**

Bilateral superior vena cavae

Bilateral sinoatrial nodes

Paired atrioventricular nodes

Bilateral morphologic right atria (appendages)

Bilateral morphologic right bronchi

Bilateral morphologic right lungs

Dextrocardia or levocardia

Asplenia

Transverse liver

Stomach right-sided or left-sided

PHYSICAL APPEARANCE

Infants with visceral heterotaxy and right isomerism are usually born at term, are normally formed, and have normal birth weights.[113] Neonatal cyanosis is invariable (see earlier) and conspicuous.

PALPATION AND PERCUSSION

Palpation of a transverse liver edge crossing the upper abdomen (see Fig. 3–31A) is presumptive evidence of visceral heterotaxy. Percussion is likely to detect a left rather than a right thoracic heart.[57,119,139] The location of the stomach is variable (see later).

THE ELECTROCARDIOGRAM

The sinus node normally resides at the junction of a morphologic right atrium and a right superior vena cava. In right isomerism, there are paired sinus nodes because each of the bilateral morphologic right atria is equipped with a junction to each of the bilateral superior vena cavae.[36,82,129,155,156] The P wave axis is usually normal, however, indicating that the *right* sinus node is the dominant atrial pacemaker.[155] A P wave axis that is directed inferior and to the *right* implies that atrial depolarization is from the *left* sinus node. The conduction system is also equipped with two atrioventricular nodes that are connected by a sling of conducting tissue.[62] Supraventricular tachycardia has been attributed to reentry between the paired atrioventricular nodes.[156] Atrioventricular block is rare in contrast to left isomerism.[115,119,129]

THE X-RAY

The x-ray is especially valuable when the upper abdomen is included (see Fig. 3–31). A transverse liver (see Fig. 3–32A) implies visceral heterotaxy but not its type. In right isomerism, the position of the stomach is variable (right, left, or occasionally central)[129,139] (see Figs. 3–31 and 3–34), and the heart can be either to the right or left of midline (see Fig. 3–31). Once visceral heterotaxy is suspected because of a transverse liver, bilateral symmetry (isomerism) is confirmed by bilaterally symmetric bronchi[119,138,152] (see Fig. 3–29). The next step is to determine whether the symmetric

Table 3–2	**Congenital Cardiac Malformations of Right Isomerism**

Common atrium

Common atrioventricular valve

Morphologic or functional single ventricle

Pulmonary stenosis or atresia

Total anomalous pulmonary venous connection

Absent coronary sinus

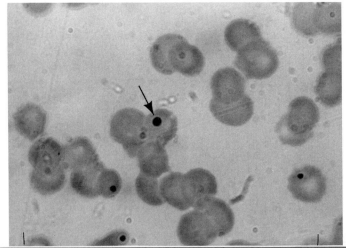

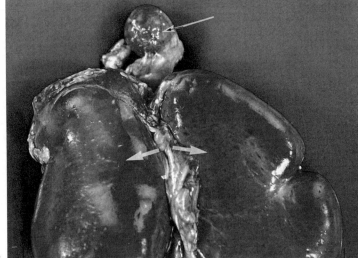

Figure 3–35
A, Peripheral blood smear in right isomerism with asplenia showing Howell-Jolly bodies (*arrow*). *B*, A normally formed sectioned spleen (*paired arrows*) with a splenule (*single arrow*).

bronchi are morphologic right or morphologic left. Overpenetrated films or tomograms serve to make this distinction (see Figs. 3–5*B,C* and 3–30).

THE ECHOCARDIOGRAM

The echocardiogram can identify morphologic right and morphologic left atrial appendages with their respective broad and narrow junctions.[127] Abdominal imaging of the liver, aorta, inferior vena cava, and hepatic veins provides a reliable basis for the diagnosis visceral heterotaxy.[12,64,65,119] The liver is transverse, and the inferior vena cava and aorta are anterior to or on the same side of the spinal column (Figs. 3–32 and 3–36). Hepatic veins drain into the inferior vena cava which joins the right-sided atrium. Imaging of the upper quadrants fails to identify a spleen. Visceral heterotaxy has been diagnosed by fetal echocardiography.[13] The largely predictable coexisting cardiac malformations are as in Table 3–2.

SUMMARY

Visceral heterotaxy with right isomerism usually comes to light because of complex cyanotic congenital heart disease

or because of the septicemia associated with asplenia. Howell-Jolly bodies on peripheral blood smears after the first week of life are evidence of asplenia. Palpation of a transabdominal liver edge in a cyanotic neonate or infant implies visceral heterotaxy but not its type. Sinoatrial nodes are bilateral, but the right sinus node is usually dominant so the P wave axis is normal. The x-ray confirms the transverse liver and may disclose bilaterally symmetric morphologic right bronchi. Abdominal echocardiography visualizes a transverse liver but no spleen. The aorta and inferior vena cava are anterior to or on the same side of the spinal column, and the inferior vena cava joins the right-sided atrium after receiving the hepatic veins.

Visceral Heterotaxy with Left Isomerism

Left isomerism as characterized in Table 3–3 is associated with the cardiovascular anomalies represented in Table 3–4. *Polysplenia* is a common but not invariable feature of left isomerism.[10,86,101,119,125] Matthew Baillie wrote,[14] "There were three spleens, nearly of the size of a pullet's egg, found adhering to the larger spleen by short adhesions, besides two other still smaller spleens which were

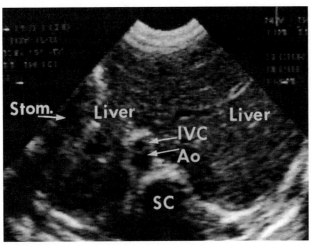

Figure 3–36
Echocardiogram from an asplenic male neonate with right isomerism. The liver is transverse, the stomach is on the right (Stom), and the aorta (Ao) and inferior vena cava (IVC) are on the same side of the spinal column (SC).

involved in the epiploon at the great end of the stomach." Baillie's *larger spleen* was accompanied by additional spleens of different size, and was an example of a normally formed spleen with *accessory spleens*. Accessory spleens or splenules are present in about 10% of the general population and are usually located in the vicinity of a normally formed spleen (see Fig. 3–35B), but may reside elsewhere in the abdomen.[38] Two well formed spleens may be accompanied by one or more splenules.[139] Because splenic tissue develops in the dorsal mesogastrium, accessory spleens tend to be located along the greater curvature of the stomach.[139] Normal single spleens are occasionally bilobed, trilobed or multilobed.[101,129] *Polysplenia* is characterized by a cluster of multiple splenules that collectively approximate the mass of one normal spleen.[101,129]

Left isomerism—bilateral left-sidedness—is characterized by bilateral morphologic left bronchi, bilateral morphologic left atrial appendages, and bilateral morphologic bilobed left lungs. The superior venae cavae are bilateral (see Fig. 3–33) and attach to morphologic left atria.[110,137] Paired morphologic left atria seemingly preclude the existence of an atrial septum, but attention has been called to a divided left-sided atrium, an intact atrial septum and a sinus venosus atrial septal defect.[50] The answer may lie in

Table 3–3 | **Characteristics of Left Isomerism**

Bilateral superior venae cavae

Bilateral morphologic left atria (appendages)

Absent or atretic sinoatrial node

Bilateral morphologic left bronchi

Bilateral morphologic left lungs

Transverse liver

Polysplenia

Stomach usually right-sided

Table 3–4 | **Congenital Cardiac Malformations of Left Isomerism**

Levocardia, less commonly dextrocardia

Common atrium

Inferior vena caval interruption with azygous continuation

Partial anomalous pulmonary venous connection

Two atrioventricular valves or a common atrioventricular valve

Atrioventricular septal defect

Ventricular–great arterial concordance

Left ventricular outflow obstruction

the nature of atrial isomerism in which the appendages are morphologically the same, but bilateral similarity (isomerism) may not include the rest of the atria.[134]

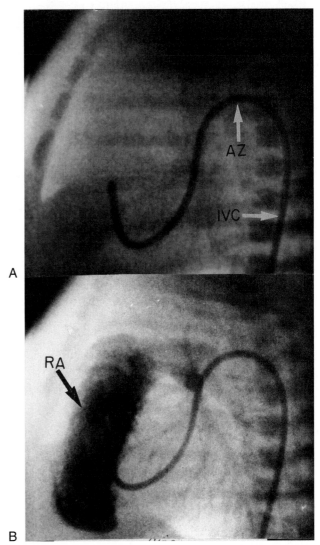

A

B

Figure 3–37
Angiocardiograms (anteroposterior projection) from a 5-month-old polysplenic female with left isomerism, inferior vena caval interruption with azygous continuation, and a right thoracic heart. *A,* The course of the catheter is through the interrupted inferior vena cava (IVC) into the azygous vein (AZ) and into the right atrium where the tip lies. *B,* Contrast material visualized the right atrium (RA).

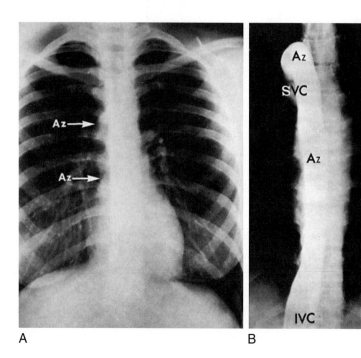

A   B

Figure 3–38

A, X-ray from a normal 28-year-old female with isolated inferior vena caval interruption and azygous continuation to a right superior vena cava. The spleen was present and single. The azygos vein (Az) ascends along the right vertebral border, forming a knuckle as it courses anterior to join the right superior cava. *B*, Inferior vena cavagram (IVC) showing the course of azygous continuation to the right superior vena cava (SVC).

However, it is *interruption of the inferior vena cava* with *azygous continuation* that is distinctive and diagnostically important.[10,101,111,113,139,146] The suprarenal segment of the inferior cava is absent, and the infrarenal segment continues as the azygos or hemiazygos vein[10] (Fig. 3–37). Rarely, isolated inferior caval interruption with azygous continuation occurs without visceral heterotaxy, without isomerism, with normal hearts, and with a normal single spleen (Fig. 3–38).[59] Even more rarely, polysplenia occurs with a normally structured heart.[33]

Anomalous pulmonary venous connection in left isomerism is partial, ventricular/great arterial alignments are concordant, and the pulmonary valve is occasionally stenotic but rarely atretic. The atrioventricular orifices are guarded by two valves or a common valve with an atrioventricular septal defect or a separate inlet ventricular septal defect.[101,113,129,139] There are two normally formed noninverted ventricles, and a moderate increase in incidence of left ventricular outflow obstruction.[144]

The most prevalent *extracardiac anomalies* in left isomerism are gastrointestinal,[37,94] and apart from the ubiquitous transverse liver, include intestinal malrotation,[50,134] biliary atresia,[3,50,60,134,145] esophageal atresia,[50] and congenital short pancreas.[109,122] Non-gastrointestinal extracardiac anomalies are analogous to those with right isomerism, namely, musculoskeletal, neurologic, and craniofacial.[50,134]

THE HISTORY

Visceral heterotaxy with *left isomerism* tends to occur in females,[50] and *right isomerism* tends to occur in males.[119] The clinical course (morbidity and mortality) of left isomerism is determined by coexisting cardiovascular malformations[9] (see Table 3–4) and by extracardiac anomalies but not by the septicemia of asplenia (see earlier). An investigation of fetal bradycardia due to complete heart block serves to identify intrauterine left isomerism.[104,121] The majority of patients present as neonates with congestive heart failure or cyanosis,[3,50,101,129] but an important minority present with symptoms related to an extracardiac malformation, especially biliary atresia.[50] Approximately 20% die as neonates and 50% survive adolescence.[50] Adult survival is uncommon but not unknown.[48,63,101,113] There are reports of familial polysplenia and familial asplenia,[35,113,118] and attention has been called to sibling

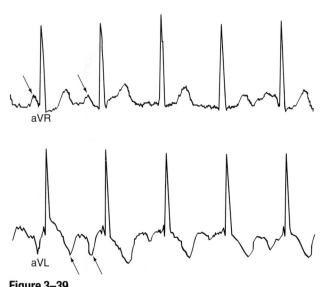

Figure 3–39

Leads aVR and aVL from a 16-month-old male with left isomerism, bilateral superior venae cavae and absent sinus node. The upright P wave in lead aVR (*arrows*) and the inverted P wave in lead aVL (*arrows*) reflect an ectopic atrial focus.

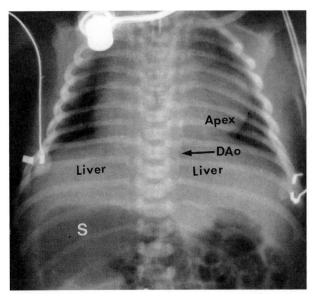

Figure 3–40
X-ray from a polysplenic female neonate with left isomerism. The liver is transverse, the apex is on the left, the stomach (S) is on the right and the descending aorta (DAo) is on the left. This opposite sided arrangement tends to occur in left isomerism.

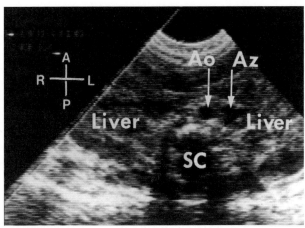

Figure 3–42
Abdominal echocardiogram from a polysplenic female infant with left isomerism. The liver is transverse. The aorta (Ao) and azygos vein (Az) are on the same side of the spinal column (SC). The inferior vena cava was interrupted with azygous continuation. A, anterior; L, left; P, posterior; R, right.

pairs in which one had polysplenia and the other had asplenia.[136]

extracardiac anomalies such as biliary atresia (jaundice), myelomeningocele, or cleft lip/palate.[50]

PHYSICAL APPEARANCE

Infants are normally formed and usually acyanotic. Abnormal physical appearance is likely to reflect the

PERCUSSION AND PALPATION

Palpation of a *transverse liver* in an *acyanotic* infant is presumptive evidence of *left* isomerism.

Figure 3–41
X-ray of conjoined twins with a single shared liver and shared intestines. Twin #1 had adequate lungs but an inadequate cardiac mass. Twin #2 had hypoplastic lungs but an adequate cardiac mass with a ventricular septal defect and pulmonary atresia.

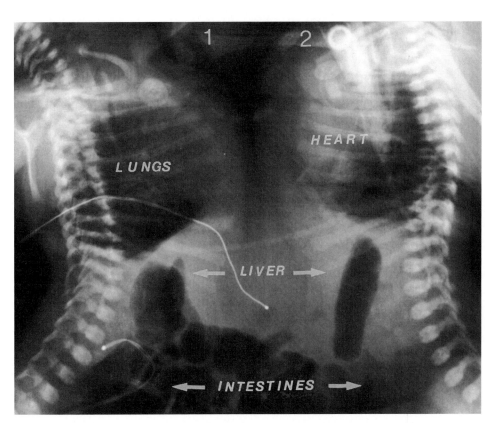

THE ELECTROCARDIOGRAM

The normal sinus node is a *right*-sided structure arising at the junction of a right superior vena cava and a morphologic right atrium (see earlier). In left isomerism, a sinus node is usually absent or hypoplastic because vena caval connection is to a morphologic *left* atrium. The atrial pacemaker is therefore ectopic (Fig. 3–39), located in the atrial wall or near the ostium of a coronary sinus,[36,82,91,111,155] so the P wave axis is abnormal.[36,47,113,129,139,155] The ectopic pacemaker may shift from one site to another[50,91] or may fire slowly (ectopic atrial bradycardia).[50] Atrial fibrillation or atrial flutter occasionally develops.[50,151] Complete atrioventricular block occurs in approximately one in five cases of left isomerism,[112] and can be present in the fetus and neonate[62,112] (see earlier) with a significant impact on morbidity and mortality.[36,47,113,129,139,146] Conduction is interrupted at the level of the penetrating bundle, producing nodoventricular discontinuity and a narrow QRS complex.[62]

THE X-RAY

A transverse liver is an important radiologic sign of visceral heterotaxy (see earlier) (Fig. 3–40), and when accompanied by symmetric morphologic left bronchi (see Fig. 3–29A), the diagnosis of heterotaxy with left isomerism is secure.[101,113,129,139,146] The heart is usually left-sided,[101,113,129] and the stomach tends to be on the side opposite the descending aorta[129] (see Fig. 3–40). A distinctive radiologic feature of left isomerism is *inferior vena caval interruption with azygous continuation* that is best seen in the frontal projection[50,111,113,146] (see Fig. 3–38). Absence of an inferior vena caval shadow in the lateral projection is not a reliable sign of interruption, because azygous continuation may create the impression of a normal uninterrupted inferior cava.[111] The lung fields usually show increased pulmonary blood flow because left-to-right shunts occur without obstruction to right ventricular outflow. A transverse liver is a feature of conjoined twins without heterotaxy (Fig. 3–41).

THE ECHOCARDIOGRAM

The echocardiogram confirms a transverse liver[64,65,127] (Fig. 3–42). The aorta and inferior vena cava lie anterior to or on the same side of the spinal column (Figs. 3–42 and 3–43). When there is inferior vena caval interruption with azygous continuation, the hepatic veins connect directly to the atria, and do not join the inferior cava (see Fig. 3–43B). Echocardiographic diagnosis can be made in the fetus.[13]

SUMMARY

Visceral heterotaxy with left isomerism presents as an acyanotic infant, usually female, with congestive heart fail-

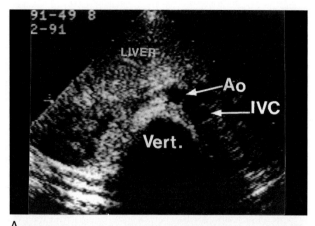

A

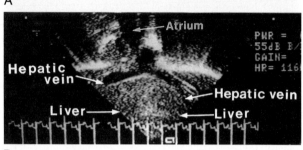

B

Figure 3–43

Abdominal echocardiogram from a polysplenic neonate with left isomerism. *A*, The liver is transverse. The aorta (Ao) and the inferior vena cava (IVC) are on the same side of the vertebral column (Vert.). *B*, Hepatic veins connect directly to an atrium because of inferior caval interruption with azygous continuation.

ure because a left-to-right shunt exists without obstruction to right ventricular outflow. Physical examination discloses a transverse liver and a left-sided heart. The x-ray confirms the transverse liver, and reveals bilaterally symmetric morphologic left bronchi. A distinctive radiologic feature is inferior vena caval interruption with azygous continuation. The electrocardiogram discloses the abnormal P wave axis of an ectopic atrial pacemaker because the sinus node is absent. A diagnostically useful electrocardiographic combination is an abnormal P wave axis, complete atrioventricular block and narrow QRS complexes. Abdominal echocardiography confirms the transverse liver and identifies an inferior vena cava and aorta anterior to or on the same side of the spinal column. When the inferior cava is interrupted, hepatic veins do not join the caval vein but instead connect to the atria.

REFERENCES

1. Abdollah H, Miliken JA: Recognition of electrocardiographic left arm/left leg lead reversal. Am J Cardiol 80:1247, 1997.
2. Abell I: Wandering spleen with torsion of the pedicle. Ann Surg 98:722, 1933.
3. Abramson SJ, Berdon WE, Altman RP, et al: Biliary atresia and noncardiac polysplenic syndrome: US and surgical consideration. Radiology 163:377, 1987.
4. Abu-Musa A, Hannoun A, Khabbaz A, Devroey P: Failure of fertilization after intracytoplasmic sperm injection in a patient with

Kartagener's syndrome and totally immobile sperm. Hum Reprod 14:2517, 1999.

5. Adams R, Churchill E: Situs inversus, sinusitis, bronchiectasis. J Thorac Surg 7:206, 1937.

6. Afzelius BA: Genetical and ultrastructural aspects of the immobile cilia syndrome. Am J Hum Genet 33:852, 1981.

7. Afzelius BA: Situs inversus and ciliary abnormalities. What is the connection? Int J Dev Biol 39:839, 1995.

8. Allen KB, Andrews G: Pediatric wandering spleen—the case for splenopexy: Review of 35 reported cases. J Pediatr Surg 24:432, 1989.

9. Amodeo A, DiDonoto R, Carotti A, et al: Pulmonary arteriovenous fistulas and polysplenia syndrome. J Thorac Cardiovasc Surg 107:1378, 1994.

10. Anderson C, Devine WA, Anderson RH, et al: Abnormalities of the spleen in relation to congenital malformations of the heart: A survey of necropsy findings in children. Br Heart J 63:122, 1990.

11. Anderson RH, Macartney FJ, Shinebourne EA, Tynan M: Terminology. In Paediatric Cardiology. Edinburgh, Churchill Livingstone, 1987, p 65.

12. Arisawa J, Morimoto S, Ikezoe J, et al: Cross sectional echocardiographic anatomy of common atrioventricular valve in atrial isomerism. Br Heart J 62:291, 1989.

13. Atkinson DE, Drant S: Diagnosis of heterotaxy syndromes by fetal echocardiography. Am J Cardiol 82:1147, 1998.

14. Baillie M: Of a remarkable transposition of the viscera. Philos Trans R Soc Lond 16:483, 1785-1790.

15. Beder SD, Gillette PC, Garson A, McNamara DG: Clinical confirmation of ECG criteria for left atrial rhythm. Am Heart J 103:848, 1982.

16. Bergstrom WH, Cook CD, Scannell J, Berenberg W: Situs inversus, bronchiectasis and sinusitis: Report of family with 2 cases of Kartagener's triad and 2 additional cases of bronchiectasis among 6 siblings. Pediatrics 6:573, 1950.

17. Bharati S, Lev M: The course of the conduction system in dextrocardia. Circulation 57:163, 1978.

18. Bigger WD, Ramirez RA, Rose V: Congenital asplenia: Immunologic assessment. Pediatrics 67:548, 1981.

19. Bleyer JM, Saphir W: Rheumatic heart disease in dextrocardia with situs inversus. Am Heart J 46:772, 1953.

20. Blieden LC, Moller JH: Analysis of the P wave in congenital cardiac malformations associated with splenic anomalies. Am Heart J 85:439, 1973.

21. Bossen PG, Van Agdent EF, Degryse HR, DeSchepper AM: Computed tomography of the polysplenia syndrome in the adult. Gastrointest Radiol 12:209, 1987.

22. Brown JW: Congenital Heart Disease. London, Staples Press, 1950.

23. Campbell M: Mode of inheritance in isolated levocardia and dextrocardia and situs inversus. Br Heart J 25:803, 1963.

24. Campbell M, Deuchar DC: Dextrocardia and isolated levocardia: I. Isolated levocardia. Br Heart J 27:69, 1965.

25. Campbell M, Deuchar DC: Dextrocardia and isolated levocardia: II. Situs inversus and isolated dextrocardia. Br Heart J 28:472, 1966.

26. Campbell M, Reynolds G: Significance of the direction of the P wave in dextrocardia and isolated levocardia. Br Heart J 14:481, 1952.

27. Caruso G, Becker AE: How to determine atrial situs? Br Heart J 41:559, 1979.

28. Casey B: Mapping of a gene for familial situs abnormalities to human chromosome Xq24-q27.1. Nat Genet 5:403, 1993.

29. Cesko I, Hajdu J, Marton T, et al: Polysplenia and situs inversus in siblings. Fetal Diagn Ther 16:1, 2001.

30. Chacko KA, Krishnaswami S, Sukumar IP, Cherian G: Isolated levocardia: Two cases with abdominal situs inversus, thoracic situs solitus and normal circulation. Am Heart J 106:155, 1983.

31. Chitayat D, Lao A, Wilson D, et al: Prenatal diagnosis of asplenia/polysplenia syndrome. Am J Obstet Gynecol 158:1085, 1988.

32. Corazza GR, Ginaldi L, Zoli G, et al: Howell-Jolly body counting as a measure of splenic function: A reassessment. Clin Lab Haematol 12:269, 1990.

33. Debich DE, Devine WA, Anderson RH: Polysplenia with normally structured hearts. Am J Cardiol 65:1274, 1990.

34. de la Cruz MV, da Rocha JP: Ontogenetic theory for explanation of congenital malformations involving truncus and concus. Am Heart J 51:782, 1976.

35. de la Monte SM, Hutchins GM: Brief clinical report: Sisters with polysplenia. Am J Med Genet 21:171, 1985.

36. Dickinson DF, Wilkinson JL, Anderson KR, et al: The cardiac conduction system in situs ambiguus. Circulation 59:879, 1979.

37. Ditchfield MR, Hutson JM: Intestinal rotational abnormalities in polysplenia and asplenia syndromes. Pediatr Radiol 28:305, 1998.

38. Dodds WJ, Taylor AJ, Erickson SJ, et al: Radiologic imaging of splenic anomalies. Am J Radiol 155:805, 1990.

39. Douard R, Feldman A, Bargy F, et al: Anomalies of lateralization in man: a case of total situs inversus. Surg Radiol Anat 22:293, 2000.

40. Eavey RD, Nadol JB, Holmes LB, et al: Kartagener's syndrome: A blinded, controlled study of cilia ultrastructure. Arch Otolaryngol Head Neck Surg 112:646, 1986.

41. Edenbrandt L, Rittner R: Recognition of lead reversals in pediatric cardiology. Am J Cardiol 82:1290, 1998.

42. Elliott LP, Jue KL, Amplatz K: A roentgen classification of cardiac malpositions. Invest Radiol 1:17, 1966.

43. Flyer DC, Buckley LP, Hellenbrand WE: Report of the New England Regional Infant Cardiac Program. Pediatrics 65:375, 1980.

44. Formigari R, Vairo U, deZorzi A, et al: Prevalence of bilateral patent ductus arteriosus in patients with pulmonic valve atresia and asplenia syndrome. Am J Cardiol 70:1219, 1992.

45. Frankl WS, Soloff LA: Left atrial rhythm. Am J Cardiol 22:645, 1968.

46. Fraser FC, Teebi AS, Walsh S, Pinsky L: Poland sequence with dextrocardia: Which comes first? Am J Med Genet 73:194, 1997.

47. Garcia OL, Mehta AV, Pickoff AS, et al: Left isomerism and complete atrioventricular block. Am J Cardiol 48:1103, 1981.

48. Gayer G, Apter S, Jonas T, et al: Polysplenia syndrome detected in adulthood: Report of eight cases and review of the literature. Abdom Imaging 24:178, 1999.

49. Gershoni-Baruch R, Gottfried E, Pery M, et al: Immotile cilia syndrome including polysplenia, situs inversus, and extrahepatic biliary atresia. Am J Med Genet 33:390, 1989.

50. Gilljam T, McCrindle BW, Smallhorn JF, et al: Outcomes of left atrial isomerism over a 28-year period at a single institution. J Am Coll Cardiol 36:908, 2000.

51. Gomez de Terreros Caro FJ, Gomez-Stern AC, Alvarez-Sala WR, et al: Kartagener's syndrome: Diagnosis in a 75 year old woman. Arch Bronchopneumol 35:242, 1999.

52. Gorgu M, Asian G, Erdooan B, et al: Goldenhar syndrome with situs inversus totalis. Int J Oral Maxillofac Surg 27:404, 1998.

53. Greenberg ML, Curtiss EI, Follansbee WP: Noninvasive diagnosis of mirror-image dextrocardia with thoraco-abdominal discordance. Am Heart J 109:172, 1985.

54. Guichard C, Harricane MC, Lafitte JJ, et al: Axonemal dynien intermediate-chain gene (DNAI 1) mutations result in situs inversus and primary ciliary dyskinesia (Kartagener syndrome). Am J Hum Genet 68:1030, 2001.

55. Harris BC, Shaver JA, Gray S, et al: Left atrial rhythm: Experimental production in man. Circulation 37:1000, 1968.

56. Harris TR, Rainey RL: Ideal isolated levocardia. Am Heart J 70:440, 1965.

57. Hashmi A, Abu-Sulaiman R, McCrindle BW, et al: Management and outcomes of right atrial isomerism: A 26-year experience. J Am Coll Cardiol 31:1120, 1998.

58. Hastreiter AR, Rodriguez-Coronel A: Discordant situs of thoracic and abdominal viscera. Am J Cardiol 22:111, 1968.

59. Heitzman ER: Radiologic appearance of the azygous vein in cardiovascular disease. Circulation 47:628, 1973.

60. Herman TE: Left-isomerism (polysplenia) with congenital atrioventricular block and biliary atresia. J Perinatal 19:155, 1999.

61. Ho SY, Cook A, Anderson RH, et al: Isomerism of the atrial appendages in the fetus. Pediatr Pathol 11:589, 1991.

62. Ho SY, Fagg N, Anderson RH, et al: Disposition of the atrioventricular conduction tissues in the heart with isomerism of the atrial appendages: Its relation to congenital complete heart block. J Am Coll Cardiol 20:904, 1992.

63. Hojo Y, Kuroda T, Yamasawa M, et al: Polysplenia accompanied by major cardiovascular anomalies with prolonged survival. Intern Med 33:357, 1994.

64. Huhta JC, Hagler DJ, Seward JB, et al: Two-dimensional echocardiographic assessment of dextrocardia: A segmental approach. Am J Cardiol 50:1351, 1982.

65. Huhta JC, Smallhorn JF, Macartney FJ: Two-dimensional echocardiographic diagnosis of situs. Br Heart J 48:97, 1982.

66. Hynes KM, Gau GT, Titus JL: Coronary heart disease in situs inversus totalis. Am J Cardiol 31:666, 1973.

67. Ivemark BI: Implications of agenesis of the spleen on the pathogenesis of conotruncus anomalies in childhood: An analysis of heart malformations in the splenic agenesis syndrome, with 14 new cases. Acta Paediatr Upps 44 (Suppl 104) L7, 1955.

68. Jacoby WJ Jr, Jacobson WA: Dextrocardia complicated by myocardial infarction. Am J Cardiol 11:119, 1963.

69. Janchar T, Milzman D, Clement M: Situs inversus: Emergency evaluations of atypical presentations. Am J Emerg Med 18:349, 2000.

70. Kalhs P, Panzer S, Kletter K, et al: Functional asplenia after bone marrow transplantation. Ann Intern Med 109:461, 1988.

71. Kaplan LC, Matsuoka R, Gilbert EF, et al: Ectopic cordis and cleft sternum: Evidence for mechanical teratogenesis following rupture of the chorion or yolk sac. Am J Med Genet 21:187, 1985.

72. Kartagener M: Zur Pathogenese der Bronchiektasien; Bronchiektasien bei Situs Viscerum Inversus. Beitr Klin Tuberk 83:489, 1933.

73. Katz M, Benzier EE, Nangeroni L, Sussman B: Kartagener's syndrome (situs inversus, bronchiectasis, and chronic sinusitis). N Engl J Med 248:730, 1953.

74. Kennedy DN, O'Craven KM, Ticho BS, et al: Structural and functional brain asymmetries in human situs inversus totalis. Neurology 53:1260, 1999.

75. Khoury MJ, Cordero JF, Rasmussen S: Ectopia cordis, midline defects and chromosome abnormalities: An epidemiologic perspective. Am J Med Genet 30:811, 1988.

76. Kirk ED Jr: Transient bundle branch block due to myocardial infarction in a patient with dextrocardia with situs inversus. Am J Cardiol 16:297, 1965.

77. Landing BH, Lawrence TK, Payne VC, Wells TR: Bronchial anatomy in syndromes with abnormal visceral situs, abnormal spleen and congenital heart disease. Am J Cardiol 28:456, 1971.

78. Lev M, Liberthson RR, Golden JG, et al: The pathologic anatomy of mesocardia. Am J Cardiol 28:428, 1971.

79. Lichtman SS: Isolated congenital dextrocardia. Arch Intern Med 48:683, 1931.

80. Losa M, Ghelfi D, Hof E, et al: Kartagener syndrome: An uncommon cause of neonatal respiratory distress? Eur J Pediatr 154:236, 1995.

81. Losekoot TG: Mirror image dextrocardia with situs solitus of the abdominal organs in a normal heart. Eur J Cardiol 1:49, 1973.

82. Macartney FJ, Zuberbuhler JR, Anderson RH: Morphological considerations pertaining to recognition of atrial isomerism. Br Heart J 44:657, 1980.

83. Malleson P, Petty RE, Nadel H, Dimmick JE: Functional asplenia in childhood onset systemic lupus erythematosus. J Rheumatol 15:1648, 1988.

84. Mandelstam ME, Reinberg SA: Die Dextrokardie. Ergeb Med Kinderheilkd 34:154, 1928.

85. Massumi RA, Tawakkol AA: Direct study of left atrial P waves. Am J Cardiol 20:331, 1967.

86. Merklin RJ: Cardiac lesions associated with visceral inversion: A study of 185 cases. J Int Coll Surg 41:597, 1964.

87. Miller BL, Medrano GA, Sodi-Pallares D: Vectorcardiogram in dextrocardia, dextroversion and dextroposition. Am J Cardiol 21:830, 1968.

88. Mirowski M, Neill CA, Bahnson HT, Taussig HB: Negative P waves in lead 1 in dextroversion-differential diagnosis from mirror-image dextrocardia. Circulation 26:413, 1962.

89. Mirowski M, Neill CA, Taussig HB: Left atrial ectopic rhythm in mirror image dextrocardia and in normally placed malformed hearts: report of twelve cases with "dome and dart" P waves. Circulation 27:864, 1963.

90. Momma K, Linde LM: Cardiac rhythms in dextrocardia. Am J Cardiol 25:420, 1970.

91. Momma K, Takao A, Shibata T: Characteristics and natural history of abnormal atrial rhythms in left isomerism. Am J Cardiol 65:231, 1990.

92. Mossberg B, Hanngren A: Kartagener's syndrome. Mt Sinai J Med 44:837, 1977.

93. Nagaratnam N, Koyagama LS: Dextrocardia, situs inversus totalis, and appendicular abscess. Postgrad Med J 33:287, 1957.

94. Nakada K, Kawaguchi F, Wakisaka M, et al: Digestive tract disorders associated with asplenia/polysplenia syndrome. J Pediatr Surg 32:91, 1997.

95. Narayan D, Krishnan SN, Upender M, et al: Unusual inheritance of primary ciliary dyskinesia (Kartagener's syndrome). J Med Genet 31:493, 1994.

96. O'Reilly RJ, Grollman JH: The lateral chest film as an unreliable indicator of azygous continuation of the inferior vena cava. Circulation 53:891, 1976.

97. Paltauf R: Dextrocardie und Dextroversio Cardis. Wien Klin Wochnschr 14:1032, 1901.

98. Pan Y, McCaskill CD, Thompson KH, et al: Paternal isodismony of chromosome 7 associated with situs inversus and immobile cilia. Am J Hum Genet 62:1551, 1998.

99. Partridge JB, Scott O, Deverall PB, Macartney FJ: Visualization and measurement of the main bronchi by tomography as an objective indicator of thoracic situs in congenital heart disease. Circulation 51:188, 1975.

100. Payne WS, Ellis FH Jr, Hunt JC: Congenital corrected transposition of great vessels with situs inversus and dextrocardia. Am J Cardiol 8:288, 1961.

101. Peoples WM, Moller JH, Edwards JE: Polysplenia: A review of 146 cases. Pediatr Cardiol 4:129, 1983.

102. Perloff JK: Physical Examination of the Heart and Circulation, 3rd ed. Philadelphia, WB Saunders, 1998.

103. Phillips DM, Jow WW, Goldstein M: Testis factors that may regulate gene expression: Evidence from a patient with Kartagener's syndrome. J Androl 16:158, 1995.

104. Phoon CK, Villegas MD, Ursell PC, Silverman NH: Left atrial isomerism detected in fetal life. Am J Cardiol 77:1083, 1996.

105. Piccolo E, Nava A, Furlanello F, et al: Left atrial rhythm: Vectorcardiographic study and electrophysiologic critical evaluation. Am Heart J 80:11, 1970.

106. Rao PS: Dextrocardia: Systematic approach to differential diagnosis. Am Heart J 102:389, 1981.

107. Reddy V, Sharma S, Cobanoglu A: What dictates the position of the diaphragm—the heart or the liver? A review of sixtyfive cases. J Thorac Cardiovasc Surg 108:687, 1994.

108. Roberts WC, Berry WB, Morrow AG: The significance of asplenia in the recognition of inoperable congenital heart disease. Circulation 26:1251, 1962.

109. Rodriguez-Recio FJ, Mainer A, Ochoa A, et al: Polysplenia with congenital short pancreas without other associated malformations. Eur J Med 2:443, 1993.

110. Roguin N, Aydinalo A: Isomeric arrangement of the left atrial appendages and visceral heterotaxy. Cardiol Young 10:668, 2000.

111. Roguin N, Hammerman H, Korman S, Riss E: Angiography of azygous continuation of inferior vena cava in situs ambiguus with left isomerism (polysplenia syndrome). Pediatr Radiol 14:109, 1984.

112. Roguin N, Pelled B, Freundlich E, et al: Atrioventricular block in situs ambiguus and left isomerism (polysplenia syndrome). PACE 7:18, 1984.

113. Rose V, Izukawa I, Moses CAF: Syndromes of asplenia and polysplenia: A review of cardiac and non-cardiac malformations in 60 cases with special reference to diagnosis and prognosis. Br Heart J 37:840, 1975.

114. Rosenbaum HD, Pellegrino ED, Treciokas LJ: Acyanotic levocardia. Circulation 26:60, 1962.

115. Rossi L, Montella S, Frescura C, Thiene G: Congenital atrioventricular block in right atrial isomerism. Chest 85:578, 1984.

116. Rubino M, Van Praagh S, Kadoba K, et al: Systemic and pulmonary venous connections in visceral heterotaxy with asplenia: Diagnostic and surgical considerations in seventy-two autopsied cases. J Thorac Cardiovasc Surg 119:641, 1995.

117. Sacks LV, Rifkin IR: Mirror image arrangement of the abdominal organs with a left-sided morphologically normal heart. Br Heart J 58:534, 1987.

118. Santoro G, Masiello P, Farina R, et al: Isolated atrial inversion in situs inversus. Ann Thorac Surg 59:1019, 1995.

119. Sapire DW, Ho SY, Anderson RH, Rigby ML: Diagnosis and significance of atrial isomerism. Am J Cardiol 58:342, 1986.

120. Schiebler GL, Edwards JE, Burchell HB, et al: Congenital corrected transposition of the great vessels. Pediatrics 27 (Suppl):851, 1961.

121. Schmidt KG, Ulmer HE, Silverman NH, et al: Prenatal outcome of fetal complete atrioventricular block. J Am Coll Cardiol 17:1360, 1991.

122. Sener RN, Alper H: Polysplenia syndrome: A case associated with transhepatic portal vein, short pancreas, and left superior vena cava with hemiazygous continuation. Abdom Imaging 19:64, 1994.

123. Shah CV, Shah KD, Ashar PN, Hanosti RC: Mirror-image dextrocardia with thoracoabdominal discordance and normal spleen. Chest 69:427, 1976.

124. Shaher RM, Johnson AM: Isolated levocardia and isolated dextrocardia: Pathology and pathogenesis. Guy's Hosp Rep 112:127, 1968.

125. Sharma S, Devine W, Anderson RH, Zuberbuhler JR: The determination of atrial arrangement by examination of appendage morphology in 1842 heart specimens. Br Heart J 60:227, 1988.

126. Sills RH: Splenic function: Physiology and splenic hypofunction. CRC Crit Rev Oncol Hematol 7:1, 1987.

127. Smallhorn J, Rigby ML, Deanfield JE: Echocardiography. In Anderson RH, Shinebourne EA, Macartney FJ, Tynan M (eds): Paediatric Cardiology. Edinburgh, Churchill Livingstone, 1987.

128. Stalsberg H: Mechanism of dextral looping of the embryonic heart. Am J Cardiol 25:265, 1970.

129. Stanger P, Rudolph AM, Edwards JE: Cardiac malpositions. Circulation 56:159, 1977.

130. Stewart PA, Becker AE, Wladimiroff JW, Essed CA: Left atrial isomerism with asplenia. J Am Coll Cardiol 4:1015, 1984.

131. Tanaka S, Kanzaki R, Yoshibayashi M, et al: Dichotic listening in patients with situs inversus: Brain asymmetry and situs asymmetry. Neuropsychologia 37:869, 1999.

132. Tek I, Dincer I, Gurlek A: Kartagener's syndrome and corrected transposition of the great arteries. Int J Cardiol 75:305, 2000.

133. Teknos TN, Metson R, Chasse T, et al: New developments in the diagnosis of Kartagener's syndrome. Otolaryngol Head Neck Surg 116:68, 1997.

134. Ticho BS, Goldstein AM, Van Praagh R: Extracardiac anomalies in the heterotaxy syndromes with focus on anomalies of midline-associated structures. Am J Cardiol 85:729, 2000.

135. Torgersen J: Familial transposition of the viscera with preliminary remarks on genetics and correlation with diseases of the respiratory tract. Acta Med Scand 126:319, 1946.

136. Toriello HV, Kokx N, Higgins JV, et al: Sibs with polysplenia developmental field defect. Am J Med Genet (Suppl) 2:31, 1986.

137. Uemura H, Ho SY, Devine WA, Anderson RH: Analysis of visceral heterotaxy according to splenic status, appendage morphology, or both. Am J Cardiol 76:846, 1995.

138. Van Mierop LHS, Eisen S, Schiebler GL: The radiographic appearance of the tracheobronchial tree as an indicator of visceral situs. Am J Cardiol 26:432, 1970.

139. Van Mierop LHS, Gessner IH, Schiebler GL: Asplenia and polysplenia syndromes. Birth Defects 8:36, 1972.

140. Van Praagh R: Terminology of congenital heart disease. Circulation 56:139, 1977.

141. Van Praagh R, Van Praagh S: Atrial isomerism in the heterotaxy syndromes with asplenia, or polysplenia, or normally formed spleen: An erroneous concept. Am J Cardiol 66:1504, 1990.

142. Van Praagh R, Van Praagh S, Vlad P, Keith JD: Anatomic types of congenital dextrocardia—diagnostic and embryologic implications. Am J Cardiol 13:510, 1964.

143. Van Praagh R, Weinberg PM, Smith SD, et al: Malpositions of the heart. In Moss AJ, Adams FH, Emmanouilides GC, Riemenschnider TA (eds): Heart Disease in Infants, Children and Adolescents, 4th ed. Baltimore, Williams & Wilkins, 1989.

144. Van Praagh S, Geva T, Freidberg DZ, et al: Aortic outflow obstruction in visceral heterotaxy: A study based on twenty postmortem cases. Am Heart J 133:558, 1997.

145. Vazquez J, Lopez Gutierrez JC, Gamez M, et al: Biliary atresia and the polysplenia syndrome. J Pediatr Surg 30:485, 1995.

146. Vaughan TJ, Hawkins IF, Elliott LP: Diagnosis of polysplenia syndrome. Diagn Radiol 101:511, 1971.

147. Vijayakumar V, Brandt T: Prolonged survival with isolated levocardia and situs inversus. Cleve Clin J Med 58:243, 1991.

148. Waldman JD, Rosenthal A, Smith AL, et al: Sepsis in congenital asplenia. J Pediatr 90:555, 1977.

149. Waller AD: On the electromotive charges connected with the beat of mammalian heart and of the human heart in particular. Philos Trans R Soc Lond 180:169, 1889.

150. Wang J, Hsieh K: Immunologic study of the asplenia syndrome. Pediatr Infect Dis J 10:819, 1991.

151. Wang TD, Tseng CD, Lee YT: Left isomerism in a middle aged woman with early onset atrial fibrillation. Int J Cardiol 58:269, 1997.

152. Winer-Muram HT, Tonkin ILD: The spectrum of heterotaxic syndromes. Radiol Clin North Am 27:1147, 1989.

153. Wittenborg MH, Aviad I: Organ influence on the normal posture of the diaphragm: A radiological study of the inversions and heterotaxies. Br J Radiol 36:280, 1963.

154. Wolfe MW, Vacek JL, Kinard RE, Bailey CG: Prolonged and functional survival with the asplenia syndrome. Am J Med 81:1089, 1986.

155. Wren C, Macartney FJ, Deanfield JE: Cardiac rhythm in atrial isomerism. Am J Cardiol 59:1156, 1987.

156. Wu M, Wang J, Lin J, et al: Supraventricular tachycardia in patients with right isomerism. J Am Coll Cardiol 32:773, 1998.

157. Yoo JHK, Orzel JA, Bagnall JW, Weiland FL: Technetium-99m red blood cell blood-pool imaging in functional asplenia due to leukemic infiltration. Clin Nucl Med 11:493, 1986.

158. Yost HJ: The genetics of midline and cardiac laterality defects. Curr Opin Cardiol 13:185, 1998.

159. Zlotogora J, Schimmel MS, Glaser Y: Familial situs inversus and congenital heart defects. Am J Med Genet 26:181, 1987.

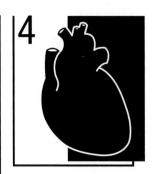

Isolated Congenital Complete Heart Block

Alfred Lewis Glabin documented atrioventricular block in humans in 1873, using an apex cardiogram.[121a] Congenital complete atrioventricular block was reported in 1901, when Morquio described familial recurrence with Stokes-Adams attacks and death in childhood.[85] In 1908, van den Heuvel published the electrocardiogram of a patient with complete heart block and syncopal episodes that dated from infancy.[123] Thirteen years later, White and Eustis[126] described slow fetal heart rate clarified at birth by electrocardiographic confirmation of complete heart block. Davis and Stecher[21] distinguished congenital from acquired complete heart block, and shortly thereafter Yater established criteria for the clinical diagnosis of the congenital form.[131–133]

Complete, or third-degree, heart block is a conduction disorder characterized by a random relationship between atrial and ventricular activation. Atrial impulses are not conducted to the ventricles, which are depolarized in response to a subsidiary pacemaker.[46] *Atrioventricular dissociation* is a disorder of both conduction and impulse formation[46,102] and is not considered in this chapter. The electrocardiogram is a simple but secure means of identifying complete heart block, which is likely to be congenital if the slow rate is known in utero or from infancy and if the QRS is narrow, indicating a normal sequence of ventricular excitation (Figs. 4–1 and 4–2). Fetal echocardiography permits an intrauterine diagnosis, in addition to which isolated complete heart block can be distinguished from cases with coexisting congenital heart disease, most commonly ventricular inversion (see Chapter 6) or left isomerism (see Chapter 3).

The incidence of congenital high-degree heart block, either complete or with more than 50% of blocked atrial impulses, has been estimated at 1 in 15,000 to 20,000 live births.[13,72,81,99,102,106] Block can be either within the atrioventricular (AV) node, within the bundle of His, or infrahisian, and discontinuity in the conduction pathways can be either anatomic or functional.[2,4,6,36,46,60] Narrow QRS complexes indicate that the subsidiary pacemaker is above the bifurcation of the bundle of His, that is, supraventricular. Morphologic abnormalities have been identified at multiple levels.[*] The connection between atrial muscle and atrioventricular node is either deficient or absent,[6,44,64,81] and the node may be congenitally absent or defective[6,36,60,62,64,81] or may be separated from the bundle of His.[61] These observations support the view that the AV node and the bundle of His originate as separate structures that are destined to join during normal early fetal development.[2,43] Disruption can be within the bundle of His,[6,63] at the origins of the bundle branches, or in the right or left bundle branch.[44,64,81] Anatomic defects occasionally exist in the AV node itself or at the junction of the AV node and atrial muscle.[43,81] Spontaneous changes from complete to incomplete heart block,[4,23,52] or even to sinus rhythm,[15,16,104] indicate that interruption of the conduction pathways is not necessarily *anatomic, complete,* or *permanent* (Fig. 4–3).

The slow heart rate, the long diastolic filling period, and the increased end-diastolic volume and fiber length augment myocardial contractile force.[100,102,104] Stroke volume increases, and basal cardiac output is maintained.[42,73,94,104,119] An increase in cardiac output with exercise is chiefly rate dependent.[42,73] Submaximal isotonic exercise generally provokes an appropriate increase in ventricular rate and cardiac output, but higher work-

---

[*]See references 2a, 6, 36, 43, 44, 59, 64, 67, 81, 125, 133.

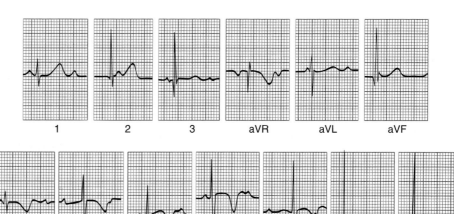

Figure 4–1

Electrocardiogram from a 7-year-old boy with isolated congenital complete heart block. P waves are independent of QRS complexes. The QRS complex is normal in configuration and duration, and its axis is normal. There are deep Q waves and tall R waves in leads V_5 and V_6. The R wave in lead V_1 is relatively tall, with an R/S ratio of 1:1. T waves are deeply inverted in right precordial leads, and are tall and peaked in left precordial leads. See Figure 4–5 for rhythm strip.

loads are accompanied by blunted hemodynamic and rate responses.[73,117] An increase in stroke volume and, to a lesser degree, an increase in arteriovenous oxygen difference partially compensate for the blunted rate response.[100] Despite compensatory mechanisms, oxygen consumption during submaximal exercise is significantly lower than in normal age- and sex-matched control subjects.[100]

An association between maternal lupus erythematosus and congenital complete heart block was reported in 1966,[40] and a decade later the association was confirmed.[*] Sinus node disease may occur in children with prenatal exposure to anti-Ro or anti-La antibodies.[79] Complete heart block in utero or at birth is strongly associated with maternal antibodies to 48-kD SSB/La, 52-kD SSA/Ro, and 60-kD SSA/Ro ribonucleoproteins and is strongly associated with the neonatal lupus syndrome.[12] The fetal sinoatrial and atrioventricular nodes may calcify.[2a] Congenital heart block has emerged as an important model of passive

autoimmunity, with cardiac injury believed to be in response to active transport of maternal IgG autoantibodies into the fetal circulation.[12]

The History

The history of congenital complete heart block begins in utero.[32,72,93,106] Fetal echocardiography establishes the diagnosis and determines whether the heart block is isolated or associated with congenital heart disease, which is usually left isomerism or ventricular inversion (see earlier). Only 14% of fetuses with coexisting congenital heart disease survive as neonates.[106] Conversely, isolated intrauterine complete heart block is only rarely accompanied by congestive failure,[32,72,106] and 85% of fetuses live beyond the neonatal period.[42a,106] This survival rate is similar to that of isolated congenital complete heart block diagnosed after birth, in which approximately 90% of infants and children are alive at long-term follow-up.[106]

The fetal cardiac rhythm may change from sinus to second-degree atrioventricular block to complete heart block, which may appear hours or weeks after birth.[106] These observations suggest that immunologic damage occurs early, develops slowly, or appears late.

There is a tendency for female preponderance in congenital complete heart block.[26,86,94,99] More than 76% of mothers of affected children are white.[12] Familial heart block is well recognized,[†] and in Morquio's original description, atrioventricular block recurred in five of eight siblings[85] (see earlier). Osler described Stokes-Adams attacks in a patient who had many relatives with slow pulses.[92] Familial heart block can be congenital, can become overt years after birth,[11,45,84] and can be characterized by right or left bundle branch block[29,41,44]; almost all

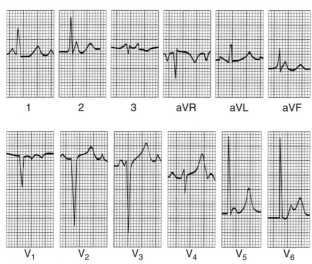

Figure 4–2

Electrocardiogram of a 25-year-old man with congenital complete heart block. P waves are independent of QRS complexes. The QRS complex is narrow, and its axis is normal. There are tall R waves and relatively tall, peaked T waves in leads V_5 and V_6.

---

*See references 9, 17, 27, 37, 40, 57, 58, 68, 69, 76, 91, 93, 98, 102, 108, 118, 128.
†See references 13, 18, 20, 31, 41, 52, 56, 71, 84, 89, 102, 103, 105, 124, 125, 128.

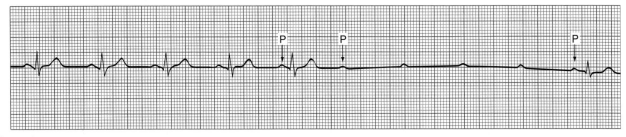

Figure 4–3
Rhythm strip from a 28-year-old man with intermittent congenital complete heart block that required a pacemaker. Sinus rhythm with normal PR intervals and normal QRS complexes is followed by sudden absence of AV conduction (see second P). The next sinus beat conducts through a slightly prolonged PR interval (see third P). (Courtesy of Dr. R.J. Burger, Fairbanks, Alaska.)

degrees and forms of heart block can be manifested by different members of the same family.[44] Four generations of a single family had right bundle branch block, left anterior fascicular block, bifascicular block, and complete heart block.[115]

Mothers with systemic lupus erythematosus who have had one child with neonatal heart block are at greater risk of having subsequent offspring with heart block.[11,33,57,58,105,116] Children of mothers with lupus may not only have congenital heart block but may also subsequently develop the overt connective tissue disease.[55] Maternal lupus may not become manifest for years after the birth of an infant with congenital complete heart block.[48,69] Long-term outcome for mothers of children with complete heart block is more reassuring, however.[9,25,78]

Congenital complete heart block usually comes to light because an inappropriately slow heart rate is discovered in an otherwise healthy, asymptomatic child (see "The Arterial Pulse"). Detection in the fetus is desirable, to distinguish the bradycardia of complete heart block from the bradycardia of fetal distress.[18,24] The distinction is more obvious when the slow regular fetal heartbeat of congenital complete heart block is recognized before the onset of labor.[24]

The key determinants of clinical stability in isolated congenital complete heart block are the ventricular rate, the hemodynamic adjustments at rest and with exercise as previously discussed, and the presence of intrinsically normal myocardium.[19,77,102] However, patients sometimes develop dilated cardiomyopathy attributed to bradycardia, although a strong relationship has been reported between SSA/Ro and SSB/La antibodies and subsequent development of cardiomyopathy.[8,25,121] Subnormal exercise performance has been reported in children and adolescents with complete atrioventricular block, but exercise tolerance is generally normal or nearly so,[14,15,22,42] and normal values for endurance performance have occasionally been observed.[100,117,127] One patient was an ardent ice hockey player,[42] and other patients have included Air Force pilots,[75,120] a cricket player,[14] a 56-year-old woman who for 20 years worked on a farm and walked 2 miles to her daily job,[16] a 38-year-old man who had won boxing matches in his youth,[16] and a 48-year-old man who experienced a normal response to a standard Royal Canadian Air

Force decompression chamber at the age of 23 years and subsequently flew jet aircraft and engaged in competitive sports.[19] High levels of physical activity are not desirable but are at least possible, despite the limitations implied by the response to exercise described earlier. Pregnancy is generally uneventful in otherwise normal women with congenital heart block,[5,26,34,35,38,87,95,110,134] but Stokes-Adams attacks occasionally occur during gestation or the puerperium.[26,95]

A substantial majority of young patients with isolated congenital complete heart block are asymptomatic, but the mortality rate even in infancy and childhood is estimated at 8%,[65,80] and the ultimate fate of large numbers of adolescents and adults is limited.[13,15,26,27,44,77,80,97,99] The heart may not respond adequately to increased circulatory demands, especially in the vulnerable neonatal period.[4,19,27,80,86,97,99,102,112] Infants with slow ventricular rates may succumb to congestive heart failure before physiologic adaptation is achieved.[20,80,86,112,124] Metabolic acidosis slows the heart rate,[114] and the stress of febrile illnesses in infancy are poorly tolerated.[89,104] Congenital complete heart block may come to light in toddlers because of night terrors or irritability[102]; the older child may experience late afternoon fatigue, and young adults may experience exercise intolerance, fatigue, faintness, or syncope.

Stokes-Adams episodes are uncommon in young patients but pose tangible hazards.[4,14,16,47,77,83,89,94,104] Complaints vary from mild dizziness, often ignored, to syncope and convulsions. Symptoms may announce themselves as a Stokes-Adams episode with sudden death in a previously asymptomatic patient (Fig. 4–4). Neurologic sequelae may follow cardiac arrest.[72,83] Fatal Stokes-Adams seizures occasionally occur in childhood,[15,83,99] but death rarely accompanies the initial episode.[89] One patient experienced recurrent Stokes-Adams episodes between 2 and 4 years of age, but the attacks gradually diminished and finally vanished, leaving him able to participate in cricket, football, and swimming.[14,15] Syncope and sudden death are usually caused by bradycardia, but ventricular tachycardia or fibrillation also play a role.[28,71,88,100] Frequent ventricular ectopic beats have been recorded during nocturnal monitoring,[65] and young patients experience unifocal, multifocal, or repetitive

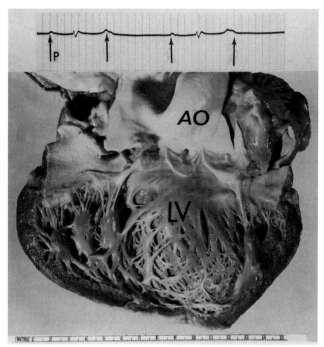

Figure 4–4

Rhythm strip and gross specimen from an 18-year-old laboratory technician with isolated congenital complete heart block who experienced a fatal Stokes-Adams episode. The rhythm strip shows broad, independent P waves and a narrow QRS. The left ventricle (LV) is dilated but otherwise normal. Ao, aorta.

ventricular ectopic beats during treadmill exercise.[127] Serious symptoms and complications are more likely to occur in patients with daytime heart rates below 50 beats per minute, wide QRS complexes, a blunted rate response to graded exercise, a disproportionate increase in left ventricular internal dimensions, or subnormal left ventricular function.[4,44,77,83,88,89,97,111]

Physical Appearance

Growth, development, and general physical appearance of patients with heart block are normal. Cyanosis may accompany congestive heart failure in bradycardic infants.[112]

The Arterial Pulse

An arterial pulse that is inappropriately slow for age often leads to the diagnosis of congenital complete heart block. At birth, the heart rate is seldom more than 90 beats per minute, and infants with complete heart block seldom have rates more than 65 or 70 beats per minute.[102] After infancy, the basal rate generally exceeds 50 beats per minute (Fig. 4–5) and not uncommonly reaches 60, 70, or even 80 beats per minute.[4,15,42,104]

Although the pulse is slow, it is relatively rapid when compared with the pulse rate associated with acquired complete heart block.[15,16] Rates of 40 to 60 beats per

minute in healthy young adults may be mistaken for sinus bradycardia.[15] The Royal Canadian Air Force veteran described by Matthewson and Harvie[75] was a case in point. The patient's slow heart rate was initially attributed to the sinus bradycardia of physical conditioning. The young man volunteered for investigations of his circulatory response to strenuous exercise, which he tolerated with no difficulty. Complete heart block believed to be congenital was subsequently recognized.

Three features other than rate deserve comment, namely, upstroke, pulse pressure, and atrial waves. The upstroke is brisk and the pulse pressure is relatively wide.[16,89] Rapid ejection of a large stroke volume from a functionally normal left ventricle increases the rate of rise and increases the systolic arterial pressure, whereas prolonged diastole permits a decline in diastolic pressure to relatively low levels.[104]

Small waves that are synchronous with atrial contraction appear on the diastolic portion of the arterial pressure pulse[39,104] and are sometimes detected by meticulous palpation. These waves are believed to result from the external impact of the left atrium on the aorta[104] and are analogous to waves that have been recorded on the pulmonary arterial pressure pulse. Sinus arrhythmia is conspicuous by its absence and weighs in favor of sinus bradycardia.

The Venous Pulse

The jugular venous pulse is in itself a reliable indication of complete heart block because of independent autonomous A waves, rapid atrial rate compared with the slower arterial pulse, and intermittent increase in amplitude (Fig. 4–6).[4,96,104] Small regular atrial A waves occur during diastole, and when timed with the carotid pulse are asynchronous and more rapid, indicating that atrial and ventricular contractions are independent. When the right atrium contracts against a tricuspid valve that is closed during ventricular systole, the A wave abruptly amplifies (see Fig. 4–6) and is called a *cannon wave*.[96] Precise timing of cannon waves assigns their maximum amplitude to isovolumetric ventricular systole.[54] The first heart sound that accompanies a cannon wave is comparatively soft because atrial systole *follows* rather than precedes ventricular contraction (see later).

Precordial Movement and Palpation

The left ventricular impulse is prominent because a large stroke volume is ejected rapidly from a volume-overloaded but functionally normal chamber.[4] A right ventricular impulse is absent despite equivalent volume overload. Variations in intensity of the first heart sound are detected by the examiner's fingertips while palpating the left ventricular impulse, and mid-diastolic distention is sensed when atrial contraction coincides with the rapid filling phase.

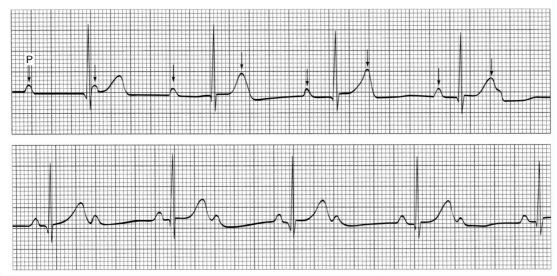

Figure 4–5
Long strip of lead 2 of the electrocardiogram shown in Figure 4–1. Independent P waves are identified by arrows. The P-P intervals are shorter when separated by a QRS complex (positive chronotropic effect). The ventricular rate is 48 to 50 beats per minute. The QRS complexes are narrow.

Auscultation

Auscultation is a means of suspecting fetal complete heart block.[24,122] The intrauterine diagnosis was made in a twin when two fetal heart rates were heard, one at 52 beats per minute and the other at 150 beats per minute.[24]

Auscultatory signs that are useful in the diagnosis of congenital complete heart block include (1) variable intensity of the first heart sound, (2) a midsystolic murmur, (3) a normally split second heart sound, (4) a third heart sound, (5) a fourth heart sound, (6) a summation sound, (7) an atrial murmur, (8) a mid-diastolic murmur, and

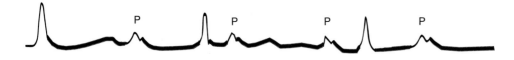

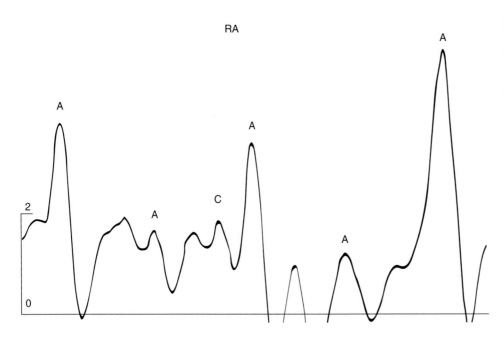

Figure 4–6
Rhythm strip (lead 2) and right atrial pressure pulse from a 13-year-old male with isolated congenital complete heart block. The A waves intermittently increase (cannon waves) when a P wave falls between QRS complex and T wave. The increase occurs because the right atrium contracts against a closed tricuspid valve. The A waves are small when a P wave falls between T wave and QRS complex, that is, when the tricuspid valve is open. RA, right atrium.

(9) vascular sounds. Variation in intensity of the first heart sound is an auscultatory hallmark of complete heart block (Figs. 4–7 through 4–10).[4,10,89,94,96,109] When the variation occurs with a slow heart rate and a regular rhythm, the diagnosis of complete heart block can be entertained with considerable confidence.

The PR relationship is an important determinant of the intensity of the first heart sound, an observation made by Wolferth and Margolies in 1930.[129] In complete heart block, the PR relationship changes from beat to beat because the atria and ventricles contract independently, so the intensity of the first heart sound varies from cycle to cycle, ranging from booming to virtual inaudibility (Figs. 4–7, 4–9, and 4–10). The first heart sound is loud—*bruit de canon*—when the PR interval is short (120 msec or less), soft when the PR interval is long (200 to 300 msec),

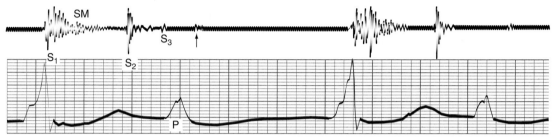

Figure 4–7

Phonocardiogram (apex) and rhythm strip (lead 2) from the 25-year-old man referred to in Figure 4–2. The first heart sound (S₁) is loud and constant because each QRS complex is immediately preceded by a P wave, to which it is fused. The independent P waves are tall and notched. There is a grade 2 of 6 systolic murmur (SM), a third heart sound (S₃), and a short, soft diastolic murmur (*arrow*) following the independent P waves.

Figure 4–8

Phonocardiogram (cardiac apex) and rhythm strip (lead 2) from the 25-year-old man whose 12-lead tracing is shown in Figure 4–2. The first heart sound (S₁) is loud (short interval between P wave and QRS complex). There is a grade 2 to 3 of 6 systolic murmur (SM) that ends well before the second heart sound (S₂). The murmur was maximum at the mid left sternal border. There is a third heart sound (S₃) and a short diastolic murmur (DM) that follows the subsequent P wave, which is notched.

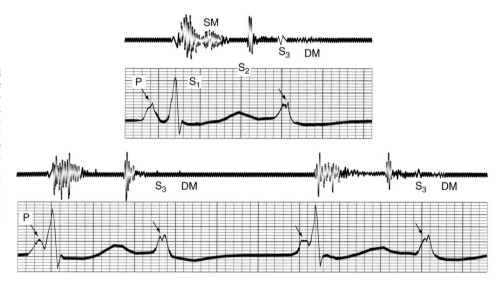

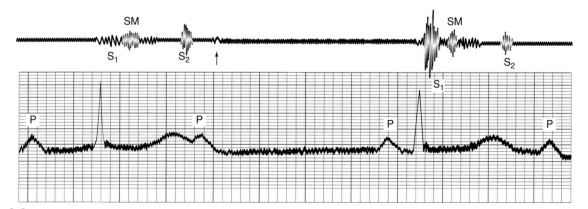

Figure 4–9

Phonocardiogram (apex) and electrocardiogram (lead 2) from a 12-year-old girl with isolated congenital complete heart block. The first heart sound (S₁) varies from soft (long PR interval) to loud (short PR interval). There is a short grade 2 of 6 midsystolic murmur (SM). A soft fourth heart sound (*arrow*) follows the second P wave.

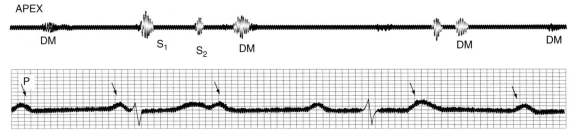

Figure 4–10

Phonocardiogram and rhythm strip (lead 2) from a 15-year-old boy with isolated congenital complete heart block. *Arrows* point to independent P waves. The first heart sound (S₁) varies from loud to soft. The short diastolic murmurs (DM) are especially prominent when atrial contraction (P wave) coincides with the rapid filling phase (shortly after the T wave).

and louder again when PR prolongation exceeds 500 msec.[10,96,109] When the PR interval is greater than 500 msec, the mitral valve reopens, followed by secondary closure at the onset of ventricular systole that results in the reappearance of the first heart sound.[10]

A grade 2 to 3 of 6 midsystolic murmur is related principally if not exclusively to rapid ejection of a large stroke volume from the right ventricle (Figs. 4–7, 4–8, and 4–9).[94] Maximum intensity is along the mid to upper left sternal border. The murmur is relatively short, occupying the first half to two thirds of systole, and always ending well before the second heart sound.[94,96,104]

Normal respiratory splitting of the second heart sound is a useful sign of congenital as opposed to acquired complete heart block.[96] Physiologic splitting implies a normal sequence of ventricular activation that is in accord with narrow QRS complexes and a subsidiary pacemaker above the bifurcation of the bundle of His (see "The Electrocardiogram").

Third heart sounds are indistinguishable from normal third heart sounds in the young (see Figs. 4–7 and 4–8). However, fourth heart sounds—aptly called *gallop du bloc* by Gallavardin[30]—are of special interest because they are *not* heard in normal young people. Timing in diastole is variable, because the atria and ventricles beat independently. The fourth sounds may have the brevity of a sound per se (see Fig. 4–9) or the prolongation of a short murmur (see Fig. 4–8). When atrial contraction coincides with rapid ventricular filling, simultaneous third and fourth heart sounds result in a summation sound, or a short mid-diastolic murmur (see Fig. 4–10). Summation sounds and mid-diastolic murmurs are detected more commonly than isolated fourth heart sounds or atrial murmurs. Systolic vascular sounds attributed to high-velocity ejection are sometimes heard over the carotid, subclavian, or femoral arteries.[4]

The Electrocardiogram

A definitive diagnosis of complete heart block depends on nothing more than an electrocardiogram. Fetal electrocardiography for prenatal diagnosis is an extension of this simple diagnostic tool.[24]

The P wave (atrial activity) and the QRS complex (ventricular activity) are completely independent, with no arithmetic relationship between the two (see Fig. 4–5). In acquired complete heart block, periods of synchronization called *accrochage* sometimes occur,[64,66,74] a phenomenon seldom witnessed in cases of congenital complete heart block (see Fig. 4–7).[104] Although atrial depolarization does not activate the ventricles, examples of change from partial to complete heart block,[23] as well as from complete to partial heart block, are occasionally encountered (see Fig. 4–3).[13,15,16,26,71] A neonate with congenital complete heart block experienced intermittent 1/1 atrioventricular conduction through a Wolff-Parkinson-White accessory pathway.[78]

The atrial rate tends to decrease with age but is rapid compared with the ventricular rate, which remains relatively constant after infancy until well into adulthood.[15,16,20] Rarely, atrial flutter coexists with congenital complete heart block.[107] The exercise electrocardiogram discloses a stepwise increase in atrial rate with slow return to normal, whereas the ventricular rate increases irregularly with a more rapid return to basal levels.[42,104] The adverse flat exercise response of the subsidiary junctional pacemaker[22,65] was mentioned earlier.

PP intervals vary in both congenital and acquired complete heart block. PP intervals that are separated by a QRS complex tend to be shorter (positive chronotropic effect), or less commonly longer (negative chronotropic effect), than PP intervals that are not separated by a QRS complex (Fig. 4–11).

Sinus P waves are tall and broad in response to volume overload (see Figs. 4–4, 4–7, and 4–8).[4] A normal QRS duration indicates a normal sequence of ventricular activation in response to a pacemaker located above the bifurcation of the bundle of His (see Figs. 4–1 and 4–2).[4,16,49,94] In acquired complete heart block, the QRS duration is prolonged because the idioventricular pacemaker is located below the bundle of His and its major branches.[46] The QRS in congenital complete heart block occasionally resembles right or left bundle branch block[34,44] because the block is infrahisian.[34,36,82] The lower the pacemaker in the conduction system, the greater the vulnerability to Stokes-Adams syncope.[83,89] When QRS prolongation coincides with a slow heart rate, Stokes-Adams attacks are likely.[44,83,89]

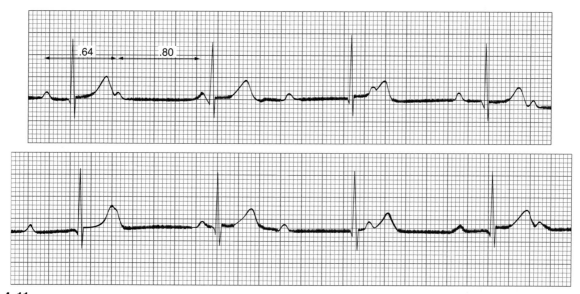

Figure 4–11

Rhythm strips of lead 2 of the electrocardiogram shown in Figure 4–1. The P waves are independent, and the ventricular rate is 47 beats per minute. The first PP interval is separated by a QRS complex and is relatively short (0.64 second, positive chronotropic effect). The second PP interval is *not* separated by a QRS complex and is relatively long (0.80 second).

In cases of familial complete heart block with adult onset, the QRS duration is prolonged and the outlook is not favorable.[103] Ambulatory electrocardiographic monitoring of uncomplicated congenital complete heart block has recorded marked nocturnal bradycardia, arrhythmias,[65] junctional exit block, exercise-related ventricular ectopic beats,[127] and blunted ventricular rate responses.[22,88]

Voltage criteria for left ventricular hypertrophy are sometimes present together with prominent left precordial Q waves of volume overload (see Figs. 4–1 and 4–2).[4,86,94,104] Right ventricular hypertrophy or biventricular hypertrophy is only occasional.[89,94]

The T-wave configuration is likely to be normal, but deep T-wave inversions or coving sometimes occur in right or midprecordial leads,[4,86] and T waves may be peaked in left chest leads (see Figs. 4–1 and 4–2).[4] QT interval prolongation increases the risk of torsades de pointes.[28,51]

Electrograms of the bundle of His in cases of congenital complete heart block shed light on the location of the conduction defect and on the site of the subsidiary pacemaker[1,7,50,80,90,101,130] (see earlier). The block is typically proximal to the site at which bundle of His potentials are recorded.[50,101,113,130] A normal HV interval and a normal QRS complex indicate a normal conduction system distal to the site of block.[101]

Bundle of His electrograms do not permit identification of where in the AV junction the escape rhythm originates,[50,101] because block proximal to the bundle of His potential can be located within the AV node, between the AV node and the atrial muscle, or in the AV node–His bundle junction.[6,101]

Escape rhythms in congenital complete heart block are likely to originate in the bundle of His because automatic-ity is a property of His/Purkinje cells but not of AV nodal cells. Origin is probably in the proximal bundle of His, in light of observations on complete heart block due to intra-His discontinuity.[7,90,101] Electrophysiologic studies have recorded split His potentials proximal and distal to the site of block,[7,90] so the escape pacemaker can be in the distal bundle of His at the site of the second of the split His potentials. The distal pacemaker is associated with a slower ventricular rate and with little or no acceleration in response to atropine.[90]

The X-Ray

The radiographic appearance of the heart, great arteries, and lungs is often normal in congenital complete heart block,[16] and ventricular chamber size tends to remain constant through adulthood.[15] However, there may be a mild to moderate increase in heart size because a slow heart rate is associated with prolonged diastolic filling periods and increased ventricular volume (Fig. 4–12, and see Fig. 4–4).[42,83,86]

The Echocardiogram

The echocardiogram with Doppler interrogation and color flow imaging confirms that the congenital complete heart block is isolated.[111] Fetal echocardiography establishes the diagnosis of intrauterine complete heart block as an isolated abnormality. Complete heart block can be diagnosed in utero by two-dimensional targeted M-mode recordings of atrial and ventricular wall movements, or by pulsed Doppler and color flow recordings of left ventricular inflow and outflow signals.[3,32,53,72,97,106]

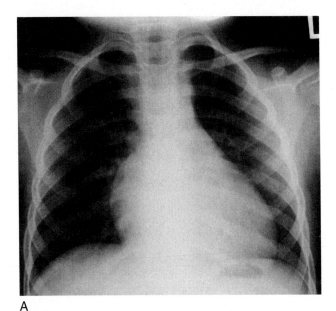

A

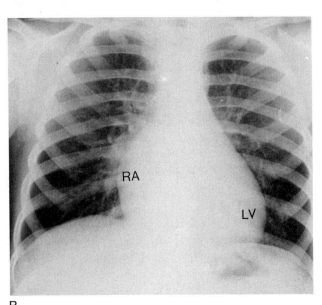

B

Figure 4–12

X-rays from the child whose electrocardiogram is shown in Figure 4–1. *A*, At the age of 4 years, the heart size was moderately increased. *B*, At the age of 7 years, there was a further increase in heart size that coincided with a decrease in heart rate to 50 beats per minute. LV, left ventricle; RA, right atrium.

Summary

Isolated congenital complete heart block is an example of passive autoimmunity, with the conduction defect or defects caused by injury from active transplacental transport of maternal IgG antibodies into the fetal circulation. The conduction defect is usually discovered incidentally in otherwise normal children, or an obstetrician may detect a slow fetal heart rate. The diagnosis of complete heart block is straightforward, based on nothing more than a standard scalar electrocardiogram. If liberal use were made of the electrocardiogram in infants and children with inappropriately slow heart rates, few or no cases would be missed. Fetal electrocardiography and echocardiography establish the intrauterine diagnosis. Stokes-Adams attacks are uncommon but occur even in the young. The arterial pulse rate is inappropriately slow for patient age, the upstroke is brisk, the pulse pressure is wide, and the rhythm is regular. The jugular venous pulse exhibits intermittent cannon waves and independent asynchronous A waves that are more rapid than the carotid pulse, indicating independent atrial and ventricular activity. The electrocardiogram records independent P waves. The QRS complexes are of normal duration because the block is above the bifurcation of the bundle of His.

REFERENCES

1. Abella JB, Teixeira OHP, Misra KP, Hastreiter AR: Changes of atrioventricular conduction with age in infants and children. Am J Cardiol 30:876, 1972.
2. Anderson RH, Weinck ACG, Losekoot TG, Becker AE: Congenital complete heart block: Developmental aspects. Circulation 56:90, 1977.
2a. Angelini A, Moreoli GS, Ruffatti A, et al: Calcification of the atrioventricular node in a fetus affected by congenital complete heart block. Circulation 105:1254, 2002.
3. Arbeille P, Paillet C, Chantepie B, et al: In utero ultrasonic diagnosis of atrioventricular block. J Cardiovasc Ultrasonogr 3:313, 1984.
4. Ayers CR, Boineau JP, Spach MS: Congenital complete heart block in children [review]. Am Heart J 72:381, 1966.
5. Barton RM, LaDue CN: Complete heart block in a case of pregnancy. Am J Med 4:447, 1948.
6. Bharati S, Lev M: Pathology of atrioventricular block. Cardiol Clin 2:741, 1984.
7. Bharati S, Lev M, Wu D, et al: Pathophysiologic correlations in two cases of split His bundle potentials. Circulation 49:615, 1974.
8. Brucato A, Gasparini M, Vignati G, et al: Isolated congenital complete heart block: Longterm outcome of children and immunogenetic study. J Rheumatol 22:541, 1995.
9. Brucato A, Franceschini F, Gasparini M, et al: Isolated congenital complete heart block: Longterm outcome in mothers, maternal antibody specificity and immunogenetic background. J Rheumatol 22:533, 1995.
10. Burggraf GW, Craige E: The first heart sound in complete heart block. Circulation 50:17, 1974.
11. Buyon J, Roubey R, Swersky S, et al: Complete congenital heart block: Risk of occurrence and therapeutic approach to prevention. J Rheumatol 15:1104, 1988.
12. Buyon JP, Heibert R, Copel J, et al: Autoimmune-associated congenital heart block: Demographics, mortality, morbidity, and recurrence rates obtained from a National Neonatal Lupus Registry. J Am Coll Cardiol 31:1658, 1998.
13. Camm AJ, Bexton RS: Congenital complete heart block. Eur Heart J 5:115, 1984.
14. Campbell M: Congenital complete heart block. Br Heart J 5:15, 1943.
15. Campbell M, Emanuel R: Six cases of congenital complete heart block followed for 34–40 years. Br Heart J 29:577, 1967.
16. Campbell M, Thorne MG: Congenital heart block. Br Heart J 18:90, 1956.
17. Chameides L, Truex RC, Vetter V, et al: Association of maternal systemic lupus erythematosus with congenital complete heart block. N Engl J Med 297:1204, 1977.
18. Connor AC, McFadden JF, Houston BJ, Finn JL: Familial congenital complete heart block [review]. Am J Obstet Gynecol 78:75, 1959.
19. Corne RA, Metthewson FAL: Congenital complete atrioventricular heart block. A 25 year follow-up study. Am J Cardiol 29:412, 1972.
20. Crittenden IH, Latta H, Ticinovich DA: Familial congenital heart block. Am J Dis Child 108:104, 1964.
21. Davis H, Stecher RM: Congenital heart block. Am J Dis Child 36:115, 1928.

22. Dewey RC, Capeless MA, Levy AM: Use of ambulatory electrocardiographic monitoring to identify high-risk patients with congenital complete heart block. N Engl J Med 316:835, 1987.
23. Dunn HG: Congenital partial heart block. Proc R Soc Med 45:456, 1952.
24. Dunn HP: Antenatal diagnosis of congenital heart block. J Obstet Gynaecol Br Emp 67:1006, 1960.
25. Eronen M: Long-term outcome of children with complete heart block diagnosed after the newborn period. Pediatr Cardiol 22:133, 2001.
26. Esscher EB: Congenital complete heart block in adolescence and adult life: A follow-up study. Eur Heart J 2:281, 1981.
27. Esscher EB: Congenital complete heart block [review]. Acta Paediatr Scand 70:131, 1981.
28. Esscher EB, Michaëlsson M: Q-T interval in congenital complete heart block. Pediatr Cardiol 4:121, 1983.
29. Esscher EB, Hardell L, Michaëlsson M: Familial, isolated, complete right bundle branch block. Br Heart J 37:745, 1975.
30. Gallavardin L: Contractions auriculaires perceptibles à l'oreille dans le bloc total. Arch Mal Coeur 7:171, 1914.
31. Gazes PC, Culler RM, Taber E, Kelly TE: Congenital familial cardiac conduction defects. Circulation 32:32, 1965.
32. Gembruch U, Hansmann M, Redel DA, et al: Fetal complete heart block: Antenatal diagnosis, significance and management. Eur J Obstet Gynecol Reprod Biol 31:9, 1989.
33. Gordon PA, Rosenthal E, Khamashta MA, Hughes GR: Absence of conduction defects in the echocardiograms of mothers with children with congenital complete heart block. J Rheumatol 28:366, 2001.
34. Griffiths SP: Congenital complete heart block. Circulation 43:615, 1971.
35. Groves AM, Allan LD, Rosenthal E: Outcome of congenital complete heart block diagnosed in utero. Heart 75: 190, 1996.
36. Hackel DB: Pathology of primary congenital complete heart block. Mod Pathol 1:114, 1988.
37. Hardy JD, Solomon S, Banwell GS, et al: Congenital complete heart block in the newborn associated with systemic lupus erythematosus and other connective tissue disorders. Arch Dis Child 54:7, 1979.
38. Harris JWS: A case of complete heart block recognized at the 38th week of pregnancy. J Obstet Gynaecol Br Emp 59:404, 1952.
39. Howarth S: Atrial waves on arterial pressure records in normal rhythm, heart block, and auricular flutter. Br Heart J 16:171, 1954.
40. Hull D, Binns BAO, Joyce D: Congenital heart block and widespread fibrosis due to maternal lupus erythematosus. Arch Dis Child 41:688, 1966.
41. Husson GS, Blackman MS, Rogers MC, et al: Familial congenital bundle branches system disease. Am J Cardiol 32:365, 1973.
42. Ikkos D, Hanson JS: Response to exercise in congenital complete A-V block. Circulation 22:583, 1960.
42a. Jaeggi ET, Hamilton RM, Silverman ED, et al: Outcome of chidren with fetal, neonatal, or childhood diagnosis of isolated congenital atrioventricular block. J Am Coll Cardiol 39:130, 2002.
43. James TN: Cardiac conduction system: Fetal and postnatal development. Am J Cardiol 25:213, 1970.
44. James TN, McKone RC, Hudspeth AS: Familial congenital heart block. Circulation 51:379, 1975.
45. James TN, Spencer MS, Kloepser JC: Adult onset syncope, with comments on the nature of congenital heart block and the morphogenesis of the human atrioventricular septal junction. Circulation 54:1001, 1976.
46. Josephson ME: Clinical Cardiac Electrophysiology, 2nd ed. Philadelphia, Lea & Febiger, 1993.
47. Kangos JJ, Griffiths SP, Blumenthal S: Congenital complete heart block. Am J Cardiol 20:632, 1967.
48. Kasinath BS, Katz AI: Delayed maternal lupus after delivery of offspring with congenital heart block. Arch Intern Med 142:2317, 1982.
49. Kay HB: Ventricular complexes in heart block. Br Heart J 10:177, 1948.
50. Kelly DT, Brodsky SJ, Mirowski M, et al: Bundle of His recordings in congenital complete heart block. Circulation 45:277, 1972.
51. Kernohan RJ, Froggatt P: Atrioventricular dissociation with prolonged QT interval and syncopal attacks in a 10 year old boy. Br Heart J 36:516, 1974.
52. Khorsandian RS, Abdol-Nabi M, Muller O: Familial congenital AV disassociation. Am J Cardiol 14:118, 1964.
53. Kleinman CS, Hobbins JC, Jaffe CC, et al: Echocardiographic studies of the human fetus: Prenatal diagnosis of congenital heart disease and cardiac dysrhythmias. Pediatrics 65:1059, 1980.
54. Lagerlof H, Werko L: Studies on circulation in man: Auricular pressure pulse. Cardiologia 13:240, 1948.
55. Lanham JG, Walport MJ, Hughes GRV: Congenital heart block and familial connective tissue disease. J Rheumatol 10:823, 1983.
56. Latta H, Crittenden IH: Acquired lesions of the conduction system in familial congenital heart block. Lab Invest 13:214, 1964.
57. Lee LA, Weston WL: New findings in neonatal lupus syndrome. Am J Dis Child 138:233, 1984.
58. Lee LA, Bias WB, Arnett FC, et al: Immunogenetics of the neonatal lupus syndrome. Ann Intern Med 99:592, 1983.
59. Lev M: Conduction system in congenital heart disease. Am J Cardiol 21:619, 1968.
60. Lev M: Normal anatomy of conduction system in man and its pathology in atrioventricular block. Ann NY Acad Sci 11:817, 1964.
61. Lev M: The anatomic basis for disturbances in conduction and cardiac arrhythmias. Prog Cardiovasc Dis 2:360, 1960.
62. Lev M, Benjamin JE, White PD: A histopathologic study of the conduction system in complete heart block of 42 years duration. Am Heart J 55:198, 1958.
63. Lev M, Cuadros H, Paul MH: Interruption of the atrioventricular bundle with congenital atrioventricular block. Circulation 43:703, 1971.
64. Lev M, Silverman J, Fitzmaurice FM, et al: Lack of connection between the atria and the more peripheral conduction system in congenital atrioventricular block. Am J Cardiol 27:481, 1971.
65. Levy AM, Camm AJ, Keane JF: Multiple arrhythmias detected during nocturnal monitoring in patients with congenital complete heart block. Circulation 55:247, 1977.
66. Levy MN, Edelstein J: The mechanism of synchronization in isorhythmic A-V dissociation. Circulation 42:689, 1970.
67. Linder E, Landtman B, Tuuteri L, Hjelt L: Congenital complete heart block. II. Histology of the conduction system. Ann Paediatr Fenn 11:11, 1965.
68. Litsey SE, Noonan JA, O'Connor WN, et al: Maternal connective tissue disease and congenital heart block. N Engl J Med 312:98, 1985.
69. Lockshin MD, Bonfa E, Elkson K, Druzin ML: Neonatal lupus risk to newborns of mothers with systemic lupus erythematosus. Arthrits Rheum 31:697, 1988.
70. Ludatscher R, Amikam S, Roguin N, et al: Electron microscopical study of myocardial biopsy material in congenital heart block. Br Heart J 37:561, 1975.
71. Lynch HT, Mohiudbin S, Moran J, et al: Hereditary progressive atrioventricular conduction defect. Am J Cardiol 36:297, 1975.
72. Machado MVL, Tynan MJ, Curry PVL, Allan LD: Fetal complete heart block. Br Heart J 60:512, 1988.
73. Manno BV, Hakki A, Eshagpour E, Iskandrian AS: Left ventricular function at rest and during exercise in congenital complete heart block. Am J Cardiol 52:92, 1983.
74. Marriott HJL: Atrioventricular synchronization and accrochage. Circulation 14:38, 1956.
75. Matthewson FAL, Harvie FH: Complete heart block in an experienced pilot. Br Heart J 19:253, 1957.
76. McCue CM, Mantakas ME, Tingelstad JB, Ruddy S: Congenital heart block in newborns of mothers with connective tissue disease. Circulation 56:82, 1977.
77. McHenry MM: Factors influencing longevity in adults with congenital complete heart block. Am J Cardiol 29:416, 1972.
78. McLeod KA, Rankin AC, Houston AB: 1:1 atrioventricular conduction in congenital complete heart block. Heart 80:525, 1998.
79. Menon A, Silverman ED, Gow RM, Hamilton RM: Chronotropic competence of the sinus node in congenital complete heart block. Am J Cardiol 82:1119, 1998.
80. Michaëlsson M, Engle MA: Congenital complete heart block: An international study of the natural history. Cardiovasc Clin 4:85, 1972.
81. Michaëlsson M, Swiderski J: High degree atrio-ventricular block in children: A preliminary report of a joint study with special reference to the natural history. Proc Assoc Eur Paediatr Cardiol 33:44, 1967.
82. Miller RA, Mehta AB, Rodriguez-Coronel A, Lev M: Congenital atrioventricular block with multiple ectopic pacemakers. Am J Cardiol 30:554, 1972.
83. Molthan ME, Miller RA, Hastreiter AR, Paul MH: Congenital heart block with fatal Adams-Stokes attacks in childhood. Pediatrics 30:32, 1962.
84. Morgans CM, Gray KE, Robb GH: A survey of familial heart block. Br Heart J 36:693, 1974.

85. Morquio L: Sur une maladie infantile et familiale caractérisée par des modifications permanentes du pouls, des attaques syncopales et epileptiforme et la mort subite. Arch Méd d'Enfants 4:467, 1901.

86. Moss AJ: Congenital complete A-V block. Clinical features, hemodynamic findings and physical working capacity. Lancet 81:542, 1961.

87. Mowbray R, Bowley CC: Congenital complete heart block complicating pregnancy. J Obstet Gynaecol Br Emp 55:438, 1948.

88. Nagashima M, Nakashima T, Asai T, et al: Study on congenital complete heart block in children by 24 hour ambulatory electrocardiographic monitoring. Jpn Heart J 28:323, 1987.

89. Nakamura FF, Nadas AS: Complete heart block in infants and children. N Engl J Med 270:1261, 1964.

90. Nasrallah AT, Gillette PC, Mullins CE: Congenital and surgical atrioventricular block within the His bundle. Am J Cardiol 36:914, 1975.

91. Nolan RJ, Shulman ST, Victoria BE: Congenital complete heart block associated with maternal mixed connective tissue disease. J Pediatr 95:420, 1979.

92. Osler W: On the so-called Stokes-Adams disease. Lancet 2:516, 1903.

93. Paredes RA, Morgan H, Lachelin GCL: Congenital heart block associated with maternal primary Sjögren's syndrome. Br J Obstet Gynaecol 90:870, 1983.

94. Paul MH, Rudolph AM, Nadas AS: Congenital complete heart block: Problems of assessment. Circulation 18:183, 1958.

95. Perloff JK: Pregnancy and congenital heart disease. In Perloff JK, Child JS (eds): Congenital Heart Disease in Adults, 2nd ed. Philadelphia, WB Saunders, 1998.

96. Perloff JK: Physical Examination of the Heart and Circulation, 3rd ed. Philadelphia, WB Saunders, 2000.

97. Pinsky WW, Gillette PC, Garson A, McNamara DG: Diagnosis, management, and long-term results of patients with congenital complete atrioventricular block. Pediatrics 69:728, 1982.

98. Reed BR, Lee LA, Harmon C, et al: Autoantibodies to SS-A/Ro in infants with congenital heart block. J Pediatr 103:889, 1983.

99. Reid JM, Coleman EN, Doig W: Congenital complete heart block: Report of 35 cases. Br Heart J 48:236, 1982.

100. Reybrouck T, Eynde BV, Dumoulin M, Van der Hauwaert LG: Cardiorespiratory response to exercise in congenital complete atrioventricular block. Am J Cardiol 64:896, 1989.

101. Rosen KM, Mehta A, Rahimtoola SH, Miller RA: Sites of congenital and surgical heart block as defined by His bundle electrocardiography. Circulation 44:833, 1971.

102. Ross BA: Congenital complete heart block. Pediatr Clin North Am 37:69, 1990.

103. Sarachek NS, Leonard JJ: Familial heart block and sinus bradycardia: Classification and natural history. Am J Cardiol 29:451, 1972.

104. Scarpelli EM, Rudolph AM: The hemodynamics of congenital heart block. Prog Cardiovasc Dis 6:327, 1964.

105. Schieb JS, Waxman J: Congenital heart block in successive pregnancies. Obstet Gynecol 73:481, 1989.

106. Schmidt KG, Ulmer HE, Silverman NH, et al: Perinatal outcome of fetal complete atrioventricular block: A multicenter experience. J Am Coll Cardiol 17:1360, 1991.

107. Schuster B, Imm CW: Congenital atrial flutter with complete heart block. Am J Cardiol 12:575, 1963.

108. Scott JS, Maddison PJ, Taylor PV, et al: Connective-tissue disease, antibodies to ribonucleoprotein, and congenital heart block. N Engl J Med 309:209, 1983.

109. Shearn MA, Tarr E, Rytand DA: Significance of changes in amplitude of the first heart sound in children with A-V block. Circulation 7:839, 1953.

110. Sherman SJ, Featherstone LS: Congenital complete heart block and successful vaginal delivery. J Perinat 17:489, 1997.

111. Sholler GF, Walsh EP: Congenital complete heart block in patients without anatomic cardiac defects. Am Heart J 118:1193, 1989.

112. Smithells RW, Outon EB: Congenital heart block. Arch Dis Child 34:223, 1959.

113. Smithen CS, Sowton E: His bundle electrograms. Br Heart J 33:633, 1971.

114. Spach MS, Scarpelli EM: Circulatory dynamics and the effects of respiration during ventricular asystole in dogs with complete heart block. Circ Res 10:197, 1962.

115. Stephan E: Hereditary bundle branch system defect. Am Heart J 95:89, 1978.

116. Stephensen O, Cleland WP, Hallidie-Smith K: Congenital complete heart block and persistent ductus arteriosus associated with maternal systemic lupus erythematosus. Br Heart J 46:104, 1981.

117. Taylor MRH, Godfrey S: Exercise studies in congenital heart block. Br Heart J 34:930, 1972.

118. Taylor PV, Scott JS, Gerlis LM, et al: Maternal antibodies against fetal cardiac antigens in congenital complete heart block. N Engl J Med 315:667, 1986.

119. Thilenius OG, Chiemmongkoltip P, Cassels DE, Arcilla RA: Hemodynamic studies in children with congenital atrioventricular block. Am J Cardiol 30:13, 1972.

120. Turner LB: Asymptomatic congenital heart block in an Army Air Force pilot. Am Heart J 34:426, 1947.

121. Udink Ten Cate FE, Breur JM, Cohen MI, et al: Dilated cardiomyopathy in isolated congenital complete atrioventricular block: Early and long-term risk in children. J Am Coll Cardiol 37:1129, 2001.

121a. Upshaw CB, Silverman ME: Alfred Lewis Galabin and the first human documentation of atrioventricular block. Am J Cardiol 88:547, 2001.

122. Valerio U: Congenital complete heart block. Clin Proc Child Hosp 14:46, 1958.

123. Van den Heuvel GCJ: De zeikte van Stokes-Adam eneen geval van aangeborenen hartblock. Groningen Proefschrift Rijks Universitait 12:142, 1908.

124. Wallgren G, Agorio E: Congenital complete atrioventricular block in three siblings. Acta Paediatr 49:49, 1960.

125. Wendkos MH, Study RS: Familial congenital complete atrioventricular heart block. Am Heart J 34:138, 1947.

126. White P, Eustis R: Congenital heart block. Am J Dis Child 22:299, 1921.

127. Winkler RB, Freed MD, Nadas AS: Exercise-induced ventricular ectopy in children and young adults with complete heart block. Am Heart J 99:87, 1980.

128. Winkler RB, Nora AH, Nora JJ: Familial congenital complete heart block and maternal lupus erythematosus. Circulation 56:1103, 1977.

129. Wolferth CC, Margolies A: The influence of auricular contraction on the first heart sound and the radial pulse. Arch Intern Med 46:1048, 1930.

130. Wolff GS, Freed MD, Ellison RC: Bundle of His recordings in congenital heart disease. Br Heart J 35:805, 1973.

131. Yater WM: Congenital heart block; review of the literature; report of case with incomplete heterotaxy; electrocardiogram in dextrocardia. Am J Dis Child 38:112, 1929.

132. Yater WM, Leamon WG, Cornall VH: Congenital heart block; report of third case of complete heart block studied by serial section through conduction system. JAMA 102:1660, 1934.

133. Yater WM, Lyon JA, McNabb PE: Congenital heart block; review and report of second case of complete heart block studied by serial sections through conduction system. JAMA 100:1831, 1933.

134. Ziegler AM: Pregnancy with complete heart block. Am J Obstet Gynecol 62:445, 1951.

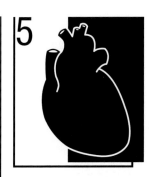

Congenital Absence of the Pericardium

Congenital absence of the pericardium was recognized by M. Realdus Columbus in 1559,[8] and by Matthew Baille in 1793,[1] but it was not until 1959 that the anomaly was diagnosed on a chest x-ray.[9] The abnormality varies from a localized defect to complete absence of the pericardium.[6,13,14,21] Morphogenesis has been attributed to premature atrophy of the left duct of Cuvier, resulting in deficient blood supply to the left pleuropericardial membrane, which normally gives rise to the left pericardium.[14,29] Necropsy incidence has been estimated at 1 in 14,000.[27] About two thirds of cases are represented by left pericardial absence that is usually partial (Fig. 5–1).[6,14,19,20,27,31] Congenital right pericardial absence or complete absence is rare (Fig. 5–2).[14,24] Approximately one third of congenital pericardial defects occur in conjunction with other congenital malformations, both cardiac (Fig. 5–3) and noncardiac.[5,13,17,23] A case in point is Cantrell syndrome, which consists of congenital malformations of the left pericardium, the heart, the sternum, the diaphragm, and the abdominal wall.[5,33]

The *peri* ("around") *cardium* ("heart") consists of two layers with nerves, lymphatics, and a blood supply. The layer that is attached to the surface of the heart is the visceral pericardium, or epicardium. The layer that is not attached to the surface of the heart is the parietal pericardium which is separated from the visceral pericardium by 20 to 30 ml of a serous ultrafiltrate of plasma. It is with the parietal pericardium that this chapter is concerned.

The parietal pericardium exerts contact stress on the heart that contributes to ventricular diastolic pressure and that limits acute dilatation.[30] The stress is greater on the relatively thin right ventricle and right atrium, the dimensions and pressures of which depend on pericardial constraint.[30] Accordingly, congenital complete absence of the parietal pericardium is accompanied by an increase in right ventricular size[30] (as measured by echocardiography) and with alterations in systemic venous return.[12]

The History

Partial or complete absence of the pericardium usually comes to light because an abnormality is identified on a routine chest x-ray of an asymptomatic patient or on a chest x-ray taken as part of the cardiovascular evaluation of a symptomatic patient with coexisting cardiac defects.[6,13,14]

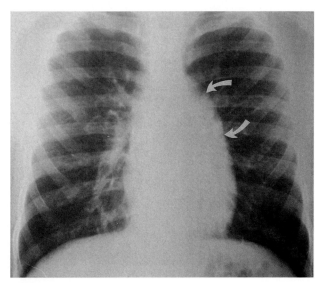

Figure 5–1

X-ray from a 12-year-old female with congenital partial absence of the pericardium. There is the typical localized convexity of a protruding left atrial appendage (*arrows*). The x-ray is otherwise normal.

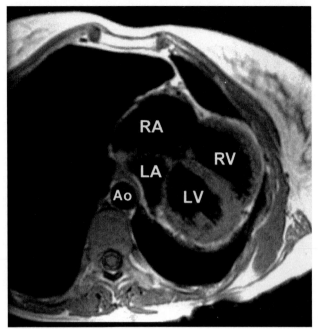

Figure 5–2

Magnetic resonance image axial view from a 38-year-old woman with congenital complete absence of the pericardium and hypoplasia of the left lower lobe and the left pulmonary artery (see Fig. 5–3). The strikingly mobile heart is displaced far into the left thoracic cavity. Ao, aorta LA/RA; left and right atrium; LV/RV, left and right ventricle.

The most common symptom is chest pain, which can appear suddenly in a previously asymptomatic adult and varies from mild and occasional to frequent, prolonged, and debilitating.[13,14] The pain is stabbing, left-sided, brief if not fleeting, unrelated to exertion but aggravated by position, especially the left lateral recumbent, awakening the patient from sleep, and relieved by an upright position.[3,6,14,24] The pain associated with partial absence of the left pericardium (see Fig. 5–1) is attributed to herniation of the left atrial appendage through the pericardial defect.[6] The pain associated with complete absence of the pericardium (see Fig. 5–2) is believed to originate from torsion of the thoracic inlet.[3,14] Myocardial ischemia is also a consideration in light of evidence of transient compression of coronary arteries.[2,14,25]

Additional symptoms include dyspnea, palpitations, dizziness, syncope, and, most ominously, sudden death.[6,14] Familial congenital partial absence of the left pericardium has been reported.[29] The male-to-female prevalence ratio is reportedly 3:1.[14] Longevity is not affected with congenital partial absence of the pericardium[3] but has not been established with congenital complete absence of the pericardium. One patient reportedly survived to the eighth decade.[15]

Physical Appearance

Patients with congenital partial absence of the left pericardium have been reported with abnormal facies and growth hormone deficiency,[4] and with VATER defects[18]

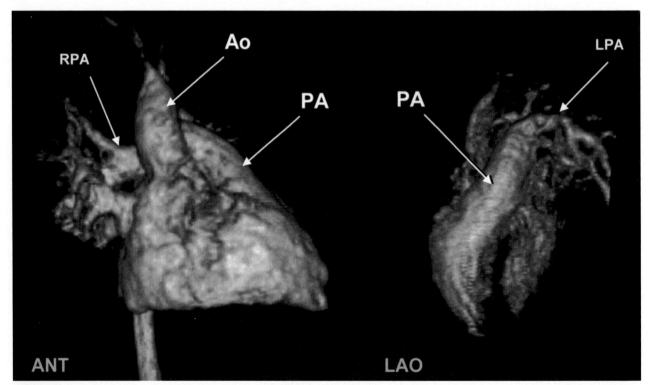

Figure 5–3

Three-dimensional reconstruction of gadolinium-enhanced magnetic resonance angiogram of the heart and great arteries from the 38-year-old woman with congenital complete absence of the pericardium with hypoplasia of the left lower lobe and left pulmonary artery (see Fig. 5–2 for magnetic resonance image). The anterior view (ANT) discloses a well-formed main pulmonary artery (PA) and a well-formed right pulmonary artery (RPA). Ao, ascending aorta. The left anterior oblique view (LAO) discloses a hypoplastic left pulmonary artery (LPA).

(V A T E R = vertebral defects, *a*nal atresia, *t*racheo-*e*sophageal fistula, and *r*adial and renal dysplasia).

The Arterial Pulse and the Jugular Venous Pulse

The arterial pulse is normal with congenital complete absence of the pericardium, despite diastolic pressure alternans.[26] The jugular venous pulse is normal with congenital partial absence of the pericardium and is normal with congenital complete absence, despite a decrease in contact stress exerted on the right atrium and right ventricle.

Precordial Movement and Palpation

With congenital partial absence of the left pericardium, the position and movements of the heart are normal. With complete pericardial absence, there is striking mobility of the heart that shifts dramatically to the left (see Fig. 5–2), a position that can be detected by percussion. Displacement is accompanied by major rotation (see Fig. 5–2),[24] so identification of a left or right ventricular impulse is not feasible.

Auscultation

Congenital complete absence of the pericardium is accompanied by torsion of the thoracic inlet and great arteries that may generate basal midsystolic murmurs, especially in the left lateral decubitus position.

The Electrocardiogram

With congenital partial absence of the left pericardium, the electrocardiogram is normal because the heart is not displaced and is inherently normal apart from the pericardial defect. With congenital complete absence of the pericardium, standard precordial lead placements show delayed transition that reflects the leftward position of the heart.[13] Axis deviation, generally right, probably results from rotation.[13,14] Incomplete right bundle branch block is frequently mentioned,[13,14,17] and there are individual reports of complete heart block[32] and sinus node dysfunction.[16]

The X-ray

The posteroanterior chest x-ray is a major key to the diagnosis and was the basis for the earliest clinical recognition of congenital absence of the pericardium.[9] Congenital partial absence of the left pericardium is accompanied by herniation of the left atrial appendage represented in the x-ray by a convexity immediately below the pulmonary trunk, or, if the herniation is larger, the convexity is in the second *and* third left interspaces (see Fig. 5–1). The heart is not displaced, and the cardiac silhouette is otherwise normal. The x-ray of an *intrapericardial* congenital aneurysm of the left atrial appendage[28] (Fig. 5–4) is similar if not indistinguishable from the x-ray of partial absence of the left pericardium (see Fig. 5–1).

A congenital pericardial cyst typically presents as a smooth homogeneous radiodensity in the right cardiophrenic angle touching the anterior chest wall and the

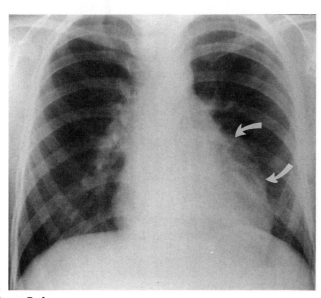
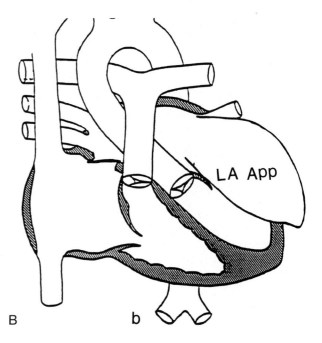

A   B

Figure 5–4

A, X-ray from a 10-year-old girl showing a relatively long left paracardiac convexity (*arrows*) caused by a congenital intrapericardial aneurysm of the left atrial appendage. *B*, Schematic illustration of the congenital intrapericardial aneurysm of the left atrial appendage (LAA App).

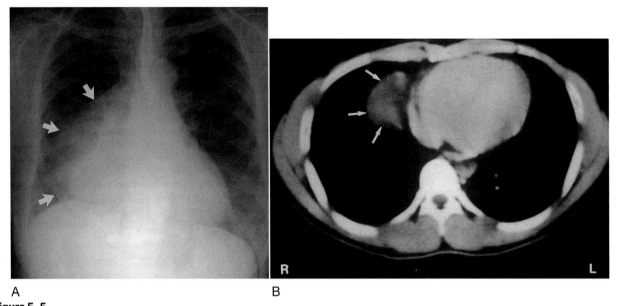

A   B

Figure 5–5

A, X-ray from a 23-year-old woman with an unusually large congenital pericardial cyst (*arrows*) that occupies the entire right cardiac border. *B,* Magnetic resonance image from an 18-year-old man with a typical congenital pericardial cyst (*arrows*) that originated at the right cardiophrenic angle.

anterior portion of the right hemidiaphragm (Fig. 5–5).[10] The distinction from congenital partial absence of the pericardium is less clear when the cyst presents along the left cardiac border above the left hemidiaphragm.[10]

Congenital complete absence of the pericardium is characterized by striking mobility of the heart that results in leftward and posterior displacement[13] (see Fig. 5–5). Displacement is even more dramatic if hypoplasia of the left pulmonary artery and left lung coexist (Fig. 5–6, and see Fig. 5–2).[17] There is no cardiac shadow to the right of the vertebral column. A tongue of lung tissue is typically interposed between the pulmonary trunk and aorta[13] (see Fig. 5–6A). The definitive clinical diagnosis is based on

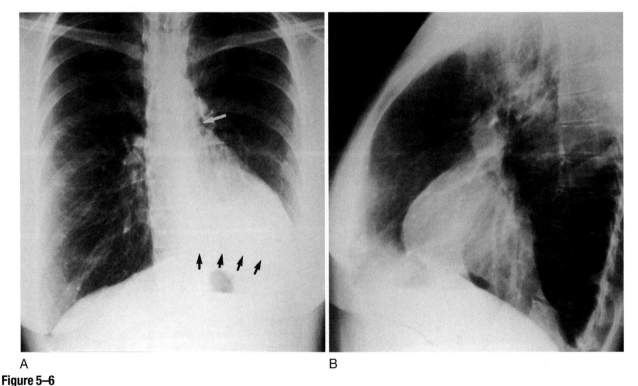

A   B

Figure 5–6

X-rays from the 38-year-old woman with congenital complete absence of the pericardium referred to in Figures 5–2 and 5–3. *A,* The frontal projection shows the marked leftward position of the mobile heart with no cardiac shadow to the right of the vertebral column. The leftward shift was exaggerated by hypoplasia of the left lung indicated by the elevated left hemidiaphragm (*black arrows*). The *white arrow* identifies a tongue of lung tissue interposed between the pulmonary trunk and aorta. *B,* The lateral projection shows the striking posterior position of the mobile heart.

thoracic magnetic resonance images in the supine and left lateral recumbent positions (see Fig. 5–2).

The Echocardiogram

The noteworthy features of the echocardiogram in congenital complete absence of the pericardium are the unorthodox windows required for imaging. There is leftward and posterior displacement together with rotation of the heart, hypermobility with an abnormal swinging movement, paradoxical motion of the ventricular septum, and enlargement of the right ventricle and right atrium.[7,13,14,22] Lack of pericardial constraint has a greater effect on the relatively thin-walled right ventricle, which accounts for right ventricular dilatation, for a selective increase in systemic venous return, and for paradoxical motion of the ventricular septum.[7,12,13] Echocardiography identifies coexisting cardiac defects.[17] Congenital partial absence of the pericardium is not an echocardiographic diagnosis. A fetal echocardiogram recognized one case of an intrapericardial aneurysm.[11]

Summary

Congenital absence of the pericardium can be partial or complete. Congenital partial absence is typically left-sided. Right-sided absence and complete absence are rare. With congenital partial absence of the pericardium, the x-ray discloses a convex shadow in the topographic location of the left atrial appendage. The clinical diagnosis is entertained when the abnormality is identified in a routine chest x-ray in an asymptomatic patient or in a patient who comes to attention because of chest pain or during evaluation of coexisting heart disease. With congenital complete absence of the pericardium, the heart is strikingly mobile and markedly displaced to the left and posteriorly.

Patients typically present in adulthood. Chest pain is left-sided, stabbing, and provoked or aggravated by position, especially the left lateral recumbent position. Additional symptoms include dyspnea, palpitations, dizziness, syncope, and, most ominously, sudden death. Thoracic magnetic resonance imaging makes a definitive diagnosis.

REFERENCES

1. Baille M: On the want of a pericardium in the human body. Trans Soc Imrov Med Chir Knowl 1:91, 1793.
2. Bennett KR: Congenital foramen of the left pericardium. Ann Thorac Surg 70:993, 2000.
3. Beppu S, Naito H, Matsuhisa M, et al: The effect of lying position on ventricular volume in congenital absence of the pericardium. Am Heart J 120:1159, 1990.
4. Boscherini B, Gallaso C, Bitti ML: Abnormal face, congenital absence of the left pericardium, mental retardation, and growth hormone deficiency. Am J Med Genet 49:111, 1994.
5. Cantrell JR, Haller JA, Ravitch MM: A syndrome of congenital defects involving the abdominal wall, sternum, diaphragm, pericardium and heart. Surg Gynecol Obstet 107:602, 1958.
6. Chapman JE, Rubin JW, Gross CM, Janssen ME: Congenital absence of pericardium: An unusual cause of atypical angina. Ann Thorac Surg 45:91, 1988.
7. Connolly HM, Click RL, Schattenberg TT, et al: Congenital absence of the pericardium: echocardiography as a diagnostic tool. J Am Soc Echocardiogr 8:87, 1995.
8. Columbus MR: De re anatomica. Vol 15. In Beurlaque N (ed): Venice 1559, p. 265.
9. Ellis K, Leeds NE, Himmelstein A: Congenital deficiencies in partial pericardium. Am J Roentgen 82:125, 1959.
10. Feigin DS, Fenoglio JJ, McAllister HA, Madewell JE: Pericardial cysts. Radiology 125:15, 1977.
11. Fountain-Dommer RR, Wiles HB, Shuler CO, et al: Recognition of left atrial aneurysm by fetal echocardiography. Circulation 102:2282, 2000.
12. Fukuda N, Oki T, Iuchi A, et al: Pulmonary and systemic venous flow patterns assisted by transesophageal Doppler echocardiography in congenital absence of the pericardium. Am J Cardiol 75:1286, 1995.
13. Gatzoulis MA, Munk MD, Merchant N, et al: Isolated congenital absence of the pericardium. Ann Thorac Surg 69:1209, 2000.
14. Gehlmann HR, van Ingen GJ: Symptomatic congenital complete absence of the left pericardium. Case report and review of the literature. Eur Heart J 10:670, 1989.
15. Hammoudeh AJ, Kelly ME, Mekhjian H: Congenital total absence of the pericardium. J Thorac Cardiovasc Surg 109:805, 1995.
16. Hano O, Baba T, Hayano M, Yano K: Congenital defect in the left pericardium with sick sinus syndrome. Am Heart J 132:1293, 1996.
17. Lonsky V, Stetina M, Habal P, Markova D: Congenital absence of the left pericardium in combination with left pulmonary artery hypoplasia, right aortic arch, and secundum atrial septal defect. Thorac Cardiovasc Surg 40:155, 1992.
18. Lu C, Ridker PM: Echocardiographic diagnosis of congenital absence of the pericardium in a patient with VATER association defects. Clin Cardiol 17:502, 1994.
19. Mehta SM, Meyers JL: Congenital heart surgery nomenclature and database project: Diseases of the pericardium. Ann Thorac Surg 69:S191, 2000.
20. Nasser WK: Congenital diseases of the pericardium. Cardiovasc Clin 7:271, 1976.
21. Nasser WK, Helman C, Tavel ME, et al: Congenital absence of the left pericardium: Clinical electrocardiographic, radiographic, hemodynamic, and angiographic findings in six cases. Circulation 41:469, 1970.
22. Oki T, Tabata H, Manabe K, et al: Cross sectional echocardiographic demonstration of the mechanisms of abnormal interventricular motion in congenital total absence of the left pericardium. Heart 77:247, 1997.
23. Rais-Bahrami K, Granholm T, Short BL, Eichelberger MR: Absence of the pericardium in an infant with congenital diaphragmatic hernia. Am J Perinatol 12:172, 1995.
24. Ratib O, Perloff JK, Williams WG: Congenital complete absence of the pericardium. Circulation 103:3154, 2001.
25. Rees AP, Risher W, McFadden PM, et al: Partial congenital defect of the left pericardium. Cath Cardiovasc Diag 28:231, 1993.
26. Shah RP: Diastolic pressure alternans: A new sign in congenital absence of the pericardium. Singapore Med J 42:78, 2001.
27. Southworth H, Stevenson CS: Congenital defects of the pericardium. Arch Intern Med 61:223, 1938.
28. Tanabe T, Ishizaka M, Ohta S, Sugie S: Intrapericardial aneurysm of the left atrial appendage. Thorax 35:151, 1980.
29. Taysi K, Hartmann AF, Shackelford GD, Sundaram V: Congenital absence of left pericardium in a family. Am J Med Genet 21:77, 1985.
30. Tyberg JV, Smith ER: Ventricular diastole and the role of the pericardium. Herz 15:354, 1990.
31. Van Son JA, Danielson GK, Schaff HV, et al: Congenital partial and complete absence of the pericardium. Mayo Clin Proc 68:743, 1993.
32. Varriale P, Rossi P, Grace WJ: Congenital absence of the left pericardium and complete heart block. Dis Chest 52:405, 1967.
33. Vasquez-Jimenez JF, Muehler EG, Daebritz S, et al: Cantrell's syndrome. Ann Thorac Surg 65:1178, 1998.

Congenitally Corrected Transposition of the Great Arteries

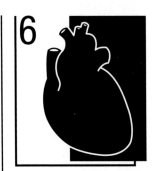

More than a century has elapsed since Karl von Rokitansky applied the term *corrected* to a hitherto undescribed form of transposition of the great arteries[64]:

The left atrioventricular valve and the left-sided ventricle resembled the usual right atrioventricular valve and right ventricle. The aorta is positioned somewhat left and anterior . . . . The right-sided ventricle . . . is finely trabeculated, as usually seen in the left-sided ventricle. The venous atrioventricular ostium has a bivalve. From the right-sided ventricle arises a somewhat right and posteriorly positioned pulmonary artery. . . . The atria are normal, a right caval atrium and a left pulmonary venous atrium.

In 1957, Anderson and coworkers described the clinical manifestations of Rokitansky's malformation,[3] and a few years later Schiebler and coworkers changed the designation from *corrected transposition* to *congenitally corrected* in order to make it clear that the correction was a gift of God and not a gift of the surgeon.[67]

Transposition of the great arteries is defined as an anatomic relationship characterized by discordant ventriculoarterial alignments (see Chapter 27). The pulmonary artery arises from a morphologic right ventricle, and the aorta arises from a morphologic left ventricle. Congenitally corrected transposition is a malformation in which ventriculoarterial alignments are discordant (transposed), but atrioventricular alignments are also discordant (Figs. 6–1 and 6–2).[1,47,67] The double discordance—ventriculoarterial *and* atrioventricular—physiologically corrects the discordance intrinsic to each malalignment (see Fig. 6–1). Blood from a morphologic right atrium reaches the pulmonary artery by traversing a morphologic mitral valve and a morphologic left ventricle, and blood from a morphologic left atrium reaches the aorta by traversing a morphologic tricuspid valve and a morphologic right ventricle (Fig. 6–3 and see Fig. 6–1).[1,47,67] The terms used in this chapter were defined in Chapter 3 and are repeated here for the reader's convenience.

Chamber designations: *Morphologic right and left atrium* and *morphologic right and left ventricle* refer to anatomic characteristics, not to positions.

The great arteries: The ascending aorta and pulmonary trunk are defined by their ventricular origins and by their lateral and anteroposterior spatial relationships.

D-Loop: Refers to the normal rightward (*dextro* = D) bend or loop in the developing straight heart tube of the embryo. A D-loop indicates that the sinus or inflow portion of the morphologic right ventricle lies to the right of the morphologic left ventricle.

L-Loop: Refers to a leftward (*levo* = L) bend or loop in the straight heart tube of the embryo. An L-loop indicates that the sinus or inflow portion of the morphologic right ventricle lies to the left of the morphologic left ventricle.

Concordant: Harmonious, appropriate.

Discordant: Disharmonious, inappropriate.

Discordant loop: An L-loop in situs solitus and a D-loop in situs inversus.

Ventriculoarterial discordance: Origin of the pulmonary artery from a morphologic left ventricle and origin of the aorta from a morphologic right ventricle.

Atrioventricular discordance: Alignment of a morphologic right atrium with a morphologic left ventricle, and alignment of a morphologic left atrium with a morphologic right ventricle.

Transposition of the great arteries: The aorta arises discordantly from a morphologic right ventricle and the pulmonary trunk arises discordantly from a morphologic left ventricle.

Congenitally corrected transposition of the great arteries: Atrioventricular discordance in conjunction with ventriculoarterial discordance. A morphologic right atrium is discordantly aligned with a morphologic left ventricle from which the pulmonary artery arises, and a morphologic left atrium is aligned discordantly with a morphologic right ventricle from which the aorta arises (see Figs. 6–1 and 6–3).

Segmental approach: Analysis of the heart according to its three major developmental segments: (1) visceroatrial situs, (2) ventricular loop, and (3) conotruncus. The atrioventricular valves and the infundibulum are the two connecting cardiac segments.

Corrected: Systemic venous blood from the right atrium finds its way into the pulmonary artery, and pulmonary venous blood from the left atrium finds its way into the aorta.

L-Transposition: An L-loop in situs solitus. The sinus or inflow portion of the morphologic right ventricle is to the left of the morphologic left ventricle.

Inversion: Reversal of position but not mirror image. *Ventricular inversion* refers to a morphologic left ventricle in the right side of the heart and a morphologic right ventricle in the left side of the heart. Morphologic tricuspid and mitral valves are concordant with morphologic right and left ventricles, so inversion of the ventricles implies inversion of the atrioventricular valves. *Ventricular inversion*, *L-transposition*, and *congenitally corrected transposition* are synonymous terms and are used interchangeably.

Congenitally corrected transposition of the great arteries[16,26,66,67] typically occurs in situs solitus in an estimated 0.5% of clinically diagnosed cases of congenital malformations of the heart or in approximately 1 in 13,000 live births.[11,20,41,56,67,69] All but 1% have coexisting cardiac malformations.[11,20,56] Atrioventricular discordance

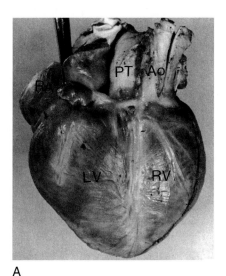

A

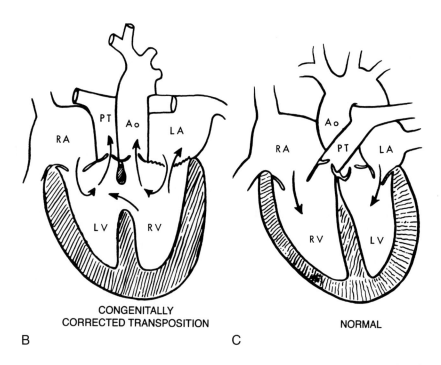

B   CONGENITALLY CORRECTED TRANSPOSITION   C   NORMAL

Figure 6–1
A, Gross specimen of congenitally corrected transposition of the great arteries illustrating ventriculoarterial discordance. The pulmonary trunk originates from the morphologic left ventricle (LV), and the aorta (Ao) originates from the morphologic right ventricle (RV). *B and C*, Illustrations of congenitally corrected transposition of the great arteries (*B*) for comparison with the normal heart (*C*). Congenitally corrected transposition is characterized by atrioventricular discordance and ventriculoarterial discordance. Blood from a morphologic right atrium (RA) traverses a morphologic mitral valve into a morphologic left ventricle (LV) and then enters a pulmonary trunk (PT) that is rightward and posterior. Blood from a morphologic left atrium (LA) traverses a morphologic tricuspid valve into a morphologic right ventricle (RV) and then enters an aorta (Ao) that is leftward and anterior. The double discordance means that right atrial blood finds its way into the pulmonary artery and left atrial blood finds its way into the aorta. Anatomic transposition of the great arteries is physiologically corrected. The great arteries run parallel to each other and do not cross as in the normal heart. Coexisting anomalies include a malformed left atrioventricular valve, a ventricular septal defect, and pulmonary stenosis. The normal heart is characterized by atrioventricular concordance, ventriculoarterial concordance, and a pulmonary artery that crosses anterior to the aorta.

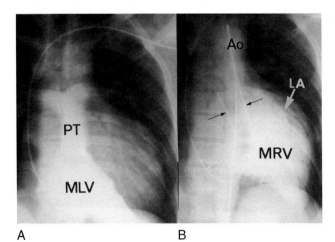

Figure 6–2

Angiocardiograms (anteroposterior) from a 34-year-old man with congenitally corrected transposition of the great arteries and a moderately incompetent left atrioventricular valve. *A*, Contrast material opacifies a morphologic left ventricle (MLV) from which a rightward and posterior pulmonary trunk arises (PT). *B*, Contrast material outlines a hump-shaped crescentic morphologic right ventricle (MRV) from which a leftward and anterior ascending aorta (Ao) arises. Catheters in the pulmonary trunk and ascending aorta (*arrows*) run parallel to each other and do not cross. The left atrium (LA) opacifies because of left atrioventricular valve regurgitation.

requires the presence of two morphologically distinct atria and two morphologically distinct ventricles. Hearts in which two morphologically distinct atria are aligned with one ventricle (univentricular atrioventricular connection) are dealt with in Chapter 26.

The coronary arteries and the ventricles are morphologically concordant in congenitally corrected transposition (Fig. 6–4 and see Chapter 32).[1,9,17,21,67,68,75] Epicardial dis-

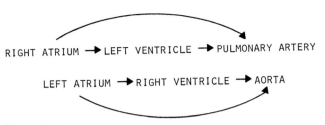

Figure 6–3

Simplified schematic illustration of the circulation in congenitally corrected transposition of the great arteries.

tribution of the coronary arteries serves as a guide to ventricular inversion because the course of the anterior descending coronary artery establishes the location of the ventricular septum. The most frequent coexisting congenital coronary anomaly is a single coronary artery (see Chapter 32).[21]

In congenitally corrected transposition of the great arteries, the anterior and leftward ascending aorta and posterior and rightward pulmonary trunk run parallel to each other and do not cross as in the normal heart (see Figs. 6–1 and 6–2).[3,67] The aorta is either convex to the left or vertical in its ascent but is not border-forming on the right. A subaortic conus is responsible for the anterior and leftward position of the ascending aorta and the posteromedial position of the pulmonary trunk.[19] *Anatomically corrected malposition* refers to an anomaly in which the ascending aorta lies anterior and to the left of the pulmonary trunk in the presence of atrioventricular and ventriculoarterial concordance.[19] *Isolated ventricular inversion* refers to atrioventricular discordance with ventriculoarterial concordance. A morphologic right atrium is aligned with a morphologic left

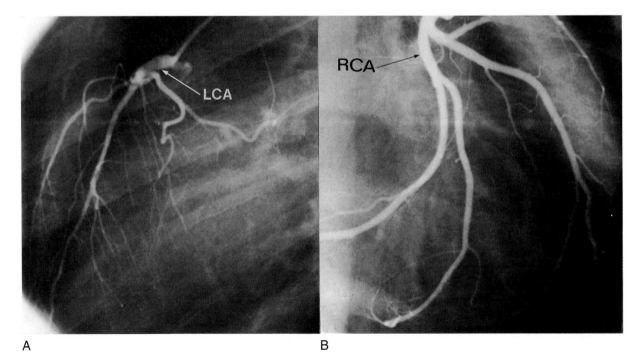

Figure 6–4

Coronary arteriograms from a 41-year-old man with congenitally corrected transposition of the great arteries. *A*, The left anterior oblique projection shows a morphologic left coronary artery (LCA) concordant with a morphologic left ventricle. *B*, The right anterior oblique projection shows a morphologic right coronary artery (RCA) concordant with a morphologic right ventricle.

ventricle that gives rise to the aorta, and a morphologic left atrium is aligned with a morphologic right ventricle that gives rise to the pulmonary trunk.[59,61,62] The physiology of the circulation is analogous to that of complete transposition of the great arteries (see Chapter 27). *Isolated infundibuloarterial inversion* refers to a rare anomaly in which the infundibulum and the great arteries are inverted, but the atria and ventricles are not inverted.[29] The inverted pulmonary trunk and its subpulmonary infundibulum originate from the morphologic left ventricle, and the inverted aorta originates from a morphologic right ventricle, so the physiology of the circulation is analogous to complete transposition of the great arteries.

Criss-cross hearts were described by Lev and Rowlatt in 1961[49] and were so named by Anderson, Shineborne, and Gerlis in 1974.[8] In normal hearts, the atrioventricular structures (inflow tracts) are parallel to each other when viewed from the front. In criss-cross hearts, the atrioventricular structures (inflow tracts) are not parallel but instead are angulated by as much as 90 degrees.[4,8,31] Criss-cross hearts result from abnormal rotation of the ventricular mass around its long axis, resulting in relationships that could not be inferred from the atrioventricular connections.[4] There are several types of criss-cross hearts.[53] Those with discordant atrioventricular alignments and concordant ventriculoarterial alignments have been called *isolated ventricular inversion* (see earlier).[62] The physiology of the circulation is analogous to that of complete transposition of the great arteries, despite ventriculoarterial concordance.[4,59] Criss-cross hearts with ventricles that are in a superoinferior or "upstairs-downstairs" relationship represent rotation of the ventricular mass along the horizontal plane of its long axis.[4,31] Criss-cross hearts and superoinferior ventricles may coexist (see Fig. 6–31) or may occur separately.[4] Recurrent morphologic patterns in criss-cross hearts include deficiency of the subpulmonary infundibulum, subpulmonary stenosis, a subaortic infundibulum, a nonrestrictive ventricular septal defect, and visceroatrial situs solitus.[38,53,62,63]

The developmental fault held responsible for atrioventricular discordance in congenitally corrected transposition resides in the L-ventricular loop of the embryonic heart tube. When the heart tube bends to the left in situs solitus, the morphologic right ventricle lies to the left of the morphologic left ventricle.[5] The developing left atrium becomes aligned with the morphologic right ventricle, and the developing right atrium becomes aligned with the morphologic left ventricle. Ventriculoarterial discordance has a less well-defined embryologic basis. One school of thought argues that the developmental fault is in the infundibular segment of the embryonic heart tube, while the other school of thought argues that the fault is in the arterial segment of the embryonic heart tube.

The physiologic consequences of congenitally corrected transposition depend on the functional adequacy of a morphologic right ventricle that is subaortic and therefore systemic, and on the coexisting congenital malformations.[1,11,21,37,67,69] The thick-walled subaortic right ventricle

is concordant with a right coronary artery that is designed to perfuse a thin-walled low-resistance subpulmonary right ventricle. A normal subpulmonary right ventricle is geometrically appropriate for the low-resistance pulmonary circulation, and the geometry remains unchanged when the subpulmonary right ventricle is inverted to the subaortic position. Regional strain and twist and radial wall motion in a subaortic right ventricle differ considerably from these indices in a subaortic left ventricle.[7] Inverted subaortic right ventricles have a high prevalence of myocardial perfusion defects and abnormalities of regional wall motion.[15] A normal subpulmonary right ventricle has a relatively high end-diastolic volume, so a normal stroke volume is achieved at the relatively low ejection fraction of 35% to 45%.[11,37] This low ejection fraction remains the same when the morphologic right ventricle is inverted into the subaortic position. The ejection fraction of an inverted right ventricle is therefore considerably less than the ejection fraction of a normal subaortic left ventricle.[11,37] The response to supine exercise of an inverted right ventricle is similar to the response of a normal noninverted right ventricle.[11,37] The response to exercise of an inverted subpulmonary left ventricle is similar to the response of a normal noninverted left ventricle.[11]

Ventricular septal defect, pulmonary stenosis, abnormalities of the left atrioventricular valve, and conduction defects have a significant impact on the function of an inherently inadequate inverted right ventricle.[1,67,71] Conduction abnormalities are discussed in the section on The Electrocardiogram.

A ventricular septal defect is present in 78% of necropsy cases (Fig. 6–5), is usually nonrestrictive perimembranous, and typically extends into the inlet septum and trabecular septum.[1,58] The inlet septum is poorly aligned with the atrial septum, resulting in a malalignment gap that is sometimes filled by tissue from the membranous septum that is considerably larger than in a normal heart.

Pulmonary stenosis or atresia occurs in 50% of cases and represents obstruction to outflow of the morphologic left ventricle.[1,3,67] The stenosis is isolated in about 20% of cases and occurs with a ventricular septal defect in the remaining 80%. Fixed subpulmonary stenosis takes several forms[1]: (1) a fibrous subpulmonary diaphragm is attached to the mitral valve, analogous to fixed subaortic stenosis in hearts with noninverted ventricles; (2) an aneurysm or fibrous tissue tags originates from the relatively large membranous septum; and (3) accessory mitral leaflet tissue.[67] Subaortic stenosis (outflow tract obstruction of the morphologic right ventricle) is caused by anterior deviation of the infundibulum septum or by hypertrophied infundibular muscle bundles.[1,64,67]

Abnormalities of the left atrioventricular valve are present in more than 90% of cases.[1] The malformed valve usually functions normally in early life, but there is an age-related increase in regurgitation. Structural abnormalities resemble Ebstein's anomaly of the right-sided tricuspid valve in hearts without ventricular inversion (Fig.

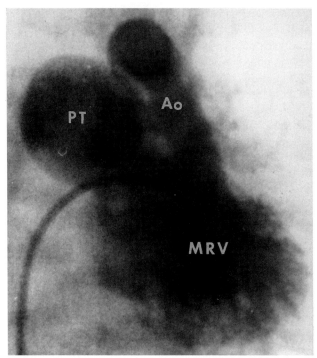

Figure 6–5

Angiocardiogram from a 4-year-old boy with congenitally corrected transposition of the great arteries and a nonrestrictive ventricular septal defect. The systemic ventricle has the shape and the coarse trabecular pattern of a morphologic right ventricle (MRV) and gives rise to an ascending aorta (Ao) that is convex to the left. An enlarged pulmonary trunk (PT) is visualized via the ventricular septal defect.

6–6A),[1,2,42,67] but the anterior leaflet of the inverted Ebstein valve is usually small and malformed,[2] and the atrialized inverted right ventricle is poorly developed.[2] Left atrioventricular valve incompetence is not necessarily caused by an Ebstein-like malformation, and the valve is occasionally obstructed rather than incompetent (see Chapter 13). Neonates with severe regurgitation of the inverted atrioventricular valve have an increased incidence of hypoplasia of the aortic arch, aortic atresia, and aortic coarctation.[18] Abnormalities of the *right-sided inverted mitral valve* have been reported in more than half of necropsy specimens.[34] These are usually functionally unimportant abnormalities that consist of multiple cusps, multiple or compound papillary muscles, anomalous chordal attachments, and a cleft valve or a common valve.[34]

The History

The male-to-female ratio is approximately 1.5:1.[3,16,39,67] The occurrence of congenitally corrected transposition and complete transposition among first-degree relatives in different families is believed to represent monogenic transmission, supporting a pathogenetic link between the two malformations.[25] Symptoms and clinical course depend chiefly on the presence and degree of coexisting malformations,[6a,51,67,69] but longevity also hinges on the vulnerabil-

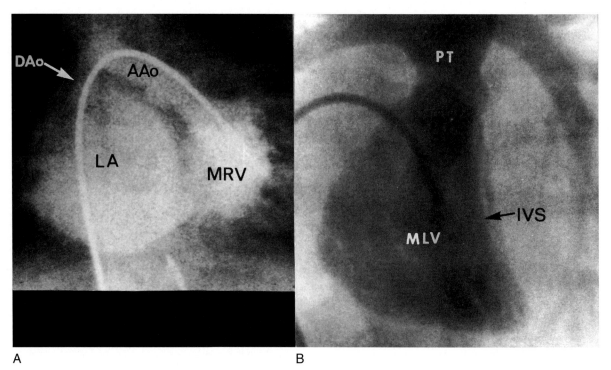

A   B

Figure 6–6

A, Angiocardiogram with contrast material injected into the small morphologic right ventricle (MRV) of a 7-month-old boy with congenitally corrected transposition of the great arteries and severe incompetence of the left atrioventricular valve. Regurgitant flow opacifies a huge left atrium (LA). The ascending aorta (AAo) originates from the morphologic right ventricle, is convex to the left, and continues as a right-sided descending aorta (DAo). *B,* Angiocardiogram with contrast material injected into the morphologic left ventricle (MLV) of a 4-year-old boy with congenitally corrected transposition of the great arteries and no coexisting malformations. The plane of the interventricular septum (IVS) is vertical and close to the left sternal border. The morphologic left ventricle is finely trabeculated and gives rise to a rightward and posterior pulmonary trunk (PT) with right and left branches at the same level.

ity of the subaortic morphologic right ventricle even when there are no coexisting malformations. Infant mortality is related to congestive heart failure. Survival is then relatively constant, with an attrition rate of approximately 1% to 2% per year.[39] Young patients with no coexisting malformations are overlooked because symptoms are absent and clinical signs are subtle.[67] The diagnosis may come to light because of subtle abnormalities on chest x-ray (Fig. 6–7), because of an abnormal electrocardiogram (see Fig. 6–20), or because of high-degree heart block (Fig. 6–8).[12,67,69]

The ventricular septal defect that accompanies congenitally corrected transposition is typically nonrestrictive, with a clinical course analogous to that of a ventricular septal defect of equivalent size in normally formed hearts[58,67] (see Chapter 17). Pulmonary stenosis exerts a protective effect by curtailing excessive pulmonary blood flow.[48,67] An inverted subpulmonary left ventricle readily adapts to systemic systolic pressure incurred by a nonrestrictive ventricular septal defect. Isolated pulmonary stenosis varies from mild to severe

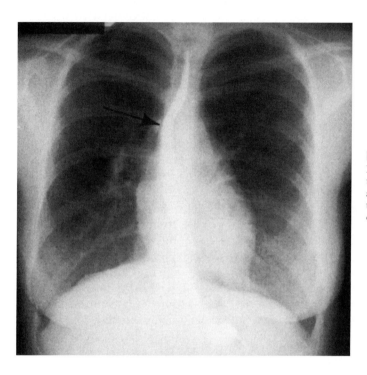

Figure 6–7
X-rays from a 23-year-old woman with congenitally corrected transposition of the great arteries and no coexisting malformations. The x-ray appears normal except for subtle evidence of an inverted ascending aorta that straightened the left superior cardiac border, and a long indentation of the barium esophagram (*unmarked black arrow*).

High-degree heart block is rarely present in utero but is occasionally present shortly after birth (see Fig. 6–8),[40,74] or may subsequently announce itself as a Stokes-Adams attack or sudden death.[35,40,73] The age-related risk of developing complete heart block is about 2% per year.[40]

Left atrioventricular valve regurgitation is closely coupled to long-term survival.[6a, 39] The incompetence is usually occult in infants who are destined to develop regurgitant flow, the late appearance of which prompts a mistaken diagnosis of acquired mitral valve regurgitation.

Survival to the sixth or seventh decade is infrequent,[6a,9,41,67,68] but two patients reached their eighth decade.[39,50] Spontaneous failure of the subaortic right ventricle is uncommon but not rare in congenitally corrected transposition with no coexisting malformations[24,56,65] and may occur during pregnancy in previously asymptomatic women.[10] Myocardial perfusion defects are prevalent,[15] and angina pectoris has been attributed to a supply-demand imbalance between a thick-walled systemic right ventricle and perfusion by a morphologic right coronary artery (see earlier).

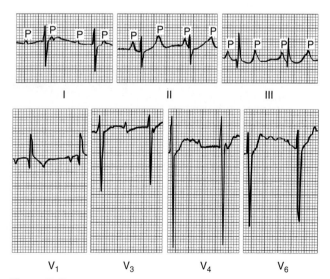

Figure 6–8
Electrocardiogram from a 20-month-old boy with congenitally corrected transposition of the great arteries and complete heart block. P waves are independent of the QRS complexes, which are narrow. Because of reversed septal depolarization, a prominent Q wave appears in lead V_1 but no Q wave appears in lead V_6.

and runs a clinical course analogous to that of equivalent pulmonary stenosis in hearts without ventricular inversion (see Chapter 11).

Physical Appearance

Retarded growth and development are restricted to infants with a large ventricular septal defects and congestive heart failure. Cyanosis and clubbing appear when pulmonary stenosis or pulmonary vascular disease reverses the shunt.[63,67]

The Arterial Pulse

The waveform is normal. The arterial pulse rate reflects the bradycardia of 2:1 heart block or complete heart block (see The Electrocardiogram).

The Jugular Venous Pulse

Prolongation of the PR interval is recognized by an increase in the interval between the jugular A wave and the carotid pulse. Two-to-one heart block is recognized by A waves that occur twice as frequently as the carotid pulse. Complete heart block is recognized by independent jugular A waves and random cannon A waves (see Chapter 4).

Pulmonary stenosis is associated with A waves that vary with severity, as in isolated pulmonary stenosis in hearts without ventricular inversion (see Chapter 11).

Pulmonary stenosis with a nonrestrictive ventricular septal defect is accompanied by a normal jugular venous pulse analogous to Fallot tetralogy (see Chapter 18).

Precordial Movement and Palpation

Precordial movements are influenced by the spatial orientation of the ventricular septum and by the anterior and leftward position of the ascending aorta. The plane of the ventricular septum faces forward, and a vertical interventricular sulcus is closely aligned with the left sternal border (see Fig. 6–6B).[44,67] Accordingly, an inverted right ventricle occupies an anterior and leftward position with its medial border adjacent to the left sternal edge and its lateral border at the apex (see Fig. 6–2B), an arrangement that accounts for the large topographic area generated by the right ventricular impulse. The impulse of the anteroapical right ventricle is accentuated by left atrioventricular valve regurgitation, because systolic expansion of the left atrium causes anterior displacement of the heart (see Fig. 6–6A). There is no retraction medial to the interventricular sulcus because the sulcus lies too close to the left sternal border (see Fig. 6–6B). The inverted left ventricle occupies a posterior and rightward position behind the sternum,[67] where it cannot be felt even in the presence of pulmonary hypertension or pulmonary stenosis (see Figs. 6–2A and 6–6B). The ascending aorta is palpated when it is dilated and convex to the left (see Fig. 6–9), and the aortic component of the second heart sound is palpated because of the anterior position of the aortic root (Fig. 6–9 and see Fig. 6–5).

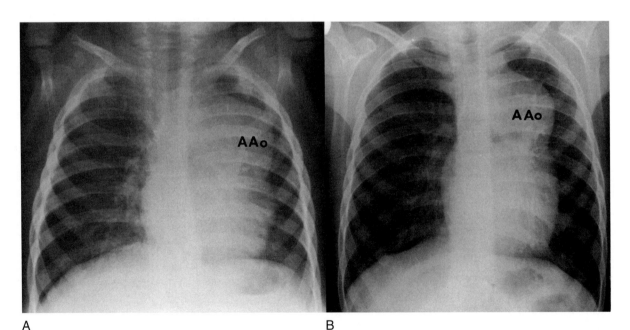

A   B

Figure 6–9

X-rays that are virtually identical at age 4 months (*A*) and at age 16 years (*B*) from a patient with congenitally corrected transposition of the great arteries, a nonrestrictive ventricular septal defect, pulmonary atresia, and reduced pulmonary blood flow. The ascending aorta (AAo) is dilated and strikingly convex to the left, but there is no vascular shadow at the right base. The heart size is normal.

Auscultation

A soft first heart sound is a sign of the PR interval prolongation of first-degree heart block. Variation in intensity of the first heart sound is a sign of complete heart block (see Chapter 4). An ejection sound at the left base (see Fig. 6–13B) originates in the anterior aorta, especially when the aortic root is dilated (see Fig. 6–9). A short, soft basal midsystolic murmur originates in the anterior aorta but may also originate in the posterior pulmonary trunk across the deeply wedged outflow tract of the morphologic left ventricle. The second heart sound is loud, because the aortic valve is anterior (see Fig. 6–13B).[3,20,67] The loudness and location of the sound invite a mistaken diagnosis of pulmonary hypertension. The pulmonary component of the second heart sound is attenuated by the posterior position of the pulmonary trunk, which makes splitting difficult to hear. When splitting is detected, it is in the second left interspace, despite the rightward position of the posterior pulmonary valve.[33] A soft, high-frequency early diastolic murmur of aortic regurgitation is occasionally heard at the mid left sternal border.[67]

The murmur of ventricular septal defect is analogous in location, configuration, and quality to the murmur of ventricular septal defect in hearts without ventricular inversion (see Chapter 17). The murmur is holosystolic (Fig. 6–10) or decrescendo (Fig. 6–11) and is absent when the shunt is reversed. A mid-diastolic murmur is generated by increased flow across the left atrioventricular valve when the left-to-right shunt is large (see Fig. 6–11). A Graham Steell murmur (see Fig. 6–10) is more likely than an early diastolic murmur of aortic regurgitation. A pulmonary ejection sound originates in the dilated hypertensive posterior pulmonary trunk (see Figs. 6–5 and 6–10A). The intensity of an inherently loud second heart sound is further augmented by pulmonary hypertension because the increased pulmonary component is synchronous with the prominent component from the anterior aortic valve (see Figs. 6–10 and 6–11).

The murmur of pulmonary stenosis is maximum in the third left intercostal space because stenosis is usually subpulmonary (Fig. 6–12) and is relatively soft for a given degree of obstruction because of the attenuating effect of the anterior aorta. Radiation of the pulmonary stenotic murmur is upward and to the right because the pulmonary trunk is oriented upward and to the right (see Fig.6–2A).[67] The loud second heart sound at the left base is aortic, not pulmonary (see Fig. 6–12).

Left atrioventricular valve regurgitation generates systolic murmurs analogous to those of mitral regurgitation in hearts without ventricular inversion (Fig. 6–13).[60] Radiation tends to be toward the left sternal edge rather than into the axilla, because the malformed tricuspid leaflets direct the jet medially within the left atrium. The first heart sound is not loud in left-sided Ebstein's anomaly because the malformed anterior tricuspid leaflet is small and poorly mobile.[2]

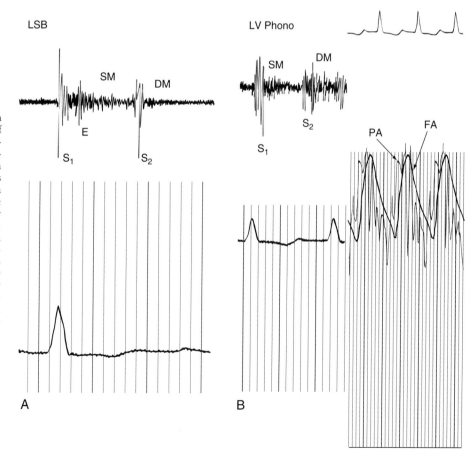

Figure 6–10

Tracings from an 8-year-old boy with congenitally corrected transposition of the great arteries, a nonrestrictive ventricular septal defect and a large left-to-right shunt. A, Phonocardiogram from the lower left sternal border (LSB) shows a pulmonary ejection sound (E), a holosystolic murmur (SM), a loud single second heart sound (S₂) and an early diastolic Graham Steell murmur (DM). B, The intracardiac phonocardiogram from the outflow tract of the subpulmonary left ventricle (LV phono) shows the ventricular septal defect murmur (SM) and the Graham Steell murmur (DM). Second panel shows equal pulmonary arterial (PA) and femoral arterial (FA) systolic pressures because the ventricular septal defect was nonrestrictive. S₁, first heart sound.

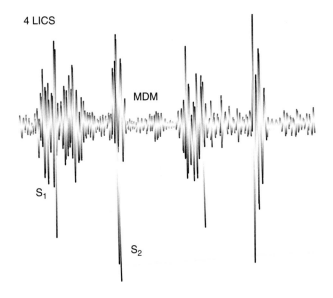

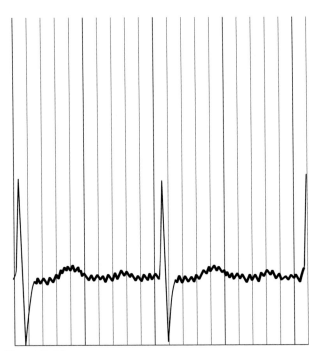

Figure 6–11
Phonocardiogram from the fourth left intercostal space (4 LICS) of a 4-month-old girl with congenitally corrected transposition of the great arteries, a nonrestrictive ventricular septal defect, and a large left-to-right shunt. A decrescendo holosystolic murmur (SM) is followed by a loud single second heart sound (S₂) and a mid-diastolic flow murmur (MDM) across the left atrioventricular valve.

The Electrocardiogram

In 1913, Monckeberg described an anterior node responsible for atrioventricular conduction in congenitally corrected transposition of the great arteries.[55] Walmsley in 1931[75] and Yater in 1933[76] established that the bundle branches were inverted. Elegant studies from Lev[48] and from Anderson[6] were major steps forward in advancing

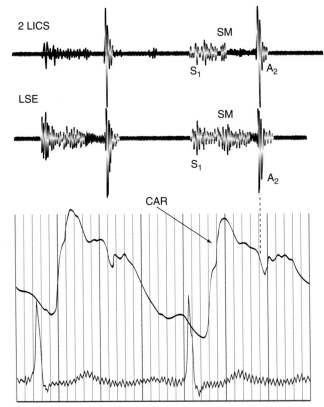

Figure 6–12
Tracings from a 15-year-old boy with congenitally corrected transposition of the great arteries and subpulmonary stenosis (gradient 20 mm Hg). The pulmonary stenotic murmur (SM) is maximum at the mid left sternal edge (LSE) rather than in the second left intercostal space (2 LICS). Aortic valve closure (A₂) is loud and single because the aorta is anterior. CAR, carotid pulse.

our knowledge of conduction tissues in hearts with ventricular inversion.

Because the atrial septum is malaligned with the inlet ventricular septum, the regular atrioventricular node does not make contact with infranodal right and left bundle branches.[6,32] Instead, there is an anomalous anterior atrioventricular node with a bundle that penetrates the atrioventricular fibrous annulus and descends onto the anterior aspect of the ventricular septum.[22] The penetrating atrioventricular bundle descends for a long distance down the septal surface before branching. The long penetrating atrioventricular bundle is well formed in the hearts of young children, but beginning in adolescence, the conduction fibers are replaced by fibrous tissue, which is responsible for atrioventricular block.[43]

Electrophysiologic studies have identified multiple levels of conduction defects that include the atrioventricular node, the penetrating bundle, and the bundle branches.[30,35,36] Complete heart block that is present at birth[22,30,63] (see Fig. 6–8) results from discontinuity between the anterior atrioventricular node and the ventricular septum.[48] A cord-like right bundle branch extends leftward to the morphologic right ventricle, and a left bundle branch descends down the septal surface of the morphologic left ventricle. The right bundle branch is concordant with the morpho-

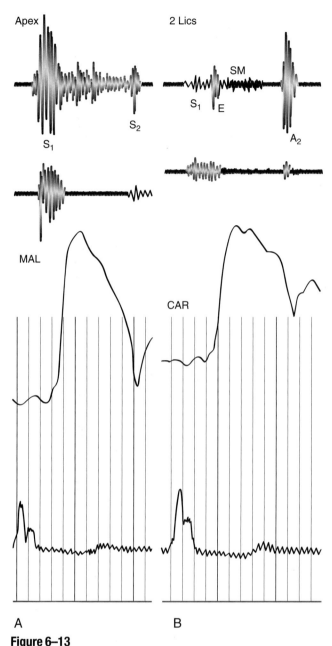

Figure 6–13
Tracings from a 34-year-old man with congenitally corrected transposition of the great arteries and moderate incompetence of the left atrioventricular valve. *A*, The apical decrescendo holosystolic murmur radiates poorly, if at all, to the midaxillary line (MAL). *B*, In the second left intercostal space (2 Lics), an aortic ejection sound (E) introduces a short systolic murmur (SM) and coincides with the onset of the carotid arterial pulse (CAR). Aortic valve closure (A_2) is loud and single because the aorta is anterior.

logic right ventricle, and the left bundle branch is concordant with the morphologic left ventricle. An Ebstein anomaly of the left atrioventricular valve with left-sided accessory pathways provides the substrate for pre-excitation between the morphologic left atrium and the morphologic right ventricle.[13,22,57] The arrhythmogenic atrialized morphologic right ventricle resides in the left side of the heart.[53]

There are three major features of the scalar electrocardiogram: (1) disturbances in conduction and rhythm, (2) QRS and T-wave patterns that reflect ventricular inversion, and

(3) modifications of the P wave, QRS, ST segment, and T wave caused by coexisting congenital heart disease. The P wave is normal in direction and configuration because the sinoatrial node is in its normal location, so the atria are normally activated. Broad notched left atrial P waves occur when the left atrium is volume overloaded by incompetence of the left atrioventricular valve or by a large left-to-right shunt through a ventricular septal defect (Fig. 6–14). Tall peaked right atrial P waves occur with pulmonary hypertension (Fig. 6–15) or pulmonary stenosis (Fig. 6–16).

Atrioventricular conduction varies from PR interval prolongation of first-degree heart block (Fig. 6–16) to complete heart block (Figs. 6–8 and 6–17). More than 75% of patients with congenitally corrected transposition exhibit varying degrees of atrioventricular block when all ages are included, and the overall incidence of complete heart block is about 30%.[6,22,30,36,39,46,67,74] Normal conduction in the surface electrocardiogram coincides with normal conduction on intracardiac electrophysiologic study and vice versa. The electrogram of the bundle of His does not necessarily localize the site of atrioventricular block, because the long course of the non-branching bundle precludes distinction between a distal atrioventricular nodal lesion and a proximal bundle of His lesion.[22] Second-degree atrioventricular block is almost always 2 to 1. The degree of block varies from time to time in the same patient, and first-degree heart block changes to intermittent 2 to 1 block to complete heart block. Complete heart block is associated with a normal sequence of ventricular activation and a normal QRS duration (see Figs. 6–8 and

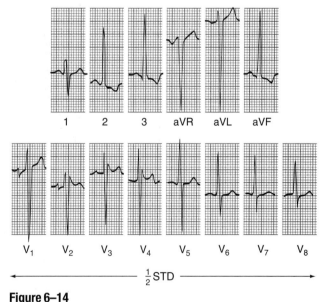

$\frac{1}{2}$ STD

Figure 6–14
Electrocardiogram from an 8-year-old boy with congenitally corrected transposition of the great arteries, a nonrestrictive ventricular septal defect and a large left-to-right shunt. Broad notched left atrial P waves appear in leads 1 and 2, and a prominent left atrial P terminal force appears in lead V_1. The QRS axis is rightward. Despite volume overload of the systemic ventricle, Q waves are absent in left precordial leads, including the lead V_8 position. T waves are upright in all precordial leads but are taller in right precordial leads. Large biphasic RS complexes of biventricular hypertrophy appear in leads V_4 and V_5.

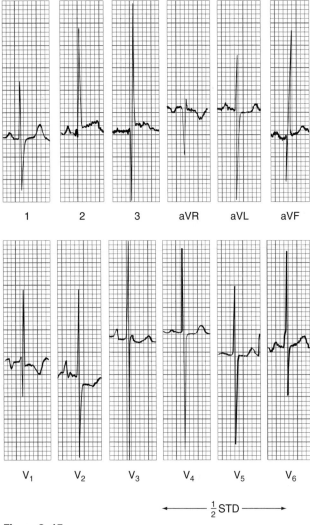

1   2   3   aVR   aVL   aVF

V₁   V₂   V₃   V₄   V₅   V₆

← ½ STD →

Figure 6–15

Electrocardiogram from a 4-month-old girl with congenitally corrected transposition of the great arteries, a nonrestrictive ventricular septal defect, and a large left-to-right shunt. Peaked right atrial P waves appear in lead 2 and in leads V_2 and V_3. The QRS axis is rightward. Q waves are prominent and are deeper in lead 3 than in lead aVF. Despite volume overload of the systemic ventricle, Q waves are absent in left precordial leads. Large biphasic RS complexes of biventricular hypertrophy appear in midprecordial leads.

6–17),[35,36] as is the case in isolated congenital complete heart block (see Chapter 4).

Accelerated conduction through bypass tracts may occur in congenitally corrected transposition with Ebstein's anomaly of the left atrioventricular valve. Delta waves in lead V_1 reflect left bypass tracts,[13,22] and fusion beats indicate dual antegrade conduction via a bypass tract and an anterior atrioventricular node.[13] When there is discontinuity beyond the anterior atrioventricular node, antegrade conduction is occasionally achieved via an accessory pathway.[13] Supraventricular tachycardia, atrial fibrillation, and atrial flutter with left-sided Ebstein's anomaly do not necessarily coincide with the presence of Wolff-Parkinson-White accessory pathways.[22,28,67] Atrial fibrillation occurs with chronic severe incompetence of the left atrioventricular valve.[67]

QRS and T-wave patterns are understood in light of the inverted right and left bundle branches[6] and in the context of coexisting cardiac malformations.[28,72] Activation of the ventricular septum in the normal heart proceeds from left to right, so Q waves appear in left precordial leads and an initial R wave appears in right precordial leads. In congenitally corrected transposition, inversion of the right and left bundle branches results in reversed septal activation that proceeds from right to left. Q waves appear in right precordial leads (Figs. 6–18 through 6–20 and see Fig. 6–16) and are consistently absent in left precordial leads (see Figs. 6–14, 6–15, and 6–18 through 6–20).[3,48,66] Absence of left precordial Q waves stands out in bold relief in the presence of volume overload of the systemic ventricle (see Figs. 6–14 and 6–15). Absence of left precordial Q waves can be confirmed by recording leads beyond the V_6 position (see Fig. 6–14). Detection of Q waves contiguous to lead V_1 benefits from recording leads V_3R and V_4R. When supplementary lead placements are used, reversed septal activation is found in all but a minority of patients. An occasional R wave in lead V_1 (see Figs. 6–14 and 6–15) should not detract from the importance of consistent absence of Q waves in left precordial leads (see Figs. 6–16 and 6–18 through 6–20). Septal

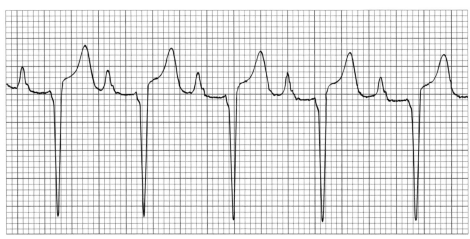

Figure 6–16

Lead V_1 from a 35-year-old woman with congenitally corrected transposition of the great arteries, a nonrestrictive ventricular septal defect, and subpulmonary stenosis. The P wave is tall and peaked (right atrial abnormality), the PR interval is 0.24 msec, and the QS wave indicates reversed septal depolarization.

V₁

Figure 6–17

Monitor leads from a 41-year-old man with congenitally corrected transposition of the great arteries whose coronary arteriograms are shown in Figure 6–4. A, The rhythm strip identifies complete disassociation between P waves and QRS complexes that are of normal duration. B, Rhythm strip after insertion of a pacemaker into the subpulmonary left ventricle. *Arrows* identify the ventricular pacemaker spikes.

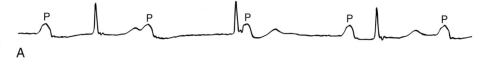

A

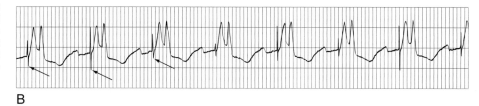

B

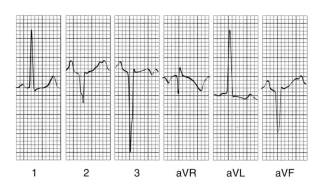

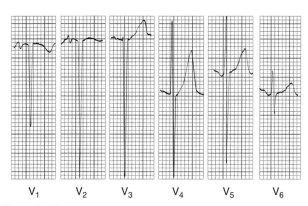

Figure 6–18

Electrocardiogram from a 2-year-old girl with congenitally corrected transposition of the great arteries, coarctation of the aorta, and systemic hypertension. There is left axis deviation. QS waves appear in leads V_1 and V_2 but no Q waves appear in lead V_6 because septal depolarization is reversed. Deep S waves in right precordial leads, a tall R wave in lead aVL, and a deep S wave in lead 3 indicate hypertrophy of the afterloaded systemic subaortic right ventricle.

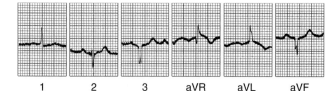

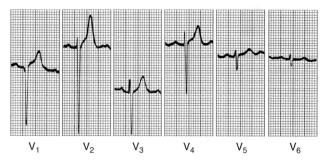

Figure 6–19

Electrocardiogram from a 15-year-old boy with congenitally corrected transposition of the great arteries and subpulmonary stenosis (gradient 25 mm Hg). There is left axis deviation. A QS complex appears in lead V_1 but Q waves do not appear in left precordial leads because septal depolarization is reversed.

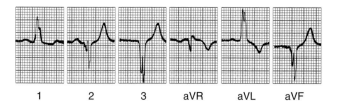

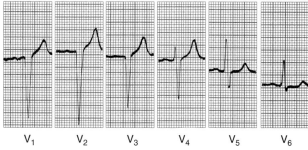

Figure 6–20

Electrocardiogram from a 34-year-old man with congenitally corrected transposition of the great arteries and mild incompetence of the left AV valve. There is left axis deviation. Prominent Q waves appear in leads 3 and aVF and in leads V_1 through V_3, but Q waves do not appear in left precordial leads because septal depolarization is reversed.

activation in a superior direction is responsible for Q waves in leads 3 and aVF and for the almost uniform absence of Q waves in leads 1 and aVL (see Figs. 6–15 and 6–18 through 6–20).[67] Q waves are consistently deeper in lead 3 than in lead aVF and not uncommonly are very deep (see Figs. 6–15 and 6–18 through 6–20).

Left axis deviation is a diagnostically significant pattern (see Figs. 6–18 through 6–20).[20,28,72] The mechanism responsible for the left superior axis is unsettled but cannot be due to left anterior fascicular block, because the left bundle branch is in the right side of the heart. Left axis deviation is most likely when systolic pressure in the subpulmonary

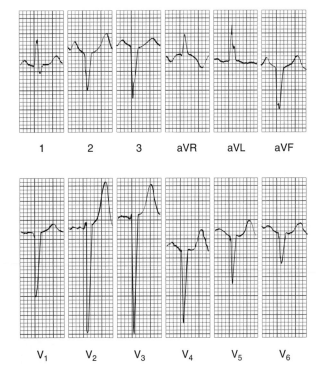

Figure 6–21

Electrocardiogram from a 23-year-old woman with congenitally corrected transposition of the great arteries and no coexisting malformations. Marked left axis deviation and marked posterior direction of ventricular depolarization result in QS waves in virtually all precordial leads.

left ventricle is not elevated (see Figs. 6–18 through 6–20) and is least likely when the subpulmonary left ventricular systolic pressure is high (see Figs. 6–14 and 6–15).[20,28,72] A left superior axis is occasionally associated with striking Q waves in leads 2, 3, and aVF and in Q waves in most if not all precordial leads (Fig. 6–21 and see Figs. 6–18 and 6–20).

Positive T waves are present in all six precordial leads in more than 80% of cases (see Figs. 6–19, 6–20, and 6–21). This distinctive feature is attributed to the side-by-side relationship of the inverted ventricles (see Fig. 6–6). The T waves are often taller in right precordial leads (Figs. 6–14, 6–17, 6–20, and 6–21).

Severe pulmonary stenosis with intact ventricular septum may produce a QR complex in lead V_1 and an RS complex in lead V_6.[72] Nonrestrictive ventricular septal defects with large left-to-right shunts are associated with large equidiphasic RS complexes in midprecordial leads and with increased R waves *without* Q waves in left precordial leads (see Figs. 6–14 and 6–15).[72]

The X-Ray

The normal heart in a posteroanterior chest x-ray is characterized by a distinctive triad of contours consisting of the ascending aorta on the right and the aortic knuckle and main pulmonary artery on the left. In congenitally corrected transposition, this triad is lost because the aorta does not ascend on the right and the pulmonary trunk is

not border forming on the left (see Fig. 6–2).[14,16,27] The most common relationship of the great arteries is side-by-side, with the ascending aorta anterior and to the left of a medially positioned posterior pulmonary trunk (see Fig. 6–2). Even when subtle, these relationships can usually be recognized as a perceptible ascending aortic shadow at the left base and by absence of an aortic shadow at the right base (Fig. 6–22 and see Fig. 6–7). The ascending aorta at the left base varies from absent (Fig. 6–23) to gently concave (see Fig. 6–22) to straight (see Fig. 6–7) to moderately convex (Fig. 6–24) to strikingly convex (see Fig. 6–9).[16,27,47] Less commonly, the ascending aorta rises vertically and anterior to the posterior pulmonary trunk, so neither great artery is border-forming (see Fig. 6–23).

The posterior and rightward pulmonary trunk tilts its right branch upward and its left branch downward, so that the two branches are at the same level (see Fig. 6–6B).[3,16,20] A dilated posterior pulmonary trunk may displace the superior vena cava to the right, forming a right basal shadow (see Fig. 6–24)[16] or may project as a right basal convexity that can be mistaken for the ascending aorta (Fig. 6–25).[47] The leftward position of the aortic arch and proximal descending aorta produce a relatively bold indentation on the left side of the esophagus (see Fig. 6–7).[16]

The silhouette of the morphologic right ventricle has two distinctive features: (1) a hump-shaped appearance caused by prominence of the inverted infundibulum[16] (see Figs. 6–2B, 6–22, and 6–23), and (2) a septal notch, which is a subtle indentation just above the left hemidiaphragm corresponding to the apical position of the interventricular groove (see Figs. 6–22 and 6–24). The hump-shaped infundibular shadow occupies the site of the left atrial appendage (see Figs. 6–2 and 6–23),[42,67] so left atrial enlargement is best identified in a lateral projection. A giant left atrium presents as a huge ball suspended below a narrow vascular pedicle (Fig. 6–26).

The Echocardiogram

Echocardiography identifies atrioventricular and ventriculoarterial discordance, the morphologic right ventricle with its tricuspid valve, the morphologic left ventricle with its mitral valve, the spatial relationships of the great arteries and their ventricles of origin, and coexisting congenital heart disease.[53,54] Echocardiographic criteria for determining the morphology of a ventricular chamber and its atrioventricular valve include the level of attachment of each valve to the ventricular septum, valve leaflet configuration (bileaflet or trileaflet), the papillary muscle arrangements, the presence of chordal attachments to the septum (tricuspid valve) or to the ventricular free wall (mitral valve), the type of ventricular trabeculations, the ventricular shape, and the presence or absence of fibrous continuity between a mitral valve and a great artery.[53,54,70] A morphologic left ventricle is recognized by its ovoid or ellipsoid shape and

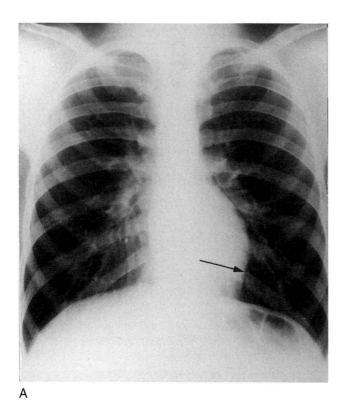

A

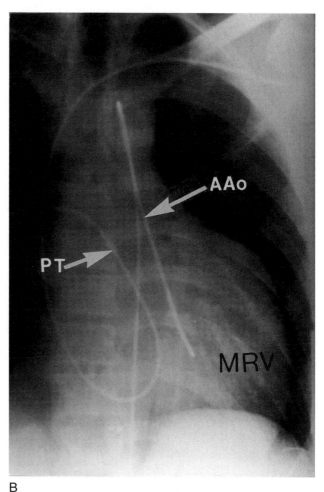

B

Figure 6–22

A, X-ray from a 15-year-old boy with congenitally corrected transposition of the great arteries and mild subpulmonary stenosis (gradient 28 mm Hg). The left cardiac silhouette has a humped appearance and a septal notch (*arrow*). The vascular pedicle is narrow because the ascending aorta is barely seen at the left base and is not seen at all at the right base. *B,* A retrograde femoral arterial catheter was advanced into a barely border-forming ascending aorta (AAo) and then into a hump-shaped subaortic morphologic right ventricle (MRV). A venous catheter was advanced into a subpulmonary morphologic left ventricle and then into the pulmonary trunk (PT). The ascending aorta and pulmonary trunk are parallel to each other and do not cross.

its fine trabecular architecture (Fig. 6–27), by an atrioventricular valve that inserts into the ventricular septum at a level more proximal than the septal insertion of the contralateral atrioventricular valve, by a bicommissural (mitral) valve with a fishmouth appearance in diastole, by paired papillary muscles, by chordae tendineae that insert only into the ventricular free wall, and by continuity between an atrioventricular valve and a great artery. A morphologic right ventricle is recognized by its crescent shape and its coarse trabecular architecture, by a moderator band, by relatively distal insertion of the atrioventricular valve into the ventricular septum, by a tricommissural (tricuspid) valve, by multiple irregular papillary muscles with chordal attachments to the ventricular septum, and by discontinuity between an atrioventricular valve and a great artery.

The crossed or spiral great arterial relationships in the normal heart (see Fig. 6–1) are imaged in the short axis as a posterior circle, which is the aorta, and an anterior sausage

shape, which is the right ventricular outflow tract and main pulmonary artery transected tangentially.[70] The transposed great arteries of congenitally corrected transposition do not cross as in the normal heart (see Fig. 6–1) and are imaged in the short axis as double circles that represent cross sections of the anterolateral aorta and posteromedial pulmonary trunk (Fig. 6–28).[53,54] Long-axis views image the aortic root and pulmonary trunk as parallel to each other. Identity of the pulmonary trunk is confirmed by its bifurcation into right and left branches (Fig. 6–29) and identity of the aorta is confirmed by its brachiocephalic branches.

A ventricular septal defect is typically nonrestrictive and perimembranous, with extension into the inlet septum (see Fig. 6–29, and see Chapter 17). A large ventricular septal defect makes the relative levels of atrioventricular valve attachments to the ventricular septum unreliable guides to ventricular inversion.[70] Malformations of the left atrioventricular valve include

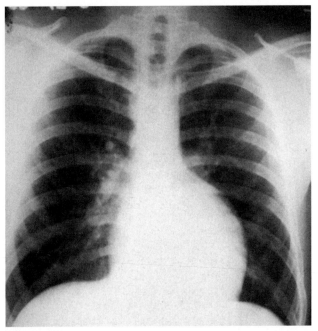

Figure 6–23

X-ray from a 34-year-old man with congenitally corrected transposition of the great arteries and mild incompetence of the left atrioventricular valve. The vascular pedicle is narrow because neither great artery is border-forming. The left cardiac silhouette is hump-shaped.

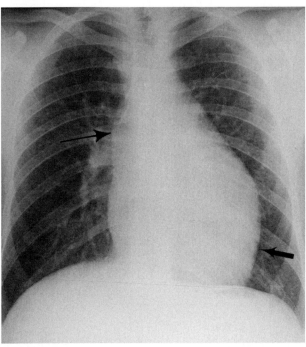

Figure 6–25

X-ray from a 22-year-old man with congenitally corrected transposition of the great arteries and severe pulmonary valve stenosis (gradient 105 mm Hg). The convexity at the right hilus (*thin arrow*) is caused by rightward projection of the dilated posterior pulmonary trunk. An inverted ascending aorta straightens the left upper cardiac border. The cardiac silhouette is hump-shaped, and there is a subtle septal notch (*arrow*).

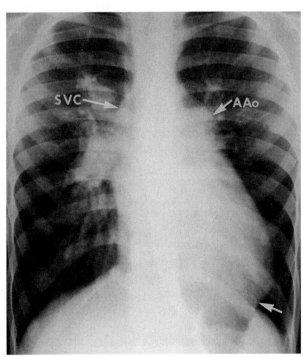

Figure 6–24

X-ray from an 8-year-old boy with congenitally corrected transposition of the great arteries, a nonrestrictive ventricular septal defect, and increased pulmonary blood flow. A septal notch (*unmarked arrow*) appears just above the left hemidiaphragm. The ascending aorta (AAo) is convex at the left base, and the dilated posterior pulmonary trunk causes rightward displacement of the superior vena cava (SVC).

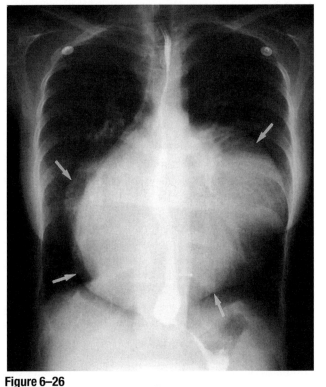

Figure 6–26

X-ray from a 17-year-old girl with congenitally corrected transposition of the great arteries and severe incompetence of the left atrioventricular valve. The cardiac silhouette resembles a huge suspended ball that consists almost entirely of a giant left atrium (*arrows*). The cause of the giant left atrium may in part have been related to childhood rheumatic fever. The vascular pedicle is narrow because neither the ascending aorta nor the pulmonary trunk is border-forming.

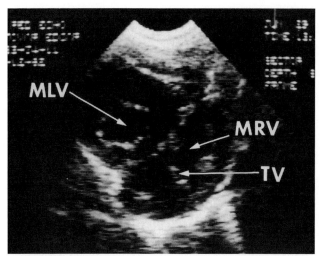

Figure 6–27
Echocardiogram (short axis) from a 4-year-old girl with congenitally corrected transposition of the great arteries. The morphologic right ventricle (MRV) is crescent-shaped and houses the tricuspid valve (TV). The morphologic left ventricle (MLV) is ovoid.

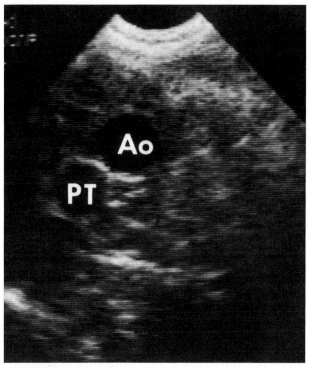

Figure 6–28
Echocardiogram (short axis) from a 4-year-old girl with congenitally corrected transposition of the great arteries. The *double circles* are cross sections of the anterior leftward aorta (Ao) and the posterior rightward pulmonary trunk (PT).

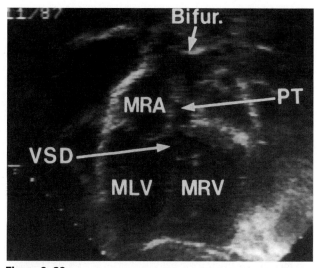

Figure 6–29
Echocardiogram (apical four chamber) from a 5-year-old girl with congenitally corrected transposition of the great arteries, a nonrestrictive ventricular septal defect (VSD), and subpulmonary stenosis. A morphologic right atrium (MRA) is aligned with a morphologic left ventricle (MLV) that gave rise to the pulmonary trunk (PT) identified by its bifurcation (Bifur.). MRV, morphologic right ventricle.

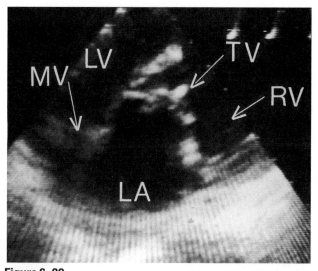

Figure 6–30
Echocardiogram (apical four chamber) from a 16-year-old girl with congenitally corrected transposition of the great arteries and Ebstein's anomaly of the left atrioventricular valve, which is displaced into the cavity of the morphologic right ventricle (RV). Compare the level of the left-sided Ebstein's tricuspid valve (TV) with the level of the right-sided mitral valve (MV). LA, morphologic left atrium; LV, morphologic left ventricle.

Ebstein's anomaly (Fig. 6–30) and multiple short chordae tendineae that attach to the septum and apex (see Chapter 13). Color flow imaging establishes the degree of left atrioventricular valve regurgitation.[23]

Echocardiography with Doppler interrogation characterizes obstruction to outflow of the subpulmonary left ventricle.[1,70] Subpulmonary stenosis can be caused by a fixed fibrous subpulmonary diaphragm, fibrous tags, a membranous septal aneurysm, or accessory mitral valve tissue.[1,70]

Echocardiography defines the different types of crisscross hearts and superoinferior ventricles (Fig. 6–31 and 6–32).[4,38,53,59] Atrioventricular discordance and ventriculoarterial discordance result in the physiology of congenitally corrected transposition.[4,38,53,59] Atrioventricular

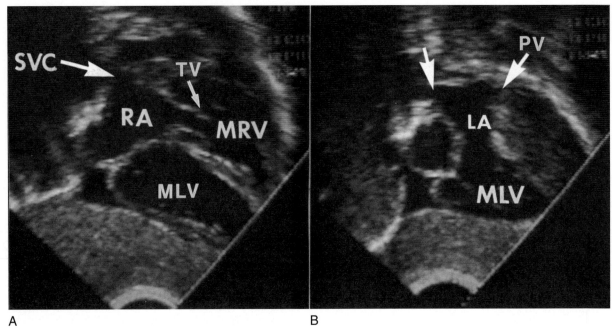

A   B

Figure 6–31
Echocardiograms (subcostal) in a criss-cross heart with superoinferior ventricles. *A*, The superior vena cava (SVC) joins a morphologic right atrium (RA) that is aligned with a concordant morphologic right ventricle (MRV) superior and to the left of a morphologic left ventricle (MLV). The tricuspid valve (TV) has a right-to-left orientation. *B*, Two pulmonary veins (PV; *arrows*) join the morphologic left atrium (LA), which is aligned with an inferior and rightward morphologic left ventricle (MLV). Atrioventricular concordance with ventriculoarterial discordance resulted in the physiology of complete transposition of the great arteries.

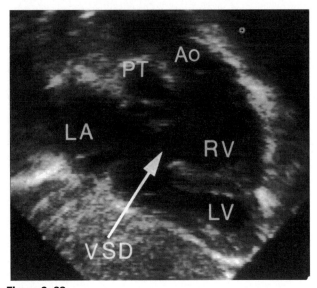

Figure 6–32
Echocardiogram from a 12-month-old girl with a criss-cross heart. The right ventricle (RV) and left ventricle (LV) are superoinferior and harbor a nonrestrictive inlet ventricular septal defect (VSD). The morphologic left atrium (LA) is concordant with a right-sided and inferior morphologic left ventricle (atrioventricular concordance). The morphologic left ventricle gives rise to the pulmonary trunk (PT), and the morphologic right ventricle gives rise to the aorta (Ao) (ventriculoarterial discordance).

concordance and ventriculoarterial discordance result in the physiology of complete transposition (see Fig. 6–31). Isolated ventricular inversion (atrioventricular discordance with ventriculoarterial concordance) results in the physiology of complete transposition of the great arteries (see Fig. 6–32).[62]

Summary

Congenitally corrected transposition of the great arteries without coexisting malformations is uncommon and initially may go unrecognized. The malformation may come to light in asymptomatic patients because of a loud second heart sound at the left base (anterior aorta); an electrocardiogram with PR interval prolongation, left axis deviation, reversed septal depolarization identified by Q waves in right precordial leads but no Q waves in left precordial leads, and deep Q waves in lead 3 and lead aVF; and an x-ray with a narrow vascular pedicle, a straight left cardiac border, or a hump-shaped left cardiac silhouette. Echocardiography establishes ventricular inversion with atrioventricular and ventriculoarterial discordance. Congenitally corrected transposition may come to light during investigation of high-degree atrioventricular block or paroxysmal rapid heart action. Two-to-one heart block is distinctive, especially when associated with intermittent complete heart block. Supraventricular tachycardia, atrial fibrillation, and atrial flutter occur with or without Ebstein's anomaly of the left atrioventricular valve. Accessory pathways are left-sided.

Ventricular septal defects are typically nonrestrictive and perimembranous and are analogous to comparable defects in hearts without ventricular inversion. Left precordial Q waves are absent despite volume overload of the systemic ventricle. The chest x-ray shows a convex shadow of the leftward ascending aorta, but the pulmonary artery segment is not border-forming despite enlargement caused by increased pulmonary blood flow. The echocardiogram identifies atrioventricular and ventriculoarterial discordance and a large perimembranous ventricular septal defect.

Left atrioventricular valve regurgitation due to an Ebstein-like malformation is seldom present in infants but is subsequently an important determinant of prognosis. A holosystolic murmur may be incorrectly diagnosed as acquired mitral regurgitation, but error is avoided when the electrocardiogram exhibits PR interval prolongation, left axis deviation, and prominent Q waves in inferior leads and in right precordial leads, with absent left precordial Q waves despite volume overload of the systemic ventricle. The chest x-ray shows a narrow vascular pedicle, a straight silhouette at the left base, and a hump-shaped inverted infundibulum that obscures enlargement of the left atrial appendage. The echocardiogram establishes the diagnosis of atrioventricular and ventriculoarterial discordance with a left-sided Ebstein's anomaly.

Pulmonary stenosis may favorably regulate the left-to-right shunt through a ventricular septal defect or may reverse the shunt. The pulmonary stenotic murmur is maximum at the middle left sternal border because of subpulmonary stenosis and radiates upward and to the right because of the rightward position and rightward course of the pulmonary trunk. A loud second heart sound in the second left intercostal space is aortic because the aortic root is anterior. The chest x-ray exhibits the smooth contour of a left basal ascending aorta or a narrow vascular pedicle, but the pulmonary trunk is not border-forming even if dilated above a stenotic pulmonary valve. The echocardiogram identifies atrioventricular and ventriculoarterial discordance and one of several types of pulmonary stenosis.

REFERENCES

1. Allwork SP, Bentall HH, Becker AE, et al: Congenitally corrected transposition of the great arteries: Morphologic study of 32 cases. Am J Cardiol 38:910, 1976.
2. Anderson KR, Zuberbuhler JR, Anderson RH, et al: Morphologic spectrum of Ebstein's anomaly of the heart. Mayo Clin Proc 54:174, 1979.
3. Anderson RC, Lillehei CW, Lester RG: Corrected transposition of great vessels of the heart: A review of 17 cases. Pediatrics 20:626, 1957.
4. Anderson RH: Criss-cross hearts revisited. Pediatr Cardiol 3:305, 1982.
5. Anderson RH, Arnold MB, Jones RS: D-Bulboventricular loop with L-transposition in situs solitus. Circulation 46:173, 1974.
6. Anderson RH, Becker AE, Arnold R, Wilkinson JL: The conduction tissues in congenitally corrected transposition. Circulation 50:911, 1974.
6a. Beauchesne LM, Warnes CA, Connolly HM, et al: Outcome of the unoperated adult with congenitally corrected transposition of the great arteries. J Am Coll Cardiol 40:285, 2002.
7. Fogel MA, Weinberg PM, Fellows KE, Hoffman EA: A study of ventriculo-ventricular interaction. Single ventricles compared with systemic right ventricles in a dual-chamber circulation. Circulation 92:219, 1995.
8. Anderson RH, Shineborne EA, Gerlis LM: Criss-cross atrioventricular relationships producing paradoxical atrioventricular concordance or discordance. Circulation 50:176, 1974.
9. Benchimol A, Tio S, Sundararajou V: Congenitally corrected transposition of the great vessels in a 58 year old man. Chest 59:634, 1971.
10. Connolly HM, Grogan M, Warnes CA: Pregnancy among women with congenitally corrected transposition of great arteries. J Am Coll Cardiol 33:1692, 1999.
11. Benson LN, Burns R, Schwaiger M, et al: Radionuclide angiographic evaluation of ventricular function in isolated congenitally corrected transposition of the great arteries. Am J Cardiol 58:319, 1986.
12. Berman DA, Adicoff A: Corrected transposition of the great arteries causing complete heart block in an adult. Am J Cardiol 24:125, 1969.
13. Bharati S, Rosen K, Steinfield L, et al: The anatomic substrate for pre-excitation in corrected transposition. Circulation 62:831, 1980.
14. Bream PR, Elliott LP, Bargeron LM: Plain film findings of anatomically corrected malposition. Radiology 126:589, 1978.
15. Hornung TS, Bernard EJ, Jeaggi ET, et al: Myocardial perfusion defects and associated systemic ventricular dysfunction in congenitally corrected transposition of the great arteries. Heart 80:322, 1998.
16. Carey LS, Ruttenberg HD: Roentgenographic features of congenital corrected transposition of the great vessels. Am J Roentgenol 92:623, 1964.
17. McKay R, Anderson RH, Smith A: The coronary arteries in hearts with discordant atrioventricular connections. J Thoracic Cardiovasc Surg 111:988, 1996.
18. Celermajer DS, Cullen S, Deanfield JE, Sullivan ID: Congenitally corrected transposition and Ebstein's anomaly of the systemic atrioventricular valve: Association with aortic arch obstruction. J Am Coll Cardiol 18:1056, 1991.
19. Colli AM, de Leval M, Somerville J: Anatomically corrected malposition of the great arteries. Am J Cardiol 55:1367, 1985.
20. Cumming GR: Corrected transposition without associated intracardiac anomalies. Am J Cardiol 10:605, 1962.
21. Dabizzi RP, Barletta GA, Caprioli G, et al: Coronary artery anatomy in corrected transposition of the great arteries. J Am Coll Cardiol 12:486, 1988.
22. Daliento L, Corrado D, Buja G, et al: Rhythm and conduction disturbances in isolated, congenitally corrected transposition of the great arteries. Am J Cardiol 58:314, 1986.
23. Lunch KP, Yan DC, Sharma S, et al: Serial echocardiographic assessment of left atrioventricular valve function in young children with ventricular inversion. Am Heart J 136:94, 1998.
24. Dimas AP, Moodie DS, Sterba R, Gill CC: Long-term function of the morphologic right ventricle in adult patients with corrected transposition of the great arteries. Am Heart J 118:526, 1989.
25. Digilio MC, Casey B, Toscano A, et al: Complete transposition of the great arteries: Patterns of congenital heart disease in familial precurrence. Circulation. 104:2809, 2001
26. Elliott LP, Jue KL, Amplatz K: A roentgen classification of cardiac malpositions. Invest Radiol 1:17, 1966.
27. Ellis K, Morgan BC, Blumenthal S, Anderson DH: Congenital corrected transposition of the great vessels. Radiology 79:35, 1962.
28. Fernandez F, Laurichesse J, Scebat L, Lenegre J: Electrocardiogram in corrected transposition of the great vessels of the bulboventricular inversion type. Br Heart J 32:165, 1970.
29. Foran RB, Belcourt C, Nanton MA, et al: Isolated infundibuloarterial inversion (S,D,I): A newly recognized form of congenital heart disease. Am Heart J 116:1337, 1988.
30. Foster JR, Damato AN, Kilne LE, et al: Congenitally corrected transposition of the great vessels: Localization of the site of complete atrioventricular block using His bundle electrograms. Am J Cardiol 38:383, 1976.
31. Freedom RM, Culham G, Rowe RD: The criss-cross and superoinferior ventricular heart. Am J Cardiol 42:620, 1978.
32. Friedman HS, Lipski J, Pantozopoulos J, et al: Bundle of His electrograms in congenital corrected transposition of the great arteries. Br Heart J 35:1307, 1973.
33. Gasul BM, Graettinger JS, Bucheleres G: Corrected transposition of the great vessels: Demonstration of a new phonocardiographic sign of this malformation. J Pediatr 55:180, 1959.
34. Gerlis LM, Wilson N, Dickinson DF: Abnormalities of the mitral valve in congenitally corrected transposition (discordant atrioventricular and ventriculoarterial connections). Br Heart J 55:475, 1986.
35. Gillette PC, Busch V, Mullins CE, McNamara DG: Electrophysiologic studies in patients with ventricular inversion and corrected transposition. Circulation 60:939, 1979.
36. Gillette PC, Reitman MJ, Mullins CE, et al: Electrophysiology of ventricular inversion. Br Heart J 36:971, 1974.

37. Graham TP, Parrish MD, Poucek RJ, et al: Assessment of ventricular size and function in congenitally corrected transposition of the great arteries. Am J Cardiol 51:244, 1983.

38. Hery E, Jimenez M, Didier D, et al: Echocardiographic and angiographic findings in superior-inferior cardiac ventricles. Am J Cardiol 63:1385, 1989.

39. Huhta JC, Danielson GK, Ritter DG, Ilstrup DM: Survival in atrioventricular discordance. Pediatr Cardiol 6:57, 1985.

40. Huhta JC, Maloney JD, Ritter DG, et al: Complete atrioventricular block in patients with atrioventricular discordance. Circulation 67:1374, 1983.

41. Ikeda U, Furuse M, Suzuki O, et al: Long-term survival in aged patients with corrected transposition of the great arteries. Chest 101:1382, 1992.

42. Jaffe RB: Systemic atrioventricular valve regurgitation in corrected transposition of the great vessels. Am J Cardiol 37:395, 1976.

43. Kangos JJ, Griffiths SP, Blumenthal S: Congenital complete heart block. Am J Cardiol 20:632, 1967.

44. Kraus Y, Yahini JH, Shem-Tov A, Neufeld H: Precordial pulsations in corrected transposition of the great vessels. Am J Cardiol 23:684, 1969.

45. Krongrad E, Ellis K, Steeg CN, et al: Subpulmonary obstruction in congenitally corrected transposition of the great arteries due to ventricular membranous septal aneurysms. Circulation 54:679, 1976.

46. Kupersmith J, Krongrad E, Gersony WM, Bowman FO: Electrophysiologic identification of the specialized conduction system in corrected transposition of the great vessels. Circulation 50:795, 1974.

47. Lester RG, Anderson RC, Amplatz K, Adams P: Roentgen diagnosis of congenital corrected transposition of the great vessels. Am J Roentgenol 83:985, 1960.

48. Lev M, Licata RH, May RC: The conduction system in mixed levocardia with ventricular inversion. Circulation 28:232, 1963.

49. Lev M, Rowlatt UF: The pathologic anatomy of mixed levocardia: A review of 13 cases of atrial or ventricular inversion with or without corrected transposition. Am J Cardiol 8:216, 1961.

50. Lieberson AD, Schumacher RR, Childress RH, Genovese PD: Corrected transposition of the great vessels in a 73 year old man. Circulation 39:96, 1969.

51. Lundstrom U, Bull C, Wyse RKH, Somerville J: The natural and "unnatural" history of congenitally corrected transposition. Am J Cardiol 65:1222, 1990.

52. Marino B, Sanders SP, Parness IA, Colan SD: Obstruction of right ventricular inflow and outflow in corrected transposition of the great arteries (S,L,L): Two-dimensional echocardiographic diagnosis. J Am Coll Cardiol 8:407, 1986.

53. Marino B, Sanders SP, Pasquini L, et al: Two-dimensional echocardiographic anatomy in crisscross heart. Am J Cardiol 58:325, 1986.

54. Meissner MD, Panidis IP, Eshaghpour E, et al: Corrected transposition of the great arteries: Evaluation by two-dimensional and Doppler echocardiography. Am Heart J 111:599, 1986.

55. Monckeberg JG: Zur Entwicklungsgeschichte des Atrioventrikular-systems. Verh Dtsch Pathol Ges 16:228, 1913.

56. Nagle JP, Cheitlin MD, McCarty RJ: Corrected transposition of the great vessels without associated anomalies. Chest 60:367, 1971.

57. Nakajima K, Bunko H, Tonami N, et al: Congenitally corrected transposition of the great arteries associated with pre-excitation syndrome. Clin Nucl Med 11:564, 1986.

58. Okamura K, Konno S: Two types of ventricular septal defect in corrected transposition of the great arteries. Am Heart J 85:483, 1973.

59. Pasquini L, Sanders SP, Parness I, et al: Echocardiographic and anatomic findings in atrioventricular discordance with ventriculoarterial concordance. Am J Cardiol 62:1256, 1988.

60. Perloff JK, Roberts WC: The mitral apparatus. Circulation 46:227, 1972.

61. Quero-Jimenez M, Raposo-Sonnenfeld I: Isolated ventricular inversion with situs solitus. Br Heart J 37:293, 1975.

62. Ranjit MS, Wilkinson JL, Mee RBB: Discordant atrioventricular connexion with concordant ventriculo-arterial connexion (so-called "isolated ventricular inversion") with usual atrial arrangement (situs solitus). Int J Cardiol 31:114, 1991.

63. Rogers JH, Roo PS: Ebstein's anomaly of the left atrioventricular valve with congenital corrected transposition of the great arteries. Chest 72:253, 1977.

64. Rokitansky KF: Die Defekte der Scheidewande des Herzens. Vienna, W. Braumuller, 1875.

65. Rotem CE, Hultgren HN: Corrected transposition of the great vessels without associated defects. Am Heart J 70:305, 1965.

66. Ruttenberg HD, Elliott LP, Anderson RC, et al: Congenital corrected transposition of the great vessels. Correlation of electrocardiograms and vectorcardiograms with associated cardiac malformations and hemodynamic states. Am J Cardiol 17:339, 1966.

67. Schiebler GL, Edwards JE, Burchell HB, et al: Congenital corrected transposition of great vessels. Pediatrics 27:851, 1961.

68. Schwartz HA, Wagner PI: Corrected transposition of the great vessels in a 55 year old woman. Chest 66:190, 1974.

69. Shea PM, Lutz JF, Vieweg WVR, et al: Selective coronary arteriography in congenitally corrected transposition of the great arteries. Am J Cardiol 44:1201, 1979.

70. Sutherland GR, Smallhorn JF, Anderson RH, et al: Atrioventricular discordance: Cross-sectional echocardiographic-morphological correlative study. Br Heart J 50:8, 1983.

71. Van Mierop LHS, Alley RD, Kausel HW, Stranahan A: Ebstein's malformation of left atrioventricular valve in corrected transposition with subpulmonary stenosis and ventricular septal defect. Am J Cardiol 8:270, 1961.

72. Victoria BE, Miller BL, Gessner IH: Electrocardiogram and vectorcardiogram in ventricular inversion (corrected transposition). Am Heart J 86:733, 1973.

73. Waldo AL, Pacifico AD, Bargeron LM, et al: Electrophysiological delineation of the specialized AV conduction system in patients with corrected transposition of the great vessels and ventricular septal defect. Circulation 52:435, 1975.

74. Walker WJ, Cooley DA, McNamara DG, Moser RH: Corrected transposition of the great vessels, atrioventricular heart block, and ventricular septal defect. Circulation 17:249, 1958.

75. Walmsley T: Transposition of the ventricles and the arterial stems. J Anat 65:528, 1931.

76. Yater WM, Lyon JA, McNabb PE: Congenital heart block: Review and report of the second case of complete heart block studied by serial sections through conduction system. JAMA 100:1831, 1933

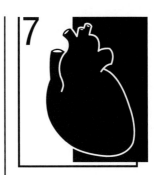

Congenital Aortic Stenosis: Congenital Aortic Regurgitation

7

In *Dorland's Illustrated Medical Dictionary*, the terms *valvular* and *valvar* are synonymous. Both are defined as "pertaining to a valve." The tendency to dismiss the term *valvular* as referring to a *valvule* is a misconception. The diminutive of *valve* is *valvula* not *valvule*. It is best to use *valve* as an unmodified term. In this chapter, aortic *valve* stenosis and *valvular* aortic stenosis are used interchangeably.

Clinical evaluation of congenital obstruction to left ventricular outflow seeks to establish the presence and degree of obstruction and the level and morphologic type.* The five varieties of congenitally abnormal aortic valves are based on the number and types of cusps and commissures (Table 7–1).[197] A *unicuspid* aortic valve is either acommissural or unicommissural.[197] An *acommissural* valve is characterized by a single leaflet with a stenotic central orifice (Fig. 7–1A, left upper).[197] Traces of three rudimentary commissures do not divide the valve.[197] This type of congenitally stenotic semilunar valve is found in the pulmonary location (see Chapter 11) but rarely in the aortic location.[197] A *unicommissural* unicuspid valve is characterized by a single commissural attachment to the aorta (Figs. 7–1A left middle and 7–2A).[60,197,198,212] The single (unicuspid) leaflet originates from a single commissural attachment, proceeds across the aortic orifice without making additional contact with the wall, bends on itself, and returns to reinsert at the same attachment site from which it originated—unicommissural.[60,197,212] When viewed from above, the orifice resembles an exclamation point (Fig. 7–1A, left middle).[197,212] Remnants of rudimentary raphes are occa-

sionally present in the single cusp.[197,198,212] The typical unicommissural valve is intrinsically stenotic, but if the free edge is sufficiently redundant and the single commissure is not fused, obstruction is initially absent but subsequently appears when mobility is reduced by fibrosis and calcification.[60]

A *bicuspid aortic valve* is the most common congenital anomaly to which that structure is subject[28,60,187,194–197,212] (Fig. 7–1A left lower group) and is the most common gross morphologic congenital abnormality of the heart or great arteries. Estimated occurrence rate is 1% to 2% of the general population with a prevalence in the United States of approximately 4 million.[13,195] Acquired calcification of a congenitally bicuspid aortic valve accounts for approximately half of surgical cases of isolated aortic stenosis in adults.[13,220] Hypercholesterolemia is a risk factor for the development of calcification.[45]

The bicuspid aortic valve was first characterized in the early 16th century by Leonardo da Vinci.[41] Three variations are based on cusp size, represented by two cusps of equal size, cusps of unequal size, and a conjoined cusp twice the size of its nonconjoined mate.[13] A false raphe can be well formed, fenestrated, calcified, or absent.[13,195] If the free edges of the bicuspid leaflets are sufficiently long, if the cusps are thin and mobile, and if the commissures are not fused, the valve is unobstructed, which is the usual condition at birth (Fig. 7–1A, left lower).[62,194–197] Conversely, if the commissures are congenitally fused,[212] or if the free edges of the cusps are not longer than the diameter of the aortic ring, the valve is inherently obstructed (Fig. 7–1A, left lower). Sclerosis of a bicuspid aortic valve begins as early as the second decade, and calcification begins as early as the fourth decade.[15] The fibrocalcific process progresses more

---

*9, 10, 28, 60, 124, 171, 183, 194–197, 212.

Table 7–1 Congenitally Abnormal Aortic Valves: The Number and Types of Cusps and Commissures

Unicuspid
    Acommissural
    Unicommissural
Bicuspid
Tricuspid
    Miniature (small aortic ring)
    Dysplastic
    Cuspal inequality with or without equal commissures
Quadricuspid
Six-cuspid

rapidly in bicuspid aortic valves with unequal cusps (maldistribution of tension during diastolic closure) and more slowly in bicuspid valves with equal cusps.[15] Rarely, a congenital bicuspid aortic valve is stenotic because of myxoid dysplasia.[44] Bicuspid aortic and bicuspid pulmonary valves coexist in the Syrian hamster[55] but not in human subjects.

A bicuspid aortic valve can remain functionally normal throughout a long lifetime,[62,195] but more often than not fibrocalcific thickening or acquired commissural fusion decrease mobility and render the valve stenotic (Figs. 7–1A, left lower group and 7–2C).[13,28,62,187,195,218] Thomas Peacock recognized this tendency in his *On Malformations of the Human Heart* (1858).[181] Abnormal mechanical stress is an important factor in promoting fibrosis and calcification of both a bicuspid bicommissural aortic valve (Fig. 7–2C) and a unicuspid unicommissural aortic valve. Another consequence of a functionally normal bicuspid aortic valve is progressive regurgitation, which may be accelerated by infective endocarditis to which a bicuspid valve is highly susceptible (see later). Rarely, a severely incompetent bicuspid aortic valve becomes stenotic with virtual loss of regurgitation.[119]

Congenital Aortic Stenosis

Trileaflet aortic valves are congenitally abnormal when three cusps and three commissures are miniaturized within a small aortic ring[190] (see Fig. 7–1A, *middle right*) or when an aortic valve has three dysplastic leaflets.[44] In a hydraulically ideal aortic valve with three equal cusps, total diastolic force is equally distributed among the three cusps and their sinus attachments. Cuspal inequality results in unequal distribution of diastolic force, and cuspal inequality is a common variation of normal (see Fig. 7–1B).[196,225] The fibrocalcific process of aging proceeds more rapidly in the cusp or cusps that bear the greatest hemodynamic stress.[13,225] Accordingly, congenital cuspal inequality enhances the aging process, converting a functionally normal trileaflet aortic valve into fibrocalcific aortic stenosis

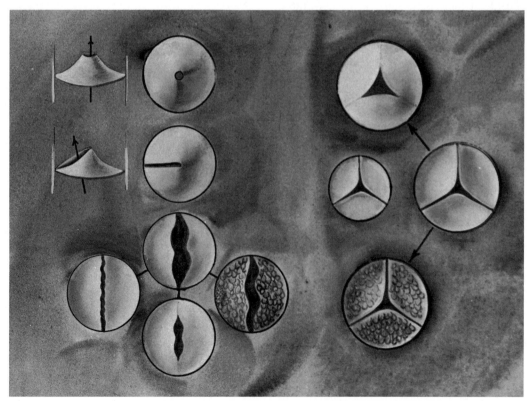

A

Figure 7–1
See legend on opposite page

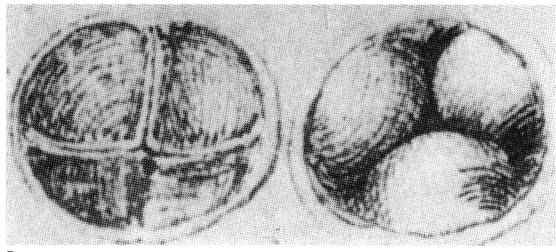

B

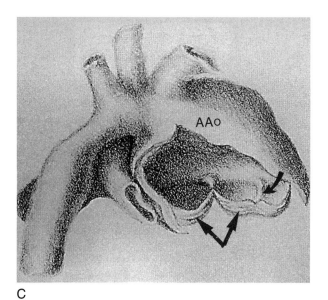

C

Figure 7–1 *Continued*

A, Illustrations of the various types of aortic valve stenosis. Illustrations on the left represent three types of congenitally abnormal aortic valves. The upper drawing shows a unicuspid acommissural valve. The middle drawing shows a unicuspid unicommissural valve with an eccentric orifice. The lower group of four drawings shows a functionally normal bicuspid aortic valve (upper center), a fibrocalcific stenotic bicuspid aortic valve (right), a bicuspid aortic valve that is inherently stenotic because the free edges are not longer than the annular diameter (left), and a bicuspid aortic valve that is inherently stenotic because of failure of commissural separation (lower center). Illustrations on the right show a normal trileaflet aortic valve with equal cusps and equal commissures (right center). A congenitally hypoplastic trileaflet aortic valve is paired beside the normal trileaflet aortic valve. A dysplastic trileaflet valve is not shown. Acquired aortic valve stenosis results from fibrosis and calcification without commissural fusion (right lower) or from rheumatic fusion of commissures (right upper). *B,* Congenital aortic cuspal inequality as represented by Leonardo da Vinci circa 1513.[41] His legend read: "Figures of the cusps (aorti) of the gateway which the left ventricle possesses when it closes itself." Drawing on the left shows the closed trileaflet valve from above. Drawing on the right shows the closed trileaflet valve from below. *C,* Dilatation of the ascending aorta (AAo) above a congenitally bicuspid aortic valve (*paired arrows*) with a false raphe (curved arrow). (As seen printed in Maude Abbott's *Atlas of Congenital Cardiac Disease* in 1936, Osler Library, McGill University.)

(see Fig. 7–1*A, lower right*).[196,225] The tendency for a bicuspid aortic valve to become fibrocalcific is related in part to the mechanical stress inherent in bicuspid inequality (see Fig. 7–2*C*). Quadricuspid aortic valves can function normally or can be incompetent (see Figs. 7–35 and 7–42) but are rarely stenotic.[151,197] Six-cuspid semilunar valves sporadically occur with truncus arteriosus (see Chapter 28).[197] Rarely, the aortic valve is absent.[11a]

Dilatation of the ascending aorta is consistently associated with a congenitally bicuspid aortic valve (Figs. 7–3 and 7–4 and see Fig. 7–1*C*). However, the term *post-stenotic* is a misnomer, because the ascending aorta is dilated due to an inherent medial abnormality, whether the bicuspid valve is stenotic, incompetent, or functionally normal.[52,97] Dilatation is identical under any of these circumstances and can express itself as an ascending aortic aneurysm with chronic aortic regurgitation (see Fig. 7–4) or dramatically as a dissecting aneurysm (see Fig. 7–5).[52,97]

Fixed *subaortic* stenosis occurs in isolation (Fig. 7–6) or with other congenital cardiac defects.[34,64,73,137,213] It is the second most common variety of congenital obstruction to left ventricular outflow[27,71,121,124,171,177,197,209] and accounts for 15% to 20% of all types of congenital aortic stenosis.[29,121] Nonfixed muscular subaortic stenosis coexists with severe aortic valve stenosis and can account for as much as half the pressure gradient.[34,56,64,73,137] This chapter deals with two principal varieties of fixed subaortic stenosis in hearts that are otherwise devoid of congenital heart disease. The first variety is characterized by a thin fibrous crescent-shaped membrane located immediately beneath the aortic valve (see Fig. 7–6*A*).[34,124,137,171,197] The membrane is occasionally relatively thick and forms a fibrous or fibromuscular collar that extends across an otherwise normal left ventricular outflow tract and inserts onto the anterior mitral leaflet. This form of fixed subaortic stenosis occurs in human hearts as well as in dogs, pigs, and cows.[188] The aortic root is not dilated.[52,54] Aortic regurgitation is associated with malformed leaflets that are

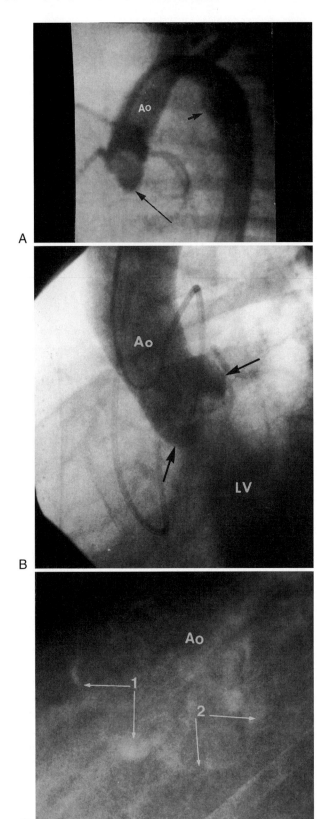

Figure 7–2

A, Lateral aortogram from a 5-day-old male with severe unicuspid unicommissural aortic stenosis (*lower arrow*). The mobile valve is in its systolic (opened) position doming upward. The aortic root (AO) is not dilated. *Upper right arrow* points to a bulge at the aortic end of a closed ductus arteriosus. *B,* Lateral aortogram from a 78-year-old man with severe bicuspid aortic stenosis and moderate aortic regurgitation. *Arrows* point to two unequal cusps. LV, left ventricle. *C,* Lateral chest radiograph from a 74-year-old man with calcific deposits in the two cusps (1 and 2) of a stenotic bicuspid aortic valve. Ao, aorta.

damaged by the proximity of the subvalvular membrane or fibromuscular collar and by the impact of the eccentric systolic jet (see Fig. 7–6B).[166,171,197,209] Tubular subaortic stenosis is the second and less common variety of fixed obstruction to left ventricular outflow and is represented by a fibromuscular channel that may occupy several centimeters within the outflow tract (Fig. 7–7).[34,64,73,124,146] A layer of fibrous tissue extends onto the ventricular surface of the anterior mitral leaflet. The aortic cusps show fibrous thickening as with discrete subaortic stenosis. The aortic root is not dilated (see Fig. 7–7).[52,54,124,146]

Fixed subaortic stenosis as just defined is not present during intrauterine cardiac morphogenesis, is therefore not *con genitus*, and accordingly is uncommon if not rare in neonates and infants.[27,64,73,137] The disorder becomes manifest after the first year of life and then changes in both severity and morphology.[121,171] In contrast to rapid progression in infants and children, fixed subaortic stenosis in adults progresses slowly.[34,64,72,121,137,146,171] Aortic regurgitation is common but is usually mild and nonprogressive (see Fig. 7–6B).[27]

Supravalvular aortic stenosis is the least common variety of congenital obstruction to left ventricular outflow. The most frequent type is a localized segmental hourglass deformity immediately above the aortic sinuses with medial thickening and fibrous intimal proliferation (Fig. 7–8A).[17,143,197] The size of the aorta distal to the obstruction is normal or reduced. The sinuses of Valsalva are typically enlarged.[106] Localized supravalvular aortic stenosis is occasionally caused by a fibrous membrane with a central opening.[17,197] An uncommon variety is represented by tubular hypoplasia of the ascending aorta beginning above the sinuses of Valsalva and is associated with narrowing of the orifices of the brachiocephalic arteries (see Fig. 7–8B).[17,66,91,170,197] The aortic leaflets are usually thickened and adherent to the supravalvular stenosing ridge,[106,197] are occasionally dysplastic,[17] and may fuse to a coronary ostium.[179,197] The aortic valve abnormalities usually cause no more than mild regurgitation.[197]

Three additional features of supravalvular aortic stenosis include (1) the anatomy of the extramural coronary arteries, (2) the condition of the aortic leaflets and aortic sinuses, and (3) the association with the characteristic facies and mental retardation of Williams syndrome. Obstruction of a coronary ostium can be caused by adherence of a distorted aortic leaflet to the supravalvular stenotic ridge,[17,150,179] by aortic medial proliferation,[17,179,201] and by the supravalvular ridge itself, which can impede diastolic flow into an ostium.[224] Because coronary ostia are proximal to the zone of supravalvular obstruction, the coronary arteries are exposed to elevated left ventricular systolic pressure[145,179,197] and become thick-walled and dilated (see Fig. 7–8A,B). The hypertension also serves as a risk factor for premature atherosclerosis.[170,179,197] Coronary artery aneurysms have been described,[88] and coronary artery abnormalities can be part of the generalized arteriopathy of Williams syndrome.

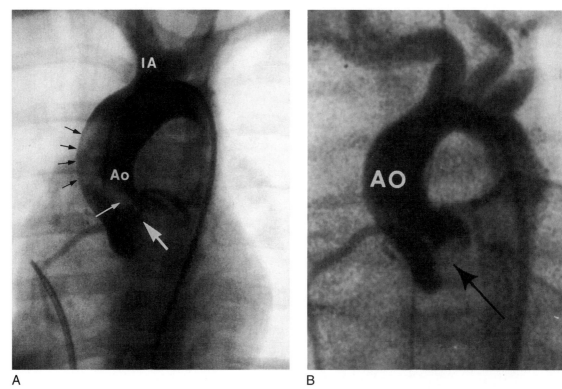

A   B

Figure 7–3

A, Aortogram from a 7-year-old boy with congenital bicuspid aortic stenosis (*large white arrow*). An eccentric jet (*small white arrow*) issues from the stenotic orifice. The jet adheres to the lateral aortic wall (*small black arrows*; Coanda effect). IA, innominate artery. The aortic root (Ao) is dilated. *B,* Left ventriculogram from a 9-year-old boy with systolic doming of a mobile bicuspid aortic valve (*arrow*).

In 1961, Williams and associates[231] described the association of supravalvular aortic stenosis with distinctive elfin facies and mental retardation. In 1962 and 1964, Beuren and coworkers[7,8] expanded the syndrome to include pulmonary artery stenosis. Williams syndrome or Williams-Beuren syndrome now includes elfin facies, mental retardation, small stature, infantile hypercalcemia, supravalvular aortic stenosis, pulmonary artery stenosis, and important vascular abnormalities, especially in adults.[111,112,163] Renal abnormalities occur in nearly half of afflicted patients and are represented by renal artery stenosis, segmental scarring, cystic dysplasia, nephrocalcinosis, marked asymmetry in kidney size, solitary kidney, and pelvic kidney.[12,111,112,152] Systemic hypertension is not necessarily related to the renovascular abnormalities,[42,112] but instead is related to stiffness of arterial walls.[67] A generalized arteriopathy is characterized by medial thickening and luminal narrowing of systemic and pulmonary arteries.[165] Long segment narrowing of the aorta may occur with or without localized coarctation.[42,112]

Involvement of cerebral arteries is responsible for strokes. Tortuous retinal arteries similar to those that accompany coarctation of the aorta (see Fig. 8–8) were described in the original report of Williams and Barratt-Boyes,[231] and in 1985 the observation was confirmed.[42]

The physiologic consequences of congenital aortic valve stenosis are reflected in the response of the left ventricle to increased afterload.[89,159] An adaptive increase in left ventricular mass in the immature heart is due chiefly to hyperplasia (replication) of cardiomyocytes, in contrast to the increase in left ventricular mass in the mature heart, whose terminally differentiated cardiomyocytes respond by hypertrophy (an increase in cell size).[184] The afterloaded immature heart is capable of capillary replication that is proportional to cardiomyocyte replication, so capillary density remains normal and coronary flow reserve remains normal.[184,189,221] The increase in left ventricular mass characterized by myocyte hyperplasia with proportionate growth in the microvascular bed sets the stage for low left ventricular systolic wall stress and supernormal ejection performance.[2,48,184] The left ventricle thickens concentrically and the cavity size is normal or small,[184] so distensibility decreases. A greater force of left atrial contraction is required to generate the end-diastolic fiber length necessary for left ventricular performance appropriate for the increased afterload without an increase in end-diastolic volume or left atrial mean pressure.

The normal trileaflet aortic valve and its annulus increase in anatomic cross-sectional area with age, even after maturity.[125] The normal trileaflet physiologic orifice, which is the cross-sectional area defined by the leaflets in systole, is flow dependent, varying directly with the volume and rate of left ventricular ejection. In the resting state, less than half the cross-sectional area of a normal trileaflet aortic valve is utilized during ejection, so a large percentage is available during high-flow states.

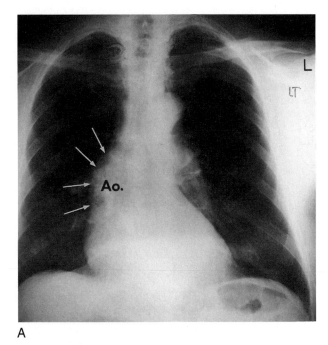

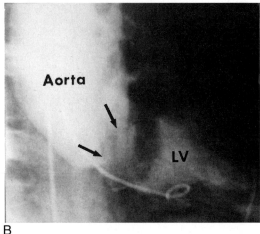

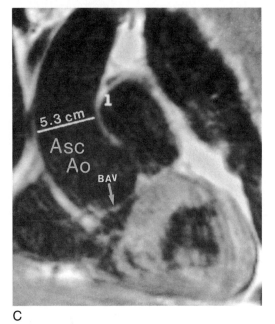

Figure 7–4

A, X-ray from a 66-year-old man with a bicuspid aortic valve, aneurysmal dilatation of the ascending aorta (Ao), and moderate aortic regurgitation. *B,* Contrast material injected into the ascending aorta identifies the aneurysmal dilatation, the bicuspid aortic valve (*paired black arrows*), and the regurgitation into the left ventricle (LV). *C,* Magnetic resonance image from a 33-year-old man with a 5.3 cm ascending aorta (AscAo) above a bicuspid aortic valve (BAV).

The physiologic consequences of congenital aortic stenosis reflect the morphology of the obstruction, the age of the patient at onset,[219] the degree of obstruction, and whether the obstruction is progressive. A functionally normal bicuspid aortic valve awaits adulthood to become stenotic as its leaflets thicken and calcify. A stenotic aortic valve in infants and young children tends to generate a pro-

gressively higher gradient because of the progressive increase in transaortic flow that accompanies the normal age-related increase in body mass, not because of a decrease in cross-sectional area of the valve itself.[57] In Williams syndrome, progressive supravalvular aortic stenosis has been assigned to inadequate growth of the sinotubular junction.[57,78] Fixed subaortic stenosis is not present in utero, but usually begins after the first year of life and undergoes a progressive decrease in cross-sectional area (see earlier).[64,72,73,137,171,209] The time course in adults is much slower.[27]

The subendocardium of the aortic stenotic left ventricle is vulnerable to ischemia because of a selective decrease in perfusion.[224] In neonates and infants with severe aortic stenosis, subendocardial ischemia is responsible for papillary muscle infarction with mitral regurgitation[224] and is responsible for endocardial fibrosis and a decrease in cavity size that depress left ventricular contractility.[21,158] A progressive rise in left ventricular filling pressure, in left atrial mean pressure, and in pulmonary arterial pressure provokes right ventricular failure.[90] Supravalvular aortic stenosis imposes the additional impediment of compromised coronary perfusion (see earlier).

The physiologic response of the neonate to severe aortic stenosis is best understood in light of the fetal circulation.[130] Intrauterine left ventricular volume is low because pulmonary blood flow is virtually nil. When the lungs expand at birth, pulmonary blood flow commences, and a severely obstructed, thick-walled left ventricle with reduced cavity size suddenly receives a sizable increment in volume.[130] Left ventricular filling pressure rises steeply, left atrial pressure rises in parallel, and a left-to-right shunt is established across a stretched valve-incompetent foramen ovale.[130] If a small left ventricular cavity is beset with

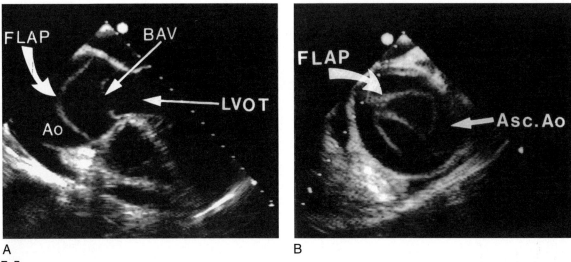

Figure 7–5
Transesophageal echocardiogram from a 37-year-old man with a bicuspid aortic valve (BAV) and a dissecting aneurysm of the ascending aorta (Ao). *A,* The flap of the aortic dissection moved freely within the dilated ascending aorta. LVOT, left ventricular outflow tract. *B,* The flap is seen again within the ascending aorta.

endocardial fibrosis or fibroelastosis (see Fig. 10–9), the hemodynamic consequences are correspondingly worse.[158] Vasoreactive pulmonary arterioles constrict, pulmonary artery pressure rises, and pressure overload is imposed on an already volume-overloaded right ventricle. Temporary patency of the ductus arteriosus diverts right ventricular blood into the aorta and delays the onset of symptoms. When the ductus closes, that advantage is lost because the entire right ventricular output enters the pulmonary circulation and the left side of the heart.[130]

Mild aortic stenosis is accompanied by a normal response to dynamic exercise, but when obstruction is severe, left ventricular stroke volume is blunted at each level of graded isotonic stress.[3,39,40,129] In congenital aortic valve stenosis, the augmented flow and increased left ventricular systolic pressure induced by exercise result in a larger computed aortic valve area, implying that the stenotic valve is sufficiently mobile to open more widely when so stressed.[3] Activation of canine left ventricular baroreceptors in response to an increase in left

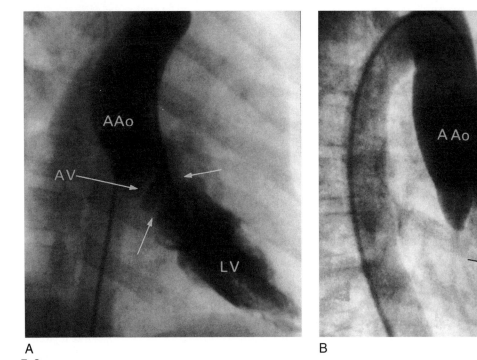

Figure 7–6
Angiocardiograms from a 3-year-old boy with fixed subaortic stenosis (gradient 40 mm Hg) and mild aortic regurgitation. *A,* Left ventriculogram (LV) shows the subaortic stenosis (*unmarked oblique arrows*) in close proximity to the aortic valve (AV). The ascending aorta (AAo) is only mildly dilated. *B,* Contrast material injected into the ascending aorta discloses mild aortic regurgitation (AR).

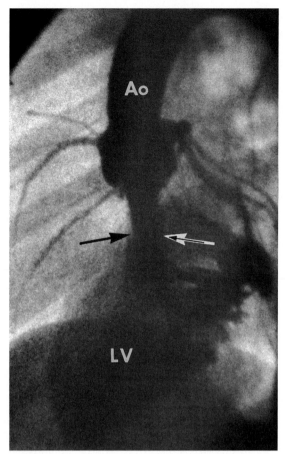

Figure 7–7
Left ventricular (LV) angiogram from a 9-year-old boy with tubular subaortic stenosis (*paired arrows*). Five years previously, the patient had undergone resection of a moderately obstructive discrete subaortic membrane. The ascending aorta (Ao) is not dilated.

ventricular pressure or stretch induces hypotension due to skeletal muscle vasodilatation.[147] In human subjects with aortic stenosis, the reflex vasodilatation and bradycardia induced by activation of left ventricular baroreceptors during isotonic exercise are responsible for hypotension and exertional syncope.[116,148]

THE HISTORY

Congenital aortic valve stenosis is considerably more common in males, with a sex ratio of approximately 4:1.[22,29,123,195] Male prevalence is less common in supravalvular aortic stenosis, depending in part on genetic transmission.[179] Discrete and tunnel subaortic stenosis both have a distinct female prevalence.[121,171,177,209] Genetically transmitted subaortic stenosis in the Newfoundland dog has an equal sex ratio.[188]

When congenital aortic stenosis is present at birth, the murmur is present at birth because the anatomic and physiologic conditions required to generate the murmur are present in the newborn.[180,185] An exception is fixed subaortic stenosis that is *not* present at birth,[64,71,72,73,121,137,171] and an additional qualification relates to specific types of congenitally malformed aortic valves.[197] As a rule, the fewer the

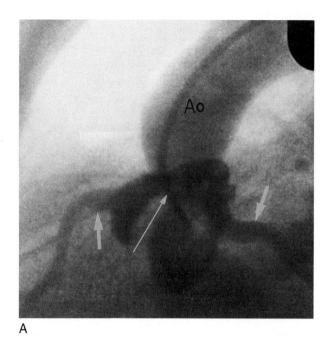

A

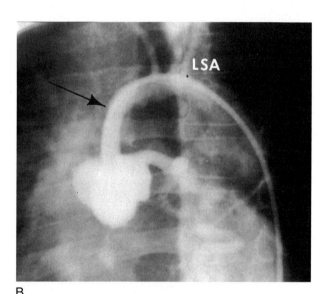

B

Figure 7–8
A, Lateral aortogram from a 15-year-old boy with supravalvular aortic stenosis. *Thin oblique arrow* points to the localized zone of obstruction just above the sinuses of Valsalva. The proximal coronary arteries are dilated (*paired thick arrows*). The size of the aortic root (AO) is normal. *B,* Aortogram from an 8-year-old boy with tubular hypoplasia (*arrow*) of the ascending and transverse aorta beginning above the sinuses and extending beyond the left subclavian artery (LSA). The origins of the brachiocephalic arteries are hypoplastic. The left coronary artery and its branches are enlarged.

cusps and commissures, the greater is the likelihood of an intrinsically stenotic valve and of a murmur at birth.[197] Intrinsically stenotic valves are usually unicuspid, unicommissural, or bicuspid,[197] but when a bicuspid aortic valve is functionally normal,[195,197] the appearance of a murmur awaits the development of fibrocalcific thickening in adulthood.[25,28,29,62,156,195,197] Stenosis of a unicommissural aortic valve occasionally follows a protracted course, similar to that of a bicuspid aortic valve.[60,220]

An impression of murmur intensity (loudness) can be inferred in the history by determining how readily a murmur was heard during follow-up examinations. A loud murmur is likely to be heard even in uncooperative infants, whereas the soft murmur of mild obstruction is likely to be overlooked or mistaken for a normal murmur in cooperative infants and older children (see Chapter 2).

Growth and development are affected in patients with Williams syndrome (see later). Supravalvular aortic stenosis may be a component of the rubella syndrome.[232] Symptoms associated with aortic stenosis, especially in children, may be absent even in the presence of severe obstruction,[22,29] and progression from mild to severe is not necessarily accompanied by symptomatic deterioration.[35,76] Effort dyspnea and fatigue reflect an inadequate increment in cardiac output and an increase in left ventricular end-diastolic pressure. *Effort syncope* arouses suspicion of aortic stenosis in an acyanotic patient with a prominent cardiac murmur dating from infancy or childhood. Syncope depends on the degree of obstruction, not on its morphologic type,[123,130,171] and is due to reflex vasodilatation and bradycardia induced by activation of left ventricular baroreceptors during isotonic exercise (see earlier).[116,147,148] Syncope can be recurrent[29,70,84,116,124,208] and sudden death looms as a threat,[84,115,123,191,208] although the risk in children is small compared to the risk in adults with aortic stenosis. Subtle cerebral symptoms consist of mild giddiness, faintness, or lightheadedness with effort. Syncope-induced hypotension may provoke electrical ventricular instability in adults with atherosclerotic coronary artery disease but seldom in young patients with aortic stenosis and normal coronary arteries.[26,43,160,224]

Angina pectoris is a feature of congenital aortic stenosis that stands out in young patients.[26,70,124,126,222] A potential disparity exists between the oxygen requirements of a hypertrophied left ventricle, and coronary blood flow and flow reserve. The disparity is aggravated by acquired coronary artery disease in adults with fibrocalcific bicuspid aortic stenosis and in children with coronary artery abnormalities that accompany supravalvular aortic stenosis.[36,150,179,222]

Inappropriate diaphoresis is sometimes recurrent and increases with the advent of congestive heart failure, especially in neonates.[101,130,158,161] In infants with severe aortic stenosis, mitral regurgitation due to papillary muscle infarction adds to the hemodynamic burden.[43,160] Nonimmunologic fetal hydrops has accompanied severe intrauterine aortic stenosis.[101]

Familial recurrence of bicuspid aortic stenosis[152] and subaortic stenosis have been reported,[80,171,188,192] but the low incidence is of questionable clinical significance. Not so with *supravalvular* aortic stenosis,[50,58,143,168,222] in which familial and nonfamilial types are the basis of the following classification: (1) familial with normal facies and normal intelligence, (2) nonfamilial with normal facies and normal intelligence, and (3) nonfamilial with Williams syndrome,[8,14,53,83,231] which results from mutation or deletion of the elastin gene located at chromosome 7q11.23.[127,131,135,142,149] Pulmonary artery stenosis in Williams syndrome tends to improve, whereas supravalvular aortic stenosis is progressive.[78] The progression has been attributed to growth failure of the sinotubular junction, which may be associated with obstruction of coronary artery ostia.[78] Supravalvular aortic stenosis has been produced experimentally in newborn rabbits by administering maternal vitamin D during gestation[75] and has occurred in human offspring when infantile hypercalcemia resulted from routine administration of vitamin D during pregnancy. Accordingly, the history should include questions regarding maternal vitamin D ingestion.

Infective endocarditis is a potential risk in all types of congenital aortic stenosis,[29,121,156,197,209] but the bicuspid aortic valve is especially vulnerable whether functionally normal, stenotic, or incompetent, an observation made by William Osler more than a century ago.[176] Dissecting aneurysm of the ascending aorta may dramatically interrupt the clinical course of bicuspid aortic stenosis (see Fig. 7–5).[79,97,133] Gastrointestinal bleeding associated with aortic stenosis, sometimes called Heyde syndrome,[206] occurs in older adults.[206] Angiodysplasia has been used to designate the offending lesions that tend to be present in the ascending colon but may be distributed throughout the gastrointestinal tract.[206] Aortic stenosis is not believed to cause the lesions but is thought to increase the likelihood that the lesions will bleed.

PHYSICAL APPEARANCE

Williams syndrome (nonfamilial supravalvular aortic stenosis) is characterized by peculiar facies, short stature, and mental retardation.[7,8,14,51,83,178,183,231,232] The chin is small (hypoplastic mandible), the mouth is large, the lips are patulous, the nose is blunt and upturned, the eyes are widely set with occasional internal strabismus, the forehead is broad, the cheeks are baggy (Fig. 7–9), the teeth are malformed, and the bite is abnormal (malocclusion) (Fig. 7–10). The patients have friendly temperaments and deep, somewhat metallic voices that further emphasize their similarities.[8] Adults with Williams syndrome are relatively short and tend to have lordosis, kyphoscoliosis, and joint abnormalities of the lower limbs that result in a stiff, awkward gait.[163] The brow is broad, with prominent supraorbital ridges. The nasal tip is broad and the nares are anteverted. Flat molar regions accentuate the prominence of a wide mouth with full lips, small jaw, and long philtrum.[163]

XO Turner syndrome (see Chapter 8) represents another distinctive physical appearance that coincides with a bicuspid aortic valve.[155] Congenital heart disease associated with Turner syndrome has been known since the first description by Morgagni and is coupled with different patterns of X monosomies.[172] Abnormal karyotypes consist of 45X mosaicism and X structural abnormalities.[173] Patients with severe dysmorphic features have a significantly higher prevalence of congenital heart disease,[173] and 45X Turner

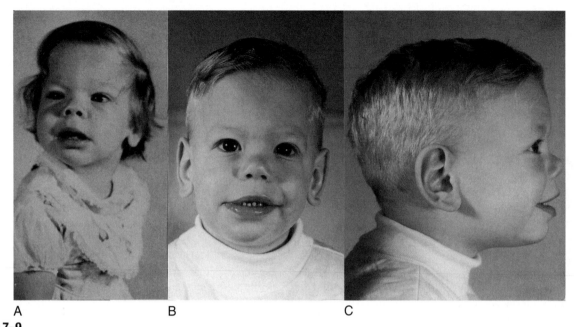

A   B   C

Figure 7–9
Typical facial appearance of a 20-month-old girl (*A*) and a 24-month-old boy (*B* and *C*) with nonfamilial supravalvular aortic stenosis and pulmonary artery stenosis (Williams syndrome). The children closely resemble each other. Both were mentally retarded and had large mouths, patulous lips, small chins, baggy cheeks, blunt upturned noses, wide-set eyes, left internal strabismus, and malformed teeth.

patients have the highest prevalence.[173] X structural abnormalities are associated with an increased prevalence of bicuspid aortic valve,[173] whereas X deletion carries no increase in the incidence of congenital heart disease.[172] In Noonan syndrome (Turner phenotype with normal genotype), obstruction to left ventricular outflow is due to hypertrophic obstructive cardiomyopathy (Fig. 7–11).

THE ARTERIAL PULSE

"It is the object of the following paragraphs to consider the aid in the diagnosis of aortic stenosis which may be supplied by a study of the pulse" (Graham Steell, *The Lancet*, November 1894). Fixed obstruction to left ventricular outflow distinctively alters the arterial pulse.[183,185,233] The pulse pressure is small, the rate of rise is slow, the peak is sustained, and the decline is gentle (Figs. 7–12 and 7–13). The typical configuration is not as frequent in children as in adults with equivalent aortic stenosis.[61,175] Children with severe obstruction may have a brachial arterial pulse that is interpreted as normal,[175] although palpation of the carotid artery improves accuracy.[1,61] A bisferiens pulse (twin peaked) implies coexisting aortic regurgitation.[185,233]

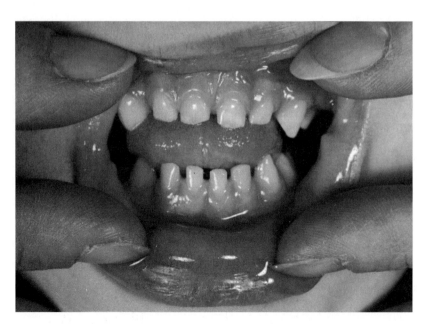

Figure 7–10
Small, widely spaced, malformed teeth from the 2-year-old boy referred to in Figure 7–9.

The right and left brachial and carotid arterial pulses are symmetric in valvular or fixed subvalvular aortic stenosis. However, in supravalvular aortic stenosis, the rate of rise, the systolic pressure, and the pulse pressure are greater in the right brachial and right carotid arteries[74,87,143,144] (see Fig. 7–13), because the hourglass deformity of supravalvular stenosis directs the high-velocity jet toward the right wall of the aorta, and the Coanda effect (affinity of a jet stream for adherence to a wall) carries the jet into the innominate artery.[74,87,144] Experimental observations utilizing an aortic arch model demonstrated that kinetic energy developed in a jet stream under conditions simulating supravalvular aortic stenosis is sufficient to account for the clinically observed differences in arterial pressure.[87] Selective narrowing of the origins of the left carotid and left subclavian arteries[69] (see Fig 7–8B) is an uncommon cause of asymmetric pulses.[74] The systolic pressure in the right arm of adults is normally 10 to 15 mm Hg higher than in the left arm.[185] Simultaneous determination of blood pressure in both arms minimizes these differences,[99] and the technique of palpation advocated in Figure 7–14 is useful in the clinical comparison of the right and left brachial pulses.[183,185]

Arterial thrills or shudders are common in the suprasternal notch and over the carotid and subclavian arteries in valvular and fixed subaortic stenosis.[1,183,185] In supravalvular aortic stenosis, the thrill is distinctly more pronounced over the right carotid artery, which exhibits an increased pulsation.[143]

THE JUGULAR VENOUS PULSE

It is seemingly inappropriate to direct attention to the amplitude of the jugular venous A wave in subjects with

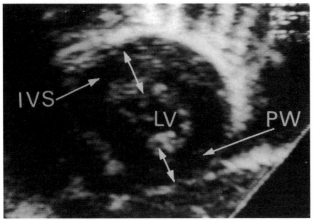

Figure 7–11
Echocardiogram (subxiphoid short axis) from a 1-month-old boy with Noonan syndrome and hypertrophic obstructive cardiomyopathy. The interventricular septum (IVS) is thicker than the posterior wall (PW). LV, left ventricle.

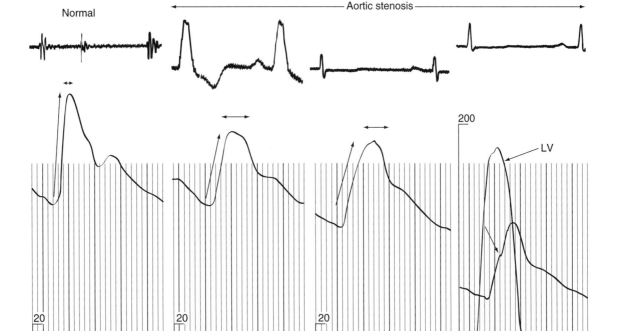

Figure 7–12
Brachial arterial pulses from a normal young adult and from three patients with aortic valve stenosis. The aortic stenotic pulses (two central panels) exhibit a slow rate of rise, a small pulse pressure, a sustained peak, and a gentle decline. In the fourth panel, there is an anacrotic notch (*arrow*) midway along the ascending limb of the arterial pulse. LV, left ventricle.

isolated obstruction to left ventricular outflow.[183,185] However, in left ventricular hypertrophy, the interventricular septum may decrease right ventricular distensibility, so the right atrium contracts with greater force.[167] Accordingly, the amplitude of the jugular venous A wave may increase severe aortic stenosis in the absence of pulmonary hypertension (Fig. 7–15).[22,183,185]

PRECORDIAL MOVEMENT AND PALPATION

Neonates with severe aortic valve stenosis have a prominent right ventricular impulse because of pulmonary hypertension and a left-to-right shunt at the atrial level.[130] An asymmetric precordial bulge is associated with right

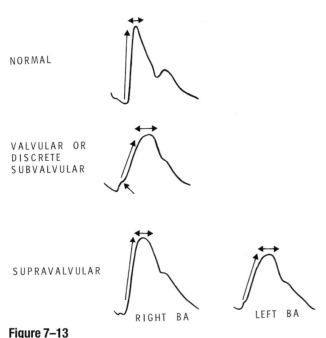

Figure 7–13
Waveforms of brachial arterial (BA) pulses in various types of congenital aortic stenosis (compare with the normal). With valvular or discrete subaortic stenosis, there is a slow rate of rise (*oblique arrow*), a reduced pulse pressure, a single sustained peak (*horizontal arrow*), and a gradual decline. The *lower unmarked arrow* identifies a small anacrotic notch. With supravalvular aortic stenosis, the pulse pressure in the right brachial artery is increased and the rate of rise brisker than in the left brachial pulse.

ventricular hypertrophy in children with aortic stenosis and pulmonary hypertension.[109] With these exceptions, the characteristic precordial impulse is left ventricular, varying from normal in cases of mild aortic stenosis to the strong sustained impulse generated by the hypertrophied left ventricle of severe aortic stenosis.[183,185] Presystolic distention of the left ventricle reflects increased force of left atrial contraction (Fig. 7–16), which is evidence that the aortic stenosis is hemodynamically significant.[32] A dilated ascending aorta rarely transmits an impulse, because the rate of ejection is blunted by the stenotic aortic valve. If an ascending aortic impulse occurs at all, it is likely to do so in patients with mild obstruction and an aortic aneurysm (see Fig. 7–4).[97,133]

Systolic thrills are trivial or absent when aortic stenosis is mild, or when severe aortic stenosis coincides with chronic left ventricular failure. The thrill radiates upward and to the right, is maximum in the second right intercostal space, and is detected in the suprasternal notch and over both carotid arteries.[185] The thrill in infants is sometimes maximum to the left of the sternum,[175] inviting a mistaken diagnosis of ventricular septal defect. Even in older children, the thrill is occasionally more pronounced in the second or third left interspace, although radiation is still upward and to the right.[185] In supravalvular aortic stenosis, the thrill is prominent below the right clavicle and in the right side of the neck.

AUSCULTATION

Normal splitting of the first heart sound must be distinguished from a first heart sound followed by an aortic ejection sound, which has considerable diagnostic significance.[183,185] The ejection sound is separated from the first heart sound by a distinct interval, is louder and higher pitched than the first sound, and is heard best at the cardiac apex (Fig. 7–17A). An aortic ejection sound is a valuable auscultatory sign of the level but not the degree of aortic stenosis.[47,59,81,98] The sound coincides with abrupt cephalad doming of a mobile stenotic valve (see Fig. 7–3B).[47,59,136,157,226,229] The ejection sound may be diffi-

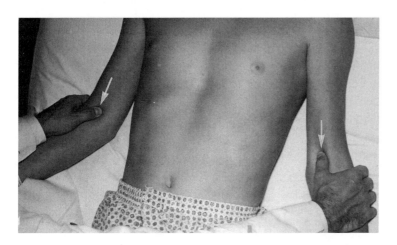

Figure 7–14
Recommended method for simultaneous palpation of right and left brachial arterial pulses. The examiner sits or stands on the patient's right.

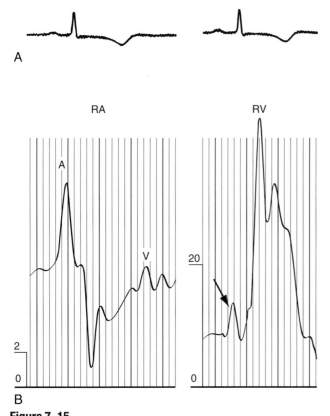

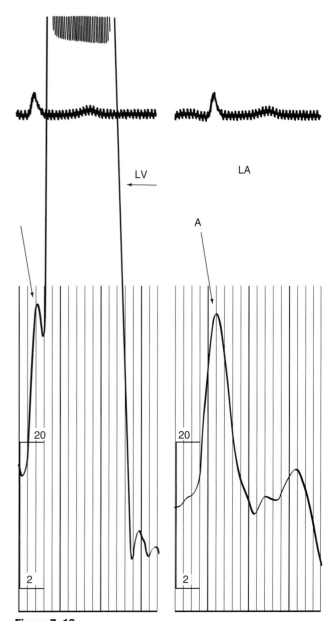

Figure 7–15
Pressure pulses from a 68-year-old man with severe calcific bicuspid aortic stenosis. The A wave in the right atrium (RA) is elevated to 12 mm Hg (first panel) with equivalent presystolic distention (*arrow*) of the right ventricle (RV; second panel).

Figure 7–16
Left ventricular (LV) and left atrial (LA) pressure pulses from a 15-year-old boy with severe bicuspid aortic stenosis. Presystolic distention of the left ventricle (*oblique arrow*; LV) was in response to the increased force of left atrial contraction reflected in the large A wave. LA, left atrium.

cult to hear in early infancy[130] and disappears in adults when fibrocalcific changes impair valve mobility (see Fig. 7–2C).[98] The ejection sound is valvular in origin, so it does not occur in fixed subaortic stenosis[98,121,124] (Fig. 7–17B) or in supravalvular aortic stenosis (Fig. 7–18).[98,179,222]

The aortic stenotic murmur is the prototype of the left-sided midsystolic murmur, beginning after the first heart sound or with the ejection sound, rising in crescendo to a systolic peak, then declining in decrescendo to end before the aortic component of the second sound (see Figs. 7–17 through 7–19).[134,183,185] The murmur is harsh, rough, and grunting, especially when loud, and may have an early systolic peak and a short duration, a relatively late peak and a prolonged duration, or all gradations in between, but the shape remains symmetric (Fig. 7–19).[18,183,185] Intensity varies from bare audibility to grade 6/6. Intensity decreases in the presence of left ventricular failure, and the murmur may alternate in a fashion analogous to pulsus alternans.[101,184,185] The Gallavardin dissociation of acquired fibrocalcific aortic stenosis differs distinctively (Fig. 7–17C).

Although configuration, length, and loudness do not necessarily correspond to the degree of obstruction, some conclusions can be drawn (see Fig. 7–19).[81] The longer and louder the murmur, and the later its symmetric systolic peak, the greater the likelihood of severe stenosis.

The shorter and softer the murmur and the earlier its symmetric peak, the greater the likelihood of mild stenosis or of a functionally normal bicuspid aortic valve.[6] Irrespective of length, the murmur remains symmetric. A late symmetric peak reflects prolonged ejection and increased severity (see Fig. 7–19), but severity does not change the shape of the aortic stenotic murmur, as is the case with congenital pulmonary valve stenosis in which the murmur becomes progressively asymmetric as severity increases (see Chapter 11).

The typical murmur of congenital aortic valve stenosis is maximal in the second right interspace with radiation upward, to the right, and into the neck, reflecting the

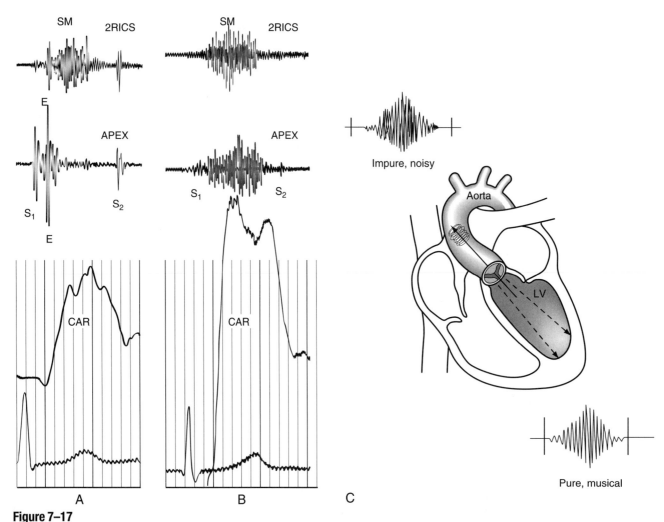

Figure 7–17

A, Recordings from a 12-year-old boy with bicuspid aortic stenosis. The phonocardiogram from the second right intercostal space (2RICS) shows a prominent aortic ejection sound (E) followed by a midsystolic murmur (SM) that ends before the prominent aortic component of the second heart sound (S_2). The ejection sound was selectively transmitted to the apex. *B*, Recordings from a 9-year-old boy with fixed subaortic stenosis of the same severity as in panel *A*. An aortic ejection sound was conspicuous by its absence, and the aortic component of the second sound (S_2) was soft. The midsystolic murmur was transmitted to the apex. CAR, carotid pulse; S_1, first heart sound. *C*, Illustration of "Gallavardin dissociation" of the two murmurs associated with fibrocalcific stenosis of a previously normal trileaflet aortic valve in older adults. The impure, noisy midsystolic murmur at the right base originates from within the aortic root because of turbulence caused by the high-velocity jet. The pure, musical midsystolic murmur at the apex originates from periodic high-frequency vibration of the three fibrocalcific but mobile aortic cusps, and radiates into the left ventricular (LV) cavity.

upward and rightward direction of the high-velocity jet within the ascending aorta (see Fig. 7–3*A*). Very loud murmurs are occasionally transmitted to the shoulders and elbows. In infants with aortic valve stenosis, the murmur may be maximum to the left of the sternum and mistaken for the murmur of ventricular septal defect,[175] but with the passage of time, maximum intensity shifts to the right base.[183] Maximum intensity in tubular subaortic stenosis is likely to be at the mid left sternal edge.[146]

When aortic stenosis is *supravalvular*, the jet may be as distal as the innominate artery, so the murmur is most prominent in the first right intercostal space (Fig 7–18) and in the right side of the neck.[143,185] A saccular aneurysm near the orifice of the innominate artery was ascribed to the jet impact.[164] Systolic murmurs in the axillae and back are likely to be caused by coexisting stenosis of the pulmonary artery and its branches.[7,8,185]

Normal supraclavicular systolic murmurs in children can be mistaken for aortic stenosis,[185] but supraclavicular murmurs are softer below the clavicles and decrease or vanish with hyperextension of the shoulders (see Chapter 2).[169,185]

An aortic stenotic midsystolic murmur at the apex must be distinguished from the holosystolic murmur of mitral regurgitation. Clear audibility of the aortic component of the second heart sound in the presence of a prominent apical murmur generally means that the murmur ends before aortic closure and is therefore not holosystolic.[134,185] An apical holosystolic murmur is likely to envelop the aortic component second sound, which is then inaudible.[134] When the aortic valve is fibrocalcific and immobile, the closure sound is soft or inaudible at the base and at the apex, so an accurate auscultatory assessment of murmur length is difficult or impossible. However, an aortic

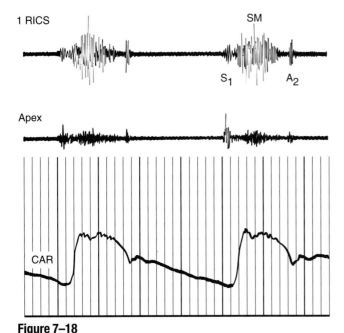

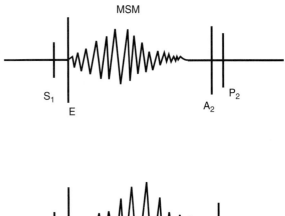

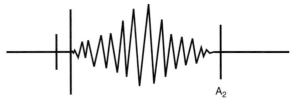

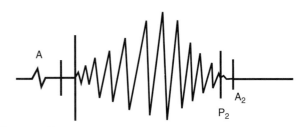

Figure 7–18
Phonocardiogram from a 7-year-old boy with supravalvular aortic stenosis (gradient 55 mm Hg). The midsystolic murmur (SM) is maximum in the first right intercostal space (1 RICS). There is no aortic ejection sound and the aortic component of the second sound (A₂) is normal.

stenotic murmur is louder in the beat after the compensatory pause that follows a premature ventricular beat, whereas the murmur of mitral regurgitation does not amplify in the post-premature beat.[186]

The second heart sound should be analyzed with regard to the intensity of the aortic component and the presence, degree, and type of splitting.[102,183,185] The mobile valve that generates an ejection sound during its abrupt cephalad movement is responsible for a well-preserved aortic component of the second sound during its abrupt caudal seating, even in the presence of appreciable obstruction (see Fig. 7–17A).[59,98,102] Clear audibility of the aortic closure sound at the apex makes it easier to judge the length of an apical systolic murmur. With subvalvular or supravalvular aortic stenosis, the aortic component of the second sound is normal, diminished, or absent, depending on the degree of stenosis (see Figs. 7–17 and 7–18).

Splitting of the second heart sound is not necessarily related to severity.[81,183,185] A delay in the aortic component results from prolonged left ventricular ejection due to an increase in duration of left ventricular systole and to a delay in the aortic incisura.[128] The incisura is delayed because of the time required for the elevated left ventricular systolic pressure to fall below the level of the low aortic root pressure, at which point the incisura is inscribed.[128] Inspiratory splitting of the second heart sound means that the duration of left ventricular ejection is not prolonged and aortic stenosis is mild (see Fig. 7–19). Paradoxical splitting or reversed sequence of semilunar valve closure (Fig. 7–20 and see Fig. 7–19) means that the duration of left ventricular ejection is prolonged and aortic stenosis is

Figure 7–19
Schematic illustrations of auscultatory and phonocardiographic signs of mild, moderate, and severe bicuspid aortic stenosis. *Mild aortic stenosis* (upper): An ejection sound (E) introduces a short symmetric midsystolic murmur (MSM) that peaks early in systole. The second sound splits normally, and the aortic component (A₂) is prominent. P₂, pulmonary component. *Moderate aortic stenosis* (middle): The ejection sound introduces a longer but still symmetric midsystolic murmur with a later systolic peak. The second sound (S₂) is single. *Severe aortic stenosis* (lower): A fourth heart sound (S₄) precedes a normal first heart sound. An aortic ejection sound introduces a long but still symmetric midsystolic murmur. The second heart sound is paradoxically split (A₂ follows P₂).

severe. Left ventricular systolic pressure is then at or near its maximum of 250 mm Hg in older children and adults, so the approximate gradient is the difference between 250 mm Hg and the cuff brachial arterial systolic blood pressure.[183,185] Reversed splitting may become evident after exercise.[81] Because paradoxical splitting is difficult to detect and because prominent inspiratory splitting is confined to mild obstruction, it follows that the majority of patients with aortic stenosis have a second sound that is single or closely split through a wide range of severity (Fig. 7–17A).

A soft early diastolic murmur of aortic regurgitation occurs in approximately 50% of cases of fixed subvalvular stenosis because of the high incidence of abnormalities of the aortic valve.[121,124,197] The murmur of aortic regurgitation is often present with mild bicuspid aortic stenosis or with a functionally normal bicuspid aortic valve because

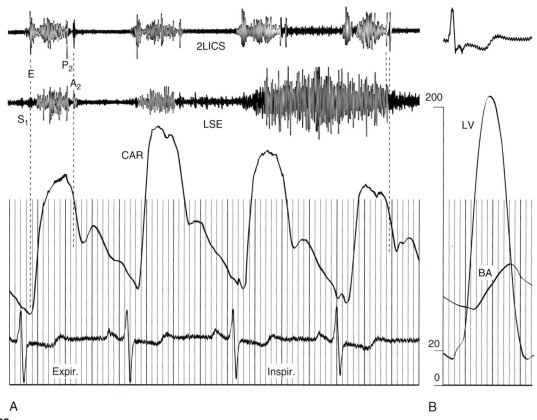

Figure 7–20

Recordings from a 62-year-old man with severe bicuspid aortic stenosis (see gradient in panel *B*). *A,* Phonocardiogram from the second left intercostal space (2LICS) recorded an aortic ejection sound (E), a midsystolic murmur, and paradoxical splitting of the second heart sound. The ejection sound and the prominent aortic component of the second sound (A$_2$) indicate that the bicuspid aortic valve is mobile. LV, left ventricle; BA, brachial artery; LSE, lower left sternal edge.

the free edges of the bicuspid leaflets must be greater than the diameter of the aortic annulus to permit unobstructed flow (see Fig. 7–1*A*). Aortic regurgitation is least likely to accompany supravalvular aortic stenosis but may do so when the cusps are malformed.[143,179,197,222]

A fourth heart sound (see Fig. 7–19) is the auscultatory counterpart of presystolic distention of the left ventricle (see Fig. 7–16), although the low-frequency fourth sound may be soft or absent despite the presence of a presystolic impulse. These signs imply an increased force of left atrial contraction required by the hypertrophied left ventricle to achieve an end-diastolic fiber length appropriate for greater contractile force (see Fig 7–16). Potain recognized this tendency in left ventricular hypertrophy when he wrote that the wall of the ventricle "is placed under tension precisely at the moment that this (the added sound) occurs."[32] Accordingly, the fourth heart sound is a feature of hemodynamically significant aortic stenosis.[32,86] However, in patients older than 40 years of age, the fourth heart sound is not a reliable sign of severity.[32]

A third heart sound appears with the advent of left ventricular failure and usually coexists with a fourth heart sound. With an increase in heart rate and an increase in PR interval, these two sounds summate or occur in close proximity, so a short, low-frequency mid-diastolic murmur is generated.[175]

THE ELECTROCARDIOGRAM

Left ventricular hypertrophy can occur with mild to moderate congenital aortic stenosis (Fig. 7–21),[22,38,105] and sudden death occasionally occurs with severe aortic stenosis and a normal or near-normal electrocardiogram.[23,191] Severity may progress without a change in the electrocardiogram, which, if initially normal, may remain so.[35] These points are noteworthy but should not detract from the value derived from careful interpretation of the scalar tracing.[94]

P waves are usually normal (Fig. 7–22, and see Fig. 7–21). Broad notched P waves are exceptional and are likely to indicate significant coexisting mitral regurgitation.[105] The QRS axis is usually normal, irrespective of severity (see Figs. 7–21 and 7–22).[16,105] Depolarization is clockwise, so Q waves appear in leads 3 and aVF (see Figs. 7–21 and 7–22). Severe congenital aortic stenosis may exhibit electrocardiographic evidence of subendocardial ischemia or infarction even in infants (Fig. 7–23).[120,139] The electrocardiogram in supravalvular aortic stenosis may reflect the ischemia of coronary ostial obstruction.[36,145,150]

Left ventricular hypertrophy is indicated by tall R waves in leads 2 and aVF, deep S waves in lead V$_1$, tall R waves in leads V$_{5-6}$, and deeply inverted and asymmetric T waves (see Figs. 7–21 through 7–23).[16,68,82,105] The T waves usually point in a direction opposite the QRS complex (wide

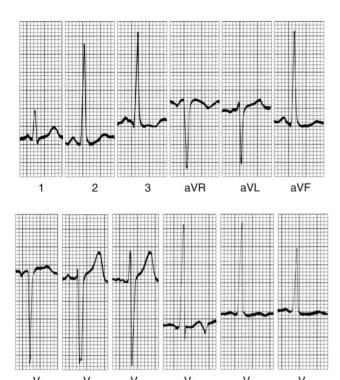

Figure 7–21

Electrocardiogram from a 19-year-old man with bicuspid aortic stenosis (gradient 35 mm Hg). The P waves and the QRS axis are normal. Left ventricular hypertrophy is indicated by the tall R waves in leads 2, 3, and aVF, the deep S waves in leads V_{1-3} and the tall R waves with biphasic or inverted T waves in leads V_{4-5}.

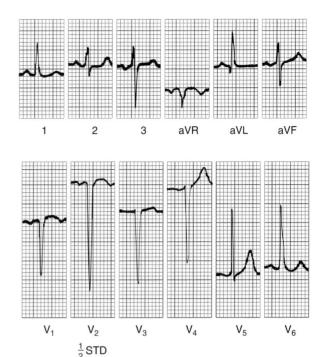

Figure 7–23

Electrocardiogram from a 13-year-old boy with severe fixed subaortic stenosis and moderate aortic regurgitation. The P waves are normal, and the QRS axis is horizontal. The R waves in leads V_{1-4} are small to absent. Deep S waves of left ventricular hypertrophy appear in right and middle precordial leads.

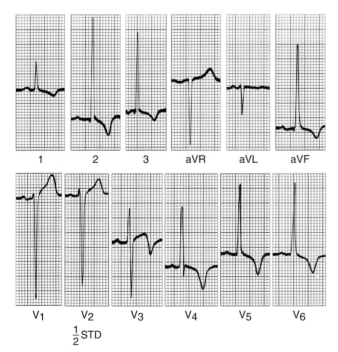

Figure 7–22

Electrocardiogram from an 18-year-old man with severe bicuspid aortic stenosis. The P waves and the QRS axis are normal. Left ventricular hypertrophy is indicated by the tall R waves and deeply inverted T waves in leads 2, 3, aVF, and V_{4-6} and the deep S waves in right precordial leads.

QRS-T angle) (see Fig. 7–22). Exercise stress tests may provoke ST-T wave abnormalities when the resting electrocardiogram is normal,[129,139] and digitalis glycosides may induce or exaggerate the ST-T patterns of left ventricular hypertrophy. Electrocardiographic evidence of right ventricular hypertrophy is reserved for neonates with pinpoint aortic valve stenosis, pulmonary hypertension, a small left ventricular cavity, and a left-to-right shunt through a patent foramen ovale (Fig. 7–24).[22,109,130] Right ventricular hypertrophy also occurs when mild to moderate supravalvular aortic stenosis occurs with severe pulmonary artery stenosis.[7,8]

THE X-RAY

Pulmonary venous congestion coincides with an increase in left ventricular filling pressure in neonates with severe aortic stenosis (Fig. 7–25).[22,130] Dilatation of the ascending aorta is an important radiologic sign of bicuspid aortic stenosis but not of its severity,[52,154] and may be the only abnormality on the x-ray when stenosis is mild (Fig. 7–26).[22,200] The ascending aorta is not dilated in fixed subvalvular aortic stenosis (Fig. 7–27),[121,124,146] is normal to small in supravalvular aortic stenosis (Fig. 7–28),[24,143,179] and is distinctly undersized when there is hypoplasia of the ascending aorta[170] (see Fig. 7–8B) or in the presence of a hypoplastic aortic annulus and a miniature valve.[146] Dilatation of the ascending aorta in cases of XO Turner

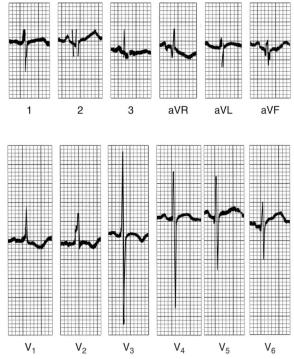

Figure 7–24

Electrocardiogram from a 5-day-old boy with severe unicuspid unicommissural aortic valve stenosis. The QRS axis is normal for age. Except for biphasic RS complexes in leads V_{3-4}, pure right ventricular hypertrophy is indicated by dominant R waves in leads aVR and V_1 and deep S waves in leads V_{5-6}.

syndrome reflects a medial abnormality that is present whether or not the aortic valve is bicuspid (see Fig. 8–9).[155]

Calcification is presumptive evidence that the stenosis is valvular, and dense calcium is evidence of severity.[28,29,200,217] A calcified bicuspid aortic valve is recognized by the bulbous or clublike configuration of a calcified raphe or by a circle or semicircle of calcium with the bulbous raphe pointing toward its center (see Fig. 7–2C).[214]

The left ventricle may attract attention because of its shape rather than its size (Figs. 7–27 through 7–29). Cardiac size can remain normal through a wide range of severity, because the adaptive response of the left ventricle is concentric hypertrophy with normal or reduced cavity size. The left ventricle enlarges downward and to the left and posterior. In the frontal view, the apex extends below the left hemidiaphragm (see Figs. 7–27B and 7–29), and in the lateral view the left ventricle extends behind the inferior vena cava. Significant left ventricular enlargement is reserved for infants with severe aortic stenosis and congestive heart failure[101] and for adults with chronic congestive heart failure whether or not the aortic stenosis is severe. An increase in left atrial size in the lateral projection is a sign of severity and coexisting mitral regurgitation.[200]

THE ECHOCARDIOGRAM

Echocardiography identifies the level, morphologic type, and severity of congenital aortic stenosis.[4,117,207] The gradient is determined by continuous-wave Doppler sonography (Fig. 7–30), the aortic orifice size can be calculated,

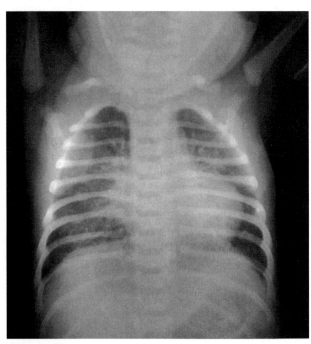

Figure 7–25

X-ray from a 48-hour-old boy with severe unicuspid unicommissural aortic valve stenosis. The ascending aorta is not border forming, the apex is occupied by a convex left ventricle, and there is pulmonary venous congestion.

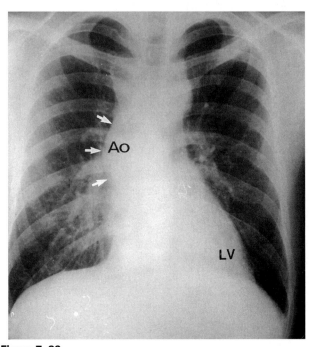

Figure 7–26

X-ray from a 28-year-old man with mild bicuspid aortic stenosis. Except for conspicuous ascending aortic dilatation (Ao), the x-ray is normal.

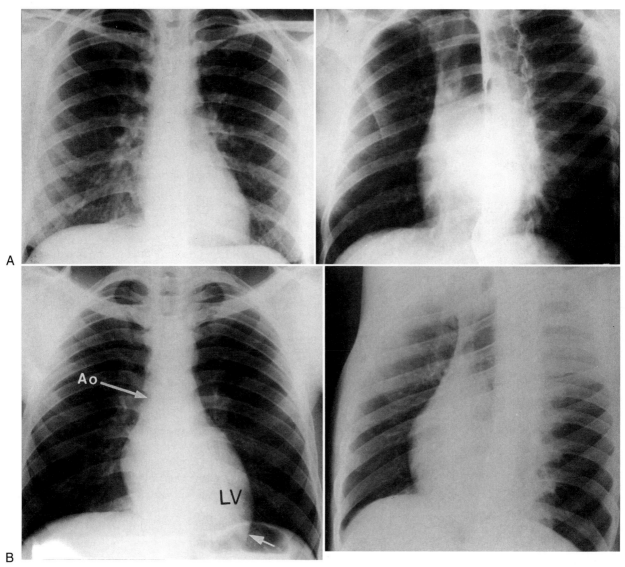

Figure 7–27
A, X-rays from a 21-year-old woman with fixed subaortic stenosis (gradient 30 mm Hg). In both views, the cardiac silhouette is normal, and the ascending aorta is not dilated. *B*, X-rays from a 22-year-old man with fixed subaortic stenosis (gradient 100 mm Hg). The ascending aorta (Ao) is not dilated in either view. An elongated left ventricular (LV) silhouette extends below the left hemidiaphragm (*arrow*).

and the two-dimensionally targeted M mode can measure septal and free wall thickness and left ventricular cavity size. Real-time imaging determines the ejection fraction.

The parasternal long-axis view identifies doming of a bicuspid aortic valve, and the parasternal short-axis view identifies a single diastolic closure line. The bicuspid valve may appear to be trileaflet because of a prominent false raphe, but error is avoided by imaging the open valve, which shows doming of two unequal leaflets with an elliptical orifice (Fig. 7–31*A*). The M-mode echocardiogram shows an eccentric diastolic closure line. The suprasternal notch view visualizes the dilated ascending aorta (Fig. 7–32*B*). A transesophageal echocardiogram confirms the bicuspid aortic valve (see Fig. 7–31) and the aortic root size and identifies a dissecting aneurysm (see Fig. 7–5). Infants with severe aortic valve stenosis usually have a unicommissural, unicuspid valve that is less mobile and more

echodense than a bicuspid valve and may be accompanied by increased reflectivity of an infarcted fibrotic mitral papillary muscle.

A subaortic membrane is imaged on the ventricular septum and the anterior mitral leaflet immediately beneath the aortic valve in the parasternal long-axis view (Fig. 7–33).[207] A subaortic fibromuscular collar or tunnel produces a dense, long ridge of echoes that attach to the ventricular septum and extend onto the anterior mitral leaflet. The M mode echocardiogram in fixed subaortic stenosis reveals distinctive, brisk early systolic closure of the aortic valve followed by marked fluttering.[202]

The hourglass deformity of supravalvular aortic stenosis is identified in the parasternal long-axis view just above the sinuses of Valsalva (Fig. 7–34).[122] Continuous-wave Doppler sonography establishes the gradient.

SUMMARY

Congenital aortic valve stenosis is much more common in males. A murmur is typically present at birth. The majority of patients are asymptomatic during childhood. The neonate with severe aortic stenosis and congestive heart failure is an exception. Deferred onset of a murmur is likely to mean progressive fibrocalcific obstruction of an initially functionally normal bicuspid aortic valve or deferred development of fixed subaortic stenosis. Symptoms reflect

cardiac failure, myocardial ischemia (angina pectoris), and cerebral ischemia (giddiness, lightheadedness, syncope). Congenital aortic stenosis is suspected when angina pectoris or syncope occurs in a young acyanotic male with a cardiac murmur dating from birth or early childhood. The risk of sudden death in children and adolescents with congenital aortic stenosis and normal coronary arteries is much less than in adults with calcific bicuspid aortic stenosis and acquired coronary artery disease. Inappropriate diaphoresis sometimes occurs and increases with the advent of congestive heart failure. Dissecting aneurysm of the ascending aorta is a distinctive and dramatic feature of a bicuspid aortic valve, which is a highly susceptible substrate for infective endocarditis. Familial recurrence is evidence of supravalvular aortic stenosis.

The following points summarize features of the physical examination, the electrocardiogram, the chest x-ray, and the echocardiogram of valvular, subvalvular, and supravalvular congenital aortic stenosis.

Congenital Aortic Valve Stenosis

The right and left brachial and carotid pulses are symmetric, with a small pulse pressure, a slow rate of rise, a sustained peak, and a gentle decline. Jugular venous A waves are increased when a hypertrophied ventricular septum decreases the diastolic distensibility of the right ventricle. A systolic thrill is maximal in the second right intercostal space with radiation to the suprasternal notch and to both sides of the neck. Severe aortic stenosis is accompanied by a prominent sustained left ventricular impulse with presystolic distension. An aortic ejection sound is loudest at the apex and is a characteristic feature of a mobile bicuspid aortic valve. The murmur is midsystolic, harsh, rough, noisy, and maximum in the second right intercostal space with

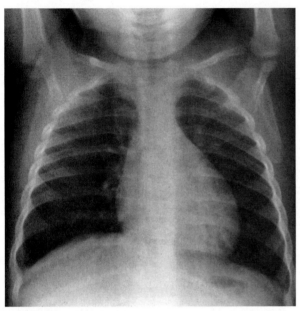

Figure 7–28
X-ray from a 4-year-old boy with supravalvular aortic stenosis (gradient 90 mm Hg) and mild pulmonary artery stenosis (gradient 10 mm Hg). The ascending aorta is not border forming. A convex left ventricle occupies the apex. Pulmonary vascularity is normal.

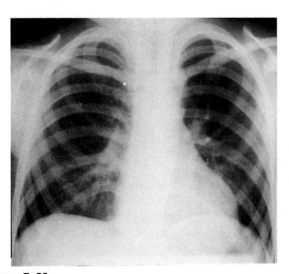
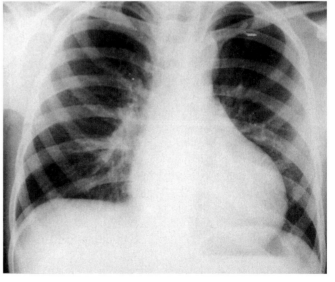

Figure 7–29
X-rays at 6 and 10 years of age from the patient shown in (Fig 7–28) with bicuspid aortic stenosis (gradient of 110 mm Hg). At the age of 10 years, the apex-forming left ventricle is more convex and extends below the left hemidiaphragm.

radiation into the neck. The second heart sound is most often single but may split normally or paradoxically. The aortic component is preserved or accentuated when the bicuspid valve is mobile and may be followed by an early diastolic murmur of aortic regurgitation in the presence of a bicuspid aortic valve or fixed subaortic stenosis. The electrocardiogram exhibits normal sinus rhythm, a normal or vertical QRS axis, and varying degrees of left ventricular hypertrophy. A dilated aortic root is a distinctive radiologic feature of a bicuspid aortic valve. The apex is occupied by the convex silhouette of concentric left ventricular hyper-

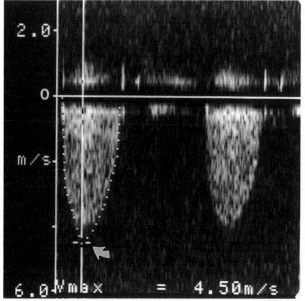

Figure 7–30
Continuous-wave Doppler from a 16-year-old man with bicuspid aortic stenosis. The peak velocity (*small curved arrow*, lower left) is 4.5 m/second, indicating a peak instantaneous gradient of 80 mm Hg.

trophy. Cardiac enlargement is reserved for infants or adults with severe aortic stenosis and congestive heart failure. Calcification establishes the valvular level of aortic stenosis, and the pattern of calcification may identify a bicuspid aortic valve. Echocardiography shows systolic doming of a mobile stenotic valve and identifies its bicuspid morphology. Unicommissural unicuspid aortic valves in symptomatic infants are relatively echo dense and less mobile. Echocardiography with Doppler interrogation establishes the gradient and permits calculation of the orifice size.

Congenital Fixed Subaortic Stenosis

The right and left brachial and carotid arterial pulses are symmetric and exhibit a slow rate of rise, a small pulse pressure, a sustained peak, and a gentle decline. A systolic thrill is maximum in the second right intercostal space with radiation into the neck, but with tunnel subaortic stenosis, the thrills are usually maximum at the midleft sternal border. The left ventricular impulse is sustained and may be accompanied by presystolic distension and a fourth heart sound. An aortic ejection sound is absent. The stenotic murmur is coarse and rough with a location and radiation that correspond to the thrill. The aortic component of the second heart sound is normal or reduced. Aortic regurgitation occurs in at least 50% of cases. The electrocardiogram is indistinguishable from that of aortic valve stenosis. The x-ray discloses a nondilated ascending aorta. Echocardiography identifies the morphologic variations of fixed subaortic stenosis.

Congenital Supravalvular Aortic Stenosis

The Williams syndrome phenotype permits the correct diagnosis at a glance. The facial appearance is characterized

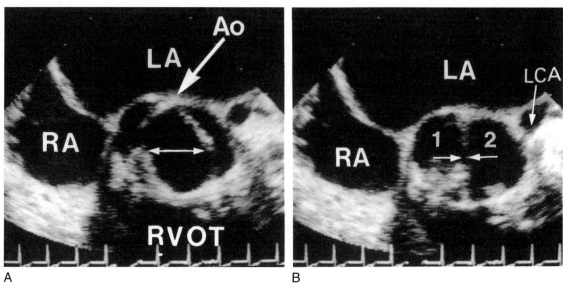

A   B

Figure 7–31
Transesophageal echocardiograms of a functionally normal bicuspid aortic valve. *A,* The valve is in its open systolic position (*unmarked horizontal arrows*). Ao, aorta; LA, left atrium; RA, right atrium; RVOT, right ventricular outflow tract. *B,* The valve is in its closed diastolic position. The two cusps (1, 2) are separated by a single linear closure line (*paired arrows*). LCA, left coronary artery.

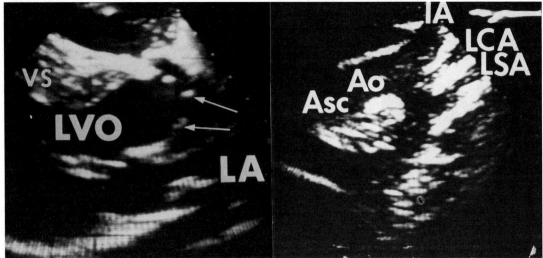

Figure 7–32

A, Echocardiogram (parasternal long-axis) from a 5-year-old boy with bicuspid aortic stenosis (gradient 90 mm Hg). *Dual arrows* point to systolic doming of the mobile bicuspid valve. The ventricular septum (VS) is thick. LVO, left ventricular outflow tract; LA, left atrium. *B,* Suprasternal notch view shows a dilated ascending aorta (Asc Ao). IA, innominate artery; LCA, left carotid artery; LSA, left subclavian artery.

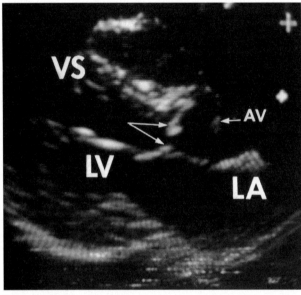

Figure 7–33

Echocardiogram (parasternal long axis) from a 19-year-old man with fixed subaortic stenosis (gradient 55 mm Hg). *Dual arrows* point to a subaortic membrane, which is attached to the ventricular septum (VS) and to the anterior mitral leaflet. AV, aortic valve; LA, left atrium; LV, left ventricle.

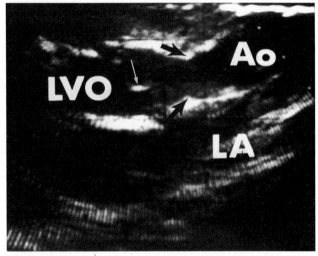

Figure 7–34

Parasternal long-axis view from an 8-year-old boy with supravalvular aortic stenosis (gradient 50 mm Hg). *Paired black arrows* point to the hourglass narrowing. The *small white arrow* identifies an echo from the aortic valve. Ao, ascending aorta; LA, left atrium; LVO, left ventricular outflow tract.

by small chin, large mouth, patulous lips, blunt upturned nose, wide-set eyes, broad forehead, baggy cheeks, malformed teeth, and abnormal bite (malocclusion). Growth can be retarded irrespective of the degree of obstruction and in the absence of heart failure. Brachial and carotid arterial pulses are asymmetric, with the pulse pressure and rate of rise greater on the right. The left ventricular impulse is sustained, with presystolic distension accompanied by a fourth heart sound. An aortic ejection sound is conspicuous by its absence, and the aortic component of the second heart sound is normal. The midsystolic stenotic murmur is prominent in the first right intercostal space with disproportionate radiation into the right side of the neck. Aortic regurgitation is uncommon if not rare. The electrocardiogram of isolated supravalvular aortic stenosis with normal coronary arteries is identical to that of congenital aortic valve stenosis. The x-ray shows a nondilated ascending aorta. Echocardiography identifies the presence and determines the severity of the supravalvular obstruction.

Congenital Aortic Regurgitation

The classic features of chronic severe aortic regurgitation have been familiar to clinicians since Corrigan's treatise in 1832 *On Permanent Patency of the Mouth of the Aorta, or Inadequacy of the Aortic Valves.*[37] The remainder of this chapter deals with pure congenital aortic regurgitation when the regurgitant flow is through an incompetent aortic valve directly into the left ventricle (Tables 7–2 and 7–3). Regurgitant flow that reaches the left ventricle through channels other than the aortic valve will be dealt with more briefly (Tables 7–2 and 7–3).[49] The causes of pure aortic regurgitation include abnormalities of the aortic valve, abnormalities of the aortic wall, and abnormalities that affect neither the valve nor the aortic wall.[9,10] Abnormalities primarily affecting the aortic valve are the most common causes of pure aortic regurgitation.

Pure congenital aortic regurgitation occurs with valves that are unicuspid unicommissural,[60] bicuspid,[199,204] tricuspid, or quadricuspid,[65,114,153,227] or that are devoid of one or more cusps,[11,31,103,113,141] or of all three cusps,[11a] and with ventricular septal defect (see Chapter 17), aortic–left ventricular tunnel,[46,92,96,104,107,118,138,205] and coronary artery to left ventricular fistula (see Chapter 22).[6,22,234] The most common cause of pure congenital aortic valve regurgitation is the bicuspid aortic valve.[195,199,204] Tricuspid aortic valves with cuspal inequality are seldom incompetent in the young but become incompetent in older patients in whom minor degrees of fibrocalcification exaggerate inherent cuspal inequality and interfere with leaflet coaptation.[185] Isolated *quadricuspid aortic valves* are rare (Fig. 7–35) and usually function normally in early life despite inherent cuspal inequality.[63,65,108,114,132,227] When quadricuspid aortic valves function abnormally, the physiologic derangement

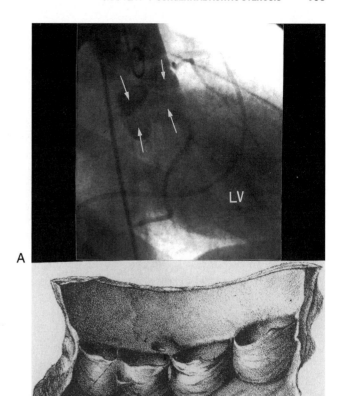

Figure 7–35

A, Aortogram from a 21-year-old man with a quadricuspid aortic valve (*four arrows*) and pure severe aortic regurgitation. LV, left ventricle. *B,* "Four leaflets at the aortic orifice from a preparation in St. Thomas's Hospital Museum." Peacock, Thomas B: On Malformations of the Human Heart. London, John Churchill, 1858.

Table 7–2	**Types of Congenital Aortic Regurgitation**

Through the aortic valve directly into the left ventricle

Through channels other than aortic valve

    Into left ventricle: aortic–left ventricular tunnel, coronary arterial fistula

    Into right atrium: ruptured sinus of Valsalva aneurysm

    Into right ventricle: ruptured sinus of Valsalva aneurysm

    Into pulmonary trunk: aortopulmonary window, truncus arteriosus

    Into pulmonary artery: patent ductus arteriosus

Table 7–3	**Malformations Associated with Pure Congenital Aortic Regurgitation**

Unicuspid unicommissural valve

Bicuspid valve

Quadricuspid valve

Congenital absence of aortic leaflet(s)

Aortic–left ventricular tunnel

Coronary artery to left ventricular fistula

is almost always pure regurgitation (see Fig. 7–35A).* Unicuspid unicommissural valves rarely have sufficient redundancy of the free edge of the single leaflet to render the mechanism incompetent.[60]

The foregoing types of congenital aortic regurgitation are characterized by regurgitant flow that is mild or absent in infancy and early childhood, but there are three types of severe aortic regurgitation that begin in the young. One or more cusps or the entire aortic valve mechanism can be congenitally absent.[11a,31,100,103,141] The deleterious effects begin in utero and continue in neonates and infants.[11a,31,103,113,141] A second form of severe aortic regurgitation that begins in infancy is an aortic–left ventricular tunnel, which is a rare malformation characterized by a vascular channel that originates immediately above the right sinus of Valsalva, tunnels through the ventricular septum, terminates in the perimembranous or infundibular septum, and enters the left ventricle immediately below the right and noncoronary cusps.[107,118] The aortic end of the tunnel is separated from the right coronary ostium (Fig. 7–36). A third and also rare form of severe aortic regurgitation that begins in infancy is a large coronary

---

*See references 63,65,108,110,114,132,174,182,211,227.

artery to left ventricular fistula (see Chapter 22).[216] Fewer than 10% of coronary artery fistulas terminate in the left ventricle. Although congestive heart failure may develop in the neonate, the magnitude of flow is usually limited, so adult survival is the rule.[216]

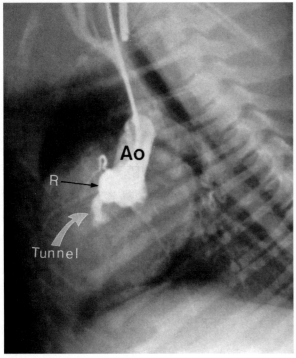

Figure 7–36
Contrast material injected into the ascending aorta (Ao) of a mixed-breed dog. The *arrow* points to a blind aortic to left ventricular tunnel. The right aortic sinus (R) is enlarged. (Courtesy of Dr. N. Sidney Moise, Cornell University College of Veterinary Medicine, Ithaca, New York.)

A functionally normal bicuspid aortic valve[62,156,195] is associated with mild aortic regurgitation (Fig. 7–37) because the free edges of bicuspid leaflets must be longer than the diameter of the aortic ring to permit unobstructed systolic flow (see Fig. 7–1A, *left panel*). Regurgitation may remain mild or may gradually or acutely increase (see Fig. 7–38).[30,62,156,162,195] Chronic severe bicuspid aortic regurgitation is caused by gradually increasing prolapse of the relatively redundant edge of the larger of the two bicuspid leaflets.[30] Regurgitation is insidious, with the fully developed hemodynamic fault awaiting adulthood.[204] However, infective endocarditis can convert a functionally normal congenital bicuspid aortic valve into the catastrophic hemodynamic fault of acute severe aortic regurgitation (see Fig. 7–38B).[30,162,195] Bicuspid aortic regurgitation is augmented by dilatation and dissection of the aortic root caused by an inherent medial abnormality of the ascending aorta above a bicuspid aortic valve (see earlier and see Fig. 7–4).[52,97,133,174]

The physiologic consequences of aortic regurgitation depend on the magnitude of regurgitant flow, the rate of its development, and the adaptive response of the volume-overloaded left ventricle. There are fundamental differ-

ences between *gradual* progression that culminates decades later in severe aortic regurgitation and the *acute* development of severe aortic regurgitation.[162,228,230] Adaptation of the left ventricle to gradual chronic aortic regurgitation was addressed in 1858 by Peacock: "This process is often so slow in its progress, that the ventricle accommodates itself to the additional exertion required; the disease becomes a source of manifest evil only after the lapse of many years."[181] Gradual development of severe aortic regurgitation permits an adaptive response of the left ventricle that is precluded if equivalent aortic regurgitation is suddenly incurred.[162]

The response of the left ventricle to a gradual increase in volume is typified by chronic severe aortic regurgitation imposed before the onset of depressed myocardial contractility (Table 7–4). The volume-overloaded ventricle achieves an adaptive increase in mass by increasing its internal dimensions (radius and base to apex) with a proportionate increase in septal and free wall thickness. The result is a magnified normal heart that is geometrically appropriate for ejecting an augmented stroke volume against normal or reduced systemic resistance.[184] The increase in ventricular mass is initially a desirable adaptive response that permits the heart to function normally at greater workloads.[184] Left ventricular end-diastolic volume and fiber length increase while end-diastolic pressure remains normal. Stroke volume and ejection fraction increase, so effective cardiac output is maintained. The velocity of ejection increases, left ventricular and aortic systolic pressures rise, aortic diastolic pressure falls, and the pulse pressure widens. Despite a considerable increase in stroke volume, the duration of left ventricular contraction remains normal because the velocity of

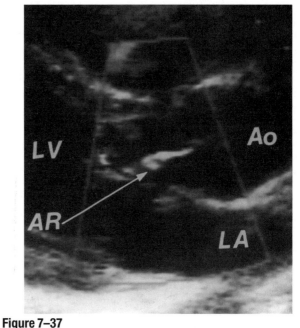

Figure 7–37
Echocardiogram (short axis) from a 13-year-old boy with a functionally normal bicuspid aortic valve. Black and white print of a color flow image (parasternal long-axis) shows mild aortic regurgitation (AR). Ao, dilated aortic root; LA, left atrium; LV, left ventricle.

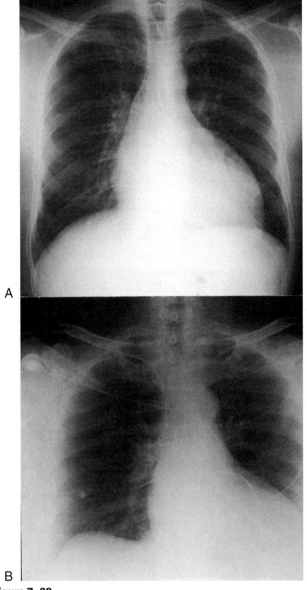

Figure 7–38

A, X-rays from a 22-year-old man with chronic severe bicuspid aortic regurgitation. The ascending aorta is dilated. A large convex left ventricle extends below the left hemidiaphragm. *B,* Portable x-rays (anteroposterior projection) from a 62-year-old woman with acute severe aortic regurgitation caused by infective endocarditis on a previously unrecognized bicuspid aortic valve. There is pulmonary venous congestion, and the left ventricle is moderately dilated.

Table 7–4	Major Hemodynamic Features of Severe Aortic Regurgitation	
	Chronic	**Acute**
LV compliance	Increased	Not increased
Regurgitant volume	Increased	Increased
LV end-diastolic pressure	Normal	Markedly increased
LV ejection velocity (dp/dt)	Markedly increased	Not significantly increased
Aortic systolic pressure	Increased	Not increased
Aortic diastolic pressure	Markedly decreased	Not significantly decreased
Systemic arterial pulse pressure	Markedly increased	Not significantly increased
Ejection fraction	Increased	Not increased
Effective stroke volume	Normal	Decreased
Effective cardiac output	Normal	Decreased
Heart rate	Normal	Increased
Peripheral vascular resistance	Normal	Increased

LV, left ventricular.

ejection is rapid and the pre-ejection period is shortened. With isotonic exercise, systemic systolic pressure rises but peripheral resistance falls, diastole shortens as heart rate increases, and regurgitant fraction per beat decreases. An appropriate increment in effective cardiac output is achieved without an increase in end-diastolic volume or end-diastolic pressure.[19] Despite these favorable adaptations, left ventricular response to isotonic or isometric exercise is not necessarily normal even in young asymptomatic patients.[19,20,85,93,95,210]

Acute severe aortic regurgitation is characterized by a dramatic rise in left ventricular end-diastolic pressure in response to the sudden increase in volume imposed upon a ventricle that is operating on the less compliant portion of its pressure-volume curve.[228,230] As stroke volume falls, heart rate accelerates in a vain attempt to maintain cardiac output. Peripheral resistance rises in an equally vain attempt to maintain systemic arterial pressure.[228] The velocity of ejection does not increase significantly, left ventricular and aortic systolic pressures are not significantly elevated, and aortic diastolic pressure cannot fall below the relatively high left ventricular end-diastolic pressure, so the systemic arterial pulse pressure remains normal or nearly so. The steep rise in left ventricular end-diastolic pressure exceeds left atrial pressure, prematurely closing the mitral valve before inscription of the P wave of the electrocardiogram.[162] The mitral valve opens later than normal because of prolonged ejection from the acutely volume-loaded left ventricle.[162] Premature closure and delayed opening of the mitral valve together with obligatory tachycardia reduce the time during which the mitral valve is open. The pulmonary arterial pressure rises in tandem with left atrial mean pressure, but competence of the mitral valve protects the left atrium from a linear transmission of the high left ventricular end-diastolic pressure into the pulmonary venous bed.[228] This protection is lost with the advent of mitral regurgitation, so left atrial pressure rises further and cardiac output reciprocally falls.[228]

THE HISTORY

Congenital aortic valve regurgitation predominates in males, a sex distribution that reflects the prevalence of bicuspid aortic valves.[195] The soft murmur of bicuspid aortic regurgitation usually goes undetected in asymptomatic infants and children. Patients with moderate to severe aortic regurgitation are often asymptomatic[193] except for awareness of neck pulsations or awareness of left ventricular premature contractions when lying in the left lateral decubitus position.[19] Vascular wall pain is occasionally experienced in the carotid and subclavian arteries and in the thoracic or abdominal aorta. Inappropriate diaphoresis sometimes begins long before the onset of congestive heart failure. When bicuspid valve infective endocarditis causes acute severe aortic regurgitation, cardiac failure is sudden and intractable.[162]

When aortic regurgitation is caused by an aortic–left ventricular tunnel, severe regurgitant flow and congestive heart failure develop early. Exceptional cases of asymptomatic survival have been reported in children and young adults.[118,138] Congenital absence of one or more aortic cusps with severe regurgitation is manifest by in utero heart failure with nonimmune fetal hydrops.[11a] Only exceptional cases of childhood or post-adolescent survival have been reported.[103,141]

THE PHYSICAL SIGNS

In 1832, Dominic Corrigan described the visible arterial pulse associated with inadequacy of the aortic valve[37]:

When a patient affected by the disease is stripped, the arterial trunks of the head, neck, and superior extremities immediately catch the eye by their singular pulsation. At each diastole the subclavian, carotid, temporal, brachial, and in some cases even the palmar arteries, are suddenly thrown from their bed, bounding up under the skin . . . though a moment before unmarked, they are at each pulsation thrown out on the surface in the strongest relief. From its singular and striking appearance, the name visible pulsation is given to this beating of the arteries.

The arterial pulse in chronic severe aortic regurgitation is characterized by a rapid rate of rise, an increased pulse pressure (high systolic, low diastolic), a single or double peak (bisferiens), and a brisk collapse.[185] The Quincke pulse (flushing and blanching of the digital capillary bed), palpable pulsations in the fingertips, and the posteroanterior head movements synchronous with systole and diastole are additional features.[185] The arterial pulse in acute severe aortic regurgitation is characterized by an unimpressive rate of rise, a moderately increased pulse pressure (systolic normal, diastolic normal, or slightly diminished), a single peak, and the pulsus alternans of left ventricular failure.

Precordial palpation in chronic severe aortic regurgitation reveals a laterally displaced hyperdynamic left ventricular impulse that imparts a rocking motion to the chest. A systolic thrill and murmur are present in the suprasternal notch and over the carotid and subclavian arteries (Corrigan's *bruit de soufflet*)[37] because of high-velocity ejection. In acute severe aortic regurgitation, the location of the left ventricular impulse is normal or moderately displaced and is not hyperdynamic.

Auscultation in chronic severe aortic regurgitation discloses a normal first heart sound, an attenuated aortic component of the second sound, and neither a third nor a fourth heart sound.[203] There is a grade 3/6 right basal aortic midsystolic murmur, a long, high-pitched aortic diastolic murmur at the midleft sternal border, and a presystolic Austin Flint murmur at the apex.[185] There is no aortic ejection sound because a severely incompetent bicuspid aortic valve does not dome.[203] Peripheral arterial auscultatory signs include the Duroziez murmur (systolic/diastolic murmur over a partially compressed femoral artery) and Traube's pistol shot sounds.[185]

In acute severe aortic regurgitation, the first heart sound is soft or absent and a fourth heart sound is precluded because of premature closure of the mitral valve. There is a third heart sound of left ventricular failure.[162] The pulmonary component of the second sound is increased in response to elevated pulmonary artery pressure. A midsystolic aortic flow murmur is less than grade 3 and is followed by an aortic diastolic murmur that is short, medium pitched, and disarmingly soft because of the relatively low velocity of regurgitant flow. It is difficult to distinguish systole from diastole because the first heart sound is soft or absent and the heart rate is rapid. Austin Flint murmurs cannot be presystolic because of premature closure of the mitral valve. There are no auscultatory signs over peripheral arteries.

An aortic–left ventricular tunnel is accompanied by systolic/diastolic to-and-fro murmurs analogous to midsystolic/early diastolic murmurs of chronic severe aortic regurgitation.[46,104,138] Doppler interrogation of flow patterns within the ascending aorta and within the tunnel identifies diastolic flow from the tunnel into the left ventricle and systolic flow from left ventricle into the tunnel.[77] The phasic flow is predominantly diastolic, which is consistent with the auscultatory observation that the diastolic murmur is loud and the systolic murmur is soft.[138] Occasionally, only the diastolic murmur is audible.[118]

THE ELECTROCARDIOGRAM

The typical electrocardiogram of chronic severe aortic regurgitation displays the voltage and repolarization criteria of left ventricular hypertrophy with prominent left precordial Q waves of chronic volume overload. Isotonic exercise even in children and young adults sometimes provokes or exaggerates ST segment depressions.[85] In acute severe aortic regurgitation, left ventricular hypertrophy is absent, the QRS voltage is normal, repolarization abnormalities are minor, and left precordial Q waves are inconspicuous.

THE X-RAY

In chronic severe bicuspid aortic regurgitation, the x-ray shows an enlarged convex left ventricle and a conspicuously dilated ascending aorta because pulsatile regurgitant flow aggregates the inherent medial abnormality (see Fig. 7–38A).[52] Pulmonary venous vascularity is normal because left ventricular filling pressure is normal. In acute severe aortic regurgitation, the left ventricular silhouette is normal or nearly so, but pulmonary venous vascularity is increased because left ventricular filling pressure is elevated (see Fig. 7–38B). In aortic regurgitation associated with aortic–left ventricular tunnel, the ascending aorta is consistently dilated and is sometimes aneurysmal.[46,77,96,138]

THE ECHOCARDIOGRAM

Echocardiography with Doppler interrogation and color flow imaging establishes the presence and degree of aortic regurgitation, determines aortic valve morphology,[33] and defines the physiologic consequences of regurgitant flow. The mild aortic regurgitation of a functionally normal bicuspid aortic valve is identified with color flow imaging (Fig. 7–37B). The regurgitant jet of bicuspid aortic regurgitation is eccentric in the left ventricular outflow tract (Fig. 7–39). Vegetations of infective endocarditis are imaged (Fig. 7–40). Continuous-wave Doppler records the profile of regurgitant flow and determines whether aortic stenosis coexists (Fig. 7–41). The four cusps of a congenitally quadricuspid aortic valve (Fig. 7–42) are better recognized on the transesophageal echocardiogram.

Two-dimensionally targeted M mode echocardiography establishes end-diastolic and end-systolic left ventricular dimensions and septal and free wall thickness. Left ventricular ejection fraction is determined from two-dimensional real time imaging.

An aortic–left ventricular tunnel can be diagnosed as the cause of aortic regurgitation, and Doppler interrogation with color flow imaging permits study of phasic directional flow within the tunnel.[5,77,92,107,215,234] An aortic–left ventricular tunnel arising from the left aortic sinus was diagnosed by echocardiography.[92]

SUMMARY

The most common cause of congenital aortic regurgitation is a bicuspid aortic valve. The degree of regurgitation varies from mild to severe. The majority of patients are males with no history of a cardiac murmur in infancy and childhood. Bicuspid aortic regurgitation progresses insidiously and usually presents in young adults with few or no symptoms despite appreciable regurgitant flow. Patients may be subjectively aware of neck pulsations and of forceful left

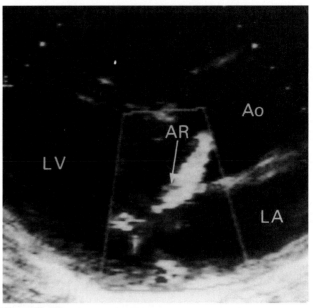

Figure 7–39
Black and white print of a color flow image from a 32-year-old man with a functionally normal bicuspid aortic valve. The eccentric jet of mild to moderate aortic regurgitation (AR) is directed toward the anterior mitral leaflet. Ao, dilated aortic root; LA, left atrium; LV, left ventricle.

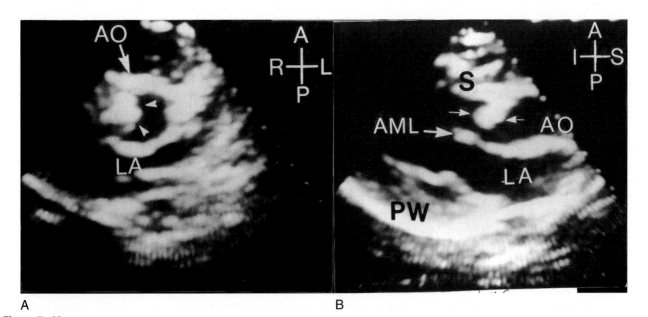

A   B

Figure 7–40
A, Echocardiogram (parasternal short axis) from an 11-year-old girl with severe bicuspid aortic regurgitation. *Paired arrowheads* point to a vegetation of healed infective endocarditis. Ao, aorta; LA, left atrium. B, Parasternal long axis shows the healed vegetation (*paired arrows*). AML, anterior mitral leaflet; PW, posterior wall; S, ventricular septum.

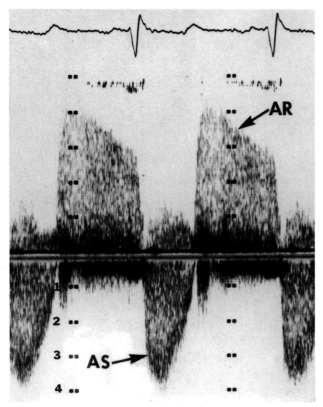

Figure 7–41

Continuous wave Doppler across a bicuspid stenotic (AS) and regurgitant (AR) aortic valve. The velocity of 3.9 m/sec indicates a peak instantaneous gradient of 60 mm Hg. The Doppler signal shows high-velocity regurgitant flow.

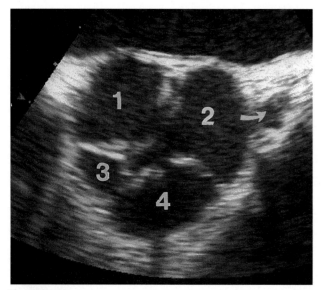

Figure 7–42

Echocardiogram (short axis) from a 66-year-old man with a congenitally quadricuspid aortic valve (1, 2, 3, 4 cusps) and severe aortic regurgitation. The left coronary artery (*arrow*) originated from the second sinus.

ventricular contractions, especially with premature beats, and may experience inappropriate diaphoresis or vascular pain over carotid arteries or over the thoracic and abdominal aorta. The systemic arterial pulse exhibits a wide pulse

pressure with a rapid rate of rise, a brisk collapse, and a bisferiens peak. The dilated hyperdynamic left ventricular impulse generates a rocking precordial motion. A systolic thrill is often present at the right base and in the suprasternal notch and neck despite the absence of aortic stenosis. The first heart sound is normal or soft. Third and fourth heart sounds are absent. A short prominent right basal midsystolic murmur radiates into the neck. The early diastolic murmur of aortic regurgitation is loud and long, and the Duroziez murmur and Traube's pistol shot sounds are heard over peripheral arteries. The electrocardiogram shows voltage and repolarization criteria of left ventricular hypertrophy. The x-ray reveals an enlarged left ventricle, a dilated ascending aorta, and normal pulmonary venous vascularity. Severe congenital aortic regurgitation typically presents in young adults with three exceptions that include severe regurgitation in neonates or infants with absence of one or more aortic cusps, an aortic–left ventricular tunnel, and a large coronary artery to left ventricular fistula.

The clinical course of a bicuspid aortic valve, whether functionally normal, stenotic, or incompetent, may suddenly be punctuated by a dissecting aortic aneurysm with an increase in preexisting aortic regurgitation. An unrecognized functionally normal bicuspid aortic valve can announce itself when infective endocarditis causes acute severe aortic regurgitation with sudden intractable heart failure. Systemic arterial pulse pressure is only moderately increased, the rate of rise is not brisk, pulsus alternans is common, and peripheral arterial signs of chronic severe aortic regurgitation are absent. The left ventricular impulse is only moderately displaced and is not hyperdynamic. The first heart sound is soft or inaudible despite tachycardia. A fourth heart sound is absent, but a third sound is prominent. The aortic midsystolic murmur is grade 3 or less, and the murmur of aortic regurgitation is short, medium pitched, and relatively soft. An Austin Flint murmur cannot be presystolic. The electrocardiogram does not show left ventricular hypertrophy. The x-ray shows a near normal or only moderately enlarged left ventricle and a conspicuous increase in pulmonary venous vascularity.

REFERENCES

1. Alpert JS, Vieweg WVR, Hagan AD: Incidence and morphology of carotid shudders and aortic valve disease. Am Heart J 92:435, 1976.
2. Assey ME, Wisenbaugh T, Spann JF, et al: Unexpected persistence into adulthood of low wall stress in patients with congenital aortic stenosis: Is there a fundamental difference in the hypertrophic response to a pressure overload present from birth? Circulation 75:973, 1987.
3. Bache RJ, Wang Y, Jorgensen CR: Hemodynamic effects of exercise in isolated valvular aortic stenosis. Circulation 44:1003, 1971.
4. Child JS: Transthoracic and transesophageal echocardiographic imaging: Anatomic and hemodynamic assessment. In Perloff JK, Child JS (eds): Congenital Heart Disease in Adults, 2nd ed. Philadelphia, WB Saunders, 1998, p 91.
5. Bash SE, Huhta JC, Nihill MR, et al: Aortico-left ventricular tunnel with ventricular septal defect: Two-dimensional Doppler echocardiographic diagnosis. J Am Coll Cardiol 5:757, 1985.
6. Bentivoglio LG, Sagarminaga J, Uricchio J, Goldberg H: Congenital bicuspid aortic valves: A clinical and hemodynamic study. Br Heart J 22:321, 1960.

7. Beuren AJ, Apitz J, Harmjanz D: Supravalvular aortic stenosis in association with mental retardation and a certain facial appearance. Circulation 26:1235, 1962.

8. Beuren AJ, Schulze C, Eberle P, et al: The syndrome of supravalvular aortic stenosis, peripheral pulmonary stenosis, mental retardation and similar facial appearance. Am J Cardiol 13:471, 1964.

9. Waller B, Howard J, Fess S: Pathology of aortic valve stenosis and pure aortic regurgitation. Part 1. Clin Cardiol 17:85, 1994.

10. Waller B, Howard J, Fess S: Pathology of aortic valve stenosis and pure aortic regurgitation. Part II. Clin Cardiol 17:150, 1994.

11. Bicoff JP, Thompson W, Arbeiter HI, et al: Severe aortic stenosis in infancy. J Pediat 63:161, 1963.

11a. Bierman FZ, Yeh M, Swersky S, et al: Absence of the aortic valve. J Am Coll Cardiol 3:833, 1984.

12. Biesecker LG, Laxova R, Friedman A: Renal insufficiency in Williams syndrome. Am J Med Genet 28:131, 1987.

13. Sabet HY, Edwards WD, Tazelaar HD, Daly RC: Congenitally bicuspid aortic valves: A surgical pathology study of 542 cases (1991 through 1996) and a literature review of 2,715 additional cases. Mayo Clin Proc 74:14, 1999.

14. Black JA, Bonham-Carter RE: Association between aortic stenosis and facies of severe infantile hypercalcemia. Lancet 2:745, 1963.

15. Beppu S, Suzuki S, Matsuda H, et al: Rapidity of progression of aortic stenosis in patients with congenital bicuspid aortic valves. Am J Cardiol 71:322, 1993.

16. Blieden LC, Allen HD, Lucas RV, Moller JH: Discrete membranous subaortic stenosis: ECG and vectorcardiographic findings. Am Heart J 107:1293, 1984.

17. Blieden LC, Lucas RV, Carter JB, et al: A developmental complex including supravalvular stenosis of the aorta and pulmonary trunk. Circulation 49:585, 1974.

18. Bonner AJ, Sacks HN, Tavel ME: Assessing the severity of aortic stenosis by phonocardiography and external carotid pulse recordings. Circulation 48:247, 1973.

19. Bonow RO, Rosing DR, McIntosh CL, et al: The natural history of asymptomatic patients with aortic regurgitation and normal left ventricular function. Circulation 68:509, 1983.

20. Borer JS, Bacharach SL, Green MV, et al: Exercise-induced left ventricular dysfunction in symptomatic and asymptomatic patients with aortic regurgitation. Am J Cardiol 42:351, 1978.

21. Rustico MA, Benettoni A, Bussani R, et al: Early fetal endocardial fibroelastosis and critical aortic stenosis. Ultrasound Obstet Gynecol 5:202, 1995.

22. Braunwald E, Goldblatt A, Aygen MM, et al: Congenital aortic stenosis. Circulation 27:426, 1963.

23. Braverman IB, Gibson S: The outlook for children with congenital aortic stenosis. Am Heart J 53:487, 1957.

24. Bristow JD: Recognition of left ventricular outflow obstruction. Circulation 31:600, 1965.

25. Brooks N: Rapid development of severe aortic stenosis from calcification of congenital bicuspid aortic valve. Br Med J 281:424, 1980.

26. Buckberg G, Eber L, Herman M, Gorlin R: Ischemia in aortic stenosis. Am J Cardiol 35:778, 1975.

27. Oliver JM, Gonzalez A, Gallego P, et al: Discrete subaortic stenosis in adults: Increased pervalence and slow rate of progression of the obstruction and aortic regurgitation. J Am Coll Cardiol 38:835, 2001.

28. Campbell M: Calcific aortic stenosis and congenital bicuspid aortic valves. Br Heart J 30:606, 1968.

29. Campbell M: The natural history of congenital aortic stenosis. Br Heart J 30:514, 1968.

30. Carter JB, Sethi S, Lee GB, Edwards JE: Prolapse of semilunar cusps as causes of aortic insufficiency. Circulation 43:922, 1971.

31. Carvalho AC, Andrade JL, Lima VC, et al: Absence of an aortic cusp, a cause of severe aortic regurgitation in infancy. Pediatr Cardiol 13:122, 1992.

32. Caulfield WH, deLeon AC, Perloff JK, Steelman RB: The clinical significance of the fourth heart sound in aortic stenosis. Am J Cardiol 28:179, 1971.

33. Chandrasekaran K, Tajik AJ, Edwards WD, Seward JB: Two-dimensional echocardiographic diagnosis of quadricuspid aortic valve. Am J Cardiol 53:1732, 1984.

34. Choi JY, Sullivan ID: Fixed subaortic stenosis: Anatomical spectrum and nature of progression. Br Heart J 65:280, 1991.

35. Cohen S, Friedman WF, Braunwald E: Natural history of mild congenital aortic stenosis elucidated by serial hemodynamic studies. Am J Cardiol 30:1, 1972.

36. Conway EE, Noonan J, Marion RW, Steeg CN: Myocardial infarction leading to sudden death in Williams syndrome: Report of three cases. J Pediatr 117:593, 1990.

37. Corrigan DJ: On permanent patency of the mouth of the aorta or inadequacy of the aortic valves. Edinburgh Med Surg J 37:225, 1832. In Willius FA, Keys TE (eds): Classics of Cardiology. Malabar, Florida, Robert E. Krieger Pub. Co., 1983.

38. Cripps T, Leech G, Leatham A: Inappropriate left ventricular hypertrophy in minor aortic valve disease: A source of error in clinical assessment. Eur Heart J 8:895, 1987.

39. Cueto L, Moller JH: Haemodynamics of exercise in children with isolated aortic valvular disease. Br Heart J 35:93, 1973.

40. Cyran SE, James FW, Daniels S, et al: Comparison of the cardiac output and stroke volume response to upright exercise in children with valvular and subvalvular aortic stenosis. J Am Coll Cardiol 11:651, 1988.

41. Da Vinci L: Leonardo on the Human Body. New York, Dover Publications, 1983.

42. Daniels SR, Loggie JMH, Schwartz DC, et al: Systemic hypertension secondary to peripheral vascular anomalies in patients with Williams syndrome. J Pediatr 106:249, 1985.

43. Davachi F, Moller JH, Edwards JE: Diseases of the mitral valve in infancy. Circulation 43:565, 1971.

44. Davis GL, McAlister WH, Friedenberg MM: Congenital aortic stenosis due to failure of histogenesis of the aortic valve (myxoid dysplasia). Am J Roentgenol 95:621, 1965.

45. Chan K, Ghani M, Woodend K, Burwash IG: Case-controlled study to assess risk factors for aortic stenosis in congenitally bicuspid aortic valve. Am J Cardiol 88:690, 2001.

46. Deuvaert FE, Goffin Y, Wellens F, et al: Aortico-left ventricular tunnel (ALVT). A diagnostic and surgical "must." Acta Cardiol 41:53, 1986.

47. Donnelly GL, Vandenberg EA: Early systolic sounds in aortic valve stenosis. Br Heart J 29:246, 1967.

48. Donner RM, Carabello BA, Black I, Spann JF: Left ventricular wall stress in compensated aortic stenosis in children. Am J Cardiol 51:946, 1983.

49. Donofrio MT, Engle MA, O'Loughlin JE, et al: Congenital aortic regurgitation: Natural history and management. J Am Coll Cardiol 20:366, 1992.

50. Dumoulin M, Van der Hauwaert L: Familial supravalvular aortic stenosis. Acta Paediatr Belg 31:129, 1978.

51. Wessel A, Pankau D, Kececioglu W, et al: Three decades of follow-up of aortic and pulmonary valve lesions in the Williams-Beuren syndrome. Am J Med Genet 52:297, 1994.

52. Niwa K, Perloff JK, Bhuta SM, et al: Structural abnormalities of great arterial walls in congenital heart disease: Light and electron microscopic analyses. Circulation 103:393, 2001.

53. Eisenberg R, Young D, Jacobson B, Boito A: Familial supravalvular aortic stenosis. Am J Dis Child 108:341, 1964.

54. El Habbal MH, Suliman RF: The aortic root in subaortic stenosis. Am Heart J 117:1127, 1989.

55. Sans-Coma V, Cardo M, Thiene G, et al: Bicuspid aortic and pulmonary valves in the Syrian hamster. Int J Cardiol 34:249, 1992.

56. Laskey WK, Kussmaul WG: Subvalvular gradients in patients with valvular aortic stenosis. Circulation 104:1019, 2001.

57. El-Said G, Galioto FM, Mullins CE, McNamara DG: Natural hemodynamic history of congenital aortic stenosis in childhood. Am J Cardiol 30:6, 1972.

58. Ensing GJ, Schmidt MA, Hagler DJ, et al: Spectrum of findings in a family with nonsyndromic autosomal dominant supravalvular aortic stenosis: A Doppler echocardiographic study. J Am Coll Cardiol 13:413, 1989.

59. Epstein EJ, Criley M, Raftery EB, et al: Cineradiographic studies of the early systolic click in aortic valve stenosis. Circulation 31:842, 1965.

60. Falcone MW, Roberts WC, Morrow AG, Perloff JK: Congenital aortic stenosis resulting from a unicommissural valve. Circulation 44:272, 1971.

61. Farrar JF, Gray RE: The pulse of aortic stenosis during childhood. Br Heart J 27:199, 1965.

62. Fenoglio JJ, McAllister HA, DeCastro CM, et al: Congenital bicuspid aortic valve after age 20. Am J Cardiol 39:164, 1977.

63. Fernicola DJ, Mann JM, Roberts WC: Congenitally quadricuspid aortic valve: Analysis of six necropsy patients. Am J Cardiol 63:136, 1989.

64. Firpo C, Azcarte MJM, Jimenez MQ, Saravalli O: Discrete subaortic stenosis (D.S.S.) in childhood: A congenital or acquired disease? Follow-up in 65 patients. Eur Heart J 11:1033, 1990.

65. Fischler D, Fitzmaurice M, Ratliff NB: Quadricuspid aortic valve. Am J Cardiovasc Pathol 3:91, 1990.

66. Folger GM: Further observations on the syndrome of idiopathic infantile hypercalcemia associated with supravalvular aortic stenosis. Am Heart J 93:455, 1977.

67. Salaymeh KH, Banerjee A: Evaluation of arterial stiffness in children with Williams syndrome: Does it play a role in evolving hypertension? Am Heart J 142:549, 2001.

68. Fowler RS: Ventricular repolarization in congenital aortic stenosis. Am Heart J 70:603, 1965.

69. Frank RH, Oran E: Asymmetric arm and neck pulses: A clue to supravalvular aortic stenosis. Circulation 28:722, 1963.

70. Frank S, Johnson A, Ross J: Natural history of valvular aortic stenosis. Br Heart J 35:41, 1973.

71. Freedom RM, Dische MR, Rowe RD: Pathologic anatomy of subaortic stenosis and atresia in the first year of life. Am J Cardiol 39:1035, 1977.

72. Freedom RM, Fowler RS, Duncan WJ: Rapid evolution from "normal" left ventricular outflow tract to fatal subaortic stenosis in infancy. Br Heart J 45:605, 1981.

73. Freedom RM, Pelech A, Brand A, et al: The progressive nature of subaortic stenosis in congenital heart disease. Int J Cardiol 8:137, 1985.

74. French JW, Guntheroth WG: An explanation of asymmetric upper extremity blood pressures in supravalvular aortic stenosis. Circulation 42:31, 1970.

75. Friedman WF, Roberts WC: Vitamin D and the supravalvular aortic stenosis syndrome. Circulation 34:77, 1966.

76. Friedman WF, Modlinger J, Morgan JR: Serial hemodynamic observations in asymptomatic children with valvular aortic stenosis. Circulation 43:91, 1971.

77. Fripp R, Werner JC, Whitman V, et al: Pulsed Doppler and two-dimensional echocardiographic findings in aortico-left ventricular tunnel. J Am Coll Cardiol 4:1012, 1984.

78. Kim YM, Yoo S, Choi JY, et al: Natural course of supravalvular aortic stenosis and peripheral pulmonary arterial stenosis in Williams' syndrome. Cardiol Young 9:37, 1999.

79. Fukuda T, Tadavarthy SM, Edwards JE: Dissecting aneurysm of the aorta complicating aortic valvular stenosis. Circulation 53:169, 1976.

80. Gale AW, Cartmill TB, Bernstein L: Familial subaortic membranous stenosis. Austr NZ J Med 4:576, 1974.

81. Gamboa R, Hugenholtz PG, Nadas AS: Accuracy of the phonocardiogram in assessing severity of aortic and pulmonic stenosis. Circulation 30:35, 1964.

82. Gamboa R, Hugenholtz PG, Nadas AS: Comparisons of electrocardiograms and vectorcardiograms in congenital aortic stenosis. Br Heart J 27:344, 1965.

83. Garcia RE, Friedman WF, Kaback MM, Rowe RD: Idiopathic hypercalcemia and supravalvular aortic stenosis. N Engl J Med 271:117, 1964.

84. Glew RH, Varghese PJ, Krovetz LJ, et al: Sudden death in congenital aortic stenosis. Am Heart J 78:615, 1969.

85. Goforth D, James FW, Kaplan S, et al: Maximal exercise in children with aortic regurgitation. Am Heart J 108:1306, 1984.

86. Goldblatt A, Aygen MM, Braunwald E: Hemodynamic-phonocardiographic correlations of the fourth heart sound in aortic stenosis. Circulation 26:92, 1962.

87. Goldstein RE, Epstein SE: Mechanism of elevated innominate artery pressures in supravalvular aortic stenosis. Circulation 42:23, 1970.

88. Yilmz AT, Arslan M, Byngol H, et al: Coronary artery aneurysm associated with adult supravalvular aortic stenosis. Ann Thorac Surg 62:1205, 1996.

89. Gorlin R, McMillan IK, Medd WE, et al: Dynamics of the circulation in aortic valvular disease. Am J Med 18:855, 1955.

90. Gould L, Venkataraman K, Goswami M, et al: Right-sided heart failure in aortic stenosis. Am J Cardiol 31:381, 1973.

91. Vaideeswar P, Shankar V, Deshpande JR, et al: Pathology of the diffuse variant of supravalvular aortic stenosis. Cardiovasc Pathol 10:33, 2001.

92. Grant P, Abrams LD, De Giovanni JV, et al: Aortico-left ventricular tunnel arising from the left aortic sinus. Am J Cardiol 55:1657, 1985.

93. Greenberg B, Massie B, Thomas D, et al: Association between the exercise ejection fraction response and systolic wall stress in patients with chronic aortic insufficiency. Circulation 71:458, 1985.

94. Griep AH: Pitfalls in the electrocardiographic diagnosis of left ventricular hypertrophy: A correlative study of 200 autopsied patients. Circulation 20:30, 1959.

95. Gumbiner CH, Gutgesell HP: Response to isometric exercise in children and young adults with aortic regurgitation. Am Heart J 106:540, 1983.

96. Guo D: Aortico-left ventricular tunnel: Diagnosis by cine angiocardiography. Am J Radiol 152:345, 1989.

97. Hahn RT, Roman MJ, Mogtader AH, Devereux RB: Association of aortic dilation with regurgitant, stenotic and functionally normal bicuspid aortic valves. J Am Coll Cardiol 19:283, 1992.

98. Hancock EW: The ejection sound in aortic stenosis. Am J Med 40:569, 1966.

99. Harrison EG, Roth GM, Hines EA: Bilateral indirect and direct arterial pulses. Circulation 22:419, 1960.

100. Hashimoto R, Miyamura H, Eguchi S: Congenital aortic regurgitation in a child with a trileaflet non-stenotic aortic valve. Br Heart J 51:358, 1984.

101. Hastreiter AR, Oshima M, Miller RA, et al: Congenital aortic stenosis syndrome in infancy. Circulation 27:1084, 1963.

102. Hirschfeld S, Liebman J, Borkat G, Bormuth C: Intracardiac pressure-sound correlates of echocardiographic aortic valve closure. Circulation 55:602, 1977.

103. Hoa T, Smolinsky A, Neufeld HN, Goor DA: Dysplastic aortic valve with absence of aortic valve cusp: An unreported cause of congenital aortic insufficiency. J Thorac Cardiovasc Surg 91:471, 1986.

104. Hovaguimian H, Cobanoglu A, Starr A: Aortico-left ventricular tunnel: A clinical review and new surgical classification. Ann Thorac Surg 45:106, 1988.

105. Hugenholtz PG, Lees MM, Nadas AS: The scalar electrocardiogram, vectorcardiogram, and exercise electrocardiogram in the assessment of congenital aortic stenosis. Circulation 26:79, 1962.

106. Stamm C, Li J, Ho SY, et al: The aortic root in supravalvular aortic stenosis. J Thorac Cardiovasc Surg 114:16, 1997.

107. Humes RA, Hagler DJ, Julsrud PR, et al: Aortico-left ventricular tunnel: Diagnosis based on two-dimensional echocardiography, color flow Doppler imaging, and magnetic resonance imaging. Mayo Clin Proc 61:901, 1986.

108. Hurwitz LE, Roberts WC: Quadricuspid semilunar valves. Am J Cardiol 31:623, 1973.

109. Husson GS, Blackman MS: Aortic stenosis with marked right ventricular hypertension. Am J Cardiol 17:273, 1966.

110. Iglesias A, Oliver J, Munoz JE, Nunez L: Quadricuspid aortic valve associated with fibromuscular aortic stenosis and aortic regurgitation. Chest 80:327, 1981.

111. Ingelfinger JR, Newburger JW: Spectrum of renal anomalies in patients with Williams syndrome. J Pediatr 119:771, 1991.

112. Ino T, Nishimoto K, Iwahara M, et al: Progressive vascular lesions in Williams-Beuren syndrome. Pediatr Cardiol 9:55, 1988.

113. Issenberg HJ, Mathew R, Kim ES, Bharati S: Congenital absence of the noncoronary aortic cusp. Am Heart J 113:400, 1987.

114. James KB, Centorbi LK, Novoa R: Quadricuspid aortic valve: Case report and review of the literature. Tex Heart Inst 18:141, 1991.

115. Suarez-Mier MP, Morentin B: Supravalvular aortic stenosis, Williams syndrome and sudden death. Forensic Sci Int 106:45, 1999.

116. Johnson AM: Aortic stenosis, sudden death and the left ventricular baroceptors. Br Heart J 33:1, 1971.

117. Dell-Agata A, Cromme-Dijkhuis Ah, Meijboom FJ, et al: Use of three-dimensional echocardiography for analysis of outflow obstruction in congenital heart disease. Am J Cardiol 83:921, 1999.

118. Kafka H, Chan KL, Leach AJ: Asymptomatic aortico-left ventricular tunnel in adulthood. Am J Cardiol 63:1021, 1989.

119. Kalan JM, McIntosh CL, Bonow RO, Roberts WC: Development of severe stenosis in a previously purely regurgitant, congenitally bicuspid aortic valve. Am J Cardiol 62:988, 1988.

120. Kangos JJ, Ferrer MI, Franciosi RA: Electrocardiographic changes associated with papillary muscle infarction in congenital heart disease. Am J Cardiol 23:801, 1969.

121. Katz NM, Buckley MJ, Liberthson RR: Discrete membranous subaortic stenosis. Circulation 56:1034, 1977.

122. Schurger D, Bartel T, Muller S, et al: Multiplane transesophageal echocardiography is the only definitive ultrasound approach in adult supravalvular aortic stenosis. Int J Cardiol 53:305, 1996.

123. Keane JF, Driscoll DJ, Gersony WM, et al: Second natural history study of congenital heart defects: Results of treatment of patients with aortic valvar stenosis. Circulation 87(Suppl I):I-16, 1993.

124. Kelly DT, Wulfsberg E, Rowe RD: Discrete subaortic stenosis. Circulation 46:309, 1972.

125. Krovetz LJ: Age-related changes in size of the aortic valve anulus in man. Am Heart J 90:569, 1975.

126. Krovetz LJ, Kurlinski JP: Subendocardial blood flow in children with congenital aortic stenosis. Circulation 54:961, 1976.

127. Dridi SM, Ghomrasseni S, Bonnet D, et al: Skin elastic fibers in Williams syndrome. Am J Med Genet 87:134, 1999.

128. Kumar S, Luisada AA: Mechanism of changes in the second heart sound in aortic stenosis. Am J Cardiol 28:162, 1971.

129. Kveselis DA, Rocchini AP, Rosenthal A, et al: Hemodynamic determinants of exercise-induced ST-segment depression in children with valvar aortic stenosis. Am J Cardiol 55:1333, 1985.

130. Lakier JB, Lewis AB, Heymann MA, et al: Isolated aortic stenosis in the neonate: Natural history and hemodynamic considerations. Circulation 50:801, 1974.

131. Morris CA: Genetic aspects of supravalvular aortic stenosis. Curr Opin Cardiol 13:214, 1998.

132. Lanzillo G, Breccia PA, Intonti F: Congenital quadricuspid aortic valve with displacement of the right coronary orifice. Scand J Cardiovasc Surg 15:149, 1981.

133. Larson EW, Edwards WD: Risk factors for aortic dissection: A necropsy study of 161 cases. Am J Cardiol 53:849, 1984.

134. Leatham A: Auscultation of the heart: Heart murmurs. Lancet 2:757, 1958.

135. Urban Z, Micheis VV, Thibodeau SN, et al: Isolated supravalvular aortic stenosis. Hum Genet 106:577, 2000.

136. Leech G, Mills P, Leatham A: The diagnosis of a non-stenotic bicuspid aortic valve. Br Heart J 40:941, 1978.

137. Leichter DA, Sullivan I, Gersony WM: "Acquired" discrete subvalvular aortic stenosis: Natural history and hemodynamics. J Am Coll Cardiol 14:1539, 1989.

138. Levy MJ, Schachner A, Blieden LC: Aortico-left ventricular tunnel: Collective review. J Thorac Cardiovasc Surg 84:102, 1982.

139. Lewis AB, Heymann MA, Stanger P, et al: Evaluation of subendocardial ischemia in valvar aortic stenosis in children. Circulation 49:978, 1974.

140. Lewis RP, Bristow JD, Griswold HE: Radiographic heart size and left ventricular volume in aortic valve disease. Am J Cardiol 27:250, 1971.

141. Lin AE, Chin AJ: Absent aortic valve: A complex anomaly. Pediatr Cardiol 11:195, 1990.

142. Von Dadelszen P, Chitayat D, Winsor EJ, et al: De novo 46 XX t(6:7)(q27;q11;23) associated with severe cardiovascular manifestations characteristic of supravalvular aortic stenosis and Williams syndrome. Am J Med Genet 90:270, 2000.

143. Logan WFWE, Jones EW: Familial supravalvular aortic stenosis. Br Heart J 27:547, 1965.

144. Lurie PR, Mandelbaum I: Mechanism of brachial pulse asymmetry in congenital aortic stenosis. Circulation 28:760, 1963.

145. Maron BJ, Sissman NJ: The electrocardiogram in supravalvular aortic stenosis. Am Heart J 82:300, 1971.

146. Maron BJ, Redwood DR, Roberts WC, et al: Tunnel subaortic stenosis. Circulation 54:404, 1976.

147. Mark AL, Abboud FM, Schmidt PG, Heistad DD: Reflex vascular responses to left ventricular outflow obstruction and activation of ventricular baroreceptors in dogs. J Clin Invest 52:1147, 1973.

148. Mark AL, Kioschos JM, Abboud FM, et al: Abnormal vascular responses to exercise in patients with aortic stenosis. J Clin Invest 52:1138, 1973.

149. Li DY, Toland AE, Boak BB, et al: Elastin point mutations cause an obstructive vascular disease, supravalvular aortic stenosis. Hum Mol Genet 6:1021, 1997.

150. Martin MM, Lemmer JH, Shaffer E, et al: Obstruction to left coronary artery blood flow secondary to obliteration of the coronary ostium in supravalvular aortic stenosis. Ann Thorac Surg 45:16, 1988.

151. McColl I: Pericarditis due to a mycotic aneurysm in subacute bacterial endocarditis: Report of a case affecting congenitally stenosed quadricuspid aortic valve. Guy Hosp Rep 107:34, 1958.

152. Pober BR, Lacro RV, Rice C, et al: Renal findings in 40 individuals with Williams syndrome. Am J Med Genet 46:271, 1993.

153. McDonald RE, Dean DC: Congenital quadricuspid aortic valve. Am J Cardiol 18:761, 1966.

154. McKusick VA, Logue B, Bahnson HT: Association of aortic valvular disease and cystic medial necrosis of the ascending aorta: Report of 4 instances. Circulation 16:188, 1957.

155. Miller MJ, Geffner ME, Lippe BM, et al: Echocardiography reveals a high incidence of bicuspid aortic valve in Turner's syndrome. J Pediatr 102:47, 1983.

156. Mills P, Leech G, Davies M, Leatham A: The natural history of non-stenotic bicuspid aortic valve. Br Heart J 40:951, 1978.

157. Mills PG, Brodie B, McLaurin L, et al: Echocardiographic and hemodynamic relationships of ejection sounds. Circulation 56:430, 1977.

158. Mocellin R, Saucer V, Simon B, et al: Reduced left ventricular size and endocardial fibroelastosis as correlates of mortality in newborns and young infants with severe aortic valve stenosis. Pediatr Cardiol 4:265, 1983.

159. Mody MR, Mody GT: Serial hemodynamic observations in congenital valvular and subvalvular aortic stenosis. Am Heart J 89:137, 1975.

160. Moller JH, Nakib A, Edwards JE: Infarction of papillary muscles and mitral insufficiency associated with congenital aortic stenosis. Circulation 44:87, 1966.

161. Morgan CL, Nadas AS: Sweating and congestive heart failure. N Engl J Med 268:580, 1963.

162. Morganroth J, Perloff JK, Zeldis S, Dunkman WB: Acute severe aortic regurgitation: Pathophysiology, clinical recognition and management. Ann Intern Med 87:223, 1977.

163. Morris CA, Leonard CO, Dilts C, Demsey CD: Adults with Williams syndrome. Am J Med Genet 6:102, 1990.

164. Morrow AG, Waldhausen JA, Peters RL, et al: Supravalvular aortic stenosis: Clinical, hemodynamic and pathologic observations. Circulation 20:1003, 1959.

165. Rein AJ, Preminger TJ, Perry SB, et al: Generalized arteriopathy in Williams syndrome. J Am Coll Cardiol 21:1727, 1993.

166. Motro M, Schneeweiss A, Shem-Tov A, et al: Correlation of distance from subaortic membrane to base of the right aortic valve cusp and the development of aortic regurgitation in mild discrete subaortic stenosis. Am J Cardiol 64:395, 1989.

167. Mounsey P: Precordial pulsations in relation to cardiac movement and sounds. Br Heart J 21:457, 1959.

168. Neilson G, Hossack KF: Supravalvular aortic stenosis in a twin. Br Heart J 40:1190, 1978.

169. Nelson WP, Hall RJ: The innocent supraclavicular arterial bruit: Utility of shoulder maneuvers in its recognition. N Engl J Med 278:778, 1968.

170. Neufeld HN, Wagenvoort CA, Ongley PA, Edwards JE: Hypoplasia of ascending aorta. Am J Cardiol 10:746, 1962.

171. Newfeld EA, Muster AJ, Paul MH, et al: Discrete subvalvular aortic stenosis in childhood. Am J Cardiol 38:53, 1976.

172. Prandstraller D, Mazzanti L, Picchio FM, et al: Turner's syndrome: Cardiologic profile according to the different chromosomal patterns and long-term clinical followup of 136 nonpreselected patients. Pediatr Cardiol 20:108, 1999.

173. Mazzanti L, Cacciari E: Congenital heart disease in patients with Turner's syndrome. J Pediatr 133:688, 1998.

174. Olson LJ, Subramanian R, Edwards WD: Surgical pathology of pure aortic insufficiency: A study of 225 cases. Mayo Clin Proc 59:385, 1984.

175. Ongley PA, Nadas AS, Paul MH, et al: Aortic stenosis in infants and children. Pediatrics 21:207, 1958.

176. Osler W: The bicuspid condition of the aortic valves. Trans Assoc Am Physicians 2:185, 1886.

177. Tentolouris K, Kontozoglou T, Trikas A, et al: Fixed subaortic revisited: Congenital abnormalities in 72 new cases and review of the literature. Cardiology 92:4, 1999.

178. Pagon RA, Bennett FC, LaVeck B, et al: Williams' syndrome: Features in late childhood and adolescence. Pediatrics 80:85, 1987.

179. Pansegrau DG, Kioshos JM, Durnin RE, Kroetz FW: Supravalvular aortic stenosis in adults. Am J Cardiol 31:635, 1973.

180. Simpson JM, Sharland GK: Natural history and outcome of aortic stenosis diagnosed prenatally. Heart 77:205, 1997.

181. Peacock TB: On Malformations of the Human Heart. London, John Churchill, 1858.

182. Peretz DI: Four-cusped aortic valve with significant hemodynamic abnormality. Am J Cardiol 23:291, 1969.

183. Perloff JK: Clinical recognition of aortic stenosis. Prog Cardiovasc Dis 10:323, 1968.
184. Perloff JK: Normal myocardial growth and the development and regression of increased ventricular mass. In Perloff JK, Child JS: Congenital Heart Disease in Adults, 2nd ed. Philadelphia, W.B. Saunders, 1998, p. 346.
185. Perloff JK: Physical Examination of the Heart and Circulation, 3rd ed. Philadelphia, W.B. Saunders, 2000.
186. Perloff JK, Roberts WC: The mitral apparatus: Functional anatomy of mitral regurgitation. Circulation 46:227, 1972.
187. Pomerance A: Pathogenesis of aortic stenosis and its relation to age. Br Heart J 34:569, 1972.
188. Pyle RL, Patterson DF, Chacko S: The genetics and pathology of discrete subaortic stenosis in the Newfoundland dog. Am Heart J 92:324, 1976.
189. Rakusan K, Flanagan MF, Geva T, et al: Morphometry of human coronary capillaries during normal growth and the effect of age in left ventricular pressure-overload hypertrophy. Circulation 86:38, 1992.
190. Reeve R Jr, Robinson SJ: Hypoplastic annulus—an unusual type of aortic stenosis: A report of three cases in children. Dis Chest 45:99, 1964.
191. Reynolds JL, Nadas AS, Rudolph AM, Gross RE: Critical congenital aortic stenosis with minimal electrocardiographic changes: A report on two siblings. N Engl J Med 262:276, 1960.
192. Richardson ME, Menahem S, Wilkinson JL: Familial fixed subaortic stenosis. Int J Cardiol 30:351, 1991.
193. Rio MT, Engle MA, O'Loughlin JE, et al: Congenital aortic regurgitation: Natural history and management. J Am Coll Cardiol 20:366, 1992.
194. Roberts WC: Anatomically isolated valvular disease: The cases against its being of rheumatic etiology. Am J Med 49:151, 1970.
195. Roberts WC: The congenitally bicuspid aortic valve: A study of 85 autopsy patients. Am J Cardiol 26:72, 1970.
196. Roberts WC: The structure of the aortic valve in clinically isolated aortic stenosis. Circulation 42:91, 1970.
197. Roberts WC: Valvular, subvalvular and supravalvular aortic stenosis. Cardiovasc Clin 5:104, 1973.
198. Roberts WC, Morrow AG: Congenital aortic stenosis produced by a unicommissural valve. Br Heart J 27:505, 1965.
199. Roberts WC, Morrow AG, McIntosh CL, et al: Congenitally bicuspid aortic valve causing severe, pure aortic regurgitation without superimposed infective endocarditis. Am J Cardiol 47:206, 1981.
200. Rockoff SD, Levine ND, Austin WG: Roentgenographic clues to the cardiac hemodynamics of aortic stenosis. Radiology 83:58, 1964.
201. Rosenkranz ER, Murphy DJ, Cosgrove DM: Surgical management of left coronary artery ostial atresia and supravalvular aortic stenosis. Ann Thorac Surg 54:779, 1992.
202. Sabbah HN, Stein PD: Mechanism of early systolic closure of the aortic valve in discrete membranous subaortic stenosis. Circulation 65:399, 1982.
203. Sabbah HN, Khaja F, Anbe DT, Stein PD: The aortic closure sound in pure aortic insufficiency. Circulation 56:859, 1977.
204. Saddee AS, Becker AE, Verheul HA, et al: Aortic valve regurgitation and the congenitally bicuspid aortic valve: A clinico-pathological correlation. Br Heart J 67:439, 1992.
205. Saylam A, Ozme S, Aslamaci S, et al: Aortico-left ventricular tunnel. Thorac Cardiovasc Surg 29:259, 1981.
206. Scheffer SM, Leatherman LL: Resolution of Heyde's syndrome of aortic stenosis and gastrointestinal bleeding after aortic valve replacement. Ann Thorac Surg 42:477, 1986.
207. Schneeweiss A, Motro M, Shem-Tov A, et al: Echocardiographic diagnosis of a discrete membranous subaortic stenosis with aneurysm of the membrane. Chest 82:194, 1982.
208. Schwartz LS, Goldfischer J, Sprague GJ, Schwartz SP: Syncope and sudden death in aortic stenosis. Am J Cardiol 23:647, 1969.
209. Shem-Tov A, Schneeweiss A, Motro M, Neufeld HN: Clinical presentation and natural history of mild discrete subaortic stenosis. Circulation 66:509, 1982.
210. Shen WF, Roubin GS, Choong CY, et al: Evaluation of relationship between myocardial contractile state and left ventricular function in patients with aortic regurgitation. Circulation 71:31, 1985.
211. Sievers HH, Regensburger D, Bernhard A: Quadricuspid aortic valve with significant insufficiency. Thorac Cardiovasc Surg 30:44, 1982.
212. Simon AL, Reis R: The angiographic features of bicuspid and unicommissural aortic stenosis. Am J Cardiol 28:353, 1971.
213. Sono J, McKay R, Arnold RM: Accessory mitral valve leaflet causing aortic regurgitation and left ventricular outflow tract obstruction: Case report and review of published reports. Br Heart J 59:491, 1988.
214. Spindola-Franco H, Fish BG, Dachman A, et al: Recognition of bicuspid aortic valve by plain film calcification. Am J Radiol 139:867, 1982.
215. Sreeram N, Franks R, Walsh K: Aortic-ventricular tunnel in a neonate: Diagnosis and management based on cross sectional and colour Doppler ultrasonography. Br Heart J 65:161, 1991.
216. Starc TJ, Bowman FO, Hordof AJ: Congestive heart failure in a newborn secondary to coronary artery-left ventricular fistula. Am J Cardiol 58:366, 1986.
217. Stein PD: A new roentgenographic assessment of anatomic deformity in calcific aortic stenosis. Am Heart J 84:321, 1972.
218. Stein PD, Sabbah HN, Pitha JV: Continuing disease process of calcific aortic stenosis: Role of microthrombi and turbulent flow. Am J Cardiol 39:159, 1977.
219. Strasburger JF, Kugler JD, Cheatham JP, McManus BM: Nonimmunologic hydrops fetalis associated with congenital aortic valvular stenosis. Am Heart J 108:1380, 1984.
220. Subramanian R, Olson LJ, Edwards WD: Surgical pathology of pure aortic stenosis: A study of 374 cases. Mayo Clin Proc 59:683, 1984.
221. Tomanek RJ: Age as a modulator of coronary capillary angiogenesis. Circulation 86:320, 1992.
222. Underhill WL, Tredway JB, D'Angelo GJ, Baay JEW: Familial supravalvular aortic stenosis: Comments on the mechanisms of angina pectoris. Am J Cardiol 27:560, 1971.
223. Varghese PJ, Izukawa T, Rowe RD: Supravalvular aortic stenosis as part of the rubella syndrome with discussion of pathogenesis. Br Heart J 31:59, 1969.
224. Vincent WR, Buckberg GD, Hoffman JIE: Left ventricular subendocardial ischemia in severe valvular and supravalvular aortic stenosis: A common mechanism. Circulation 49:326, 1974.
225. Vollebergh FEMG, Becker AE: Minor congenital variations of cusp size in tricuspid aortic valves. Br Heart J 39:1006, 1977.
226. Waider W, Craige E: First heart sound and ejection sounds. Echocardiographic and phonocardiographic correlation with valvular events. Am J Cardiol 35:346, 1975.
227. Waller BF, Taliercio CP, Dickos DK, et al: Rare or unusual causes of chronic, isolated, pure aortic regurgitation. Clin Cardiol 13:577, 1990.
228. Welch GH, Braunwald E, Sarnoff SJ: Hemodynamic effects of quantitatively varied experimental aortic regurgitation. Circ Res 5:546, 1957.
229. Whittaker AV, Shaver JA, Gray S, Leonard JJ: Sound-pressure correlates of the aortic ejection sound. Circulation 29:475, 1969.
230. Wigle ED, Labrosse CJ: Sudden severe aortic insufficiency. Circulation 32:708, 1965.
231. Williams IC, Barratt-Boyes BG, Lowe IB: Supravalvular aortic stenosis. Circulation 24:1311, 1961.
232. Williams RL, Azouz EM: Aortic anomalies in an adolescent with the Williams' elfin facies syndrome. Pediatr Radiol 14:122, 1984.
233. Wood P: Aortic stenosis. Am J Cardiol 1:553, 1958.
234. Wu J, Huang T, Chen Y, et al: Aortico-left ventricular tunnel: Two-dimensional echocardiographic and angiocardiographic features. Am Heart J 117:697, 1989.

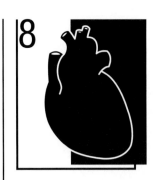

Coarctation of the Aorta

8

Coarctation of the Aorta

In 1760, the Prussian anatomist Johann Friedreich Meckel characterized coarctation of the aorta as an "extraordinary dilatation of the heart which came from the fact that the aortic conduit was too narrow."[104] Jarcho's informative historical papers underscored the clarity of early accounts of this congenital malformation.[103–107]

Coarctation of the aorta is typically located near the aortic attachment of the ligamentum arteriosum or patent ductus arteriosus (Figs. 8–1A and 8–2). An obtuse indentation in the posterolateral wall of the aorta corresponds to the location of an internal ridge or shelf that eccentrically narrows the aortic lumen, hence the term *coarctatus* (L), which means "contracted, tightened, or pressed together." The ridge that forms the coarctation consists of smooth muscle, fibrous tissue, and elastic tissue similar in composition to a muscular arterial ductus (see Chapter 20).[66,188] Intimal proliferation distal to the ridge culminates in nar-

rowing of the lumen.[66,188] The junction between the ductus and the elastic aorta is clearly defined, and extension of ductal tissue into the aortic wall does not exceed 30% of the aortic circumference.[188] However, in coarctation of the aorta, especially preductal coarctation, ductal tissue forms a circumferential sling that extends around the aorta.[188] In juxtaductal coarctation, ductal tissue is not a significant part of the aortic wall.[138] The coarctation ridge is thought to represent the original wall of the distal left sixth aortic arch (the ductus arteriosus; see Chapter 20). The neural crest is believed to play a role in the pathogenesis of some forms of coarctation.[138]

The common form of coarctation of the aorta is represented by a localized constriction containing the ridge or shelf, as just described.[66] Less commonly, a relatively long segment of constriction extends beyond the left subclavian artery. *Tubular hypoplasia* refers to uniform narrowing within the aortic arch.[66] Localized coarctation and tubular hypoplasia can coexist or occur independently.

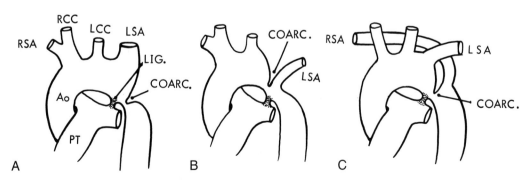

Figure 8–1
A, Typical coarctation of the aorta showing the localized obstruction is just *distal* to the left subclavian artery (LSA). Ao, ascending aorta; LCC, left common carotid artery; LIG, ligamentum arteriosum; PT, pulmonary trunk; RCC, right common carotid artery; RSA, right subclavian artery. *B,* Coarctation is immediately proximal to the left subclavian artery. *C,* The right subclavian artery (RSA) arises anomalously distal to the coarctation.

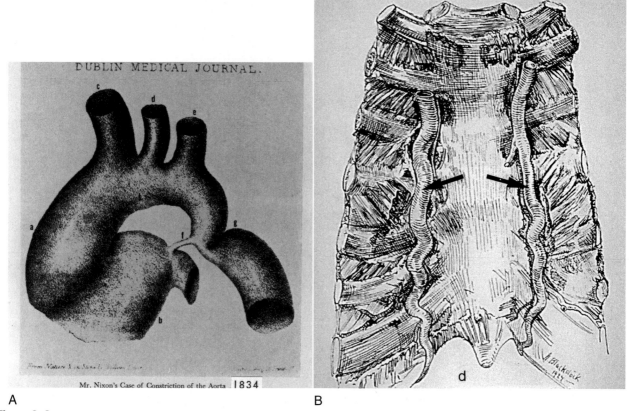

A   **B**

Figure 8–2

A, An anatomic drawing of coarctation of the aorta published in 1834. (From Nixon RL: Dublin J Med. In Chem Sci 5:386–400, 1834; courtesy of Dr. Saul Jarcho). *B,* Anatomical drawing of retrosternal internal mammary artery collaterals (*arrows*) in coarctation of the aorta. (*B,* As seen printed in Maude Abbott's *Atlas of Congenital Cardiac Disease* in 1936, Osler Library, McGill University.)

The mechanisms responsible for the location of coarctation take into account a number of variables: (1) the quantitative morphology and growth of the aortic arch in the normal fetus[96,123,153]; (2) the site of the aortic orifice of the ductus arteriosus; (3) the presence of ductal tissue in the coarctation[66,188]; (4) constriction of ductal tissue immediately after birth; (5) the occurrence of coarctation in the presence of a widely patent ductus in the fetus[3,4]; and (6) the occurrence of coarctation in the presence of a widely patent ductus after birth.[66] Current consensus favors an interplay between aortic growth and blood flow.[96,123,153] High-resolution echocardiographic imaging in the normal fetus has disclosed progressive tapering of the diameter of the aortic arch at all gestational ages, with the smallest diameter consistently at the isthmus.[96] Tapering is believed to reflect the relative proportion of fetal cardiac output traversing each aortic segment. The smallest proportion traverses the isthmus, which retains its smaller dimension relative to the remainder of the aortic arch well into postnatal life, especially in premature infants.[96] Neonatal coarctation is characterized by relative hypoplasia of the transverse aorta in the presence of a relatively large pulmonary trunk, a combination that is believed to reflect an in utero decrease in aortic arch flow together with an increase in flow through the main pulmonary artery and the ductus.[153]

The coarctation ridge is located either immediately proximal to the aortic insertion of the ductus, or opposite the aortic insertion (juxtaductal), or immediately distal to the aortic insertion.[66,186,224] Infants with a juxtaductal coarctation show no signs of aortic obstruction as long as a widely patent ductus ensures unobstructed pulmonary trunk–ductus–descending aortic continuity. When the ductus closes, the coarctation becomes apparent immediately and dramatically, and the femoral pulses disappear.

The left subclavian artery is dilated because coarctation is located immediately distal to the subclavian origin (Figs. 8–3D and 8–4A, and see Fig. 8–1A) However, coarctation may lie at or proximal to the left subclavian orifice, compromising the lumen (see Figs. 8–1B and 8–27).[98,109] Exceptionally, the right subclavian artery arises distal to the coarctation (see Fig. 8–1C) or the coarctation resides in a right aortic arch.[125]

Coarctation of the abdominal aorta can be part of a systemic vascular disorder such as Takayasu arteritis or von Recklinghausen disease but can also be congenital and is therefore an appropriate topic for inclusion here.[12,20,31,47,89,126,178,182,237] Abdominal coarctation is rare, accounting for 0.5% to 2% of all varieties of aortic coarctation.[126] The percentage of cases that are congenital is unknown. Abdominal coarctation can be suprarenal, infrarenal, or inter-renal,[126] and systemic hypertension is

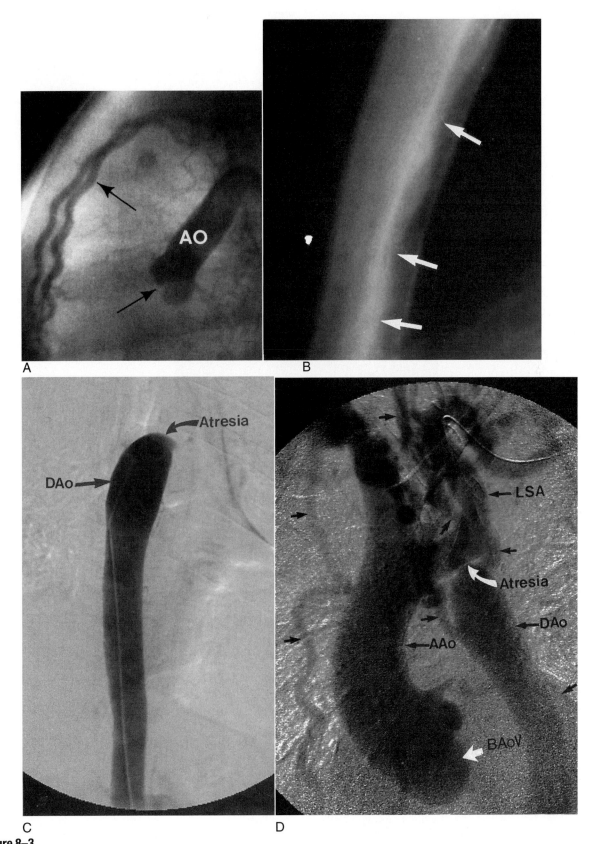

Figure 8–3

A, Lateral view of large retrosternal internal mammary arteries (*upper left arrow*) in a 9-year-old boy with coarctation of the aorta. The ascending aorta (AO) is moderately dilated above a bicuspid aortic valve (*lower arrow*). *B*, Close-up of the lateral chest x-ray showing retrosternal notching (*arrows*). *C*, Retrograde descending aortogram (DAo) of a 65-year-old man with coarctation of the aorta and atresia at the coarctation site. *D*, Lateral ascending aortogram showing the coarctation atresia (*curved white arrow*), proximal to which the left subclavian artery (LSA) is dilated. The descending aorta (DAo) opacified through abundant collaterals (*unmarked arrows*). Internal mammary collaterals (*two left arrows*) were responsible for retrosternal notching. The ascending aorta (AAo) is dilated above a bicuspid aortic valve (BaoV).

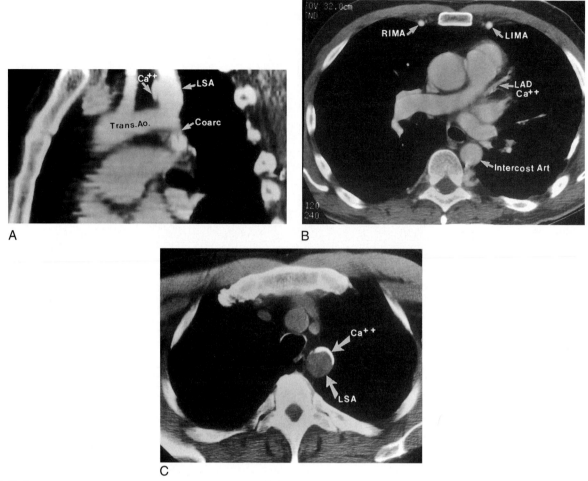

A

B

C

Figure 8–4
Magnetic resonance imaging scans from a 62-year-old woman. *A,* Sagittal plane shows the site of coarctation (coarc) distal to a dilated left subclavian artery (LSA) that is calcified (Ca^{++}). Trans Ao, transverse aorta. *B,* Transverse plane shows the right internal mammary (RIMA) and left internal mammary artery collaterals (LIMA), a large intercostal arterial collateral (Intercost Art), and calcium in the left anterior descending coronary artery (LAD Ca^{++}). *C,* Calcified dilated left subclavian artery (LSA).

believed to reflect renal artery involvement.[182] Congenital origin is based on the combination of a localized hourglass deformity with an intraluminal membrane, occurrence at a young age, absence of a systemic vascular disorder, and slow progression with development of extensive collaterals.[182]

Pseudocoarctation refers to a rare anomaly characterized by buckling or kinking of the aorta in the vicinity of the ligamentum arteriosum, resulting in elongation, tortuosity, and dilatation of the distal aortic arch and the proximal descending aorta (Fig. 8–5).[*] "Pseudo" correctly implies absence of a gradient at the site of the localized external deformity, absence of collaterals, and absence of systemic hypertension. The femoral pulses are occasionally reduced because of the damping effect of sharp angulation of the aortic arch (see Fig. 8–5).[21] Pseudocoarctation is not necessarily benign and is not necessarily "pseudo." Thin-walled saccular aneurysms may form in the distal segment,[13] spontaneous rupture and dissection have been

reported in the proximal descending thoracic aorta[63] and in the ascending aorta,[121,235] and true coarctation may coexist with *pseudo*coarctation.[52] A bicuspid aortic valve has been reported with pseudocoarctation[9] that occasionally involves the abdominal aorta.[68]

Certain congenital cardiac and vascular malformations tend to be associated with coarctation of the aorta. The strongest association is with a bicuspid aortic valve that is either functionally normal, stenotic, or incompetent (Fig. 8–6B, and see Chapter 7).[1,16,36,62,71,113] The bicuspid valve that accompanies coarctation is equally bicuspid, with the orifice positioned centrally between two equal sinuses of Valsalva.[71] A decrease in left ventricular interpapillary muscle distance is common[30,51,73] and culminates in the single papillary muscle of a parachute mitral valve (see Chapter 9).[16,38,41,183,184,202] The endocardial fibroelastosis associated with coarctation is patchy rather than confluent.[151,164] Two shunt lesions accompany coarctation of the aorta, namely, patent ductus arteriosus[15,36,77,93] and ventricular septal defect.[8,15,77,148,158,212] The ventricular septal defect is usually characterized by leftward malalignment that

---

[*]13, 21, 59, 86, 95, 124, 156, 214, 217, 235, 242

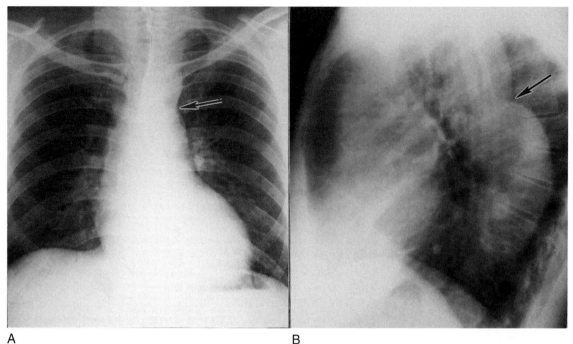

Figure 8–5

A, Anteroposterior x-ray from a 62-year-old man with pseudocoarctation characterized by buckling of the aorta (*arrows*) in the vicinity of the ligamentum arteriosum. The aortic lumen is not narrowed at the site of the external deformity. *B,* Lateral x-ray from a 68-year-old woman with pseudocoarctation illustrating the buckled aorta.

curtails the amount of left ventricular blood reaching the aortic isthmus.[8,148,212,229]

A variety of vascular disorders occur with coarctation of the aorta. Dissecting aneurysm with hemopericardium was reported in 1830.[57] The substrate for aneurysm formation is the inherent abnormality of medial smooth muscle and extracellular matrix that is a consistent feature of the proximal and distal paracoarctation aorta.[99,159] Aneurysms of the circle of Willis set the stage for fatal intracranial hemorrhage (Fig. 8–7, and see further discussion under The History). A large aneurysm of the left subclavian artery can acutely dissect.[120] Relatively benign aneurysms occasionally develop in intercostal arteries.[232]

Arterial collaterals are important vascular sequelae of coarctation of the aorta and depend for their development on subclavian artery patency (see Figs 8–3 and 8–6*A*). When coarctation obstructs the orifice of the left subclavian artery, collaterals fail to develop on that side (see Fig 8–27). A subclavian steal may be caused by retrograde flow down the ipsilateral vertebral artery.[53]

Retinal arterioles are the site of a benign and unexplained vascular pattern.[110] In 1948 at the annual meeting of the Swedish Ophthalmological Society, Professor K.O. Granstrom stated, "As in other cases of hypertension, these patients are sent as a matter of routine for examination to the eye department. As soon as I had seen a few such cases, it became evident that the retinal picture in coarctation of the aorta is often somewhat characteristic, the principal feature being pronounced tortuosity of the arteries. . . . I therefore expressed the opinion that it should be possible . . . to distinguish between coarctation of the aorta and other cases of juvenile hypertension by means of ophthalmoscopy."[133] The U-shaped tortuous retinal arterioles (Fig. 8–8) may be accompanied by serpentine pulsations that are synchronous with the arterial pulse.[110] Granstrom correctly concluded that the distinctive retinal abnormality in coarctation was benign, and that hypertensive retinopathy was conspicuous by its absence. "Other retinal changes usually present in hypertensive disorders . . . are almost entirely lacking."[133]

Coarctation of the aorta can contribute to the formation of a vascular ring associated with a double aortic arch,[161] a right aortic arch, a left ligamentum arteriosum, or an aberrant subclavian artery.[10,45,101] A double aortic arch with coarctation of one of the limbs of the double arch has been responsible for a vascular ring.[67] An anomalous retroesophageal right subclavian artery occasionally accompanies coarctation of the aorta (see Fig. 8–1*C*) but does not cause tracheoesophageal compression.

The pathogenesis of systemic hypertension in coarctation of the aorta has been the subject of three theories. The mechanical theory focuses on resistance at the site of obstruction. This theory in itself cannot be sustained, but it is central to the neural theory that involves the distensibility characteristics of the precoarctation aorta and the sensitivity of carotid sinus baroreceptors.[146,193] Elastic properties of the normal aorta decrease with distance from the aortic root. In coarctation of the aorta, the proximal aortic segment is characterized by an increase in collagen and a decrease in smooth muscle[19,193] that are responsible for an increase in stiffness and a decrease in distensibility.[155] The relatively noncompliant precoarctation aorta is responsible for the elevation of systolic blood pressure at rest and the

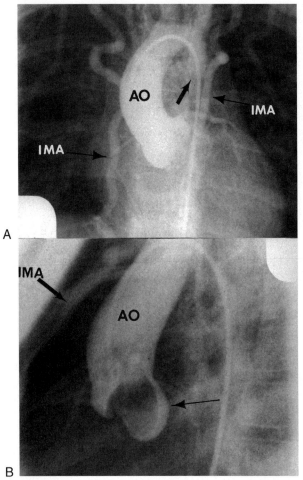

Figure 8–6

Aortograms (AO) from a 9-year-old boy with coarctation of the aorta and a bicuspid aortic valve. *A,* The *thick oblique arrow* points to the coarctation. The *two thin arrows* identify internal mammary artery collaterals (IMA). *B,* Lateral aortogram showing the bicuspid aortic valve (*unmarked arrow*) above which the aorta (AO) is dilated. There is a large retrosternal internal mammary artery collateral (IMA).

disproportionate rise during isotonic exercise[165] and is also held responsible for resetting the carotid sinus baroreceptors to operate at higher pressures.[97,193]

The renal theory of pathogenesis takes into account a unique feature of coarctation hypertension, namely, that the elevated blood pressure is confined to the upper extremities. Accordingly, the renal arteries are exposed to the neurohumoral effects of hypertension without being exposed to the hydraulic effects of elevated blood pressure.[6,11,33] The coarctation gradient increases during isotonic exercise and is accompanied by a disproportionate increase in systolic pressure,[49] which is an exaggeration of the inherent disproportionate systolic hypertension related to rigidity of the precoarctation aortic wall. The mean blood pressure response to exercise in coarctation is approximately the same as in control subjects.[60] Hypertension has been produced when experimental constriction of the aorta consigns the renal arteries to the distal low pressure zone.[5] When experimental aortic constriction is placed *below* the renal arteries, blood pres-

sure remains normal.[5,234] Coarctation hypertension is seldom accompanied by vascular disease. Toxemia of pregnancy is not a feature of coarctation hypertension.[198] Eye grounds do not exhibit hypertensive retinopathy[5,65,231] but instead exhibit the distinctive retinal arterioles of coarctation (see Fig. 8–8).[65,110,231]

The increase in left ventricular mass induced by the afterload of coarctation is characterized by myocyte replication rather than myocyte hypertrophy,[168] which is believed to account for reduced end-systolic wall stress and enhanced left ventricular ejection performance.[26,56]

THE HISTORY

The male-to-female ratio of coarctation ranges from 1.4:1 to 3:1.[35,36,69,77] Familial recurrence has been reported in siblings, in monozygotic twins, in parent and child,[36,82,154,184, 192,207,226,238] and as an autosomal dominant trait in four generations.[17] True coarctation and pseudocoarctation have been reported in siblings.[115] Turner syndrome (see Physical Appearance) results in sterility and cannot be transmitted. However, seven women in three generations of one family had Turner syndrome attributed to loss of the short arm of one X chromosome that permitted transmission from phenotypically normal female carriers with a balanced X-1 translocation.[127] A peak seasonal incidence of coarctation has been observed in September through November and in January through March.[141] The stated rarity of coarctation in black Americans is open to question.[90,228] Hypoplasia of the abdominal aorta (abdominal coarctation) has been described in offspring of mothers with rubella (see earlier).

Coarctation of the aorta tends to produce significant symptoms in early infancy[10,69,91,108,128,225] and after the age of 20 or 30 years.[34] Neonates with severe juxtaductal coarctation become acutely symptomatic when the ductus closes. The majority of those who survive the potential hazards of infancy reach adulthood, although more than a quarter die by 20 years of age, half by 30 years of age, and more than three quarters by 50 years of age.[1,34,35,177] Figures 8–24 and 8–26 are from patients aged 54 years, 62 years, and 70 years. Survival has been reported at ages 74 years[88] and 76 years.[116] Isolated atresia of the aortic arch was surgically repaired in a patient 65 years of age.[144] The longest recorded survival with coarctation was Raynaud's account (1828) in a 92-year-old man.[106] Raynaud's remarkable anatomic illustrations are even more noteworthy. However, these examples of exceptional longevity should not obscure the inherent risk of coarctation that results in death at an average age of 33 years.

Mild coarctation of the aorta does not necessarily have a benign long-term outlook, underscoring that coarctation is more than a mechanical disorder. Except for symptomatic infants, patients tend to be clinically well when the diagnosis is first made.[77] Initial suspicion requires little more than attention to upper and lower extremity arterial pulses and blood pressure (see The Arterial Pulse). Nevertheless, delayed recognition is not unusual,[220,233] and the diagnosis has been made by chance as late as the fifth decade.[28] Minor

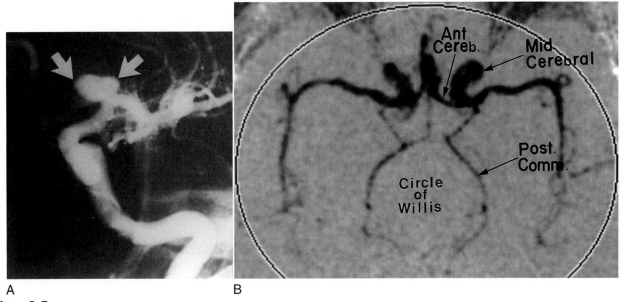

A
B

Figure 8–7

A, Cerebral arteriogram from a 28-year-old woman. There is an 11-mm aneurysm of the circle of Willis (*paired arrows*). *B,* Normal circle of Willis showing the delicate posterior communicating artery (Post Comm). The middle cerebral artery and anterior cerebral artery are not parts of the circle of Willis.

symptoms include epistaxis and leg fatigue. Muscular fatigue involving the left arm occurs when the orifice of the left subclavian artery is compromised by coarctation in left-handed patients. Leg fatigue occurs in about half of patients,[77] but claudication is reserved for abdominal coarctation. Patients are sometimes subjectively aware of arterial pulsations in the neck, especially after effort or excitement. Dysphagia may occur when a retroesophageal right subclavian artery originates distal to the coarctation and passes behind the esophagus[205] (see Fig. 8–1C) or when coarctation is a component of a vascular ring.

Major symptoms are related to four eventualities: (1) congestive heart failure, (2) rupture or dissection of the aorta, (3) infective endarteritis or endocarditis, and (4) cerebral hemorrhage.[18,34,61,128,200] Hypertension is chiefly responsible for morbidity and mortality with advancing age.[128] The incidence of cardiac failure is highest in infants[69,83,91,209] and is high again after the fourth decade.[35] In a review of 234 patients with coarctation of the aorta, aged 1 day to 72 years, congestive heart failure occurred in 67% of patients younger than 1 year of age and in 67% of patients older than 40 years of age but in only 4% of patients between 1 year and 40 years of age.[128] Many, if not most, of the neonates and infants who experience congestive heart failure have a coexisting ventricular septal defect or patent ductus arteriosus.[16,84,158,201] The corollary is that little or no difficulty is experienced by the more than 90% of infants and children with uncomplicated coarctation.[91]

When coarctation is juxtaductal or proximal to the neonatal ductus, continuity between the pulmonary trunk and descending aorta is maintained and the femoral arterial pulses remain palpable.[66,83] When the ductus closes, femoral pulses disappear, pulmonary blood flow is diverted into the lungs, the left ventricle is suddenly volume overloaded, and the blood pressure and blood flow proximal to the coarctation suddenly increase. A high left atrial pressure opens the pliant valve of the foramen ovale, initiating a left-to-right shunt that imposes volume load on the already pressure-overloaded pulmonary hypertensive right ventricle.[108] Initial closure of the pulmonary arterial end of the ductus may temporarily leave the aortic end of the ductus sufficiently patent to permit the proximal aorta to decompress.[224] When the aortic end of the ductus closes, the isthmus is suddenly obstructed; distal aortic pressure, flow, and renal perfusion fall; and the renin-angiotensin system is activated.[5,11,14]

Rupture or dissection of the aorta is a dramatic complication of coarctation with peak incidence in the third and fourth decades.[35,61,128,177] Rupture originates in either a paracoarctation aneurysm because of an inherent medial abnormality[61,99,159,236] or in the ascending aorta above a coexisting bicuspid aortic valve because of an inherent medial abnormality at that site (see Chapter 7).[35,61,159]

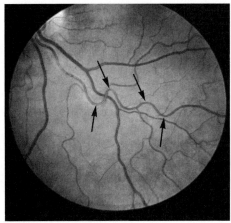

Figure 8–8

Typical U-shaped corkscrew retinal arterioles (*arrows*) in a 22-year-old woman with coarctation of the aorta.

Rupture of a post-coarctation aneurysm may be accompanied by bleeding into the esophagus that is announced by hematemesis and melena.[236] In XO Turner syndrome (see Physical Appearance), rupture or dissection of an ascending aortic aneurysm occurs because of an inherent medial abnormality[159] whether or not coarctation of the aorta or a bicuspid aortic valve coexists (Fig. 8–9).[7,80,129,132,219] Aneurysms of intercostal arteries are almost always occult and therefore relatively benign.[232] Pseudocoarctation has been regarded as a disorder that incurs little or no risk, but the malformation is not necessarily benign and is not necessarily "pseudo" (see earlier). Pseudocoarctation has been reported with Turner syndrome.[119] Cerebral arterial aneurysms are discussed under cerebrovascular accidents (see later).

Infective endarteritis or endocarditis is a major complication of coarctation of the aorta, although the more susceptible site is a coexisting bicuspid aortic valve (see Chapter 7).[34,35,128] Saccular septic aneurysms may be sequelae of infective endarteritis.[61]

Cerebrovascular accidents are the fourth major eventuality in coarctation of the aorta.[18,35,128,200] Hypertension is not a necessary precondition, because cerebral complications occur in normotensive patients long after successful repair. An aneurysm of the circle of Willis first described in 1927[243] is the chief offender (see Fig. 8–7) and sets the stage for rupture and cerebral hemorrhage.[94] Less commonly but not less importantly, aneurysms occur in other cerebral arteries.[18] Bicuspid aortic valve infective endocarditis can give rise to septic cerebral aneurysms that rupture.[35] Rarely, an unruptured intracranial aneurysm has triggered musical hallucinations.[145]

Coarctation hypertension is a risk factor for premature atherosclerotic coronary artery disease (see Fig. 8–4B and earlier discussion).[128,189,230] There is also evidence of structural abnormalities of terminal intramural coronary arteries.[189] Gonadal dysgenesis of Turner syndrome reportedly increases atherosclerotic cardiovascular risk.[135]

Pregnancy is accompanied by blood pressure fluctuations that are similar in direction to fluctuations in uncomplicated pregnancy but from a higher baseline.[35,170,198] In pregnant women with coarctation, which is not a resistance vessel disease, the incidence of toxemia is lower than in pregnant women with other forms of hypertension.[170,198] Pregnancy increases the risk of aortic rupture

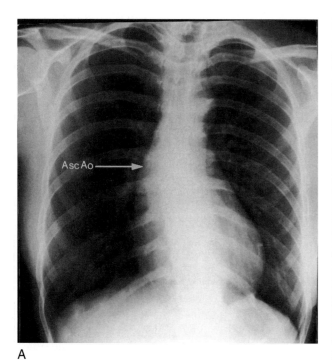

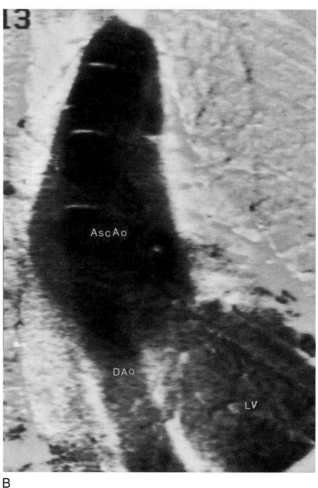

A   B

Figure 8–9

A, X-ray from a 28-year-old woman with 45XO Turner syndrome, an aneurysm of the ascending aorta (Asc Ao), and a bicuspid aortic valve. *B,* Digital vascular image angiogram after injection of contrast material into the superior vena cava. The ascending aortic aneurysm ruptured 8 weeks later. DAo, descending aorta; LV, left ventricle.

and the risk of intracranial hemorrhage, because gestational changes in connective tissue reinforce the inherent medial abnormalities in the arterial walls.[35,159,170,198]

PHYSICAL APPEARANCE

An athletic appearance of the chest and shoulders contrasts with narrow hips and thin legs in patients with coarctation of the aorta.[35] When coarctation compromises the origin of the left subclavian artery, the left arm may be smaller than normal. General growth and development are impaired in infants with congestive heart failure.

XO Turner syndrome, with its distinctive physical appearance (Figs. 8–10 and 8–11), prompts suspicion of coarctation of the aorta.[35,36,79,162] Chromosomal patterns 45XO, X-mosaicism, and X-structural abnormalities are coupled with other cardiac expressions.[40,46,87,139,142] Aortic rupture or dissection in Turner syndrome was mentioned earlier (see Fig. 8–9).[7,64,80,129,218,219,241] The typical XO Turner phenotypic female (see Fig. 8–10) is of short stature with webbing of the neck, absent or scanty auxiliary and pubic hair (ovarian dysgenesis), broad chest with widely spaced hypoplastic or inverted nipples, low anterior and posterior hairlines, small chin, prominent ears because

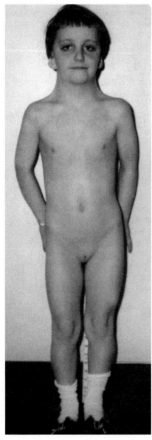

Figure 8–10
Thirteen-year-old girl with 45XO Turner syndrome and coarctation of the aorta. Physical appearance is characterized by short stature, webbing of the neck, absent pubic hair, wide-set nipples, and small chin. Bangs obscure a low anterior hair line.

of large auricles, cubitus valgus, short fourth metacarpals and metatarsals, distal palmar triaxial radii, narrow hyperconvex nails, and pigmented cutaneous nevi.[162,227] Infants with Turner syndrome exhibit lymphedema with loose skin of the neck, puffiness of the dorsum of the hands and feet, and low hairlines.[131,162] Congenital heart disease is much more frequent in patients with Turner syndrome with webbing of the neck than in patients with Turner syndrome without webbing,[40,131] and coarctation of the aorta is eight times as frequent when Turner syndrome is accompanied by webbing of the neck.[131] Noonan syndrome (Turner phenotype with normal genotype) (see Fig. 8–11) is only occasionally accompanied by coarctation of the aorta[163] and rarely by ascending aortic aneurysm.[162,195,204]

THE ARTERIAL PULSE

Forceful carotid and suprasternal notch pulsations become increasingly apparent with age and exercise because of the disproportionate systolic hypertension associated with stiffness of the precoarctation aortic wall (see earlier).[97,165,193] Abnormal differences in upper and lower extremity arterial pulses and blood pressure are hallmarks of coarctation of the aorta. If proper attention were paid to these physical signs, few or no diagnoses would be missed.[169,233] Two methods have been advocated for comparing upper and lower extremity pulses. One method compares femoral and radial pulses. The other method compares femoral and brachial pulses. Radial and femoral pulses are normally sensed as synchronous, so that *any* femoral delay is considered abnormal. Positioning the patient's wrist next to the groin is believed to facilitate comparison. In infants and newborns, palpation of the brachial artery (Fig. 8–12*B*) is technically easier than palpating the tiny radial artery, which is surrounded by subcutaneous fat pads. I therefore recommend comparative palpation of brachial and femoral pulses, which is accomplished by placing a thumb on each (see Fig. 8–12*A*).[169]

The slight delay in perceived arrival time of the normal femoral pulse (15 msec in adults, less in infants and children) is easily established as a norm against which even slight deviations can be judged. When the examiner is palpating the femoral pulse in an infant, the baby must be allowed to relax its legs voluntarily, because restraint can decrease or abolish a normal femoral pulse. What is sensed as the abnormal femoral delay associated with aortic coarctation is not a delay in arrival time of the pulse, but instead the slow rate of rise of the pulse to a delayed peak (Fig. 8–13). When the femoral arterial pulse is unequivocally reduced, diagnostic differences between upper and lower extremities are also unequivocal. A normal femoral pulse effectively eliminates all but mild coarctation provided the aortic valve is functioning normally (see later). Palpation begins by focusing separately on the brachial and femoral arterial pulse, applying to each the amount of digital pressure required to elicit the maximum systolic impact.[169]

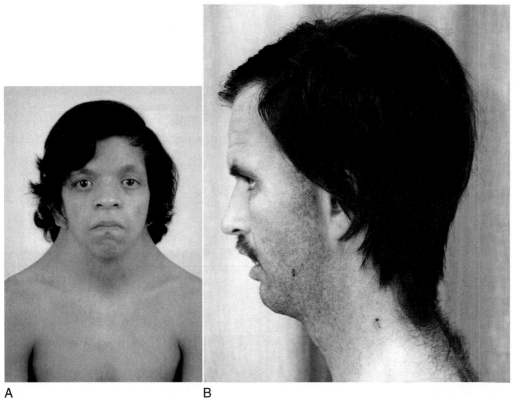

A   B

Figure 8–11

A, Eighteen-year-old man with Noonan syndrome (Turner phenotype with normal genotype). There is typical webbing of the neck. Long hair obscures low anterior and posterior hair lines. *B*, Twenty-four-year-old man with Noonan syndrome (Turner phenotype with normal genotype) and dissecting aneurysm of the ascending aorta. There is a low posterior hairline, low-set auricles, and micrognathia.

Bicuspid aortic regurgitation reinforces the femoral pulse, which can be misjudged as normal unless properly compared with the brachial pulse (Fig. 8–14*A*).[77] Bicuspid aortic stenosis can be misjudged by the brachial arterial pulse because coarctation amplifies the ascending aortic and brachial arterial systolic pressure (see Fig. 8–14*B*).[77] Conversely, aortic stenosis damps the ascending aortic systolic pressure and may obscure evidence of coarctation (Fig. 8–14*C*).[77]

The right and left brachial arteries should be compared by palpation and by blood pressure determinations (see Fig. 8–12*B*). A decreased or absent left brachial arterial pulse indicates that the coarctation has compromised the lumen of the left subclavian artery (see Fig. 8–1*B*) or is proximal to its origin.[35,109] Comparison of the two brachial pulses recognizes that systolic pressure is normally 10 to 15 mm Hg lower in the left arm.[169] Diminution or absence of the right brachial pulse implies that the right subclavian artery originates distal to the coarctation (see Fig. 8–1*C*). Absence of *both* brachial arterial pulses signifies that coarctation is compromising the lumen of the left subclavian artery while the right subclavian artery arises distal to the coarctation.[221] Femoral arterial pulses are temporarily palpable at birth if the coarctation is juxtaductal, if the ductus is distal to the coarctation, or if the aortic end of the ductus is patent.[66,83] The abdominal aorta is readily palpable proximal to an abdominal coarctation but is not palpable in the presence of coarctation of the aortic isthmus. Pseudocoarctation leaves the arterial pulses normal because there is no aortic obstruction, although angulation at the level of the ligamentum arteriosum occasionally damps the distal aortic and femoral pulses (see Fig. 8–5).[21]

Collateral arterial pulsations must be specifically sought by having patients who are old enough stand and bend forward with arms hanging at the sides while the examiner scrutinizes the patient's back, especially around and between the scapulae.[37] A tangential light in a darkened room highlights subcutaneous collaterals in shadowed relief. Collateral arteries occasionally appear around the shoulders, along the right and left sternal borders, and, rarely, over the upper abdominal wall.

Cuff blood pressure is an important supplement to the information derived from palpation of the arterial pulses. Blood pressure should be measured in the right and left arms and in a leg. Correct cuff size is mandatory, because improper cuff size results in inaccurate readings.[24,117,136,157,167,169] An undersized cuff overestimates and an oversized cuff underestimates intra-arterial blood pressure by as much as 10 to 30 mm Hg.[167] The American Heart Association recommendations for cuff size are shown in Table 8–1.[117] References to cuff size apply to the width and length of the inner inflatable bladder, not to the cloth covering. Cuff size is determined by limb circumference, not by patient age. The width of the inflatable bladder within the cuff should be 40% of the circumference of the midpoint of the limb. The

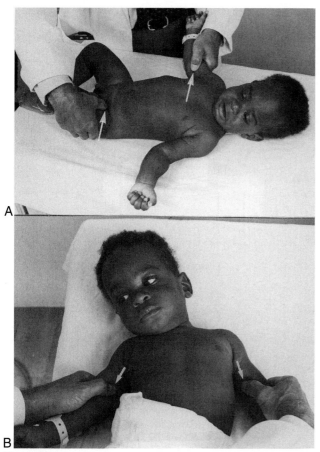

Figure 8–12

A, Palpation of brachial and femoral arteries as illustrated here is a useful way of comparing upper and lower extremity pulses. Application of the thumbs allows either simultaneous or sequential palpation, which permits detection of subtle differences in amplitude and timing. *B,* Recommended method of simultaneous palpation of right and left brachial arterial pulses (*arrows*).

length of the inflatable bladder must be sufficient to encircle the limb without overlapping.[24,117]

The examining room should be quiet, with the patient comfortable and reassured. Sufficient time should elapse for recovery from recent activity or apprehension. When an infant is quieted with a bottle or a pacifier, blood pressure can be obtained by the usual auscultatory method. An alternative is the flush method, which requires two examiners.[24] An uninflated cuff is applied to the forearm, which is elevated, while the limb distal to the cuff is massaged to induce blanching. The cuff is inflated above anticipated systolic pressure while the arm remains elevated and blanched. The arm is then slowly lowered into a horizontal position while the cuff is slowly deflated. The point at which the blanched hand becomes flushed is an estimate of the mean arterial pressure. Doppler ultrasonic or oscillometric techniques accurately determine systolic and diastolic blood pressure and can be accomplished by a single examiner.[24,201,233]

Upper extremity blood pressure in infants and adults is usually recorded in the supine position, but a comfortable sitting position is acceptable in infants and young children. Lower extremity blood pressure is best determined from the popliteal artery with the patient prone.[169] While the

popliteal artery is being palpated, a thigh cuff is applied and inflated slowly to avoid discomfort. The cuff is inflated until the popliteal pulse vanishes at a level just above the brachial arterial systolic pressure. Systolic and diastolic pressures are then estimated by auscultation of popliteal Korotkoff sounds. Only systolic Korotkoff sounds may be heard. Diagnostic differences in arm and leg blood pressures are based on systolic levels. Diastolic pressure is important in confirming accuracy, because diastolic pressures are not significantly different in the upper and lower extremities (see Fig. 8–13). When intra-arterial brachial and femoral pressures are compared in normal persons, there is no significant difference in systolic, diastolic, or mean pressure, although the femoral auscultatory systolic pressure is about 10 mm Hg higher than the direct femoral arterial pressure.[167] Differences between arm and leg systolic pressures in coarctation are exaggerated by exercise, which causes an increase in brachial arterial pressure but either no change or a reduction in femoral arterial pressure.[50]

Measurement of the blood pressure should be a routine part of the physical examination after infancy and is desirable in infants on at least one occasion.[24,233] Normal arterial pressure is based on age and sex.[24,54,143] The average systolic blood pressure in females rises to a plateau at around 14 years of age and remains almost constant during the early reproductive years.[54] The average systolic blood pressure in males may not plateau until around 20 years of age.[24,54,143] Diastolic pressure differences are in the same direction but are smaller in degree.

From birth to 6 months of age, normal upper extremity blood pressure averages 80/45 mm Hg. From 2 years of age to puberty, the average upper extremity blood pressure is 90/60 to 100/60 mm Hg,[24,54] with the diastolic pressure more consistent than the systolic pressure. Coarctation of the aorta is accompanied by a progressive age-related increase in blood pressure, especially systolic, so the pulse pressure widens.[35,97,193]

In pregnant women with coarctation, the directional changes in blood pressure are similar to those in normal pregnant women but from an initially higher level with a fall during the second trimester and a rise toward term.[170] In Turner syndrome, systemic hypertension may occur without coarctation.[219] Systemic hypertension in patients with abdominal coarctation is likely to be caused by renal artery stenosis rather than by the coarctation.[182]

THE JUGULAR VENOUS PULSE

Prominent arterial pulsations must be distinguished from the jugular venous pulse, which is normal except in patients with coarctation and biventricular failure.

PRECORDIAL MOVEMENT AND PALPATION

The left ventricular impulse varies from normal to the sustained heaving impulse of pressure overload hypertrophy.[169] In symptomatic infants with biventricular failure,

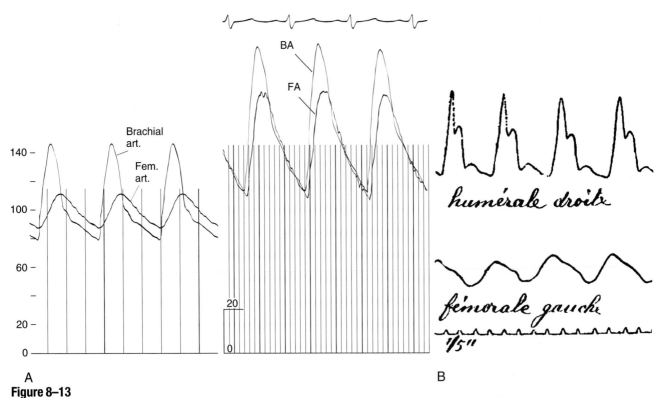

Figure 8–13

A, Simultaneous direct brachial and femoral arterial pressure pulses from a 10-year-old boy and from a 4-year-old boy with coarctation of the aorta. The femoral arterial pulses (Fem art) were palpable but smaller than the brachial arterial pulses (Brachial art). The diastolic pressures virtually coincide. The important differences are systolic, not diastolic. There is no delay in arrival time of the femoral arterial pulse. *B,* The right brachial arterial pulse (*humerale droite*) and the left femoral arterial pulse (*femorale gauche*) are representative of coarctation of the aorta. (*B,* As seen printed in Maude Abbott's *Atlas of Congenital Cardiac Disease* in 1936, Osler Library, McGill University.)

the right ventricular impulse is dynamic because of pressure overload (pulmonary hypertension) and volume overload (left-to-left shunt through the foramen ovale). Suprasternal notch systolic thrills are frequent in cases of uncomplicated coarctation. Precordial thrills are generated by coexisting bicuspid aortic stenosis.

AUSCULTATION

Coarctation of the aorta is associated with systolic, diastolic, or continuous murmurs (Fig. 8–15). An ejection sound is an auscultatory sign of a coexisting bicuspid aortic valve (Fig. 8–16). Systolic murmurs originate from three sources (see Fig. 8–15): (1) arterial collaterals, (2) the coarctation itself, and (3) the brachiocephalic arteries. The origin of murmurs in collateral arteries is based on observations that localized superficial collateral murmurs are abolished by compression and that murmurs have been recorded from the surfaces of surgically exposed collateral arteries.[215] A murmur cannot be generated across coarctation when obstruction is complete (see Fig. 8–3B), yet murmurs are prominent because arterial collaterals are well developed (see Fig. 8–3A,C).[215] The widespread anatomic distribution of the collateral arterial circulation accounts for the widespread thoracic distribution of the accompanying murmurs.[27,118] Collateral murmurs are crescendo-decrescendo and are delayed in onset and termination because they originate at a distance from the heart (Figs. 8–17 and 8–18, and see Fig. 8–15).[215]

Although widespread thoracic murmurs constitute presumptive evidence of collateral circulation, collaterals in young children may be well developed without generating murmurs, and an occasional adult with abundant collaterals has inconspicuous murmurs.

The coarctation itself is responsible for a systolic murmur[215] that correlates with the size of the coarctation, and the localized posterior position over the thoracic spine correlates with the site of the coarctation (see Figs. 8–15 and 8–18B). Infants are best examined prone. Older patients are examined prone or sitting in a relaxed position that minimizes the interference of muscle tremor. Posterior auscultation begins in the midline at the upper thoracic spine and then descends to the mid-thoracic and lumbar spine. A murmur overlying the coarctation is soft and high frequency, so detection is best achieved with the stethoscopic diaphragm or firm pressure with the bell. Typical isthmic coarctation generates a posterior murmur at the level of the fourth or fifth thoracic spinous process (see Figs. 8–15 through 8–18).[215] Murmurs are usually absent in infants except in this posterior location. Heart failure causes the coarctation murmur to decrease or disappear. As severity of coarctation increases, the short posterior thoracic systolic murmur lengthens (see Figs. 8–15 and 8–18B) and continues into diastole (see Figs. 8–15 through 8–17). When the coarctation diameter decreases to 2.5 mm, the murmur occupies all of the cardiac cycle.[215]

The continuous murmur is soft and high frequency, so assessment requires a quiet room, a cooperative patient,

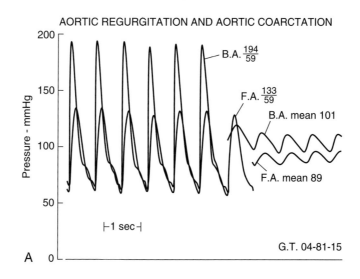

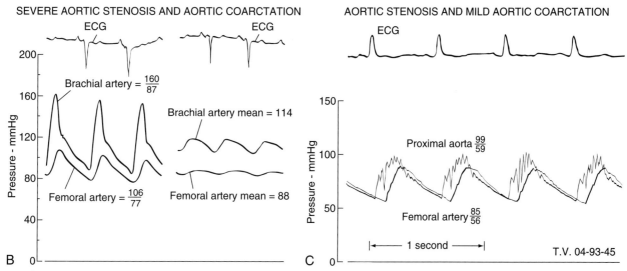

Figure 8–14

A, Pressure pulses from a 19-year-old man with severe coarctation of the aorta and bicuspid aortic regurgitation. The brachial arterial pressure (BA) is higher than the femoral arterial pressure (FA), although the brisk femoral arterial pulse and wide pulse pressure do not suggest coarctation. *B,* Thirty-eight-year-old man with coarctation of the aorta and severe bicuspid aortic stenosis. The brachial pulse is amplified by the coarctation and does not suggest aortic stenosis. *C,* Five-year-old boy with moderately severe bicuspid aortic stenosis and mild coarctation of the aorta. The proximal aortic and therefore brachial arterial systolic pressure is damped by aortic stenosis, but the femoral arterial systolic pressure is preserved because the coarctation was mild. (From Glancy DL, Morrow AG, Simon AL, Roberts WC: Juxtaductal coarctation. Am J Cardiol 51:537, 1983; with permission.)

Table 8–1	**Recommended Bladder Dimensions for Blood Pressure Cuff**	
Arm Circumference at midpoint,* cm	**Bladder Width, cm**	**Bladder Length, cm**
5–7.5 Newborn	3	5
7.5–13 Infant	5	8
13–20 Child	8	13
17–26 Small adult	11	17
24–32 Average adult	13	24
32–42 Large adult	17	32
42–50 Thigh	20	42

* Midpoint is defined as half the distance from the acromion to the olecranon.

From Kirkendall WM, Feinleib M, Freis ED, Mark AL: AHA Committee Report: Recommendations for human blood pressure determinations by sphygmomanometers. Circulation 62:1146A, 1980; reprinted with permission of the American Heart Association.

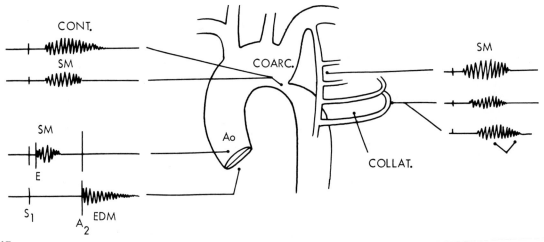

Figure 8–15

Illustration of the principal murmurs that accompany coarctation of the aorta (COARC, Ao). At the lower left are auscultatory events associated with a bicuspid aortic valve, namely, an aortic ejection sound (E), a short midsystolic murmur (SM), and an early diastolic murmur (EDM) of aortic regurgitation. Shown at the upper left are the continuous murmur (CONT) and the delayed systolic murmur (SM) that originate at the coarctation site and are heard posteriorly over the thoracic spine. Shown on the right are collateral arterial murmurs (COLLAT) that are crescendo-decrescendo and delayed in onset and termination because of origin in arteries that are distant from the heart. Collateral murmurs are illustrated here on one side as a matter of convenience. A_2, aortic second sound; S_1, first heart sound.

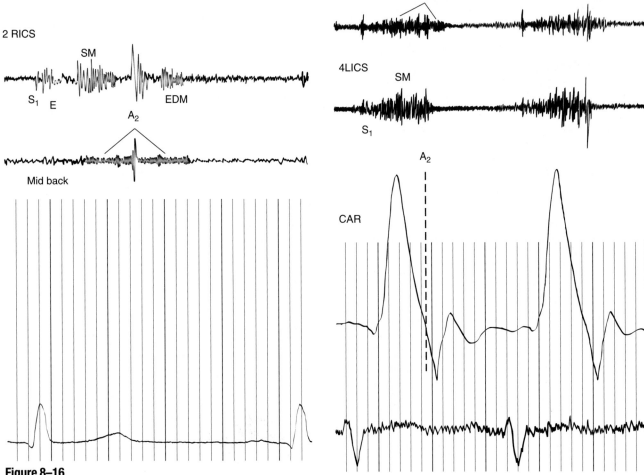

Figure 8–16

Phonocardiograms from a 10-year-old boy with coarctation of the aorta and a bicuspid aortic valve. In the second right intercostal space (2 RICS) there is an aortic ejection sound (E), a short midsystolic murmur (SM), and an early diastolic murmur (EDM) of aortic regurgitation. The tracing from the middle of the back was recorded over the site of coarctation and shows a continuous murmur that is delayed in onset and extends into diastole (*paired arrows*).

Figure 8–17

Tracings from a 22-year-old man with coarctation of the aorta. The phonocardiogram from the middle of the back over the site of coarctation shows a systolic murmur that is delayed in onset and continues into diastole (*paired arrows*). The systolic murmur in the fourth left intercostal space (4 LICS) originated in a left internal mammary collateral (see Fig. 8–3). CAR, carotid.

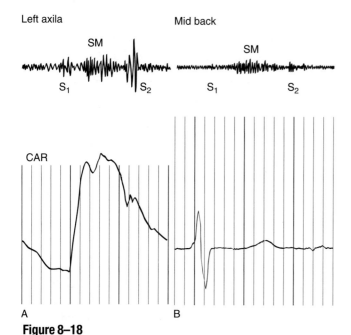

Figure 8–18

Tracings from a 6-year-old boy with coarctation of the aorta. *A*, The phonocardiogram in the left axila shows a delayed systolic murmur (SM) that originated in arterial collaterals. *B*, The phonocardiogram in the middle back over the vertebral column shows a delayed systolic murmur at the site of coarctation. CAR, carotid pulse; S_1, first heart sound; S_2, second heart sound.

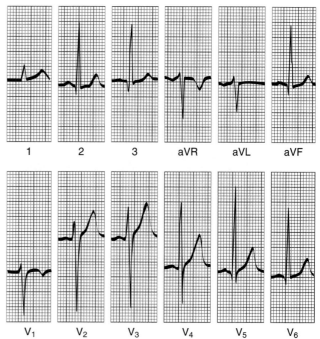

Figure 8–19

Electrocardiogram from a 23-year-old man with coarctation of the aorta. The QRS axis is normal. Broad left atrial P waves are present in leads 2 and aVF. Left ventricular hypertrophy is suggested by the sum of the S wave in V_1 and the R wave in V_5.

and the stethoscopic diaphragm or firm pressure with the bell. Rarely, the coarctation murmur is loud enough to radiate to the anterior chest.[215] A loud brachiocephalic systolic murmur accompanied by a thrill is commonly heard in the suprasternal notch, and prominent systolic murmurs are heard over the right and left subclavian arteries. A short, low- to medium-frequency diastolic murmur over the left ventricular impulse is caused by a decrease in interpapillary distance, which culminates in the single papillary muscle of a parachute mitral valve (see Chapter 9).[30,41] The murmur of abdominal coarctation is heard posteriorly over the lower thoracic or lumbar spine and anteriorly in the epigastrium or just below.[20,88,182] Pseudocoarctation generates a systolic murmur posteriorly over the site of the aortic kink (see Fig. 8–5).[86,156]

The second heart sound in coarctation of the aorta is either single or normally split, with increased intensity of the aortic component. A loud single second sound in the second left interspace is due to augmented aortic valve closure (see Fig. 8–16). In symptomatic infants with pulmonary hypertension, the loud single second sound is the summation of aortic and pulmonary components.

Fourth heart sounds reflect the afterload-induced left ventricular hypertrophy of coarctation. Third heart sounds or summation sounds occur especially in infants with heart failure and a rapid heart rate.

THE ELECTROCARDIOGRAM

Electrocardiographic patterns fall into two age groups, namely, symptomatic neonatal coarctation and coarctation after childhood. Left atrial P wave abnormalities occur in adults (Fig. 8–19) and right atrial P wave abnormalities occur in symptomatic infants (Fig. 8–20). The mean QRS axis is normal, although a leftward axis is occasionally found in older patients (Fig. 8–21). Right axis deviation with right ventricular hypertrophy is typical of the electro-

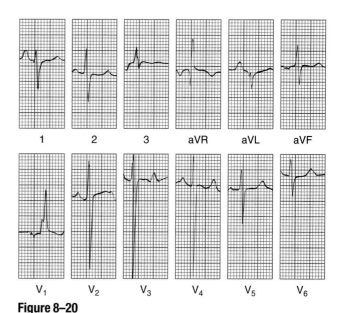

Figure 8–20

Electrocardiogram from a 6-year-old male with coarctation of the aorta and congestive heart failure in infancy (see Fig. 8–18). The electrocardiogram still shows a prominent right atrial P wave in lead 1 with right axis deviation and right ventricular hypertrophy manifested by a tall R wave in lead V_1 and deep S waves in left precordial leads.

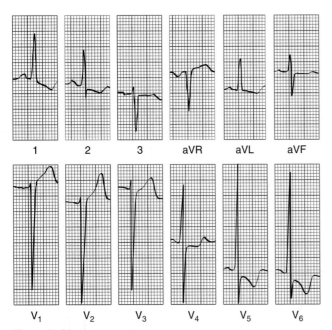

Figure 8–21

Electrocardiogram from a 41-year-old man with coarctation of the aorta. The QRS axis is horizontal. Bifid left atrial P waves appear in leads 1 and 2. Left ventricular hypertrophy is manifested by deep S waves in right precordial leads and tall R waves with ST segment depressions and T wave inversions in left precordial leads. There is a wide QRS-T angle in the frontal plane.

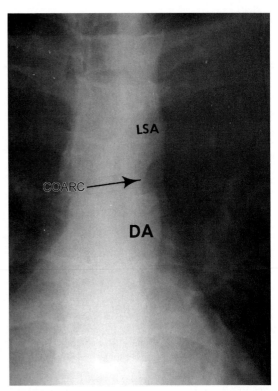

Figure 8–22

X-ray from a 3-year-old boy with coarctation of the aorta (COARC). The child was too young to have developed rib notching, but the radiologic diagnosis can be suspected because the descending aorta (DA) is convex to the left and the left subclavian artery (LSA) is dilated—the figure-3 sign.

cardiogram in symptomatic infants with right ventricular pressure overload (pulmonary hypertension) and right ventricular volume overload (left-to-right shunt across a patent foramen ovale). Right ventricular hypertrophy that persists beyond infancy is rare in cases of uncomplicated coarctation (see Fig. 8–20).

Left ventricular hypertrophy is characterized by tall R waves and low, flat, or inverted T waves in left precordial leads (see Fig. 8–21).[77] Prominent coved ST segment depressions with deeply inverted T waves are exceptional (see Fig. 8–21) and suggest coexisting bicuspid aortic stenosis. Prominent left precordial Q waves suggest the volume overload of bicuspid aortic regurgitation.

THE X-RAY

The x-ray varies from normal to pathognomonic. In asymptomatic infants and young children, the x-ray is likely to be read as normal. The descending thoracic aorta in normal children and young adults is a straight line that runs parallel to the vertebral column. However, the post-coarctation descending thoracic aorta in children and young adults has a distinctive leftward convexity that is accompanied by dilatation of the left subclavian artery (Fig. 8–22).[76] The x-ray in symptomatic infants with coarctation discloses pulmonary venous congestion and dilatation of the right ventricle and of the right and left atrium (Fig. 8–23). Left ventricular size remains normal or nearly so.

Notching of the ribs is a classic radiologic sign of coarctation of the aorta caused by collateral flow through dilated, tortuous, pulsatile posterior intercostal arteries (Figs. 8–24 and 8–25). The notches vary from rib to rib and from patient to patient and may be single, multiple, shallow, deep, broad, or narrow.[15,25] Because notching originates in posterior intercostal arteries that run in intercostal grooves, the anterior ribs are spared because anterior intercostal arteries do not run in intercostal grooves.[25] Because notching involves the undersurfaces of posterior ribs within intercostal grooves (see Fig. 8–24), the inferior margins of the posterior ribs are spared.[58] Rarely, the superior margin of a rib is notched because of contact with an overhanging intercostal artery.[210] Rib notching seldom appears before 6 years of age, although exceptional examples have been described as early as 2 years of age.[15,22,58]

Typical coarctation distal to the left subclavian artery results in bilateral notching between the third and the eighth posterior ribs (see Fig. 8–25).[25] Notching is rare above the third or below the ninth rib.[25] Anatomic variations of the coarctation site are accompanied by variations in these typical radiologic patterns. The development of arterial collaterals depends on patency of the ipsilateral subclavian artery. When the left subclavian lumen is compromised by the coarctation, ipsilateral collaterals fail to develop. Unilateral rib notching is confined to the right hemithorax (Fig. 8–27).[25,35,58,109] Anomalous origin of the right subclavian artery distal to the coarctation (see Fig. 8–1C) results in failure of collateral development in the right hemithorax, so unilateral notching is confined to

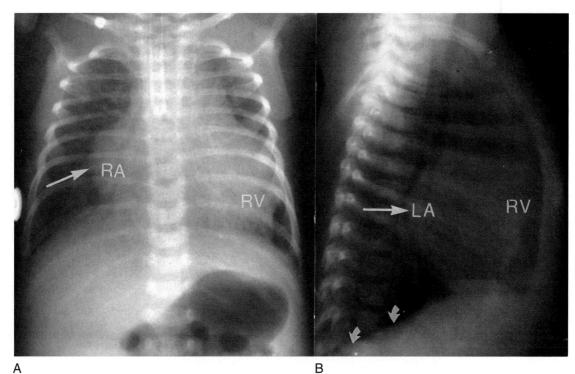

A B

Figure 8–23

A, X-ray from a 1-month-old boy with coarctation of the aorta, congestive heart failure, and a left-to-right shunt through a patent foramen ovale. There is pulmonary venous congestion. An enlarged right ventricle (RV) occupies the apex, and a dilated right atrium (RA) forms the right lower cardiac border. *B,* Lateral chest x-ray from a 4-month-old girl with 45XO Turner syndrome, coarctation of the aorta, congestive heart failure, and a left-to-right shunt through a foramen ovale. The left atrium (LA) is enlarged. The retrosternal space is occupied by a dilated right ventricle (RV), but the left ventricle is not enlarged. The crural portions of the diaphragm are flat (*unmarked white arrows*) because the lungs were hyperinflated.

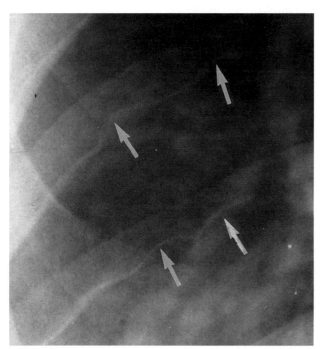

Figure 8–24

Close-up showing irregular scalloped notching of the inferior margins of posterior ribs in a 54-year-old man with coarctation of the aorta.

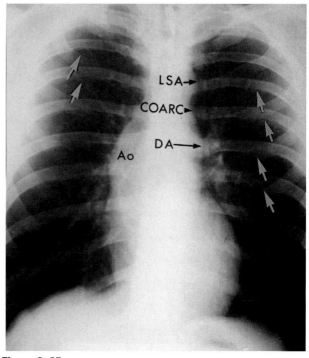

Figure 8–25

X-ray from a 23-year-old man with coarctation of the aorta (COARC). *Arrows* point to notching on the undersurfaces of the posterior ribs. The ascending aorta (Ao) is dilated. The left subclavian artery (LSA) is dilated above the coarctation, and the descending aorta (DA) is dilated below the coarctation forming a figure-3.

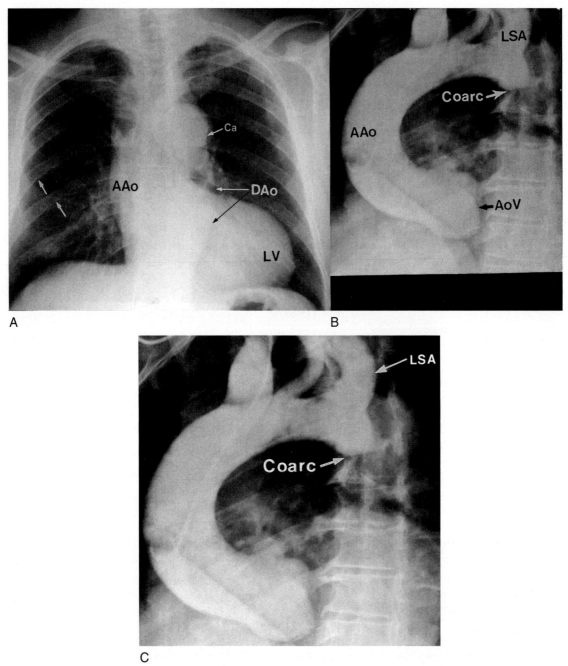

Figure 8–26

A, X-ray from a 62-year-old man with coarctation of the aorta distal to the left subclavian artery. *Unmarked arrows* in the right hemithorax identify subtle rib notching. The ascending aorta (AAo) is dilated, and calcium (Ca) appears in the aortic knuckle. The descending thoracic aorta (DAo) is convex to the left, which in part is age related. An enlarged convex left ventricle (LV) occupies the apex. *B,* Thoracic aortogram shows a dilated and elongated ascending aorta (AAo) and complete obstruction at the coarctation site (Coarc). The aortic valve (AoV) is trileaflet. LSA, left subclavian artery. *C,* Lateral aortogram from a 70-year-old woman with complete obstruction at the site of aortic coarctation (Coarc). LSA, left subclavian artery.

the left hemithorax.[58,205] Lateral x-rays show retrosternal notching or scalloping caused by dilated tortuous internal mammary arteries (see Fig. 8–3*A,B*).[15,22,77] When coarctation is in the abdominal aorta, notching, if present at all, is confined to the lower ribs.[20]

The ascending aorta in older children and adults with coarctation is moderately to markedly dilated (see Figs. 8–25 and 8–26).[22,77] In patients with XO Turner syndrome, the ascending aorta may be aneurysmal (see Fig. 8–9). The paracoarctation aorta is typically dilated (see

Fig. 8–2).[15,76,77,159] Postcoarctation aortic dilatation is sometimes aneurysmal,[77] and calcification is occasionally visible in the wall of the aneurysm. The combination of a dilated left subclavian artery proximal to the coarctation and a dilated aorta distal to the coarctation produces a distinctive figure-3 silhouette on the x-ray (see Fig. 8–25).[15,76,77] The mirror image of the figure-3 sign is seen when the left subclavian artery and descending aorta indent a barium esophagram (Fig. 8–28).[15,22] The left subclavian artery cannot enlarge when its lumen is compromised

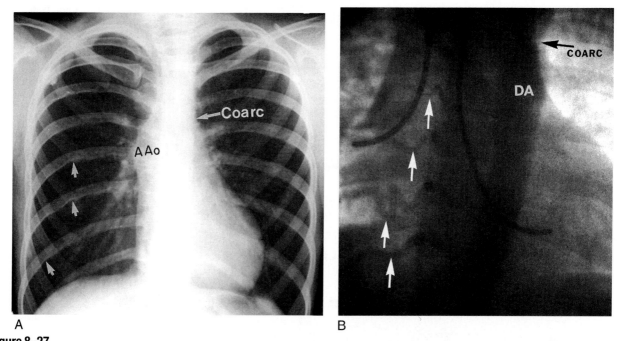

Figure 8–27

A, X-ray from a 14-year-old boy with coarctation of the aorta (Coarc) that obstructed the orifice of the left subclavian artery, which is not dilated above the coarctation site, but the ascending aorta (AAo) is dilated. *Arrows on the right* point to unilateral notching of the ribs. *B*, Aortogram opacified unilateral collateral arteries on the right (*arrows*). *Black arrow* identifies the coarctation site. The descending aorta (DA) is convex to the left.

by the coarctation, so dilatation of the distal paracoarctation aorta exists alone (see Fig. 8–27). A retroesophageal aberrant right subclavian artery is sometimes identified as a posterior indentation of the barium esophagram.[25]

The kinked aorta of pseudocoarctation[114,115,156,214,217] has a transverse arch and a descending aorta that form a large figure-3 sign above and below the kink (see Fig. 8–5).[114,115,156,214,217] Pseudocoarctation is conspicuous, but rib notching is conspicuous by its absence (see Fig. 8–5).

THE ECHOCARDIOGRAM

Transthoracic and transesophageal echocardiography with Doppler interrogation and color flow imaging (Figs. 8–29, 8–30, and 8–31) permit segment-by-segment analysis of the ascending aorta, the aortic arch, the brachiocephalic arteries, the aortic isthmus, and the proximal descending aorta from birth to maturity.[44,48,208] An echocardiographic diagnosis of coarctation can be made in utero.[3] The suprasternal notch window with color flow imaging identifies the coarctation as a zone of localized accelerated flow and by providing the target through which the continuous wave Doppler beam can be aligned to determine the gradient (see Figs. 8–29A,B, 8–30, and 8–31).[44,208] Peak systolic velocity reflects the maximum systolic gradient, and persistent high velocity diastolic forward flow reflects severity (see Figs. 8–29B and 8–31B).[39,44,147,208] The Doppler pattern across the coarctation is affected by reduced proximal aortic compliance.[81] Color flow identifies the precise level at which laminar flow becomes turbulent (see Fig. 8–29C). In the fetus and neonate, normal tapering of the aortic isthmus[96] can be mistaken for isthmic obstruction, and the artifacts from the duc-

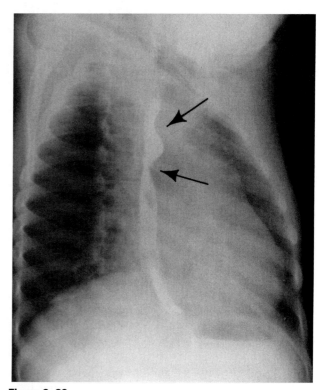

Figure 8–28

Right anterior oblique x-ray from a 6-year-old boy with coarctation of the aorta. The barium esophagram exhibits the figure-E sign (*arrows*) caused by compression from the dilated left subclavian artery above and the dilated descending aorta below. The figure-E sign is the mirror image of the figure-3 sign (see Fig. 8–25).

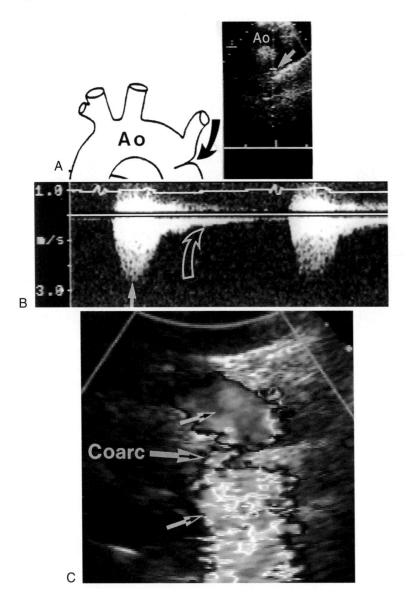

Figure 8–29

A, Images from a 5-year-old boy with coarctation of the aorta. The two-dimensional echocardiogram (*upper right*) identifies the coarctation, which is schematically illustrated to the left (*curved arrow*). Ao, aorta. *B,* Continuous wave Doppler shows systolic turbulence across the coarctation (*vertical white arrow*) that continued through most of diastole (*large curved arrow*). *C,* Black and white print of a color flow image from a 3-year-old boy shows abrupt change at the coarctation site (Coarc) from laminar flow (*upper arrow*) to turbulent flow (*lower arrow*).

tus insertion sometimes make interpretation difficult.[208] A long segment of luminal narrowing can be identified.[188] The relationship between the site of coarctation and the aortic insertion of the ligamentum arteriosum establishes preductal, juxtaductal or postductal location.[208]

SUMMARY

Coarctation of the aorta will not be overlooked if attention is paid to the upper and lower extremity arterial pulses and blood pressure during routine physical examination. The diagnosis is entertained in patients with systemic hypertension and reduced or absent femoral pulses. Disproportionate systolic hypertension heightens suspicion. Minor symptoms include headache, epistaxis, and leg fatigue. Major complications include congestive heart failure, especially in infants, rupture or dissection of the paracoarctation aorta, infective endarteritis, and cerebral hemorrhage due to rupture of an aneurysm of the circle of Willis. The physical appearance of patients with XO Turner

syndrome increases the probability of coarctation. Pulse pressure proximal to the coarctation increases with age, resulting in conspicuous carotid and suprasternal notch pulsations. Collateral arterial pulsations should be sought beneath the skin, especially around the scapulae. Tortuous retinal arterioles are distinctive. A left ventricular impulse occupies the apex. A right ventricular impulse is reserved for symptomatic infants with heart failure, pulmonary hypertension, and a left-to-right shunt across a patent foramen ovale. Auscultatory signs include widespread delayed systolic murmurs through collateral arteries and a systolic or continuous murmur over the coarctation site. Systolic murmurs are especially prominent in the suprasternal notch and along the left sternal border over internal mammary collaterals. Auscultatory signs in infants are limited to the posterior interscapular murmur over the coarctation. Electrocardiographic criteria for left ventricular hypertrophy reflect the left ventricular afterload. Right ventricular hypertrophy characterizes the electrocardiogram of symptomatic infants. Notching of the third to

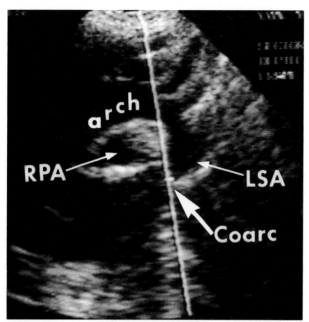

Figure 8–30
Echocardiogram (suprasternal notch) from a 10-month-old boy with coarctation of the aorta. The coarctation (Coarc) is represented by a localized shelf or ridge that narrows the aortic lumen distal to the left subclavian artery (LSA). RPA, right pulmonary artery. Doppler sample volume at the coarctation site detects the flow disturbance.

eighth posterior ribs is a radiologic feature of major diagnostic importance but is seldom present before 6 years of age. Dilatation of the left subclavian artery and the proximal descending aorta are useful radiologic signs, especially in children too young to have developed rib notching. The transthoracic and transesophageal echocardiogram with Doppler interrogation and color flow imaging identify the coarctation and determine its severity.

Interruption of the Aortic Arch

The thoracic aorta lends itself to segmental analysis of the ascending portion, the arch, the isthmus, and the descending portion. This chapter has dealt so far with obstruction of the aortic isthmus—coarctation. Atresia, or complete interruption of the aortic arch, can be considered the ultimate expression of obstructive thoracic aortic anomalies that begin with coarctation.[229] The embryogenesis of these anomalies is similar, if not identical.[229]

Interruption of the aortic arch was first described in the 18th century by Raphael Steidele of the University of Vienna.[216] *Steidele's complex* is occasionally applied as an eponym to this rare malformation,[130,223] which is characterized by complete anatomic discontinuity or by an atretic fibrous strand between the aortic arch and the descending aorta (Fig. 8–32).[23,42,150,180] The classification of complete interruption by Celoria and Patton[42] refers to one of three sites,[74,130,180,223] two of which were described in 1927 by Maude Abbott.[2] Interruption between the left common carotid and left subclavian arteries (type B) (Fig. 8–33; see also Fig. 8–32) is more common than interruption distal to the left subclavian artery (type A). The least common site is between the innominate artery and the left carotid artery (type C) (Fig. 8–34).[42,100,102] Subtypes are based on anomalous origin of the right subclavian artery.[100,122,221] Rarely, interruption involves a right-sided aortic arch.[191]

Interruption of the aortic arch seldom occurs as an isolated anomaly.[55,92,112,179] Patent ductus arteriosus and ventricular septal defect are in a physiologic sense inherent components upon which tenuous neonatal survival depends. The clinical picture in infants is largely determined by patency of the ductus arteriosus which provides nonrestrictive flow from the pulmonary trunk into the

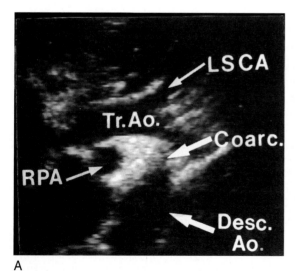 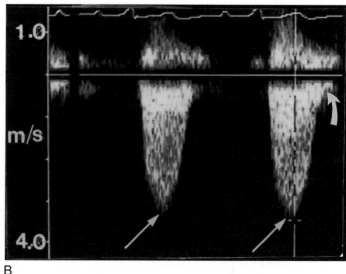

A   B

Figure 8–31
A, Echocardiogram from a 12-year-old boy with coarctation of the aorta (Coarc) distal to the left subclavian artery (LSCA). The transverse aorta tapers toward the isthmus. The descending aorta (Desc. Ao.) distal to the coarctation is dilated. B, Continuous wave Doppler from a 27-year-old man with coarctation of the aorta. The peak systolic velocity estimated the gradient at 45 mm Hg. Flow into early diastole is identified by the *curved arrow* at the upper right.

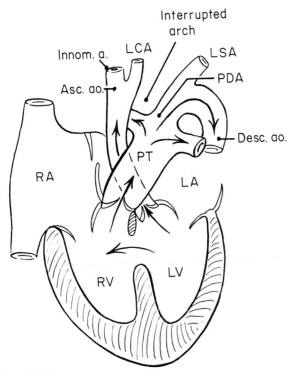

Figure 8–32

Illustration of the anatomic and circulatory derangements in the most common variety of complete interruption of the aortic arch (type B). The ascending aorta (Asc ao) gives rise to the innominate artery (Innom a) and to the left carotid artery (LCA). The left subclavian artery (LSA) arises from the descending aorta (Desc. ao), which is continuous with the pulmonary trunk (PT) via a nonrestrictive patent ductus arteriosus (PDA). A large ventricular septal defect provides the left ventricle with access to the descending aorta via pulmonary trunk–ductus–descending aortic continuity. LA, left atrium; LV, left ventricle; RA, right atrium; RV, right ventricle.

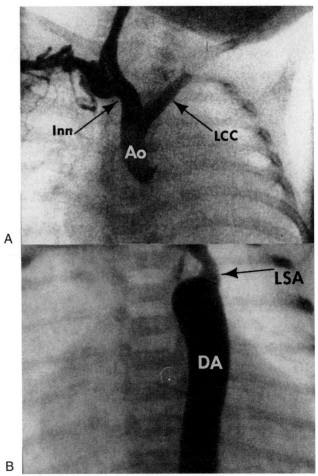

Figure 8–33

A, Aortogram from a female neonate with complete interruption of the aortic arch distal to the left common carotid artery (LCC). The innominate artery (Inn) gives rise to the right common carotid artery and to the right subclavian artery. Ao, ascending aorta. *B,* Aortogram from a 3-day-old boy with complete interruption of the aortic arch distal to the left common carotid artery. The left subclavian artery (LSA) originates from the descending aorta (DA). Compare with Figure 8–32.

descending aorta–pulmonary trunk–ductus–descending aortic continuity (see Fig. 8–32).[130,150,180]

The propensity of the ductus to constrict or remain patent is crucial. In the majority of patients with interrupted aortic arch, the ductus is histologically mature with prominent intimal cushions that prefigure constriction. In a minority of patients, an immature ductus is devoid of intimal cushions and has marked elastification that sets the stage for persistent patency. A ventricular septal defect almost invariably coexists with interruption between the left carotid and left subclavian arteries (type B) and in about 50% of cases with interruption distal to the left subclavian artery (type A).[8,74,92,100,130,150,180] A posterior malaligned ventricular septal defect is the rule when the interrupted arch is between the left carotid and left subclavian arteries (type B).[23,74,187] Posterior deviation of the infundibular septum encroaches on the left ventricular outflow tract and causes subaortic obstruction.[8,74] Defects in the perimembranous and muscular septum are uncommon.[8] An intact ventricular septum is even less common, but when the septum is intact, a physiologically equivalent aortopulmonary window is almost always present,[29,43] and the interrupted arch is distal to the left subclavian artery (type A).[29]

Theories regarding pathogenesis have focused on the role of reduced aortic flow during early morphogenesis,

analogous to the theories proposed for the pathogenesis of coarctation of the aorta (see earlier).[29,122] The malaligned ventricular septal defect in type B interruption encroaches on the left ventricular outflow tract, reducing aortic blood flow[122] and favoring pulmonary blood flow.[74,122,229] These anatomic arrangements are in keeping with the small caliber of the ascending aorta in response to the paucity of aortic blood flow during fetal development.[8] The unique vascular morphology of the fourth aortic arches has been implicated in the pathogenesis of type B interruption with anomalous right subclavian artery.[213] An unresolved morphogenic point is the relatively rare occurrence of interruption between the innominate artery and the left common carotid artery (type C, 4% of cases), implying that this segment of the arch is less vulnerable to decreased flow or depends on a separate developmental defect. Aortic arch interruption distal to the left subclavian artery (type A) and coarctation of the aorta are believed to be morphogenetically related.[229]

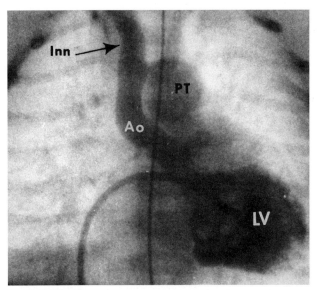

Figure 8–34

Left ventriculogram (LV) in a female neonate with complete interruption of the aortic arch distal to the innominate artery (Inn). The ascending aorta (Ao) ascends vertically and is small compared to the dilated pulmonary trunk (PT). The left common carotid artery and left subclavian artery originated from the descending aorta. Compare with Figure 8–32.

The physiologic consequences of interrupted aortic arch with patent ductus arteriosus and ventricular septal defect reflect ascending aortic blood flow derived directly from the left ventricle and descending aortic blood derived directly from the pulmonary trunk through the ductus (see Fig. 8–32).[92,150] The left-to-right interventricular shunt is reinforced by resistance to left ventricular outflow caused by the malaligned ventricular septal defect. The magnitude of the right-to-left shunt through the ductus arteriosus depends on the relative resistances in the pulmonary and systemic vascular beds. Constriction of the ductus is catastrophic, suddenly abolishing flow into the descending aorta and diverting virtually all pulmonary blood flow into the already flooded lungs.[190] Nevertheless, interruption or atresia of the aortic arch *without* a patent ductus is compatible with life,[102, 152] even adult survival,[144,190,199,240] provided that both subclavian arteries arise from the descending aorta, an arrangement that potentially permits retrograde flow to the entire body except for the head.[102,152,199] A variation on this theme is the congenital subclavian steal that occurs when both subclavian arteries arise distal to the interruption.[53,75,171] Constriction of the ductus prompts a fall in pressure in the subclavian arteries and a steal *into* those arteries through collateral channels from ascending to descending aorta via the circle of Willis and the vertebral arteries.[75]

THE HISTORY

Complete interruption of the aortic arch occurs in 19 per million live births according to the New England Regional Infant Cardiac Program.[70] Males and females are equally represented.[130,180,223] Recurrence has been reported in siblings,[32,166,175,181] and a 2.5% recurrence rate of congenital heart disease has been reported in siblings of patients with type B interruption.[172]

The typical clinical picture is represented by a neonate who becomes acutely ill as the ductus closes.[55,180,223] Symptoms reflect the sudden increase in pulmonary blood flow and the sudden decrease in circulation to the trunk and lower limbs. The result is cardiac shock, severe acidosis, renal failure, intracranial hemorrhage,[190] and a mean survival of 4 to 10 days.[74,180,223] Three quarters of unoperated infants are dead by 1 month, and only 10% reach their first birthday.[78,130,180] Occasional survival into childhood, adolescence, and young adulthood has been reported,[92,140,152,173,199] with three patients surviving to their early or mid-30s.[176,206,223,240] Interruption of the aortic arch or aortic arch atresia without patent ductus arteriosus or ventricular septal defect resembles severe coarctation of the aorta.[55,144,199] Symptoms await post-adolescence or young adulthood. Rupture of an intracranial aneurysm was reported in a teenager[197] and in an adult.[174]

PHYSICAL APPEARANCE

Cyanosis is inconspicuous until the advent of acute congestive heart failure. Differential cyanosis caused by right-to-left ductal flow into the descending aorta is, with rare exception, canceled by the left-to-right shunt through the ventricular septal defect (see Fig. 8–32),[92,130,150,180] a mechanism that was recognized in 1852 by Greig,[85] who wrote:

The additional complication . . . of such a large aperture between the ventricles must have established complete admixture of the blood of the two sides of the heart before it was sent into the aorta and pulmonary artery, so that, independent of subsequent abnormalities of the vessels, all parts of the body would be supplied with blood of the same quality.

Deletion at 22q 11.2 and the DiGeorge syndrome (see Fig. 28–6), which consists of hypoplastic mandible, defective ears, short philtrum, and aplasia or hypoplasia of the thymus and parathyroid glands, are associated with type A or type B interruption.[111,134,149,179,196,229,239]

THE ARTERIAL PULSE

Femoral arterial pulses are maintained because of continuity between the pulmonary trunk, ductus, and descending aorta (see Fig. 8–32).[92,140,180] A reduction in femoral pulses signifies ductal constriction, which initially may be intermittent.[92] When the left subclavian artery originates from the descending aorta (type B), ductal constriction reduces the left brachial pulse in addition to the femoral pulse. Anomalous origin of the right subclavian artery places the right brachial pulse in the distal low pressure zone.[122] On the rare occasion of interruption of the aortic arch or arch atresia *without* patent ductus or ventricular septal defect, palpation of the systemic arterial pulses is analogous to palpation in coarctation of the aorta.[55,92,112,152,199,221] When interruption occurs proximal to both subclavian arteries (anomalous origin of the right subclavian), the carotid pulses are bounding but the brachial and femoral pulses are diminished or absent.[112,199,221] If either or both subclavian arteries originate proximal to the interruption, the arms will be hypertensive, the carotid pulses will be bounding, and the femoral pulses will be weak or absent.[55,199]

PRECORDIAL MOVEMENT AND PALPATION

An isolated *right ventricular impulse* is palpated in infants with interruption of the aortic arch because of obligatory pulmonary hypertension associated with a nonrestrictive patent ductus arteriosus and ventricular septal defect. A left ventricular impulse is absent despite a left-to-right shunt at the ventricular level because blood entering the pulmonary trunk is diverted through the ductus into the descending aorta rather than through the pulmonary circulation into the left side of the heart (see Fig. 8–32). Interruption of the aortic arch without patent ductus or ventricular septal defect results in a left ventricular impulse analogous to coarctation of the aorta.[199]

AUSCULTATION

Murmurs are unimpressive or absent.[180] The ductus is silent because the shunt is entirely right-to-left through a single nonrestrictive arterial conduit formed by continuity of the pulmonary trunk, ductus, and descending aorta. Systolic murmurs originating through the ventricular septal defect are early systolic, decrescendo, and grade 3/6 or less.[140,222] A continuous murmur has been attributed to collateral circulation that connects the ascending and descending aorta.[140] Diastolic murmurs are due to pulmonary hypertensive pulmonary regurgitation[180] and are introduced by a loud pulmonary component of the second heart sound. Interruption of the aortic arch without a ductus or ventricular septal defect presents with auscultatory signs that are similar to imperforate coarctation of the aorta, with widespread collateral murmurs[211] that include the entire head but are especially located behind the ears.[55,199]

THE ELECTROCARDIOGRAM

Peaked right atrial P waves and right ventricular hypertrophy are electrocardiographic features in the neonate with interruption of the aortic arch, ventricular septal defect, and patent ductus arteriosus (Fig. 8–35).[222] Biventricular hypertrophy emerges in response to left ventricular volume overload and persistent right ventricular pressure overload (Fig. 8–36).[180] Interruption *without* patent ductus or ventricular septal defect results in right ventricular hypertrophy in infants[221] but left ventricular hypertrophy in older patients.

THE X-RAY

The cardiac silhouette enlarges and pulmonary venous congestion develops rapidly when closure of the ductus

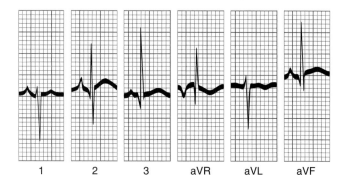

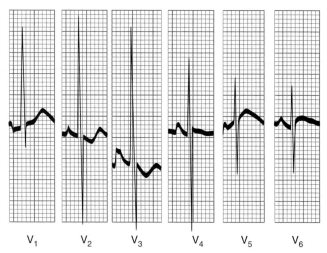

Figure 8–35

Electrocardiogram from a 3-day-old boy with complete interruption of the aortic arch. A tall peaked right atrial P wave appears in lead 2. Right ventricular hypertrophy is represented by the tall monophasic R wave in lead V_1 and the deep S wave in lead V_6. Biventricular hypertrophy is represented by the large biphasic RS complexes in the mid-precordial leads.

arteriosus causes a sudden increase in pulmonary blood flow and volume overload of the left ventricle. The aortic knuckle is absent because the ascending aorta is small and ascends vertically (Figs. 8–37 and 8–38).[100] The trachea is not deviated by an aortic arch and is therefore midline.[100] The x-ray shows an increase in pulmonary venous and pulmonary arterial vascularity with enlargement of the left ventricle (see Figs. 8–37 and 8–38).[140,222] Isolated interruption of the aortic arch *without* a ductus or a ventricular septal defect is radiologically similar to coarctation of the aorta, including rib notching.[55,102,211] Whether the notching is bilateral or unilateral depends on the site of interruption, the origin of the subclavian arteries, and the length of survival.[100,102]

THE ECHOCARDIOGRAM

Echocardiography with Doppler interrogation and color flow imaging identifies the major segments of the thoracic aorta, visualizes the patent ductus and the ventricular septal defect, and distinguishes interruption of the aortic arch from coarctation with tubular hypoplasia. In type C interruption, echocardiography identifies antegrade flow in the

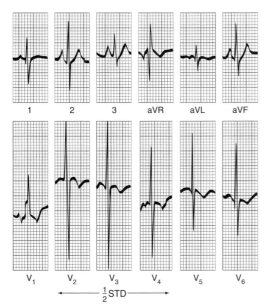

Figure 8–36

Electrocardiogram from a 6-month-old girl with complete interruption of the aortic arch. Tall peaked right atrial P waves appear in leads 2, 3, and aVF. Right ventricular hypertrophy is represented by the tall notched R wave in lead V_1 and by the deep S wave in lead V_6. The prominent Q wave and well-developed R wave in lead V_6 are evidence of left ventricular volume overload. Biventricular hypertrophy is represented by large equidiphasic RS complexes in leads V_{2-4}, which are half standardized.

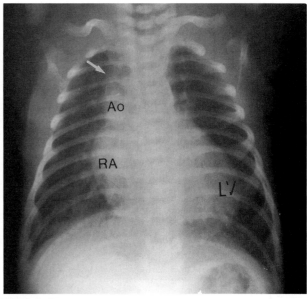

Figure 8–37

X-ray from a 2-day-old boy with complete interruption of the aortic arch. There is pulmonary venous congestion. The patient is slightly rotated to the left, increasing the prominence of the ascending aorta (Ao) and right atrium (RA) and decreasing the prominence of the left ventricle (LV). The density at the right thoracic inlet is thymus (*arrow*).

right carotid and basilar arteries but retrograde flow in the left carotid artery.[185] Echocardiography has identified type B interruption of a right aortic arch[194] and has diagnosed aortic arch interruption in utero.[137]

A normal aorta exhibits a continuous smooth curvature from its ascending to its descending portion, but when the arch is interrupted distal to the left carotid artery (type B), the ascending aorta rises vertically, exhibits little curvature, and bifurcates into the innominate and left carotid arteries,[179] with the carotid artery appearing as an index finger pointing toward the neck (Fig. 8–39). When the arch is interrupted distal to the left subclavian artery (type A), the ascending aorta exhibits a slight curvature and gives off three branches—the innominate, the left carotid, and the left subclavian arteries[179]

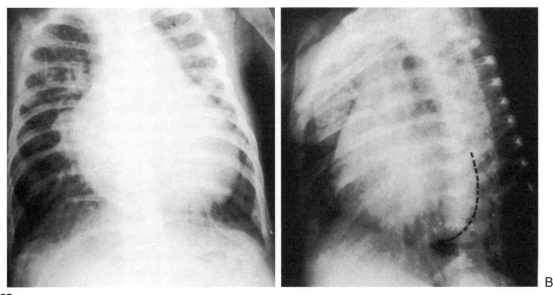

Figure 8–38

X-rays from the 6-month-old girl whose electrocardiogram is shown in Figure 8–36. *A*, Prominent pulmonary soft tissue densities represent venous congestion and increased pulmonary arterial vascularity. The pulmonary trunk is dilated in contrast with the inconspicuous ascending aorta, and the right atrium is markedly dilated. *B*, In the left anterior oblique projection, the right ventricle and left ventricle (dotted line) were both enlarged.

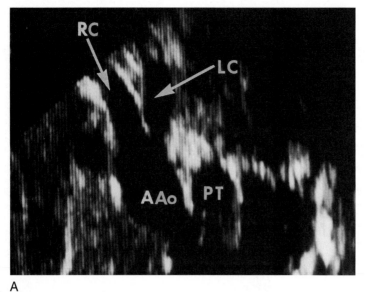
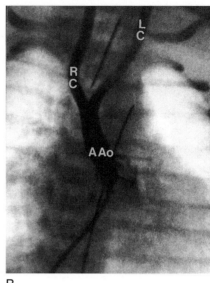

A   B

Figure 8–39

A, Echocardiogram from a neonate with complete interruption of the aortic arch distal to the left carotid artery. The ascending aorta (AAo) rises vertically, exhibits no curvature, and branches as the right carotid (RC) and left carotid artery (LC). PT, pulmonary trunk. *B*, The aortogram shows a small ascending aorta that rises vertically and exhibits no curvature. The right carotid artery (RC) and the left carotid artery (LC) are shown as in the echocardiogram.

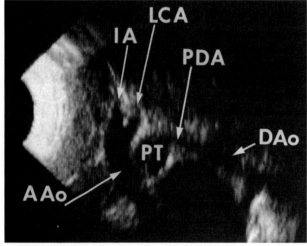

Figure 8–40

Echocardiogram from a 7-month-old girl with complete interruption of the aortic arch. The ascending aorta (AAo) gives rise to the innominate artery (IA) and to the left carotid artery (LCA) distal to which the arch was interrupted. The pulmonary trunk (PT) is continuous with the descending aorta (DAo) via a patent ductus arteriosus (PDA).

(Fig. 8–40)—because the right subclavian artery is prone to anomalous origin.

A useful echocardiographic observation is the discrepancy between the small caliber of the ascending aorta and conspicuous dilatation of the pulmonary trunk. The image created by continuity of the pulmonary trunk, ductus, and descending aorta superficially resembles an uninterrupted aortic arch, but identification of the origins of the right and left pulmonary arterial branches, together with absence of brachiocephalic branches, prevents this diagnostic error (see Fig. 8–40).[179]

Characterization of the ventricular septal defect is an important part of the echocardiographic examination. A malaligned ventricular septal defect is associated with posterior and leftward deviation of the conal septum and varying degrees of subaortic narrowing.[160,179,187,203] An intact ventricular septum with an interrupted aortic arch prompts search for an aortopulmonary window.[179]

SUMMARY

The typical clinical picture of interruption of the aortic arch is an acyanotic neonate who initially appears well but who suddenly becomes ill when the ductus arteriosus constricts and deprives the trunk and lower limbs of arterial circulation and diverts pulmonary arterial blood into the lungs and into the left side of the heart. Tachypnea and symmetric cyanosis develop, the femoral pulses disappear, and the chest x-ray exhibits pulmonary venous congestion with progressive cardiac enlargement. When the interruption is proximal to the left subclavian artery, the left brachial arterial pulse disappears as well. There is either no murmur at all or an inconspicuous early systolic decrescendo murmur through the ventricular septal defect. The electrocardiogram shows peaked right atrial P waves and right ventricular hypertrophy, but if survival permits, biventricular hypertrophy emerges. Echocardiography identifies the interrupted arch. The ascending aorta may take a straight cephalad course and is small compared with the dilated pulmonary trunk. A smooth unbroken contour represents continuity between pulmonary trunk, ductus, and descending aorta. A leftward and posterior malaligned ventricular septal defect is the rule when interruption is between the left carotid and left subclavian arteries. An aortopulmonary window is likely to be present if the ventricular septum is intact.

REFERENCES

1. Abbott ME: Coarctation of the aorta of adult type; statistical study and historical retrospect of 200 recorded cases with autopsy; of stenosis or obliteration of descending arch in subjects above age of two years. Am Heart J 3:574, 1928.
2. Abbott ME: Congenital cardiac disease. In Osler's Modern Medicine, 3rd ed. Philadelphia, Lea & Febiger, 1927.
3. Allan LD, Chita SK, Anderson RH, et al: Coarctation of the aorta in prenatal life: An echocardiographic, anatomical, and functional study. Br Heart J 59:356, 1988.
4. Allan LD, Crawford DC, Tynan M: Evolution of coarctation of the aorta in intrauterine life. Br Heart J 52:471, 1984.
5. Alpert BS, Bain HH, Balfe JW, et al: Role of the renin-angiotensin-aldosterone system in hypertensive children with coarctation of the aorta. Am J Cardiol 43:828, 1979.
6. Amsterdam EA, Albers WH, Christlieb AR, et al: Plasma renin activity in children with coarctation of the aorta. Am J Cardiol 23:396, 1969.
7. Anabtawi IN, Ellison RG, Yeh TJ, Hall DP: Dissecting aneurysm of aorta associated with Turner's syndrome. J Thorac Cardiovasc Surg 47:750, 1964.
8. Anderson RH, Lenox CC, Zuberbuhler JP: Morphology of ventricular septal defect associated with coarctation of the aorta. Br Heart J 50:176, 1983.
9. Angelini GD, Kulatilake ENP, Hayward M, Ruttley MSR: Pseudocoarctation of the aortic arch associated with bicuspid aortic valve lesion: Is it a surgical entity. Thorac Cardiovasc Surg 33:36, 1985.
10. Backer CL, Ilbawi MN, Idriss FS, DeLeon SY: Vascular anomalies causing tracheoesophageal compression: Review of experience in children. J Thorac Cardiovasc Surg 97:725, 1989.
11. Bagby SP, Moss RD: Abnormality of the renin/body-fluid-volume relationship in serially-studied inbred dogs with neonatally-induced coarctation hypertension. Hypertension 2:631, 1980.
12. Bahabozorgui S, Nemir P Jr: Coarctation of the abdominal aorta. Am J Surg 111:224, 1966.
13. Bahabozorgui S, Bernstein RG, Frater RWM: Pseudo coarctation of aorta associated with aneurysm formation. Chest 60:616, 1971.
14. Baile MD, Donoso VS, Gonzalez NC: Role of the renin-angiotensin system in hypertension after coarctation of the aorta. J Lab Clin Med 104:553, 1984.
15. Baron MG: Obscuration of the aortic knob in coarctation of the aorta. Circulation 43:311, 1971.
16. Becker AE, Becker MJ, Edwards JE: Anomalies associated with coarctation of the aorta. Circulation 41:1067, 1970.
17. Beekman RH, Robinow M: Coarctation of the aorta inherited as an autosomal dominant trait. Am J Cardiol 56:818, 1985.
18. Schievink WI, Mokri B, Offogras DG, Gittenberger-de Groot AC: Intracranial aneurysms and cervicocephalic arterial dissections associated with congenital heart disease. Neurosurgery 39:685, 1996.
19. Bell DR, Bohr DF: Endothelium in functional aortic changes of coarctation hypertension. Am J Physiol 260:H1187, 1991.
20. Ben-Shoshan M: Coarctation of abdominal aorta. Arch Pathol 95:221, 1973.
21. Bilgic A, Ozer S, Atalay S: Pseudocoarctation of the aorta. Jpn Heart J 31:875, 1990.
22. Björk L, Friedman R: Routine roentgenographic diagnosis of coarctation of the aorta in the child. Am J Roentgenol 95:636, 1965.
23. Blake HA, Manion WC, Spencer FC: Atresia or absence of the aortic isthmus. J Thorac Cardiovasc Surg 43:607, 1962.
24. Blumenthal S: Report of the task force on blood pressure control in children. Pediatrics 59:797, 1977.
25. Boone ML, Swenson BE, Felson B: Rib notching: Its many causes. Am J Roentgenol 91:1075, 1964.
26. Borow KM, Colan SD, Neumann A: Altered left ventricular mechanics in patients with valvular aortic stenosis and coarctation of the aorta: Effects on systolic performance and late outcome. Circulation 72:515, 1985.
27. Bousvaros GA: Diagnostic auscultatory complex in coarctation of the aorta. Br Heart J 29:443, 1967.
28. Braimbridge MV, Yen A: Coarctation in the elderly. Circulation 31:209, 1965.
29. Braulin E, Peoples WM, Freedom RM, et al: Interruption of the aortic arch with aorticopulmonary septal defect. Pediatr Cardiol 3:329, 1982.
30. Bruno E, Juaneda E, Moreyra E, Alday LE: The mitral mid-diastolic rumble in isolated coarctation of the aorta: Cross-sectional and Doppler echocardiographic study. J Cardiovasc Technology 9:143, 1990.
31. Brust AA, Howard JM, Bryant MR, Godwin JT: Coarctation of the abdominal aorta with stenosis of the renal arteries and hypertension: Clinical and pathologic study of 2 cases and review of the literature. Am J Med 27:793, 1959.
32. Burch J, Wennevold A, Efsen F, Andersen GE: Interrupted aortic arch in two siblings. Acta Paediatr Scand 69:783, 1980.
33. Burford TH, Ferguson TB, Goldring D, Behrer MR: Coarctation of the aorta in infants: A clinical and experimental study. J Thorac Cardiovasc Surg 39:47, 1960.
34. Campbell M: Natural history of coarctation of the aorta. Br Heart J 32:633, 1970.
35. Campbell M, Baylis JH: Course and prognosis of coarctation of aorta. Br Heart J 18:475, 1956.
36. Campbell M, Poloni PE: The aetiology of coarctation of the aorta. Lancet 1:463, 1961.
37. Campbell M, Suzman S: Coarctation of the aorta. Br Heart J 9:185, 1947.
38. Carey LS, Sellers RD, Shone JD: Radiologic findings in the developmental complex of parachute mitral valve, supravalvular ring of left atrium, subaortic stenosis, and coarctation of aorta. Radiology 82:1, 1964.
39. Carvalho JS, Redington AN, Shinebourne EA, et al: Continuous wave Doppler echocardiography and coarctation of the aorta: Gradients and flow patterns in the assessment of severity. Br Heart J 64:133, 1990.
40. Mazzanti L, Cacciari E: Congenital heart disease in patients with Turner's syndrome. J Pediatr 133:686, 1998.
41. Celano V, Pieroni DR, Morera JA, et al: Two-dimensional echocardiographic examination of mitral valve abnormalities associated with coarctation of the aorta. Circulation 69:924, 1984.
42. Celoria GC, Patton RB: Congenital absence of the aortic arch. Am Heart J 58:407, 1959.
43. Chiemmongkoltip O, Moulder PV, Cassels DE: Interruption of the aortic arch with aorticopulmonary septal defect and intact ventricular septum in a teenage girl. Chest 60:324, 1971.
44. Child JS: Transthoracic and transesophageal echocardiographic imaging: Anatomic and hemodynamic assessment. In Perloff JK, Child JS: Congenital Heart Disease in Adults. Philadelphia, WB Saunders, 1998.
45. Chun K, Colombani PM, Dudgeon DC, Haller JA: Diagnosis and management of congenital vascular rings: A 22-year experience. Ann Thorac Surg 53:597, 1992.
46. Prandstrailer D, Mazzanti L, Picchio FM, et al: Turner's syndrome: Cardiologic profile according to the different chromosomal patterns and long term clinical follow-up of 136 nonselected patients. Pediatr Cardiol 20:108, 1999.
47. Cohen JR, Biernbaum E: Coarctation of the abdominal aorta. J Vasc Surg 8:160, 1988.
48. Gopal AS, Arora NS, Vardanian S, Messineo FC: Utility of transesophageal echocardiography for the characterization of cardiovascular anomalies associated with Turner's syndrome. J Am Soc Echocardiogr 14:60, 2001.
49. Cumming GR, Mir GH: Exercise haemodynamics of coarctation of the aorta. Br Heart J 32:365, 1970.
50. Dahlback O, Dahn I, Westling H: Hemodynamic observations in coarctation of the aorta, with special reference to the blood pressure above and below the stenosis at rest and during exercise. Scand J Clin Lab Invest 16:339, 1964.
51. Davachi F, Moller JH, Edwards JE: Diseases of the mitral valve in infancy. Circulation 48:565, 1971.
52. Yamada M, Horigome H, Ishil S: Pseudocoarctation of the aorta coexistent with coarctation. Eur J Pediatr 155:993, 1996
53. Deeg KH, Singer H: Doppler sonographic diagnosis of subclavian steal in infants with coarctation of the aorta and interrupted aortic arch. Pediatr Radiol 19:163, 1989.
54. deMan SA, Andre J, Bachmann H, et al: Blood pressure in childhood: Pooled findings in six European studies. J Hypertension 9:109, 1991.
55. Dische MR, Tsai M, Baltaxe HA: Solitary interruption of the arch of the aorta. Am J Cardiol 35:271, 1975.
56. Donner R, Black I, Spann JF, Carabello BA: Left ventricular wall stress and function in childhood coarctation of the aorta. J Am Coll Cardiol 5:1161, 1985.
57. Doyle L: Coarctation of the aorta with dissecting aneurysm and haemopericardium: An account by Joseph Jordan, Manchester, 1830. Thorax 46:268, 1991.

58. Drexler CJ, Stewart JR, Kincaid OW: Diagnostic implications of rib notching. Am J Roentgenol 91:1064, 1964.

59. Taneja K, Kawira S, Sharma S, Rajani M: Pseudocoarctation of the aorta: Complementary findings on plain film x-ray, CT, DSA, and MRI. Cardiovasc Intervent Radiol 21:430, 1998.

60. Earley A, Joseph MC, Shinebourne EA, de Siviet M: Blood pressure and effect of exercise in children before and after surgical correction of coarctation of the aorta. Br Heart J 44:411, 1980.

61. Edwards JE: Aneurysms of the thoracic aorta complicating coarctation. Circulation 48:195, 1973.

62. Edwards JE: The congenital bicuspid aortic valve. Circulation 23:485, 1961.

63. Ikonomidis JS, Robbins RC: Cervical aortic arch with pseudocoarctation: presentation with spontaneous rupture. Ann Thorac Surg 67:248, 1999.

64. Edwards WE, Leaf DS, Edwards JE: Dissecting aortic aneurysm associated with bicuspid aortic valve. Circulation 57:1022, 1978.

65. Eisalo A, Raitta C, Kala R, Holonen PI: Fluorescence angiography of the fundus vessels in aortic coarctation. Br Heart J 32:71, 1970.

66. Elzenga NJ, Gittenberger-de Groot AC: Localized coarctation of the aorta. Br Heart J 49:317, 1983.

67. Ettedgui JA, Lorber A, Anderson D: Double aortic arch associated with coarctation. Int J Cardiol 12:258, 1986.

68. Schellhammer F, von den DP, Gaitzsch A: Pseudocoarctation of the abdominal aorta. Vasa 26:308, 1997.

69. Gutgesell HP, Barton DM, Elgin KM: Coarctation of the aorta in the neonate. Am J Cardiol 88:457, 2001.

70. Flyer DC, Buckley LP, Hellenbrand WE, Cohn HE: Report of the New England regional infant cardiac program. Pediatrics 65 (Suppl) :376, 1980.

71. Folger GM, Stein PD: Bicuspid aortic valve morphology when associated with coarctation of the aorta. Cathet Cardiovasc Diagn 10:17, 1984.

72. Seifert BL, DesRochers K, Ta M, et al: Accuracy of Doppler methods for estimating peak-to-peak instantaneous gradients across coarctation of the aorta: An in vitro study. J Am Soc Echocardiogr 12:744, 1999.

73. Freed MD, Keane JF, van Praagh R, et al: Coarctation of the aorta with congenital mitral regurgitation. Circulation 49:1175, 1974.

74. Freedom RM, Bain HH, Esplugas E, et al: Ventricular septal defect in interruption of aortic arch. Am J Cardiol 39:572, 1977.

75. Garcia OL, Hernandez FA, Tamer D, et al: Congenital bilateral subclavian steal. Am J Cardiol 44:101, 1979.

76. Garman JE, Hinson RE, Eyler WR: Coarctation of the aorta in infancy: Detection on chest x-rays. Radiology 85:418, 1965.

77. Glancy DL, Morrow AG, Simon AL, Roberts WC: Juxtaductal coarctation. Am J Cardiol 51:537, 1983.

78. Gokcebay TM: Complete interruption of the aortic arch. Am J Radiol 114:362, 1972.

79. Goldberg MD, Scully AL, Solomon IL, Steinbach HL: Gonadal dysgenesis in phenotypic female subjects. Am J Med 45:529, 1968.

80. Goldberg SM, Pizzarello RA, Goldman MA, Padmanabhan VT: Aortic dilatation resulting in chronic severe aortic regurgitation and complicated by aortic dissection in a patient with Turner's syndrome. Clin Cardiol 7:233, 1984.

81. Tacy TA, Baba K, Cape EG: Effect of aortic compliance on Doppler diastolic flow pattern in coarctation of the aorta. J Am Soc Echocardiogr 12:636, 1999.

82. Gough JH: Coarctation of the aorta in father and son. Br J Radiol 4:670, 1961.

83. Graham TP, Atwood GF, Boerth RC, et al: Right and left heart size and function in infants with symptomatic coarctation. Circulation 56:641, 1977.

84. Graham TP, Burger J, Boucek RJ, et al: Abnormal left ventricular volume loading in infants with coarctation of the aorta and a large ventricular septal defect. J Am Coll Cardiol 14:1545, 1989.

85. Greig D: Case of malformation of the heart and blood vessels of the fetus: Pulmonary artery giving off descending aorta and left subclavian artery. Mthly J Med Soc Bd 15:28, 1852.

86. Griffin JF: Congenital kinking of the aorta (pseudocoarctation). N Engl J Med 271:726, 1964.

87. Gunning JF, Oakley CM: Aortic valve disease in Turner's syndrome. Lancet 1:389, 1970.

88. Haldane JH: Coarctation of the aorta in an elderly man. Can Med Assoc J 128:1298, 1983.

89. Hallett JW, Brewster DC, Darling RC, O'Hara PJ: Coarctation of the abdominal aorta. Ann Surg 191:430, 1980.

90. Hernandez FA, Miller RH, Schiebler GL: Rarity of coarctation of the aorta in the American Negro. J Pediatr 74:623, 1969.

91. Hesslein PS, Gutgesell HP, McNamara DG: Prognosis of symptomatic coarctation of the aorta in infancy. Am J Cardiol 51:299, 1983.

92. Higgins CB, French JW, Silverman JF, Wexler L: Interruption of the aortic arch: Pre-operative and postoperative clinical, hemodynamic and angiographic features. Am J Cardiol 39:563, 1977.

93. Ho SY, Anderson RH: Coarctation, tubular hypoplasia and the ductus arteriosus. Br Heart J 41:268, 1979.

94. Hodes HL, Steinfeld L, Blumenthal S: Congenital cerebral aneurysms and coarctation of the aorta. Arch Pediatr 76:28, 1959.

95. Hoeffel JC, Henry M, Mentre B, et al: Pseudo coarctation or congenital kinking of the aorta: Radiologic considerations. Am Heart J 89:428, 1975.

96. Hornberger LK, Weintraub RG, Pesonen E, et al: Echocardiographic study of the morphology and growth of the aortic arch in the human fetus. Observations related to the prenatal diagnosis of coarctation. Circulation 86:741, 1992.

97. Igler FO, Boerboom LE, Werner PH, et al: Coarctation of the aorta and baroreceptor resetting. Circ Res 48:365, 1981.

98. Inada K, Yokoyama T, Ryoichi N: Atypical coarctation of the aorta. Angiology 14:506, 1963.

99. Isner JM, Donaldson RF, Fulton D, et al: Cystic medial necrosis in coarctation of the aorta: A potential factor contributing to adverse consequences observed after percutaneous balloon angioplasty of coarctation sites. Circulation 75:689, 1987.

100. Jaffe RB: Complete interruption of the aortic arch: Characteristic radiographic findings in 21 patients. Circulation 52:714, 1975.

101. Jaffe RB: Radiographic manifestations of congenital anomalies of the aortic arch. Radiol Clin North Am 29:319, 1991.

102. Jaffe RB: Complete interruption of the aortic arch. Circulation 53:161, 1976.

103. Jarcho S: Aortic coarctation and aortic stenosis (Nixon, 1834). Am J Cardiol 11:238, 1963.

104. Jarcho S: Coarctation of the aorta (Meckel, 1750; Paris, 1791). Am J Cardiol 7:844, 1961.

105. Jarcho S: Coarctation of the aorta (Otto, 1824; Bertin, 1824). Am J Cardiol 8:843, 1961.

106. Jarcho S: Coarctation of the aorta (Reynaud, 1828). Am J Cardiol 9:591, 1962.

107. Jarcho S: Coarctation of the aorta (Legrand, 1833). Am J Cardiol 10:266, 1962.

108. Jentsch E, Liersch R, Bourgeois M: Prolapsed valve of the foramen ovale in newborns and infants with coarctation of the aorta. Pediatr Cardiol 9:29, 1988.

109. Johansson BW, Hall P, Krook H, et al: Aortic anomaly with atypical coarctation: A report of 3 cases presenting coarctation between the origin of the left carotid and the left subclavian artery. Am J Cardiol 7:853, 1961.

110. Johns KL, Johns JA, Feman SS: Retinal vascular abnormalities in patients with coarctation of the aorta. Arch Ophthalmol 109:1266, 1991.

111. Johns RA: Interrupted aortic arch. Curr Opin Cardiol 3:776, 1988.

112. Judez VM, Maitre MJ, de Artaza M, et al: Interruption of aortic arch without associated cardiac abnormalities. Br Heart J 36:313, 1974.

113. Wessel A, Pankau R, Kececioglu D, et al: Three decades of follow-up of aortic and pulmonary vascular lesions in the Williams-Beuren syndrome. Am J Med Genet 52:297, 1994.

114. Kavanagh-Gray D, Chiu P: Kinking of the aorta (pseudo coarctation). Can Med Assoc J 103:717, 1970.

115. Keller HI, Cheitlin MD: The occurrence of mild coarctation of the aorta (pseudocoarctation) and coarctation in one family. Am Heart J 70:115, 1965.

116. Miro O, Jimenez S, Gonzalez J, et al: Highly effective compensatory mechanisms in a 76 year old man with coarctation of the aorta. Cardiology 92:284, 1999.

117. Kirkendall WM, Feinleib M, Freis ED, Mark AL: AHA Committee Report: Recommendations for human blood pressure determinations by sphygmomanometers. Circulation 62:1146A, 1980.

118. Kirks DR, Currarino G, Chen JTT: Mediastinal collateral arteries: Important vessels in coarctation of the aorta. Am J Radiol 146:757, 1986.

119. Klein LW, Levin JL, Weintraub WS, et al: Pseudocoarctation of the aortic arch in a patient with Turner's syndrome. Clin Cardiol 7:621, 1984.

120. Henderson RA, Ward C, Campbell C: Dissecting left subclavian artery aneurysm: An unusual presentation of coarctation of the aorta. Int J Cardiol 40:69, 1993.
121. Safir J, Kerr A, Morehouse H, et al: Magnetic resonance imaging of dissection in pseudocoarctation of the aorta. Cardiovasc Intervent Radiol 16:180, 1993.
122. Kutsche LM, van Mierop LHS: Cervical origin of the right subclavian artery in aortic arch interruption. Am J Cardiol 53:892, 1984.
123. Langille BL, Brownlee RD, Adamson SL: Perinatal aortic growth in lambs: Relation to blood flow changes at birth. Am J Physiol 259:H1247, 1990.
124. Lavin N, Mehta S, Liberson M, Pouget JM: Pseudocoarctation of the aorta. Am J Cardiol 24:584, 1969.
125. McMahon CJ, Vick GW, Nihill MR: Right aortic arch and coarctation. Heart 85:492, 2001.
126. Bergamini TM, Bernard JD, Mavroudis C, et al: Coarctation of the abdominal aorta. Ann Vasc Surg 9:352, 1995.
127. Leichtman DA, Schmickel RD, Gelehrter TD, et al: Familial Turner syndrome. Ann Intern Med 89:473, 1978.
128. Liberthson RR, Pennington DG, Jacobs ML, Daggett WM: Coarctation of the aorta: Review of 234 patients. Am J Cardiol 43:835, 1979.
129. Lie JT: Aortic dissection in Turner's syndrome. Am Heart J 103:1077, 1982.
130. Lie JT: The malformation complex of the absence of the arch of the aorta—Steidele's complex. Am Heart J 73:615, 1967.
131. Lin AE, Garver KL: Monozygotic Turner syndrome twins: Correlation of phenotype severity and heart defect. Am J Med Genet 29:529, 1988.
132. Lin AE, Lippe BM, Geffner ME, et al: Aortic dilatation, dissection, and rupture in patients with Turner syndrome. J Pediatr 109:820, 1986.
133. Granstrom KO: Retinal changes in coarctation of the aorta. Br J Ophthal 35:143, 1951.
134. Lodewik HS, van Mierop MD, Kutsche LM: Cardiovascular anomalies in DiGeorge syndrome and importance of neural crest as a possible pathogenetic factor. Am J Cardiol 58:133, 1986.
135. Cracowski JL, Vanzetto G, Douchin S, et al: Myocardial infarction and Turner syndrome. Clin Cardiol 22:245, 1999.
136. Manning DM, Kuchirka C, Kaminski J: Miscuffing: Inappropriate blood pressure cuff application. Circulation 68:763, 1983.
137. Marasini M, Pongiglione G, Lituania M, et al: Aortic arch interruption: Two-dimensional echocardiographic recognition in utero. Pediatr Cardiol 6:147, 1985.
138. Kappetein AP, Gittenberger-de Groot AC, Zwinderman AH, et al: The neural crest as a possible pathogenetic factor of coarctation of the aorta and bicuspid aortic valve. J Thorac Cardiovasc Surg 102:830, 1991.
139. McCrindle BW: Coarctation of the aorta. Curr Opin Cardiol 14:448, 1999.
140. Merrill DL, Webster CA, Samson PC: Congenital absence of the aortic isthmus. J Thorac Cardiovasc Surg 33:311, 1957.
141. Miettinen OA, Reiner ML, Nadas AS: Seasonal incidence of coarctation of the aorta. Br Heart J 32:103, 1970.
142. Miller MJ, Geffner ME, Lippe BM, et al: Echocardiography reveals a high incidence of bicuspid aortic valve in Turner syndrome. J Pediatr 102:47, 1983.
143. Miller RA, Shekelle RB: Blood pressure in tenth grade students: Results from the Chicago Heart Association Pediatric Heart Screening Project. Circulation 54:993, 1976.
144. Milo S, Massini C, Goor DA: Isolated atresia of the aortic arch in a 65 year old man. Br Heart J 47:294, 1982.
145. Roberts DL, Tatini U, Zimmerman RS, et al: Musical hallucinations associated with seizures originating from an intracranial aneurysm. Mayo Clin Proc 76:423, 2001.
146. Jinping X, Shiota T, Omoto R, et al: Intravascular ultrasound assessment of regional aortic wall stiffness, distensibility, and compliance in patients with coarctation of the aorta. Am Heart J 134:93, 1997.
147. Tacy TA, Baba K, Cape EG: Effect of aortic compliance on Doppler diastolic flow pattern in coarctation of the aorta. J Am Soc Echocardiogr 12:636, 1999.
148. Moene RJ, Gittenberger-DeGroot AC, Oppenheimer-Dekker A, Bartelings MM: Anatomic characteristics of ventricular septal defect associated with coarctation of the aorta. Am J Cardiol 59:952, 1987.
149. Moerman P, Dumoulin M, Lauweryns J, Van Der Hauwaert LG: Interrupted right aortic arch in DiGeorge syndrome. Br Heart J 58:274, 1987.
150. Moller JH, Edwards JE: Interruption of the aortic arch: Anatomic patterns and associated cardiac malformations. Am J Roentgenol 95:557, 1965.
151. Moller JH, Lucas RV, Adams P, et al: Endocardial fibroelastosis. Circulation 30:759, 1964.
152. Morgan JR, Forker AD, Fosburg RG, et al: Interruption of the aortic arch without a patent ductus arteriosus. Circulation 42:961, 1970.
153. Morrow WR, Huhta JC, Murphy DJ, McNamara DG: Quantitative morphology of the aortic arch in neonatal circulation. J Am Coll Cardiol 8:616, 1986.
154. Moss AJ: Coarctation of the aorta in siblings. J Pediatr 46:707, 1955.
155. Brili S, Dernellis J, Aggeli C, et al: Aortic elastic properties in patients with repaired coarctation of the aorta. Am J Cardiol 82:1140, 1998.
156. Nasser WK, Helman C: Kinking of the aortic arch (pseudocoarctation): Clinical, radiographic, hemodynamic, and angiographic finding in 8 cases. Ann Intern Med 64:971, 1966.
157. Falkner B, Chair, Working Group: Update on the 1987 task force report on high blood pressure in children and adolescents. Pediatrics 98:649, 1996.
158. Neches WH, Park SC, Lenox CC, et al: Coarctation of the aorta with ventricular septal defect. Circulation 55:189, 1977.
159. Niwa K, Perloff JK, Bhuta SM, et al: Structural abnormalities of great arterial walls in congenital heart disease. Circulation 103:393, 2001.
160. Kreutzer J, Van Praagh R: Comparison of left ventricular outflow tract obstruction in interruption of the aortic arch and in coarctation of the aorta, with diagnostic, developmental, and surgical implications. Am J Cardiol 86:856, 2000.
161. Brockmeier K, Demirakca S, Metzner R, Floemer F: Double aortic arch. Circulation 102:e93, 2000.
162. Nora JJ, Torres FG, Sinhas AK, McNamara DG: Characteristic cardiovascular anomalies of XO Turner syndrome, XX and XY phenotype and XO/XX Turner mosaic. Am J Cardiol 25:639, 1970.
163. Digilio MD, Marino B, Picchio F, et al: Noonan syndrome and aortic coarctation. Am J Med Genet 80:160, 1998.
164. Oppenheimer EH: The association of adult-type coarctation of the aorta with endocardial fibroelastosis in infancy. Bull Johns Hopkins Hosp 93:309, 1953.
165. O'Rourke MF, Cartmill TB: Influence of aortic coarctation on pulsatile hemodynamics in the proximal aorta. Circulation 44:281, 1971.
166. Pankau R, Funda J, Wessel A: Interrupted aortic arch type B1 in a brother and sister: Suggestion of a recessive gene. Am J Med Genet 36:175, 1990.
167. Park MK, Guntheroth WG: Direct blood pressure measurements in brachial and femoral arteries in children. Circulation 41:321, 1970.
168. Perloff JK: Normal myocardial growth and the development and regression of increased ventricular mass. In Perloff JK, Child JS (eds): Congenital Heart Disease in Adults, 2nd ed. Philadelphia, W.B. Saunders, 1998, p 357.
169. Perloff JK: Physical Examination of the Heart and Circulation, 3rd ed. Philadelphia, W.B. Saunders, 1998.
170. Perloff JK: Pregnancy in congenital heart disease: The mother and the fetus. In Perloff JK, Child JS (eds): Congenital Heart Disease in Adults, 2nd ed. Philadelphia, W.B. Saunders, 1998, p 144.
171. Pieroni DR, Brodsky ST, Rowe RD: Congenital subclavian steal. Am Heart J 84:801, 1972.
172. Pierpont MEA, Gobel JW, Moller JH, Edwards JE: Cardiac malformations in relatives of children with truncus arteriosus or interruption of the aortic arch. Am J Cardiol 61:423, 1988.
173. Pierpont MEA, Zollikofer CL, Moller JH, Edwards JE: Interruption of the aortic arch with right ascending aorta. Pediatr Cardiol 2:153, 1982.
174. Hu WY, Sevick RJ, Tranmer BI, et al: Aortic arch interruption associated with ruptured cerebral aneurysm. Can Assoc Radiol J 47:20, 1996.
175. Gobel JW, Pierpont ME, Moller JH, et al: Familial interruption of the aortic arch. Pediatr Cardiol 14:110, 1993.
176. Karkar P, Dalvi B, Kate P: Interrupted aortic arch with associated cardiac anomalies: Survival to adulthood. Chest 103:279, 1993.
177. Reifenstein GH, Levine SA, Gross RE: Coarctation of the aorta: A review of 104 autopsied cases of the "adult-type," two years of age or older. Am Heart J 33:146, 1947.
178. Riemenschneider TA, Emmanouilides GC, Hirose R, Linde LM: Coarctation of the abdominal aorta in children. Pediatrics 44:716, 1969.

179. Riggs TW, Berry TE, Aziz KV, Paul MH: Two-dimensional echocardiographic features of interruption of the aortic arch. Am J Cardiol 50:1385, 1982.

180. Roberts WC, Morrow AC, Braunwald E: Complete interruption of the aortic arch. Circulation 26:39, 1962.

181. Nakada T, Yonesaka S: Interruption of aortic arch type A in two siblings. Acta Pediatr Jpn 38:83, 1996.

182. Roques X, Bourdeau'dhui A, Choussat A, et al: Coarctation of the abdominal aorta. Ann Vasc Surg 2:138, 1988.

183. Rosenquist GC: Congenital mitral valve disease associated with coarctation of the aorta: A spectrum that includes parachute deformity of the mitral valve. Circulation 49:985, 1974.

184. Rowen MJ: Coarctation of the aorta in father and son. Am J Cardiol 4:540, 1959.

185. Thomson PS, Teele RL: Reversal of left carotid arterial blood flow as a sign of type C interruption of the aortic arch. Pediatr Radiol 24:300, 1994.

186. Rudolph AM, Heymann MA, Spitznas U: Hemodynamic considerations in the development of narrowing of the aorta. Am J Cardiol 30:514, 1972.

187. Al Marsafawy HM, Ho SY, Redington AN, Anderson RH: The relationship of the outlet septum to the outflow tract in hearts with interruption of the aortic arch. J Thorac Cardiovasc Surg 109:1225, 1995.

188. Russell GA, Berry PJ, Watterson K, et al: Patterns of ductal tissue in coarctation of the aorta in the first three months of life. J Cardiovasc Surg 102:596, 1991.

189. Schneeweiss A, Scherf L, Lehrer E, et al: Segmental study of the terminal coronary vessels in coarctation. Am J Cardiol 49:1996, 1982.

190. Schumacher G, Schreiber R, Meisner H, et al: Interrupted aortic arch: Natural history and operative results. Pediatr Cardiol 7:89, 1986.

191. Mishaly D, Birk E, Katz J, Vidne BA: Interruption of right sided aortic arch. J Cardiovasc Surg (Torino) 36:277, 1995.

192. Sehested J: Coarctation of the aorta in monozygotic twins. Br Heart J 47:619, 1982.

193. Sehested J, Baandrup U, Mikkelson E: Different reactivity and structure of the prestenotic and poststenotic aorta in human coarctation. Circulation 65:1060, 1982.

194. Geva T, Gagarski RJ: Echocardiographic diagnosis of type B interruption of a right aortic arch. Am Heart J 129:1042, 1995.

195. Shachter N, Perloff JK, Mulder DG: Aortic dissection in Noonan's syndrome. Am J Cardiol 54:464, 1984.

196. Takahashi K, Kuwahara T, Nagatsu M: Interruption of the aortic arch at the isthmus with DiGeorge syndrome and 22q11.2 deletion. Cardiol Young 9:516, 1999.

197. Baysai T, Kutlu R, Sarac K, Karaman I: Ruptured intracranial aneurysm associated with isolated aortic arch interruption. Neuroradiology 42:842, 2000.

198. Shanahan WR, Romney SL, Currens JH: Coarctation of the aorta and pregnancy: Report of 10 cases with 24 pregnancies. JAMA 167:275, 1958.

199. Sharratt GP, Carson P, Sanderson JM: Complete interruption of aortic arch, without persistent ductus arteriosus in an adult. Br Heart J 37:221, 1975.

200. Shearer WT, Rutman JY, Weinberg WA, Goldring D: Coarctation of the aorta and cerebrovascular accident. J Pediatr 77:1004, 1970.

201. Shinebourne EA, Tam ASY, Elseed AM, et al: Coarctation of the aorta in infancy and childhood. Br Heart J 38:375, 1976.

202. Shone JD, Anderson RC, Amplatz K, et al: Pulmonary venous obstruction from two separate coexistent anomalies. Am J Cardiol 11:525, 1963.

203. Kruetzer J, Van Praagh R: Comparison of left ventricular outflow tract obstruction in interruption of the aortic arch and in coarctation of the aorta. Am J Cardiol 86:856, 2000.

204. Siggers DC, Polani PE: Congenital heart disease in male and female subjects with somatic features of Turner's syndrome and normal sex chromosomes (Ullrich's and related syndromes). Br Heart J 34:41, 1972.

205. Silander T: Anomalous origin of the right subclavian artery and its relation to coarctation of the aorta. Acta Chir Scand 124:412, 1962.

206. Rangei A, Chavez E, Espinosa I: Interruption of the aortic arch in adults. Arch Inst Cardiol Mex 69:144, 1999.

207. Simon AB, Zloto AE, Perry BL, Sigmann JM: Familial aspects of coarctation of the aorta. Chest 66:687, 1974.

208. Simpson IA, Sahn DJ, Valdez-Cruz LM, et al: Color flow Doppler mapping in patients with coarctation of the aorta. Circulation 77:736, 1988.

209. Sinha SN, Kandatyke ML, Cole RB, et al: Coarctation of the aorta in infancy. Circulation 40:385, 1969.

210. Sloan RD, Cooley RN: Coarctation of the aorta: The roentgenologic aspects of 125 surgically confirmed cases. Radiology 61:701, 1953.

211. Starreveld JS, van Rossum AC, Hruda J: Rapid formation of collateral arteries in a neonate with interruption of the aortic arch. Cardiol Young 11:464, 2001.

212. Smallhorn JF, Anderson RH, Macartney FJ: Morphological characterisation of ventricular septal defects associated with coarctation of aorta by cross-sectional echocardiography. Br Heart J 49:485, 1983.

213. Bergwerff M, DeRuiter MC, Hall S, et al: Unique vascular morphology of the fourth aortic arches: Possible implications for the pathogenesis of type B aortic arch interruption and anomalous right subclavian artery. Cardiovasc Res 44:185, 1999.

214. Smyth PT, Edwards JE: Pseudocoarctation, kinking or buckling of the aorta. Circulation 46:1027, 1972.

215. Spencer MP, Johnston FR, Meredith JH: The origin and interpretation of murmurs in coarctation of the aorta. Am Heart J 56:722, 1958.

216. Steidele RJ: Sammlung Verschiedener in der chirurgisch Praktik. Lehrschule Germachten Beobb 2:114, 1777–88.

217. Steinberg I: Anomalies (pseudocoarctation) of the arch of the aorta: Report of eight new and review of eight previously published cases. Am J Roentgenol 88:73, 1962.

218. Cracowski JL, Vanzetto G, Douchin S, et al: Myocardial infarction and Turner syndrome. Clin Cardiol 22:245, 1999.

219. Strader WJ, Wachtel HL, Lundberg GD: Hypertension and aortic rupture in gonadal dysgenesis. J Pediatr 79:473, 1971.

220. Strafford MA, Griffiths SP, Gersony WM: Coarctation of the aorta: A study in delayed detection. Pediatrics 69:159, 1982.

221. Subramanian AR: Coarctation or interruption of aorta proximal to origin of both subclavian arteries. Br Heart J 34:1225, 1972.

222. Tabakin BS, Hanson JS: Congenital absence of the aortic arch associated with ventricular septal defect. Am J Cardiol 6:689, 1960.

223. Takashina T, Ishikura Y, Yamane K, et al: The congenital cardiovascular anomalies of interruption of the aorta—Steidele's complex. Am Heart J 83:93, 1972.

224. Talner NS, Berman MA: Postnatal development of obstruction in coarctation of the aorta: Role of the ductus arteriosus. Pediatrics 56:562, 1975.

225. Tawes RL, Aberdeen E, Waterson DJ, Bonham-Carter RE: Coarctation of the aorta in infants and children. Circulation 39(Suppl. 1):173, 1969.

226. Taylor RR, Pollock BE: Coarctation of the aorta in three members of a family. Am Heart J 45:470, 1953.

227. Turner HH: A syndrome of infantilism, congenital webbed neck, and cubitus valgus. Endocrinology 23:566, 1938.

228. Van der Horst RL, Gotsman MS: Racial incidence of coarctation of aorta. Br Heart J 34:289, 1972.

229. van Mierop LH, Kutsche LM: Interruption of the aortic arch and coarctation of the aorta: Pathogenetic relations. Am J Cardiol 54:829, 1984.

230. Vlodaver Z, Neufeld HN: Coronary arteries in coarctation of the aorta. Circulation 37:449, 1968.

231. Walker GL, Stanfield TF: Retinal changes associated with coarctation of the aorta. Trans Am Ophthalmol Soc 50:407, 1952.

232. Wallace RB, Nast EP: Postcoarctation mycotic intercostal arterial pseudoaneurysm. Am J Cardiol 59:1014, 1987.

233. Ward KE, Pryor RW, Matson JR, et al: Delayed detection of coarctation in infancy: Implications for timing of newborn-follow-up. Pediatrics 86:972, 1990.

234. Warren DJ, Smith RS, Naik RB: Inappropriate renin secretion and abnormal cardiovascular reflexes in coarctation of the aorta. Br Heart J 45:733, 1981.

235. Weiner SN, Bernstein RG, Shapiro M: Dissecting aneurysm in a patient with pseudocoarctation of the aorta. N Y State J Med 83:988, 1983.

236. Whyte D, Lu AT: Coarctation of the aorta with aneurysm and rupture into the esophagus: Report of a case and review of the literature. J Pediatr 49:461, 1956.

237. Wiest JW, Traverso LW, Dainko EA, Barker WF: Atrophic coarctation of the abdominal aorta. Ann Surg 191:224, 1980.

238. Wilson DI, Cross IE, Goodship JA, et al: DiGeorge syndrome with isolated aortic coarctation and isolated ventricular septal defect in three sibs with a 22q11 deletion of maternal original. Br Heart J 66:308, 1991.

239. Woltman HW, Shelden WD: Neurologic complications associated with congenital stenosis of isthmus of aorta: Case of cerebral aneurysm with rupture and case of intermittent lameness presumably related to stenosis of isthmus. Arch Neurol Psychiatr 17:303, 1927.

240. Wong C, Cheng C, Lau C, et al: Interrupted aortic arch in an asymptomatic adult. Chest 96:678, 1989.

241. Youker JE, Benson BR: Aneurysm of the aortic sinuses and ascending aorta in Turner's syndrome. Am J Cardiol 23:89, 1969.

242. Young MW, Lau SH, Stein E, Damato AN: Pseudocoarctation of the aorta. Am Heart J 77:259, 1969.

243. Wolman HW, Shelden WD: Neurologic complications associated with congenital stenosis of isthmus of aorta: Case of cerebral aneurysm with rupture and case of intermittent lameness presumably related to stenosis of isthmus. Arch Neurol Psychiatr 17:303, 1927.

Congenital Obstruction to Left Atrial Flow: Mitral Stenosis, Cor Triatriatum, Pulmonary Vein Stenosis

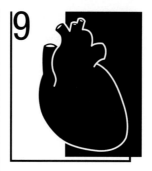

Congenital obstruction to left atrial flow can originate at or near the junction of pulmonary veins and left atrium (pulmonary vein stenosis), within the left atrium (cor triatriatum), immediately above the mitral valve (supravalvular ring), or within the mitral apparatus (mitral stenosis) (Fig. 9–1, Table 9–1). Pure or relatively pure forms of each defect are emphasized in this chapter, although a variety of anomalies can coexist.[14,84] Pulmonary veno-occlusive disease is covered in Chapter 14, total anomalous pulmonary venous connection with obstruction is covered in Chapter 15, and hypoplastic left heart with a hypoplastic mitral orifice is covered in Chapter 31.

Congenital Mitral Stenosis

Congenital mitral stenosis resides in the annulus, the leaflets, the chordae tendineae, the papillary muscles, or immediately above and contiguous with the annulus. The incidence of congenital mitral stenosis has been estimated at 0.6% of necropsy cases of congenital heart disease and 0.21% to 0.42% of clinical cases of congenital heart disease.[10] Congenital mitral stenosis with a functionally adequate left ventricle includes the following malformations in approximate order of frequency (see Table 9–1)[7,28,31,48,60,81,87]:

1. Short chordae tendineae with reduction in or obliteration of interchordal spaces and a decrease in interpapillary muscle distance (Fig. 9–2A)[14,67];
2. Parachute mitral valve with a single eccentric papillary muscle into which all chordae tendineae insert from both leaflets (Fig. 9–3, and see Fig. 9–2B).[14,69,74,84]
3. Anomalous mitral arcade characterized by a band of fibrous tissue that runs adjacent to the free margins of the mitral leaflets with short or absent chordae tendineae and

multiple contiguous papillary muscles.[12,33,50] This valve mechanism can function normally[31] or can be incompetent when chordae tendineae are well-formed.[30,31,42,50,62] Rarely, an anomalous mitral arcade coexists with a tricuspid arcade and incompetence of *both* atrioventricular valves.[50]

4. Supravalvular stenosing ring represented by a circumferential diaphragm at the base of the atrial surfaces of the mitral leaflets (see Fig. 9–2C).[18,69,74,77,81] The supravalvular ring has been reported with mitral regurgitation.[36,67]
5. Accessory mitral valve tissue.[18]
6. Anomalous left ventricular muscle bundles or anomalous obstructing papillary muscles.[18,73]
7. Double orifice mitral valve that can be stenotic, incompetent, or functionally normal.[16,32,41]

Flow across a normal mitral orifice is between the leaflets (interleaflet) and between the chordae tendineae (interchordal). Flow across a parachute mitral valve cannot be interleaflet because all chordae tendineae insert into a single papillary muscle (absence of a papillary muscle or fusion of the two papillary muscles), and interchordal flow is compromised because of reduced or obliterated interchordal spaces (see Figs. 9–2B and 9–3).[69] A parachute mitral valve becomes incompetent when elongated chordae tendineae are not significantly fused.

The parachute mitral valve is usually one component of a developmental complex consisting of four obstructive lesions, namely, supravalvular stenosing ring, parachute mitral valve, subaortic stenosis, and coarctation of the aorta—Shone's complex (see Fig. 9–3).[14,77,79,84] All four obstructive lesions are not necessarily significant or even present.[68,69,84] The supravalvular mitral ring can be

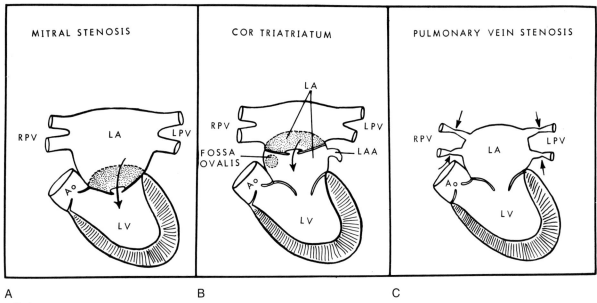

Figure 9–1

A, Illustration of congenital obstruction to left atrial flow involving the mitral apparatus or immediately above or contiguous with the mitral annulus. Ao, aorta; LA, left atrium; LV, left ventricle; LPV, left pulmonary veins; RPV, right pulmonary veins. *B,* Illustration of typical cor triatriatum. A fibrous or fibromuscular diaphragm partitions the left atrium. The proximal compartment receives the pulmonary veins and is a high-pressure zone. The distal compartment contains the fossa ovalis and the left atrial appendage (LAA) and is a low-pressure zone. *C,* Illustration of pulmonary vein stenosis in which there is narrowing of one or more pulmonary veins near their left atrial junction.

rudimentary (see Fig. 9–3*C*), can bridge the mitral orifice as a stenosing diaphragm (see Fig. 9–3*B*),[18,81] or, rarely, can occur as an isolated obstructive lesion.[79,93]

The functional consequences of congenital mitral stenosis are analogous to acquired mitral stenosis.[17,88] The elevated left atrial pressure is transmitted into pulmonary veins and pulmonary artery as pulmonary hypertension.

THE HISTORY

In congenital mitral stenosis there is a male predilection,[14] in contrast to a female predilection in acquired rheumatic

Table 9–1 | Congenital Obstruction to Left Atrial Flow With Functionally Adequate Left Ventricle

---

Congenital mitral stenosis

   Obstruction within the mitral apparatus: short chordae tendineae with decreased interpapillary muscle distance and reduced or obliterated interchordal spaces

   Parachute mitral valve

   Anomalous mitral arcade

   Accessory mitral valve tissue

   Anomalous left ventricular muscle bundles or obstructing papillary muscles

   Double orifice mitral valve

   Supravalvular stenosing ring

Cor triatriatum

Pulmonary vein stenosis

mitral stenosis. Familial recurrence has not been reported in congenital mitral stenosis. If stenosis is severe, symptoms begin shortly after birth when pulmonary blood flow is established and suddenly received by the obstructed left atrium.[74,88] Fifty percent of symptomatic infants die within 6 months,[88] but an occasional infant is asymptomatic, and a few remain relatively free of symptoms for years.[17] A parachute mitral valve or a supravalvular mitral ring permits better longevity (median 10 years and 5.5 years, respectively), whereas short chordae tendineae, obliterated interchordal spaces, and contiguous papillary muscles result in death at a median age of 6 months.[69,81] Anomalous mitral arcade or double-orifice mitral valve permits adult survival when the mitral apparatus functions normally or is purely regurgitant.[7,41,62]

Orthopnea, dyspnea, tachypnea, and paroxysmal cough result from pulmonary edema interspersed with recurrent lower respiratory infections.[14,17,23,78] Congenital mitral stenosis is occasionally associated with syncope[17] but seldom with hemoptysis.[78] Aphonia has been attributed to compression of the recurrent laryngeal nerve by a dilated hypertensive pulmonary trunk, analogous to hoarseness in adults with pulmonary hypertension and rheumatic mitral stenosis.[88] Infective endocarditis is rare.[14]

PHYSICAL APPEARANCE

Mild cyanosis is related to congestive heart failure.[17,23] Recurrent lower respiratory infections and the catabolic effects of heart failure account for physical underdevelopment.[17,23,78]

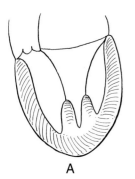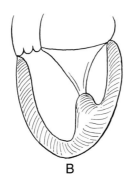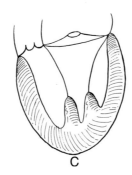

Figure 9–2

Illustrations of three anatomic types of congenital mitral stenosis involving the mitral apparatus. *A,* The typical form is characterized by decreased interpapillary muscle distance and reduction in interchordal spaces. *B,* Parachute mitral valve with a single eccentric papillary muscle. *C,* Supravalvular stenosing mitral ring.

THE ARTERIAL PULSE, THE JUGULAR VENOUS PULSE, AND PRECORDIAL MOVEMENT AND PALPATION

The arterial pulse is normal and confirms normal sinus rhythm, which is the rule in congenital mitral stenosis.[17,23] The jugular venous pulse discloses an increased A wave of pulmonary hypertension (Fig. 9–4). A precordial bulge is common,[78] and a right ventricular impulse is palpable at the lower left sternal border and subxiphoid area.[17,78]

AUSCULTATION

A loud first heart sound and an opening snap require abrupt closing and opening movements of the belly of a mobile anterior mitral leaflet. These two auscultatory signs of rheumatic mitral stenosis are not features of congenital mitral stenosis because mitral leaflet morphology does not provide the necessary preconditions (Figs. 9–5 and 9–6).[6,12,14,17,23,28,69,78,88] A holosystolic murmur at the apex or lower left sternal edge with a parachute mitral valve[48] or a supravalvular ring[36,67] is due to mitral regurgitation or pulmonary hypertensive tricuspid regurgitation.[23] An apical mid-diastolic murmur with presystolic accentuation (see Figs. 9–5 and 9–6) is exceptional because the rapid heart rate in infants shortens diastole[14,17,23,48,78,88] and because a dilated hypertensive right ventricle displaces the left ventricle from the apex.[63,64] The pulmonary component second heart sound is loud because of pulmonary hypertension that sets the stage for the Graham Steele murmur of high pressure pulmonary regurgitation.[14,18,88]

THE ELECTROCARDIOGRAM

Atrial fibrillation is exceptional, in contrast to rheumatic mitral regurgitation.[14,48] Pulmonary hypertension results in right atrial P wave abnormalities,[17,23,48,88] right axis deviation,[14,23,48,88] and right ventricular hypertrophy (Fig. 9–7).[14,17,23,88]

THE X-RAYS

In the chest x-ray, pulmonary venous congestion, including Kerley lines, can be seen at the bases (Fig. 9–8).[14,17,78]

Mild to moderate left atrial enlargement is recognized in the lateral view (see Fig. 9–8B). Straightening of the left cardiac border (Fig. 9–9) by an enlarged left atrial appendage is much less common than in rheumatic mitral stenosis.[14,17,23,48,88] Calcification of the mitral valve is absent histologically and on the x-ray.[66] The pulmonary trunk, right ventricle, and right atrium are enlarged because of pulmonary hypertension (see Figs. 9–8 and 9–9).[17]

THE ECHOCARDIOGRAM

Congenital mitral stenosis is characterized by two well-formed papillary muscles with reduced interpapillary distance.[69] A parachute mitral valve is characterized by a single papillary muscle onto which all chordae tendineae converge (Fig. 9–10, and see Fig. 9–3B,C).[33,79,80,90] The effective orifice size cannot be determined by two-dimensional echocardiography because flow is interchordal and the valve is eccentric (see Fig. 9–10B), but Doppler interrogation determines the gradient and the orifice size (see Fig. 9–10C,D). A supravalvular ring is identified more readily when it is unattached to the mitral leaflets (see Figs. 9–3B and 9–10A),[31,81] but when the supravalvular ring is attached to the mitral leaflets, it may be seen only in diastole.[81] An anomalous mitral arcade has multiple papillary muscles and little or no chordae tendineae interposed between the arcade and mitral leaflets.[31,33] The relative size of the two orifices of a double-orifice mitral valve can be determined, the chordal insertions can be characterized, and the functional state of the valve can be established as normal, stenotic, or incompetent.[41,87]

SUMMARY

Congenital mitral stenosis is a rare form of obstruction to left atrial flow that becomes manifest in infancy with pulmonary edema and pulmonary hypertension. Symptoms usually begin shortly after the newborn lungs inflate and pulmonary blood flow commences. Dyspnea, tachypnea, and cough are provoked by pulmonary venous congestion. The physical signs of pulmonary hypertension and right ventricular failure are overt, but the auscultatory signs of mitral stenosis are muted. The electrocardiogram exhibits right atrial P waves, right axis deviation, and right ventricular hypertrophy. The x-ray exhibits pulmonary venous

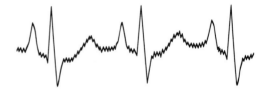

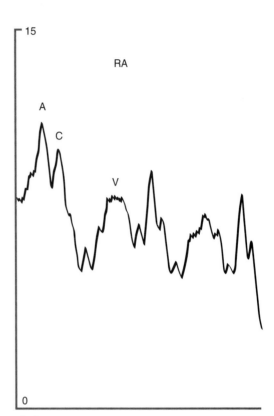

Figure 9–4
Right atrial pressure pulse (RA) showing a prominent A wave in a 3-year-old girl with congenital mitral stenosis.

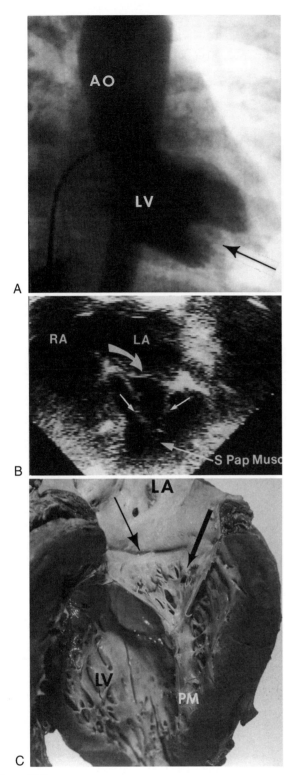

Figure 9–3
A, Left ventriculogram (LV) from an 8-year-old girl with a parachute mitral valve identified by the single papillary muscle (*arrow*, wedge of negative contrast). AO, ascending aorta. *B*, Echocardiogram (apical four-chamber) from a 10-year-old boy with Shone complex, a supravalvular stenosing ring (*unmarked curved arrow*), a parachute mitral valve (*smaller unmarked oblique arrows*), and an eccentric single papillary muscle (S Pap Musc). LA, left atrium; RA, right atrium. *C*, Necropsy specimen from a 14-year-old boy with a parachute mitral valve, obstructing interchordal slits, and insertion into a single eccentric papillary muscle (PM). A supravalvular ring is identified by the *upper left arrow*. Compare to the echocardiogram in part *B*. LA, left atrium; LV, left ventricle.

congestion, left atrial enlargement, and dilatation of the pulmonary trunk, right ventricle, and right atrium. Echocardiography establishes the anatomic type of congenital mitral stenosis and the degree of obstruction.

Cor Triatriatum

Partition of the left atrium into two compartments was recognized by Andral in 1829.[5] Four decades later, Church published the first detailed pathologic description of the malformation[13] that Borst (1905) called *cor triatriatum*.[9] The anomaly is rare, with a prevalence of about 0.1% of cases of congenital heart disease.[60,85]

Cor triatriatum is characterized by a membrane that partitions the left atrium into a proximal accessory chamber that receives the pulmonary veins and a distal true left atrial chamber that contains the left atrial appendage and the fossa ovalis (Fig. 9–11, and see Fig. 9–1*B*).[10,27,39,45,49,51,85,89,94] The malformation results from failure of incorporation of the common pulmonary vein into the left atrium,[21,49,89] a

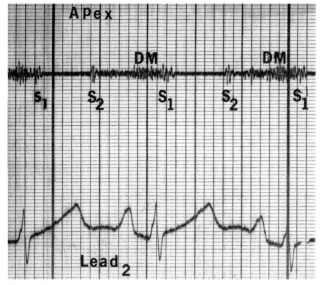

Figure 9–5

Phonocardiogram from a 2-year-old girl with Shone complex (supravalvular stenosing ring, parachute mitral valve, coarctation of the aorta) and a patent ductus arteriosus with pulmonary vascular disease and reversed shunt. The first heart sound (S_1) is soft. There is no opening snap. A soft mid-diastolic murmur is followed by presystolic accentuation. DM, diastolic murmur; S_2, second heart sound.

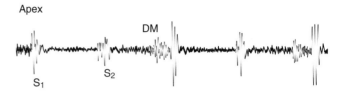

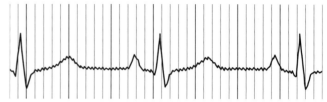

Figure 9–6

Phonocardiogram from the 3-year-old girl with congenital mitral stenosis referred to in Figure 9–4. The first heart sound (S_1) is loud but there is no opening snap. A soft mid-diastolic murmur (DM) is followed by presystolic accentuation.

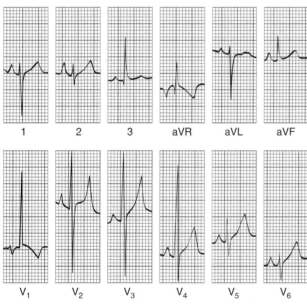

Figure 9–7

Electrocardiogram from the 2-year-old girl with Shone complex and pulmonary vascular disease referred to in Figure 9–5. Tall peaked right atrial P waves are present in leads 1, 2, and V_2. There is marked right axis deviation. Right ventricular hypertrophy is manifested by the tall monophasic R wave in lead V_1 and the deep S wave in lead V_6. Large RS complexes in lead V_2 and V_3 suggest biventricular hypertrophy for which coarctation of the aorta was responsible.

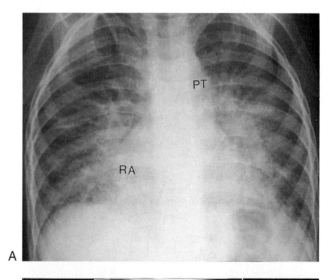

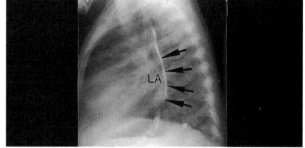

Figure 9–8

X-rays from the 2-year-old girl with Shone complex whose phonocardiogram is shown in Figure 9–5. A, Pulmonary venous congestion is striking. The pulmonary trunk (PT) and right atrium (RA) are dilated. B, The lateral film shows displacement of the barium esophagram by an enlarged left atrium (LA).

process that begins at about the fifth week of gestation and proceeds through subsequent stages of embryogenesis.[49] The proximal accessory chamber, which cannot be identified externally,[49] therefore represents persistence of the common pulmonary vein of the embryo. Anatomic varia-

tions of cor triatriatum are referred to as *diaphragmatic, hourglass,* and *tubular*.[49,85] In the diaphragmatic type, which is the most representative, the proximal accessory chamber and the distal true left atrial chamber are sepa-

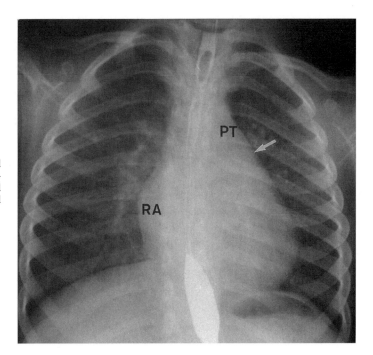

Figure 9–9
X-ray from the 3-year-old girl with congenital mitral stenosis referred to in Figures 9–4 and 9–6. Hilar pulmonary venous congestion is bilateral. The right atrium (RA) and pulmonary trunk (PT) are dilated, and the left cardiac border is straightened by an enlarged left atrial appendage (*arrow*).

rated by a fibrous or fibromuscular diaphragm (see Fig. 9–11) that contains either a single opening or multiple openings, the size of which determines the degree of obstruction.[49,57] Functionally insignificant nonobstructive ridges of tissue go unrecognized or are incidental findings at necropsy.[24,44,57,61,83] At the other extreme, no communication exists between the accessory chamber and the true left atrium (atresia of the common pulmonary vein).[19,46,58]

Tubular cor triatriatum is the most primitive and least common variety.[49] The proximal chamber retains the shape of the common pulmonary vein, which is the

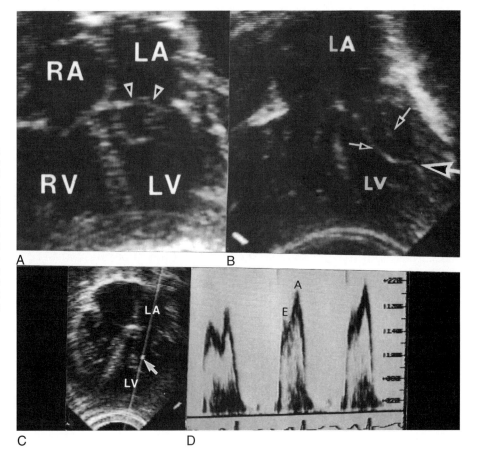

Figure 9–10
Echocardiograms (apical four chamber) with Doppler interrogation from a 3-year-old boy with Shone complex. *A, Unmarked paired arrowheads* point to a supravalvular stenosing ring. LA, left atrium; LV, left ventricle; RA, right atrium; RV, right ventricle. *B, Paired oblique arrows* identify a parachute mitral valve with chordae tendineae that insert into a single eccentric papillary muscle (*large right unmarked arrow*). *C,* The Doppler sample volume within the parachute mitral valve (*arrow*). *D,* The peak presystolic velocity across the parachute mitral valve (A) was 2.2 m/sec and the estimated gradient was 18 mm Hg. E, peak mid-diastolic flow.

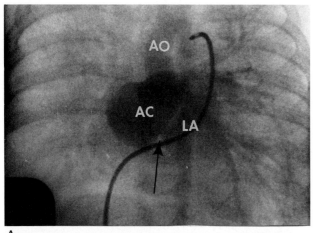

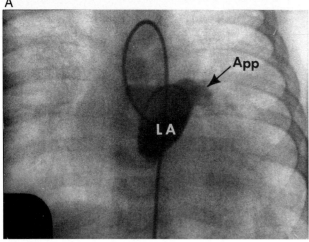

Figure 9–11

A, Levophase angiocardiogram following injection of contrast material into the pulmonary trunk in the typical diaphragmatic type of cor triatriatum. *Arrow* points to a linear zone of negative contrast that represents the diaphragm that separates the proximal accessory chamber (AC) from the left atrium proper (LA). AO, ascending aorta. *B,* Contrast material outlines the distal compartment (LA), the upper margin of which is sharply delineated by the diaphragm. The left atrial appendage (App) lies within the distal chamber.

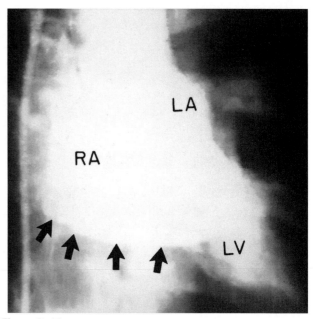

Figure 9–12

Angiocardiogram from a 22-year-old woman with cor triatriatum dexter. Contrast material filled an enlarged proximal right atrial chamber (RA; *arrows*) and opacified the left atrium through a sinus venosus atrial septal defect. The superior vena cava drained anomalously into the left atrium (LA) through the sinus venosus atrial septal defect. LV, left ventricle. (Courtesy of Dr. Irving R. Tessler, St. Vincent's Medical Center, Los Angeles, CA.)

anatomic basis of the tubular configuration, the distal end of which joins the left atrium directly without an intervening membrane.[49]

The hourglass type of cor triatriatum is developmentally intermediate between the diaphragmatic and tubular types. The constriction projects inward as an obstructing shelf, which is seen externally as an hourglass deformity at the junction of the accessory chamber and the true left atrium.[49]

An interatrial communication usually takes the form of a valve-incompetent foramen ovale positioned between the right atrium and the distal true left atrium.[49] Alternatively, an ostium secundum atrial septal defect communicates with the true left atrium or, exceptionally, with the accessory chamber.[49]

Cor triatriatum dexter is a rare type of triatrial heart (Fig. 9–12).[3,11,34,52,70,86] During early cardiogenesis, the

right horn of the sinus venosus is guarded by two valves. The smaller left valve becomes incorporated into the septum secundum. The larger right valve initially divides the right atrium into two chambers and then regresses between the ninth and the 15th week of gestation.[3] A persistent embryonic right valve of the sinus venosus becomes the septating membrane of cor triatriatum dexter. The venae cavae and the coronary sinus are on one side of the membrane, and the right atrial appendage and tricuspid orifice are on the other side. One or more perforations in the membrane permit communication from one side to the other. Septation ranges from partial to complete.

The physiologic consequences of cor triatriatum are analogous to other forms of congenital obstruction to left atrial flow with the following unique qualification.[49,53–55] In cor triatriatum, the pressure is elevated in the accessory chamber that is proximal to the obstruction, while the pressure is normal in true left atrium that is distal to the obstruction. Accordingly, the stenotic orifice remains open throughout the cardiac cycle so blood flow across the obstructing partition is continuous.

THE HISTORY

Mild asymptomatic cor triatriatum is diagnosed incidentally during routine echocardiography[83] or discovered incidentally at necropsy.[44] An echocardiographic diagnosis was made in a 70-year-old woman during routine investigation of a murmur.[53] Severe cor triatriatum announces itself in neonates and young children as dyspnea, tachypnea, paroxysmal cough, irritability, poor feeding, and failure to thrive.[27,54] However, symptoms may be delayed until adolescence or adulthood, and severe obstruction occasionally remains virtually asymptomatic until announced by acute pulmonary edema.[49,53] Sudden deterioration sometimes follows years of good health. Massive recurrent hemoptysis may be the precipitating cause of death,[53] in contrast to congenital mitral stenosis, in which hemoptysis is uncommon (see earlier).

PHYSICAL APPEARANCE

Physical appearance is normal except for failure to thrive in chronically symptomatic infants and young children.[40,54]

THE ARTERIAL PULSE, THE JUGULAR VENOUS PULSE, PRECORDIAL MOVEMENT, AND PALPATION

Atrial fibrillation is uncommon if not rare.[72] The jugular venous pulse reflects pulmonary hypertension that is responsible for increased A waves accompanied by large V waves with the advent of tricuspid regurgitation and right ventricular failure. Pulmonary hypertension is responsible for right ventricular and pulmonary trunk impulses and a palpable pulmonary component of the second sound.

AUSCULTATION

The first heart sound is not increased because diastolic pressure is not exerted against the belly of the anterior mitral leaflet, so its systolic excursion is not brisk (Fig. 9–13). The second heart sound is closely split or single with a loud pulmonary component that reflects pulmonary hypertension (see Fig. 9–13).[40] An opening snap is rare for the same reason that the first sound is not loud.[72]

The stenosing diaphragm of cor triatriatum is responsible for systolic, diastolic or continuous murmurs or no murmur at all (Fig. 9–14, and see Fig. 9–13).[6,22,38,47,53,54,72] The undulating membrane moves toward the mitral valve during diastole, reflecting a diastolic gradient, and moves away from the mitral valve during systole, reflecting reversal of the gradient as left ventricular contraction exerts pressure on the membrane through the closed mitral valve.[60,72] Systolic and diastolic thrills over the left atrium at surgery are in accord with these pressure/flow relationships and coincide with the systolic/diastolic murmurs heard at the bedside.[22] A continuous murmur reflects continuous flow across the partitioning diaphragm and is the result of a systolic murmur that continues into diastole and is reinforced as left ventricular pressure falls below the pressure in the true left atrium. A high-frequency holosystolic murmur of tricuspid regurgitation is in response to pulmonary hypertension (see Fig. 9–14).[38] When the enlarged right ventricle occupies the apex, the tricuspid systolic murmur radiates to the apex but should not be mistaken for mitral regurgitation. A high-frequency early diastolic murmur at the mid-left sternal edge is the Graham Steell murmur of pulmonary hypertension.

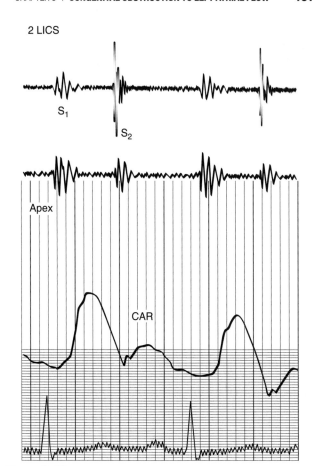

Figure 9–13

Tracings from an 18-year-old man with cor triatriatum and suprasystemic pulmonary vascular resistance. The single second heart sound (S_2) was loud because of the loud pulmonary component. There were no murmurs. CAR, carotid; 2 LICS, second left intercostal space.

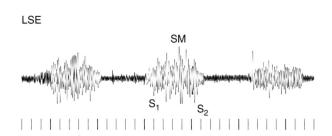

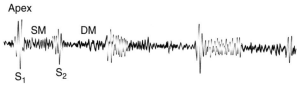

Figure 9–14

Phonocardiogram from a 17-month-old boy with cor triatriatum. Pulmonary artery systolic pressure was 115 mm Hg and systemic systolic pressure was 90 mm Hg. A high-frequency holosystolic murmur (SM) of pulmonary hypertensive tricuspid regurgitation was loudest at the lower left sternal edge (LSE) with radiation to the apex where a mid-diastolic/presystolic murmur (DM) and a prominent first heart sound (S_1) were recorded. S_2, second heart sound.

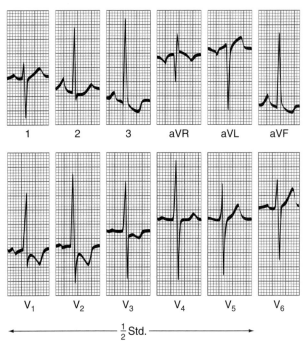

Figure 9–15

Electrocardiogram from an 18-year-old man with cor triatriatum and suprasystemic pulmonary vascular resistance referred to in Figure 9–13. Pulmonary hypertension is indicated by tall peaked right atrial P wave in lead 2, right axis deviation, and striking evidence of right ventricular hypertrophy with tall R waves and ST-T wave abnormalities in right precordial leads and deep S waves in the left precordium.

THE ELECTROCARDIOGRAM

Peaked right atrial P waves are common (Fig. 9–15). Broad notched left atrial P waves have been ascribed to prolonged conduction in the proximal accessory chamber.[22,54] Right axis deviation and right ventricular hypertrophy are typical features of the electrocardiogram (see Fig. 9–15).[72]

THE X-RAY

The lung fields exhibit pulmonary venous congestion with a diffuse hazy ground-glass appearance (Figs. 9–16 through 9–18), and Kerley lines may be present (see Fig. 9–17). Radiologic hemosiderosis has been verified at necropsy and is in accord with a history of hemoptysis (see earlier).[16] The configuration of the heart varies from normal or nearly so to conspicuous enlargement of the right ventricle, right atrium, and pulmonary trunk in response to pulmonary hypertension (see Figs. 9–16 through 9–18). The radiologic appearance of the left atrium is of special interest because the size of the true distal left atrium is normal. The combination of pulmonary venous congestion without left atrial enlargement is therefore a radiologic feature of cor triatriatum. The left atrial appendage resides in the distal low-pressure compartment and is not seen on the x-ray (see Figs. 9–11, 9–16, and 9–17).[53] Slight enlargement of the proximal accessory compartment should not be mistaken for enlargement of the left atrium proper (see Fig. 9–16).[53,54] Calcium has been found in specimens of the stenosing diaphragm but not on the x-ray.[53]

THE ECHOCARDIOGRAM

Echocardiography identifies an essential anatomic feature of cor triatriatum—the thin undulating intra-atrial membrane—which is characterized by diastolic movement toward the mitral funnel and systolic movement away

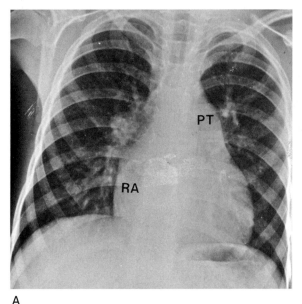
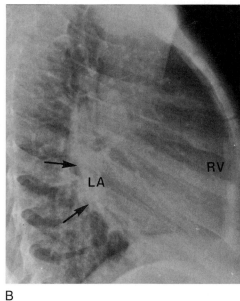

Figure 9–16

X-rays from a 6-year-old boy with a severely obstructing membrane of cor triatriatum. *A,* Pulmonary venous congestion is conspicuous. The pulmonary trunk (PT) and the right atrium (RA) are dilated, but the left atrial appendage is not visible. *B,* The proximal accessory left atrial compartment is enlarged (LA). An enlarged right ventricle (RV) occupies the retrosternal space.

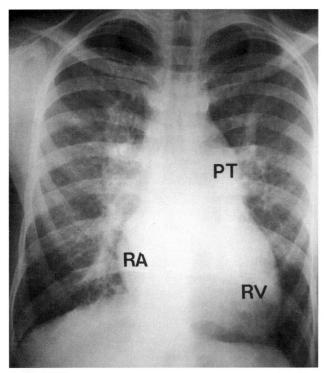

Figure 9–17
X-ray from an 18-year-old man with cor triatriatum and suprasystemic pulmonary vascular resistance whose phonocardiogram is shown in Figure 9–13. Pulmonary venous congestion is striking. The pulmonary trunk (PT), right atrium (RA), and right ventricle (RV) are dilated. The left atrial appendage is conspicuous by its absence.

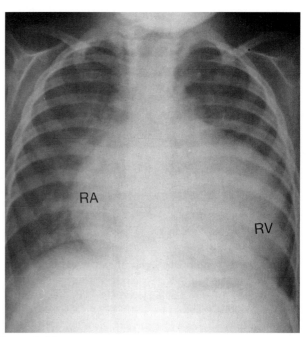

Figure 9–18
X-ray from a 17-month-old boy with cor triatriatum and suprasystemic vascular resistance whose phonocardiogram is shown in Figure 9–14. There is moderate pulmonary venous congestion. The right atrium (RA) is huge. The pulmonary trunk is obscured by the dilated outflow tract of a huge right ventricle (RV). A left atrial appendage is not seen.

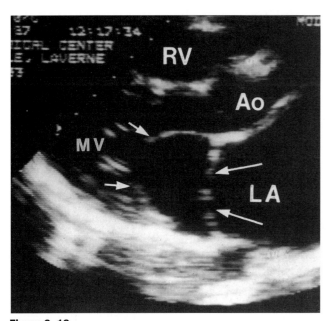

Figure 9–19
Echocardiogram (parasternal long axis) from a 21-year-old woman with cor triatriatum. The *paired arrows* on the right point to a membrane distal to the moderately enlarged accessory left atrial chamber (LA). A normal mitral valve (MV) had just begun to open. The membrane was a large, thin, mobile curtain during real-time imaging.

(Figs. 9–19 and 9–20).[37,47,60,72,92,93] When the membrane is imaged relative to the left atrial appendage, the appendage lies within the distal compartment (see Fig. 9–20), thus distinguishing cor triatriatum from a supravalvular mitral ring.[60,72,80] The position of the left atrial appendage is best determined during ventricular systole when the membrane moves away from the mitral orifice (see Fig. 9–20). The mitral valve itself is normal in cor triatriatum except for high-frequency diastolic oscillations,[47,60] in contrast to a supravalvular stenosing ring, which is accompanied by a deformed mitral valve (see earlier). Color flow imaging and continuous wave Doppler interrogation disclose continuous flow across the membrane with peak flow higher during diastole.[4] The true distal left atrium is normal, but the proximal accessory chamber may be slightly dilated (see Fig. 9–19).

Echocardiography can also diagnose cor triatriatum dexter and the location, size, and attachment site of the anomalous remnant of the valve of the right sinus venosus (see Fig. 9–12).[3,11,86]

SUMMARY

Cor triatriatum is characterized by obstruction to left atrial flow and pulmonary hypertension. Murmurs originating at the site of obstruction are systolic, diastolic, or continuous, but more often than not there is no murmur at all. When obstruction is mild or moderate, symptoms may await adolescence or adulthood or remain absent altogether. Severe obstruction comes to light in infants and young children because of dyspnea, tachypnea, paroxysmal cough, and hemoptysis. The physical signs are typical of pulmonary hypertension. The electrocardiogram exhibits right atrial

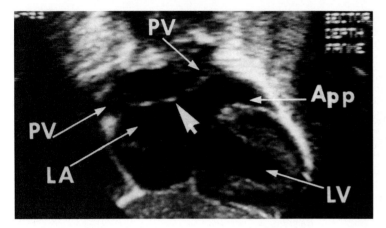

Figure 9–20
Echocardiogram (subxiphoid) from a 1-year-old boy with cor triatriatum. The membrane (*large central arrow*) inserts proximal to the left atrial appendage (App) and distal to the pulmonary veins (PV). LA, left atrium; LV, left ventricle.

P waves with right ventricular hypertrophy. The x-ray shows pulmonary venous congestion without enlargement of the left atrium but with enlargement of the right atrium, right ventricle, and pulmonary trunk. The proximal accessory chamber may dilate slightly and reveal itself on the lateral chest x-ray. The left atrial appendage does not enlarge and does not reveal itself on the x-ray because it is in the distal low-pressure compartment. Echocardiography with color flow imaging and Doppler interrogation identify the anatomic and physiologic features of cor triatriatum. The undulating membrane is proximal to the left atrial appendage and the mitral valve, features that distinguish cor triatriatum from a supravalvular stenosing ring.

Congenital Pulmonary Vein Stenosis

The incidence of congenital stenosis of pulmonary veins is estimated at 0.4% to 0.6% of pediatric cardiac necropsies.[21,26] Isolated pulmonary vein stenosis is much rarer.[2,9,56,91] The abnormality is characterized by hypoplasia of one or more pulmonary veins or by focal narrowing at or near their left atrial junction (see Fig. 9–1C).[2,8,20,26,40,57,65,75,91] Hypoplasia varies from slight narrowing to atresia of individual pulmonary veins or of a common pulmonary vein.[17,35,43,46,59,82] Focal narrowing is caused by a circumferential collar of fibrous intimal thickening or by a membranous diaphragm.[45,56,76] Focal stenosis, hypoplasia, and atresia may coexist with involvement of most or all pulmonary veins.[55] Congenital pulmonary vein stenosis is believed to be a developmental fault of the common pulmonary vein, a structure that is normally incorporated into the left atrium as four separate venous channels (see earlier).[21,35,59]

The following comments deal with pulmonary vein stenosis as an isolated cause of congenital obstruction to left atrial inflow, although the disorder coexists with a number of other congenital malformations.[2,20,40,56,91] The physiology of the circulation resembles congenital mitral stenosis or cor triatriatum, but left atrial pressure is normal. Except for stenosis or atresia of the common pulmonary vein,[35,43] high pulmonary venous pressure is not distributed uniformly within the lungs because of variation in the location and severity of the sites of stenosis.[57]

CLINICAL MANIFESTATIONS

Pulmonary vein stenosis causes dyspnea, orthopnea, cough, hemoptysis, and lower respiratory infections.[9,20,26,56,76,82] Lifespan occasionally extends into the middle or late teens, but only a minority of patients survive childhood.[20] Precordial palpation detects a right ventricular and pulmonary trunk impulse and a loud pulmonary component of the second heart sound.[26] Murmurs are absent except for high-pressure pulmonary regurgitation or tricuspid regurgitation.[56,76] The electrocardiogram reflects pulmonary hypertension with right atrial P wave abnormalities, right axis deviation, and right ventricular hypertrophy.[26,59,76] Left atrial P wave abnormalities are uniformly absent. Pulmonary vascular patterns in the x-rays are determined by which of the four pulmonary veins are stenosed and by the degree of stenosis.[2,8,43,59,82] Regional differences are characterized by asymmetry between the right and left lungs and by nonuniform distribution within each lung.[2,8,43,59,82] Left atrial size remains normal because pulmonary vein stenosis is proximal to the left atrium.[40,57,65,76] The heart tends to shift toward the side of major involvement, which is usually the left hemithorax.[2,8,15] The echocardiogram excludes congenital mitral stenosis or cor triatriatum as the cause of obstruction to left atrial flow. Color flow imaging and Doppler interrogation disclose continuous turbulent flow with normal velocities in the involved pulmonary veins.[91] Interrogation of each pulmonary vein is required because focal and long-segment stenoses are associated with different flow patterns.[91] Atresia of the common pulmonary vein has been diagnosed by fetal echocardiography.[71]

SUMMARY

The clinical manifestations of congenital pulmonary vein stenosis resemble congenital mitral stenosis and cor triatriatum, but there are important differences. In congenital pulmonary vein stenosis, electrocardiographic and radiologic signs of left atrial enlargement are absent. Pulmonary venous congestion is not uniformly distributed in the x-ray because pulmonary vein stenosis varies among the four pulmonary veins. The echocardiogram rules out congenital mitral stenosis or cor triatriatum and focuses on abnormal flow patterns in the pulmonary veins as the cause of obstruction to left atrial inflow.

REFERENCES

1. Lee D, Ha J, Chung B, et al: Double orifice mitral valve. Clin Cardiol 22:425, 1999.
2. Adey CK, Soto B, Shin MS: Congenital pulmonary vein stenosis: A radiologic study. Radiology. 161:113, 1986
3. Alboliras ET, Edwards WD, Driscoll DJ, Seward JB: Cor triatriatum dexter: Two-dimensional echocardiographic diagnosis. J Am Coll Cardiol 9:334, 1987.
4. Alwi M, Hamid ZAA, Zambahari R: A characteristic continuous wave Doppler signal in cor triatriatum? Br Heart J 68:6, 1992.
5. Andral G: Précis d'anatomie pathologique. Paris, Gabon, 2:313, 1829.
6. Baker CG, Benson PF, Joseph MC, Ross DN: Congenital mitral stenosis. Br Heart J 24:498, 1962.
7. Bano-Rodrigo A, van Praagh S, Trowitzsch E, van Praagh R: Double-orifice mitral valve: 8. A study of 27 postmortem cases with developmental, diagnostic and surgical considerations. Am J Cardiol 61:152, 1988.
8. Belcourt CL, Roy DL, Nanton MA, et al: Stenosis of individual pulmonary veins: Radiologic findings. Radiology 161:109, 1986.
9. Borst M: Ein Cor Triatriatum. Zentralbl Pathol 16:812, 1905.
10. Godoy I, Tantibhedhyankul W, Karp R, Lang R: Cor triatriatum. Circulation 98:2781, 1998.
11. Burton DA, Chin A, Weinberg PM, Pigott JD: Identification of cor triatriatum dexter by two-dimensional echocardiography. Am J Cardiol 60:409, 1987.
12. Castaneda AR, Anderson RC, Edwards JE: Congenital mitral stenosis resulting from anomalous arcade and obstructing papillary muscles. Am J Cardiol 24:237, 1969.
13. Church WS: Congenital malformation of the heart: Abnormal septum in the left auricle. Trans Pathol Soc Lond 19:188, 1868.
14. Collins-Nakai RL, Rosenthal A, Castaneda AR, et al: Congenital mitral stenosis: A review of 20 years' experience. Circulation 56:1039, 1977.
15. Cullens S, Deasy PF, Tempany E, Duff DF: Isolated pulmonary vein atresia. Br Heart J 63:350, 1990.
16. Darke CS, Emery JL, Lorber J: Triatrial heart. Br Heart J 23:329, 1961.
17. Dauod G, Kaplan S, Perrin EV, et al: Congenital mitral stenosis. Circulation 27:185, 1963.
18. Davachi F, Moller JH, Edwards JE: Diseases of the mitral valve in infancy. Circulation 43:565, 1971.
19. Deshpande JR, Kinare SG: Atresia of the common pulmonary vein. Int J Cardiol 30:221, 1991.
20. Driscoll DJ, Hesslein PS, Mullins CE: Congenital stenosis of individual pulmonary veins. Am J Cardiol 49:1767, 1982.
21. Edwards JE: Congenital stenosis of pulmonary veins. Pathologic and developmental considerations. Lab Invest 9:46, 1960.
22. Ehrich DA, Vieweg WVR, Alpert JS, et al: Cor triatriatum. Am Heart J 94:217, 1977.
23. Elliott LP, Anderson RC, Amplatz K, et al: Congenital mitral stenosis. Pediatrics 30:552, 1962.
24. Feld H, Shani J, Rudansky HW, et al: Initial presentation of cor triatriatum in a 55 year old woman. Am Heart J 124:788, 1992.
25. Fisher T: Two cases of congenital disease of the left side of the heart. Br Med J 1:639, 1902.
26. Geggel RL, Fried R, Tuuri DT, et al: Congenital pulmonary vein stenosis. J Am Coll Cardiol 3:193, 1984.
27. Gheissari A, Malm JR, Bowman FO, Bierman FZ: Cor triatriatum sinistrum: One institution's 28-year experience. Pediatr Cardiol 13:85, 1992.
28. Glancy DL, Chang MY, Borney ER, Roberts WC: Parachute mitral valve. Am J Cardiol 27:309, 1971.
29. Glaser J, Yakirevich V, Vidne BA: Preoperative echocardiographic diagnosis of supravalvular stenosing ring of the left atrium. Am Heart J 108:169, 1984.
30. Gopinathan K, Esguerra O, Kozam RL: Congenital mitral regurgitation. Am J Cardiol 24:241, 1969.
31. Grant VS, Fripp RR, Whitman V, et al: Anomalous mitral arcade. Pediatr Cardiol 4:163, 1983.
32. Greenfield WS: Double mitral valve. Trans Pathol Soc London 27:128, 1876.
33. Grenadier E, Sahn DJ, Valdez-Cruz LM, et al: Two-dimensional echo Doppler study of congenital disorders of the mitral valve. Am Heart J 107:319, 1984.
34. Hansing CE, Young WP, Rowe CC: Cor triatriatum dexter: Persistent right sinus venosus valve. Am J Cardiol 30:559, 1972.
35. Hawker RD, Celermajer JM, Gengos DC, et al: Common pulmonary vein atresia. Circulation 46:368, 1972.
36. Isner JM, Salem DN, Seaver PR, et al: Supravalvular stenosing ring of the left atrium associated with bilateral atrioventricular valvular regurgitation. Am Heart J 106:1150, 1983.
37. Jacobstein MD, Hirschfeld SS: Concealed left atrial membrane. Am J Cardiol 49:780, 1982.
38. Jegier W, Gibbons JE, Wiglesworth FW: Cor triatriatum: Clinical, hemodynamic and pathological studies. Surgical correction in early life. Pediatrics 31:255, 1963.
39. Jorgensen R, Ferlic RM, Varco RL, et al: Cor triatriatum. Circulation 36:101, 1967.
40. Kingston HM, Patel RG, Watson GH: Unilateral absence or extreme hypoplasia of pulmonary veins. Br Heart J 49:148, 1983.
41. Kron J, Standerfer RJ, Starr A: Severe mitral regurgitation in a woman with a double orifice mitral valve. Br Heart J 55:109, 1986.
42. Layman TE, Edwards JE: Anomalous mitral arcade. Circulation 35:389, 1967.
43. Ledbetter MK, Wells DH, Connors DM: Common pulmonary vein atresia. Am Heart J 96:580, 1978.
44. Loeffler E: Unusual malformation of left atrium: Pulmonary sinus. Arch Pathol 48:371, 1949.
45. Lucas RV Jr, Anderson RC, Amplatz K, et al: Congenital causes of pulmonary venous obstruction. Pediatr Clin North Am 10:781, 1963.
46. Lucas RV Jr, Woolfrey BF, Anderson RC, et al: Atresia of the common pulmonary vein. Pediatrics 29:729, 1962.
47. Ludomirsky A, Erickson C, Vick GW, Cooley DA: Transesophageal color flow Doppler evaluation of cor triatriatum in an adult. Am Heart J 120:451, 1990.
48. Macartney FJ, Scott O, Ionescu MI, Deverall TB: Diagnosis and management of parachute mitral valve and supravalvular mitral ring. Br Heart J 36:641, 1974.
49. Marin-Garcia J, Tandon R, Lucas RV, Edwards JE: Cor triatriatum: Study of 20 cases. Am J Cardiol 35:59, 1975.
50. Matsushima AY, Park J, Szulc M, et al: Anomalous atrioventricular valve arcade. Am Heart J 121:1824, 1991.
51. Maxwell GM, Young WP, Rowe GG, Connors DM: Cor triatriatum. J Pediatr 50:71, 1957.
52. Mazzucco A, Bortolotti U, Gallucci V, et al: Successful repair of symptomatic cor triatriatum dexter in infancy. J Thorac Cardiovasc Surg 85:140, 1983.
53. McGuire LB, Nolan TB, Reeve R, Dammann JF: Cor triatriatum as a problem of adult heart disease. Circulation 31:263, 1965.
54. Miller GAH, Ongley PA, Anderson MW, et al: Cor triatriatum: Hemodynamic and angiocardiographic diagnosis. Am Heart J 68:298, 1964.
55. Mori K, Dohi T: Mitral and pulmonary vein blood flow patterns in cor triatriatum. Am Heart J 117:1167, 1989.
56. Mortensson W, Lundstrom N: Congenital obstruction of the pulmonary veins at their atrial junctions. Am Heart J 87:359, 1974.
57. Nakib A, Moller JH, Kanjuh VI, Edwards JE: Anomalies of the pulmonary veins. Am J Cardiol 20:77, 1967.
58. Nash FW, MacKinnon D: Cor triatriatum: Congenital stenosis of common pulmonary vein. Arch Dis Child 31:222, 1956.
59. Nasrallah AT, Mullins CE, Finger D, et al: Unilateral pulmonary vein atresia. Am J Cardiol 36:969, 1975.
60. Ostman-Smith I, Silverman NH, Oddershaw P, et al: Cor triatriatum sinistrum. Br Heart J 51:211, 1984.
61. Patel AK, Ninnerman RW, Rahko PS: Surgical resection of cor triatriatum in a 74 year old man: Review of echocardiographic findings with emphasis on Doppler and transesophageal echocardiography. J Am Soc Echocardiogr 3:402, 1990.
62. Perez JA, Herzberg AJ, Reimer KA, Bashore TM: Congenital mitral insufficiency secondary to anomalous mitral arcade in an adult. Am Heart J 114:894, 1987.

63. Perloff JK: Auscultatory and phonocardiographic manifestations of pulmonary hypertension. Progr Cardiovasc Dis 9:303, 1967.

64. Perloff JK: Physical Examination of the Heart and Circulation, 3rd ed. Philadelphia, W.B. Saunders, 2000.

65. Reid JM, Jamieson MPG, Cowan MD: Unilateral pulmonary vein stenosis. Br Heart J 55:599, 1986.

66. Rodan BA, Chen JTT, Kirks DR, Benson DW: Mitral valve calcification in congenital mitral stenosis. Am Heart J 105:514, 1983.

67. Rogers HM, Waldron BR, Murphey DFH, Edwards JE: Supravalvular stenosing ring of left atrium in association with endocardial sclerosis (endocardial fibroelastosis) and mitral insufficiency. Am Heart J 50:777, 1955.

68. Rosenquist CG: Congenital mitral valve disease associated with coarctation of the aorta: A spectrum that includes parachute deformity of the mitral valve. Circulation 49:985, 1974.

69. Ruckman RN, van Praagh R: Anatomic types of congenital mitral stenosis. Am J Cardiol 42:592, 1978.

70. Runcie J: A complicated case of cor triatriatum dexter. Br Heart J 30:729, 1968.

71. Samuel N, Sirotta L, Bar-Ziv J, et al: The ultrasonic appearance of common pulmonary vein atresia in utero. J Ultrasound Med 7:25, 1988.

72. Schluter M, Langenstein BA, Thier W, et al: Transesophageal two-dimensional echocardiography in the diagnosis of cor triatriatum in the adult. J Am Coll Cardiol 2:1011, 1983.

73. Schrivastava S, Moller JH, Tadavarthy M, et al: Clinical pathologic conference: Anomalous muscle bundles of left ventricle causing mitral valvular obstruction. Am Heart J 91:513, 1976.

74. Sethia B, Sullivan ID, Elliott MJ, et al: Congenital left ventricular inflow obstruction: Is the outcome related to the site of the obstruction? Eur J Cardiothorac Surg 2:312, 1988.

75. Sherman FE, Stengel WF, Bauersfeld SR: Congenital stenosis of pulmonary veins at their atrial junctions. Am Heart J 56:908, 1958.

76. Shone JD, Amplatz K, Anderson RC, et al: Congenital stenosis of individual pulmonary veins. Circulation 26:574, 1962.

77. Shone JD, Sellers RD, Anderson RC, et al: The developmental complex of "parachute mitral valve," supravalvular ring of left atrium, subaortic stenosis, and coarctation of aorta. Am J Cardiol 11:714, 1963.

78. Singh SP, Gotsman MS, Abrams LD, et al: Congenital mitral stenosis. Br Heart J 29:83, 1967.

79. Smallhorn J, Tommasini G, Deanfield J, et al: Congenital mitral stenosis. Br Heart J 45:527, 1981.

80. Snider RA, Roge CL, Schiller NB, Silverman NH: Congenital left ventricular inflow obstruction evaluated by two-dimensional echocardiography. Circulation 61:848, 1980.

81. Sullivan ID, Robinson PJ, de Leval M, Graham TP: Membranous supravalvular mitral stenosis: A treatable form of congenital heart disease. J Am Coll Cardiol 8:159, 1986.

82. Swischuk LE, L'Heureux P: Unilateral pulmonary vein atresia. AJR 135:667, 1980.

83. Tanaka F, Itoh M, Esaki H, et al: Asymptomatic cor triatriatum incidentally revealed by computed tomography. Chest 100:272, 1991.

84. Tandon R, Moller JH, Edwards JE: Anomalies associated with the parachute mitral valve: A pathologic analysis of 52 cases. Can J Cardiol 2:278, 1986.

85. Thilenius OG, Bharati S, Lev M: Subdivided left atrium: An expanded concept of cor triatriatum sinistrum. Am J Cardiol 37:743, 1976.

86. Trakhtenbroit A, Majid P, Rokey R: cor triatriatum dexter: Antemortem diagnosis in an adult by cross sectional echocardiography. Br Heart J 63:314, 1990.

87. Trowitzsch E, Bano-Rodrigo A, Burger BM, et al: Two-dimensional echocardiographic findings in double orifice mitral valve. J Am Coll Cardiol 6:383, 1985.

88. Van der Horst RL, Hastreiter AR: Congenital mitral stenosis. Am J Cardiol 20:773, 1967.

89. van Praagh R, Corsini I: Cor triatriatum: Pathologic anatomy and a consideration of morphogenesis based on 13 postmortem cases and a study of normal development of the pulmonary vein and atrial septum in 83 human embryos. Am Heart J 78:379, 1969.

90. Vitarelli A, Landolina G, Gentile R, et al: Echocardiographic assessment of congenital mitral stenosis. Am Heart J 108:523, 1984.

91. Webber SA, de Souza E, Patterson MWH: Pulsed wave and color Doppler findings in congenital pulmonary vein stenosis. Pediatr Cardiol 13:112, 1992.

92. Vuocolo LM, Stoddard MF, Longaker RA: Transesophageal two-dimensional and Doppler echocardiographic diagnosis of cor triatriatum in the adult. Am Heart J 124:791, 1992.

93. Weindorf S, Goldberg H, Goldman M, Dietman M: Diagnosis of cor triatriatum by two-dimensional echocardiography. J Clin Ultrasound 9:97, 1981.

94. van Sen JAM, Danielson GK, Schaff HV, et al: Cor triatriatum: Diagnosis, operative approach, and late results. Mayo Clin Proc 68:854, 1993.

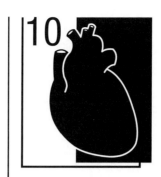

Endocardial Fibroelastosis

Endocardial fibroelastosis, a self-defining term introduced in 1943 by Weinberg and Himmelfarb,[74] is characterized by an opaque, pearly-white thickening (Fig. 10–1) due to proliferation of collagen and elastic fibers.[12, 16, 32, 46, 48, 77] Isolated endocardial fibroelastosis resides in the endocardium of a dilated, hypertrophied left ventricle,[32, 48] hence the term *primary endocardial fibroelastosis of the dilated type.* Conversely, albeit rarely, the left ventricular cavity is small, hence the term *endocardial fibroelastosis of the contracted type.*[32, 48] Another type of endocardial fibroelastosis designated as *secondary* accompanies certain types of congenital malformations of the heart,[19, 48] especially aortic stenosis,[14] coarctation of the aorta,[25, 52] anomalous origin of the left coronary artery from the pulmonary trunk,[51] and hypoplastic left heart.[50] Pathogenesis must take into account the gross and histologic endocardial abnormalities as well as the left ventricular hypertrophy that characterizes primary endocardial fibroelastosis of the dilated type. Fibroelastosis per se is a response to a variety of endocardial stimuli, with intrauterine endocardial injury as the common denominator.[11, 21, 36, 41, 58, 60–63, 75] Fibroelastosis occurs in infants and adults after myocardial infarction,[7, 30, 66] underscoring the endocardial response to injury.

Primary dilated endocardial fibroelastosis is the type that occurs in infants.[5,27,46,53,65,67,70] Beyond infancy, endocardial fibroelastosis is patchy and is associated with myocardial fibrosis.[65] The relationship between the infantile, the adolescent, and the adult form of the disease is unclear.[4, 5, 26–28, 45, 53, 65, 67, 70] Endocardial fibrosis is a substrate for mural thrombosis, which sets the stage for systemic emboli.[9, 15, 66, 70] The endocardium occasionally calcifies.[70]

Primary endocardial fibroelastosis of the dilated type principally involves the left ventricle.[3,17,32,34,42,43,46,48,56,65] The left atrium, right atrium, and right ventricle are only occasionally affected.[6,10,32,65,70] The relationship between the dilated and nondilated types has not been established.[7,11,12,16,24,48,61,68,69]

Mitral regurgitation usually coexists with the dilated type[13,16,48,70] because the papillary muscles originate high on the left ventricular wall—from the upper third—and accordingly exert undesirable lateral axes of tension on the chordae tendineae and mitral cusps, provoking faulty leaflet apposition.[3,16,48] Chordae tendineae are short and thick as well as laterally aligned,[10,13] and the papillary muscles tend to be small, with histologic changes resembling infarction.[13] Aortic incompetence is rare.[1]

The physiologic consequences of primary endocardial fibroelastosis of the dilated type reflect from the basic disorder of left ventricular endocardium in concert with mitral regurgitation (Figs. 10–2 and 10–3). Endocardial thickening restricts contraction of the dilated left ventricle and is responsible for global hypokinesis (see Figs. 10–1 and 10–2).[38,42,45,56] Elevated left atrial, pulmonary venous, and pulmonary arterial pressures are in response to high left ventricular filling pressure and mitral regurgitation.[42] Pulmonary hypertension is especially pronounced in the nondilated form of the disease because of the high filling pressure of the small left ventricle.[18,42,68]

The History

Primary endocardial fibroelastosis of the dilated type is equally distributed between the sexes[17,32,60,65] and has been reported in siblings, in identical twins,[22,35,40,55,64] and in more than one generation.[18,26,32,39,47,49,54,59,71,75] The disease manifests itself in the first 6 to 12 months of life.[17,19,32,44,48,60,65] The majority of affected children do not live beyond their second birthday.[17,19,32] Prognosis is especially poor in neonates.[75] Symptoms can begin

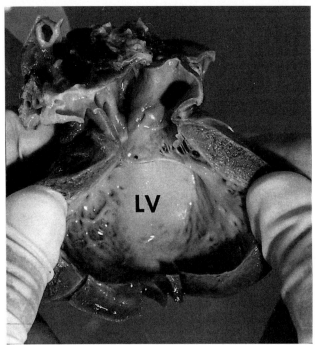

Figure 10–1
Necropsy specimen from a 2-month-old boy. The left ventricle (LV) is markedly dilated, the walls are hypertrophied, and the endocardium exhibits typical diffuse pearly-white opaque thickening of endocardial fibroelastosis.

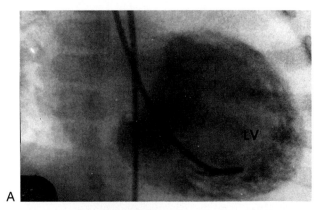

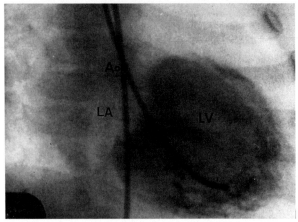

Figure 10–2
Angiocardiogram in a 15-month-old boy with primary endocardial fibroelastosis of the dilated type. *A*, The diastolic frame shows the typical spherically dilated left ventricle (LV). *B*, The systolic frame shows a trivial decrease in left ventricular size, reflecting striking global hypokinesis. The left atrium (LA) filled because of mitral regurgitation. Visualization of the aorta (Ao) was faint because of the low stroke volume.

suddenly, the disorder can run a protracted course,[2,32,72] or death can be sudden and unexpected.[17] Systemic emboli from left ventricular mural thrombi result in serious neurologic sequelae and death.[9,32]

Physical Appearance

The catabolic effects of chronic congestive heart failure are responsible for poor growth and development. Arterial oxygen unsaturation is related to cardiac failure.

The Arterial Pulse

The rate of rise reflects impaired left ventricular contractility.[45] Sinus tachycardia and the pulsus alternans are reflections of heart failure.[32,73]

The Jugular Venous Pulse

High systemic venous pressure results in hepatomegaly and a liver pulse, but the jugular pulse cannot be analyzed in symptomatic infants.

Precordial Movement and Palpation

The impulse of the dilated left ventricle is hypodynamic because endocardial restriction impairs contractility. Mid-

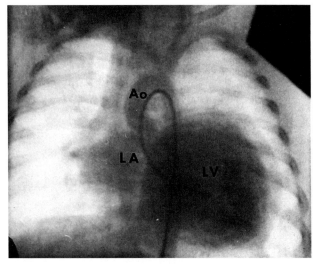

Figure 10–3
Angiocardiogram in a 4-month-old boy with primary endocardial fibroelastosis of the dilated type. The spherical left ventricle (LV) is strikingly dilated. The left atrium (LA) filled because of mitral regurgitation. Visualization of the aorta (Ao) was faint because of the low stroke volume.

diastolic distention represents a palpable third heart sound or summation sound generated by rapid flow into a non-compliant left ventricle. Mid-diastolic distention is more pronounced when mitral regurgitation coexists. Systolic expansion of an enlarged left atrium in response to mitral regurgitation produces systolic anterior precordial movement that can be mistaken for an intrinsic right ventricle. The relatively dynamic impulse of a dilated failing right ventricle may eclipse the impulse of a hypokinetic left ventricle.

Auscultation

Left ventricular hypokinesis diminishes the murmur of mitral regurgitation despite appreciable regurgitant flow (Fig. 10–4).[4,19,32,38,56,60] Elevated pulmonary artery pressure augments the pulmonary component of the second heart sound and narrows the splitting. A third heart sound reflects the decrease in left ventricular distensibility[4,32,42,60] and is especially prominent when mitral regurgitation coexists. Third and fourth heart sounds summate to produce a triple rhythm or a short mid-diastolic murmur (see Fig. 10–4).

The Electrocardiogram

The electrocardiogram records a variety of disturbances in rhythm and conduction, including paroxysmal atrial, junctional, or ventricular tachycardia and neonatal atrial fibrillation.[6,19,23,33,48,55,57,70,73] Complete heart block has been detected in utero[29,32,55] and raises the question of a relationship between maternal antibodies, congenital complete heart block, and endocardial fibroelastosis (see Chapter 4).[41,63] P waves show left atrial, biatrial, or right atrial abnormalities (Fig. 10–5), especially in the presence of mitral regurgitation and elevated pulmonary artery pressure.[48,60,73] The PR interval is normal or slightly increased,[48,60,73] except in sporadic cases with Wolff-Parkinson-White accessory pathways.[3,23,73]

The QRS axis is normal, although rightward or leftward axes occasionally occur.[60,73] Left ventricular hypertrophy is an important feature of primary dilated endocardial fibroelastosis (Fig. 10–6 and see Fig. 10–5).[20,31,60] Right ventricular or biventricular hypertrophy is reserved for infants with left ventricular failure and reactive pulmonary hypertension.[31,37,42,48,73] Isolated

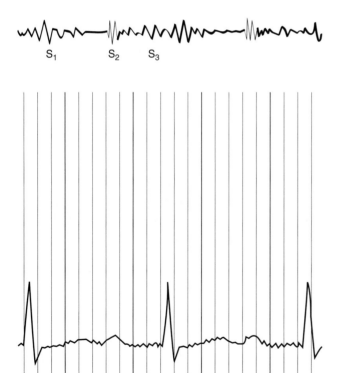

Figure 10–4

Phonocardiogram from the cardiac apex of a 6-month-old girl with primary endocardial fibroelastosis of the dilated type. The third heart sound (S_3) is followed by a short mid-diastolic murmur. A systolic murmur was absent despite angiographic mitral regurgitation because regurgitant flow was hypokinetic. S_1, first heart sound; S_2, second heart sound.

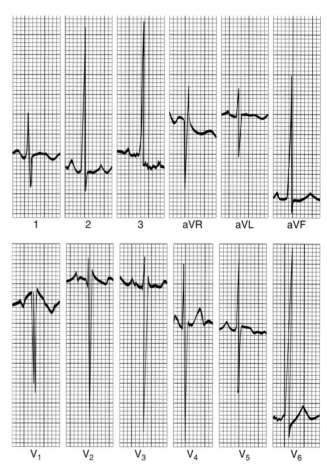

Figure 10–5

Electrocardiogram from a 2-month-old boy with primary endocardial fibroelastosis of the dilated type. Notched P waves in leads V_{2-5} reflect a left atrial abnormality and the tall, peaked wave in lead 2 reflects a right atrial abnormality. Left ventricular hypertrophy is indicated by tall R waves in leads 2, 3, aVF and in lead V_6.

right ventricular hypertrophy is a feature of the nondilated form of primary endocardial fibroelastosis.[7,42,60,68] Q waves are common in left precordial leads of the dilated form because of the volume overload of mitral regurgitation (see Fig. 10–6).[31,60] An infarct pattern is a feature of

endocardial fibroelastosis associated with an anomalous origin of the left coronary artery from the pulmonary trunk (see Chapter 21).[40] Should an infarct pattern occur in primary endocardial fibroelastosis, the Q waves are in right precordial leads,[4,40] not in leads 1 and aVL (see Chapter 21).

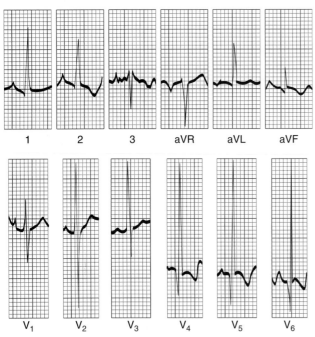

Figure 10–6
Electrocardiogram recorded the day before the death of a 4-month-old girl with endocardial fibroelastosis of the dilated type. Left precordial leads exhibit the tall R waves and inverted T waves of left ventricular hypertrophy. There are prominent Q waves in leads V$_{4-6}$ despite the absence of mitral regurgitation.

The X-Ray

Cardiomegaly in the dilated form of primary endocardial fibroelastosis reflects enlargement of the left ventricle and left atrium (Figs. 10–7 and 10–8).[20,56,60] Calcification of the thickened endocardium is occasionally found at necropsy but rarely on the x-ray.[70] Mitral regurgitation is associated with left atrial enlargement that can be massive.[48,60] The ascending aorta and pulmonary trunk are inconspicuous compared with the striking increase in heart size (see Figs. 10–7 and 10–8).

The Echocardiogram

The dilated type of primary endocardial fibroelastosis is imaged as spherical left ventricular enlargement with striking global hypokinesis.[58] Distinctive bright echoes originate in the thickened endocardium (see Figs. 10–1 and 10–9). Septal and free wall thicknesses are increased because of left ventricular hypertrophy (Fig. 10–9). The left atrium is dilated, and color flow imaging determines the degree of mitral regurgitation. The echocardiogram permits an intrauterine diagnosis.[8,11,61]

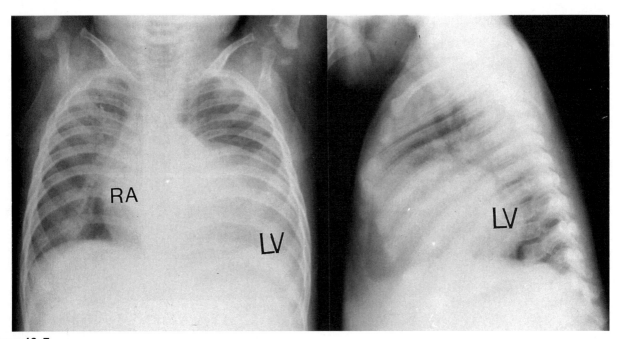

Figure 10–7
X-rays from the 2-month-old boy whose electrocardiogram is shown in Figure 10–5. The left ventricle (LV) is strikingly dilated in both projections, and the right atrium (RA) is enlarged. The great arteries are inconspicuous. The lung fields exhibit pulmonary venous congestion.

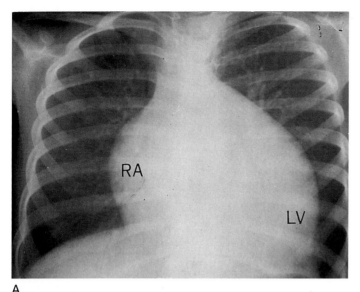

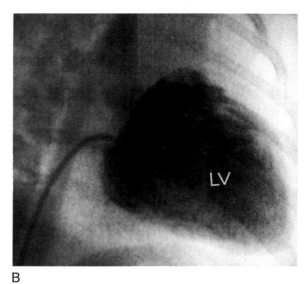

A   B

Figure 10–8

A, X-ray from the 6-month-old girl whose phonocardiogram is shown in Figure 10–4. The left ventricle (LV) and the right atrium (RA) are strikingly dilated. The large cardiac silhouette stands out in contrast to the inconspicuous great arteries. There is pulmonary venous congestion. *B,* Angiogram shows the dilated hypokinetic left ventricle (LV).

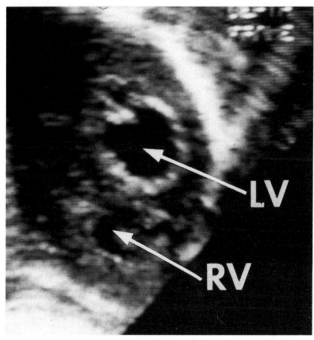

Figure 10–9

Echocardiogram (short axis) from a 1-day-old boy with critical aortic valve stenosis. The figure illustrates the highly echogenic endocardium of fibroelastosis in the hypertrophied left ventricle (LV). RV, right ventricle.

Summary

Primary endocardial fibroelastosis of the dilated type is characterized by (1) congestive heart failure in infancy accompanied by mitral regurgitation; (2) hypokinesis of the left ventricle despite its large size and hypertrophied wall; (3) absent or inconspicuous cardiac murmurs despite mitral regurgitation; (4) electrocardiographic signs of left ventricular hypertrophy; (5) striking left ventricular and left atrial dilatation on the x-ray with comparatively inconspicuous great arteries; and (6) an echocardiogram that images a spherically dilated, hypertrophied but hypokinetic left ventricle with distinctive bright echoes arising from the thickened endocardium.

REFERENCES

1. Ainger LE: Mitral and aortic valve incompetence in endocardial fibroelastosis. Am J Cardiol 28:309, 1971.
2. Alter BP, Czapek EE, Rowe RD: Sweating in congenital heart disease. Pediatrics 41:123, 1968.
3. Angelov A, Kulova A, Gurdevsky M: Endocardial fibroelastosis: Clinico-pathologic study of 38 cases. Pathol Res Pract 178:384, 1984.
4. Auld WH, Watson H: Fibroelastosis of the heart in adolescence. Br Heart J 19:186, 1957.
5. Bharati S, Strasberg B, Bilitch M, et al: Anatomic substrate for preexcitation in idiopathic myocardial hypertrophy with fibroelastosis of the left ventricle. Am J Cardiol 48:47, 1981.
6. Bjorkhem G, Lundstrom N: Endocardial fibroelastosis with predominant involvement of the left atrium. Br Heart J 46:331, 1981.
7. Bleiden LC, Schneeweiss A, Deutsch V, Neufeld HN: Contracted form of endocardial fibroelastosis. Pediatr Cardiol 4:281, 1983.
8. Bovicelli L, Picchio FM, Pilu G, et al: Prenatal diagnosis of endocardial fibroelastosis. Prenat Diagn 4:67, 1984.
9. Branch CL, Castle RF: Thromboembolic complications in primary endocardial fibroelastosis. J Pediatr 69:250, 1966.
10. Burke EC, von Bernuth G, Holley KE: Pediatric clinicopathologic conference. Mayo Clin Proc 45:467, 1970.
11. Carceller AM, Maroto E, Fouron JC: Dilated and contracted forms of primary endocardial fibroelastosis: A single fetal disease with two stages of development. Br Heart J 63:311, 1990.
12. Chen SC, Thompson MW, Rose V: Endocardial fibroelastosis. J Pediatr 79:385, 1971.
13. Davachi F, Moller JH: Diseases of the mitral valve in infancy. Circulation 43:565, 1971.
14. DuShane JW, Edwards JE: Congenital aortic stenosis in association with endocardial sclerosis of the left ventricle. Proc Staff Meet Mayo Clin 29:102, 1954.
15. Dyson BC, Decker JP: Endocardial fibroelastosis in the adult. AMA Arch Pathol 66:190, 1958.

16. Edwards JE, Carey LS, Neufeld HN, Lester RG: Congenital Heart Disease. Philadelphia, W.B. Saunders, 1965.

17. Fisher JH: Primary endocardial fibroelastosis: A review of 15 cases. Can Med Assoc J 87:105, 1962.

18. Fixler DE, Cole RB, Paul MH, et al: Familial occurrence of the contracted form of endocardial fibroelastosis. Am J Cardiol 26:208, 1970.

19. Forfar JO, Miller RA, Bain AD, Macleod W: Endocardial fibroelastosis. Br Med J 2:7, 1964.

20. Freundlich E, Munk J, Griffel B, Steinlauf J: Primary myocardial disease in infancy. Am J Cardiol 13:721, 1964.

21. Gersony WM, Katz SL, Nadas AS: Endocardial fibroelastosis and the mumps virus. Pediatrics 37:430, 1966.

22. Greaves JL, Wilkins PSW, Pearson S: Endocardial fibroelastosis in identical twins. Arch Dis Child 29:447, 1954.

23. Gueron M, Cohen W: Anomalous left ventricular chordae tendineae and preexcitation: Unusual cause of praecordial pansystolic murmur in a baby with fibroelastosis. Br Heart J 34:966, 1972.

24. Guraieb SR, Rigdon RH: Fibroelastosis in adults: A review of the literature and report of a case. Am Heart J 52:138, 1956.

25. Hallidie-Smith KA, Olsen EGJ: Endocardial fibroelastosis, mitral incompetence, and coarctation of the abdominal aorta. Br Heart J 30:850, 1968.

26. Hanukoglu A, Fried D, Somekh E: Inheritance of familial primary endocardial fibroelastosis. Clin Pediatr 25:272, 1986.

27. Hashimoto T, Yano K, Matsumoto Y, Hashiba K: Contracted form of primary endocardial fibroelastosis in a young adult without congestive heart failure. Jpn Heart J 29:121, 1988.

28. Hoffman FG: Adult endocardial fibroelastosis associated with dextrocardia and situs inversus. Circulation 22:437, 1960.

29. Hung W, Walsh BJ: Congenital auricular fibrillation in a newborn infant with endocardial fibroelastosis. J Pediatr 61:65, 1962.

30. Hutchins G, Bannayan GA: Development of endocardial fibroelastosis following myocardial infarction. Arch Pathol 91:113, 1971.

31. Keith J: Endocardial fibroelastosis. In Cassels DE, Ziegler RF (eds): Electrocardiography in Infants and Children. New York, Grune & Stratton, 1966.

32. Kelly J, Andersen DH: Congenital endocardial fibroelastosis: Clinical and pathologic investigation of those cases without associated cardiac malformations including report of 2 familial instances. Pediatrics 18:539, 1956.

33. Lambert EC, Shumway CN, Terplan K: Clinical diagnosis of endocardial fibrosis. Pediatrics 11:255, 1953.

34. Larson JE, McManus BM, Hofschire PJ, et al: Isolated endocardial fibroelastosis of the right ventricle associated with pulmonary hypertension. Am Heart J 107:1286, 1984.

35. Lee MH, Liebman J, Steinberg AG, et al: Familial occurrence of endocardial fibroelastosis in 3 siblings including identical twins. Pediatrics 52:402, 1973.

36. Liang Y, Ni S, Cong Y, Li P: Clinico-pathological study on primary endocardial fibroelastosis. Acta Paediatr Jpn 29:13, 1987.

37. Linde LM, Adams FH: Prognosis in endocardial fibroelastosis. Am J Dis Child 105:329, 1963.

38. Linde LM, Adams FH, O'Loughlin BJ: Endocardial fibroelastosis: Angiocardiographic studies. Circulation 17:40, 1958.

39. Lindenbaum RH, Andrews PS, Kahn ASSI: Two cases of endocardial fibroelastosis; possible X-linked determination. Br Heart J 35:38, 1973.

40. Lintermans JP, Kaplan EL, Morgan BC, et al: Infarction patterns in endocardial fibroelastosis. Circulation 33:202, 1966.

41. Litsey SE, Noonan JA, O'Connor WN, et al: Maternal connective tissue disease and congenital heart block. N Engl J Med 312:98, 1985.

42. Lynfield J, Gasul BM, Luan LL, Dillon RF: Right and left heart catheterization and angiocardiographic findings in idiopathic cardiac hypertrophy with endocardial fibroelastosis. Circulation 21:386, 1960.

43. Manning JA, Keith JD: Fibroelastosis in children. Progr Cardiovasc Dis 7:172, 1964.

44. Manning JA, Sellers FJ, Bynum RS, Keith JD: Medical management of clinical endocardial fibroelastosis. Circulation 29:60, 1964.

45. Miller GAH, Rahimtoola SH, Ongley PA, Swan HJC: Left ventricular volume and volume change in endocardial fibroelastosis. Am J Cardiol 15:631, 1965.

46. Mitchell SC, Froehlich LA, Banas JS, Gilkeson MR: An epidemiologic assessment of primary endocardial fibroelastosis. Am J Cardiol 18:859, 1966.

47. Moller JH, Fisch RO, Fromm AHL, Edwards JE: Endocardial fibroelastosis occurring in a mother and son. Pediatrics 38:918, 1966.

48. Moller JH, Lucas RV, Adams P, et al: Endocardial fibroelastosis. Circulation 30:759, 1964.

49. Nielsen JS: Primary endocardial fibroelastosis in three siblings. Acta Med Scand 177:145, 1965.

50. Noonan JA, Nadas AS: The hypoplastic left heart syndrome. Pediatr Clin North Am 5:1029, 1958.

51. Noren GR, Raghib G, Moller JH, et al: Anomalous origin of the left coronary artery from the pulmonary trunk with special reference to the occurrence of mitral insufficiency. Circulation 30:171, 1964.

52. Oppenheimer EH: Association of adult type coarctation of aorta with endocardial fibroelastosis in infancy. Bull Johns Hopkins Hosp 93:309, 1953.

53. Rafinski T, Folenia A, Wozneiwicz B, Wlad S: Familial endocardial fibroelastosis. J Pediatr 10:574, 1967.

54. Rios B, Castaneda P, Simpson JW: Endocardial fibroelastosis occurring in a mother and daughter. Texas Heart Inst J 11:296, 1984.

55. Rios B, Duff J, Simpson JW: Endocardial fibroelastosis with congenital complete heart block in identical twins. Am Heart J 107:1290, 1984.

56. Ronderos A: Endocardial fibroelastosis. Am J Roentgenol 84:442, 1960.

57. Santoro EV: Congenital endocardial fibroelastosis and total heart block: Report of a case. Arch Pediatr 73:94, 1956.

58. Schryer MJT, Karnauchow PN: Endocardial fibroelastosis: Etiologic and pathogenetic considerations in children. Am Heart J 88:557, 1974.

59. Seibold H, Mohr W, Lehmann WD, et al: Fibroelastosis of the right ventricle in two brothers of triplets. Pathol Res Pract 170:402, 1980.

60. Sellers FJ, Keith JD, Manning JA: The diagnosis of primary endocardial fibroelastosis. Circulation 29:49, 1964.

61. Sharland GK, Chita SK, Fagg NIK, et al: Left ventricular dysfunction in the fetus: Relation to aortic valve anomalies and endocardial fibroelastosis. Br Heart J 66:419, 1991.

62. Shone JD, Muñoz Armas S, Manning JA, et al: The mumps antigen skin test in endocardial fibroelastosis. Pediatrics 37:423, 1966.

63. Singsen BH, Akhter JE, Weinstein MM, Sharp GC: Congenital complete heart block and SSA antibodies: Obstetric implications. Am J Obstet Gynecol 152:655, 1985.

64. Stadler HE: Endocardial fibroelastosis in one of monozygotic twins. Am Heart J 61:116, 1961.

65. Still WJS: Endocardial fibroelastosis. Am Heart J 61:579, 1961.

66. Thomas WA, Lee KT, McGavran MH, Rabin ER: Endocardial fibroelastosis in infants associated with thrombosis and calcification of arteries and myocardial infarcts. N Engl J Med 255:464, 1956.

67. Thomas WA, Randall RV, Bland EF, Castleman B: Endocardial fibroelastosis: A factor in heart disease of obscure etiology—A study of 20 autopsied cases in children and adults. N Engl J Med 251:327, 1954.

68. Tingelstad JB, Shiel FO, McCue CM: The electrocardiogram in the contracted type of primary endocardial fibroelastosis. Am J Cardiol 27:304, 1971.

69. Ursell PC, Neill CA, Anderson RH, et al: Endocardial fibroelastosis and hypoplasia of the left ventricle in neonates without significant aortic stenosis. Br Heart J 51:492, 1984.

70. Van Buchem FS, Arends A, Schroder EA: Endocardial fibroelastosis in adolescents and adults. Br Heart J 21:229, 1959.

71. Vestermark S: Primary endocardial fibroelastosis in siblings. Acta Paediatr 51:94, 1962.

72. Vestermark S: Primary endocardial fibroelastosis. Cardiologia (Basel) 48:520, 1966.

73. Vlad P, Rowe RD, Keith JD: The electrocardiogram in primary endocardial fibroelastosis. Br Heart J 17:189, 1955.

74. Weinberg T, Himmelfarb AJ: Endocardial fibroelastosis. Bull Johns Hopkins Hosp 72:299, 1943.

75. Westwood M, Harris R, Burn JL, Barson AJ: Heredity in primary endocardial fibroelastosis. Br Heart J 37:1077, 1975.

76. Yoshida T, Nimura Y, Sakakibara H, et al: A diffuse endocardial fibroelastosis with markedly dilated right atrium observed in an adult. Jpn Heart J 5:85, 1964.

77. Zanker T, Fisher RS: Endocardial fibroelastosis. Maryland Med J 9:60, 1960.

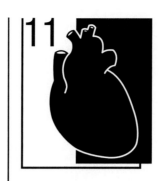

Congenital Pulmonary Stenosis

Congenital obstruction to right ventricular outflow in hearts with two noninverted ventricles can originate in, below, or above the pulmonary valve. Stenosis originating in the pulmonary valve consists of three morphologic types[12]: (1) typical mobile dome-shaped, (2) dysplastic, and (3) bicuspid.

Dome-shaped pulmonary valve stenosis was described in 1761 by John Baptist Morgagni[77] and is characterized by a thin mobile valve mechanism with a narrow central opening at its apex (Fig. 11–1). Three rudimentary raphes extend from the central opening to the wall of the pulmonary artery, but separate leaflets and separate commissures cannot be identified. Pinpoint dome-shaped pulmonary valve stenosis in neonates is sometimes referred to as functional pulmonary atresia (Fig. 11–1C, D). The pulmonary trunk is consistently dilated because of an inherent medial abnormality that is coupled with the morphology of the mobile dome-shaped valve, not with its functional state (see Fig. 11–1).[5] The jet from the stenotic valve breaks up upon striking the apex of the pulmonary trunk, and the pressure component of total energy increases with a proportionat pressure in the left branch (see Fig. 11–37A).[80] The physics of jet dispersion is believed to account for the disparity in size between left and right branches. Calcification of a dome-shaped stenotic pulmonary valve is exceptional and is reserved for older patients (see The X-ray).[3,38,100]

Dysplastic pulmonary valve stenosis is a much less common variety. Obstruction is caused by myomatous thickening of three separate but poorly mobile leaflets without commissural fusion (Fig. 11–2, Table 11–1).[56,63,89,106]

Bicuspid pulmonary valve stenosis is a feature of Fallot's tetralogy (see Chapter 18). Isolated bicuspid pulmonary valves are rare and are of little or no functional significance.

Subvalvular pulmonary stenosis can be infundibular or subinfundibular. The infundibular variety is caused by anterior and rightward deviation (malalignment) of the infundibular septum and is dealt with in Chapter 18. Secondary hypertrophic infundibular pulmonary stenosis accompanies severe pulmonary valve stenosis (Fig. 11–3, and see Fig. 11–38). Stenosis of the ostium of the infundibulum is a rare form of fixed obstruction to right ventricular outflow (see Figs. 11–31 and 11–36).[13] Subinfundibular stenosis, or double-chambered right ventricle, was described in 1858 by Thomas Peacock and is also a rare form of congenital obstruction to right ventricular outflow.[90] Obstructing muscle bundles within the right ventricular cavity were the subject of Sir Arthur Keith's Hunterian lecture in 1909.[54] The right ventricle is divided into a high-pressure inlet portion and a low-pressure outlet portion by normal or anomalous muscle bundles[39,65,88,96,103,115,116] or by apical trabecular muscle sequestered from the rest of the right ventricle.[31] The degree of obstruction varies from nil to severe to virtual atresia.[96] Double-chambered right ventricle has a strong tendency to coexist with ventricular septal defect.[65,96]

Supravalvular or pulmonary artery stenosis, described by Oppenheimer in 1938,[87] is caused by narrowing of the pulmonary trunk, its bifurcation, or its primary or intrapulmonary branches (Figs. 11–4 and 11–5).[36] Stenosis of the pulmonary artery and its branches is usually an isolated malformation[9,36,114] and can be unilateral or bilateral,[2] single or multiple,[60] and either segmental or prolonged, culminating in tubular hypoplasia (see Figs. 11–4 and 11–5).[23,36,44] Intrapulmonary arteries distal to the stenoses tend to be dilated (see Figs. 11–4 and 11–5). Rarely, a membranous form of obstruction occurs immediately above the valve.[4,36,110]

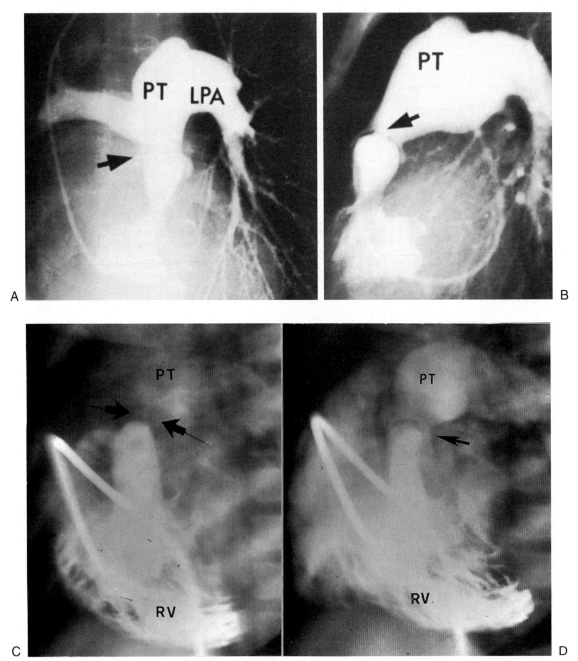

Figure 11–1

A and *B*, Angiocardiograms with contrast material injected into the right ventricle of a 47-year-old woman with pulmonary valve stenosis (gradient 106 mm Hg). *A, Arrow* points to the level of the stenotic pulmonary valve. A dilated pulmonary trunk (PT) continues as a dilated left branch (LPA). *B,* Lateral projection. The stenotic pulmonary valve is mobile and domed (*arrow*), and the pulmonary trunk (PT) is conspicuously dilated. There is an hourglass systolic narrowing of the ostium of the infundibulum. *C* and *D,* Angiocardiograms with contrast material injected into the right ventricle (RV) of a 10-month-old girl with pinpoint pulmonary valve stenosis. *C,* A wisp of contrast crosses the pin-point valve (*arrow*) and faintly visualizes a dilated pulmonary trunk (PT). *D,* The mobile stenotic valve is dome-shaped (*arrow*), and the pulmonary trunk (PT) is conspicuously dilated.

Normal neonates, especially premature neonates, exhibit a disparity between the size of the pulmonary trunk and its proximal branches, with angulations at the origins of the branches. These arrangements cause a physiologic drop in systolic pressure in the absence of morphologic pulmonary artery stenosis (see Chapter 2, Fig. 2–4).[26,101] The small pulmonary trunk and proximal branches of Fallot's tetralogy are discussed in Chapter 18. Bilateral stenosis of pulmonary artery branches is associated with supravalvular

aortic stenosis in Williams syndrome (see Chapter 7).[11] Pulmonary stenosis can incur anatomic and functional changes in the developing pulmonary vascular bed.[61] Experimental constriction of the pulmonary trunk in fetal lambs results in thin-walled intrapulmonary resistance vessels.[61]

In 1941, McAlister Gregg, an Australian ophthalmologist, described a relationship between maternal rubella and congenital abnormalities in offspring.[45] Stenosis of the

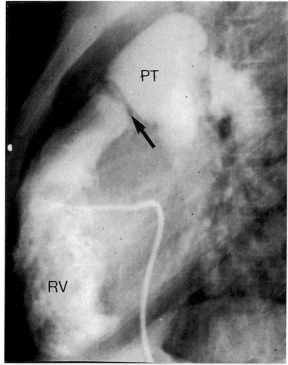

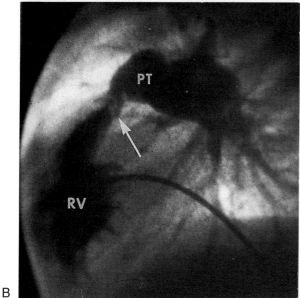

Figure 11–2

A, Right ventriculogram (RV) from a 6-year-old girl with a thickened immobile dysplastic pulmonary valve (*arrow*). The pulmonary trunk (PT) is only moderately dilated. *B*, Right ventriculogram (lateral projection) from a 3-year-old boy with a thickened dysplastic pulmonary valve (*arrow*). The pulmonary trunk (PT) and its left branch are moderately dilated.

pulmonary artery and its branches[22,37,72,79,102,112] and patent ductus arteriosis[37,79] are features of what came to be known as the *rubella syndrome*. Maternal viremia is a prerequisite for placental and fetal infection during initial exposure to rubella.[37] Maternal rubella can have serious noncardiac effects, including spontaneous abortion, stillbirth, mental retardation, cataracts, and deafness.[37] Fetal risk is small when infection occurs later than the 16th

Table 11–1	Congenitally Dysplastic Pulmonary Valve

Three immobile cusps without commissural fusion

Noonan syndrome

Family history

Growth retardation

Absent ejection sound

Absent pulmonary component of the second heart sound

Nondilated pulmonary trunk

week of gestation.[37,79] A worldwide rubella epidemic in 1962 prefigured the 1964/65 rubella epidemic in the United States that affected an estimated 12.5 million patients and caused 11,000 fetal deaths.[22] An estimated 2100 of approximately 20,000 infants born with the rubella syndrome died as neonates.[22]

The physiologic consequences of pulmonary stenosis result from increased resistance to right ventricular outflow. Systolic pressure is elevated proximal to the stenosis and is normal or low distal to the stenosis. Pulmonary artery stenosis causes systolic hypertension in the pulmonary trunk proximal to the obstruction (see Fig. 11–19),[126] whereas the converse is the case when pulmonary stenosis is valvular or subvalvular.

The adaptive response of the right ventricle to an increase in afterload is characterized by an increase in thickness of the free wall and the ventricular septum[93]

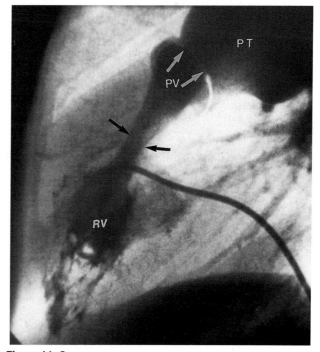

Figure 11–3

Right ventriculogram in the lateral projection (RV) from a 37-year-old man with severe stenosis of a mobile dome pulmonary valve (PV) and secondary hypertrophic subpulmonary stenosis (*paired black arrows*). The pulmonary trunk (PT) is conspicuously dilated.

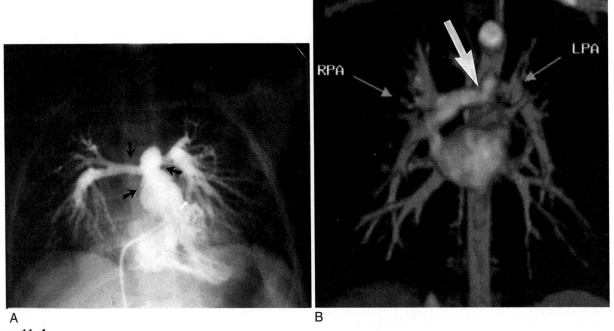

Figure 11–4

A, Angiocardiogram from a 2-year-old girl with stenosis of the pulmonary artery and its branches (gradient 46 mm Hg). *Left lower arrow* points to a normal pulmonary valve. *Left upper arrow* points to tubular hypoplasia of the proximal right pulmonary artery. The *right middle arrow* identifies stenosis of the pulmonary trunk. Tubular hypoplasia of the proximal left pulmonary artery is not shown. The intrapulmonary arteries are dilated distal to the stenoses. *B,* Gadolinium-enhanced magnetic resonance angiogram from a 32-year-old woman with the rubella syndrome status post ductal ligation. There is moderate segmental stenosis (*large arrow*) of the proximal left pulmonary artery (LPA). RPA, right pulmonary artery.

with normal cavity size.[83] In neonates with pinpoint pulmonary stenosis, cavity size is diminished (see Fig. 11–28). Right ventricular pressure overload is responsible for systolic and diastolic dysfunction of the left ventricle.[124,125] Systolic dysfunction has been ascribed to chronic underfilling of the left ventricle, and diastolic dys-

function (reduced left ventricular compliance) has been ascribed to displacement of the hypertrophied septum into the left ventricular cavity.

Children and young adults with mild to moderate pulmonary valve stenosis have normal or near normal right ventricular function and are capable of increasing their

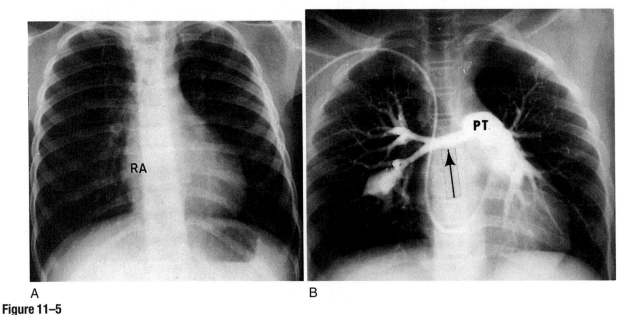

Figure 11–5

A, X-ray from a 7-year- old boy with stenosis of the pulmonary arterial branches. The pulmonary trunk is not dilated. The right atrium is prominent, and a convex right ventricle occupies the apex. *B,* Pulmonary angiogram (PT) discloses tubular hypoplasia of the right pulmonary artery with distal dilatation. Tubular hypoplasia of the left pulmonary artery is not shown.

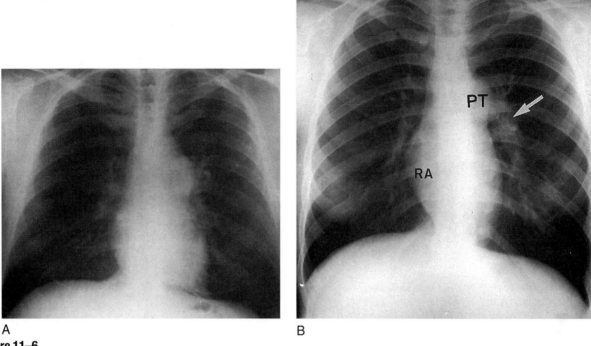

A   B

Figure 11–6
X-rays from a 39-year-old father (A) and his 14-year-old daughter (B), both of whom had typical mobile dome-shaped pulmonary valve stenosis with gradients of 22 mm Hg and 67 mm Hg, respectively. Both x-rays show conspicuous dilatation of the pulmonary trunk (PT) and its left branch (*arrow*) and mild convexity of the right atrium (RA).

cardiac output with exercise.[113] Analogous patients with severe pulmonary valve stenosis have a fixed stroke volume, a fixed cardiac output, and an increase in right ventricular end-diastolic pressure.[76] Systolic contraction of hypertrophied infundibular muscle in severe pulmonary valve stenosis (see Fig. 11–3) is reinforced by exercise.[113]

The History

Typical mobile dome-shaped pulmonary valve stenosis is a relatively common malformation with a prevalence as high as 10% of cases of congenital heart disease.[1,18] Sex distribution is equal[18] or has a female prevalence[30] and is also equal with dysplastic pulmonary valve stenosis.[104]

The murmur of pulmonary stenosis is usually discovered at birth because the anatomic and physiologic conditions necessary for its production are present at birth. Parents are told that their newborn has congenital heart disease before discharge. However, the murmur of pinpoint pulmonary stenosis (see Fig. 11–1C,D) is disarmingly soft, and the non-precordial thoracic murmurs accompanying pulmonary artery stenosis in neonates and infants are easily overlooked or lost in the rapid breath sounds. A history of first-trimester maternal rubella arouses suspicion of pulmonary artery stenosis. Murmur intensity can be estimated by asking parents how readily a murmur was reconfirmed by different examiners.

Familial recurrence of mobile dome-shaped pulmonary valve stenosis is uncommon if not rare (Fig. 11–6).[17,55,69] The converse is the case in dysplastic pulmonary valve stenosis.[56] Some family members have a dysplastic valve whereas others have a mobile dome-shaped valve.[56] Similar observations have been made in the hereditary canine pulmonary valve dysplasia of beagles,[89] with dysplastic pulmonary stenosis and dome-shaped pulmonary stenosis occurring in litter mates.[89] Familial Noonan syndrome is relatively frequent, with dysplastic pulmonary valve stenosis recurring in three generations.[6,71] Familial pulmonary artery stenosis occurs as an isolated anomaly or with coexisting supravalvular aortic stenosis.[4] Members of the same family may have either or both anomalies.[4]

Normal birth weights and normal growth and development are characteristic of mobile dome-shaped pulmonary valve stenosis. However, growth and development are poor in patients with Noonan syndrome with dysplastic pulmonary valve stenosis,[56,63,71,85,104] and low birth weights and retarded physical and mental development in patients with the rubella syndrome[4,22,37,117] and with Williams syndrome are associated with pulmonary artery stenosis (see Chapter 7).

Neonates with pinpoint pulmonary valve stenosis confront rapidly progressive cardiac failure and early death. However, the majority of patients with mobile dome-shaped pulmonary valve stenosis experience little or no difficulty in infancy and childhood.[49] In a review of 69 cases, the average age at death was 26 years; 7 patients survived to age 50 years, and 3 survived to 70 and 75 years. In 21 adults, the average follow-up period was 50 years.[53] There are examples of survival into the sixth, seventh, and eighth decade,[42,43,118,119] with one patient reaching age 78 years.[42] Longevity depends on three variables: (1) the initial severity of stenosis, (2) whether a given degree of stenosis remains constant or progresses, and (3) whether the function of the afterloaded right ventricle is preserved.[49,76,111] Mild pulmonary valve stenosis in infancy usually remains mild, but moderate to severe pulmonary stenosis may progress.[74] Stenosis of the pulmonary artery and its branches is usually nonprogressive. A normal pulmonary valve orifice increases linearly with age and body surface area.[66] The orifice of a mobile dome-shaped stenotic pulmonary valve increases with age, but the increase does not necessarily keep pace with somatic growth.[25,49,66,75] In older adults, fibrous thickening and occasionally calcification may be responsible for increasing the degree of stenosis.[3,100]

Equivalent degrees of pulmonary stenosis may handicap one patient in childhood yet leave another relatively free of symptoms in adulthood. It is not surprising that mild pulmonary stenosis is asymptomatic, but it is surprising that an appreciable number of patients with moderate to severe pulmonary stenosis claim to be virtually asymptomatic. Patients with right ventricular systolic pressures between 50 and 100 mm Hg include a New Zealand long-distance swimmer, a long-distance runner, and an English hockey captain.[122] My patients include a 17-year-old boy who played baseball despite a right ventricular systolic pressure of nearly 200 mm Hg, a 32-year-old man who had run the quarter mile in high school despite a right ventricular systolic pressure of 75 mm Hg, and a woman who worked full-time with a right ventricular pressure of nearly 200 mm Hg and who had recurrent ascites for 7 years before death at the age of 60 years. Dyspnea and fatigue are mild as long as the right ventricle maintains a normal stroke volume at rest and augments its stroke volume with exercise.[76,111] However, patients with few or no symptoms may deteriorate rapidly. Cardiac output becomes inadequate even at rest when the hemodynamic burden imposed on the right ventricle leads to right ventricular failure, which is the most common cause of death.[43]

Giddiness and light-headedness with effort prefigure syncope.[122] Children as well as adults occasionally experience the chest pain of right ventricular myocardial ischemia.[9,15,57,64,119] A 3-year-old with severe pulmonary artery stenosis and angina pectoris died during an episode of chest pain and at necropsy had infarction of the right ventricular free wall and interventricular septum. Sudden death has been associated with right ventricular infarction and abnormal right ventricular intramural coronary arteries.[21] Rupture of dilated thin-walled intrapulmonary artery aneurysms distal to stenoses of pulmonary artery branches (see Fig. 11–5B) results in hemoptysis, which can be intermittent and mild or recurrent and brisk.[36]

Severe pulmonary stenosis generates giant jugular venous A waves (see Fig. 11–8) that patients may be subjectively aware of, especially during effort or excitement. These neck pulsations can be seen in the mirror when a young man shaves or when a young woman sits at her vanity. A 13-year-old girl with pulmonary valve stenosis and congenital complete heart block was unpleasantly aware of intermittent amplification of A waves as her right atrium randomly contracted against a closed tricuspid valve, and a 15-year-old boy was unpleasantly aware of intermittent amplification of jugular venous A waves caused by premature ventricular beats.

Mobile dome-shaped pulmonary valve stenosis is a substrate for infective endocarditis[74] that results in a medical valvotomy when the infection interrupts valve tissue and increases orifice size.[122] Pulmonary artery stenosis causes jet lesions that can serve as substrates for infective endarteritis.[36]

Physical Appearance

Five physical appearances are relevant in patients with pulmonary stenosis and include those in patients with (1) mobile dome-shaped pulmonary valve stenosis in infancy, (2) Noonan syndrome, (3) the rubella syndrome, (4) Williams syndrome, and (5) Alagille syndrome (arteriohepatic dysplasia).

Infants with dome-shaped pulmonary valve stenosis occasionally have chubby, round, bloated faces with highly colored cheeks (Fig. 11–7A) and well-developed fat deposits.[122] The digits may be erythematous or frankly red in response to a small or intermittent right-to-left shunt through a patent foramen ovale (see Chapter 16).

Noonan syndrome[27,28,85,86] (see Fig. 11–7C–E) is characterized by short stature, webbed neck, pterygium colli, ptosis, hypertelorism, lymphedema, low-set ears, low anterior and posterior hairlines, flat or shield chest, pectus excavatum or carinatum, hyperelastic skin, inguinal hernia, nevi, dystrophic nails, micrognathia, hypospadias, and small undescended or cryptorchid testes.[28,71] Approximately one third of Noonan syndrome patients are mentally retarded, and approximately two thirds have congenital heart disease,[28,71,104,121] especially dysplastic pulmonary valve stenosis (60%) or hypertrophic cardiomyopathy (20%).[24,28,52,71,85,91,104] Successful pregnancy is possible in women with Noonan syndrome.[27]

The rubella syndrome is characterized by cataracts, retinopathy, deafness, hypotonia, dermatoglyphic abnormalities, and mental retardation.[37] Height and weight are usually normal for age despite intrauterine growth retardation. Patent ductus arteriosis (see Chapter 20) and stenosis of the pulmonary artery and its branches are the most frequent types of coexisting congenital heart disease.[37]

Williams syndrome is characterized by mental retardation and small chin, large mouth, patulous lips, blunt upturned

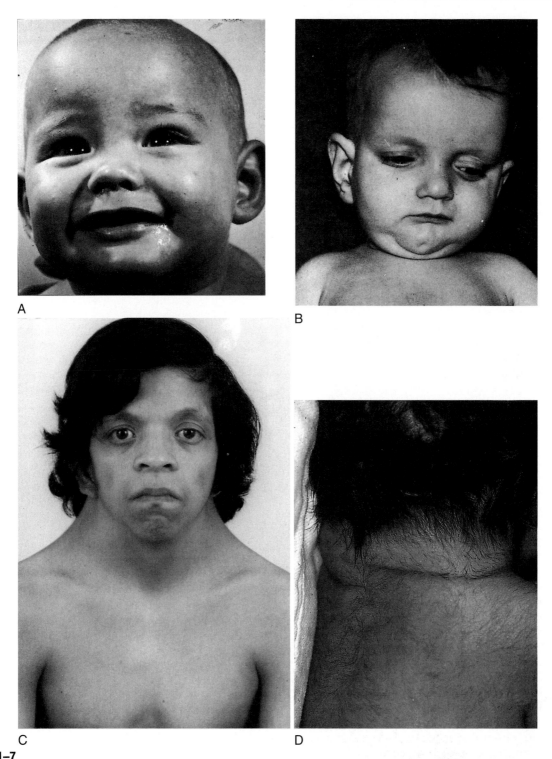

Figure 11–7

A, The chubby round bloated face of an infant with typical mobile dome-shaped pulmonary valve stenosis. *B,* Facial appearance of arteriohepatic dysplasia (Alagille syndrome) characterized by deeply set eyes, prominent overhanging forehead, and small pointed chin. *C,* Noonan syndrome in an 18-year-old phenotypic male with webbing of the neck, low-set ears, abnormal auricles, hypertelorism, and a small chin. *D,* Low posterior hair line of a neonate with Noonan syndrome. *Illustration continued on following page*

nose, wide-set eyes, broad forehead, baggy cheeks, and malformed teeth (see Chapter 7). The most frequent coexisting congenital heart disease is pulmonary artery stenosis with supravalvular aortic stenosis (see Chapter 7).

Alagille syndrome, also referred to as arteriohepatic dysplasia or the Alagille-Watson syndrome, is an autosomal dominant disorder with abnormalities of heart, liver, eyes, kidneys, and skeleton.[14,18] Facial appearance is characterized by a prominent overhanging forehead, deep-set eyes, and a small pointed chin (see Fig. 11–7B).[14,18,62,120] The most frequent type of coexisting congenital heart disease is stenosis of the pulmonary artery and its branches.[18]

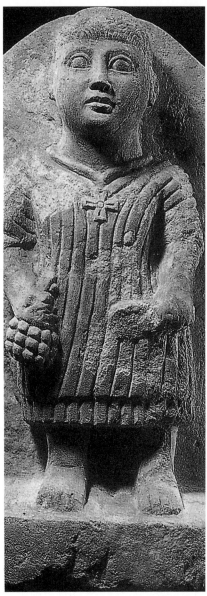

E

Figure 11–7
E, Fourth-century grave stele of a young phenotypic male with the short stature and broad neck of Noonan syndrome.

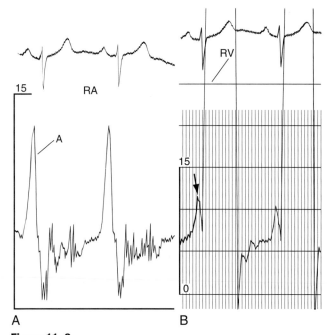

A   **B**

Figure 11–8
Pressure pulses from the 47-year-old woman with severe pulmonary valve stenosis referred to in Figure 11–1. *A,* There is a large A wave in the right atrium (RA). *B,* Presystolic distention (*arrow*) of the right ventricle (RV) coincided with the large right atrial A wave.

The Arterial Pulse

The arterial pulse is reduced when severe pulmonary stenosis is accompanied by right ventricular failure and left ventricular dysfunction. Asymmetry of right and left brachial and carotid arterial pulses (right greater than left) is a feature of supravalvular aortic stenosis that may accompany stenosis of the pulmonary artery and its branches (see Chapter 7).

The Jugular Venous Pulse

The jugular venous A wave gets progressively larger as the severity of pulmonary stenosis increases (Figs. 11–8*A* and

11–9). Exercise and excitement increase the A wave still further. The giant A wave that "leaps to the eye, towering above and dwarfing the other waves of the venous pulse"[1] is even more impressive when compared to the normal or small arterial pulse. Powerful right atrial contraction gen-

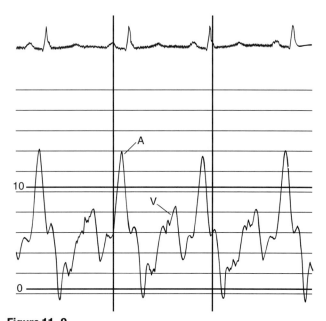

Figure 11–9
Prominent right atrial A wave in a 4-year-old girl with pulmonary valve stenosis and a peak systolic gradient of 50 mm Hg.

erates a giant jugular venous A wave and a presystolic liver pulse. With the advent of right ventricular failure and tricuspid regurgitation, the V wave increases, the Y descent becomes brisk, and the liver manifests presystolic *and* systolic pulsations.

Precordial Movement and Palpation

Chest asymmetry is rarely prominent. Thrills reflect the location, radiation, and intensity of accompanying murmurs (see Auscultation). The thrill associated with pulmonary valve stenosis is maximum in the second left intercostal space with radiation upward and to the left because the intrapulmonary jet is directed upward and toward the left pulmonary artery (see Fig. 11–37A).[80] The thrill is maximum in the third or fourth left intercostal space when secondary hypertrophic subpulmonary stenosis coexists (see Fig. 11–3). A left parasternal or left basal thrill sometimes accompanies stenosis at the bifurcation of the main pulmonary artery.

A right ventricular impulse is more readily palpated when the fingertips are applied between the ribs during full held exhalation or by applying a fingertip against the diaphragm in the subxiphoid area.[50,94] The later technique is especially useful in infants because respiratory excursions may interfere with parasternal palpation. Mild pulmonary valve stenosis is associated with a gentle right ventricular impulse best palpated after exercise or in infants after feeding or crying. The right ventricular impulse in severe pulmonary valve stenosis is forceful and sustained and is detected up to and including the third intercostal space.[50,82,94] Infundibular pulmonary stenosis relegates the high-pressure zone to the inflow portion of the right ventricle, so the accompanying impulse is assigned to the fourth and fifth left intercostal spaces. Subinfundibular stenosis is accompanied by a deceptively unimpressive right ventricular impulse confined to the fifth interspace or subxiphoid area.

A systolic impulse over the pulmonary trunk is absent irrespective of the level or morphologic type of pulmonary stenosis. Pulmonary valve stenosis puts a brake on the rate of right ventricular ejection, so there is little or no systolic expansion of the pulmonary trunk, which is not palpated despite dilatation. With stenosis of the pulmonary artery and its branches, the pulmonary trunk is not dilated and therefore does not transmit an impulse.

A presystolic impulse along the lower left sternal border or in the subxiphoid area (Fig. 11–8B) reflects presystolic distention of the right ventricle in response to the increased force of right atrial contraction that is responsible for the large jugular venous A wave (Fig. 11–8A). A prominent pulmonary ejection sound is occasionally palpable in the second left intercostal space during held exhalation.

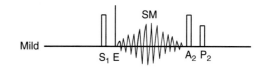

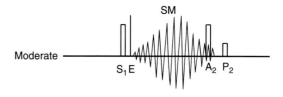

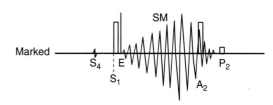

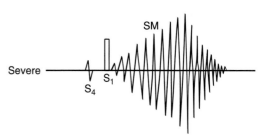

Figure 11–10
Schematic phonocardiograms illustrating mild to severe mobile dome-shaped pulmonary valve stenosis. A$_2$, aortic component of the second sound; E, pulmonary ejection sound; P$_2$, pulmonary component of the second sound; S$_1$, first heart sound; S$_4$, fourth heart sound; SM, midsystolic murmur.

Auscultation

An ejection sound coincides with the abrupt cephalad excursion of a mobile dome-shaped pulmonary valve (see Figs. 11–1B and 11–3) and is therefore important in the auscultatory characterization of right ventricular outflow obstruction (Fig. 11–10).[59,94] Ejection sounds do not occur with dysplastic pulmonary valves, which move poorly if at all,[56,63] or with fixed subvalvular stenosis[94] or pulmonary artery stenosis in which the valve mechanism is normal. An analogous sound has been attributed to a functionally normal bicuspid pulmonary valve.[70] The ejection sound is recognized by its high-pitched clicking quality, by its maximum intensity in the second left intercostal space, and by its distinctive selective decrease during inspiration (Figs. 11–11 through 11–13).[51,58,94] Respiratory variation is related to the amount of cephalad movement available to the mobile valve as the right ventricle contracts.[51] The increase in right atrial contractile force during inspiration

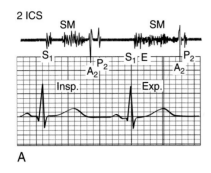

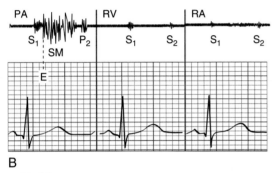

Figure 11–11

Phonocardiograms from a 9-year-old girl with mobile dome-shaped pulmonary valve stenosis and a gradient of 25 mm Hg. *A*, In the second left intercostal space (2 ICS), a pulmonary ejection sound is absent during inspiration (Insp.) and is present (E) during expiration (EXP). A midsystolic murmur (SM) diminishes before the aortic component of the second heart sound (A₂). The pulmonary component of the second sound (P₂) is clearly evident and delayed. The split widened further during inspiration and narrowed but persisted during expiration. *B*, Intracardiac phonocardiogram from within the main pulmonary artery (PA) shows an amplified midsystolic murmur (SM) that promptly vanished when the catheter microphone was withdrawn into the right ventricle (RV). RA, right atrium.

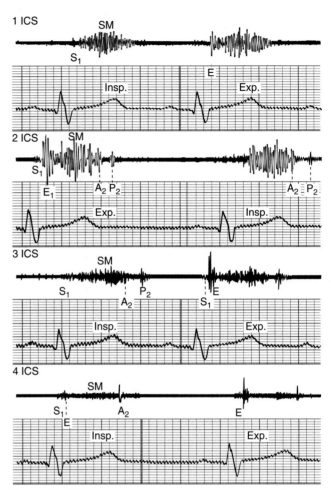

Figure 11–12

Phonocardiograms from the first through the fourth left intercostal spaces (1 ICS through 4 ICS) of a 12-year-old boy with mobile dome-shaped pulmonary valve stenosis and a gradient of 50 mm Hg. The midsystolic murmur goes up to the aortic component of the second sound (A₂), is maximum in the second intercostal space, and radiated upward and to the left. The pulmonary ejection sound vanishes during inspiration and is prominent during expiration. The second sound is widely split because of a delayed soft pulmonary component (P₂). The splitting increased further during inspiration.

is transmitted into the right ventricle and onto the undersurface of the mobile pulmonary valve, which moves into a relatively cephalad position.[99] Additional cephalad movement is therefore reduced, so the ejection sound softens or vanishes altogether.[51] Conversely, the decrease in right atrial contractile force during expiration leaves the mobile pulmonary valve in a slack position, so right ventricular contraction induces maximum cephalad excursion and maximum intensity of the ejection sound.[51]

The interval between the first heart sound and the ejection sound varies inversely with the degree of stenosis (see Fig. 11–10).[40,59] As severity increases, the rate of right ventricular contraction increases, the pulmonary valve opens earlier, and the ejection sound occurs earlier and merges with the first heart sound[40,115] (see Fig. 11–10) but retains its distinctive respiratory variation that distinguishes it from a loud first heart sound.[115] A pulmonary ejection sound that occurs at a well-defined interval after the first heart sound is a sign of mild pulmonary stenosis, and an ejection sound that merges with the first heart sound is a sign of severe pulmonary stenosis. Fibrosis and calcification impair mobility, so the ejection sound decreases or disappears.[3]

The murmur of pulmonary valve stenosis was recognized in 1858 by Peacock.[90] The maximum precordial intensity is in the second left intercostal space (see Figs. 11–11 through 11–13), which topographically overlies the pulmonary trunk and coincides with the location of the murmur recorded by intracardiac phonocardiography[94] (see Fig. 11–11B). Prominence of the murmur in the third left intercostal space is due to secondary hypertrophic subpulmonary stenosis (Fig. 11–14B, and see Fig. 11–3). The murmur radiates upward and to the left (see Fig. 11–12) because the intrapulmonary jet is directed upward and to the left (see Fig. 11–37A). Loud systolic murmurs radiate to the suprasternal notch and to the base of the neck, especially the left side of the neck. Intensity varies directly with the degree of obstruction, but intensity per se is not necessarily an index of severity. The murmur is deceptively soft in neonates with pinpoint pulmonary stenosis (Fig. 11–1C, D). Grade 3/6 murmurs are features of mild

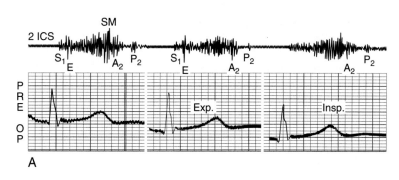

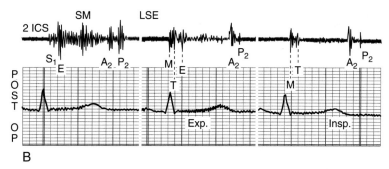

Figure 11–13

Phonocardiograms from a 21-year-old woman with mobile dome-shaped pulmonary valve stenosis and a gradient of 80 mm Hg. *A*, Before pulmonary valvotomy was performed PRE OP, the systolic murmur (SM) peaked late and enveloped the aortic component of the second sound (A$_2$), the soft pulmonary component (P$_2$) was delayed, and a pulmonary ejection sound was recorded during expiration and was absent during inspiration. *B*, After valvotomy POST OP, the gradient was 20 mm Hg, and the phonocardiogram resembles that of mild pulmonary valve stenosis (see Figs. 11–10 and 11–11). M, mitral component of the first sound; T, tricuspid component.

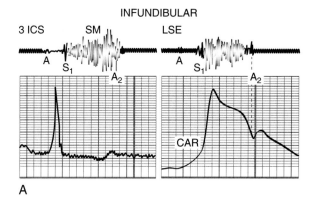

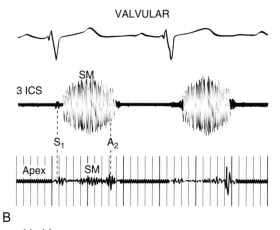

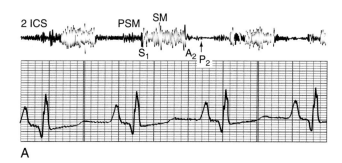

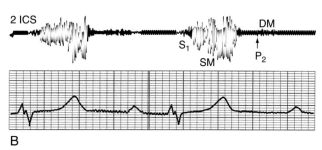

Figure 11–14

A, Phonocardiogram from a 34-year-old man with infundibular pulmonary stenosis and a gradient of 140 mm Hg. A long systolic murmur (SM) enveloped the aortic component of the second sound (A$_2$) and was equally prominent in the third intercostal space (3 ICS) and at the lower left sternal edge (LSE). CAR, carotid pulse; S$_4$, fourth heart sound. *B*, Phonocardiogram from a 14-year-old boy with mobile dome-shaped pulmonary valve stenosis and a gradient of 115 mm Hg. The systolic murmur envelops the aortic component of the second sound (A$_2$) and is prominent in the third left intercostal space (3 ICS) because of secondary hypertrophic subpulmonary stenosis.

Figure 11–15

A, Phonocardiogram from a 10-month-old girl with mobile dome-shaped pulmonary valve stenosis and a gradient of 95 mm Hg. A right atrial A wave of 17 to 20 mm Hg coincided with the presystolic murmur (PSM). A long systolic murmur (SM) encroached upon the aortic component of the second heart sound (A$_2$). The faint pulmonary component (P$_2$) is considerably delayed. *B*, Phonocardiogram in the second intercostal space (2 ICS) of a 6-year-old boy with mobile dome-shaped pulmonary valve stenosis and a gradient of 100 mm Hg. A soft diastolic murmur (DM) began with a markedly delayed pulmonary component of the second heart sound (P$_2$). The systolic murmur is long and kite-shaped and enveloped the aortic component of the second sound.

pulmonary stenosis (see Fig. 11–11), and murmurs of grade 3/6 to 6/6 are features of moderate to severe pulmonary stenosis (see Figs. 11–12 through 11–14). Exercise, feeding, crying, and amyl nitrite increase intensity.

The severity determines the duration of right ventricular ejection, which in turn determines the length of the systolic murmur. The length of the pulmonary systolic murmur relative to the aortic component of the second heart sound permits comparison of the relative durations of right and left ventricular ejection (see Fig. 11–10). When pulmonary stenosis is mild, right ventricular ejection is not prolonged, so the symmetric systolic murmur ends before registration of the aortic component of the second sound (see Figs. 11–10 and 11–11).[115] When stenosis is moderate, the murmur ends at or slightly after the aortic component of the second sound, which remains audible (see Figs. 11–10 and 11–12).[115] When stenosis is severe, the murmur extends beyond the aortic component of the second sound, which is partially or completely obscured (see Figs. 11–10, 11–13, and 11–14).[115] With a further increase in severity, the murmur lengthens and peaks later in systole and assumes an asymmetric kite shape.[40,68,115] Figure 11–10 illustrates the relationship between the duration and configuration of the systolic murmur and the degree of pulmonary stenosis.

Stenosis of the ostium of the infundibulum (see Figs. 11–31 and 11–36) is accompanied by a lower precordial location of the murmur that is maximum in the third and fourth intercostal spaces (see Fig. 11–14).[1,115] Subinfundibular

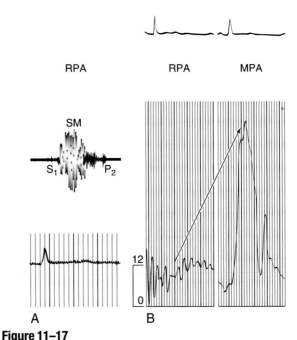

Figure 11–17

Tracings from a 19-year-old man with pulmonary artery stenosis. *A,* Intracardiac phonocardiogram from the distal right pulmonary artery (RPA) recorded a crescendo-decrescendo systolic murmur (SM) that is delayed in onset. *B,* As the catheter was withdrawn from the distal right pulmonary artery to the main pulmonary artery (MPA), a gradient was recorded (*oblique arrow*), and the distinctive contour of the main pulmonary artery pressure pulse emerged (see Fig. 11–16A). The gradient is systolic and does not continue into diastole, so the murmur is confined to systole.

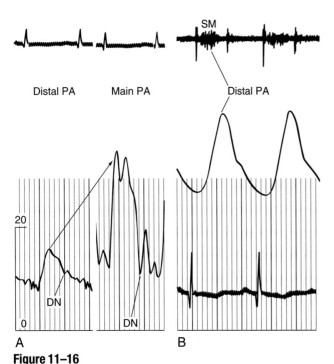

Figure 11–16

Tracings from a 4-year-old girl with stenosis of the pulmonary artery and its branches. *A,* Pressure pulses recorded from the distal and main pulmonary arteries (PA) establish the systolic gradient and illustrate the distinctive contour of the main pulmonary arterial pressure pulse, which is characterized by a rapid rise and a rapid descent to a low dicrotic notch (DN). *B,* Intracardiac phonocardiogram from a distal pulmonary artery (PA) recorded a crescendo-decrescendo systolic murmur (SM).

stenosis assigns the murmur to the fourth or fifth left intercostal space.[88] The holosystolic murmur of tricuspid regurgitation with right ventricular failure is distinguished by its high frequency, its lower left or right sternal edge location, and its selective increase during inspiration.

Several types of diastolic murmurs occur in patients with pulmonary valve stenosis, although rarely. A low-intensity atrial systolic murmur is attributed to presystolic flow across the pulmonary valve (Fig. 11–15A).[59] Powerful right atrial contraction generates an A wave that exceeds the diastolic pressure in the pulmonary trunk, so the pulmonary valve opens before the onset of ventricular contraction, permitting presystolic flow and a presystolic murmur (see Fig 11–38).[59,94,115] Prolonged vibrations of a fourth heart sound occasionally generate a presystolic murmur,[92] and soft diastolic murmurs have been attributed to low-pressure pulmonary regurgitation (see Figs. 11–15B, 11–37B, and 11–38).[59,115] Dysplastic[63] or calcific pulmonary valves[3,100] are rarely incompetent.

Murmurs associated with pulmonary artery stenosis are typically confined to systole (Figs. 11–16 and 11–17) but exceptionally are continuous.[36,46,81,95] Thoracic distribution is determined by the locations of the stenotic segments, which are usually multiple and involve the pulmonary trunk and the proximal and distal branches (see Figs. 11–4 and 11–5B). The accompanying systolic murmurs are heard centrally in the vicinity of the second left and right intercostal spaces and peripherally in the axillae and back (Fig. 11–18).[36] The interpretation of nonprecordial thoracic murmurs requires a judgment as to

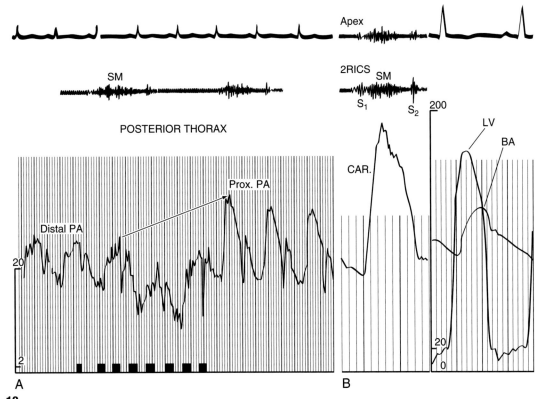

Figure 11–18

Recordings from a 7-year-old boy with pulmonary artery stenosis and supravalvular aortic stenosis. *A,* The phonocardiogram from the posterior thorax shows the peripheral pulmonary stenotic murmur (SM). As the catheter was withdrawn from distal to proximal pulmonary artery (PA), a systolic gradient was recorded (*oblique arrow*) together with the distinctive contour of the proximal pulmonary artery pressure pulse. *B,* Phonocardiogram at the right base shows the supravalvular aortic stenotic murmur (SM). 2 RICS, second right intercostal space. The left ventricular (LV) and brachial arterial (BA) pressure pulses reflect the supravalvular gradient. CAR, carotid pulse.

whether they originate peripherally or radiate from a loud central murmur. Peripheral pulmonary systolic murmurs due to high flow accompany uncomplicated atrial septal defect and are difficult to distinguish from murmurs of coexisting pulmonary artery stenosis.[95] Normal neonates, especially premature neonates, experience a physiologic drop in systolic pressure from pulmonary trunk to proximal branches that is accompanied by peripheral pulmonary systolic murmurs that vanish within a few months (see Chapter 2).[26,101]

Systolic murmurs of pulmonary artery stenosis are crescendo-decrescendo (see Figs. 11–16 and 11–17) with delayed onset because of their relatively distal origins (see Fig. 11–17). Stenoses that originate at or near the bifurcation of the pulmonary trunk generate murmurs that occasionally reach grade 4/6 in the second left intercostal space,[4] but as a rule the central precordial murmur is grade 3/6 and the peripheral murmurs are softer. When the intensity of precordial and non-precordial murmurs is equal, the widespread non-precordial murmurs originate peripherally. Intrapulmonary phonocardiograms confirm that systolic murmurs originate distal to stenoses in the pulmonary trunk or in the proximal pulmonary arterial branches (see Figs. 11–16 through 11–18). Peripheral pulmonary systolic murmurs are often overlooked because of their low intensity and because auscultation is not systematically conducted at non-precordial sites. The difficulty is

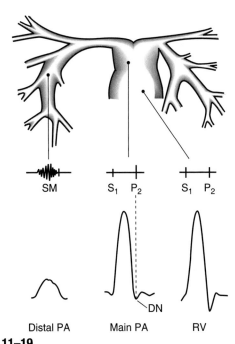

Figure 11–19

Illustrations of the anatomic, intracardiac phonocardiographic and hemodynamic features of pulmonary artery stenosis. A systolic murmur (SM) originates in the pulmonary artery distal to the stenosis. The pressure pulse in the main pulmonary artery (PA) is characterized by a rapid rise, an elevated peak, and a rapid descent to a low dicrotic notch (DN). The systolic gradient does not continue into diastole, so the accompanying murmur is confined to systole. The pulmonary component of the second heart sound (P_2) is not increased because the pulmonary valve closes at a low pressure.

compounded in infants with rapid respiratory rates, because the frequency composition of breath sounds is close to the frequency composition of peripheral pulmonary systolic murmurs. The diaphragm of the stethoscope should be applied with the patient in supine, prone, and sitting positions and during held respiration, age permitting.

Continuous murmurs imply continuous gradients across the stenotic sites, but recordings of pressure pulses proximal and distal to the zones of stenosis show that systolic gradients seldom continue into diastole.[33] The central pulmonary artery pulse is characterized by an elevated systolic pressure but a rapid fall to diastolic levels that are normal or nearly so (Fig. 11–19, and see Fig. 11–17).[2] Gradients are confined to systolic, so the accompanying murmur is confined to systole (see Figs. 11–17 and 11–19).[33] Why, then, do continuous murmurs occur at all? It has been postulated that systolic expansion of the high-pressure pulmonary trunk proximal to the stenosis sets the stage for brisk diastolic flow across the distal segments as the expanded proximal segment recoils.[33] Modest diastolic flow following a large systolic gradient may explain the occasional occurrence of a soft, low-frequency diastolic murmur that follows a prominent systolic murmur.[33] Pulmonary artery stenosis may also give rise to increased flow through bronchial arterial collaterals,[34] and angiographically demonstrated bronchial collaterals are believed to be responsible for a continuous murmur.[60]

Splitting of the second heart sound and the intensity of the pulmonary component are important signs in the auscultatory characterization of obstruction to right ventricular outflow. In typical mobile dome-shaped pulmonary valve stenosis, the intensity of the pulmonary component varies from normal to inaudible as severity increases (Figs. 11–10 through 11–15). However, timing is more important than intensity in assessing severity.[40,59] The more severe the stenosis, the longer the duration of right ventricular ejection, the later the timing of pulmonary valve closure, and the wider the split (see Fig. 11–10). With mild stenosis, splitting is mild to moderate (see Fig. 11–11).[109] With severe stenosis, splitting may be as great as 120 to 140 msec (see Fig. 11–15) and, if heard at all, is fixed because right ventricular stroke volume is fixed.[109] The aortic component of the second sound is obscured by the long murmur of severe pulmonary stenosis, and the pulmonary component may be inaudible (see Figs. 11–10 and 11–14).[59,108,109] When stenosis is mild, the pulmonary component tend to be delayed by the increased capacitance of the pulmonary vascular bed associated with dilatation of the pulmonary trunk and its proximal branches.[107,108,109,115] These qualifications not withstanding, a slight increase in splitting with normal intensity of the pulmonary component favors mild stenosis (see Fig. 11–11), and a marked increase in splitting with a faint or inaudible pulmonary component favors severe stenosis (see Figs. 11–14 and 11–15).

Factors that influence the behavior of the second heart sound in pulmonary artery stenosis differ from those that

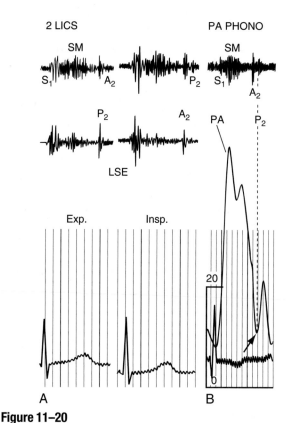

Figure 11–20

Recordings from a 4-year-old girl with pulmonary artery stenosis. *A*, Phonocardiograms in the second left intercostal space (2 LICS) show a midsystolic murmur (SM) followed by normal splitting of the second heart sound with normal intensity of the pulmonary component. *A₂*, aortic component of the second sound; LSE, left sternal edge; Exp., expiration; Insp., inspiration; P₂, pulmonary component of the second sound. *B*, Intracardiac phonocardiogram (PHONO) and pressure pulse from the proximal pulmonary artery (PA). The pulmonary component of the second heart sound (P_2) is soft because the valve closed at a low pressure despite systolic hypertension. A short systolic murmur (SM) was recorded in the pulmonary trunk.

influence the second sound in valvular or subvalvular stenosis.[95] Stenosis of the pulmonary artery and its branches is unique among causes of pulmonary hypertension because it elevates systolic but not diastolic pressure in the pulmonary trunk. Accordingly, the valve closes at a normal or near normal pressure,[2,92,95] so the intensity of the pulmonary component of the second sound is normal (see Figs. 11–19 through 11–21).[4,36,95] However, the cusps might bulge abruptly toward the right ventricle during isometric relaxation, suddenly increasing the volume capacity of the pulmonary trunk,[2] so the intensity of the pulmonary component may be influenced by the abruptness with which the leaflets seat. The intensity of the pulmonary second sound remains unchanged as severity increases,[95] in contrast to mobile dome-shaped pulmonary valve stenosis or fixed subvalvular stenosis in which the intensity of the pulmonary component varies inversely with the degree of stenosis.

The timing of pulmonary valve closure in pulmonary artery stenosis cannot be judged by criteria that apply to valvular or fixed subvalvular pulmonary stenosis, both of which prolong right ventricular ejection. Potential prolon-

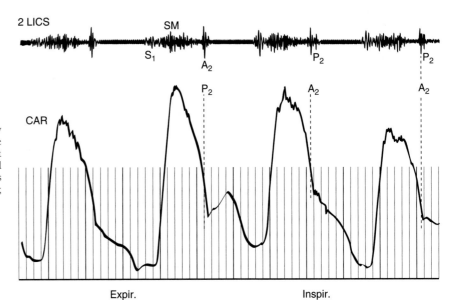

Figure 11–21

Recordings from a 5-year-old boy with pulmonary artery stenosis and a gradient of 63 mm Hg. There is a midsystolic murmur (SM) in the second left intercostal space (2 LICS). The second sound splits normally. The pulmonary component (P_2) is neither increased nor delayed. CAR, carotid pulse; Expir., expiration; Inspir., inspiration.

gation of right ventricular ejection in pulmonary artery stenosis is countered by the rapidity with which the pulmonary artery pressure falls from its systolic peak (see Fig. 11–17).[2] The second heart sound is normally split even in the presence of appreciable obstruction,[95] and the degree of splitting varies appropriately with respiration (Figs. 11–20 and 11–21).[95]

Abrahams and Wood drew attention to the fourth heart sound in pulmonary stenosis,[1] reasoning that "strong right atrial contraction in presystole helps the hypertrophied right ventricle to generate a high systolic pressure." This was considered "an example of Starling's law of the heart, strong atrial systole augmenting late diastolic distention of the right ventricle so that the chamber contracts more

forcibly." Presystolic distension of the right ventricle and fourth heart sounds are features of severe pulmonary stenosis because these physiologic conditions prevail when obstruction to right ventricular outflow is severe (Fig. 11–22, and see Figs. 11–8B and 11–10).[59,123]

The Electrocardiogram

As severity increases, P waves become tall and peaked (Fig. 11–23). Giant P waves occasionally appear, especially in lead 2 (Fig. 11–24). The P wave in lead V_1 may be entirely

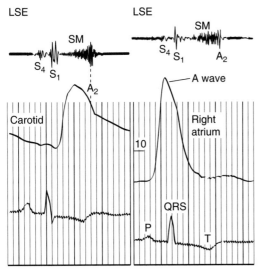

Figure 11–22

Recordings from a 23-year-old woman with mobile dome-shaped pulmonary valve stenosis and a gradient of 118 mm Hg. A prominent fourth heart sound (S_4) at the lower left sternal edge (LSE) coincides with the large A wave in the right atrium. The soft systolic murmur (SM) at the lower sternal edge was Grade 4 in the second left interspace.

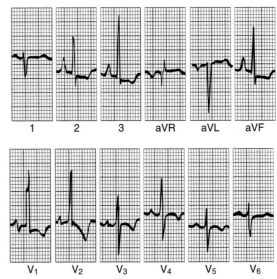

Figure 11–23

Electrocardiogram from a 43-year-old woman with mobile dome-shaped pulmonary valve stenosis and a gradient of 135 mm Hg. Tall peaked right atrial P waves appear in leads 2, 3, and aVF. Right ventricular hypertrophy is manifested by right axis deviation, tall monophasic R waves in right precordial leads indicating suprasystemic right ventricular systolic pressure, coved ST segments with inverted T waves in right/mid-precordial leads, and deep S waves in the left precordium.

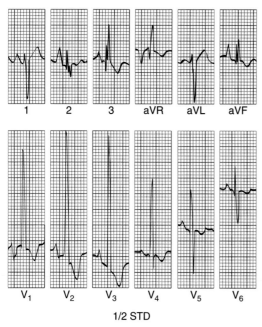

Figure 11–24

Electrocardiogram from an 8- month-old girl with mobile dome-shaped pulmonary valve stenosis and suprasystemic right ventricular pressure. A tall peaked right atrial P wave is present in lead 2. The right atrial P wave abnormality in lead V_1 is almost entirely negative (compare to lead aVR). Right ventricular hypertrophy is manifested by right axis deviation, striking monophasic R waves, and deeply inverted T waves in right precordial leads and deep S waves in left precordial leads. This pattern is typical of suprasystemic right ventricular pressure.

negative because the P terminal force is written by right atrial dilatation (see Fig. 11–24).[67] PR interval prolongation has been attributed to an increase in right atrial size that prolongs the transit time from sinus node to atrioventricular node (Fig. 11–25).[67,123] Right axis deviation tends to vary directly with right ventricular systolic pressure (Figs. 11–23 through 11–26).[25,123] Superior orientation of

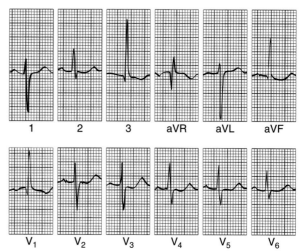

Figure 11–25

Electrocardiogram from a 16-year-old girl with mobile dome-shaped pulmonary valve stenosis and a gradient of 70 mm Hg. The PR interval is 200 msec. Right ventricular hypertrophy is manifested by right axis deviation and a monophasic R wave in lead V_1. The qR complex in lead V_1 is similar to the qR complex in lead aVR and is evidence of right atrial enlargement.

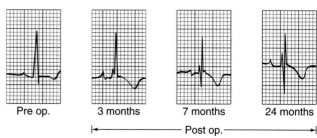

Figure 11–27

Pre- and postoperative lead V_1 in a 6-year-old girl with mobile dome-shaped pulmonary valve stenosis and a gradient of 100 mm Hg before pulmonary valvotomy. The postoperative sequence reflects electrocardiographic regression of right ventricular hypertrophy. The tall monophasic preoperative R wave became an rR′, an rsR′, and 24 months later an rSr′ where it remained.

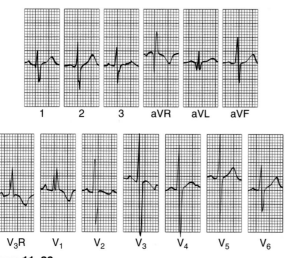

Figure 11–26

Electrocardiogram from a 2-year-old girl with stenosis of the pulmonary artery and a gradient of 46 mm Hg. Right ventricular hypertrophy is manifested by the rightward, superior, and anterior direction of the QRS axis, the tall R wave in lead aVR, the rR′ in lead V_3R and the deep S waves in left precordial leads.

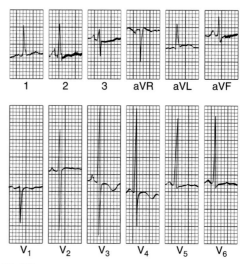

Figure 11–28

Electrocardiogram from a 9-day-old male with pinpoint pulmonary valve stenosis and a thick-walled right ventricle with a small cavity. Peaked right atrial P waves appear in leads 2 and V_3. The QRS axis and the r wave in lead V_1 are normal.

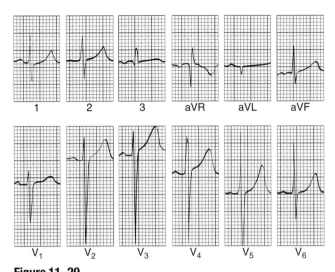

Figure 11–29

Electrocardiogram from a 5-year-old boy with mobile dome-shaped pulmonary valve stenosis and a gradient of 25 mm Hg. The tracing is normal except for upright right precordial T waves.

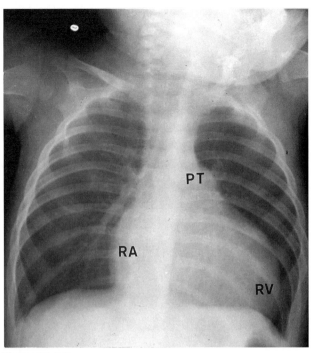

Figure 11–30

X-ray from a 10-month-old girl with mobile dome-shaped pulmonary valve stenosis and suprasystemic right ventricular pressure. Pulmonary vascularity is reduced, the pulmonary trunk (PT) is dilated, the right atrium (RA) is enlarged, and a dilated convex right ventricle (RV) occupies the apex.

the QRS axis has been reported in infants with pulmonary artery stenosis and the rubella syndrome.[47]

Severity is closely coupled to R wave amplitude in lead V_1 and R/S ratio in leads V_1 and V_6 (Figs. 11–23 through 11–27).[8,25,98] After infancy, the R wave in lead V_1 is normally less than 8 mm, and in children an R wave amplitude greater than 10 mm is exceptional.[123] With severe pulmonary stenosis, the R wave in lead V_1 is tall and monophasic, and lead V_6 exhibits a reciprocally deep S wave (see Figs. 11–23 and 11–24). Children tend to generate higher R waves in lead V_1 than adults with similar gradients.

The configuration of the QRS in lead V_1 varies (see Fig. 11–27). In mild pulmonary stenosis, an rSr′ is difficult to distinguish from normal.[16,34,35] With a greater degree of stenosis, the terminal R wave becomes taller, writing an rsR pattern (see Fig. 11–26),[34] or a small r wave appears as a notch on the upstroke of a tall R′ (see Figs. 11–26 and 11–27). The pattern in lead V_1 in severe pulmonary stenosis is either a monophasic R wave (see Figs. 11–23 and 11–24) or a qR, with the q wave reflecting right atrial enlargement (see Fig. 11–25). The neonate with pinpoint pulmonary stenosis and a small right ventricular cavity has an electrocardiogram that resembles pulmonary atresia with intact ventricular septum, namely a normal QRS axis and adult progression in precordial leads (Fig. 11–28).[73] A feature of subinfundibular pulmonary stenosis (double-chambered right ventricle) is a degree of right ventricular hypertrophy in leads V_{1-3} that is appreciably less than anticipated based on the severity of stenosis because less of the right ventricle is in the high-pressure hypertrophied proximal compartment.[88,103]

Upright right precordial T waves in normal neonates become inverted by 4 days of age. In infants and children with mild pulmonary stenosis, upright right precordial T waves may persist as the only electrocardiographic sign

(Fig. 11–29).[19] In severe pulmonary stenosis, the T wave direction shifts leftward superiorly and posteriorly as the QRS axis shifts to the right and anteriorly. The QRS-T angle

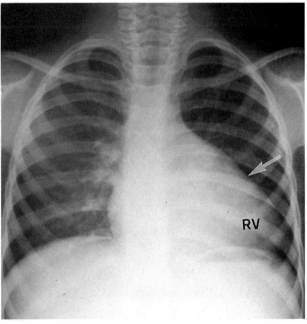

Figure 11–31

X-ray from a 5-year-old girl with severe fixed stenosis of the ostium of the infundibulum (*arrow*) distal to which the infundibulum is moderately convex. An enlarged right ventricle (RV) occupies the apex. Hypovascularity of the upper lobe of the left lung was due to unilateral stenosis of the left pulmonary artery.

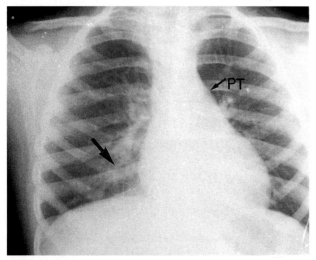

Figure 11–32
X-ray from a 5-year-old girl with pulmonary artery stenosis and a gradient of 40 mm Hg. Vascular densities (*arrow*) adjacent to the right lower cardiac border are dilated intrapulmonary arteries distal to the pulmonary artery stenoses. The pulmonary trunk (PT) is virtually normal.

widens, so inverted T waves appear in leads 2, 3, and aVF and in the right precordial leads (see Figs. 11–23 and 11–24). Deeply inverted T waves that cove upward on their descending limbs and are accompanied by ST segment depressions extending beyond lead V_2 are features of severe pulmonary stenosis (see Figs. 11–23 and 11–24).[123]

Noonan syndrome with dysplastic pulmonary valve stenosis has an electrocardiographic pattern that differs from the patterns just described. Axis deviation may be extreme,[56,63,97,104] the QRS tends to be splintered and pro-

longed, and a QS pattern appears in inferior and left precordial leads.[104]

The X-Ray

Pulmonary vascularity remains normal even in severe pulmonary stenosis until the right ventricle fails and blood flow declines (Fig. 11–30). Flow to the right lung is occasionally less than flow to the left lung (unequal distribution).[20,80] Pulmonary artery stenosis may be associated with zones of segmental hypovascularity that correspond to the locations of the arterial obstructions.[9] Multiple fusiform areas of intrapulmonary dilatation are signs of pulmonary artery stenosis (Figs. 11–32, and see Figs. 11–4 and 11–5).[9,36]

Typical mobile dome-shaped pulmonary valve stenosis is consistently accompanied by dilatation of the pulmonary trunk, which is an important radiologic feature (Figs. 11–33 and 11–34, and see Figs. 11–1, 11–3, 11–6, and 11–30).[1] Dilatation is present at an early age (see Figs. 11–1 and 11–30) and may reach aneurysmal proportions (see Fig. 11–34).[1,5,7,32] Conversely, dysplastic pulmonary valve stenosis is accompanied by comparatively little dilatation of the pulmonary trunk, discounting turbulent flow as an essential cause of dilatation. (Fig. 11–35).[5,56,106] Dilatation of the pulmonary trunk above a mobile dome-shaped pulmonary valve is attributed to intrinsic abnormalities of the media that are coupled to the specific congenital morphology of the valve, not to its functional state.[5] Disproportionate dilatation of the left branch often accompanies dilatation of the pulmonary trunk (see Fig. 11–1A, B).[41] The jet from the stenotic valve breaks up as it strikes

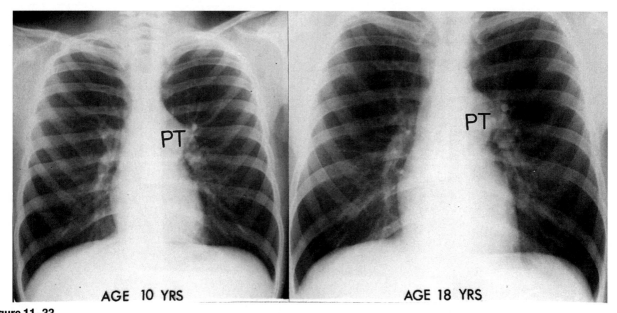

Figure 11–33
Identical cardiac silhouettes at 10 years and 18 years of age in a male patient with mobile dome-shaped pulmonary valve stenosis and a 25 mm Hg gradient at both ages. The x-rays are normal except for conspicuous dilatation of the pulmonary trunk (PT) and proximal branches.

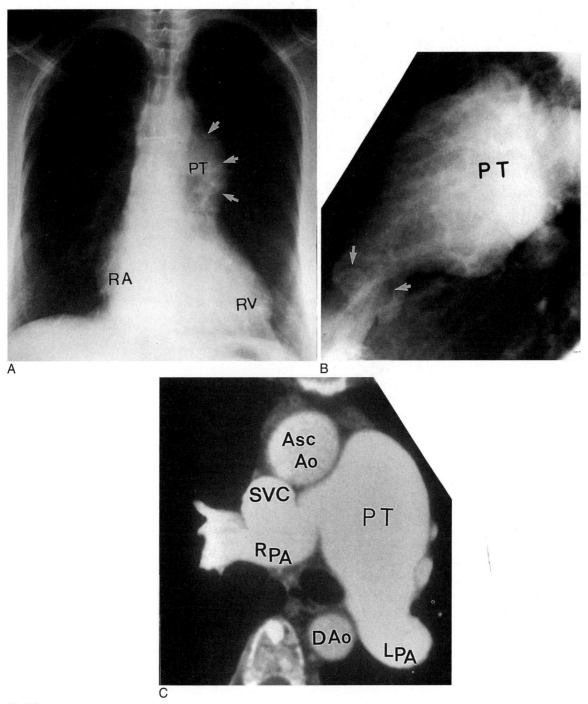

Figure 11–34

A, X-ray from a 61-year-old woman with mobile dome-shaped pulmonary valve stenosis and a gradient of 35 mm Hg. The pulmonary trunk (PT) is aneurysmal. A convex right atrial shadow (RA) occupies the lower right cardiac border, and the apex is occupied by a moderately enlarged right ventricle (RV). *B*, Lateral angiogram visualizes the aneurysmal pulmonary trunk (PT) and the mobile dome-shaped pulmonary valve (*arrows*). *C*, Computed tomographic angiogram showing the aneurysmal pulmonary trunk and the dilated right and left pulmonary artery branches (RPA, LPA).

the dome of the pulmonary trunk (see Fig. 11–37*A*), whose left branch is a smooth geometric continuation of the dilated trunk.[80] Calcification of a dome-shaped stenotic pulmonary valve is rare and is reserved for older adults,[3,38,100] although calcific deposits can be sequelae of infective endocarditis.[3]

Stenosis of the ostium of the infundibulum is characterized by slight indentation of the ostium above which there may be moderate convexity of the infundibular chamber (see Fig. 11–31). Pulmonary artery stenosis is accompanied by dilatation of intrapulmonary branches beyond the zones of stenosis (see Figs. 1–4, 11–5*B*, and 11–32).[4,9]

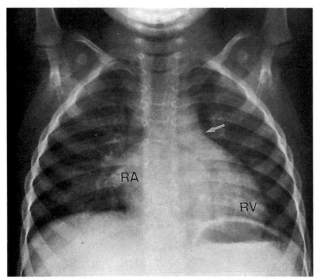

Figure 11–35

X-ray from a 3-year-old boy with dysplastic pulmonary valve stenosis (see Fig. 11–2B). The pulmonary trunk is conspicuous by its absence. A convex right atrial (RA) silhouette occupies the right lower cardiac border, and an enlarged right ventricle (RV) ccupies the apex.

A conspicuous increase in right atrial and right ventricular size is a radiologic sign of severity, especially if the enlargement appears at an early age (see Fig. 11–30). The dilated right ventricle is rounded rather than boot-shaped and its apex is above the left hemidiaphragm (see Fig. 11–30).

The aortic arch is left-sided, with rare exception (Fig. 11–36).[15,48] In Noonan syndrome, in contrast to Turner syndrome, ascending aortic dilatation is rare (see Chapter 7).[78,105]

The Echocardiogram

Color flow imaging in patients with typical mobile dome-shaped pulmonary valve stenosis discloses a high-velocity jet directed toward the left pulmonary artery (Fig. 11–37A).[84] Continuous-wave Doppler determines the velocity across the stenotic pulmonary valve from which the peak instantaneous gradient can be estimated (see Fig. 11–37B).[127,84] The mobile pulmonary valve domes briskly cephalad as a single unit during right ventricular systole. In severe pulmonary stenosis, the increased force of right atrial contraction is transmitted via the right ventricle to the undersurface of the mobile pulmonary valve, which opens in presystole, generating a Doppler signal (Fig. 11–38). Secondary hypertrophic subpulmonary stenosis is recognized as an envelope within the major continuous-wave Doppler signal (see Fig. 11–38). Mild pulmonary regurgitation is occasionally detected in the presence of pulmonary valve stenosis (see Figs. 11–37B and 11–38).

The position of the atrial septum can be established as concave to the left, reflecting a high right atrial pressure. Color flow imaging detects a right-to-left interatrial shunt via a patent foramen ovale. Right atrial size can be estimated, and the size, function, and degree of right ventricular hypertrophy can be established.[84] The ventricular septum thickens and flattens when pulmonary stenosis is severe.[84] Color flow imaging determines the presence and

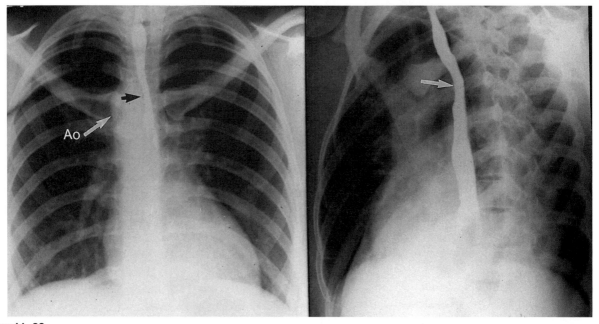

Figure 11–36

Posteroanterior and left anterior oblique x-rays from a 22-year-old woman with isolated stenosis of the ostium of the infundibulum and a gradient of 40 mm Hg. The pulmonary trunk is not border forming. A right aortic arch displaces the barium-filled esophagus to the left and then descends along the right vertebral border. The oblique projection shows the posterior displacement of the barium-filled esophagus by the right aortic arch.

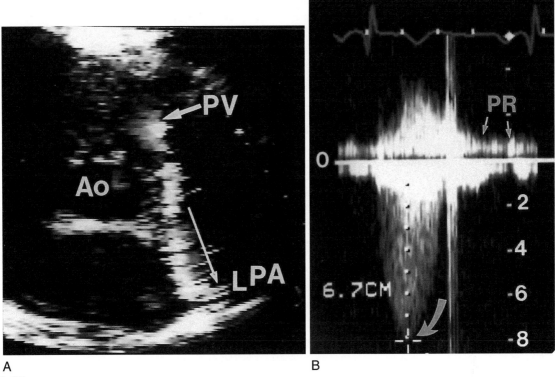

A   B

Figure 11–37
Echocardiogram with color flow imaging and Doppler interrogation from a 39-year-old woman with severe mobile dome-shaped pulmonary valve stenosis. *A,* Black and white rendition of a color flow image in the short axis shows a high-velocity jet originating at the stenotic pulmonary valve (PV) and entering the left pulmonary artery (LPA). Ao, aorta. *B,* Continuous-wave Doppler across the stenotic pulmonary valve. The velocity was 6.7 cm (*unmarked curved arrow*), reflecting a peak instantaneous gradient of 180 mm Hg. There was mild pulmonary regurgitation (PR).

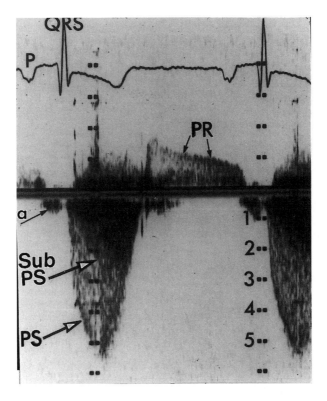

Figure 11–38
Continuous-wave Doppler from a 32-year-old man with severe mobile dome-shaped pulmonary valve stenosis (PS) and secondary hypertrophic subpulmonary stenosis (compare to Fig. 11–3). The velocity across the stenotic pulmonary valve was 5.4 cm, reflecting a peak instantaneous gradient of 117 mm Hg. The asymmetric profile within the envelope of the continuous-wave Doppler signal represents the gradient across the zone of secondary hypertrophic subpulmonary stenosis (Sub PS). Mild pulmonary regurgitation (PR) was inaudible. The small presystolic Doppler signal (a, upper left) was caused by opening of the mobile pulmonary valve as powerful right atrial contraction was transmitted to its undersurface.

degree of tricuspid regurgitation from which right ventricular systolic pressure can be estimated by the velocity of the continuous wave regurgitant jet. Systolic and diastolic function of the left ventricle should be established because right ventricular pressure overload influences the physiologic properties of the left ventricle (see earlier).[124,125]

Dysplastic pulmonary valve stenosis is identified by thickened leaflets that move little, if at all. The pulmonary trunk is not significantly dilated, in contrast to dome-shaped pulmonary valve stenosis.

Stenosis of the ostium of the infundibulum and subinfundibular stenosis (double-chambered right ventricle) can be identified and physiologically assessed. Pulmonary artery stenosis is accompanied by a normal-sized pulmonary trunk and by small proximal pulmonary arteries. Doppler interrogation records the velocities across the sites of branch stenosis and distinguishes fixed pulmonary artery stenosis from the normal neonatal physiologic drop in systolic pressure between the pulmonary trunk and its proximal branches.[101]

Summary

Mobile dome-shaped pulmonary valve stenosis is characterized by a murmur that dates from birth. The physical appearance in infancy is sometimes represented by a round bloated face and well-developed fat pads. There is a prominent jugular venous A wave, a right ventricular impulse that includes the third left intercostal space, a pulmonary ejection sound, a midsystolic systolic murmur and thrill maximum in the second left interspace with radiation upward and to the left, and a delayed soft pulmonary component of the second heart sound. The electrocardiogram shows right atrial P wave abnormalities and varying degrees of right ventricular hypertrophy. The chest x-ray discloses normal or reduced pulmonary blood flow with dilatation of the pulmonary trunk and its left branch. The echocardiogram identifies the mobile dome-shaped pulmonary valve, and continuous-wave Doppler estimates the right ventricular systolic pressure and the gradient.

Dysplastic pulmonary valve stenosis occurs in patients with Noonan syndrome that is recognized by its distinctive phenotype. A pulmonary ejection sound and a pulmonary component of the second heart sound are absent. Echocardiography identifies the thickened dysplastic cusps that exhibit little or no motion.

Stenosis of the ostium of the infundibulum is represented by a right ventricular impulse below the third left intercostal space, by absence of a pulmonary ejection sound, and by a midsystolic murmur that is maximum in the third left intercostal space. The x-ray shows a slight indentation at the ostium above which the infundibular chamber may be convex, but the pulmonary trunk is not dilated.

Subinfundibular stenosis (double-chambered right ventricle) is represented by a right ventricular impulse confined to the lower left sternal border or subxiphoid area, a midsystolic murmur below the third left intercostal space, absence of an ejection sound, a nondilated pulmonary trunk, an electrocardiogram that shows less right ventricular hypertrophy than anticipated for the estimated degree of stenosis, and an echocardiogram that images obstructing muscle bundles within the right ventricular cavity with a Doppler flow disturbance within the right ventricle.

Pulmonary artery stenosis is accompanied by a murmur that is not necessarily recognized at birth. There may be a history of maternal rubella, occasional familial recurrence, hemoptysis from rupture of thin-walled intrapulmonary aneurysms distal to the sites of stenoses, and the physical appearance of the rubella syndrome or Williams syndrome. A pulmonary ejection sound is absent, there is normal intensity and splitting of the second heart sound, and there are widespread systolic murmurs in the axillae and back. The x-ray shows no dilatation of the pulmonary trunk but instead areas of dilatation of intrapulmonary arteries.

REFERENCES

1. Abrahams DG, Wood P: Pulmonary stenosis with normal aortic root. Br Heart J 13:519, 1951.
2. Agustsson MH, Arcilla RA, Gasul BM, et al: The diagnosis of bilateral stenosis of the primary pulmonary artery branches based on characteristic pulmonary trunk pressure curves. Circulation 26:421, 1962.
3. Alday LE, Morey RAE: Calcific pulmonary stenosis. Br Heart J 35:887, 1973.
4. Arvidsson H, Carlsson E, Hartmann A, et al: Supravalvular stenosis of the pulmonary arteries. Acta Radiol 56:466, 1961.
5. Niwa K, Perloff JK, Bhuta S, et al: Structural abnormalities of great arterial walls in congenital heart disease: Light and electron microscopic observations. Circulation 103:393, 2001.
6. Baird PA, De Jong BP: Noonan's syndrome (XX and XY Turner phenotype) in three generations of a family. J Pediatr 80:110, 1972.
7. Shindo T, Kuroda T, Watanabe S, et al: Aneurysmal dilatation of the pulmonary trunk with mild pulmonic stenosis. Int Med 34:199, 1995.
8. Bassingthwaighte JB, Parkin TW, DuShane JW, et al: The electrocardiographic and hemodynamic findings in pulmonary stenosis with intact ventricular septum. Circulation 28:893, 1963.
9. Baum D, Khoury GH, Ongley PA, et al: Congenital stenosis of the pulmonary artery branches. Circulation 29:680, 1964.
10. Beck W, Schrire V, Vogelpoel L, et al: Hemodynamic effects of amyl nitrite and phenylephrine on the normal human circulation and their relation to changes in cardiac murmurs. Am J Cardiol 8:341, 1961.
11. Beuren AJ, Schulze C, Eberle P, et al: The syndrome of supravalvular aortic stenosis, peripheral pulmonary stenosis, mental retardation and similar facial appearance. Am J Cardiol 13:471, 1964.
12. Waller BF, Howard J, Fess S: Pathology of pulmonic stenosis and pure regurgitation. Clin Cardiol 18:45, 1995.
13. Blount SG Jr, Vigoda PS, Swan H: Isolated infundibular stenosis. Am Heart J 57:684, 1959.
14. Berrocal T, Gamo E, Navalon J, et al: Syndrome of Alagille: Radiological and sonographic findings: A review of 37 cases. Eur Radiol 7:115, 1997.
15. Bressie JL: Pulmonary valvular stenosis with intact ventricular septum and right aortic arch. Br Heart J 26:155, 1964.
16. Camerini F, Davis LG: Secondary R waves in right chest leads. Br Heart J 17:28, 1955.
17. Campbell M: Factors in the aetiology of pulmonary stenosis. Br Heart J 24:625, 1962.
18. Krantz ID, Piccoli DA, Spinner NB: Alagille syndrome. J Med Genet 34:152, 1997.
19. Celermajer MB, Izukawa T, Varghese PJ, Rowe RD: Upright T wave in V1: A useful diagnostic sign of mild pulmonic valve stenosis in children. J Pediatr 74:413, 1969.
20. Chen JTT, Robinson AE, Goodrich JK, Lester RG: Uneven distribution of pulmonary blood flow between left and right lungs in isolated valvular pulmonary stenosis. Am J Radiol 107:343, 1969.

21. Sharani J, Zafari AM, Roberts WC: Sudden death, right ventricular infarction, and abnormal right ventricular intramural coronary arteries in isolated congenital valvular pulmonic stenosis. Am J Cardiol 72:368, 1993.

22. Cochi SL, Edmonds LE, Dyer K, et al: Congenital rubella syndrome in the United States, 1970–1985. On the verge of elimination. Am J Epidemiol 129:349, 1989.

23. Coelho E, DePaiva E, Nunes A: Malformations of the pulmonary artery and its branches, including two cases of absence of the right pulmonary artery. Am J Cardiol 13:462, 1964.

24. Collins E, Turner G: The Noonan syndrome: A review of the clinical and genetic features of 27 cases. J Pediatr 83:941, 1973.

25. Danilowicz D, Hoffman JIE, Rudolph AM: Serial studies of pulmonary stenosis in infancy and childhood. Br Heart J 37:808, 1975.

26. Danilowicz DA, Rudolph AM, Hoffman JIE, Heymann M: Physiologic pressure differences between main and branch pulmonary arteries in infants. Circulation 45:410, 1972.

27. Cullimore AJ, Smedstad KG, Brennan BG: Pregnancy in women with Noonan syndrome. Obstet Gynecol 93:813, 1999.

28. Burch M, Sharland M, Shinbourne E, et al: Cardiologic abnormalities in Noonan syndrome: phenotypic diagnosis and echocardiographic assessment of 118 patients. J Am Coll Cardiol 22:1189, 1993.

29. Deverall PB, Roberts NK, Stark J: Arrhythmias in children with pulmonary stenosis. Br Heart J 32:472, 1970.

30. Greech V: History, diagnosis, surgery and epidemiology of pulmonary stenosis in Malta. Cardiol Young 8:337, 1998.

31. Yoo SJ, Kim YM, Bae EJ, et al: Rare variants of divided right ventricle with sequestered apical trabecular component. Int J Cardiol 60:249, 1997.

32. Tami LF, McEldry MW: Pulmonary aneurysm due to severe congenital pulmonic stenosis. Angiology 45:383, 1994.

33. Eldridge F, Selzer A, Hultgren H: Stenosis of a branch of the pulmonary artery: An additional cause of continuous murmurs over the chest. Circulation 15:865, 1957.

34. Ellison RC, Miettinen OS: Interpretation of RSR prime in pulmonic stenosis. Am Heart J 88:7, 1974.

35. Fowler RS: Terminal QRS conduction delay in pulmonary stenosis in children. Am J Cardiol 21:669, 1968.

36. Franch RH, Gay BB Jr: Congenital stenosis of the pulmonary artery branches. Am J Med 35:512, 1963.

37. Freij BJ, South MA, Sever JL: Maternal rubella and the congenital rubella syndrome. Clin Perinatol 15:247, 1988.

38. Gabriele OF, Scatliff JH: Pulmonary valve calcification. Am Heart J 80:299, 1970.

39. Gale GE, Heimann KW, Barlow JB: Double-chambered right ventricle. Br Heart J 31:291, 1968.

40. Gamboa R, Hugenholtz PG, Nadas AS: Accuracy of the phonocardiogram in assessing severity of aortic and pulmonic stenosis. Circulation 30:35, 1964.

41. Gay BB Jr, Franch RH: Pulsations in the pulmonary arteries as observed with roentgenoscopic image amplification. Am J Roentgenol 83:335, 1960.

42. Genovese PD, Rosenbaum D: Pulmonary stenosis with survival to the age of 78 years. Am Heart J 41:755, 1951.

43. Geraci JE, Burchell HB, Edwards JE: Cardiac Clinics. CXL. Congenital pulmonary stenosis with intact ventricular septum in persons more than 50 years of age: Report of two cases. Proc Staff Meet Mayo Clin 28:346, 1953.

44. Gluck MC, Moser KM: Pulmonary artery agenesis. Circulation 41:859, 1970.

45. Gregg NM: Congenital cataract following German measles in the mother. Trans Opthalmol Soc Aust 3:35, 1941.

46. Gross DR, Lu P, Dodd KT, Hwang NHC: Physical characteristics of pulmonary artery stenosis murmurs in calves. Am J Physiol 238:H876, 1980.

47. Halloran KH, Sanyal SK, Gardner TH: Superiorly oriented electrocardiographic axis in infants with the rubella syndrome. Am Heart J 72:600, 1966.

48. Hastreiter AR, D'Cruz IA, Cantez T: Right-sided aorta. Br Heart J 28:722, 1966.

49. Hayes CJ, Gersony WM, Driscoll DJ, et al: Second natural history study of congenital heart defects. Results of treatment of patients with pulmonary valvar stenosis. Circulation 87(Suppl I):128, 1993.

50. Holt JH Jr, Eddleman EE Jr: The precordial movements in adults with pulmonic stenosis. Circulation 35:492, 1967.

51. Hultgren HN, Reeve R, Cohn K, McLeod R: The ejection click of valvular pulmonic stenosis. Circulation 40:631, 1969.

52. Johansson BW, Mandahl N: Ullrich-Noonan syndrome. Acta Med Scand 207:505, 1980.

53. Johnson LW, Grossman W, Dalen J, Dexter L: Pulmonic stenosis in the adult-long term follow-up study. N Engl J Med 23:287, 1972.

54. Keith A: Malformations of the heart. Lancet 2:359, 1909.

55. Klinge T, Laursen HB: Familial pulmonary stenosis with underdeveloped or normal right ventricle. Br Heart J 37:60, 1975.

56. Koretzky ED, Moller JH, Korns ME, et al: Congenital pulmonary stenosis resulting from dysplasia of the valve. Circulation 40:43, 1969.

57. Lasser RP, Genkins G: Chest pain in patients with isolated pulmonic stenosis. Circulation 15:258, 1957.

58. Leatham A, Vogelpoel L: The early systolic sound in dilatation of the pulmonary artery. Br Heart J 16:21, 1954.

59. Leatham A, Weitzman D: Auscultatory and phonocardiographic signs of pulmonary stenosis. Br Heart J 19:303, 1957.

60. Lees MH, Dotter CT: Bronchial circulation in severe multiple peripheral pulmonary artery stenosis. Circulation 31:759, 1965.

61. Levin DL, Heymann MA, Rudolph AM: Morphological development of the pulmonary vascular bed in experimental pulmonic stenosis. Circulation 59:179, 1979.

62. Levin SE, Zarvos P, Miller S, Schmaman A: Arteriohepatic dysplasia: Association of liver disease with pulmonary arterial stenosis as well as facial and skeletal abnormalities. Pediatrics 66:876, 1980.

63. Linde LM, Turner SW, Sparkes RS: Pulmonary valvular dysplasia: A cardiofacial syndrome. Br Heart J 35:301, 1973.

64. Lowance MI, Jones EC, Matthews WB, Dunstan EM: Congenital pulmonary stenosis. Am Heart J 35:820, 1948.

65. Lucas RV Jr, Varco RL, Lillehei CW, et al: Anomalous muscle bundles of the right ventricle: Hemodynamic consequences and surgical considerations. Circulation 25:443, 1962.

66. Lueker RD, Vogel JHK, Blount SC: Regression of valvular pulmonary stenosis. Br Heart J 32:779, 1970.

67. Macruz R, Perloff JK, Case RB: A method for the electrocardiographic recognition of atrial enlargement. Circulation 17:882, 1958.

68. Mannheimer E, Jonsson B: Heart sounds and murmurs in congenital pulmonary stenosis with normal aortic root. Acta Paediatr 100(Suppl):167, 1954.

69. McCarron WE, Perloff JK: Familial congenital valvular pulmonic stenosis. Am Heart J 88:357, 1974.

70. Mehlman DJ, Troncoso P, Hay R, Glagov S: Midsystolic click accompanying isolated bicuspid pulmonic valve. Am Heart J 103:145, 1982.

71. Mendez HMM, Opitz JM: Noonan syndrome: A review. Am J Med Genet 21:493, 1985.

72. Miller E, Cradock-Watson JE, Pollock TM: Consequences of confirmed maternal rubella at successive stages of pregnancy. Lancet 2:781, 1982.

73. Miller GAH, Restifo M, Shinebourne EA, et al: Pulmonary atresia with intact ventricular septum and critical pulmonary stenosis. Br Heart J 35:9, 1973.

74. Mody MR: The natural history of uncomplicated valvular pulmonic stenosis. Am Heart J 90:317, 1975.

75. Moller JH, Adams P Jr: Natural history of pulmonary valvular stenosis. Serial cardiac catheterization in 21 children. Am J Cardiol 16:654, 1965.

76. Moller JH, Rao S, Lucas RV: Exercise hemodynamics of pulmonary valvular stenosis: Study of 64 children. Circulation 46:1018, 1972.

77. Morgagni JB: The Seats and Causes of Diseases Investigated by Anatomy. Padua, 1761. Translated from the Latin by Benjamin Alexander. London, Millar, Cadell, Johnson and Payne.

78. Morgan JM, Coupe MO, Honey M, Miller GAH: Aneurysms of the sinuses of Valsalva in Noonan's syndrome. Eur Heart J 10:190, 1989.

79. Munro ND, Smithells RW, Sheppard S, et al: Temporal relations between maternal rubella and congenital defects. Lancet 2:201, 1987.

80. Muster AJ, van Grondelle A, Paul MH: Unequal pressures in the central pulmonary arterial branches in patients with pulmonary stenosis. Pediatr Cardiol 2:7, 1982.

81. Myers JD, Murdaugh HV, McIntosh HD, Blaisdell RK: Observations on continuous murmurs over partially obstructed arteries. Arch Intern Med 97:726, 1956.

82. Nagle RE, Tamara FA: Left parasternal impulse in pulmonary stenosis and atrial septal defect. Br Heart J 29:735, 1967.

83. Nakazawa M, Marks RA, Isabel-Jones J, Jarmakani JM: Right and left ventricular volume characteristics in children with pulmonary stenosis and intact ventricular septum. Circulation 53:884, 1976.

84. Nishimura RA, Pieroni DR, Bierman FZ, et al: Second natural history study of congenital heart defects. Pulmonary stenosis: Echocardiography. Circulation 87(Suppl I):I-73, 1993.

85. Noonan JA: Hypertelorism with Turner's phenotype: A new syndrome with associated congenital heart disease. Am J Dis Child 116:373, 1968.

86. Noonan JA, Ehmke DA: Associated noncardiac malformations in children with congenital heart disease. J Pediatr 63:468, 1963.

87. Oppenheimer EH: Partial atresia of main branches of pulmonary artery occurring in infancy and accompanied by calcification of pulmonary artery and aorta. Bull Johns Hopkins Hosp 63:261, 1938.

88. Patel R, Astley R: Right ventricular obstruction due to anomalous muscle bands. Br Heart J 35:890, 1973.

89. Patterson DF, Haskins ME, Schnarr WR: Hereditary dysplasia of the pulmonary valve in beagle dogs. Am J Cardiol 47:631, 1981.

90. Peacock TB: On Malformations of the Human Heart. London, J. Churchill and Sons, 1858.

91. Pearl W: Cardiovascular anomalies in Noonan's syndrome. Chest 71:677, 1977.

92. Perloff JK: Auscultatory and phonocardiographic manifestations of pulmonary hypertension. Progr Cardiovasc Dis 9:303, 1967.

93. Perloff JK: The increase and regression of ventricular mass. In Perloff JK, Child JS (eds): Congenital Heart Disease in Adults. Philadelphia, W.B. Saunders, 1991.

94. Perloff JK: Physical Examination of the Heart and Circulation, 3rd ed. Philadelphia, W.B. Saunders, 2000.

95. Perloff JK, LeBauer EJ: Auscultatory and phonocardiographic manifestations of isolated stenosis of the pulmonary artery and its branches. Br Heart J 31:314, 1969.

96. Perloff JK, Ronan JA Jr, DeLeon AC: Ventricular septal defect with "two-chambered right ventricle." Am J Cardiol 16:894, 1965.

97. Rasmussen K, Sorland SJ: Electrocardiogram and vectorcardiogram in Turner phenotype with normal chromosomes and pulmonary stenosis. Br Heart J 35:937, 1973.

98. Rasmussen K, Sorland SJ: Prediction of right ventricular systolic pressure in pulmonary stenosis from combined vectorcardiographic data. Am Heart J 86:318, 1973.

99. Riggs TW, Weinhouse E: Respiratory influence on Doppler estimation of valvar gradients in congenital pulmonic stenosis. Am J Cardiol 70:956, 1992.

100. Roberts WC, Mason DT, Morrow AG, Braunwald E: Calcific pulmonic stenosis. Circulation 37:973, 1968.

101. Rodriguez RJ, Riggs TW: Physiologic peripheral pulmonic stenosis in infancy. Am J Cardiol 66:1478, 1990.

102. Rowe RD: Maternal rubella and pulmonary artery stenosis. Pediatrics 32:180, 1963.

103. Rowland TW, Rosenthal A, Castaneda AR: Double chamber right ventricle. Am Heart J 89:455, 1975.

104. Sanchez-Cascos A: The Noonan syndrome. Eur Heart J 4:223, 1983.

105. Schachter N, Perloff JK, Mulder DG: Aortic dissection in Noonan's syndrome (46XY Turner). Am J Cardiol 54:464, 1984.

106. Schneeweiss A, Blieden LC, Shem-Tov A, et al: Diagnostic angiocardiographic criteria in dysplastic stenotic pulmonic valve. Am Heart J 106:761, 1983.

107. Schrire V, Vogelpoel L: The role of the dilated pulmonary artery in abnormal splitting of the second heart sound. Am Heart J 63:501, 1962.

108. Shaver JA, Nadolny RA, O'Toole JD, et al: Sound pressure correlates of the second heart sound. Circulation 49:316, 1974.

109. Singh SP: Unusual splitting of the second heart sound in pulmonary stenosis. Am J Cardiol 25:28, 1970.

110. Smith WG: Pulmonary hypertension and a continuous murmur due to multiple peripheral stenoses of the pulmonary arteries. Thorax 13:194, 1958.

111. Stone FM, Bessinger FB, Lucas RV, Moller JH: Pre- and postoperative rest and exercise hemodynamics in children with pulmonary stenosis. Circulation 49:1102, 1974.

112. Tang JS, Kauffman SL, Lynfield J: Hypoplasia of the pulmonary arteries in infants with congenital rubella. Am J Cardiol 27:491, 1971.

113. Truccone NJ, Steeg CN, Dell R, Gersony WM: Comparison of the cardiocirculatory effects of exercise and isoproterenol in children with pulmonary or aortic valve stenosis. Circulation 56:79, 1977.

114. Vermillion MB, Leight L, Davis LA: Pulmonary artery stenosis. Circulation 17:55, 1958.

115. Vogelpoel L, Schrire V: Auscultatory and phonocardiographic assessment of pulmonary stenosis with intact ventricular septum. Circulation 22:55, 1960.

116. Von Doenhoff LJ, Nanda NC: Obstruction within the right ventricular body: Two-dimensional echocardiographic features. Am J Cardiol 51:1498, 1983.

117. Wasserman MP, Varghese PJ, Rowe RD: The evolution of pulmonary arterial stenosis associated with congenital rubella. Am Heart J 76:638, 1968.

118. White PD, Hurst JW, Fennell RH: Survival to the age of 75 years with congenital pulmonary stenosis and patent foramen ovale. Circulation 2:558, 1950.

119. Wild JB, Eckstein JW, Van Epps EF, Culbertson JW: Three patients with congenital pulmonic valvular stenosis surviving for more than 57 years. Am Heart J 53:393, 1957.

120. Wolfish NM, Shanon A: Nephropathy in arteriohepatic dysplasia (Alagille's syndrome). Child Nephrol Urol 9:169, 1988.

121. Wong C, Cheng C, Lau C, Leung W: Congenital coronary artery anomalies in Noonan's syndrome. Am Heart J 119:396, 1990.

122. Wood P: Diseases of the Heart and Circulation, 2nd ed. Philadelphia, JB Lippincott, 1956.

123. Ziegler RF: Electrocardiographic Studies in Normal Infants and Children. Springfield, Ill, Charles C Thomas, 1951.

124. Kelly DT, Spotnitz HM, Beiser GD, et al: Effects of chronic right ventricular volume and pressure loading on left ventricular performance. Circulation 44:403, 1971.

125. Stenberg RG, Fixler DE, Taylor AL, et al: Left ventricular dysfunction due to chronic right ventricular pressure overload. Am J Med 84:157, 1988.

126. Falkenbach KH, Zheutlin N, Dowdy AH, O'Louglin BJ: Pulmonary hypertension due to pulmonary arterial coarctation. Radiology 73:575, 1959.

127. Childs JS: Transthoracic and transesophageal echocardiographic imaging. In Perloff JC, Child JS (eds): Congenital Heart Disease in Adults. Philadelphia, WB Saunders, 1998, p 91.

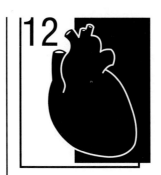

Congenital Pulmonary Valve Regurgitation

In *The Principles and Practice of Medicine* (1892), William Osler described pulmonary insufficiency[45]: "This rare affection is occasionally due to a congenital malformation, particularly fusion of the two segments. . . . The condition is extremely rare and of little practical significance." In 1910, the distinctive diastolic murmur of low-pressure pulmonary regurgitation was characterized,[26] and in 1936, isolated congenital pulmonary regurgitation was reported with a review of the literature.[33] Maude Abbott's necropsy study of 1000 cases of congenital heart disease included two examples of isolated congenital pulmonary valve regurgitation,[1] and in 1955, the first clinical diagnosis was made in an asymptomatic 24-year-old medical student.[32] The morphology of the congenitally malformed valve is variable.[14,16,25,33,34,57,62] One, two, or three cusps may undergo faulty development,[7,29,57,58] all three cusps may be rudimentary,[7,29] one cusp may be absent and the other two rudimentary,[62] or there may be no valve tissue at all—congenital absence of the pulmonary valve[4,49,50,58]—which was reported by Chevers in 1846.[10] The anomaly rarely occurs in isolation[2,29,35,37,50,57,60] but instead coexists with Fallot's tetralogy (see Chapter 18) and only sporadically with other malformations.[5,11,61,62]

A bicuspid pulmonary valve is rare as an isolated anomaly and is occasionally incompetent.[18,23,34] A quadricuspid pulmonary valve can occur as an isolated congenital malformation[6] or with truncus arteriosus (see Chapter 28). If the four cusps are equal, the valve functions normally, but if there is cuspal inequality or if there is a supernumerary cusp, the valve is rendered incompetent, especially if pulmonary artery pressure is elevated.[6,28] This chapter is concerned with pulmonary valve regurgitation as an isolated congenital malformation. Regurgitation associated with pulmonary hypertension and a normal pulmonary valve is dealt with in Chapter 14 on primary pulmonary hypertension.

The diagnosis of congenital pulmonary valve regurgitation takes into account the relatively high incidence of normal or physiologic pulmonary regurgitation identified by color flow echocardiography and Doppler interrogation in individuals with normal hearts.[9,12,40,57] The prevalence of trivial, mild, or moderate pulmonary regurgitation based on color flow imaging and Doppler echocardiography in normal hearts from birth to age 14 years disclosed an age-related incidence—nil under 1 year of age, with a peak incidence of 42% between 6 and 11 years of age.[9] The mature right ventricle is a low-pressure, low-resistance pump that readily adapts to augmented volume,[25,36,50] although the degree and duration of regurgitant flow are important determinants of this response.[36] The physiologic consequences of pulmonary regurgitation are especially dramatic in utero because systemic pressure in the pulmonary trunk augments regurgitant flow, even more so if there is agenesis of the fetal ductus.[7,57] Acquired elevation of pulmonary artery pressure in adults with bronchopulmonary disease or left ventricular failure is analogous but less dramatic.[18,22]

The History

Isolated congenital pulmonary valve regurgitation is suspected because of a murmur or because of a dilated pulmonary arterial trunk on a chest x-ray. Sex distribution is about equal.[3,19,51] Diagnosis is usually delayed because a murmur present at birth goes undetected until years later,[7] and routine chest x-rays are seldom done before adulthood.

Clinical manifestations of isolated congenital pulmonary valve regurgitation fall into three categories. The first and largest category consists of asymptomatic children, adolescents, and young adults[3,14,37,51] who tolerate the anomaly through middle age[13,31] and occasionally into the sixth[24,59] or even eighth decade.[35,37] Exceptional examples of isolated congenital absence of the pulmonary valve have been reported at age 69 years[58] and 73 years.[49]

The second and much smaller category consists of adults in whom heart failure occurs after decades of stability.[3,18,22] Severe pulmonary valve regurgitation per se can cause right ventricular failure,[20,25] but moderate regurgitation produces little or no ill effect unless the degree of regurgitant flow is significantly increased by adult-acquired elevation in pulmonary artery pressure due to bronchopulmonary disease[25,58] or left ventricular failure.[18,22] Infective endocarditis is a low-probability cause of increased regurgitation.[23,27,38,41]

A third and rare category of congenital pulmonary valve regurgitation becomes manifest in the fetus[56] or neonate[3,7,29] when elevated pulmonary arterial pressure augments the volume of regurgitation across a congenitally malformed or absent pulmonary valve.[3,56] In utero patency of the ductus is desirable because ductal agenesis increases resistance to right ventricular discharge and increases regurgitant flow.[2,21] The converse is the case with ductal patency after birth, which adds to the burden of the right ventricle by allowing diastolic flow to proceed from the aorta through the ductus into the pulmonary artery and across the incompetent pulmonary valve into the right ventricle.[3,21,37,59]

Physical Appearance, the Arterial Pulse, and the Jugular Venous Pulse

Physical appearance and the arterial pulse are normal. The A wave, V wave, and mean jugular venous pressure rise with the advent of right ventricular failure.

Precordial Movement and Palpation

The right ventricular impulse is gentle when pulmonary regurgitation is mild or moderate and may be detected only in the subxiphoid area during held inspiration. Severe regurgitation that accompanies congenital absence of the pulmonary valve generates a hyperdynamic impulse at the left sternal border and subxiphoid area in addition to an impulse in the second left intercostal space caused by systolic expansion of a dilated pulmonary trunk (see Fig. 12–7).[3,24,51,56]

Auscultation

The first heart sound is normal and is occasionally followed by an ejection sound into the dilated pulmonary

trunk. The pulmonary component of the second heart sound is absent when the leaflets are rudimentary or absent.[3,52] The pulmonary component is soft when cusps are present but defective, although audibility per se confirms the presence of valve tissue.[30] The split may be wide because of a delay in the pulmonary component caused by increased capacitance of the pulmonary vascular bed and slow elastic recoil.[30,53–55] The occasional occurrence of complete right bundle branch block may delay the pulmonary component of the second sound (Fig. 12–1). The degree of splitting increases with inspiration unless the right ventricle has failed.[30] Narrow splitting sometimes occurs because rapid right ventricular ejection coupled with brisk decline in the descending limb of the pulmonary artery pressure pulse cancels a potential delay in pulmonary valve closure.

The hallmark of congenital pulmonary valve regurgitation is the distinctive diastolic murmur of low-pressure, low-velocity regurgitant flow.[8] The murmur is maximum in the second or third left intercostal space, medium- to low-pitched, crescendo-decrescendo, delayed in onset, and short in duration, ending well before the subsequent first heart sound (Figs. 12–1 and 12–2).[3,13,15,25,27,39,48] The murmur begins immediately after the right ventricular and pulmonary arterial pressure pulses diverge in early diastole and is loudest when the diastolic gradient is maximum, which is at the time of an early diastolic dip (Fig. 12–3A).[25] When the pulmonary component of the second heart sound is soft or absent, there is a silent interval between the aortic component and the onset of the diastolic murmur (see Fig. 12–2).[46] Equilibration of pulmonary artery and right ventricular pressures in latter diastole reduces or eliminates the regurgitant gradient and abolishes the murmur (Figs. 12–4 and 12–5, and see Fig. 12–3A).[46] The normally low diastolic pressure in the pulmonary trunk

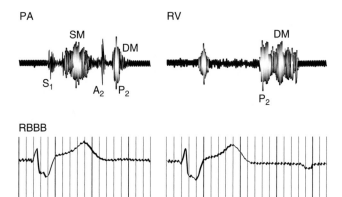

Figure 12–1

Intracardiac phonocardiograms from a 17-year-old boy with congenital pulmonary valve regurgitation. A prominent midsystolic murmur (SM) was recorded in the main pulmonary artery (PA), and a short diastolic murmur (DM) issued from the delayed pulmonary component of the second sound (P₂). The second sound is widely split due to complete right bundle branch block (RBBB). The diastolic murmur was most prominent in the right ventricle (RV) just beneath the pulmonary valve. A₂, aortic component of the second sound; S₁, first heart sound.

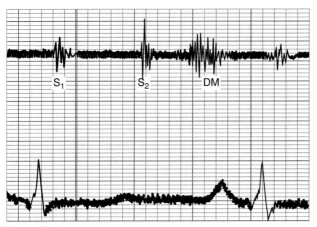

Figure 12–2
Phonocardiogram at the third left intercostal space of a 36-year-old woman with congenital pulmonary valve regurgitation. A short, medium-frequency mid-diastolic murmur (DM) begins well after the aortic component of the second sound (S_2) and ends well before the subsequent first sound (S_1).

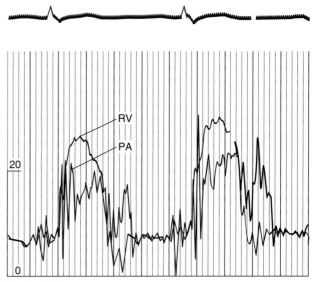

Figure 12–4
Right ventricular (RV) and pulmonary artery (PA) pressure pulses from an 18-year-old man with severe congenital pulmonary valve regurgitation. A small regurgitant gradient appears immediately after the pressure pulses diverge. The gradient is rapidly abolished as the pressure pulses equilibrate (compare to Fig. 12–3A).

is responsible for a low rate of regurgitant flow and a correspondingly low- to medium-pitched murmur.[46] With pulmonary hypertensive pulmonary regurgitation, maximal instantaneous flow velocity is maintained at about the same strength throughout diastole, which is appropriate for the high-frequency holodiastolic Graham Steell

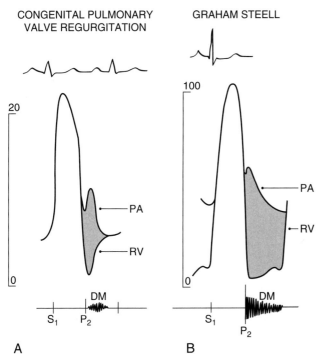

Figure 12–3
Line drawings from actual pressure pulses and phonocardiograms in cases of congenital pulmonary valve regurgitation (*A*) and hypertensive pulmonary regurgitation (*B*). *A*, Low pulmonary artery diastolic pressure is exerted against the incompetent pulmonary valve. The diastolic murmur (DM) begins shortly after the right ventricular (RV) and pulmonary artery (PA) pressure pulses diverge and is loudest when the diastolic gradient (*shaded area*) is maximal at the early diastolic dip in right ventricular pulse. Equilibration of pulmonary artery and right ventricular pressures later in diastole abolishes the regurgitant gradient and eliminates the murmur. *B*, High pulmonary artery diastolic pressure is exerted against the incompetent pulmonary valve. The large regurgitant gradient (*shaded area*) diminishes but persists throughout diastole because the PA and RV diastolic pressure pulses do not equilibrate. The accompanying murmur begins in early diastole and is holodiastolic, decrescendo, and high frequency (Graham Steell).

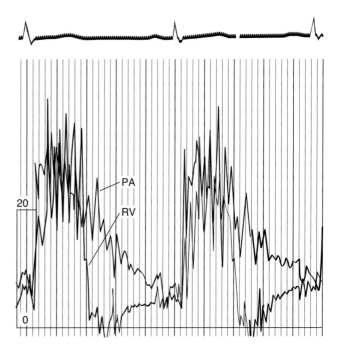

Figure 12–5
Pulmonary artery (PA) and right ventricular (RV) pressure pulses from a 23-year-old man with congenital pulmonary valve regurgitation. The diastolic pressures in the PA and RV do not equilibrate until the end of diastole because the regurgitation was mild.

murmur (see Fig. 12–3*B*).[42,47,48] With low-pressure pulmonary regurgitation, peak velocity is in early diastole with a gradual decline toward end-diastole,[42] which is appropriate for the low- to medium-frequency diastolic murmur that ends well before the subsequent first heart sound (see Fig. 12–3*A*). When mild congenital pulmonary regurgitation permits the low diastolic pressure in the pulmonary trunk to remain higher than the diastolic pressure in the right ventricle, the murmur extends throughout diastole but remains of low to medium frequency (see Fig. 12–5).[46]

The intensity of the diastolic murmur varies from grade 1 to 3/6 but exceptionally is sufficiently loud and rough to generate a thrill.[13,23–25,51] During inspiration, the early diastolic dip in the right ventricular pressure pulse falls more rapidly than the corresponding diastolic pressure in the pulmonary trunk, so the regurgitant gradient transiently increases and the loudness of the murmur increases correspondingly.[15,27,56,57]

Midsystolic murmurs with congenital pulmonary valve regurgitation are due to rapid ejection of an increased right ventricular stroke volume into a dilated pulmonary trunk (Fig. 12–1).[3,23,56] The systolic murmur is short and crescendo-decrescendo, ending well before both components of the second heart sound (see Fig. 12–1). Rarely, a low-frequency presystolic murmur assigned to vibrations of the tricuspid valve is believed to represent a right-sided Austin Flint murmur.[3,48]

The Electrocardiogram

The electrocardiogram is normal when congenital pulmonary regurgitation is mild to moderate.[13,23,24,50] Atrial fibrillation is exceptional even with congenital absence of the pulmonary valve.[59] The most common change in the QRS pattern reflects volume overload of the right ventricle and is represented by terminal r waves in leads V_1 and aVR and S waves in leads 1 and V_{5-6} (Fig. 12–6).[3,55] The rSr′ in lead V_1 is analogous to the rSr′ with right ventricular volume overload of an atrial septal defect (see Chapter 15). Right bundle branch block is uncommon (see Fig. 12–1).[14]

The X-Ray

Dilatation of the pulmonary trunk is the most consistent feature of the x-ray (Figs. 12–7 and 12–8).[13,17,23,24,56] The degree of dilatation varies considerably, sometimes reaching aneurysmal proportions[4,56] (see Fig. 12–7) and has been ascribed to coexisting medial abnormalities.[44] Right ventricular enlargement corresponds to the degree of volume overload. Vigorous pulsations of the pulmonary trunk and its proximal branches are seen flouroscopically[3,13,23,24] or with real time echocardiography (see next section).

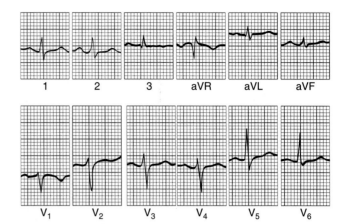

Figure 12–6

Electrocardiogram from a 34-year-old woman with mild to moderate congenital pulmonary valve regurgitation. The terminal forces of the QRS point to the right and superior, writing a terminal r in lead aVR and small s waves in leads 1, 2, aVL, aVF, and V_6.

Occasionally, a chest x-ray fortuitously records striking intermittent changes in pulmonary arterial size (see Fig. 12–7).[24]

The Echocardiogram

Echocardiography with color flow imaging and Doppler interrogation establishes the diagnosis of congenital pulmonary valve regurgitation. The trivial to mild pulmonary regurgitation that frequently occurs in normal subjects is not accompanied by the diastolic murmur of low-pressure pulmonary regurgitation.[9,12] Color flow imaging with Doppler interrogation characterizes the depth, width, duration, and peak velocity of the diastolic jet (Fig. 12–9), which differs from pulmonary hypertensive pulmonary regurgitation (Fig. 12–10). Echocardiography defines the size of the pulmonary trunk and its proximal branches and the vigor of pulsations in response to rapid ejection of the regurgitant volume.[24] The physiologic consequences of congenital pulmonary valve regurgitation are reflected in the size and contractility of the right ventricle and in paradoxical motion of the ventricular septum.

Summary

Congenital pulmonary valve regurgitation comes to light in healthy asymptomatic individuals in whom diastolic/systolic murmurs are discovered or who exhibit dilatation of the pulmonary trunk in a routine chest x-ray. An exception is the neonate with severe isolated congenital pulmonary valve regurgitation or complete absence of the pulmonary valve. Precordial palpation detects a right ventricular impulse that corresponds to the degree of regurgitation. Systolic expansion of the pulmonary trunk imparts an

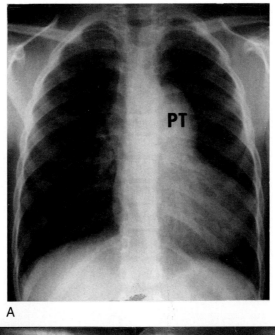

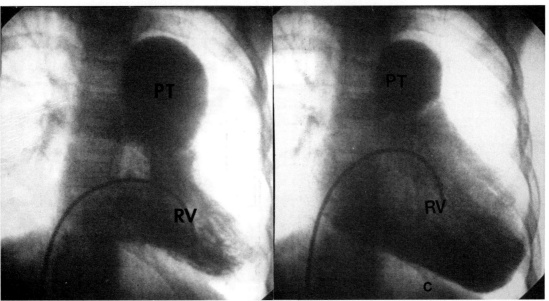

Figure 12–7
X-ray (*A*) and right ventriculogram (RV) (*B*) from a 7-year-old boy with severe congenital pulmonary valve regurgitation. Fluoroscopy and real time echocardiography disclosed striking systolic expansion of the dilated pulmonary trunk (PT). (*Left, systole; right, diastole.*)

impulse in the second left intercostal space. Auscultation reveals a distinctive diastolic murmur that is maximum in the second or third left interspace, is low to medium frequency, crescendo-decrescendo, delayed in onset, short in duration, and occasionally louder during inspiration. A pulmonary midsystolic flow murmur is usually present. The second heart sound is normal or widely split, the pulmonary component is soft or inaudible, and the split may be persist-

ent but not fixed. The electrocardiogram is either normal or exhibits signs of volume overload of the right ventricle with an rSr′ in lead V_1. The x-ray shows dilatation of the pulmonary trunk that is occasionally aneurysmal and dilatation of the right ventricle. Echocardiography with color flow imaging and Doppler interrogation establishes the presence and degree of pulmonary regurgitation and the physiologic consequences of the regurgitant flow.

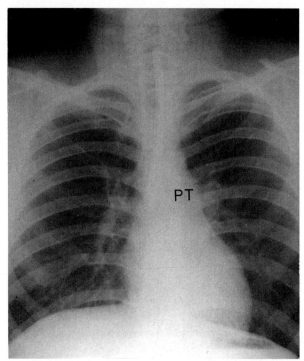

Figure 12–8

X-ray from a 10-year-old boy with moderate congenital pulmonary valve regurgitation. The pulmonary trunk (PT) is moderately dilated. The x-ray is otherwise normal.

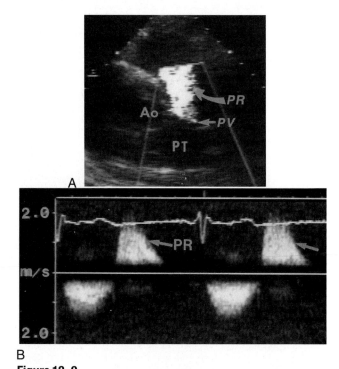

Figure 12–9

A, Black and white print of a color flow image (short axis) from an 11-year-old boy with moderate congenital pulmonary valve regurgitation (PR) that begins at the level of the pulmonary valve (PV). The pulmonary trunk (PT) is moderately dilated. Ao, aorta. B, Continuous-wave Doppler across the right ventricular outflow tract shows low-pressure low-velocity pulmonary regurgitation (PR). The systolic signal is low velocity because there was no gradient across the pulmonary valve.

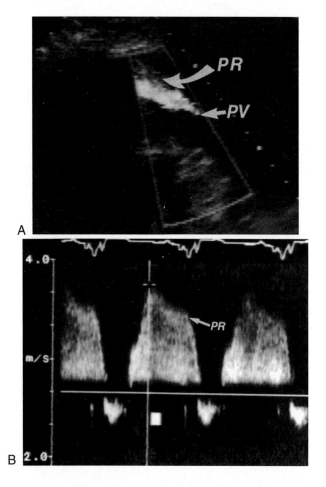

Figure 12–10

Echocardiograms from an 18-year-old woman with primary pulmonary hypertension. A, Black and white print of a color flow image (short axis) shows the high-velocity jet of pulmonary hypertensive pulmonary regurgitation (PR) beginning at the pulmonary valve (PV). B, Continuous-wave Doppler across the right ventricular outflow tract shows high-pressure, high-velocity pulmonary regurgitation (PR) with a peak of just over 3 m/sec. Compare with Figure 12–9.

REFERENCES

1. Abbott ME: Atlas of Congenital Cardiac Disease. New York, American Heart Association, 1936.
2. Alpert BS, Moore HV: "Absent" pulmonary valve with atrial septal defect and patent ductus arteriosus. Pediatr Cardiol 6:107, 1985.
3. Ansari A: Isolated pulmonary valvular regurgitation: Current perspectives. Prog Cardiovasc Dis 33:329, 1991.
4. Attie F, Rijlaarsdam M, Chuquiure E: Isolated absence of the pulmonary valve. Circulation 99:455, 1999.
5. Baker WP, Kelminson LL, Turner WM, Blount SA: Absence of the pulmonary valve associated with double outlet right ventricle. Circulation 36:452, 1967.
6. Becker AE: Quadricuspid pulmonary valve. Acta Morphol Neerl Scand 10:299, 1972.
7. Berman W, Fripp RR, Rowe SA, Yabek SM: Congenital isolated pulmonary valve incompetence: Neonatal presentation and early natural history. Am Heart J 124:248, 1992.
8. Bousvaros CA, Deuchar DC: The murmur of pulmonary regurgitation which is not associated with pulmonary hypertension. Lancet 2:962, 1961.
9. Brand A, Dollberg S, Keren A: The prevalence of valvular regurgitation in children with structurally normal hearts: A color Doppler echocardiographic study. Am Heart J 123:177, 1992.
10. Chevers N: A collection of facts illustrative of the morbid conditions of the pulmonary artery, as bearing upon the treatment of cardiac and pulmonary diseases. London Med Gazette 38:828, 1846.
11. Chiemmongkoltip P, Replogle RL, Gonzalez-Lavin L, Arcilla RA: Congenital absence of the pulmonary valve with atrial septal defect surgically corrected. Chest 62:100, 1972.
12. Choong CY, Abascal VM, Weyman J, et al: Prevalence of valvular regurgitation by Doppler echocardiography in patients with structurally normal hearts by two-dimensional echocardiography. Am Heart J 117:636, 1989.
13. Collins NP, Braunwald E, Morrow AG: Isolated congenital pulmonary valvular regurgitation. Am J Med 28:159, 1960.
14. Cortes FM, Jacoby WJ: Isolated congenital pulmonary valvular insufficiency. Am J Cardiol 10:287, 1962.
15. Criscitiello MG, Harvey WP: Clinical recognition of congenital pulmonary valve insufficiency. Am J Cardiol 20:765, 1967.
16. D'Cruz IA, Miller RA: Norman Chevers: A description of congenital absence of pulmonary valve and supravalvular aortic stenosis in the 1840's. Br Heart J 26:723, 1964.
17. Deshmukh M, Guvenc S, Bentivoglio L, Goldberg H: Idiopathic dilatation of the pulmonary artery. Circulation 21:710, 1960.
18. Dickens J, Raber GT, Goldberg H: Dynamic pulmonary regurgitation associated with a bicuspid valve. Ann Intern Med 48:851, 1958.
19. Edwards JE, Carey LS, Neufeld HM, Lester RG: Congenital Heart Disease. Philadelphia, W.B. Saunders, 1965.
20. Ehrenhaft JL: Discussion. In Ellison RG, Brown WJ Jr, Hague EE Jr, Hamilton WF: Physiologic observations on experimental pulmonary insufficiency. J Thorac Cardiovasc Surg 30:633, 1955.
21. Ettedgui JA, Sharland GK, Chita SK, et al: Absent pulmonary valve syndrome with ventricular septal defect: Role of the arterial duct. Am J Cardiol 66:233, 1990.
22. Fish RG, Takaro T, Crymes T: Prognostic considerations in primary isolated insufficiency of the pulmonic valve. N Engl J Med 261:739, 1959.
23. Ford AB, Hellerstein HK, Wood C, Kelly HB: Isolated congenital bicuspid pulmonary valve. Am J Med 20:474, 1956.
24. Goldberg E, Katz I: Isolated pulmonary regurgitation with intermittent pulmonary artery dilatation. Am J Cardiol 9:619, 1962.
25. Hambry RI, Gulotta SJ: Pulmonic valvular insufficiency: Etiology, recognition, and management. Am Heart J 74:110, 1967.
26. Hirschfelder AD: Diseases of the Heart and Aorta. Philadelphia, J.B. Lippincott, 1910.
27. Holmes JC, Fowler NO, Kaplan S: Pulmonary valvular insufficiency. Am J Med 44:851, 1968.
28. Hurwitz LE, Roberts WC: Quadricuspid semilunar valve. Am J Cardiol 31:623, 1973.
29. Ito T, Engle MA, Holswade GR: Congenital insufficiency of the pulmonic valve: A rare cause of neonatal heart failure. Pediatrics 28:712, 1961.
30. Jacoby WJ Jr, Tucker DH, Summer RG: The second heart sound in congenital pulmonary valvular insufficiency. Am Heart J 69:603, 1965.
31. Kelly DT: Isolated congenital pulmonary incompetence. Br Heart J 27:777, 1965.
32. Kezdi P, Priest WS, Smith JM: Pulmonic regurgitation. Q Bull Northwestern U Med School 29:368, 1955.
33. Kissin M: Pulmonary insufficiency with supernumerary cusp in pulmonary valve: Report of a case and review of the literature. Am Heart J 12:206, 1936.
34. McAleer E. Rosenzweig BP, Katz FS, et al: Unusual echocardiographic views of bicuspid and quadricuspid pulmonic valves. J Am Soc Echo 10:1036, 2001.
35. Laneve SA, Uesu CT, Taguchi JT: Isolated pulmonary valvular regurgitation. Am J Med Sci 244:446, 1962.
36. Lau K, Cheung HH, Mok C: Congenital absence of the pulmonary valve, intact ventricular septum, and patent ductus arteriosus: Management in a newborn infant. Am Heart J 120:711, 1990.
37. Lendrum BL, Shaffer AB: Isolated congenital pulmonic valve regurgitation. Am Heart J 57:298, 1959.
38. Levin HS, Runco V, Wooley CF, Ryan JM: Pulmonic regurgitation following staphylococcal endocarditis: An intracardiac phonocardiographic study. Circulation 30:411, 1964.
39. Maciel BC, Simpson IA, Valdes-Cruz LM, et al: Color flow Doppler mapping studies of "physiologic" pulmonary and tricuspid regurgitation: Evidence for true regurgitation as opposed to a valve closing volume. J Am Soc Echocardiogr 4:589, 1991.
40. Massumi RA, Just H, Tawakkol A: Pulmonary valve regurgitation secondary to bacterial endocarditis in heroin addicts. Am Heart J 73:308, 1967.
41. Miyatake K, Okamoto M, Kinoshita N, et al: Pulmonary regurgitation studied with the ultrasonic pulsed Doppler technique. Circulation 65:969, 1982.
42. Morton RF, Stern TN: Isolated pulmonary valvular regurgitation. Circulation 14:1069, 1956.
43. Nemickas R, Roberts J, Gunnar RM, Tobin JR Jr: Isolated congenital pulmonary insufficiency. Am J Cardiol 14:456, 1964.
44. Niwa K, Perloff JK, Bhuta SM, et al: Structural abnormalities of great arterial walls in congenital heart disease: Light and electron microscopic analyses. Circulation 103:393, 2001.
45. Osler W: The Principles and Practice of Medicine. New York, D. Appleton and Company, 1892, p. 620.
46. Perloff JK: Auscultatory and phonocardiographic manifestations of pulmonary hypertension. Prog Cardiovasc Dis 9:303, 1967.
47. Perloff JK: Physical Examination of the Heart and Circulation, 3rd ed. Philadelphia, W.B. Saunders, 2000.
48. Podzimkova J, Hickey MS, Slavik Z, et al: Absent pulmonary valve syndrome with intact ventricular septum. Int J Cardiol 61:109, 1997.
49. Pouget JM, Kelly CE, Pilz CG: Congenital absence of the pulmonic valve: Report of a case in a 73 year old man. Am J Cardiol 19:732, 1967.
50. Price BO: Isolated incompetence of the pulmonic valve. Circulation 23:596, 1961.
51. Rogers WM, Simandl E, Bhonslay SB, Deterling RA: The pulmonary valve in direct phonocardiography. Circulation 18:992, 1958.
52. Sanyal SK, Hipona FA, Browne MJ, Talner NS: Congenital insufficiency of the pulmonary valve. J Pediatr 64:728, 1964.
53. Schrire V, Vogelpoel L: The role of the dilated pulmonary artery in abnormal splitting of the second heart sound. Am Heart J 63:501, 1962.
54. Shaver JA, Nadolny RA, O'Toole JD, et al: Sound pressure correlates of the second heart sound. Circulation 49:316, 1974.
55. Sloman G, Keng Por Wee MB: Isolated congenital pulmonary valve incompetence. Am Heart J 66:532, 1963.
56. Smith RD, DuShane JW, Edwards JE: Congenital insufficiency of the pulmonary valve: Including a case of fetal cardiac failure. Circulation 20:554, 1959.
57. Takao S, Miyatake K, Izumi S, et al: Clinical implications of pulmonary regurgitation in healthy individuals: Detection by cross sectional pulsed Doppler echocardiography. Br Heart J 59:542, 1988.
58. Tanabe Y, Takahashi M, Kuwano H, et al: Long-term fate of isolated congenital absent pulmonary valve. Am Heart J 124:526, 1992.
59. Thanopoulos D, Fisher EA, Hastreiter AR: Large ductus arteriosus and intact ventricular septum associated with congenital absence of the pulmonary valve. Br Heart J 55:602, 1986.
60. Venables AW: Absence of pulmonary valve with ventricular septal defect. Br Heart J 24:293, 1962.
61. Vlad P, Weidman M, Lambert EC: Congenital pulmonary regurgitation: A report of 6 autopsied cases. Am J Dis Child 100:640, 1960.
62. Wennevold A, Jacobsen JR, Efsen F: Spontaneous change from pulmonic stenosis to pulmonic regurgitation. Am Heart J 108:608, 1984.

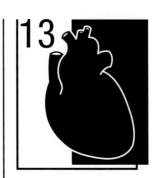

Ebstein's Anomaly of the Tricuspid Valve

Ebstein's Anomaly

In June 1864, a 19-year-old laborer was admitted to the All-Saints Hospital in Breslau (now Wroclaw) Poland, where he died 10 days later. Wilhelm Ebstein, assistant physician and prosector, subsequently wrote a scholarly account of the clinical and necropsy findings entitled "On a Very Rare Case of Insufficiency of the Tricuspid Valve Caused by a Severe Congenital Malformation of the Same."[41] The correlation of pathology with clinical notes and the hypotheses of pathophysiology resulted in a landmark publication. English translations are available and repay study.[81,115,143] Quality not withstanding, Ebstein's original report was overlooked[81] until 1937, when Yater and Shapiro published radiologic and electrocardiographic observations on Ebstein's anomaly.[139] In 1949, Tourniaire, Deyrieux, and Tartulier diagnosed the anomaly in a living subject,[129] and in 1950, Engle analyzed data from three patients who died with Ebstein's anomaly and asserted that clinical recognition was possible.[43] In the same year, Kerwin and Reynolds published the first English-language account of cases recognized during life,[68,104] and the following year Soloff, Stauffer, and Zatuchni made the clinical diagnosis in a 34-year-old patient[126] and confirmed the diagnosis at necropsy 6 years later.[127] The anomaly that Ebstein described occurs in approximately 1 in 20,000 live births,[90,143] has a prevalence of 0.3% to 0.7% of all cases of congenital heart disease,[109,122] and represents about 40% of congenital malformations of the tricuspid valve.[60]

Normal tricuspid leaflets consist of basal attachments to the annulus (right atrioventricular sulcus), peripheral zones into which chordae tendineae insert, and clear zones that lie between the basal attachments and the peripheral zones.[121] The semicircular or quadrangular anterior leaflet is the largest of the three.[121] The posterior leaflet is scalloped. The septal leaflet attaches chiefly to the ventricular septum, as the name indicates, but part of its basal attachment is to the posterior wall of the right ventricle.[121] The septal leaflet normally exhibits a slight but distinct apical displacement of its basal attachment compared to the mitral valve—15 mm in children and 20 mm in adults.[56]

Ebstein wrote, "When we turn our attention to the description of the right ventricle, we see at once an extremely abnormal appearance of the tricuspid valve" (Fig. 13–1).[41,81,115,130]

The septal and posterior leaflets do not attach normally to the tricuspid annulus, so the valve orifice is displaced downward into the right ventricular cavity at the junction of the inlet and trabecular components of the right ventricle.[2,4,56,75,130] The right side of the heart therefore consists of three morphologic components: the right atrium proper, the inlet portion of the right ventricle, which is thin-walled and functionally integrated with the right atrium, and the trabecular and outlet portion, which constitute the functional right ventricle.[130] The greater the apical displacement of the posterior and septal leaflets, the larger the atrialized right ventricle and the smaller the functional right ventricle (Fig. 13–2). Downward displacement of the septal tricuspid leaflet is associated with discontinuity of the central fibrous body and the septal atrioventricular ring, creating a potential substrate for accessory pathways and preexcitation.[130] The leaflets and tensile apparatus of the normal tricuspid valve are believed to be formed chiefly by a process of delamination of the inner layers of the inlet zone of the right ventricle.[130] Downward displacement of the tricuspid leaflets suggests that delamination of the inlet portion of the right ventricle fails to occur in Ebstein's anomaly.[130,135]

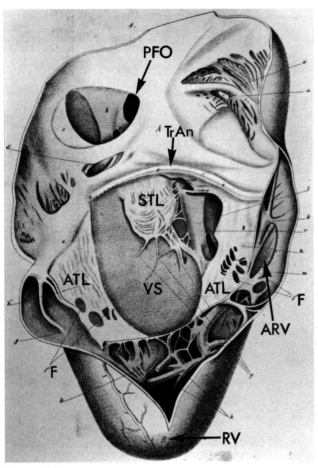

Figure 13–1

Illustration from Ebstein's original 1866 paper. The essential anatomic features of Ebstein's anomaly are indicated by my lettering: ARV, atrialized right ventricle; ATL, anterior tricuspid leaflet; F, fenestrations; PFO, patent foramen ovale; RV, functional right ventricle; STL, septal tricuspid leaflet; TrAn, tricuspid annulus; VS, ventricular septum.

The morbid anatomy encompasses a broad range of severity,[117,124] but certain features are relatively constant.[2,4,31,73,105,108,142] The anterior leaflet is almost always normally attached to the atrioventricular junction.[4,73,75,108] A salient anatomic feature is the level of the hinge points of the septal and posterior leaflets, which are characterized by apical displacement of their basal attachments[56] and impaired movement because of short chordae tendineae and nodular fibrotic thickening (see Fig. 13–1).[105,108] When the septal leaflet is absent, the posterior leaflet arrangement serves to distinguish Ebstein's anomaly from a congenitally unguarded tricuspid orifice (see later).[108] The anterior leaflet differs appreciably from the septal and posterior leaflets. The basal attachment of the anterior leaflet is at the level of the atrioventricular sulcus (annulus).[2,4,75,108] The large and potentially mobile anterior leaflet[105,108] contains muscular strands instead of consisting entirely of a fibrous membrane as in the normal tricuspid valve.[2,4] Mobility can be impaired by thickening, modularity, and fibrosis or by multiple short chordae.[105,108]

Displaced insertions of the malformed septal and posterior leaflets allow free communication between the proximal (atrialized) and distal (functional) parts of the right

ventricle. Alternatively, communication between the atrialized and functional right ventricle is confined to slits or perforations in the anterior tricuspid leaflet as Ebstein originally described, or the proximal and distal right ventricular compartments are separated by a muscular partition or shelf (see Fig. 13–32) that restricts flow to the commissure between the anterior leaflet and the displaced septal leaflet.[73] When the anteromedial commissure is fused and the anterior leaflet is intact, the tricuspid orifice is imperforate.[4,73,142]

The thin-walled atrialized right ventricle has isolated islands of myocytes, is typically dilated, often aneurysmally, and expands paradoxically during ventricular systole. Morphometric analyses of the trabecular and infundibular portions of the functional right ventricle disclose an absolute decrease in the number of myocytes and an increase in fibrous content, deficits that may be responsible for infundibular dilatation.[2-4,31] The majority of hearts with Ebstein's anomaly have a patent foramen ovale (see Figs. 13–1 and 13–2).[130] Ebstein believed that "Regurgitation of blood into the right atrium caused its dilatation and prevented complete closure of the valve of the foramen ovale."[41] In more than one third of cases, the interatrial communication is an ostium secundum atrial septal defect.[2-4] Rarely, a morphologic mitral valve has anatomical features of Ebstein's anomaly, and one report described the anomaly in both the tricuspid *and* mitral valves. Ebstein's anomaly of an inverted tricuspid valve is dealt with in Chapter 6 on Congenitally Corrected Transposition of the Great Arteries.

Tricuspid regurgitation due to a *congenitally unguarded tricuspid orifice*[5,6,13,55,66] or to *tricuspid valve dysplasia* differs fundamentally from Ebstein's anomaly.[15,64,72] A congenitally unguarded tricuspid orifice is characterized by absence of all three leaflets,[5,64] or by a muscular partition or shelf that leaves the atrioventricular orifice unguarded (see Fig. 13–32).[142] The tricuspid leaflets in Ebstein's anomaly are occasionally dysplastic,[105] but *congenital dysplasia of the tricuspid valve* refers to nodular thickening and rolling of the edges of the leaflets without downward displacement.[72]

Idiopathic dilatation of the right atrium has been reported in children without Ebstein's anomaly.[16,118] Transient tricuspid regurgitation of the newborn does not have a discernible anatomical basis and resolves within a few weeks.[51] Uhl's anomaly is discussed separately at the end of this chapter.

Abnormalities of the left side of the heart in Ebstein's anomaly consist of derangements of left ventricular geometry and impairment of systolic and diastolic function.[14,18,87,110] Superior systolic displacement of the mitral valve (prolapse) occurs because mitral leaflets with normal areas and chordal lengths are housed in a left ventricular cavity that is geometrically altered and reduced in size (see Fig. 13–31).[18,26,29,31,87,106,130] Depressed left ventricular systolic function is due to a combination of abnormal shape, impaired diastolic filling, and increased fibrous content of the free wall and ventricular septum.[3,30,31,130]

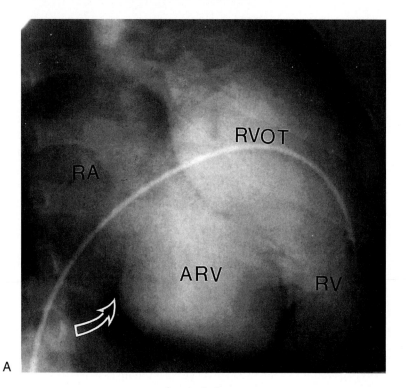

A

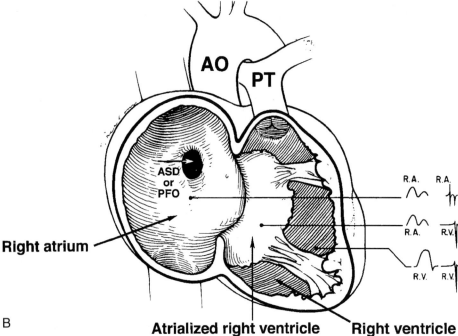

B

Right atrium

Atrialized right ventricle   **Right ventricle**

Figure 13–2

A, Angiocardiogram from a 10-year-old acyanotic boy with Ebstein's anomaly and an ostium secundum atrial septal defect. The tricuspid annulus (*arrow*) separates the right atrium proper (RA) from the atrialized right ventricle (ARV). The functional right ventricle lies between the ARV and the large right ventricular outflow tract (RVOT). *B,* Schematic illustration of the anatomic, functional, and electrophysiologic features of Ebstein's anomaly for comparison with part *A.* In the right atrium (RA), the pressure pulse and intracardiac electrogram are both right atrial. In the functional right ventricle (RV), the pressure pulse and the intracardiac electrogram are both right ventricular. In the atrialized right ventricle, the pressure pulse is atrial but the intracardiac electrogram is ventricular. ASD, atrial septal defect; PFO, patent foramen ovale.

The physiologic consequences of Ebstein's anomaly are determined by the condition of the tricuspid leaflets, by the hemodynamic burden imposed on an inherently flawed right ventricle, by left ventricular function, and by atrial rhythm. The tricuspid orifice is typically incompetent, occasionally stenotic, and rarely imperforate.[2,52,73,142] Functional impairment of the right ventricle depends on the severity of tricuspid regurgitation and on the ratio of the combined areas of the right atrium and atrialized right ventricle relative to the areas of the functional right ventricle and left ventricle.[30] The thin-walled atrialized right ventricle either behaves passively during the cardiac cycle or behaves as an aneurysm that expands paradoxically during systole as an active functional impediment.[57,58,105] Exercise intolerance has been ascribed to an inadequate increment in pulmonary blood flow and a fall in systemic arterial oxygen saturation.[11,38] Atrial tachyarrhythmias have serious physiologic consequences, especially the rapid heart actions associated with accessory pathways (see The Electrocardiogram and The History).

The functionally inadequate right ventricle is especially vulnerable in utero and at birth. High neonatal pulmonary

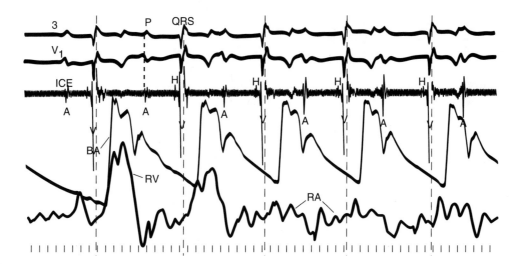

Figure 13–3

The electrophysiologic abnormalities of Ebstein's anomaly identified with a filtered bipolar system. Lead 3, lead V_1, and an intracardiac electrogram (ICE) are shown with a right ventricular (RV) and then a right atrial (RA) pressure pulse. In the intracardiac electrogram (ICE), atrial depolarization (A) coincides with P waves in lead 3 and lead V_1, and ventricular depolarization (V) coincides with the QRS complex in lead 3 and V_1. BA, brachial arterial pulse. In the first two cycles, the intracardiac electrogram recorded right ventricular depolarization with a right ventricular pressure pulse (RV). In the subsequent three cycles, the intracardiac electrogram continued to record right ventricular depolarization, but the pressure pulse was right atrial (RA) because the recording was over the atrialized right ventricle.

vascular resistance increases right ventricular afterload, augments tricuspid regurgitation, increases right atrial pressure, and establishes a right-to-left shunt across a patent foramen ovale or an atrial septal defect.[100] The process is reversed as neonatal pulmonary vascular resistance falls and right ventricular afterload normalizes.[100] The enlarging right atrium becomes sufficiently compliant to accommodate a large volume of regurgitant flow with little or no increase in pressure (see Fig. 13–5),[52] but right ventricular filling pressure may rise again in older patients, provoking a parallel rise in right atrial pressure with re-establishment of the right-to-left interatrial shunt.

Ebstein's original case was an example of obstruction at the tricuspid orifice (see Fig. 13–1).[41] He wrote, "The membrane divided the right ventricle into two halves. These two halves communicated with each other in two ways: one through the oval opening which leads into the right conus arteriosus, and two through the already described multiple openings in the fenestrated membrane."[41] The elevation of right atrial pressure in Ebstein's anomaly with a stenotic or imperforate tricuspid orifice is

determined by the degree of obstruction. The A wave is often giant, and a right-to-left shunt at atrial level persists after the fall in neonatal pulmonary vascular resistance.

The electromechanical properties of the right atrium, the atrialized right ventricle, and the functional right ventricle provided the first secure basis for the clinical diagnosis of Ebstein's abnormality (Figs. 13–2 and 13–3).[61,78,86,125,136,140] The right atrium proper generates a right atrial pressure pulse and an intracavitary atrial electrogram. The functional right ventricle generates a right ventricular pressure pulse and a right ventricular intracavitary electrogram. The atrialized right ventricle generates an intracavitary right ventricular electrogram but an atrial pressure pulse (see Figs. 13–2 and 13–3). Because the atrialized right ventricle contains right ventricular muscle fibers, mechanical stimulation provokes a right ventricular electrogram and risks inducing polymorphic ventricular tachycardia[12,76] that rapidly degenerates into ventricular fibrillation (Fig. 13–4) because isolated islands of myocytes cannot anchor reentrant spiral/scroll waves, which break up immediately.[145]

Figure 13–4

Continuous tracing of lead 1 (L1). A catheter tip in the atrial-ized right ventricle induced ventricular fibrillation (*vertical arrow*) that abated and then recurred (*horizontal arrow*) without preceding ventricular tachycardia.

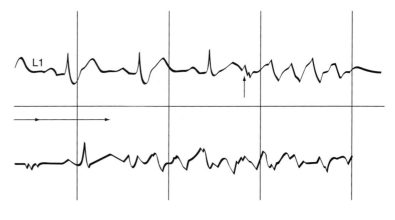

The geometric configuration and the function of the right and left ventricles are closely coupled in Ebstein's anomaly.[18,29,87,110] Leftward displacement of the ventricular septum (see Fig.13–31) results in impaired left ventricular diastolic filling and in a reduction in ejection fraction. Exercise provokes an increase in left ventricular ejection fraction because end-systolic volume decreases with little or no change in end-diastolic volume. The right ventricular free wall contributes feebly to forward flow, which is materially assisted by paradoxical movement of the ventricular septum that functions as part of the right ventricle, as in Uhl's anomaly (see later). Left ventricular function is adversely impacted by the combined effects of the diastolic position of the ventricular septum, geometric distortion of the ventricle (see Fig. 13–31), reduced end-diastolic volume, paradoxical septal motion, and an increase in fibrous tissue and a decrease in cardiomyocytes in the free wall and septum.[30,31,87,110]

THE HISTORY

Males and females are equally affected.[21,50,100,111,112,132,137] Familial Ebstein's anomaly has been reported,[*] and one patient with Ebstein's anomaly of a noninverted right-sided tricuspid valve had a cousin with congenitally corrected transposition of the great arteries and Ebstein's anomaly of an inverted left-sided atrioventricular valve.[21] A novel mutation has been held responsible for the genetic syndrome of ventricular preexcitation and conduction system disease of childhood onset,[94] but these observations cannot be extrapolated to the general population of patients with preexcitation, or to patients with Ebstein's anomaly in the absence of preexcitation.

The Danish Registry estimated that the relative risk of Ebstein's anomaly was increased 500-fold in offspring exposed to in utero lithium carbonate, a drug commonly used for the treatment of bipolar disorders.[48,90,93,141] The probability of occurrence of Ebstein's anomaly in the general population is 1:20,000, so the likelihood of the malformation occurring spontaneously in a pregnant woman is low.[141] It is currently estimated that the increased lithium risk is not more than 28-fold, considerably less than estimates from the Danish Registry.[90,93,141]

The clinical course of Ebstein's anomaly ranges from intrauterine death to asymptomatic survival to late adulthood.[†] The most common age-related presentations are (1) detection of the anomaly in a routine fetal echocardiogram, (2) neonatal cyanosis, (3) heart failure in infancy, (4) murmur in childhood, and (5) arrhythmias in adolescents and adults.[8,21,50,52,86,112] The outlook for fetal Ebstein's anomaly has been aptly characterized as "appalling."[8] With rare exception, fetal hydrops is fatal.[102,128] Neonates not only confront a high risk of mortality but also confront a signifi-cant continuing risk of morbidity and later death if they survive infancy.[30] Neonates with symptoms that resolve in the first month of life may die suddenly,[30] but transient neonatal cyanosis that recurs a decade or more later is an occasional and distinctive feature of Ebstein's anomaly.[8] An early right-to-left interatrial shunt disappears as neonatal pulmonary vascular resistance normalizes, but the shunt reappears later as filling pressure rises in the functionally abnormal right ventricle.[100] Tachyarrhythmic sudden death is a threat regardless of severity of the anomaly[49,107] and is held responsible for the drop-off in survival in the fifth decade.[49] Isolated Wolff-Parkinson-White syndrome in otherwise normal individuals carries an estimated risk of sudden cardiac death of 0.02%.[24] Atrial flutter or fibrillation with accelerated conduction via accessory pathways in Ebstein's anomaly provokes an increase in cyanosis, pallor, diaphoresis, weakness, lightheadedness, syncope, and an increase in the risk of sudden death.[50,71,91,112] Stimulation of the arrhythmogenic atrialized right ventricle initiates polymorphic ventricular tachycardia that is promptly followed by ventricular fibrillation (see Fig. 13–4) (see earlier). Spontaneous ventricular tachycardia/fibrillation originating in the atrialized right ventricle looms as a potential risk. The degree of cyanosis does not necessarily correlate with symptoms, but once symptoms and cyanosis develop, disability tends to be progressive even in patients who were relatively asymptomatic before adolescence or adulthood.[50,71] The onset of chronic atrial fibrillation predicts death within 5 years.[49]

Despite legitimate qualifications, there are legendary accounts of astonishing longevity in patients with Ebstein's anomaly, with survivals into the eighth and ninth decades.[21,27,71,80,132,137] Ebstein's anomaly was discovered at necropsy in a 75-year-old man who as a youth had been a lumberjack working on log booms.[59] He was reportedly asymptomatic until his 50s, when he was obliged to outrun an irate female bear.[59] At necropsy 25 years later, his right atrium was thin-walled and greatly dilated, and the tricuspid valve was characteristically malformed.[59] The oldest recorded patient with Ebstein's anomaly lived to 85 years without cardiac symptoms until the age of 79 years.[116]

The chest pain that occasionally occurs with Ebstein's anomaly is an enigma.[21,50,112,132] The pain is retrosternal, epigastric, or in the right or left anterior chest. The quality is sharp, stabbing, or shooting. Certain features suggest serous surface origin from pericardium overlying the atrialized right ventricle (see Auscultation).[50,112]

Important, although less frequent, symptoms are the result of paradoxical emboli or brain abscess.[50,71,112,132] Infective endocarditis is uncommon because regurgitant flow across the malformed tricuspid valve is low velocity with low turbulence.[50] Pregnancy confronts the gravid woman with risks inherent in a functionally inadequate volume-overloaded right ventricle that copes poorly with the additional hemodynamic burden of gestation.[37,100] Paroxysmal atrial tachyarrhythmias are potential hazards during pregnancy, especially with the rapid rates associated

---

[*]9, 21, 36, 42, 54, 71, 77, 85, 97, 113, 122, 137.

[†]28, 30, 46, 47, 49, 50, 52, 71, 84, 91, 100, 109, 132, 137.

with accessory pathways. Cyanosis may first become manifest during pregnancy because of a rise in filling pressure of the functionally inadequate volume-overloaded right ventricle. Hypoxemia increases the risk of fetal wastage.[37] A right-to-left interatrial shunt poses puerperal risk of paradoxical embolization.

PHYSICAL APPEARANCE

Growth and development are normal in patients who were asymptomatic as neonates and infants.[50,52,84,112] Persistent cyanosis or intermittent exercise-induced cyanosis occurs in more than 50% of cases.[21,50,71,112] Precordial asymmetry is usually due to left parasternal prominence, but occasionally the right anterior chest is prominent, presumably because of the large right atrium.[52,112]

THE ARTERIAL PULSE

The arterial pulse is normal but diminishes as left ventricular stroke volume falls.[112, 132]

THE JUGULAR VENOUS PULSE

The jugular pulse is normal except for a prominent C wave that coincides with mobility of the anterior tricuspid leaflet (Figs. 13–5 and 13–6, first panel).[50,52,71] The interval between the jugular A wave and the carotid pulse is often prolonged because of prolongation of the PR interval (see The Electrocardiogram). Prominent A waves are seldom seen in the jugular pulse, but atrial contraction sometimes generates presystolic waves in the pulmonary arterial pressure pulse.[50,71] An attenuated X descent and a systolic venous V wave of tricuspid regurgitation seldom appear in the jugular pulse despite severe regurgitant flow because of the damping effect of the compliant right atrium and the thin-walled toneless atrialized right ventricle, and because tricuspid regurgitation is low pressure and hypokinetic (Figs. 13–5 and 13–6).[50,71] Right ventricular failure induces a rise in mean jugular venous pressure and a rise in the A and V waves crest, but systolic pulsations of the liver are generally inconspicuous because the right ventricle is hypokinetic.[84,91] A stenotic or imperforate tricuspid orifice is accompanied by A waves that may be giant.

PRECORDIAL MOVEMENT AND PALPATION

A right ventricular impulse and a tricuspid systolic thrill are reserved for neonates prior to normalization of pulmonary vascular resistance.[21,50,71,100,112] With this exception, absence of a systolic impulse over the inflow portion of the right ventricle is an important negative sign in the clinical diagnosis of Ebstein's anomaly.[21,35,50,71] An undulating rippling motion over the atrialized right ventricle is sometimes seen in older patients.[50] Enlargement of the infundibular portion of the functional right ventricle is accompanied by a systolic impulse in the third left inter-

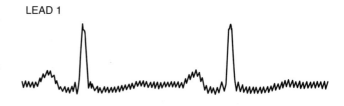

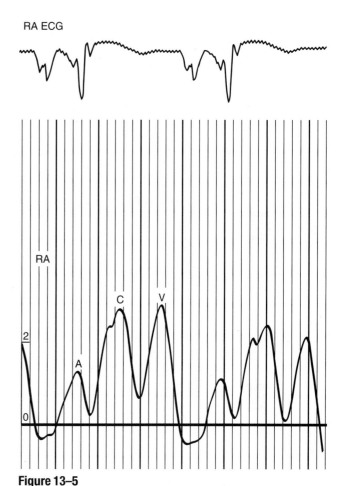

Figure 13–5

Tracings from a 14-year-old boy with Ebstein's anomaly. The electrode catheter in the right atrium recorded an intracardiac atrial electrogram (RA ECG) and a right atrial pressure pulse (RA). A and V waves in the right atrial pressure pulse (RA) are normal, and the X descent is preserved despite severe tricuspid regurgitation, but the C wave is prominent because of a large mobile anterior tricuspid leaflet.

costal space.[98] Ebstein described a gentle left ventricular impulse, stating that[41] "the cardiac apex was visible under the sixth rib somewhat outside the mammary line." Ebstein also percussed the enlarged right atrium[41]: "...the cardiac dullness extended for two centimeters beyond the right border of the sternum at the level of the fourth rib and for three centimeters at the level of the sixth rib, where it merged with the liver dullness, which was normal in extent."

The initial component of a widely split first heart sound coincides with mitral valve closure, and the second delayed component coincides with closure of the large anterior

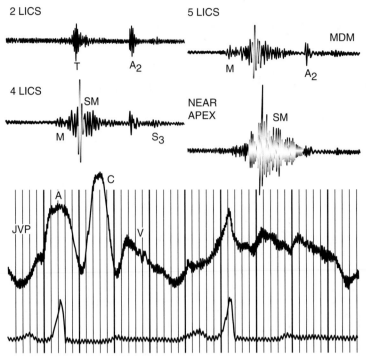

Figure 13–6

Phonocardiograms and jugular venous pulse (JVP) from a 17-year-old acyanotic boy with Ebstein's anomaly. The A and V waves are normal despite severe tricuspid regurgitation, but the C wave is prominent because of a large mobile anterior tricuspid leaflet. The loud sound labeled T was generated by the mobile anterior tricuspid leaflet. The soft preceding sound (M) is mitral. A decrescendo systolic murmur (SM) is loudest near the cardiac apex over the displaced tricuspid valve. The second heart sound is single (A₂, aortic component). There is a third heart sound (S₃) in the fourth left intercostal space (4 LICS) and a short mid-diastolic murmur (MDM) in the fifth left intercostal space (5 LICS). 2 LICS, second left intercostal space.

tricuspid leaflet (Figs. 13–6 through 13–9).[35, 45, 98, 112, 138] The delay in tricuspid valve closure is not simply due to complete right bundle branch block and a hypokinetic right ventricle, but instead is due to the large size and increased excursion of the anterior leaflet, which requires longer to reach its tense, fully closed position.[138] The increased tension developed by the large anterior leaflet as it reaches the limits of its systolic excursion accounts for the loudness of the tricuspid component of the first heart sound—the sail sound—which is an important auscultatory sign of anterior leaflet mobility (see Fig. 13–30).[45,96] A long PR interval softens the mitral component, so the first heart sound is then represented by a loud single tricuspid component. Preexcitation of the right ventricle buries the mitral component of the first sound in the early loud tricuspid component (Fig. 13–10).[70]

The systolic murmur of tricuspid regurgitation is typically grade 2 or 3/6, is maximum over the displaced tricuspid valve, and is therefore heard in a relatively leftward location toward the apex (see Figs. 13–6 and 13–9).[112] Intensity of the murmur does not increase during inspiration because the functionally inadequate right ventricle cannot increase its stroke volume and regurgitant flow. The murmur is impure, medium frequency, and decrescendo in response to low-velocity regurgitant flow from a hypokinetic low-pressure right ventricle (see Figs. 13–7 through 13–10).[35,50,52,71] An early systole decrescendo murmur is a recognized feature of low-pressure tricuspid regurgitation because regurgitant flow diminishes in latter systole as the

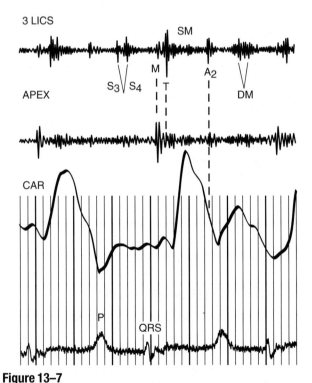

Figure 13–7

Phonocardiograms and carotid pulse (CAR) from an acyanotic 22-year-old woman with Ebstein's anomaly. The first heart sound is widely split. The tricuspid component (T) is prominent in the third left intercostal space (3 LICS) rather than at the apex. M, mitral component. There is a soft decrescendo tricuspid systolic murmur (SM). A third heart sound (S₃) and a fourth sound with duration (S₄) are separately recorded in the first cycle. In the second cycle, the third and fourth heart sounds fuse to form a short mid-diastolic murmur (DM).

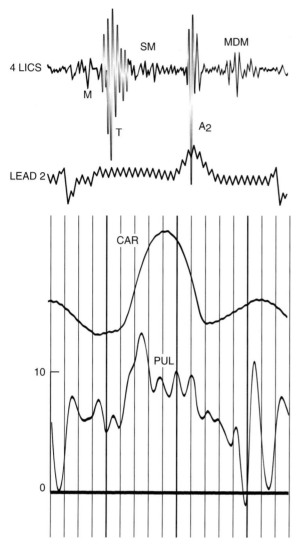

Figure 13–8

Phonocardiogram (4 LICS, fourth left intercostal space), electrocardiogram (lead 2), carotid pulse (CAR), and pulmonary artery pulse (PUL) from an 18-year-old cyanotic man with Ebstein's anomaly. The first heart sound is widely split with a loud tricuspid component (T) caused by a large mobile anterior tricuspid leaflet. The tricuspid systolic murmur (SM) is soft and decrescendo. A short mid-diastolic murmur (MDM) represents fusion of a third and fourth heart sound. A_2, aortic component of the second heart sound; M, mitral component of the first heart sound.

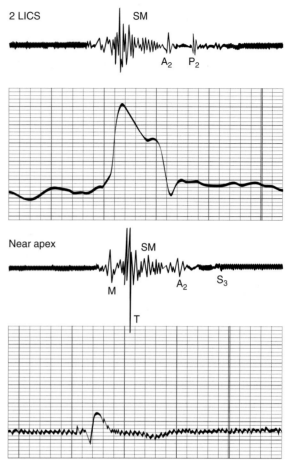

Figure 13–9

Phonocardiograms from a 37-year-old acyanotic woman with Ebstein's anomaly. The first heart sound is widely split, and the tricuspid component (T) is prominent in the second left intercostal space (2 LICS) and near the apex. M, mitral component. The tricuspid systolic murmur (SM) is decrescendo. The second heart sound is widely split (A_2, aortic component; P_2, pulmonary component). A soft third heart sound (S_3) was recorded near the apex.

right atrial V wave reaches the height of normal right ventricular systolic pressure.[95] In neonates with Ebstein's anomaly, the tricuspid regurgitant murmur is holosystolic because right ventricular systolic pressure is elevated.[100]

Wide splitting of the second heart sound is due to a delay in the pulmonary component caused by complete right bundle branch block (see Fig. 13–9).[35] However, the second sound is often single because pulmonary closure is inaudible owing to low pressure in the pulmonary trunk (see Figs. 13–6 and 13–7).[21,35,52] The split changes little if at all with respiration[35] but can be paradoxical when an accessory pathway prematurely activates the right side of the ventricular septum.[98]

Third and fourth heart sounds produce a distinctive triple or quadruple rhythm (Figs. 13–6, 13–7, and 13–9),[35,50,52,71] often summate because of PR interval prolongation, and may increase during inspiration because of origin in the right side of the heart.[112] Third and fourth heart sounds are sometimes sufficiently prolonged to produce short diastolic murmurs[71,84,132] (Fig. 13–11, and see Figs. 13–8 and 13–10), especially when the sounds occur in close proximity or when they summate (see Fig. 13–7).

Early diastolic sounds with the timing of opening snaps have been described in cases of Ebstein's anomaly and attributed to opening movements of the large mobile anterior tricuspid leaflet.[35,50,132]

The timing and quality of systolic and diastolic murmurs occasionally create the impression of a pericardial friction rub (Fig. 13–12).[50,112,132] A fibrinous pericardium has been found at necropsy over the atrialized right ventricle.[112] The distinctive cadence created by a rublike systolic murmur and a rublike mid-diastolic and presystolic murmur resembles the rhythmic chugging of a locomotive engine as it gathers speed (see Fig. 13–12).

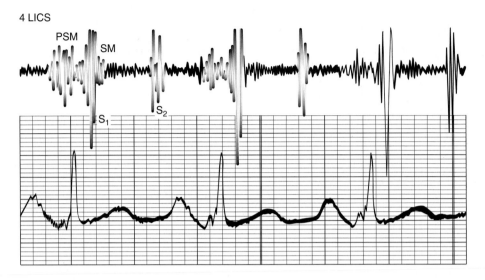

Figure 13–10
Tracings from an acyanotic 21-year-old man with Ebstein's anomaly. The phonocardiogram in the fourth left intercostal space (4 LICS) shows a loud presystolic murmur (PSM), a prominent first heart sound (S_1), and a soft tricuspid early systolic murmur (SM). The loud tricuspid component of the first heart sound occurred early because of a short PR interval associated with preexcitation of the right ventricle. The electrocardiogram (lead 2) shows the short PR interval and the delta wave of type B Wolff-Parkinson-White preexcitation. S_2, second heart sound.

THE ELECTROCARDIOGRAM

A confident diagnosis of Ebstein's anomaly can sometimes be based on the electrocardiogram per se.[71,78,79] The electrocardiogram is seldom normal even when the anomaly is mild (Fig. 13–13; see also Fig. 13–15), but rarely and oddly, the tracing is normal even when the anomaly is severe.[78] The major electrophysiologic abnormalities in Ebstein's anomaly are summarized in Table 13–1.

P waves are abnormal in height, duration, and configuration (Figs. 13–14, 13–17, and 13–19).[21,67,79] Taussig aptly characterized the tall peaked P waves as *Himalayan*,[21] patterns that have been ascribed to prolonged aberrant conduction in the enlarged right atrium.[67,79] Permanent atrial standstill, which has been reported in familial Ebstein's anomaly,[97] is a rare and distinctive electrophysiologic abnormality in which atrial myocardium is unresponsive to electrical or mechanical stimulation and P waves are absent in scalar and transesophageal electrocardiograms.

The PR interval is prolonged (see Figs. 13–14, 13–15, and 13–16), sometimes markedly so (see Fig. 13–19).[79,132] The duration of the PR interval and the width of the P wave

RA PHONO

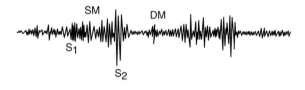

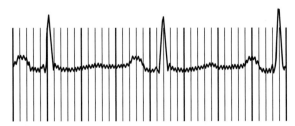

Figure 13–11
Right atrial intracardiac phonocardiogram (RA Phono) from a 17-year-old boy with Ebstein's anomaly. The tricuspid systolic murmur (SM) is holosystolic at its intracardiac site but decrescendo at its thoracic wall site (see Fig. 13–6). DM is a short tricuspid mid-diastolic murmur.

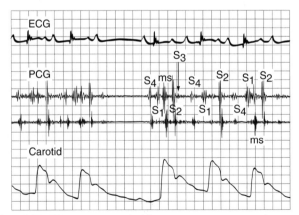

Figure 13–12
Phonocardiogram (PCG) from a 20-year-old man with Ebstein's anomaly. Auscultatory signs suggested a three-component friction rub because prolonged impure third and fourth heart sounds (S_3, S_4) were accompanied by an impure short midsystolic murmur (ms), and because these three auscultatory events were brought closer to the chest wall by the dilated atrialized right ventricle.

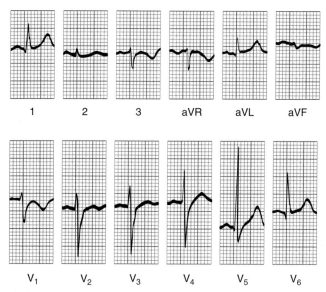

Figure 13–13

Electrocardiogram from an 11-year-old girl with mild Ebstein's anomaly. The tracing is normal except for a short PR interval (120 msec) and a horizontal QRS axis. The diagnosis was confirmed by transesophageal echocardiography.

Table 13–1	Major Electrophysiologic Abnormalities in Ebstein's Anomaly

Intra-atrial conduction disturbance: right atrial P wave abnormalities, PR interval prolongation

Atrioventricular nodal conduction: PR interval prolongation

Infranodal conduction

    Intra- or infra-His conduction abnormalities

    Right bundle branch block

    Bizarre second QRS attached to preceding normal QRS

Type B Wolff-Parkinson-White preexcitation

Supraventricular tachycardia

Atrial fibrillation or flutter

Arrhythmogenic atrialized right ventricle

Deep Q waves in leads V_{1-4} and in inferior leads

Figure 13–14

Electrocardiogram from an 11-month-old girl with Ebstein's anomaly and recurrent supraventricular tachycardia. Tall peaked right atrial P waves appear in leads 1, 2, and V_{2-4}. The PR interval is prolonged for age. Delta waves are positive in lead aVL and in leads V_{2-6}, and are negative in leads 2, 3, and aVF. These limb lead patterns, together with an abrupt transition from an isoelectric delta wave in lead V_1 (rsR) to a positive delta wave in lead V_2 (slurred Rs) suggest a right posterior septal accessory pathway. The prolonged terminal force of the QRS points to the right, superior, and anterior because of a right ventricular conduction defect.

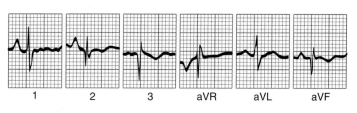

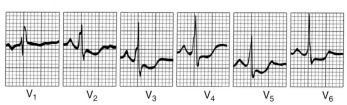

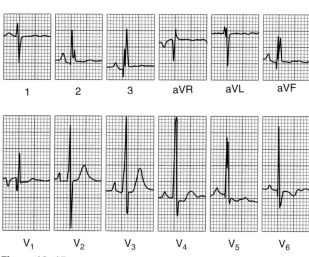

Figure 13–15

Electrocardiogram from a moderately cyanotic female neonate with Ebstein's anomaly. The PR interval is prolonged for age. A right atrial abnormality is indicated by tall peaked P waves in lead 2 and V_{2-3}, a deep broad P terminal force in lead V_1 and a Q wave in lead V_1, that is similar to the pattern aVR. The QRS is splintered and the terminal force is prolonged. The relatively tall R wave in lead V_1 suggests unanticipated right ventricular hypertrophy.

correlate with prolonged conduction in the large right atrium.[67,79] In the presence of preexcitation, the PR interval is usually (see Fig. 13–17) but not necessarily (see Fig. 13–14) short because of early inscription of the delta wave. However, a short PR interval occasionally occurs without a delta wave and without a history of paroxysmal rapid heart action (see Fig. 13–13).

Electrophysiologic studies have identified intra-His and infra-His delay in Ebstein's anomaly.[67] Prolonged HV intervals have been ascribed to lengthened and impaired conduction within the atrialized right ventricle,[67,120] conclusions that are in accord with the observation that complete heart block is rare despite prolongation of the PR interval and HV interval (see Fig. 13–19).[99]

The QRS is characterized by a right ventricular conduction defect of the right bundle branch type in 75% to 95% of cases (see Fig. 13–16).[22,50,52,67,71] QRS prolongation is largely if not exclusively due to prolonged activation of the atrialized right ventricle, and is less fully developed in infants (see Fig. 13–14).[50,71,112] The conduction defect is therefore *distal* to the right bundle branch,[67] and is

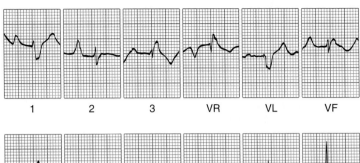

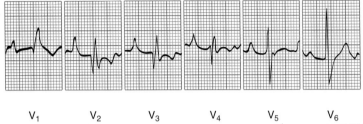

Figure 13–16

Electrocardiogram from an 18-year-old acyanotic man with Ebstein's anomaly. The typical electrocardiogram includes PR interval prolongation, tall peaked right atrial P waves in lead 2 and V_{2-5}, complete right bundle branch block, and QR complexes in leads V_{1-4}.

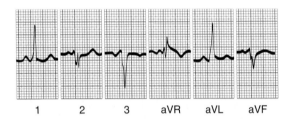

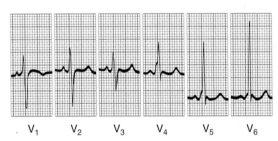

Figure 13–17

Electrocardiogram from a 17-year-old boy with Ebstein's anomaly. Low-amplitude P waves are peaked in leads V_{1-3} but are otherwise normal. A short PR interval is followed by delta waves that are positive in leads 1, aVL, and V_{4-6} and negative in leads 2, 3, and aVF. These patterns suggest a right posterior septal accessory pathway. The delta wave is isoelectric in leads V_1 and V_2, which is presumptive evidence of the accessory pathway in the right posterolateral free wall.

sometimes present despite a septal accessory pathway (see Fig. 13–14). A distinctive *second* QRS complex attached to the preceding *normal* QRS complex originates in the atrialized right ventricle according to intracardiac mapping (Fig. 13–20).[50,67]

The QRS axis is inferior, although a splintered polyphasic QRS sometimes makes the axis difficult to determine. Left axis deviation represents type B preexcitation (see Fig. 13–18), but a horizontal QRS axis occasionally occurs in the absence of accessory pathways (see Fig. 13–15).[44,50,112] Initial force abnormalities apart from delta waves are important features of the electrocardiogram. Deep Q waves appear in leads 2, 3, and aVF (see Fig. 13–19),[22,44] but more important are precordial Q waves in lead V_1 (see Fig. 13–16) or in leads V_{1-4} (see Figs. 13–17 and 13–19).[22,71] This distinctive precordial Q wave pattern occurs because the precordial surface leads record right ventricular intracavitary potentials unusually far to leftward owing to the large right atrium.[22] For the same reason, QRS patterns are similar if not identical in lead V_1 and lead aVR (see Figs. 13–17 and 13–19). Prominent Q waves in right precordial leads can be misleading when adults with Ebstein's anomaly present with chest pain (see The History).

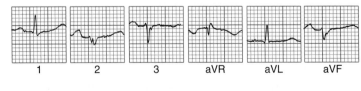

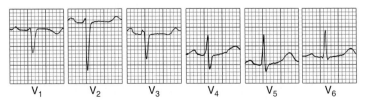

Figure 13–18

Electrocardiogram from a 39-year-old woman with a mild form of Ebstein's anomaly and a patent foramen ovale confirmed by transesophageal echocardiography. She came to medical attention because of a cerebral ischemic event caused by a paradoxical embolus. Her x-ray is shown in Figure 13–21. The P waves are normal, the PR interval is 200 msec, and there is left axis deviation but without delta waves. The terminal R wave in aVR is slightly prolonged.

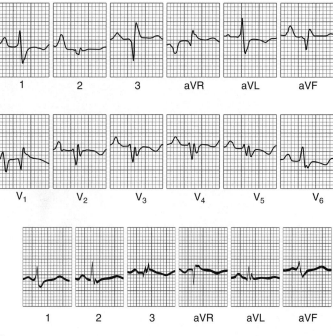

Figure 13–19

Electrocardiogram from a 58-year-old woman with acyanotic Ebstein's anomaly. The PR interval is 220 msec. There are tall peaked right atrial P waves in leads 1, 2, and aVF and in leads V_{2-5}. Prominent Q waves appear in leads 2, 3, and aVF and in leads V_{1-4}. Recurrent Mobitz II atrioventricular block progressed to complete heart block that required a pacemaker, which was implanted onto the left ventricular epicardium.

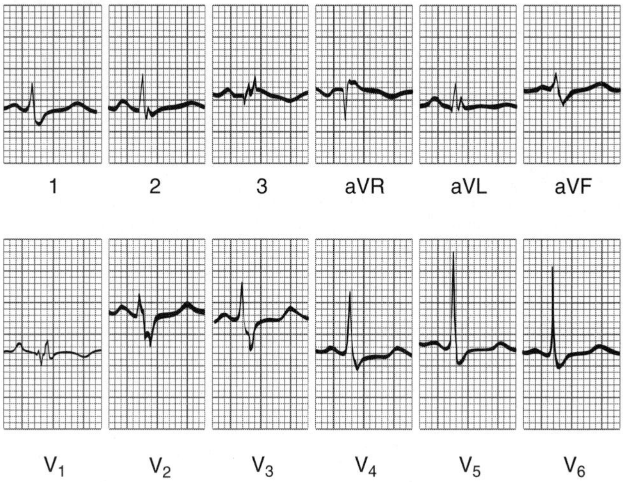

Figure 13–20

Electrocardiogram from an acyanotic 30-year-old woman with Ebstein's anomaly. A bizarre second QRS complex is attached to the preceding normal QRS complex. The PR interval and the P waves are normal.

Supraventricular tachycardia, atrial fibrillation, and atrial flutter occur in 25% to 30% of cases.[*] Ebstein reported that his patient "has always been troubled with palpitations."[41] Wide QRS tachycardia via bypass tracts must be distinguished from ventricular tachycardia, which is uncommon if not rare as a spontaneous tachyarrhythmia (see Fig. 13–4).[76,123] Right bundle branch block is a feature of Brugada syndrome, which occurs with ST segment elevations in leads V_{1-2} and ventricular fibrillation, but without structural heart disease.[69,74,146,148]

Wolff-Parkinson-White preexcitation, which was described in 1930[63] and characterized electrophysiologically in 1967,[83] is an important feature of Ebstein's anomaly that is present in 5% to 25% of the electrocardiograms (see Fig. 13–17).[21,22,67,112,132,137] Downward displacement of the septal tricuspid leaflet is accompanied by discontinuity between the central fibrous body and the septal atrioventricular ring, creating a substrate for preexcitation (see earlier).[130] Ebstein's anomaly is the only congenital cardiac malformation consistently associated with preexcitation that is uniformly via a right bypass tract, that is, type B Wolff-Parkinson-White (see Fig. 13–17). Patients with preexcitation may never experience rapid heart action, and atrial tachyarrhythmias are not confined to patients with accessory atrioventricular conduction.[50,52] Nevertheless, the combination of type B preexcitation and cyanosis constitutes presumptive evidence of Ebstein's anomaly. Accessory conduction can be intermittent or permanent,[112] delta waves can occur with normal PR intervals, or short PR intervals can occur without delta waves (see Fig. 13–13).[44]

Tachyarrhythmias in patients with Ebstein's anomaly have recurred over a 60-year time span.[50] Type B bypass conduction is associated with a left superior QRS axis (see Fig. 13–17), but a left superior axis is not always associated with delta waves (see Fig. 13–18). The direction of the delta wave vector and the QRS configuration make it possible to assign the accessory atrioventricular pathway to the right posterolateral free wall or to the right posterior septum. (see Figs. 13–14 and 13–18).[123] When accessory pathways are multiple, as they are in more than one third of patients with Ebstein's anomaly, conduction tends to be over the septal pathway.[123] Mahaim nodoventricular fibers are likely to be present when a left bundle branch block pattern occurs during sinus rhythm or during an episode of tachycardia.[123]

THE X-RAY

The cardiac silhouette varies from near normal (Figs. 13–21 and 13–22) to diagnostic (Figs. 13–23 through 13–27).[21,50,52,71,88,112] Heart size in symptomatic infants may be immense (Figs. 13–28 and 13–29).[100,112] Normal

---

[*]21,50,52,67,71,78,79,107,112,123,132

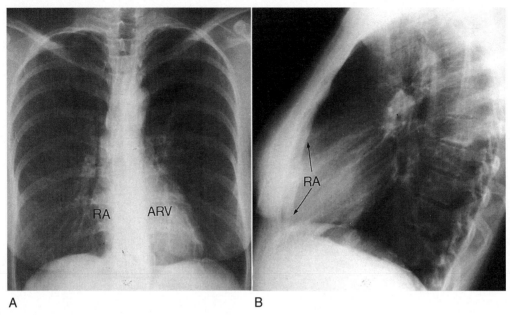

Figure 13–21

X-rays from the 39-year-old woman with mild Ebstein's anomaly whose electrocardiogram is shown in Figure 13–18. *A*, The size and configuration of the heart are normal, but the ascending and transverse aorta are relatively prominent for age and sex. ARV, atrialized right ventricle; RA, right atrium. *B*, In the lateral projection, the retrosternal right atrium (RA) reveals itself.

pulmonary vascularity accompanies mild acyanotic Ebstein's anomaly (see Figs. 13–21 and 13–22), and reduced pulmonary blood flow accompanies severe cyanotic Ebstein's anomaly (see Figs. 13–25, 13–26, and 13–27).[50,52,71,84,88,132] The infundibulum either straightens the left cardiac border[52] (see Figs. 13–22, 13–23, and 13–24) or forms a conspicuous convex shoulder[52] (see

Figs. 13–25, 13–26, and 13–27). The most consistent and dramatic feature of the x-ray is the right atrial silhouette, which is almost invariably enlarged (see Figs. 13–23 through 13–25), sometimes dramatically so (see Figs. 13–26 through 13–29), and is seldom normal even when the cardiac silhouette is otherwise normal (see Figs. 13–21 and 13–22A). Marked rightward convexity

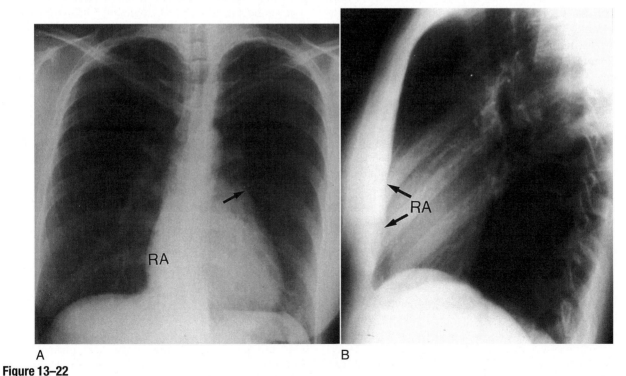

Figure 13–22

X-rays from a 33-year-old woman with mild Ebstein's anomaly. *A*, The left cardiac border is straightened by the infundibulum (*arrow*). The right atrial contour is only slightly prominent (RA). *B*, Retrosternal right atrial enlargement (*arrows*) is more apparent in the lateral projection.

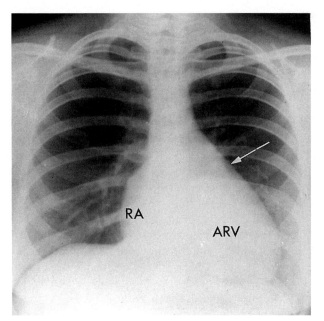

Figure 13–23

X-ray from an acyanotic 23-year-old woman with Ebstein's anomaly who came to medical attention because of recurrent paroxysmal rapid heart action without electrocardiographic evidence of an accessory pathway. The infundibulum is border forming (*arrow*), the right atrium (RA) is prominent, and the vascular pedicle is narrow. ARV, atrialized right ventricle.

of the enlarged right atrium with marked leftward convexity of the enlarged infundibulum accounts for a box-like configuration (see Figs. 13–26 and 13–27).[21,52,71] The vascular pedicle is narrow because the pulmonary trunk is not border forming and the ascending aorta is inconspicuous or absent (see Figs. 13–22 through 13–27), with rare exception (see Fig. 13–21).

THE ECHOCARDIOGRAM

Echocardiography with color flow imaging and Doppler interrogation establishes the diagnosis and severity of Ebstein's anomaly.[30,72,100,101,108,109] The diagnosis can be made in utero.[64,102,105,128] Apical displacement of the septal tricuspid leaflet exceeds 15 mm in children and 20 mm in adults (Fig. 13–30).[56,101] The right atrium proper lies proximal to the anatomic tricuspid annulus, and the atrialized right ventricle occupies the interval between the anatomic tricuspid annulus and the distally displaced septal tricuspid leaflet (see Fig. 13–30).[108] The displaced tethered septal tricuspid leaflet moves little if at all, in contrast to the large elongated anterior leaflet, which may exhibit brisk sail-like movements by real-time imaging (Fig. 13–31, and see Fig. 13–30).[108] Rarely, a broad echogenic band separates the atrialized right ventricle from the distal functional right ventricle, and the proximal annulus is unguarded by tricuspid leaflet tissue (Fig. 13–32).[73,142] Echocardiography defines left ventricular geometry and cavity size, and real-time imaging identifies displacement of the ventricular septum into the left ventricular cavity with paradoxical motion of the septum (see Fig. 13–31).[18,110] Superior systolic displacement (prolapse) occurs because normal-sized mitral leaflets and chordae tendineae are housed in a left ventricular cavity that is reduced in size and altered in shape (see Fig. 13–31).[18] The right ventricular outflow tract in the short axis is dilated, in contrast to the adjacent normal or small aortic root. Color flow imaging and Doppler interrogation quantify tricuspid regurgitation and establish the relatively low velocity of regurgitant flow, which begins at the level of the displaced septal and posterior leaflets and courses through the atrialized right ventricle into the right atrium proper (Figs. 13–33 and 13–34).

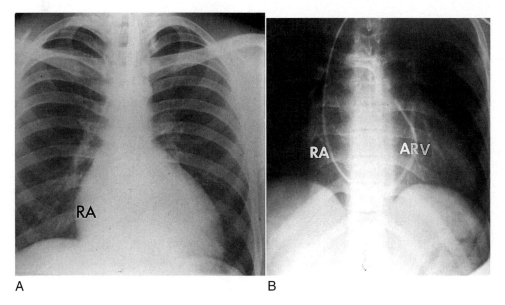

A   B

Figure 13–24

X-rays from an 18-year-old cyanotic man with Ebstein's anomaly. *A*, The increase in heart size is due to enlargement of the right atrium (RA) and atrialized right ventricle. The vascular pedicle is narrow. *B*, The loop of the catheter outlines the right atrium (RA) and contiguous atrialized right ventricle (ARV).

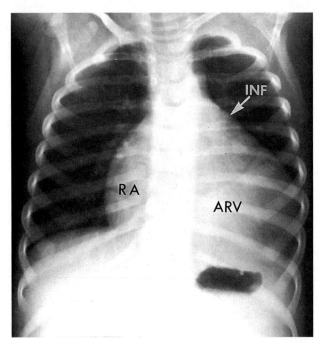

Figure 13–25
X-ray from a 19-month-old acyanotic girl with Ebstein's anomaly. The lung fields are oligemic. The infundibulum (INF) is prominent, but neither the pulmonary trunk nor the ascending aorta is border forming. Cardiac enlargement is due to a huge right atrium (RA) and the atrialized right ventricle (ARV).

Echocardiography identifies a patent foramen ovale or an ostium secundum atrial septal defect, and color flow imaging with Doppler interrogation confirms the presence of the interatrial communication and determines whether a right-to-left shunt coexists.

SUMMARY

Cyanosis with normal or reduced pulmonary blood flow and a dominant left ventricle is a useful combination in the clinical diagnosis of Ebstein's anomaly. When these features are supplemented by type B Wolff-Parkinson-White preexcitation, the diagnosis is virtually secure. Outlook is poorest in symptomatic newborns, but neonatal cyanosis occasionally regresses only to recur years later. The crests of the A and V waves and the mean jugular venous pressure are normal. An enlarged infundibulum is palpable in the third left intercostal space, but a right ventricular inflow impulse is conspicuous by its absence. The first heart sound is widely split, and the tricuspid component is loud and delayed. The low-pressure tricuspid regurgitation murmur is early systolic, decrescendo, medium frequency, and maximum toward the apex over the displaced tricuspid valve. Triple or quadruple rhythms are caused by third and fourth heart sounds that may fuse to form short middiastolic or presystolic murmurs, especially when the PR interval is prolonged. The electrocardiogram is characterized by tall broad right atrial P waves, a prolonged PR interval, right bundle branch block, and deep Q waves in right precordial leads. The x-ray shows normal or decreased pulmonary vascularity, a narrow vascular pedicle, a prominent infundibulum, and a large right atrium. In symptomatic neonates, the cardiac silhouette may occupy virtually the entire chest. Echocardiography, color flow imaging, and Doppler interrogation identify abnormalities of the three tricuspid leaflets and identify the atrialized right ventricle, paradoxical motion of the ventricular septum, the size and shape of the left ventricle, the degree of

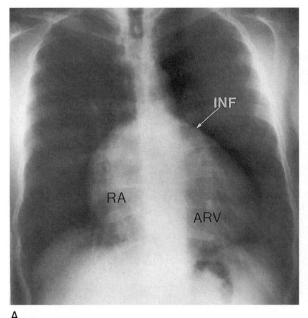

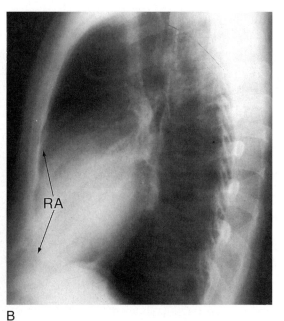

A   B

Figure 13–26
X-rays from an acyanotic 41-year-old man with Ebstein's anomaly and exercise-induced hypoxemia. The lung fields are oligemic, although the film is overpenetrated. *A,* The infundibulum (INF) is prominent but the vascular pedicle is narrow because neither the ascending aorta nor the pulmonary trunk is border forming. Cardiac enlargement is due to a huge right atrium (RA) and the atrialized right ventricle (ARV). The x-ray bears a striking resemblance to Figure 13–25 from the 19-month-old acyanotic girl with Ebstein's anomaly. *B,* The retrosternal space is occupied by the enlarged right atrium (RA; *arrows*).

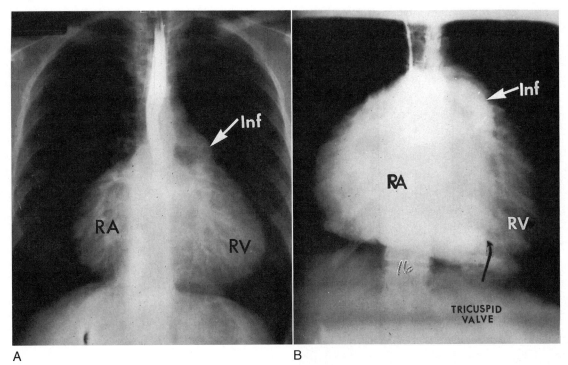

A

B

Figure 13–27

X-ray and angiocardiogram from a 32-year-old acyanotic woman with Ebstein's anomaly. *A,* The infundibulum (Inf) is prominent but the vascular pedicle is narrow because neither the ascending aorta nor the pulmonary trunk is border forming. Cardiomegaly is due to enlargement of the right atrium (RA) and atrialized right ventricle. (RV, functional right ventricle). The lung fields are remarkably clear, although the x-ray is overpenetrated. *B,* Angiocardiogram shows the huge right atrium and contiguous atrialized right ventricle with the displaced tricuspid valve *(arrow).* The cardiac silhouette is boxlike because of the prominent infundibulum and the large right atrium.

tricuspid regurgitation, and the presence of a patent foramen ovale or an atrial septal defect.

Uhl's Anomaly

Parchment heart was so designated by Osler in 1905[92] and was redescribed by Segall in 1950.[114] Two years later,

Uhl reported "almost total absence of myocardium of the right ventricle."[131] Uhl's anomaly consists of aplasia or hypoplasia of most if not all of the myocardium in the trabecular portions of the right ventricle in the presence of a

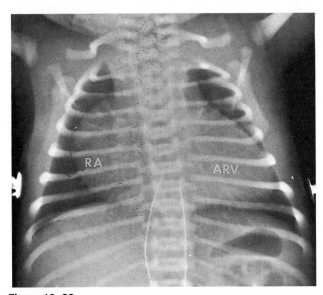

Figure 13–28

X-ray from a symptomatic cyanotic female neonate with Ebstein's anomaly. The huge cardiac silhouette covers all but a fraction of oligemic lung fields. Cardiomegaly is due to a huge right atrium (RA) and the atrialized right ventricle (ARV). Diagnosis was confirmed at necropsy.

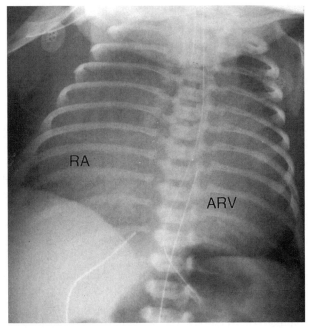

Figure 13–29

X-ray from a symptomatic cyanotic male neonate with Ebstein's anomaly. Striking cardiomegaly was due to a huge right atrium (RA) and atrialized right ventricle (ARV). Thymus occupies the thoracic inlet. Compare to Figure 13–28. Diagnosis was confirmed at necropsy.

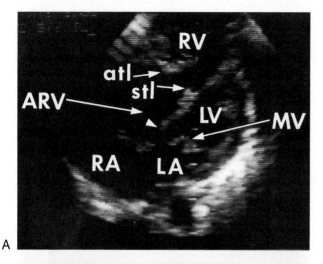

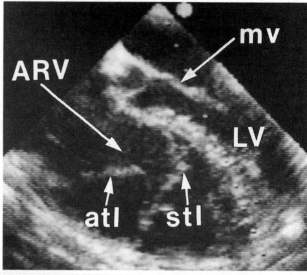

Figure 13–31

Transesophageal echocardiogram from the 41-year-old man whose x-rays are shown in Figure 13–26. An immobile septal tricuspid leaflet (stl) is apically displaced. The large nondisplaced anterior tricuspid leaflet (atl) was highly mobile on real-time imaging. The size and configuration of the left ventricle (LV) are abnormal because of encroachment by the ventricular septum. ARV, atrialized right ventricle; mv, mitral valve.

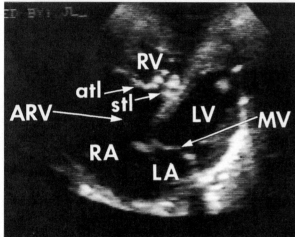

Figure 13–30

Echocardiograms (apical four-chamber) from a 5-year-old female with acyanotic Ebstein's anomaly. The septal tricuspid leaflet (stl) is displaced into the right ventricle and tethered to the septum. The large anterior tricuspid leaflet (atl) was highly mobile in real-time imaging and is shown here in diastole (A) and in systole (B). A, The atrialized right ventricle (ARV) lies between the displaced septal tricuspid leaflet and the anatomic tricuspid anulus (*unmarked arrowhead*). The functional right ventricle (RV) lies distally, and the anatomic right atrium (RA) lies proximally. LA, left atrium; LV, left ventricle; MV, mitral valve.

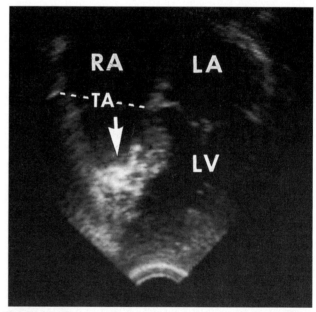

Figure 13–32

Echocardiogram (four-chamber view) from an 8-week-old girl with cyanotic Ebstein's anomaly. *Unmarked arrow* points to a broad echogenic band that completely divided the atrialized right ventricle from the functional right ventricle. At necropsy, the thick muscular partition was partially calcified. The tricuspid annulus (TA) above the partition was devoid of tricuspid leaflet tissue. LA, left atrium; LV, left ventricle; RA, right atrium.

structurally normal and functionally competent tricuspid valve.[7,19,32,34,53,103,133] The parchment right ventricle of Uhl's anomaly has been characterized as *inexcitable,* in contrast to the arrhythmogenic atrialized right ventricle of the Ebstein's anomaly heart.[20] Uhl's anomaly has been reported in identical twins[62] and has been diagnosed in utero.

The basic hemodynamic fault in Uhl's anomaly is lack of right ventricular contraction. The chamber functions as a passive conduit through which right atrial blood is channeled on its way to the pulmonary trunk.[32] The thin-walled right ventricle balloons aneurysmally with each systole.[32] The morphologically uninvolved ventricular septum exhibits vigorous paradoxical systolic motion and functions as part of the right ventricle, contributing materially to forward flow.[32]

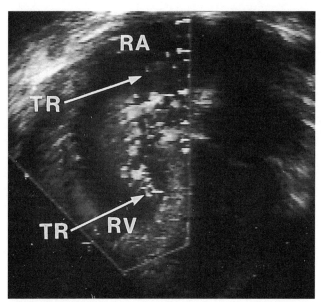

Figure 13–33
Echocardiograms from a 3-month-old girl with Ebstein's anomaly. Black and white print of a color flow image shows the jet of tricuspid regurgitation (TR) originating at the junction of the functional right ventricle (RV) and the atrialized right ventricle. RA, right atrium.

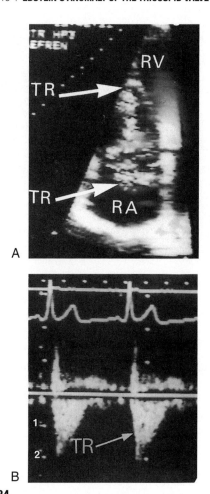

Figure 13–34
A, Black and white print of a color flow image from a 19-year-old man with acyanotic Ebstein's anomaly. The jet of tricuspid regurgitation (TR) originates within the right ventricular cavity at the junction of the functional right ventricle (RV) and the atrialized right ventricle. RA, right atrium. *B,* Continuous-wave Doppler shows the low-velocity tricuspid regurgitant jet (TR).

Survival into adulthood is expected despite the functionally inadequate right ventricle. The jugular venous pulse is normal because the tricuspid valve is competent and because the force of right atrial contraction is not increased despite the parchment right ventricle. An elevation in right ventricular end-diastolic pressure and mean right atrial pressure rarely causes a right-to-left shunt through a patent foramen ovale.[32] A left ventricular impulse occupies the apex, but a right ventricular impulse is absent by definition. A right ventricular third heart sound is generated by passive flow into the poorly compliant right ventricle. The second heart sound is widely split even though the right ventricular conduction defect is believed to be peripheral (Fig. 13–35). The electrocardiogram shows right atrial P waves (see Fig. 13–35) because the right atrium tends to be larger than normal despite a

competent tricuspid valve (Fig. 13–36).[32] The PR interval is normal, and preexcitation is unknown. The x-ray shows normal pulmonary vascularity and an increase in heart size due chiefly to the dilated right ventricle (see Fig. 13–36).

Figure 13–35
Electrocardiogram from a 25-year-old woman with Uhl's anomaly. A right atrial abnormality is indicated by the deep broad P terminal force in lead V_1 and the tall peaked P wave in lead V_2. The QRS duration is prolonged because of what appears to be a right ventricular conduction defect despite absence of right ventricular myocardium.

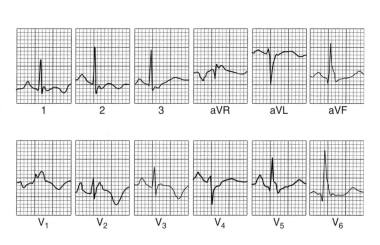

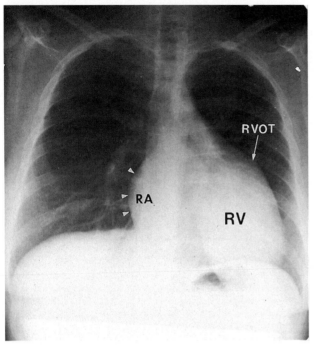

Figure 13–36

X-ray from a 25-year-old woman with Uhl's anomaly. The heart is enlarged because of dilatation of the right ventricle (RV) and right atrium (RA). The right ventricular outflow tract (RVOT) is hump-shaped. The ascending aorta is inconspicuous.

ventricular septum, and normal tricuspid leaflets (Fig. 13–37). Doppler echocardiography with color flow imaging confirms the competence of the tricuspid valve.

Arrhythmogenic right ventricular dysplasia varies from mild focal lesions detected histologically to widespread segmental transmural involvement of the free wall of the right ventricle and infundibulum.[23,25,39,82,89,133,134] Biventricular involvement occurs infrequently.[40,147] Prevalence has been estimated at 1 in 5000.[145] Dysplasia is represented by focal replacement of myocardium with fibrous and adipose tissue, not by focal congenital absence of the myocardium.[82,89] The lesions can be detected by magnetic resonance imaging[23] and by low-amplitude endocardial electrograms that identify replaced myocardium.[17]

Familial recurrence of right ventricular dysplasia[82] has been confirmed in a study of nine families.[89] The echocardiogram discloses segmental and generalized abnormalities of right ventricular wall motion, abnormal trabecular architecture, and areas of saccular dilatation.[10,89] Isolated noncompaction of left ventricular myocardium or Barth syndrome is arrhythmogenic and is characterized morphologically by numerous prominent trabeculations and conspicuous intertrabecular recesses that penetrate deeply into the left ventricular myocardium.[33,65]

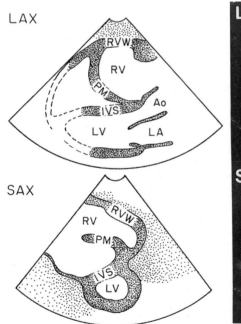

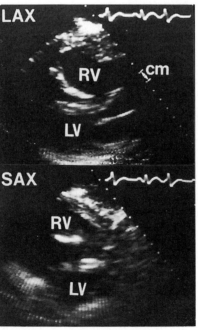

Figure 13–37

Echocardiograms (parasternal long-axis, LAX, and short-axis, SAX) from the 25-year-old woman with Uhl's anomaly whose x-ray is shown in Fig. 13–36. The right ventricle (RV) is dilated and its cavity contains a large refractile papillary muscle (PM) shown in the short axis sketch. The interventricular septum (IVS, labeled in the sketches) exhibited brisk paradoxical systolic motion in real time, whereas the right ventricular wall (RVW, labeled in the sketch) was akinetic. Ao, aorta; LA, left atrium. (From Child JS, Perloff JK, et al: Uhl's anomaly [parchment right ventricle]. Am J Cardiol 53:635, 1984.)

The right atrial silhouette is rounded but unimpressive compared with Ebstein's anomaly (see Fig. 13–36). The morphologically spared infundibulum presents as a hump-shaped convexity at the upper left cardiac border (see Fig. 13–36). Echocardiography identifies a large right ventricle with an akinetic free wall, brisk paradoxical motion of the

REFERENCES

1. Adams JCL, Hudson R: Case of Ebstein's anomaly surviving to age of seventy-nine. Br Heart J 18:129, 1956.
2. Anderson KR, Lie JT: Pathologic anatomy of Ebstein's anomaly of the heart revisited. Am J Cardiol 41:739, 1978.
3. Anderson KR, Lie JT: Right ventricular myocardium in Ebstein's anomaly. Mayo Clin Proc 54:181, 1979.

4. Anderson KR, Zuberbuhler JR, Anderson RH, et al: Morphologic spectrum of Ebstein's anomaly of the heart. Mayo Clin Proc 54:174, 1979.

5. Anderson RH, Silverman NH, Zuberbuhler JR: Congenitally unguarded tricuspid orifice: Its differentiation from Ebstein's malformation in association with pulmonary atresia and intact ventricular septum. Pediatr Cardiol 11:86, 1990.

6. Antra AU, Osunkoya BO: Congenital tricuspid incompetence. Br Heart J 31:664, 1969.

7. Arcilla RA, Gasul BM: Congenital aplasia or marked hypoplasia of the myocardium of the right ventricle (Uhl's anomaly). J Pediatr 58:381, 1961.

8. Celermajor DS, Bull C, Till JA, et al: Ebstein's anomaly: Presentation and outcome from fetus to adult. J Am Coll Cardiol 23:170, 1994.

9. Balaji S, Dennis NR, Keeton BR: Familial Ebstein's anomaly: A report of 6 cases in two generations associated with mild skeletal abnormalities. Br Heart J 66:26, 1991.

10. Baran A, Falkoff M, Barold SS, Gallagher JJ: Two-dimensional echocardiographic detection of arrhythmogenic right ventricular dysplasia. Am Heart J 103:1066, 1982.

11. Barber G, Danielson GK, Heise CT, Driscoll DJ: Cardiorespiratory response to exercise in Ebstein's anomaly. Am J Cardiol 56:509, 1985.

12. Obio-Ngwa O, Milliez P, Richardson A, et al: Ventricular tachycardia in Ebstein's anomaly. Circulation 104:92, 2001.

13. Barritt DW, Urich H: Congenital tricuspid incompetence. Br Heart J 18:133, 1956.

14. Bashour TT, Saalouke M, Yazji ZI: Apical left ventricular diverticulum with Ebstein malformation. Am Heart J 115:1332, 1988.

15. Becker AE, Becker MJ, Edwards JE: Pathologic spectrum of dysplasia of the tricuspid valve: Features in common with Ebstein's malformation. Arch Pathol 91:167, 1971.

16. Beder SD, Nihill MR, McNamara DG: Idiopathic dilatation of the right atrium in a child. Am Heart J 103:134, 1982.

17. Boulos M, Lashevsky I, Reisner S, Gepstein L: Electroanatomic mapping of arrhythmogenic right ventricular dysplasia. J Am Coll Cardiol 38:2020, 2001.

18. Benson LN, Child JS, Schwaiger M, et al: Left ventricular geometry and function in Ebstein's anomaly of the tricuspid valve. Circulation 75:353, 1987.

19. Berwick DJ, Chandler BM, Montagne TJ: Dilated right ventricular cardiomyopathy: Uhl's anomaly. Chest 90:300, 1986.

20. Bharati S, Ciraulo DA, Bilitch M, et al: Inexcitable right ventricle and bilateral bundle branch block in Uhl's disease. Circulation 57:636, 1978.

21. Bialostozky D, Horitz S, Espino-Vela J: Ebstein's malformation of the tricuspid valve: A review of 65 cases. Am J Cardiol 29:826, 1972.

22. Bialostozky D, Medrano GA, Munoz L, Contrera S: Vectorcardiographic study and anatomic observations in 21 cases of Ebstein's malformation of the tricuspid valve. Am J Cardiol 30:354, 1972.

23. Candinas R, Duru F: Unusual clinical presentation of a patient with an extreme form of right ventricular dysplasia. Circulation 104:848, 2001.

24. Fitzsimmons PJ, McWhirter PD, Peterson DW, Kruyer WR: The natural history of Wolff-Parkinson-White syndrome in 228 aviators: A long-term follow-up of 22 years. Am Heart J 142:530, 2001.

25. Ouyang F, Fotuhi P, Goya M, et al: Ventricular tachycardia around the tricuspid annulus in right ventricular dysplasia. Circulation 103:913, 2001.

26. Cabin HS, Roberts WC: Ebstein's anomaly of the tricuspid valve and prolapse of the mitral valve. Am Heart J 101:177, 1981.

27. Cabin HS, Wood TP, Smith JO, Roberts WC: Ebstein's anomaly in the elderly. Chest 80:212, 1981.

28. Hong YM, Moller JH: Ebstein's anomaly: A long-term study of survival. Am Heart J 125:1419, 1993.

29. Castaneda-Zuniga W, Nath HP, Moller JH, Edwards JE: Left-sided anomalies in Ebstein's malformation of the tricuspid valve. Pediatr Cardiol 3:181, 1982.

30. Celermajor DS, Cullen S, Sullivan ID, et al: Outcome in neonates with Ebstein's anomaly. J Am Coll Cardiol 19:1041, 1992.

31. Celermajor DS, Dodd SM, Greenwald SE, et al: Morbid anatomy in neonates with Ebstein's anomaly of the tricuspid valve: Pathophysiologic and clinical implications. J Am Coll Cardiol 19:1049, 1992.

32. Child JS, Perloff JK, Francoz R, et al: Uhl's anomaly (parchment right ventricle): Clinical, echocardiographic, radionuclear, hemodynamic and angiocardiographic features. Am J Cardiol 53:635, 1984.

33. Chin TK, Perloff JK, Williams RG, et al: Isolated noncompaction of left ventricular myocardium. Circulation 82:507, 1990.

34. Cote M, Davignon A, Fouron J: Congenital hypoplasia of the right ventricular myocardium (Uhl's anomaly). Am J Cardiol 31:658, 1973.

35. Crews TL, Pridie RB, Benham R, Leatham A: Auscultatory and phonocardiographic findings in Ebstein's anomaly: Correlation of first heart sound with ultrasonic records of tricuspid valve movement. Br Heart J 34:681, 1972.

36. Donegan CC, Moore MM, Wiley TM, et al: Familial Ebstein anomaly of the tricuspid valve. Am Heart J 75:375, 1968.

37. Donnelly JE, Brown JM, Radford DJ: Pregnancy outcome and Ebstein's anomaly. Br Heart J 66:368, 1991.

38. Driscoll DJ, Mottram CD, Danielson GK: Spectrum of exercise intolerance in 45 patients with Ebstein's anomaly and observations on exercise tolerance in 11 patients after surgical repair. J Am Coll Cardiol 11:831, 1988.

39. Dungan WT, Garson A, Gillette PC: Arrhythmogenic right ventricular dysplasia: A cause of ventricular tachycardia in children with apparently normal hearts. Am Heart J 102:745, 1981.

40. Pinamonti B, Pagnan L, Bussani R, et al: Right ventricular dysplasia with biventricular involvement. Circulation 98:1943, 1998.

41. Ebstein W: On a very rare case of insufficiency of the tricuspid valve caused by a severe congenital malformation of the same. Arch F Anat Physiol Wissensch Med Leipz 238, 1866. Translated by Schiebler GL, Gravenstein JS, Van Mierop LHS: Am J Cardiol 22:867, 1968.

42. Emanuel R, O'Brien K, Ng R: Ebstein's anomaly: Genetic study of 26 families. Br Heart J 38:5, 1976.

43. Engle MA, Payne TPB, Bruins C, Taussig HB: Ebstein's anomaly of the tricuspid valve: Report of three cases and analysis of clinical syndrome. Circulation 1:1246, 1950.

44. Follath F, Hallidie-Smith KA: Unusual electrocardiographic changes in Ebstein's anomaly. Br Heart J 34:513, 1972.

45. Fontana ME, Wooley CF: Sail sound in Ebstein's anomaly of the tricuspid valve. Circulation 46:155, 1972.

46. Attie F, Rosas M, Rijlaarsdam M, et al: The adult patient with Ebstein anomaly: Outcome in 72 unoperated patients. Medicine 79:27, 2000.

47. Yefman AT, Freedom RM, McCrindle BW: Outcome in cyanotic neonates with Ebstein's anomaly. Am J Cardiol 81:749, 1998.

48. Gellenberg AJ: Lithium efficacy and adverse effects. J Clin Psychiatry 49:8, 1988.

49. Gentles TL, Calder AL, Clarkson PM, Neutze JM: Predictors of long-term survival with Ebstein's anomaly of the tricuspid valve. Am J Cardiol 69:377, 1992.

50. Genton E, Blount SG Jr: The spectrum of Ebstein's anomaly. Am Heart J 73:395, 1967.

51. Gewillig M, Dumoulin M, van der Hanwaert LG: Transient neonatal tricuspid regurgitation. Br Heart J 60:446, 1988.

52. Giuliani ER, Fuster V, Brandenberg RO: Ebstein's anomaly. Mayo Clin Proc 54:163, 1979.

53. Gould L, Guttman AB, Carrasco J, Lyon AF: Partial absence of the right ventricular musculature. Am J Med 42:636, 1968.

54. Gueron M, Hirsch M, Stern J, et al: Familial Ebstein's anomaly with emphasis on the surgical treatment. Am J Cardiol 18:105, 1966.

55. Gussenhoven EJ, Essed CE, Bos E: Unguarded tricuspid orifice with two-chambered right ventricle. Pediatr Cardiol 7:175, 1986.

56. Gussenhoven EJ, Stewart PA, Becker AE, et al: "Offsetting" of the septal tricuspid leaflet in normal hearts and in hearts with Ebstein's anomaly. Am J Cardiol 54:172, 1984.

57. Hallali P, Iung B, Davido A, et al: Congenital diverticulum of the right ventricle: Report of two cases associated with other congenital heart defects. Am Heart J 117:957, 1989.

58. Hamaoka K, Onaka M, Tanaka T, Onouchi Z: Congenital ventricular aneurysm and diverticulum in children. Pediatr Cardiol 8:169, 1987.

59. Harris RHD: Ebstein's anomaly: Discovered in a seventy-five year old subject in the dissecting laboratory. Can Med Assoc J 83:653, 1960.

60. Hauck AJ, Freeman DP, Ackermann DM, et al: Surgical pathology of the tricuspid valve: A study of 363 cases spanning 25 years. Mayo Clin Proc 63:851, 1988.

61. Hernandez FA, Rochkind R, Cooper HR: Intracavitary electrocardiogram in the diagnosis of Ebstein's anomaly. Am J Cardiol 1:181, 1958.

62. Hoback J, Adicoff A, From AHL, et al: A report of Uhl's disease in identical adult twins. Chest 79:306, 1981.

63. Wolff L, Parkinson J, White PD: Bundle-branch block with short P-R interval in healthy young people prone to paroxysmal tachycardia. Am Heart J 5:685, 1930.

64. Hornberger LK, Sahn DJ, Kleinman CS, et al: Tricuspid valve disease with significant tricuspid insufficiency in the fetus: Diagnosis and outcome. J Am Coll Cardiol 17:167, 1991.

65. Ichida F, Tsubata S, Boles KR, et al: Novel gene mutations in patients with left ventricular noncompaction or Barth syndrome. Circulation 103:1256, 2001.

66. Kanjuh VI, Stevenson JE, Amplatz K, Edwards JE: Congenitally unguarded tricuspid orifice with co-existent pulmonary atresia. Circulation 30:911, 1964.

67. Kastor JA, Goldreyer BN, Josephson ME, et al: Electrophysiological characteristics in Ebstein's anomaly of the tricuspid valve. Circulation 52:987, 1975.

68. Kerwin AJ: Ebstein's anomaly: Report of a case diagnosed during life. Br Heart J 17:109, 1955.

69. Scheinman MM: Brugada syndrome. Baylor Univ Med Center Proc 14:127, 2001.

70. Koiwaya Y, Narabayashi H, Koyanagi S, et al: Early closure of the tricuspid valve in a case of Ebstein's anomaly with Type B Wolff-Parkinson-White syndrome. Circulation 60:446, 1979.

71. Kumar AE, Flyer DC, Miettinen OS, Nadas AS: Ebstein's anomaly: Clinical profile and natural history. Am J Cardiol 28:84, 1971.

72. Lang D, Oberhoffer R, Cook A, et al: Pathologic spectrum of malformations of the tricuspid valve in prenatal and neonatal life. J Am Coll Cardiol 17:1161, 1991.

73. Leung ME, Baker EJ, Anderson RH, Zuberbuhler JR: Cineangiographic spectrum of Ebstein's malformation: Its relevance to clinical presentation and outcome. J Am Coll Cardiol 11:154, 1988.

74. Surawicz B: Brugada syndrome: Manifest, concealed, "asymptomatic," suspected and simulated. J Am Coll Cardiol 38:775, 2001.

75. Lev M, Liberthson RR, Joseph RH, et al: The pathologic anatomy of Ebstein's anomaly. Arch Pathol 90:334, 1970.

76. Lo H, Lin F, Jong Y, et al: Ebstein's anomaly with ventricular tachycardia: Evidence for the arrhythmogenic role of the atrialized ventricle. Am Heart J 117:959, 1989.

77. Lo KS, Loventhal JP, Walton JA: Familial Ebstein's anomaly. Cardiology 64:246, 1979.

78. Lowe KG, Emslie-Smith D, Robertson PGC, Watson H: Scalar, vector, and intracardiac electrocardiograms in Ebstein's anomaly. Br Heart J 30:617, 1968.

79. Macruz R, Tranchesi J, Ebaird M, et al: Ebstein's disease: Electrovectorcardiographic and radiologic correlations. Am J Cardiol 21:653, 1968.

80. Makous N, Vander Veer JB: Ebstein's anomaly and life expectancy: Report of a survival to over seventy-nine. Am J Cardiol 18:100, 1966.

81. Mann RJ, Lie JT: The life story of Wilhelm Ebstein (1836–1912) and his almost overlooked description of a congenital heart disease. Mayo Clin Proc 54:197, 1979.

82. Marcus FI, Fontaine GH, Guiraudon G, et al: Right ventricular dysplasia: A report of 24 adult cases. Circulation 65:384, 1982.

83. Durrer D, Roos JP: Epicardial excitation of the ventricles in a patient with Wolff-Parkinson-White syndrome (type B). Circulation 35:15, 1967.

84. Mayer FE, Nadas AS, Ongley PA: Ebstein's anomaly: Presentation of ten cases. Circulation 16:1057, 1957.

85. McIntosh N, Chitayat D, Bardanis M, Fouron J: Ebstein's anomaly: Report of a familial occurrence and prenatal diagnosis. Am J Med Genet 42:307, 1992.

86. Moles SS, Jacoby WJ Jr, McIntosh HD: Ebstein's malformation: Discordant intracavitary electrocardiographic and pressure relationship. Am J Cardiol 14:720, 1964.

87. Monibi AA, Neches WH, Lenox CC, et al: Left ventricular anomalies associated with Ebstein's malformation of the tricuspid valve. Circulation 57:303, 1978.

88. Mu-Sheng T, Partridge J, Radford D: A plain chest radiograph in uncomplicated Ebstein's disease. Clin Radiol 37:551, 1986.

89. Nava A, Thiene G, Canciani B, et al: Familial occurrence of right ventricular dysplasia: A study involving 9 families. J Am Coll Cardiol 12:1222, 1988.

90. Nora JJ, Nora AH, Toews WH: Lithium, Ebstein's anomaly and other congenital heart defects. Lancet 2:594, 1974.

91. Oldenburg FA, Nichol AD: Ebstein's anomaly in the adult. Ann Intern Med 52:710, 1960.

92. Osler W: The Principles and Practice of Medicine, 6th ed. New York, Appleton-Century-Crofts, 1905, p. 820.

93. Park JM, Sridaromont S, Ledbetter EO, Terry WM: Ebstein's anomaly of the tricuspid valve associated with prenatal exposure to lithium carbide. Am J Dis Child 134:703, 1980.

94. Gollob MH, Seger JJ, Gollob TN: Novel PRKAG 2 mutation responsible for the genetic syndrome of ventricular preexcitation and conduction system disease with childhood onset and absence of cardiac hypertrophy. Circulation 104:3030, 2001.

95. Perloff JK: Physical Examination of the Heart and Circulation, 3rd ed. Philadelphia, W.B. Saunders, 2000.

96. Oki T, Fukuda N, Tabata T, et al: The sail sound and tricuspid regurgitation in Ebstein's anomaly: The value of echocardiography in evaluating their mechanisms. L Heart Valve Dis 6:189, 1997.

97. Pierard LA, Henard L, Demoulin J: Persistent atrial standstill in familial Ebstein's anomaly. Br Heart J 53:594, 1985.

98. Pocock WA, Tucker RBK, Barlow JB: Mild Ebstein's anomaly. Br Heart J 31:327, 1969.

99. Price JE, Amsterdam EA, Vera Z, et al: Ebstein's disease associated with complete atrioventricular block. Chest 73:542, 1978.

100. Radford DJ, Graff RF, Neilson GH: Diagnosis and natural history of Ebstein's anomaly. Br Heart J 54:517, 1985.

101. Ammash NM, Warnes CA, Connolly HM, et al: Mimics of Ebstein's anomaly. Am Heart J 134:508, 1997.

102. Hsieh YY, Lee CC, Chang CC, et al: Successful prenatal digoxin therapy for Ebstein's anomaly with hydrops fetalis. J Reprod Med 43:710, 1998.

103. Reeve R, Macdonald D: Partial absence of right ventricular musculature-partial parchment heart. Am J Cardiol 14:415, 1964.

104. Reynolds G: Ebstein's disease: A case diagnosed clinically. Guy's Hosp Rep 99:276, 1950.

105. Roberson DA, Silverman NH: Ebstein's anomaly: Echocardiographic and clinical features in the fetus and neonate. J Am Coll Cardiol 14:1300, 1989.

106. Roberts WC, Glancy DL, Seningen RP, et al: Prolapse of the mitral valve (floppy valve) associated with Ebstein's anomaly of the tricuspid valve. Am J Cardiol 38:377, 1976.

107. Rossi L, Thiene G: Mild Ebstein's anomaly associated with supraventricular tachycardia and sudden death: Clinicomorphologic features in three patients. Am J Cardiol 53:332, 1984.

108. Rusconi PG, Zuberbuhler JR, Anderson RH, Rigby ML: Morphologic-echocardiographic correlates of Ebstein's malformation. Eur Heart J 12:784, 1991.

109. Saxena A, Fong LV, Tristam M, et al: Late noninvasive evaluation of cardiac performance in mildly symptomatic older patients with Ebstein's anomaly of the tricuspid valve: Role of radionuclide imaging. J Am Coll Cardiol 17:182, 1991.

110. Saxena A, Fong LV, Tristam M, et al: Left ventricular function in patients greater than 20 years of age with Ebstein's anomaly of the tricuspid valve. Am J Cardiol 67:217, 1991.

111. Samanek M: Boy:girl ratio in children born with different forms of cardiac malformation: A population-based study. Pediatr Cardiol 15:53, 1994.

112. Schiebler GL, Adams P Jr, Anderson RC, et al: Clinical study of 23 cases of Ebstein's anomaly of the tricuspid valve. Circulation 19:165, 1959.

113. Correa-Villasenor A, Ferenz C, Neill CA, et al: Ebstein's malformation of the tricuspid valve: Genetic and environmental factors. The Washington-Baltimore infant study group. Teratology 50:137, 1994.

114. Segall HN: Parchment heart (Osler). Am Heart J 40:948, 1950.

115. Sekelj P, Bensey BG: Historical landmarks: Ebstein's anomaly of the tricuspid valve. Am Heart J 88:108, 1974.

116. Seward JB, Tajik AJ, Feist DJ, Smith HC: Ebstein's anomaly in an 85 year old man. Mayo Clin Proc 54:193, 1979.

117. Choi YH, Park JH, Choe YH, Yoo SJ: Magnetic resonance imaging of Ebstein's anomaly of the tricuspid valve. Am J Roentgenol 163:539, 1994.

118. Sheldon WC, Johnson DC, Favaloro RG: Idiopathic enlargement of the right atrium. Am J Cardiol 23:278, 1969.

119. Kahn IA, Cohen RA: Ebstein's anomaly of the tricuspid valve associated with congenital deafmutism. Int J Cardiol 70:219, 1999.

120. Ho SY, Goltz D, McCarthy K, et al: The atrioventricular junctions in Ebstein's malformation. Heart 83:444, 2000.

121. Silver MD, Lam JHC, Ranganathan N, Wigle ED: Morphology of the human tricuspid valve. Circulation 43:333, 1971.

122. Simcha A, Bonham-Carter RE: Ebstein's anomaly: Clinical study of 32 patients in childhood. Br Heart J 33:46, 1971.

123. Smith WM, Gallagher JJ, Kerr CR, et al: The electrophysiologic basis and management of symptomatic recurrent tachycardia in patients with Ebstein's anomaly of the tricuspid valve. Am J Cardiol 49:1223, 1982.

124. Dearini JA, Danielson GK: Congenital heart surgery nomenclature and database project: Ebstein's anomaly and tricuspid valve disease. Ann Thorac Surg 69:106, 2000.
125. Sodi-Pallares D, Marsico F: Importance of electrocardiographic patterns in congenital heart disease. Am Heart J 49:202, 1955.
126. Soloff LA, Stauffer HM, Zatuchni J: Ebstein's disease: Report of the first case diagnosed during life. Am J Med Sci 222:554, 1951.
127. Soloff LA, Stauffer HM, Zatuchni J: Ebstein's disease: Description of the heart of the first case diagnosed during life. Am J Med Sci 233:23, 1957.
128. Pavlova M, Fouron JC, Drblik SP, et al: Factors affecting the prognosis of Ebstein's anomaly during fetal life. Am Heart J 135:1081, 1998.
129. Tourniaire M, Deyrieux F, Tartulier M: Maladie d'Epstein. Arch Mal Coeur 42:1211, 1949.
130. Frescura C, Angelini A, Daliento L, Thiene G: Morphologic aspects of Ebstein's anomaly in adults. Thorac Cardiovasc Surg 48:203, 2000.
131. Uhl HSM: Previously undescribed congenital malformation of the heart: Almost total absence of myocardium of the right ventricle. Bull Johns Hopkins Hosp 91:197, 1952.
132. Vacca JB, Bussmann DW, Mudd JG: Ebstein's anomaly: Complete review of 108 cases. Am J Cardiol 2:210, 1958.
133. Vecht RJ, Carmichael DJS, Gopal R, Philip G: Uhl's anomaly. Br Heart J 41:676, 1979.
134. Virmani R, Rabinowitz M, Clark MA, McAllister HA: Sudden death and partial absence of right ventricular myocardium. Arch Pathol Lab Med 106:163, 1982.
135. Benson DW, Silberbach GM, Kavanaugh-McHugh A, et al: Mutations in the cardiac transcription factor NKX2.5 affect diverse cardiac developmental pathways. J Clin Invest 104:1567, 1999.
136. Watson H: Electrode catheters and the diagnosis of Ebstein's anomaly of the tricuspid valve. Br Heart J 28:161, 1966.
137. Watson H: Natural history of Ebstein's anomaly of tricuspid valve in childhood and adolescence: An international cooperative study of 505 cases. Br Heart J 36:417, 1974.
138. Willis PW, Craige E: The first heart sound in Ebstein's anomaly. J Am Coll Cardiol 2:1165, 1983.
139. Yater WM, Shapiro MJ: Congenital displacement of tricuspid valve (Ebstein's disease): Review and report of case. Ann Intern Med 11:1043, 1937.
140. Yim BJB, Yu PN: Value of an electrode catheter in diagnosis of Ebstein's disease. Circulation 17:543, 1958.
141. Zalzstein E, Koren G, Einarson T, Freedom RM: A case-control study on the association between first trimester exposure to lithium and Ebstein's anomaly. Am J Cardiol 65:817, 1990.
142. Zuberbuhler JR, Becker AE, Anderson RH, Lenox CC: Ebstein's malformation and the embryological development of the tricuspid valve. Pediatr Cardiol 5:289, 1984.
143. Van Son JA, Konstantinov IE, Zimmerman V: Wilhelm Ebstein and Ebstein's malformation. Eur J Cardiothorac Surg 20:1082, 2001.
144. Xie F, Qu Z, Garfinkle A: Dynamics of reentry around a circular obstacle in cardiac tissue. Physiol Rev 58:6355, 1998.
145. Gemayel C, Pelliccia A, Thompson PD: Arrhythmogenic right ventricular dysplasia. J Am Coll Cardiol 38:1773, 2001.
146. Wichter I, Matheja P, Eckardt L, Kies P: Cardiac autonomic dysfunction in Brugada syndrome. Circulation 105:702, 2002.
147. McCrohon JA, John AS, Lorenz CH, et al: Left ventricular involvement in arrhythmogenic right ventricular cardiomyopathy. Circulation 105:1394, 2002.
148. Priori SG, Napolitano C, Gasparini M, et al: Natural history of Brugada syndrome. Circulation 105:1342, 2002.

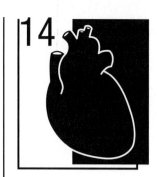

Primary Pulmonary Hypertension

Pulmonary arterial pressure was measured in 1852,[6] but a century then elapsed before cardiac catheterization set the stage for studying the physiology of lesser circulation. Elevated pulmonary arterial pressure, or *pulmonary hypertension*, results from disorders of the pulmonary vascular bed, the pulmonary parenchyma, and ventilation (Table 14–1).[60] This chapter focuses on the pulmonary vascular bed, specifically on primary pulmonary hypertension, a disorder that originates in the terminal muscular pulmonary arteries and arterioles.

The earliest description of idiopathic pulmonary hypertension was an 1891 report of the cardiac pathology in a patient with pulmonary artery sclerosis and right ventricular hypertrophy of unknown cause.[107] *Primary pulmonary hypertension*, a term coined by Dresdale in 1951, referred to an idiopathic disorder residing in the terminal pulmonary arteries and arterioles of three young women.[23] These age and sex patterns—young and female—have been borne out. A year after Dresdale's report, Wood characterized the clinical manifestations of primary pulmonary hypertension.[131] In 1973, the World Health Organization proposed a classification based on three histopathologic patterns: plexogenic pulmonary arteriopathy, microthrombotic pulmonary arteriopathy, and pulmonary veno-occlusive disease.[45] In 1981, the National Heart, Lung, and Blood Institute established

Table 14–1   **Etiologic Classification of Pulmonary Hypertension**

The pulmonary vascular bed: prearteriolar, arteriolar, venous

The pulmonary parenchyma: airway, interstitium

Alveolar hypoventilation: respiratory center depression, upper airway obstruction, chest bellows

a primary pulmonary hypertension registry designed to collect information in accordance with a uniform database.[99]

Primary pulmonary hypertension refers to a disorder with no identifiable cause in which pulmonary artery pressure at rest is above the normal of 30 mm Hg systolic and 18 mm Hg diastolic in adults at sea level. The definition, which was recommended by the World Health Organization, remains in current use,[45] and the histopathologic classification retains its credibility.[*]

The pulmonary vascular bed consists of an elaborately branched system of arteries, arterioles, capillaries, venules, and veins that accommodate the cardiac output at low flow pressures. Approximately 17 generations of arterial vascular channels separate the main pulmonary artery from the pulmonary arterioles. The pulmonary arteriole in the fetus is structurally analogous to the systemic arteriole and is designed to meet the full force of systemic pressure the moment the neonatal lungs expand and pulmonary blood flow commences. The thick-walled neonatal pulmonary arterioles rapidly involute, and the pulmonary vascular bed remodels, establishing the low-resistance lesser circulation. Remodeling continues for 1 or 2 months as the lungs adapt to extrauterine life, and then proceeds slowly as the pulmonary vascular bed matures throughout childhood.[46] The major airways and the major pulmonary arterial branches are formed by 16 weeks of gestation.[51]

An understanding of the density of small peripheral pulmonary arteries per unit area relative to alveolar density is crucial to an understanding of normal and abnormal fetal and postnatal pulmonary arterial development.[21,51,52,68,125] The number of peripheral acinar units increases in proportion to

---

[*]7, 13, 34, 50, 53, 56, 86, 97, 99, 101, 127, 129, 132.

the number of intra-acinar arteries until lung growth is completed at 8 to 10 years of age. Two thirds of the normal number of intra-acinar arteries are formed by 18 months and most of the remainder are formed by 5 years of age.[21,51,52] Also important is normal age-related distal extension of medial smooth muscle.[21,52] At birth, the vascular channels beyond the terminal bronchioles are devoid of medial smooth muscle, but within 2 to 3 years, medial smooth muscle extends to the junction of respiratory bronchioles and alveolar ducts and by the mid-teens extends among alveoli into precapillary vessels. The essential role of the pulmonary circulation is to receive oxygen passively and to eliminate carbon dioxide passively, in contrast to the systemic circulation, which delivers oxygen selectively to metabolizing tissues and therefore requires vasoreactive arterioles that regulate regional blood flow in accordance with local metabolic needs.

Heath and Edwards, in 1958, published elegant descriptions of the histopathology of pulmonary vascular disease together with a comprehensive classification.[49,128] The earliest identified abnormality was muscular thickening of small pulmonary arteries due to medial hyperplasia followed by intimal thickening (hyperplasia) that ranged from minimal to virtual luminal occlusion. The end-stage was the plexiform lesion that represents one of the three major histopathologic types of primary pulmonary hypertension in the World Health Organization classfication.[45]

Plexogenic pulmonary arteriopathy characterizes advanced pulmonary vascular disease irrespective of cause. The abnormality resides in small muscular arteries 100 to 200 μm in diameter and is a complex process that involves intimal cell proliferation, migration of medial smooth muscle cells, recruitment of inflammatory cells, and deposition of extracellular matrix proteins.[13,84,92,97,99,101] Intimal proliferation is disproportionate to medial hypertrophy and culminates in complete luminal obliteration. Plexiform lesions are found in upwards of 70% of patients with primary pulmonary hypertension.[97]

Microthrombotic pulmonary arteriopathy accounts for 20% to 50% of cases of primary pulmonary hypertension[97] and is represented by recanalized in situ microthrombi that consist of fibrous webs with eccentric intimal fibrosis together with medial hypertrophy but without plexiform lesions.[13,69,84,92,97,99,101]

Pulmonary veno-occlusive disease accounts for less than 7% of cases of primary pulmonary hypertension[97] and is characterized by intimal proliferation and fibrosis of intrapulmonary venules, culminating in complete obliteration of venous channels that tend to recanalize.[13,84,92,97,99,101]

Studies of pulmonary vascular pathophysiology employing light and electron microscopy have confirmed and extended the above observations (Table 14–2).[133] The clinical manifestations of primary pulmonary hypertension do not distinguish among these histopathologic types. Early vasoreactivity ultimately becomes fixed,[15,62,86,110,124,127] but once the disorder is established, it rarely regresses.[10,32,34,49,97,127,128]

Table 14–2	**Pulmonary Hypertension**

PULMONARY VASCULAR PATHOPHYSIOLOGY

Endothelium/subendothelium

Subendothelial migration of smooth muscle cells

Muscularization of nonmuscular intrapulmonary arteries

Medial hypertrophy of intrinsically muscular intrapulmonary arteries

PULMONARY VEINS

Migration of smooth muscle cells with a decrease in pulmonary vein compliance

Intimal proliferation with fragmentation of elastin and increased collagen

Modified from Ye C, Rabinovitch M: New developments in the pulmonary circulation in children. J Am Coll Cardiol 114:821, 1964.

Advances in pulmonary vascular biology continue to shed light on the pathogenesis of primary pulmonary hypertension.[1,25,84,98,100,116] Endothelial abnormalities have been identified (vasoconstrictor endothlin-1 homeostasis[3,4,5,151]) together with defects in voltage-gated potassium channels,[23,30] abnormalities in metalloproteinase and elastase activity,[30] in transforming growth factor-β,[143,144]and in bone morphogenetic protein.[29] Specific genetic molecular mechanisms are believed to be associated with familial as well as sporadic cases of primary pulmonary hypertension (see The History).[29,30,139–142]

Persistent fetal circulation or persistent pulmonary hypertension of the newborn is a disorder of unknown origin first described in 1969.[37] Muscularization of small pulmonary arteries in the fetal lung and high neonatal pulmonary vascular resistance do not regress in the neonate, so right-to-left shunts persist through the ductus arteriosus and foramen ovale.[36,37,42,47,81,95,114] A relationship between persistent fetal circulation and primary pulmonary hypertension is tenuous.

Portal hypertension may be associated with pulmonary hypertension because the pulmonary vascular bed is presumably exposed to vasoreactive substances normally metabolized by the liver.[17,103,109] An association between human immunodeficiency infection and hypertensive pulmonary arteriopathy has also been reported.[117] Alveolar hypoventilation and sleep apnea caused by chronic upper airway obstruction of hypertrophied tonsils and adenoids in children may result in an increase in pulmonary vascular resistance (see Table 14–1).[2,8,12,76] High-altitude pulmonary hypertension clinically and histologically resembles primary pulmonary hypertension, which is more common at high altitudes than at sea level, and low partial pressure of oxygen aggravates primary pulmonary hypertension (see The History).[63,82,113]

The physiologic consequences of primary pulmonary hypertension are direct reflections of the increased resistance to blood flow through the lesser circulation. The elevated pulmonary artery pressure can exceed systemic levels (see Fig. 14–3). Pulmonary vasoreactivity diminishes and ultimately is completely lost. Resting pulmonary blood flow and cardiac output fall below normal and either fail to increase during exercise or fall further.[83] Asymptomatic gene carriers for primary pulmonary hypertension have been identified by abnormal responses to exercise.[85]

Forceful right atrial contraction generates a large A wave and an increase in right ventricular end-diastolic segment length. The afterloaded right ventricle ultimately fails under its unrelenting burden. Right ventricular end-diastolic pressure rises, right atrial mean pressure rises, and a right-to-left shunt may be established through a patent foramen ovale that may be widely stretched. Systemic venous pressure may be sufficiently elevated to cause impaired choroidal perfusion and venous stasis retinopathy.[58,59]

The atrial natriuretic peptide system is highly activated in patients with primary pulmonary hypertension.[19] Atrial natriuretic peptide levels are significantly correlated with right ventricular preload and afterload and may protect from right ventricular failure.[19] Conversely, brain natriuretic peptide levels increase in proportion to right ventricular dysfunction.[14]

A mild albeit significant reduction in total lung capacity occurs in females with primary pulmonary hypertension, and a reduction in forced vital capacity is present in both males and females.[99] Hypoxemia and hypocapnia are almost invariable because of a ventilation-perfusion mismatch, not because of a right-to-left shunt across a patent foramen ovale.[99] The diffusing capacity for carbon monoxide is significantly less than predicted.[99] Nocturnal hypoxemia is common.[61]

The ventricular septum encroaches abnormally on the left ventricular cavity, sometimes appreciably (see Fig. 14–21). End-systolic and early diastolic deformation of the left ventricular cavity result in impaired filling in early diastole and in redistribution of filling in late diastole.[73,119] Early diastolic filling of the right ventricle is also encroached upon because high pulmonary vascular resistance prolongs the duration of right ventricular systole and prolongs isovolumetric relaxation.[119]

The time course of pulmonary hypertension can be determined from the histology of the pulmonary trunk relative to the histology of the aortic root.[33,35,38,48,105,127,128] When pulmonary hypertension begins at birth, the histology of the pulmonary trunk and aortic root are virtually indistinguishable (Fig. 14–1C,D). When pulmonary hypertension begins after birth, the histology of the pulmonary trunk and aortic root differ significantly (Fig. 14–1A,B). Primary pulmonary hypertension is only exceptionally present at birth (con genitas),[33,48,105,121,127,128] but the disorder is included here because it represents a model of pure pulmonary hypertension[98] that serves as a backdrop against which pulmonary hypertension associated with congenital heart disease can be related.[129]

The History

The relative frequency of primary pulmonary hypertension in young females was pointed out as early as 1927,[16] with a female-to-male ratio as high as 3:1.[7,34,56] Oral contraceptives are an important consideration in light of evidence that birth control pills may aggravate if not initiate pulmonary vascular disease.[65] However, in the National Institutes of Health Registry, the sex incidence in children was equal, and the adult female-to-male ratio was 1.7 to 1, with a relatively constant incidence decade by decade.[99] Variations in sex incidence may in part reflect differences among the three histopathologic subgroups. Plexogenic pulmonary arteriopathy has a female-to-male ratio of 3:1, and this subgroup is the most frequent of the three histopathologic types of primary pulmonary hypertension (see earlier).[92,99] In the less common subgroup with microthrombotic pulmonary hypertension, the female-to-male ratio is approximately equal,[92] and the veno-occlusive subgroup, which accounts for less than 7% of cases, is associated with a slight male predominance.[97]

Familial primary pulmonary hypertension is well recognized (see Fig. 14–12A) and occasionally recurs in more than one generation.[*] Inheritance is autosomal dominant with incomplete penetrance.[72,85] The genetic basis has been assigned to mutations in the bone morphogenetic protein receptor.[135–138]

The mean patient age of primary pulmonary hypersion in three large studies was 21 to 30 years, with a range of 2 to 56 years.[7,27,80,126,127] In the National Institutes of Health Registry, only 8% of patients were between 61 and 70 years of age.[11,99] Primary pulmonary hypertension of long duration has been reported,[15] and regression has been suspected, albeit rarely.[10,32] Right ventricular failure is the most common cause of death.[7,20,96,108] Longevity and morbidity are significantly influenced by lifestyle. Abrupt, strenuous, or isometric exercise should be strictly avoided, and isotonic exercise should cease at the very onset of dyspnea, light-headedness, dizziness, or chest pain. High altitude is an avoidable risk, and certain constraints are appropriate for air travel. A commercial jetliner flying at 33,000 to 36,000 feet has cabin atmospheric conditions that are the altitude equivalents of approximately 6000 to 8000 feet, which is comparable to breathing 15% oxygen at sea level.[149] Airline passengers normally experience a significant decrease in arterial P_{O_2} but experience only a mild decrease in arterial oxygen saturation.[149] Low humidity causes dehydration and an undesirable fall in systemic blood pressure. Just as important are the risks of non-flight-related stress and travel fatigue. Rushing at the last minute, carrying heavy luggage, flying at peak periods, and transferring from one aircraft to another at large busy airports are risks that should be minimized, if not avoided.

The most common symptoms associated with primary pulmonary hypertension are effort dyspnea, fatigue, light-headedness, and chest pain. Hyperventilatory dyspnea due to an increase in ventilatory response to exercise is a consistent finding attributed chiefly to a ventilation/perfusion

---

[*]9, 18, 31, 34, 41, 43, 54, 57, 64, 67, 71, 72, 79, 87, 106, 122, 123.

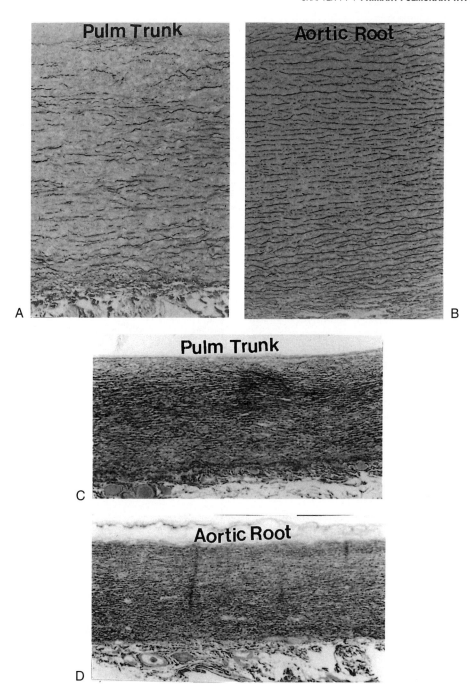

Figure 14–1

A and B, Histology of the pulmonary trunk and aortic root in an 11-year-old girl with primary pulmonary hypertension. *A,* Elastic fibers in the media of the pulmonary trunk are widely spaced, short, irregular, sparse, and branched. *B,* Elastic fibers in the media of the aortic root are long, uniform, and parallel. The differences in media of the pulmonary trunk and aortic root indicate that primary pulmonary hypertension was not present at birth. *C and D,* Histology of the pulmonary trunk and aortic root in a 46-year-old woman with a nonrestrictive ventricular septal defect and Eisenmenger syndrome. The media of the pulmonary trunk and aortic root are identical, indicating that pulmonary hypertension was present at birth.

mismatch.[83,97] Dyspnea is provoked by effort and excitement and occurs without orthopnea.[131] Muscle fatigue is attributed to a reduction in the rate of aerobic regeneration of ATP.[83] A surprisingly high prevalence of hypothyroidism has been reported in primary pulmonary hypertension,[70] a diagnostic possibility that should be considered in patients with inappropriate fatigue. Stress-related or exercise-related light-headedness, giddiness, dizziness, or faintness indicates an inability to maintain sufficient cardiac output

and systemic blood pressure to sustain cerebral blood flow. Myocardial ischemic chest pain originates in the hypertrophied hypoperfused right ventricle.[134] Histologic evidence of right ventricular infarction has been found in patients with primary pulmonary hypertension and normal coronary arteries. Myocardial ischemia has also been attributed to compression of the left main coronary artery by the dilated hypertensive pulmonary trunk.[78,93] Syncope is usually provoked by effort or excitement, is ominous, and can herald sudden death.[7,23,24,55,97,99,152] Seemingly innocuous stress has preceded sudden death, which has occurred during cardiac catheterization[96] and after a seemingly uncomplicated bone marrow aspiration.[121] Surgery, anesthesia, and even sedatives are poorly tolerated.

The risk of pregnancy warrants special emphasis because the maternal mortality rate is as high as 50%.[22,28,77,90,104,120] Symptoms may first appear during pregnancy.[22,77] Fixed pulmonary vascular resistance blunts or precludes adaptive responses to the hemodynamic fluctuations during gestation, labor, delivery, and the puerperium. The hypercoagulable state in the third trimester serves to reinforce the preexisting propensity for in situ thromboses in small terminal pulmonary arteries (see earlier).

Hemoptysis is not a feature of primary pulmonary hypertension as it is in Eisenmenger syndrome (see Chapter 17).[56] Raynaud phenomenon is occasionally associated with primary pulmonary hypertension and calls attention to autoimmunity (see earlier).[100,115,130] Hoarseness, or Ortner syndrome, results from vocal cord weakness caused by compression of the left recurrent laryngeal nerve by the dilated hypertensive pulmonary trunk.[97,106] Patients may be subjectively aware of neck pulsations caused by giant jugular A waves that may be unpleasantly visible (Fig. 14–2).

Physical Appearance

Mild dusky hues of the face, nose, ears, and extremities are peripheral and are related to low cardiac output and reduced skin blood flow. A right-to-left shunt through a patent foramen ovale causes a decrease in systemic arterial oxygen saturation and central cyanosis.

The Arterial Pulse and the Jugular Venous Pulse

The systemic arterial pulse is small and the pulse pressure is narrow (Fig. 14–3) because left ventricular stroke volume is reduced.[131] The small arterial pulse is in striking contrast to the large if not giant jugular venous A wave (see Figs. 14–2 and 14–4A), which Paul Wood aptly described[131]: "This presystolic venous pulse is abrupt and collapsing in quality; is little influenced by change in posture and may be more noticeable on inspiration. Thus it is best seen when the patient sits bolt upright or stands up, when the V wave usually disappears altogether." An increase in V wave awaits the advent of tricuspid regurgitation, which attenuates the X descent and exaggerates the Y trough. The jugular venous pulse exhibits two prominent crests, A and V. Giant V waves reached the mandible in a 25-year-old man with primary pulmonary hypertension and a ruptured tricuspid papillary muscle.[66]

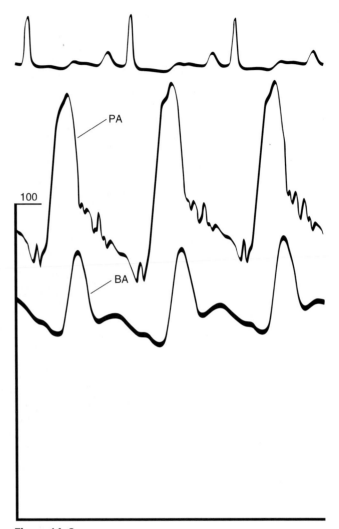

Figure 14–2
Pressure pulses from an 18-year-old man with primary pulmonary hypertension. Pulmonary arterial (PA) pressure exceeds brachial arterial (BA) pressure. The low systemic arterial pressure and narrow pulse pressure result from depressed systemic stroke volume.

Precordial Movement and Palpation

Prominence of a right ventricular impulse varies with the severity and duration of pulmonary hypertension and with the size and function of the right ventricle. Presystolic distention caused by an increased force of right atrial contraction is palpated at the lower left sternal edge and subxiphoid (Figs. 14–4 and 14–5). An enlarged right ventricle displaces the left ventricle from the apex. Palpation in the second left intercostal space detects a dilated hypertensive pulmonary trunk, a loud pulmonary ejection sound, and ". . . the closure of the semilunar valve being generally perceptible to the hand placed over the pulmonary area as a sharp thud" (Graham Steell).[118]

Auscultation

The auscultatory signs are pure reflections of pulmonary hypertension.[88,89] Eight auscultatory signs include the

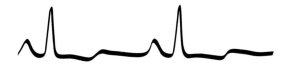

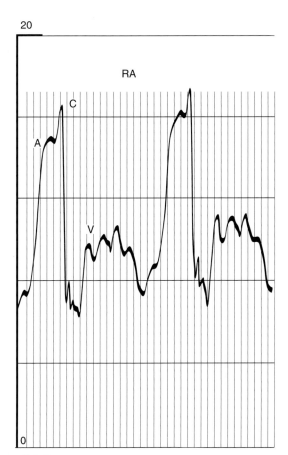

Figure 14–3

Right atrial pressure pulse from the 18-year-old man referred to in Figure 14–2 showing A waves of 14 to 16 mm Hg.

pulmonary ejection sound, the pulmonary midsystolic murmur, the tricuspid holosystolic murmur, the second heart sound, the Graham Steell murmur, the fourth heart sound, the third heart sound, and a mid-diastolic/presystolic murmur (Fig. 14–6). The pulmonary ejection sound is identified by its high-pitched sharp clicking quality; its maximum intensity in the second left intercostal space; and occasionally but distinctively by selective decrease during inspiration (Figs. 14–6, 14–7, and 14–8A). The onset of the ejection sound is determined by the interval between the onset of right ventricular systole and the opening of the pulmonary valve (isovolumetric contraction). The slower the rate of right ventricular contraction and the higher the pulmonary arterial diastolic pressure, the later the ejection sound (see Figs. 14–7 and 14–8A).[88] A loud ejection sound radiates to the lower left sternal edge and apex, especially when the right ventricle occupies the apex.

A pulmonary midsystolic murmur results from ejection into the dilated pulmonary trunk (see Figs. 14–6 and 14–7). The murmur is symmetric and short, is confined to the second left intercostal space, is impure grade 1/6 or 2/6, and is introduced by the pulmonary ejection sound. The murmur of tricuspid regurgitation is maximum at the lower left sternal edge (Figs. 14–6, 14–7 and 14–8B). When the right ventricle occupies the apex, the murmur is well heard at the apex, and when the right atrium is enlarged, the murmur is well heard to the right of the sternum.

The tricuspid murmur is holosystolic and high pitched because regurgitant flow is holosystolic and high velocity.[89] Intensity may be sufficient to generate a thrill or may be barely sufficient to achieve audibility. An increase in intensity during active inspiration—Rivero-Carvallo sign—is diagnostically important (Fig. 14–6),[88,89,102] and the murmur may be audible only during deep inspiration. Amplification depends on whether the right ventricle is functionally capable of converting the inspiratory increase in venous return into an increase in stroke volume and regurgitant flow.[88] This capacity is lost with advanced right ventricular failure, so the Rivero-Carvallo sign disappears.[89]

The pulmonary component of the second heart sound is altered regarding its timing, intensity, and precordial location.[88,89] The degree of splitting is the net effect of two variables: (1) decreased capacitance and increased resistance in the pulmonary vascular bed serve to narrow the split, and (2) prolongation of right ventricular systole serves to increase the split.[91,111,112] When right ventricular function is normal, inspiratory splitting is normal or close (see Fig. 14–6).[112] A depressed right ventricle cannot increase its stroke volume with inspiration, so the split becomes fixed.[91,112] A loud pulmonary component in the second left interspace may obscure a closely preceding aortic component (see Figs. 14–7 and 14–8), but auscultation at the right base, lower left sternal edge or apex permits analysis of the transmitted but attenuated pulmonary component and allows detection of splitting (Fig. 14–9, and see Fig. 14–8B).[88] Of all the auscultatory signs of pulmonary hypertension, the loud pulmonary component of the second sound is the most distinctive (Fig. 14–10, and see Figs. 14–6 through 14–9). Graham Steell wrote that "accentuation of the pulmonary second sound is always present, the closure of the semilunar valves being generally perceptible to the hand placed over the pulmonary area as a sharp thud" (see Precordial Palpation).[118] Detection of the loud pulmonary component at the apex is a useful sign of elevated pressure in the pulmonary artery.[88]

"There is occasionally heard over the pulmonary area . . . and below this region for the distance of an inch or two along the left border of the sternum, and rarely over the lowest part of the bone itself, a soft blowing diastolic murmur immediately following or more exactly running off the accentuated second sound, while the usual indications of aortic regurgitation afforded by the pulse, etc., are absent. When the second sound is reduplicated, the murmur

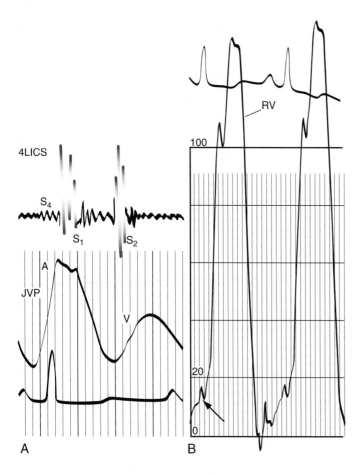

Figure 14–4

Recordings from the 18-year-old man referred to in Figure 14–2. *A*, A fourth heart sound (S$_4$) was present in the fourth left intercostal space (4 LICS), and the jugular venous pulse (JVP) exhibits a correspondingly prominent A wave. S$_1$, first heart sound; S$_2$, second heart sound. *B*, An increased force of right atrial contraction resulted in presystolic distention of the right ventricle (*thin arrow*, lower left). RV, right ventricle.

proceeds from its latter part. That such a murmur as I have described does exist, there can, I think, be no doubt."[118] Graham Steell made this auscultatory observation with a light boxwood monaural stethoscope of unusual length.[145] The Graham Steell murmur is typically located in the second and third left intercostal spaces adjacent to the sternum (see Figs. 14–6 and 14–7), but when loud is heard at the lower left sternal edge or even to the right of the sternum. Elevated diastolic pressure is exerted on the incompetent pulmonary valve at the dichotic notch as the right ventricular and pulmonary arterial pressure pulses diverge, so the murmur begins with or immediately after the accentuated pulmonary component of the second sound (Figs. 14–10 and 14–11). The marked difference in diastolic pressures between right ventricle and pulmonary artery exist from the beginning to the end of diastole, so the accompanying murmur is high frequency and prolonged (see Figs. 14–10 and 14–11). The configuration is decrescendo (see Figs. 14–7 and 14–11), but vibrations may be almost equal throughout diastole, or the murmur may be crescendo-decrescendo (see Fig. 14–10). Intensity may be sufficient to generate a thrill or may be soft and variable to the point of inaudibility. Steell was adept at detecting these murmurs despite his monaural boxwood stethoscope because of the "absolute quiet which prevailed during his lengthy round."[75]

Fourth heart sounds accompany presystolic distention of the right ventricle (see Figs. 14–4 and 14–6) and are best detected at the lower left sternal edge but are heard at the apex when the apex is formed by the right ventricle. Fourth heart sounds are distinguished from split first heart sounds or pulmonary ejection sounds by their quality, precordial location, and response to respiration.[88,89] The low-frequency fourth sound may be more readily palpated than heard, a feature recognized by Potain, who stated that "if one applies the ear to the chest, it affects the tactile sensation more than the auditory sense."[94] Right-sided fourth sounds become louder and earlier during inspiration (see Fig. 14–6), because the greater force of right atrial contraction is translated into earlier and more vigorous presystolic filling of the right ventricle.

Third heart sounds occur during the rapid filling phase of the cardiac cycle and are signs of right ventricular failure (see Fig. 14–6).[89] With the advent of tricuspid regurgitation, third sounds intensify because high right atrial V waves are followed by more accelerated atrioventricular flow. The third heart sounds are low-frequency events of variable intensity best detected with the bell of the stethoscope applied over the body of the right ventricle, but these sounds are audible at the apex when the apex is occupied by the right ventricle.

In 1931, MacCallum described a mid-diastolic rumbling murmur in a young woman with pulmonary hypertension,[74] and the occasional occurrence of mid-diastolic/presystolic murmurs has been confirmed (see Figs. 14–6 and 14–12).[88,89] These murmurs represent prolonged vibrations of third or

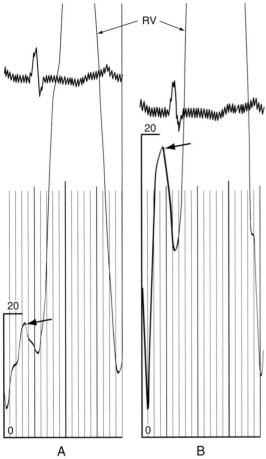

Figure 14–5
Readily palpable presystolic distention of the right ventricle (*thin oblique arrows*) recorded at different sensitivities in a 29-year-old woman with primary pulmonary hypertension.

fourth heart sounds and may increase during inspiration (see Fig. 14–6).[88] Mid-diastolic murmurs are more apt to occur when the tricuspid valve is incompetent and the rate of atrioventricular flow is rapid (Fig. 14–12A). Right-sided Austin Flint mid-diastolic/presystolic murmurs have been described in the presence of pulmonary hypertensive pulmonary regurgitation.[40]

Evans and coworkers, in a 1957 article on solitary pulmonary hypertension, remarked that "a sound that resembles a mitral opening snap was heard in early diastole."[26] McKusick recorded an "early diastolic snap" in a patient with necropsy-confirmed primary pulmonary hypertension and assigned the sound to the tricuspid valve. One of my patients had a soft early diastolic sound that was recorded but not heard (see Fig. 14–8B).[88]

The Electrocardiogram

The electrocardiogram is a reflection of right ventricular hypertrophy that is acquired after birth (Fig. 14–13).[97] Abnormal P waves show pure right atrial configurations (see Fig. 14–13).[121] Atrial fibrillation is exceptional.[97] The PR interval is normal or slightly prolonged. The QRS axis varies from normal to right axis deviation, and the QRS duration is normal or slightly increased (see Fig. 14–13).

The degree of right ventricular hypertrophy is determined by the severity and duration of pulmonary hypertension. At one end of the spectrum, the electrocardiogram shows no more than a rightward shift of the QRS axis. At the other end of the spectrum is right axis deviation with right precordial leads that exhibit tall monophasic R waves with ST segment depressions and asymmetric T wave inversions, and left precordial leads that exhibit deep S waves (see Fig. 14–13).

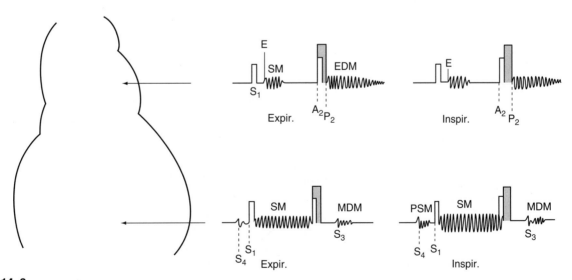

Figure 14–6
Composite drawing of the auscultatory features of pulmonary hypertension. A₂, aortic component of the second heart sound; E, pulmonary ejection sound; EDM, early diastolic murmur; EXPIR, expiration; INSPIR, inspiration; MDM, mid-diastolic murmur; P₂, pulmonary component of the second heart sound; PSM, presystolic murmur; S₁, first heart sound; S₃, third heart sound; S₄, fourth heart sound; SM, systolic murmur.

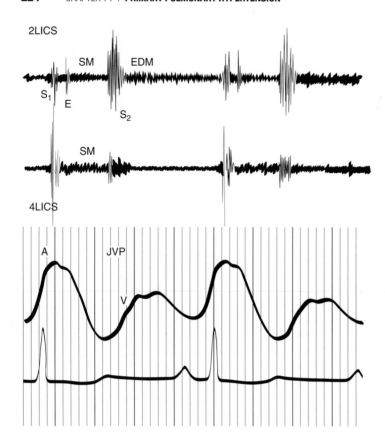

Figure 14–7

Phonocardiograms with jugular venous pulse (JVP) from the 18-year-old man with primary pulmonary hypertension referred to in Figure 14–2. In the second left intercostal space (2 LICS), a pulmonary ejection sound (E) begins at a long interval after the first heart sound and introduces a soft, short, midsystolic murmur (SM). The single second heart sound (S_2) is prolonged and loud because the pulmonary component was of great amplitude. A soft early diastolic murmur (EDM) issues from the loud second sound. A high-frequency holosystolic murmur of tricuspid regurgitation appears in the fourth left intercostal space (4 LICS). The A wave in the jugular venous pulse is prominent.

The X-Ray

Enlargement of the pulmonary trunk and its proximal branches is characteristic and varies from moderate to marked but is seldom aneurysmal (Figs. 14–14 through 14–16).[97] The lucent pruned appearance of the peripheral lung fields stands out in sharp contrast to the prominence of the pulmonary trunk and its central branches (see Figs. 14–15 and 14–16). Pulmonary venous congestion is reserved for the occasional patient with veno-occlusive primary pulmonary hypertension.[97] The ascending aorta is inconspicuous compared with the dilated pulmonary trunk (see Figs. 14–14 and 14–15). Enlargement of the hypertensive right ventricle reflects the degree and chronicity of right ventricular failure (see Fig. 14–15). Right atrial enlargement varies from a slight convexity at the right lower cardiac border (see Fig. 14–14) to striking enlargement provoked by right ventricular failure and tricuspid regurgitation (Fig. 14–17, and see Figs. 14–15 and 14–16).

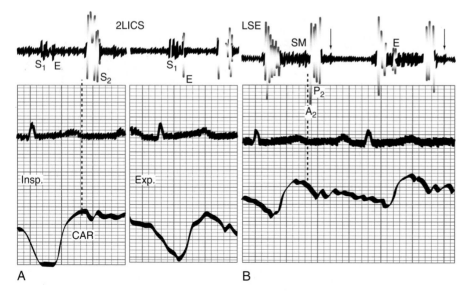

Figure 14–8

Phonocardiograms from a 21-year-old woman with primary pulmonary hypertension. *A*, The first heart sound (S_1) in the second left intercostal space (2 LICS) is followed by a pulmonary ejection sound (E) that selectively decreased during inspiration (INSP) and was transmitted to the lower left sternal edge (LSE). The second heart sound (S_2) is loud and prolonged because of increased intensity of the pulmonary component. CAR, carotid. *B*, A holosystolic murmur of tricuspid regurgitation (SM) is present at the lower left sternal edge (LSE). The loud transmitted pulmonary component of the second heart sound (P_2) permitted identification of both components at the left sternal edge (LSE). A_2, aortic component. A low-amplitude early diastolic sound with the timing of an opening snap was recorded but not heard (*thin vertical arrows*).

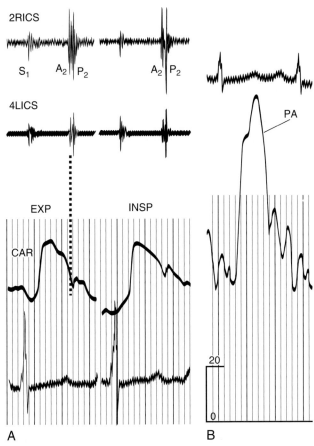

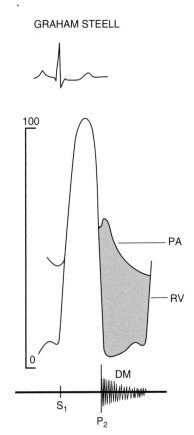

GRAHAM STEELL

Figure 14–9

Recordings from a 21-year-old woman with primary pulmonary hypertension. *A,* The upper phonocardiograms show a loud pulmonary component of the second heart sound (P_2) that was transmitted to the second right intercostal space (2 RICS). The second sound was closely split during expiration. 4 LICS, fourth left intercostal space. *B,* The pulmonary arterial (PA) pressure was at systemic level (120 mm Hg). CAR, carotid.

Figure 14–11

Drawings from pulmonary arterial (PA) and right ventricular (RV) pressure pulses with phonocardiogram illustrating an early diastolic Graham Steell murmur (DM). High pressure is exerted against the incompetent pulmonary valve throughout diastole (*shaded area*), so high-velocity regurgitant flow is associated with a high-frequency holodiastolic murmur.

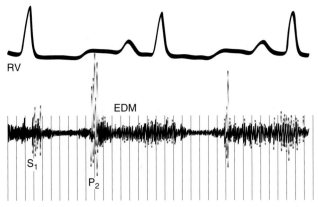

Figure 14–10

Intracardiac phonocardiogram from the right ventricular (RV) outflow tract of the 18-year-old man with primary pulmonary hypertension referred to in Figure 14–2. A high-frequency early diastolic Graham Steell murmur (EDM) begins with the loud pulmonary component of the second sound (P_2). The murmur lasts throughout diastole, and the configuration varies from beat to beat.

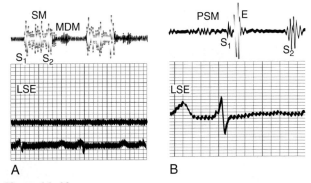

Figure 14–12

A, Phonocardiogram from a 20-year-old man with primary pulmonary hypertension whose younger sister also had primary pulmonary hypertension. The tracing at the lower left sternal edge (LSE) shows a holosystolic murmur of tricuspid regurgitation and a short middiastolic murmur (MDM). *B,* Phonocardiogram from the 29-year-old woman referred to in Figure 14–5. A short presystolic murmur (PSM) and a prominent pulmonary ejection sound (E) are shown at the lower left sternal edge. S_2, second heart sound.

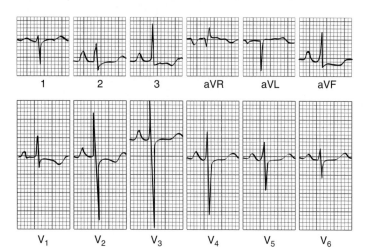

Figure 14–13

Electrocardiogram from a 27-year old woman with primary pulmonary hypertension. Tall peaked right atrial P waves appear in leads 2 and aVF and in the mid-precordium. Right ventricular hypertrophy is manifested by right axis deviation, a monophasic R wave in lead V_1, and a prominent S wave in lead V_6.

The Echocardiogram

Transthoracic and transesophageal echocardiography with Doppler interrogation and color flow imaging exclude coexisting congenital or acquired heart disease that might cause pulmonary hypertension and establish the physiologic and morphologic consequences of elevated pressure in the lesser circulation.[39,148,150]Intravascular ultrasonography has been introduced as a method of assessing the pulmonary circulation in pulmonary hypertension.[146]

Echocardiography defines the size of the right atrium and right ventricle, characterizes right ventricular free wall motion, provides an estimate of right ventricular ejection fraction, establishes the position and motion of the ventricular septum, and determines the effect of ventricular septal position on the diastolic size and shape of the left ventricle (Fig. 14–18).[147] Color flow imaging establishes the presence and degree of pulmonary and tricuspid regurgitation (see Figs. 14–19 through 14–21). Continuous-wave Doppler across the right ventricular outflow tract and

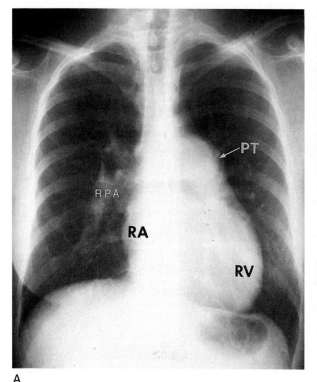

A

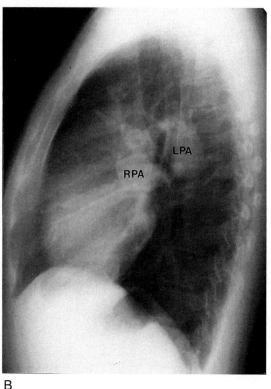

B

Figure 14–14

X-rays from a 31-year-old woman with primary pulmonary hypertension. *A*, Pulmonary vascularity is reduced. The pulmonary trunk (PT) and right pulmonary artery (RPA) are dilated, but the ascending aorta is not border forming. A convex right ventricle (RV) occupies the apex, but the right atrial (RA) silhouette is not prominent. *B*, The right pulmonary artery (RPA) and left pulmonary artery (LPA) are dilated. The right ventricle and right atrial appendage do not encroach on the retrosternal space.

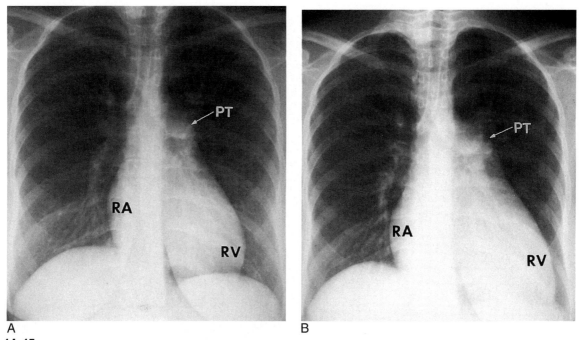

Figure 14–15

A, X-ray from a 24-year-old woman with primary pulmonary hypertension. Pulmonary vascularity is reduced. The pulmonary trunk (PT) is dilated, but the ascending aorta is not border forming. A convex right ventricle (RV) occupies the apex, and the right atrium (RA) is moderately enlarged. *B*, X-ray from the same patient 28 months later, after the onset of right ventricular failure and tricuspid regurgitation. The pulmonary trunk, right atrium, and right ventricle have considerably increased in size.

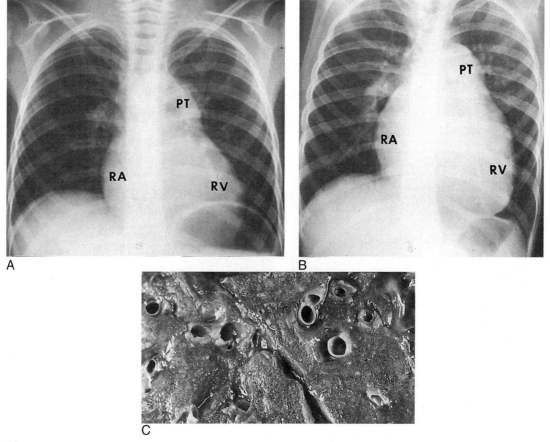

Figure 14–16

A, X-ray at 6 years of age from the patient with primary pulmonary hypertension referred to in Figure 14–1. Pulmonary vascularity is reduced. The pulmonary trunk (PT) is dilated, the right atrial silhouette (RA) is increased, and a dilated convex right ventricle (RV) occupies the apex and extends below the left hemidiaphragm. *B*, X-ray at 10 years of age after the onset of right ventricular failure shows a striking increase in size of the pulmonary trunk, right atrium, and right ventricle. *C*, The patient died at 11 years of age. Cross-section of the lung at necropsy shows thick-walled intrapulmonary arteries that rise above the surface. See also Figure 14–1.

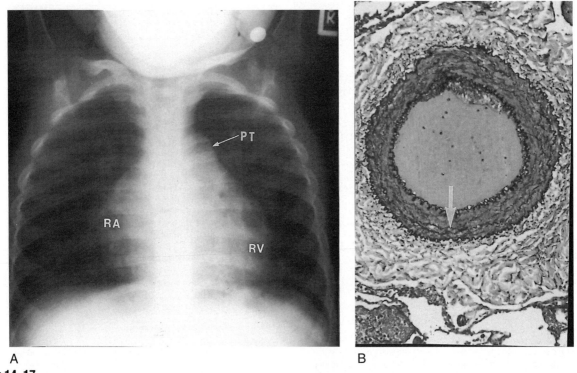

Figure 14–17

A, X-ray from a 3-year-old girl with primary pulmonary hypertension. Pulmonary vascularity is reduced. The pulmonary trunk (PT), right atrium (RA) and right ventricle (RV) are considerably enlarged. *B*, Histology of a pulmonary artery at necropsy shows medial hypertrophy (*arrow*).

tricuspid valve permit estimates of the pulmonary artery diastolic pressure and the right ventricular systolic pressure (see Figs. 14–19 through 14–21). The ventricular septum flattens toward the left ventricular cavity at end-systole and in early diastole.[73] The resulting deformation of the left ventricular cavity is associated with an impaired left ventricle in early diastole and redistribution of filling into later diastole (see Figs. 14–18 and 14–21).[73,119]

Summary

The typical patient with primary pulmonary hypertension is an otherwise healthy young acyanotic female who presents with effort dyspnea, fatigue, light-headedness, syncope, and chest pain but with no history of heart disease. Physical signs include a small arterial pulse, a large jugular venous A wave, a palpable right ventricle and a

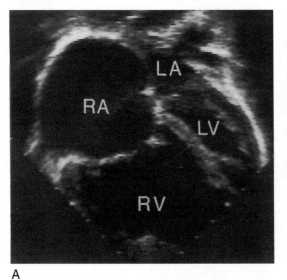

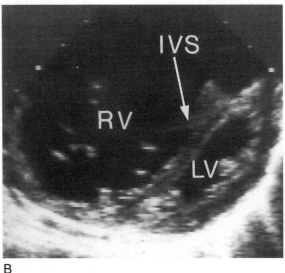

Figure 14–18

Echocardiograms 2 months before death of the 11-year-old girl with primary pulmonary hypertension referred to in Figures 14–1 and 14–16. *A*, The four-chamber view shows striking dilatation of the right atrium (RA) and right ventricle (RV). The left ventricular cavity size (LV) is considerably reduced. *B*, Short-axis showing the dilated right ventricle (RV) and the flat interventricular septum (IVS) that encroaches on the cavity of the left ventricle (LV) and markedly reduces its size.

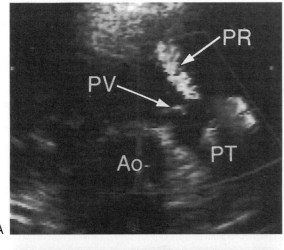

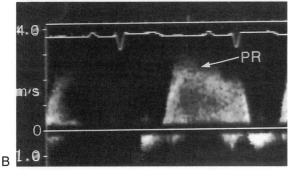

Figure 14–19
Black and white print of a color flow image from an 18-year-old woman with primary pulmonary hypertension. *A*, A high-velocity diastolic jet of pulmonary regurgitation (PR) originates at the pulmonary valve (PV). The pulmonary trunk is dilated (PT). Ao, aorta. *B*, Continuous-wave Doppler across the pulmonary valve records a peak regurgitant velocity (PR) that indicates a pulmonary artery diastolic pressure of 40 mm Hg.

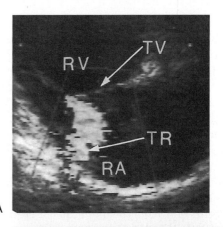

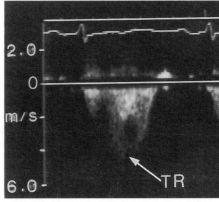

Figure 14–20
Black and white print of a color flow image from a woman with primary pulmonary hypertension who died at the age of 21 years. *A*, A high-velocity regurgitant (TR) jet originates at the tricuspid valve (TV) and enters an enlarged right atrium (RA). The right ventricle is dilated (RV). *B*, Continuous-wave Doppler across the tricuspid valve records a peak velocity that indicates a right ventricular systolic pressure of 75 mm Hg.

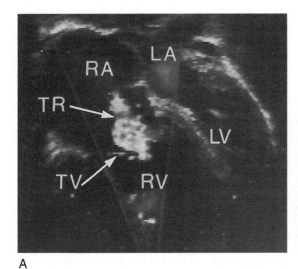

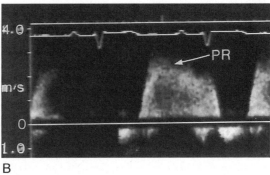

Figure 14–21
A, Black and white print of a color flow image from the 11-year-old girl with primary pulmonary hypertension referred to in Figures 14–1, 14–16, and 14–18. A high-velocity regurgitant jet (TR) originates at the tricuspid valve (TV) and enters an enlarged right atrium (RA). A dilated right ventricle (RV) encroaches on the left ventricular cavity (LV). LA, left atrium. *B*, Continuous-wave Doppler signal across the pulmonary valve records a peak velocity of pulmonary regurgitation (PR) that indicates a diastolic pressure of 45 mm Hg. Peak velocity across the tricuspid valve (not shown) indicated a right ventricular systolic pressure of 100 mm Hg.

palpable pulmonary trunk, presystolic distention of the right ventricle that coincides with a right ventricular fourth heart sound, a pulmonary ejection sound, a short pulmonary midsystolic murmur, a loud pulmonary component of the second heart sound, the murmur of tricuspid regurgitation, and a Graham Steell murmur. The electrocardiogram is characterized by a right atrial P wave abnormality, right axis deviation, and pure right ventricular hypertrophy. The chest x-ray discloses dilatation of the pulmonary trunk and its proximal branches, clear peripheral lung fields, and enlargement of the right ventricle and right atrium. Echocardiography with color flow imaging and Doppler interrogation excludes coexisting congenital or acquired heart disease as causes of pulmonary hypertension, and establishes the anatomic and physiologic consequences of elevated pressure in the lesser circulation. Echocardiography establishes the size of the right atrium and right ventricle, assesses right ventricular freewall motion, estimates the right ventricular ejection fraction, and defines the abnormal position and movement of the ventricular septum and the abnormal size and shape of the left ventricular cavity. Color flow imaging determines the presence and degree of tricuspid and pulmonary regurgitation, and continuous wave Doppler permits an estimate of right ventricular systolic pressure and pulmonary artery diastolic pressure. Pulsed Doppler characterizes the physiologic abnormalities of left ventricular inflow.

REFERENCES

1. Abman SH, Chatfield BA, Hall SL, McMurtry IV: Role of endothelium-derived relaxing factor during transition of pulmonary circulation at birth. Am J Physiol 259:H1921, 1990.
2. Ainger LE: Large tonsils and adenoids in small children with cor pulmonale. Br Heart J 30:356, 1968.
3. Chen YF, Oparil S: Endothelin and pulmonary hypertension. J Cardiovasc Pharmacol 35:S49, 2000.
4. Mikhail G, Chester AH, Gibbs SR, et al: Role of vasoactive mediators in primary and secondary pulmonary hypertension. Am J Cardiol 82:254, 1998.
5. Lopes AA, Maeda NY, Goncalves RC, Bydlowski SP: Endothelial cell dysfunction correlates differentially with survival in primary and secondary pulmonary hypertension. Am Heart J 139:618, 2000.
6. Beutner A: Z F Rat Med 2:97, 1852.
7. Bjornsson J, Edwards WD: Primary pulmonary hypertension. Mayo Clin Proc 60:16, 1985.
8. Bland JW, Edwards FK: Pulmonary hypertension and congestive heart failure in children with chronic upper airway obstruction. Am J Cardiol 23:830, 1969.
9. Boiteau GM, Libanoff AJ: Primary pulmonary hypertension: Familial incidence. Angiology 14:260, 1963.
10. Bourdillon PDV, Oakley CM: Regression of primary pulmonary hypertension. Br Heart J 38:264, 1976.
11. Braman SS, Eby E, Kuhn C, Rounds S: Primary pulmonary hypertension in the elderly. Arch Intern Med 151:2433, 1991.
12. Brouillette RT, Fernbach SK, Hunt CE: Obstructive sleep apnea in infants and children. J Pediatr 100:31, 1982.
13. Burke AP, Farb A, Virmani R: The pathology of primary pulmonary hypertension. Mod Pathol 4:269, 1991.
14. Nagaya N, Nishikimi T, Uemarsu M, et al: Plasma brain natriuretic peptide as a prognostic indicator in patients with primary pulmonary hypertension. Circulation 102:865, 2000.
15. Charters AD, Baker W deC: Primary pulmonary hypertension of unusually long duration. Br Heart J 32:130, 1970.
16. Clarke RC, Coombs CF, Hadfield G, Todd AT: Certain abnormalities, congenital and acquired, of the pulmonary artery. Q J Med 21:51, 1927.
17. Cohen N, Mendelow H: Concurrent "active juvenile cirrhosis" and "primary pulmonary hypertension." Am J Med 39:127, 1965.
18. Coleman PN, Edmunds AWB, Tregillus J: Primary pulmonary hypertension in three sibs. Br Heart J 21:81, 1959.
19. Wiedermann R, Ghofrani A, Weissman N, et al: Atrial natriuretic peptide in severe primary and nonprimary pulmonary hypertension. J Am Coll Cardiol 38:1130, 2001.
20. D'Alonzo GE, Barst RJ, Ayres SM, et al: Survival in patients with primary pulmonary hypertension: Results from a national prospective registry. Ann Intern Med 115:343, 1991.
21. Davies G, Reid L: Growth of the alveoli and pulmonary arteries in childhood. Thorax 25:669, 1970.
22. Dawkins KD, Burke CM, Billingham ME, Jamieson SW: Primary pulmonary hypertension and pregnancy. Chest 89:383, 1986.
23. Dresdale DT, Schultz M, Michton RJ: Primary pulmonary hypertension. 1. Clinical and hemodynamic study. Am J Med 11:686, 1951.
24. Dressler W: Effort syncope as an early manifestation of primary pulmonary hypertension. Am J Med Sci 223:131, 1952.
25. Yuan JX, Aldinger AM, Juhaszova M, et al: Dysfunctional voltage-gated K+ channels in pulmonary smooth muscle cells of patients with primary pulmonary hypertension. Circulation 98:1400, 1998.
26. Evans W, Short DS, Bedford DE: Solitary pulmonary hypertension. Br Heart J 19:93, 1957.
27. Farrar JF, Reye RDK, Stuckey D: Primary pulmonary hypertension in childhood. Br Heart J 23:605, 1961.
28. Feijen HWH, Hein PR, van Lakwijk-Vondrovicova EL, Nijhuis GMM: Primary pulmonary hypertension and pregnancy. Eur J Obstet Gynecol Reprod Biol 15:159, 1983.
29. Michado RD, Pauciulo MW, Thompson JR, et al: BMRP2 haploinsufficiency as the inherited molecular mechanism for primary pulmonary hypertension. Am J Hum Genet 68:92, 2001.
30. Archer S, Rich S: Primary pulmonary hypertension: A vascular biology and translational research "work in progress." Circulation 102:2781, 2000.
31. Fleming H: Primary pulmonary hypertension in 8 patients including a mother and her daughter. Aust Ann Med 9:18, 1960.
32. Fujii A, Rabinovitch M, Matthews EC: A case of spontaneous resolution of idiopathic pulmonary hypertension. Br Heart J 46:574, 1981.
33. Fujinami M, Nishikawa T, Kajita A, Takao A: Primary pulmonary hypertension in infancy: Report of two autopsy cases. Acta Cardiol 40:19, 1989.
34. Fuster V, Steele PM, Edwards WD, et al: Primary pulmonary hypertension. Circulation 70:581, 1984.
35. Tredal SM, Carter JB, Edwards JE: Cystic medial necrosis of the pulmonary artery: Association with pulmonary hypertension. Arch Pathol 97:183, 1974.
36. Gersony WM: Neonatal pulmonary hypertension: Pathophysiology, classification, and etiology. Clin Perinatol 11:517, 1984.
37. Gersony WM, Duc GV, Sinclair JC: "P.F.C." syndrome (persistent of the fetal circulation). Circulation 40:III-87, 1969.
38. Roberts WC: The histologic structure of the pulmonary trunk in patients with "primary" pulmonary hypertensin. Am Heart J 65:230, 1963.
39. Goodman DJ, Harrison DC, Popp RL: Echocardiographic features of primary pulmonary hypertension. Am J Cardiol 33:438, 1974.
40. Green EW, Agruss NS, Adolph RJ: Right-sided Austin Flint murmur. Am J Cardiol 32:370, 1973.
41. Galle N, Manes A, Uguccioni L, et al: Primary pulmonary hypertension: Insights into pathogenesis from epidemiology. Chest 114:184S, 1998.
42. Hageman JR, Adams MA, Gardner TH: Persistent pulmonary hypertension in the new-born. Am J Dis Child 138:592, 1984.
43. Fishman AP: Etiology and pathogenesis of primary pulmonary hypertension. Chest 114:242S, 1998.
44. Harris A: The second heart sound in health and in pulmonary hypertension. Am Heart J 79:145, 1970.
45. Hatano S, Strasser T (eds): Primary Pulmonary Hypertension Report on a WHO Meeting. Geneva, World Health Organization, 1975.
46. Haworth SG: Pulmonary vascular remodeling in neonatal pulmonary hypertension. Chest 93:133S, 1988.
47. Haworth SG, Reid L: Persistent fetal circulation: Newly recognized structural features. J Pediatr 88:614, 1976.
48. Heath D, Edwards JE: Configuration of elastic tissue of pulmonary trunk in idiopathic pulmonary hypertension. Circulation 21:59, 1960.
49. Heath D, Edwards JE: Pathology of hypertensive pulmonary vascular disease. Circulation 18:533, 1958.

50. Heath D, Smith P, Gosney J, et al: The pathology of the early and late stages of primary pulmonary hypertension. Br Heart J 58:204, 1987.

51. Hislop A, Reid LM: Intrapulmonary arterial development during fetal life-branching pattern and structure. J Anat 113:35, 1972.

52. Hislop A, Reid LM: Pulmonary arterial development during childhood: Branching pattern and structure. Thorax 28:129, 1973.

53. Hogg JC: Primary pulmonary hypertension: Aspen lung conference. Chest 93:172S, 1988.

54. Hood WB, Spencer H, Loss RW, Daley R: Primary pulmonary hypertension: Familial occurrence. Br Heart J 30:336, 1968.

55. Howarth S, Lowe JB: Mechanism of effort syncope in primary pulmonary hypertension and cyanotic congenital heart disease. Br Heart J 15:47, 1953.

56. Hughes JD, Rubin LJ: Primary pulmonary hypertension: An analysis of 28 cases and a review of the literature. Medicine 65:56, 1986.

57. Husson GS, Wyatt TC: Primary pulmonary hypertension in siblings. Am J Dis Child 92:506, 1956.

58. Bhan A, Rennele IG, Higenbottam TW: Central retinal veniocclusion associated with primary pulmonary hypertension. Retina 21:83, 2001.

59. Saran BR, Brucker AJ, Brandello F, Verougstraete C: Familial primary pulmonary hypertension and associated ocular findings. Retina 21:34, 2001.

60. Gaine S: Pulmonary hypertension. JAMA 284:3160, 2000.

61. Rafanan AL, Golish JA, Dinner DS, et al: Nocturnal hypoxemia is common in primary pulmonary hypertension. Chest 120:894, 2001.

62. Kanemoto N: Natural history of pulmonary hemodynamics in primary pulmonary hypertension. Am Heart J 114:407, 1987.

63. Khoury GH, Hawes CR: Primary pulmonary hypertension in children living at high altitudes. J Pediatr 62:177, 1963.

64. Kingdon HS, Cohen LS, Robert WC, Braunwald E: Familial occurrence of primary pulmonary hypertension. Arch Intern Med 118:422, 1966.

65. Kleiger RE, Boxer M, Ingham RE, Harrison DC: Pulmonary hypertension in patients using oral contraceptives. Chest 69:143, 1976.

66. Kunhali K, Cherian G, Bakthaviziam A, et al: Rupture of a papillary muscle of the tricuspid valve in primary pulmonary hypertension. Am Heart J 99:225, 1980.

67. Langleben D, Heneghan JM, Batten AP, et al: Familial pulmonary capillary hemangiomatosis resulting in primary pulmonary hypertension. Ann Intern Med 109:106, 1988.

68. Levin DL, Rudolph AM, Heymann MA, Phibbs RH: Morphologic development of the pulmonary vascular bed in fetal lambs. Circulation 53:144, 1976.

69. Levin DL, Weinberg AG, Perkin RM: Pulmonary microthrombi syndrome in newborn infants with unresponsive persistent pulmonary hypertension. J Pediatr 102:299, 1983.

70. Curnock AL, Dweik RA, Higgins BH, et al: High prevalence of hypothyroidism in patients with primary pulmonary hypertension. Am J Med Sci 318:289, 1999.

71. Lloyd JE, Atkinson JB, Pietra GG, et al: Heterogeneity of pathologic lesions in familial primary pulmonary hypertension. Am Rev Respir Dis 138:952, 1988.

72. Lloyd JE, Primm RK, Newman JH: Familial primary pulmonary hypertension. Am Rev Respir Dis 129:194, 1984.

73. Louie EK, Rich S, Brundage BH: Doppler echocardiographic assessment of impaired left ventricular filling in patients with right ventricular pressure overload due to primary pulmonary hypertension. J Am Coll Cardiol 8:1298, 1986.

74. MacCallum WG: Obliterative pulmonary arteriosclerosis. Bull Johns Hopkins Hosp 49:37, 1931.

75. Major RH: Classic Descriptions of Disease. Springfield, Ill, Charles C Thomas, 1948.

76. Mauer KW, Staats BA, Olsen KD: Upper airway obstruction and disordered breathing in children. Mayo Clin Proc 58:349, 1983.

77. McCaffrey RM, Dunn LJ: Primary pulmonary hypertension in pregnancy. Obstet Gynecol Surv 19:567, 1964.

78. Patrat JF, Jondeau G, Dudourg O, et al: Left main coronary artery compression during primary pulmonary hypertension. Chest 112:842, 1997.

79. Melmon KL, Braunwald E: Familial pulmonary hypertension. N Engl J Med 269:770, 1963.

80. Lilienfeld DE, Rubin LJ: Mortality from primary pulmonary hypertension in the United States 1979–1996. Chest 117:796, 2000.

81. Murphy JD, Rabinovitch M, Goldstein JD, Reid LM: The structural basis of persistent pulmonary hypertension of the newborn infant. J Pediatr 98:962, 1981.

82. Neill DO, Morton R, Kennedy JA: Progressive primary pulmonary hypertension in a patient born at high altitude. Br Heart J 45:725, 1981.

83. Sun X, Hansen JE, Oudiz RJ, Wasserman K: Exercise pathophysiology in patients with primary pulmonary hypertension. Circulation 104:429, 2001.

84. Newman JH, Ross JC: Primary pulmonary hypertension: A look at the future. J Am Coll Cardiol 14:551, 1989.

85. Grunig E, Janssen B, Mereles D, et al: Abnormal pulmonary artery pressure response in asymptomatic carriers of primary pulmonary hypertension gene. Circulation 102:1145, 2000.

86. Palevsky HI, Schloo BL, Pietra GG, et al: Primary pulmonary hypertension: Vascular structure, morphometry, and responsiveness to vasodilator agents. Circulation 80:1207, 1989.

87. Parry WR, Verel D: Familial primary pulmonary hypertension. Br Heart J 28:193, 1966.

88. Perloff JK: Auscultatory and phonocardiographic manifestations of pulmonary hypertension. Prog Cardiovasc Dis 9:303, 1967.

89. Perloff JK: The Physical Examination of the Heart and Circulation, 3rd ed. Philadelphia, W.B. Saunders, 2000.

90. Perloff JK: Pregnancy in congenital heart disease: The mother and the fetus. In Perloff JK, Child JS (eds): Congenital Heart Disease in Adults, 2nd ed. Philadelphia, W.B. Saunders, 1998.

91. Perloff JK, Harvey WP: Mechanism of fixed splitting of the second heart sound. Circulation 18:998, 1958.

92. Pietra GG, Edwards WD, Kay JM, et al: Histopathology of primary pulmonary hypertension: A qualitative and quantitative study of pulmonary blood vessels from 58 patients in the National Heart, Lung, and Blood Institute, primary pulmonary hypertension registry. Circulation 80:1198, 1989.

93. Kawat SM, Silvestry FE, Ferrari VA, et al: Extrinsic compression of the left main coronary artery by the pulmonary artery in patients with long-standing pulmonary hypertension. Am J Cardiol 83:984, 1999.

94. Potain PCE: Concerning the cardiac rhythm called gallop rhythm. Bull Mém Soc Méd d'Hôp Paris 12:137, 1876.

95. Reece EA, Moya F, Yazigi R, et al: Persistent pulmonary hypertension: Assessment of perinatal risk factors. Obstet Gynecol 70:696, 1987.

96. Rhodes J, Barst RJ, Garofano RP, et al: Hemodynamic correlates of exercise function in patients with primary pulmonary hypertension. J Am Coll Cardiol 18:1738, 1991.

97. Rich S: Primary pulmonary hypertension. Prog Cardiovasc Dis 31:205, 1988.

98. Rich S, Brundage BH: Pulmonary hypertension: A cellular basis for understanding the pathophysiology and treatment. J Am Coll Cardiol 14:545, 1989.

99. Rich S, Dantzker DR, Ayres SM, et al: Primary pulmonary hypertension: A national prospective study. Ann Intern Med 107:216, 1987.

100. Rich S, Kieras K, Hart K, et al: Antinuclear antibodies in primary pulmonary hypertension. J Am Coll Cardiol 8:1307, 1986.

101. Rich S, Levitsky S, Brundage BH: Pulmonary hypertension from chronic pulmonary thromboembolism. Ann Intern Med 108:425, 1988.

102. Rivero-Carvallo JM: New diagnostic sign of tricuspid insufficiency. Arch Inst Cardiol Mex 16:531, 1946.

103. Robalino BD, Moodie DS: Association between primary pulmonary hypertension and portal hypertension: Analysis of its pathophysiology and clinical, laboratory and hemodynamic manifestations. J Am Coll Cardiol 17:492, 1991.

104. Roberts NV, Keast PJ: Pulmonary hypertension and pregnancy—a lethal combination. Anaesth Intens Care 18:366, 1990.

105. Roberts WC: The histologic structure of the pulmonary trunk in patients with "primary" pulmonary hypertension. Am Heart J 65:230, 1963.

106. Rogge JD, Mishkin ME, Genovese PD: Familial occurrence of primary pulmonary hypertension. Ann Intern Med 65:672, 1966.

107. Romberg E: Ueber Sklerose der Lungenarterie. Dtsch Arch Klin Med 48:197, 1891.

108. Rozkovec A, Montanes P, Oakley CM: Factors that influence the outcome of primary pulmonary hypertension. Br Heart J 55:449, 1986.

109. Ruttner JR, Bartschi JP, Niedermann R, Schneider J: Plexogenic pulmonary arteriopathy and liver disease. Thorax 35:133, 1980.

110. Satyanarayana Rao BN, Moller JH, Edwards JE: Primary pulmonary hypertension in a child. Circulation 40:583, 1969.

111. Shapiro S, Clark TJH, Goodwin JF: Delayed closure of the pulmonary valve in obliterative pulmonary hypertension. Lancet 2:1207, 1965.

112. Shaver JA, Nadolny RA, O'Toole JD, et al: Sound pressure correlates of the second heart sound. Circulation 49:316, 1974.

113. Sime F, Banchero N, Penaloza D, et al: Pulmonary hypertension in children born and living at high altitudes. Am J Cardiol 11:143, 1963.

114. Siassi B, Goldberg SJ, Emmanouilides GC, et al: Persistent pulmonary vascular obstruction in newborn infants. J Pediatr 78:610, 1971.

115. Smith WM, Kroop IG: Raynaud's disease in primary pulmonary hypertension. JAMA 165:1245, 1957.

116. Snyder SH: Nitric oxide: First in a new class of neurotransmitters? Science 257:494, 1992.

117. Speich R, Jenni R, Opravil M, et al: Primary pulmonary hypertension in HIV infection. Chest 100:1268, 1991.

118. Steell G: The murmur of high pressure in the pulmonary artery. Med Chron 9:182, 1888.

119. Stojnic BB, Brecker SJD, Xiao HB, et al: Left ventricular filling characteristics in pulmonary hypertension: A new mode of ventricular interaction. Br Heart J 68:16, 1992.

120. Takeuchi T, Nishii O, Okamura T, Yaginuma T: Primary pulmonary hypertension in pregnancy. Int J Gynecol Obstet 26:145, 1988.

121. Thilenius OG, Nadas AS, Jockin H: Primary pulmonary vascular obstruction in children. Pediatrics 36:75, 1965.

122. Thompson P, McRae C: Familial pulmonary hypertension. Evidence of autosomal dominant inheritance. Br Heart J 32:758, 1970.

123. Van Epps EF: Primary pulmonary hypertension in brothers. Am J Roentgenol 78:471, 1957.

124. van Hooft IMS, Grobbee DE, Waal-Manning HJ, Hofman A: Hemodynamic characteristics of the early phase of primary pulmonary hypertension. Circulation 87:1100, 1993.

125. Villaschi S, Pietra G-G: Alveolar capillary membrane in primary pulmonary hypertension. Appl Pathol 4:132, 1986.

126. Wagenvoort CA: Lung biopsy specimens in the evaluation of primary pulmonary vascular disease. Chest 77:614, 1980.

127. Wagenvoort CA, Wagenvoort N: Primary pulmonary hypertension. Circulation 42:1163, 1970.

128. Wagenvoort CA, Heath D, Edwards JE: The Pathology of the Pulmonary Vasculature. Springfield, Ill, Charles C Thomas, 1963.

129. Waldman JD, Lamberti JJ, Mathewson JW, et al: Congenital heart disease and pulmonary hypertension. J Am Coll Cardiol 2:1158, 1983.

130. Winters WL, Joseph RR, Learner N: "Primary" pulmonary hypertension and Raynaud's phenomenon. Arch Intern Med 114:821, 1964.

131. Wood P: Pulmonary hypertension. Br Med Bull 8:348, 1952.

132. Yamaki S, Wagenvoort CA: Plexogenic pulmonary arteriopathy. Am J Pathol 105:70, 1981.

133. Ye C, Rabinovitch M: New developments in the pulmonary circulation in children. Curr Opin Cardiol 7:124, 1992.

134. Gomez A, Bialostozky D, Zajarias A, et al: Right ventricular ischemia in patients with primary pulmonary hypertension. J Am Coll Cardiol 38:1137, 2001.

135. Deng Z, Morse JH, Slager SL, et al: Familial primary pulmonary hypertension (gene PPH1) is caused by mutations on the bone marrow morphogenetic protein receptor gene. Am J Hum Genet 67:737, 2000.

136. SoRelle R: Gene for familial primary pulmonary hypertension identified. Circulation 102:E9010, 2000.

137. Morse JH, Jones AC, Barst RJ, et al: Familial primary pulmonary hypertension locus mapped to chromosome 2q31-q32. Chest 114:57S, 1998.

138. Newman JH, Wheeler L, Lane KB, et al: Mutation in the gene for bone morphogenetic protein receptor as a cause of primary pulmonary hypertension in a large kindred. N Engl J Med 345:319, 2001.

139. Geraci MW, Moore M, Gesell T, et al: Gene expression patterns in the lungs of patients with primary pulmonary hypertension. Circ Res 88:555, 2001.

140. Thomson JR, Trembath RC: Primary pulmonary hypertension: the pressure rises for a gene. J Clin Pathol 53:899, 2000.

141. Krohn BG: The enigma of primary pulmonary hypertension. J Am Coll Cardiol 37:1476, 2001.

142. Loscalzo J: Genetic clues to the cause of primary pulmonary hypertension. N Engl J Med 345:367, 2001.

143. Morrell NW, Yang X, Upton PD, et al: Altered growth responses of pulmonary artery smooth muscle cells from patients with primary pulmonary hypertension to transforming growth factor beta and bone morphogenetic proteins. Circulation 104:790, 2001.

144. Yeager ME, Halley GR, Golpon HA, et al: Microsatellite instability of endothelial cell growth and apoptosis genes within plexiform lesions in primary pulmonary hypertension. Circ Res 88:E2, 2001.

145. Silverman BD: Graham Steele: Profiles in Cardiology. Clin Cardiol 18:54, 1995.

146. Ivy DD, Neish SR, Knudson OA, et al: Intravascular ultrasonic characteristics and vasoreactivity of the pulmonary vasculature in children with pulmonary hypertension. Am J Cardiol 81:740, 1998.

147. Marcus JT, Vonk NA, Roeleveld RJ, et al: Impaired left ventricular filling due to right ventricular pressure overload in primary pulmonary hypertension. Chest 119:1761, 2001.

148. Bossone E, Duong TH, Paciocco G, et al: Echocardiographic features of primary pulmonary hypertension. J Am Soc Echocardiogr 12:655, 1999.

149. Harinck E, Hutter PA, Hoorntje TM, et al: Air travel in adults with cyanotic congenital heart disease. Circulation 93:272, 1996.

150. Child JS: Transthoracic and Transesophageal Imaging: Anatomic and Hemodynamic Assessment. In Perloff JK, Child JS (eds): Congenital Heart Disease in Adults, 2nd ed. Philadelphia, WB Saunders, 1998, p. 91.

151. Rich S: Clinical insights into the pathogenesis of primary pulmonary hypertension. Chest 114:237S, 1998.

152. Mikhail GW, Gibbs JS, Yacoub MH: Pulmonary and systemic arterial pressure changes during syncope in primary pulmonary hypertension. Circulation 104:1326, 2001.

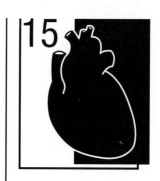

Atrial Septal Defect: Simple and Complex

Galen knew of the foramen ovale and its normal postnatal closure.[123] Leonardo da Vinci wrote, "I have found from left auricle to right auricle the perforating channel," and his subsequent account a true atrial septal defect is believed to be the first record of a congenital malformation of the human heart.[145] Botallo described a persistent foramen ovale after birth but without understanding its function in the fetus.[123] Gassendi composed an entire treatise based on observations of a patent foramen ovale in an adult cadaver.[123] In 1875, Karl von Rokitansky published superb observations on the pathological anatomy of atrial septal defects together with their presumed embryologic basis, and distinguished septum primum from septum secundum defects.[359] In 1921, Assmann described the radiologic features of atrial septal defects that paved the way for clinical recognition.[22] In 1934, Roesler analyzed 62 necropsy cases, only one of which had been correctly diagnosed during life.[357] Bedford, Papp and Parkinson defined the clinical features of atrial septal defects in a landmark publication in 1941,[36] and Hudson's 1955 description of the normal and abnormal interatrial septum[227] was confirmed and refined in 1979 by Sweeney and Rosenquist.[413] These accounts have been supplemented by superb studies of the anatomy of the interatrial septum based on transesophageal echocardiography.[376]

The normal atrial septum viewed from its right side is a blade-shaped structure with a superior-anterior margin that reflects the curvature of the ascending aorta, an inferior margin that borders the mitral annulus, and a posterior margin that is convex.[413] The left side of the septum has a network of trabeculations that are remnants of the septum primum. The fossa ovalis is bordered by a limbus and guarded by a valve (see Fig 15–46C) and constitutes approximately 28% of the septal area irrespective of age.[413] The fetal patent foramen ovale closes after birth by fusion of its valve with the limbus of the fossa ovalis when left atrial pressure exceeds right atrial pressure. The incidence of persistent patency of the foramen ovale declines from approximately one third during the first three decades of life to approximately one fourth during the fourth through eighth decades.[199] The morphogenetic sequence of normal intrauterine formation and closure of the atrial septum is illustrated in Figure 15–1.[227] Redundancy of the valve of the foramen ovale can result in an atrial septal aneurysm (see Fig 15–48).[39,58,205,331,353,390,391]

The most common type of atrial septal defect is in the *ostium secundum* or fossa ovalis location (Figs. 15–2 and 15–3).[34] The defect results either from shortening of the valve of the foramen ovale, excessive resorption of the septum primum, or deficient growth of the septum secundum (Figs. 15–1, 15–2 and see Fig. 15–46C). An ostium secundum atrial septal defect lies in a folded area rather than in a flat plane, and its anatomy is more complex on its right side than on its left side.[122] Next in frequency are *ostium primum* atrial septal defects that represent absence of the atrioventricular septum and are therefore located in the inferior portion of the atrial septum (Figs. 15–1 and 15–2). *Sinus venosus* atrial septal defects are uncommon but not rare, constituting 2% to 3% of interatrial communications.[110] During normal embryogenesis, the right horn of the sinus venosus incorporates the inferior vena cava and the right superior vena cava. Faulty resorption of the sinus venosus results in an interatrial communication near the orifice of either the superior or the inferior vena cava. The right valve of the sinus venosus is a broad membrane that almost partitions the developing right atrium, with the two cavas located on its left side. The principle variety of sinus venosus defect was described in 1868 as a "free communication between the auricles by deficiency of the upper part of the septum auricularum."[431] Superior vena caval sinus venosus

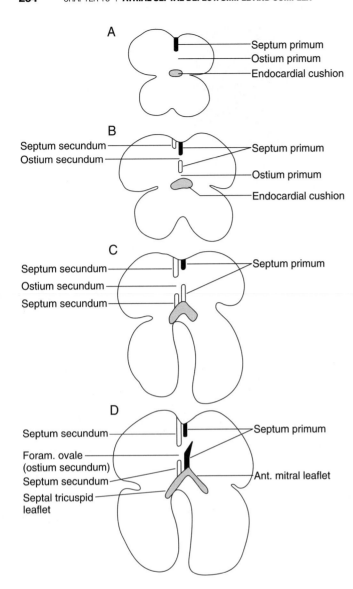

Figure 15–1

Schematic illustrations of sequential changes during the formation of the atrial septum. (Modified from Hudson R: Normal and abnormal interatrial septum. Br Heart J 17:489, 1955; and from Van Mierop LHS. In: Feldt RH. Atrioventricular Canal Defects. Philadelphia, WB Saunders, 1976.)

defects vary from small to nonrestrictive and are located immediately inferior to the junction of the superior cava and right atrium (Fig. 15–2 and see Fig. 15–47A), with the orifice of the superior vena cava overriding the defect which is therefore biatrial.[151] *Inferior vena caval* sinus venosus defects are located below the foramen ovale and merge with the floor of the inferior cava (Fig. 15–2 and see Fig. 15–47B).[34,174] As the valve resorbs, its rudiment becomes the eustachian valve that directs inferior vena caval blood across the fetal foramen ovale. Persistence of a large eustachian valve (see Fig. 15–10) channels inferior vena caval blood across an ostium secundum atrial septal defect (see Fig 15–9) or across an inferior vena caval sinus venosus defect (see Figure 15–47B).[174,421] A *coronary sinus atrial septal defect* is uncommon but not rare, and as the name implies is located at the site normally occupied by the right atrial ostium of the coronary sinus (Fig. 15–2).[55,261,285,319,347] The defect is characterized either by an opening in the wall of the distal end of the coronary sinus,[55,285] or by *unroofing* caused by absence of the partition between the coronary sinus and the left atrium.

Coronary sinus atrial septal defects are accompanied by a left superior vena cava that inserts into the upper left corner of the left atrium.[55,285] A relatively rare combination of anomalies consists of absence of the coronary sinus, a defect in the atrial septum in the location of the ostium of the coronary sinus, and a left superior vena cava that is connected to the left atrium.[347] The combination is cyanotic because blood from the left superior vena caval enters the left atrium directly. Atrial septal defects are usually located in only one of the foregoing locations, but separate ostium secundum, sinus venosus, and ostium primum defects occasionally coexist.[407]

Spontaneous closure of an ostium secundum atrial septal defect refers to sealing of a true tissue defect in the atrial septum and not to cessation of a left-to-right shunt through a valve-incompetent foramen ovale.* Ostium secundum atrial septal defects are seldom symptomatically manifest in infants and young children (see Fig. 15–46B), but when they are so manifest, approximately one third reportedly

---

*See references 23, 58, 79, 91, 101, 169, 185, 210, 221, 306.

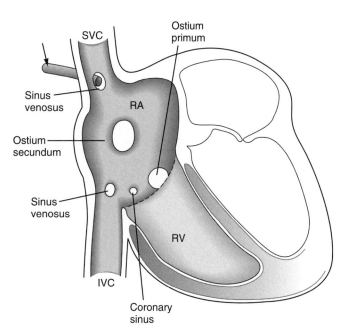

Figure 15–2

The locations of an ostium secundum atrial septal defect, an ostium primum atrial septal defect, a superior vena caval (SVC) and an inferior vena caval (IVC) sinus venosus atrial septal defect, and a coronary sinus defect. RV, right ventricle. Unmarked arrow upper left identifies the right superior pulmonary vein.

close spontaneously between one and two years of age.[91,185,306] The mechanism(s) responsible for spontaneous closure remain to be established.[23,58,390]

Anatomic connections and physiologic drainage of pulmonary veins are important features of atrial septal defects. *Connection* refers to a pulmonary vein that is *anatomically* contiguous with a morphologic left atrium or a morphologic right atrium.[138,290,410] *Drainage* refers to the *physiologic* pathway of blood from pulmonary veins into the left atrium or right atrium. Pulmonary veins that connect normally can drain normally or anomalously, but pulmonary veins that connect anomalously drain anomalously. Normal right pul-

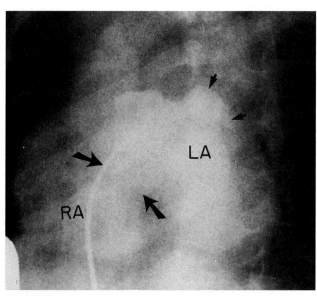

Figure 15–3

Angiocardiogram (*shallow left oblique*) in an 8-year-old boy with an ostium secundum atrial septal defect. Contrast material outlines the left atrium (LA) including its appendage (*small paired arrows*). Contrast material crossed a nonrestrictive ostium secundum atrial septal defect (*large arrow*) and filled the right atrium (RA).

monary veins connect to the left atrium close to the rim of ostium secundum atrial septal defects,[138,410,411] so a substantial portion of right pulmonary venous blood preferentially drains into the right atrium even though the veins connect anatomically to the left atrium (Fig. 15–4). *Partial* anomalous pulmonary venous connection exists when one or more but not all pulmonary veins connect anomalously to the right atrium.[8,14,37,110,193,290,318,396,404] *Total* anomalous pulmonary venous connection applies when *all four* pulmonary veins connect anomalously to the right atrium either indirectly or directly. Ten to fifteen percent of ostium secundum atrial septal defects are associated with partial anomalous pulmonary venous connections.[193] Eighty to ninety percent of superior vena caval sinus venosus defects are associated with anomalous connection of the right superior pulmonary vein to right atrium or superior vena cava (Figs. 15–2 and 15–5).[110,151] Approximately 90% of partial anomalous pulmonary venous connections join the right upper or middle lobe pulmonary veins to the right atrium or superior vena cava.[290,396,404] Partial anomalous connection of right pulmonary veins is usually associated with an ostium secundum atrial septal defect,[166] is exceptionally associated with an intact atrial septum, and may go unrecognized when associated with a restrictive sinus venosus defect (Fig. 15–5).[61,110] Anomalous connection of *left* pulmonary veins is far less prevalent (about 10%) as anomalous connection of right pulmonary veins, and is represented by anomalous connections to the innominate vein or to a persistent left superior vena cava that attaches to the innominate vein. *Bilateral* partial anomalous pulmonary venous connections are rare.

The *scimitar syndrome*, described in 1836 by Chassinat,[81] is a rare anomaly characterized by connection of all of the right pulmonary veins to the inferior vena cava, and usually by hypoplasia of the ipsilateral lung and pulmonary artery[72,133,322] (Figs. 15–6 through 15–8). The term *scimitar*

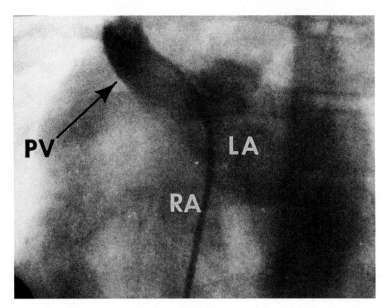

Figure 15–4

Angiocardiogram (shallow left oblique) from an 11-year-old girl with an ostium secundum atrial septal defect. Contrast material from left atrium (LA) flows into right atrium (RA) across the nonrestrictive atrial septal defect. The right superior pulmonary vein (PV) connects normally to the left atrium (LA, catheter tip).

refers to an x-ray shadow that resembles the shape of a Turkish sword (Fig. 15–6C). The lower portion of the right lung is perfused by systemic arteries from the abdominal aorta.[72,133,286] The scimitar syndrome rarely involves the left lung.[114,286]

Anatomical studies of the mitral, tricuspid and pulmonary valves in ostium secundum atrial septal defects have disclosed morphologic and architectural modifications.[94] Mitral valve abnormalities consist of thickening and fibrosis of leaflets and chordae tendineae attributed to traumatic cusp movements resulting from left ventricular cavity deformity.[54,316] The lesions are believed to be the basis for mitral regurgitation that develops with age in patients with an ostium secundum atrial septal defect.[54,113,172,236,316,435] Superior systolic displacement of the mitral leaflets (mitral valve prolapse) occurs because leaflets with normal areas and chordal lengths are housed in a left ventricular cavity that is reduced in size and abnormally shaped by the position of the ventricular septum (see Fig. 15–46B).[113]

In cyanotic patients with nonrestrictive atrial septal defects and pulmonary vascular disease, the hypertensive proximal pulmonary arteries develop aneurysmal dilatation, massive intraluminal thrombus, and mural calcification (see Fig. 15–12).[71,149,374,379] Abnormalities of medial smooth muscle, elastin, collagen, and ground substance reside in the walls of these pulmonary arteries and are held responsible for dilatation that is out of proportion to hemodynamic or morphogenetic expectation.[152] Aneurysmal proximal pulmonary arteries may rupture.[152,379]

The *physiologic consequences* of atrial septal defects depend on the magnitude and chronicity of the left-to-right shunt and on the behavior of the pulmonary vascular bed. When the defect is *restrictive*, size plays a role in determining the magnitude of the shunt.[60] When the defect is *nonrestrictive*, there is no pressure difference between the right and left atrium, so shunt volume is determined by the

relative compliance of the two ventricles.[120,364] All four cardiac chambers are in common communication during diastole. Accordingly, blood can flow from the *left atrium* through the atrial septal defect into the right atrium and across the tricuspid valve into the right ventricle or directly into the left ventricle across the mitral valve, or blood can flow from the *right atrium* across the atrial septal defect into the left atrium across the mitral valve into the left ventricle or directly into the right ventricle across the tricuspid valve. The right ventricle is thinner and more compliant than the left ventricle in an ostium secundum atrial septal defect, so the flow of blood is from left atrium through the atrial septal defect across the tricuspid valve into the relatively compliant right ventricle, establishing a left-to-right shunt.[120,364] A transient right-to-left shunt coincides with the onset of ventricular systole (Fig. 15–9B). The left-to-right shunt reaches its peak in late systole and early diastole, diminishes throughout diastole, and is supplemented in late diastole by atrial contraction (Fig. 15–9B).[7,240] Clinical and experimental studies of instantaneous flow across atrial septal defects have confirmed these patterns.[7]

The fetal circulation is not disturbed by an atrial septal defect because normal *in utero* interatrial flow is from right-to-left through a patent foramen ovale (see Fig. 15–46C). There is little or no shunt in either direction across an atrial septal defect at birth because the compliance of the right and left ventricles is virtually identical.[292,360,430] In response to the fall in neonatal pulmonary vascular resistance, the right ventricle becomes thinner and more compliant than the left ventricle, so left atrial blood then flows across the atrial septal defect into the relatively compliant right ventricle.[269] Pulmonary blood flow that is received by the *right* pulmonary veins is channeled into the right atrium because of proximity of the right pulmonary veins to the rim of the atrial septal defect (Fig. 15–4). Pulmonary blood flow that is received by the *left* pulmonary veins is

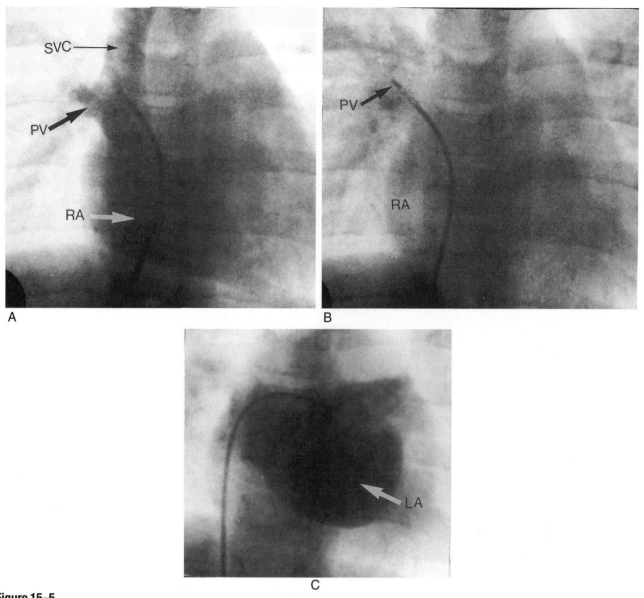

Figure 15–5

Angiocardiograms from a 10-year-old boy with a restrictive superior vena caval (SVC) sinus venosus atrial septal defect and anomalous pulmonary venous connection (PV) to the right atrium (RA). *A,B,* The catheter tip is in the right superior pulmonary vein (PV) that was entered from the right atrium (RA). *C,* The opacified left atrium (LA) was entered across the sinus venosus atrial septal defect. There was no left-to-right shunt.

channeled into the left atrium and is then shunted across the atrial septal defect. Accordingly, the right ventricle is volume overloaded and the left is volume underloaded. The mature right ventricle is a highly compliant pump that readily adapts to volume overload and ejects an increased stroke volume into the low resistance pulmonary vascular bed.[269] Right ventricular function is usually maintained through the fourth decade.[269] Ischemic heart disease and systemic hypertension conspire to reduce left ventricular compliance and to increase the left-to-right shunt.[2,120,423] Excessive volume overload of the right atrium provokes atrial fibrillation and atrial flutter, which augment the left-to-right shunt and result in congestive heart failure (Fig. 15–11).

Left ventricular end-diastolic volume, stroke volume, ejection fraction and cardiac output are decreased in infants through adults with an atrial septal defect,[51,52, 159,194,292,343,369,423] and ejection fraction tends to decrease with exercise.[51,117] Diminished left ventricular functional reserve is related to the mechanical effects of right ventricular volume overload, which displaces the ventricular septum into the left ventricular cavity, reducing its size and changing its shape from ovoid to crescentic (Fig. 15–46C).[51,52,117,159,236,369] In addition, coronary reserve may be compromised in the volume overloaded right ventricle when the left main coronary artery is compressed by a dilated pulmonary trunk.[142]

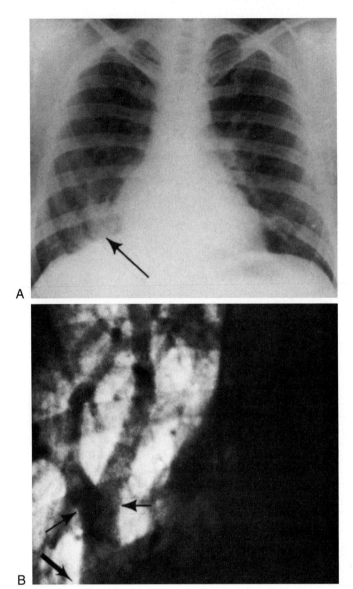

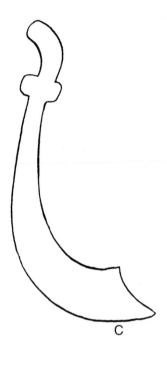

Figure 15–6

A, X-ray from a 28-year-old man with anomalous pulmonary venous connection of the entire right lung–*scimitar syndrome.* Right pulmonary veins converge to form a vascular trunk (*arrow*) that drained into the inferior vena cava. The right lung was not hypoplastic. *B,* Levophase following injection of contrast material into the pulmonary trunk shows the common pulmonary venous channel (scimitar, *paired arrows*) and the entrance site (*left lower arrow*). *C,* Turkish sword or scimitar.

An important and poorly understood deviation from the prevailing pattern of asymptomatic onset of the left-to-right shunt across an atrial septal defect is the occasional infant who develops a large shunt and right ventricular failure (Fig. 15–46B).[66,91,125,185,232] Initiation of a left-to-right shunt before right ventricular compliance increases has been attributed to more complete emptying of the right ventricle (reduced resistance to discharge), which preferentially fills during diastole. Right ventricular failure ensues because of volume overload of the neonatal right ventricle before involution of its free wall thickness.[160] Although right ventricular failure is occasionally intractable, there is a surprising propensity for clinical improvement because of spontaneous closure of the atrial septal defect.[91,185,306]

The paucity of pulmonary vascular disease in patients with nonrestrictive atrial septal defects has been ascribed to the timing of the large left-to-right shunt after pulmonary artery pressure has normalized. The shunt transverses a low-resistance low-pressure pulmonary vascular bed that accommodates to an appreciable increment in blood flow without an increase in pressure.[70,100,219] Pulmonary vascular disease with a right-to-left shunt occurs in less than 10% of patients with an atrial septal defect. High pulmonary vascular resistance is believed to represent the coincidence in young females of primary pulmonary hypertension and an ostium secundum atrial septal defect (see Fig. 15–13 and see Chapter 14).[100,109,181,369] Older adults experience moderate increases in pulmonary artery pressure but with persistence of the left-to-right shunt. Thus, pulmonary hypertension with nonrestrictive atrial septal defect is bimodal, and is represented by young females who have coexisting primary pulmonary hyper-

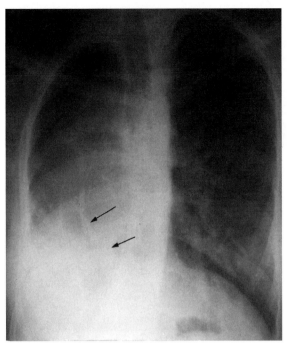

Figure 15–7

X-ray from a 16-year-old girl with anomalous pulmonary venous connection of the entire right lung (scimitar sign, *upper arrow*) that drained into the inferior vena cava (*lower arrow*). The heart was displaced into the right hemithorax and the right hemidiaphragm was elevated because the right lung was hypoplastic. An ostium secundum atrial septal defect coexisted.

tension and a small or reversed shunt, or by older males or females who have moderate pulmonary hypertension with a persistent left-to-right shunt.

Atrial septal defects with pulmonary hypertension are relatively common in patients born at high altitude.[104,105,250]

Increased resistance to right ventricular discharge can result from massive occlusive thrombus in dilated proximal pulmonary arteries (see Figs. 15–12*B* and 15–42).

The physiologic consequences of partial anomalous pulmonary venous connection associated with an atrial septal defect are similar if not identical to an isolated atrial septal defect with an equivalent net shunt because the hemodynamic fault remains a left-to-right shunt at atrial level.[14,16,37,151,193] However, flow through anomalous pulmonary veins into right atrium is obligatory and is therefore established earlier than left-to-right shunts across an atrial septal defect. When partial anomalous pulmonary venous connection occurs with an *intact* atrial septum, flow is increased in the segment of lung with the anomalous pulmonary veins because right atrial pressure is lower than left atrial pressure (intact atrial septum). The pressure gradient across the anomalously draining lung is therefore greater than across the normally draining lung.[8,166,404]

Anomalous *systemic venous drainage* from a normally aligned inferior vena cava results in cyanosis with *increased* pulmonary blood flow. Small amounts of inferior vena caval blood transiently stream across an ostium secundum atrial septal defect in early systole, a pattern appropriate for the normal direction of fetal blood from inferior vena cava across a foramen ovale.[176] A large persistent eustachian valve sometimes extends from the orifice of the inferior vena cava to the margin of an *ostium secundum* atrial septal defect (Fig. 15–10), selectively channeling inferior caval blood into the left atrium in sufficient amounts to cause cyanosis.[31,174,284,442] A large eustachian valve in the presence of an *inferior vena caval sinus venosus* atrial septal

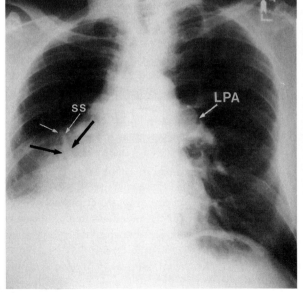

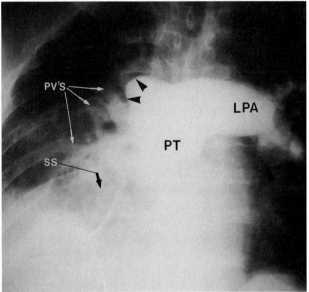

Figure 15–8

A, X-ray from a 66-year-old man with anomalous pulmonary venous connection of the entire right lung that drained into the inferior vena cava–scimitar syndrome (SS). The right lung was hypoplastic, the heart was displaced into the right hemithorax, the right hemidiaphragm was elevated, and there was proximity of the posterior ribs. The left pulmonary artery (LPA) is prominent because of a left-to-right shunt through an ostium secundum atrial septal defect and elevated pulmonary artery pressure. *B,* Pulmonary arteriogram showing absence of the right pulmonary artery (*unmarked black arrow heads*). The pulmonary trunk (PT) and left pulmonary artery (LPA) are dilated. The levophase visualizes the right pulmonary veins (PVs) and faintly visualizes the scimitar sign (SS).

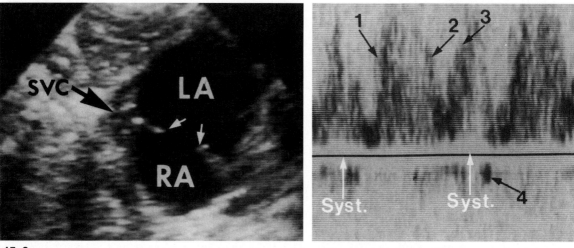

Figure 15–9

A, Echocardiogram (subcostal) showing an ostium secundum atrial septal defect (*paired white arrows*) in the midportion of the atrial septum remote from the superior vena cava (SVC). RA, right atrium; LA, left atrium. *B,* Pulsed Doppler within the atrial septal defect shows signals that are positive and maximum in late systole (1) and in early diastole (2) and then continue throughout diastole with presystolic reinforcement caused by atrial contraction (3). A negative early systolic Doppler signal (4) was caused by a transient right-to-left shunt.

defect channels inferior caval blood directly into the left atrium (Fig. 15–47B).[174]

THE HISTORY

The female-to-male ratio is at least 2:1 in patients with an ostium secundum atrial septal defect,[160] while sinus venosus atrial septal defects have sex ratios that are approximately equal.[110] Ostium secundum atrial septal defects are sometimes familial, occasionally recur in several generations,[111,226,241,279,321,354] have been described in identical twins,[294] and familial scimitar syndrome has been reported.[95,320] Autosomal dominant inheritance is a feature of atrial septal defect with Holt-Oram syndrome (see Physical Appearance).[173,291,345,392,402] Autosomal dominant inheritance tends to occur in ostium secundum defects and prolonged atrioventricular conduction,[43,44,147,332] with some members in a given family having an atrial septal defect with PR interval prolongation, others having PR prolongation with intact atrial septum,[43] and still others experiencing sudden death.[147]

Atrial septal defects may go unrecognized for decades because symptoms are mild or absent and physical signs are subtle. The soft pulmonary midsystolic murmur in children and young adults is often overlooked or discounted as an innocent murmur (see Chapter 2). An atrial septal defect may first come to light on a routine chest x-ray.[378] An important exception is the symptomatic infant with an ostium secundum atrial septal defect (Fig. 15–46B) in whom congestive heart failure may be followed by spontaneous closure (see earlier).*

Approximately half of patients with the *scimitar* syndrome are asymptomatic or only mildly symptomatic when the diagnosis is made, despite varying degrees of hypoplasia of the right lung (Figs. 15–6 through 15–8).[72,322] A small but important group of scimitar syndrome patients consists of symptomatic infants with cyanosis and pulmonary hypertension.[72] Older children and young adults with the scimitar syndrome come to light because of an x-ray that discloses the scimitar sign and the hypoplastic right lung, or because of an atrial tachyarrhythmia, or recurrent lower respiratory infections or a murmur.[72,141,322]

Paul Wood remarked, "In any series of geriatric necropsies atrial septal defect is always represented." Ostium secundum atrial septal defects are among the commonest congenital cardiac malformations in adults, accounting for 30% to 40% of unoperated patients over 40 years of age.[68,253,256,288,334,346] Many patients survive to advanced age, but life expectancy is not normal. Three quarters of patients are alive through the third decade, but three quarters of these are dead by age 50 years, and 90% are dead by age 60 years.[68] Sporadic survivals have been recorded beyond age 70 years, and there are rare examples of patients in their eighties or nineties (see Fig. 15–43B).[2,18,105,253,256,334,346] An exceptional patient died three months before his ninety-fifth birthday (see Fig. 15–43A).[334] Death is often unrelated to the malformation, but when a relationship exists, cardiac failure is the commonest cause.[2,100,109]

The clinical course of ostium secundum atrial septal defects spans the reproductive years, and the majority of patients are female. It is therefore reassuring that despite the gestational increase in cardiac output and stroke volume, young gravida with an atrial septal defect generally endure pregnancy—even multiple pregnancies—without tangible ill effects.[336] However, hemorrhage during deliv-

*See references 2, 4, 79, 91, 124, 125, 160, 169, 185, 221, 306.

ery provokes a rise in systemic vascular resistance and a fall in systemic venous return, a combination that augments the left-to-right shunt, sometimes appreciably.[336] There is a peripartum risk of paradoxical embolization from leg veins or pelvic veins because emboli carried by the inferior vena cava tend to traverse the atrial septal defect and enter the systemic circulation.[336]

Dyspnea and fatigue are the earliest symptoms of an ostium secundum atrial septal defect.[100,109,181,288,369] The large left-to-right shunt is responsible for a decrease in pulmonary compliance and an increase in the work of breathing. Orthopnea may be experienced because the supine position increases the work of breathing in patients with reduced lung compliance. Platypnea-orthodeoxia is a rare syndrome characterized by orthostatic provocation of a right-to-left shunt across an atrial septal defect or a patent foramen ovale.[74, 381] Platypnea (dyspnea induced by the upright position and relieved by recumbency) and orthodeoxia (arterial desaturation in the upright position with improvement during recumbency) are the essential features of this rare disorder. Clinical suspicion may originate from the patient's observation that dyspnea is provoked by standing upright.

Recurrent lower respiratory infections are common especially in children.[19,100] The pulmonary valve is theoretically susceptible to infective endocarditis owing to the rapid rate of ejection, but only a single case has been reported.[177]

Older patients deteriorate chiefly on three counts. First, a decrease in left ventricular distensibility associated with aging, ischemic heart disease, systemic hypertension, or acquired calcific aortic stenosis augments the left-to-right shunt.[2, 10,120,346,423] Second, the age related increase in prevalence of paroxysmal atrial tachycardia, atrial fibrillation, and atrial flutter precipitates congestive heart failure (Fig. 15–11 and Fig. 15–45).[100,254] Third, mild-to-moderate pulmonary hypertension in older adults occurs in the face of a persistent left-to-right shunt, so the aging right ventricle is doubly beset by both pressure and volume overload.[109,181,369] Pulmonary vascular disease with reversed shunt is believed to represent the coincidence of primary pulmonary hypertension with an ostium secundum atrial septal defect in young females who are predisposed to both lesions (Fig. 15–13, see earlier).[100,105,120,219] Importantly, the outlook is better when primary pulmonary hypertension occurs with an atrial septal defect or a patent foramen ovale because the right heart can decompress (see Chapter 14).

A *patent foramen ovale* is the most common remnant of the fetal circulation (Fig. 15–46C), occurring in 10% to 15% of the normal adult population and in 20% to 30% of normal hearts at postmortem.[66,75,199] The patent foramen ovale varies in anatomical and functional size and has been implicated in paradoxical embolization, transient ischemic attacks, venoarterial gas embolism, decompression sickness, and platypnea-orthodeoxia.[13,66,211,312,405]

An *atrial septal aneurysm* is a congenital malformation characterized by a protrusion beyond the plane of the atrial septum and by rapid even dramatic phasic cardiorespiratory oscillations (Fig. 15–48).[13,38,39,56,96,121,131,157,205,331] Cerebral emboli originate from fibrin-platelet aggregates that form on the left atrial side of the aneurysm and are dislodged by the phasic excursions.[13,56,131,157] Atrial septal aneurysms have been incriminated as a cause of atrial arrhythmias in children and adults as well as in the fetus.[353] An atrial septal defect may coexist.

PHYSICAL APPEARANCE

Children with an atrial septal defect may have a delicate gracile habitus with weight more affected than height (Fig. 15–14A), and may have a left precordial bulge with Harrison's grooves (Fig. 15–14A and B).[19] Newborns who subsequently manifest an atrial septal defect are on an average smaller than their normal siblings.[69] *Symptomatic* infants may be cyanotic and reflect the catabolic effects of congestive heart failure.[91, 125,232] Cyanosis also occurs when a large eustachian valve selectively channels inferior vena caval blood into the left atrium through an ostium secundum atrial septal defect (Fig. 15–10) or through an inferior vena caval sinus venosus defect (see Fig. 15–47B).[31,174,176]

Holt-Oram syndrome is a distinctive physical appearance that heightens suspicion of an ostium secundum atrial septal defect (Figs. 15–15 and 15–16).[143,173,224,291,305,345,392,402] The thumb is hypoplastic with an accessory phalanx that results in triphalangism and a crooked appearance and difficulty in apposition of thumb to fingertips. The abnormality becomes more obvious when the palms are supinated (Fig. 15–15). The thumb may be rudimentary or absent, and the metacarpal bone may be small or absent with hypoplasia extending to the radius (Fig. 15–16). The bony anomaly ranges from minor changes perceptible only on x-ray to

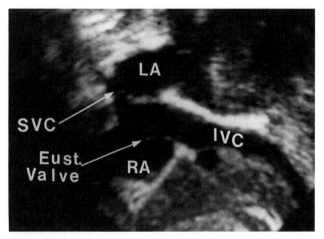

Figure 15–10
Echocardiogram (subcostal) showing a eustachian valve (Eust Valve highlighted) that extended from the inferior vena cava (IVC) and directed inferior vena caval blood toward the midportion of the atrial septum. LA, left atrium; RA, right atrium; SVC, superior vena cava.

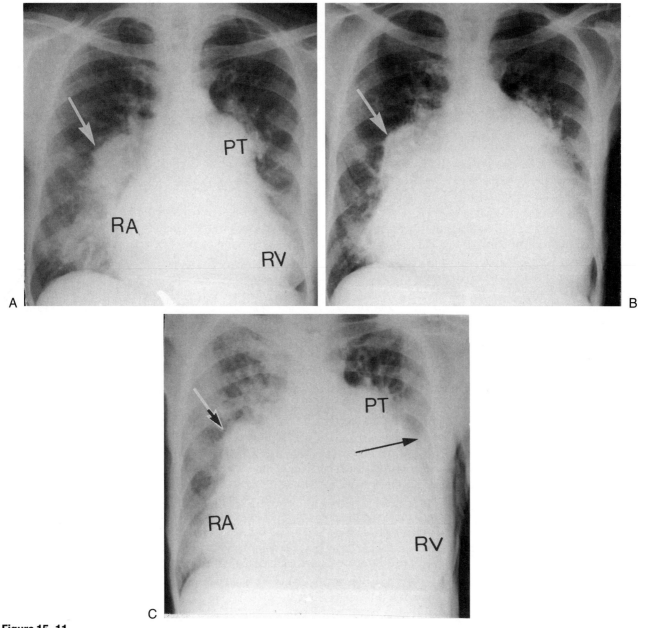

Figure 15–11

X-rays from a 71-year-old woman in sinus rhythm with a nonrestrictive ostium secundum atrial septal defect. *A,* Pulmonary arterial vascularity is increased, the pulmonary trunk (PT) and right branch (*arrow*) are enlarged, a prominent right atrium (RA) occupies the lower right cardiac border, and a large right ventricle (RV) occupies the apex. *B,* X-ray from the same patient 5 months after the onset of atrial fibrillation. *C,* At age 73 years, the cardiac silhouette is immense because of striking dilatation of the right ventricle (RV) and right atrium (RA). An aneurysmal pulmonary trunk (PT) is encroached upon by the right ventricular outflow tract (*black arrow*). The lungs show venous vascularity.

absence of the arm (abrachia) or absent arms with persistent underdeveloped hands (phocomelia).[222,272,345] An ostium secundum atrial septal defect is the commonest associated cardiac anomaly[112,143,173,224,291,305,345,392,402] and may coexist with an ostium primum atrial septal defect.[305] Other cardiac malformations occur without prevailing patterns.[291,305,392] Mutations in a gene on chromosome 12q2 play an important role in skeletal and cardiac development, and produce a wide range of partial phenotypes of the Holt-Oram syndrome.[85]

Patau syndrome (trisomy 13) is characterized by polydactyly, flexion deformities of the fingers, palmar crease, microcephaly, holoprosencephaly, cleft lip, cleft palate and low-set malformed ears. *Edward syndrome* (trisomy 18) is characterized by clenched fists, rocker bottom feet, prominent occiput, low-set malformed ears, and micrognathia (see Fig. 19–5 and Fig. 20–11). The most common congenital cardiac malformations in trisomy 13 and in trisomy 18 are atrial septal defect, ventricular septal defect, and patent ductus arteriosus.[314]

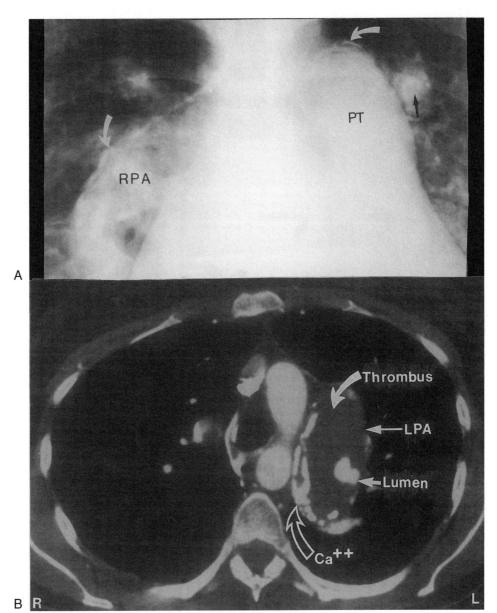

Figure 15–12

A, Close-up x-ray of the central pulmonary arteries of a 38-year-old cyanotic woman with a nonrestrictive ostium secundum atrial septal defect and pulmonary vascular disease. The hypertensive pulmonary trunk (PT) and right pulmonary artery (RPA) are dilated and calcified (*curved arrows*). The *black arrow* at the upper right identifies a dilated end-on intrapulmonary artery. *B,* Pulmonary computed tomographic angiogram from a 36-year-old cyanotic woman with a nonrestrictive ostium secundum atrial septal defect and pulmonary vascular disease. The dilated left pulmonary artery (LPA) is extensively calcified (Ca⁺⁺) and virtually occluded by massive thrombus, leaving a small lumen.

THE ARTERIAL PULSE

The arterial pulse is normal even though left ventricular ejection fraction tends to be decreased. During the Valsalva maneuver, left ventricular output is maintained despite a fall in systemic venous return because of the large volume of blood pooled in the lungs. Tachycardia is less pronounced during the straining phase, and there is a smaller decrease in pulse pressure. Bradycardia is less pronounced after cessation of straining, and there is a smaller systolic overshoot.[203] These abnormal responses to the Valsalva maneuver can be identified by palpating the brachial arterial pulse.[203]

THE JUGULAR VENOUS PULSE

There is left atrialization of the jugular venous wave form.[328] The crests of the jugular venous A and V waves tend to be equal (Fig. 15–17) because the two atria are in

common communication (nonrestrictive atrial septal defect). A wave amplitude varies with heart rate as in normal subjects.[419] When left ventricular compliance decreases, left atrial pressure rises and with it the right atrial pressure.[120,328,419,423] Pulmonary vascular disease results in an increased force of right atrial contraction and a dominant if not giant A wave (Fig. 15–18).

PRECORDIAL MOVEMENT AND PALPATION

In 1934, Roesler called attention to the conspicuous thrust of the right ventricle in atrial septal defect.[357] The impulse is hyperdynamic but not sustained because the volume-overloaded right ventricle contracts vigorously and empties rapidly into a low resistance pulmonary vascular bed.[136,317,335] The impulse is especially prominent at the left sternal border during held exhalation, and in the subxiphoid area during held inspiration.[335] Anterior

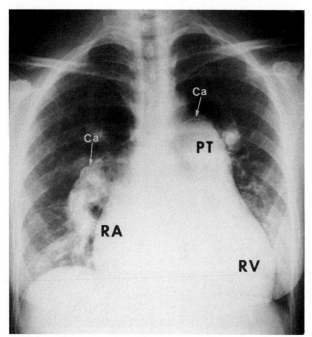

Figure 15–13
X-ray from a 32-year-old cyanotic woman with an ostium secundum atrial septal defect, pulmonary vascular disease, and reversed shunt. Pulmonary vascularity is decreased above the breast shadows. The pulmonary trunk (PT) and its right branch are dilated and contain eggshell calcium (Ca). The right atrium (RA) is enlarged, and a dilated right ventricle (RV) occupies the apex.

movement at the left sternal border is accompanied by retraction at the apex because the enlarged right ventricle occupies the apex.[36,335] A dilated pulsatile pulmonary trunk is palpable in the second left intercostal space, but a systolic thrill is seldom present despite hyperkinetic right ventricular ejection into a dilated pulmonary trunk.

AUSCULTATION

Auscultatory signs are the same in all varieties of isolated nonrestrictive atrial septal defects.[156,260,274,342,352, 371] The first heart sound is split at the lower left sternal edge and apex, and the tricuspid component is loud (Fig 15–19).[260,274,335,352,371,417] Increased diastolic flow across the tricuspid valve depresses the bellies of the tricuspid leaflets into the right ventricle, and vigorous right ventricular contraction causes abrupt cephalad excursion of the leaflets, generating a loud tricuspid component of the first heart sound.[156,417,432] A pulmonary ejection sound is uncommon despite dilatation of the pulmonary trunk (see Fig. 15–23).[29,342]

The pulmonary systolic murmur begins immediately after the first heart sound because right ventricular isovolumetric contraction is short. The murmur is crescendo-decrescendo, peaks in early or mid-systole, and ends well before the second heart sound (Figs. 15–20 and 15–21).[19,26,36,156,260,283] Origin in the pulmonary trunk has been confirmed by intracardiac phonocardiography[156] (Fig. 15–21) and by intraoperative phonocardiograms recorded from the surface of the pulmonary trunk.[283] The murmur is grade 2/6 to 3/6, is maximum in the second left intercostal space over the pulmonary trunk, and is impure and superficial because of proximity of the dilated pulmonary trunk to the chest wall.

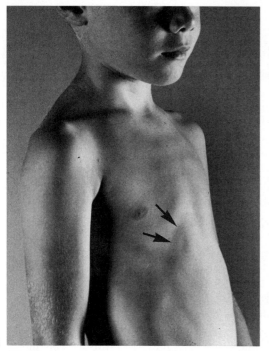

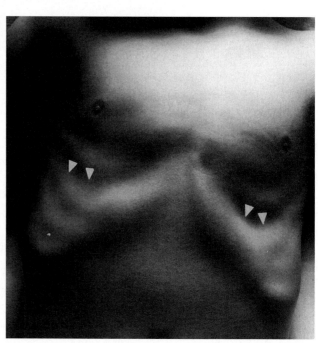

Figure 15–14
A, Five-year-old boy with a nonrestrictive ostium secundum atrial septal defect and a delicate frail gracile appearance with weight more affected than height. Harrison's grooves caused by chronic dyspnea are identified by the *arrows*. B, Six-year-old girl with a nonrestrictive ostium secundum atrial septal defect and Harrison's grooves (*paired arrowheads*).

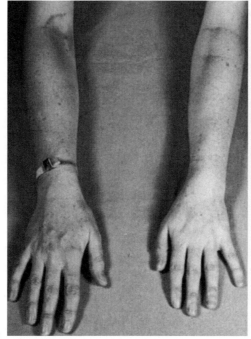
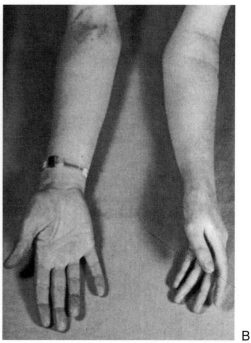

Figure 15–15
Thirty-four-year-old woman with Holt-Oram syndrome and an ostium secundum atrial septal defect. *A,* The left thumb is hypoplastic, and the left arm is shorter than the right. *B,* Supination was prevented by radial hypoplasia, but the crooked appearance of the hypoplastic triphalangeal thumb becomes apparent. Fingertips of the supinated right hand are erythematous because of a small right-to-left shunt.

The murmur radiates to the apex because the right ventricle occupies the apex.[260] A louder murmur is reserved for coexisting pulmonary valve stenosis (see Chapter 16). Systolic murmurs widely distributed in the right chest, axillae, and back are generated by rapid flow through peripheral pulmonary arteries (Fig. 15–20).[295,338]

The pulmonary component of the second sound is prominent because of proximity of the dilated pulmonary trunk to the chest wall and because of brisk elastic recoil

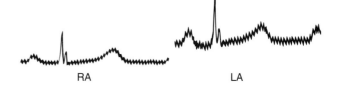

RA   LA

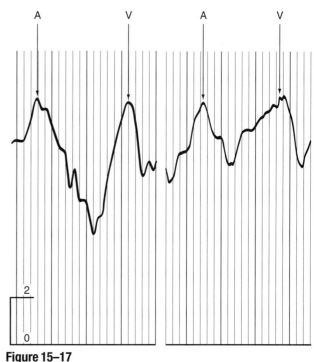

Figure 15–17
Sequential pressure pulses recorded as a catheter was withdrawn from right atrium (RA) to left atrium (LA) of an 11-year-old girl with a nonrestrictive ostium secundum atrial septal defect. The crests of the right atrial and left atrial A wave and V waves are identical because the atrial septal defect was nonrestrictive.

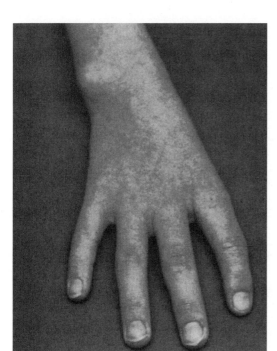

Figure 15–16
Photograph of a 26-year-old woman with Holt-Oram syndrome and absent thumb. An ostium secundum atrial septal defect coexisted.

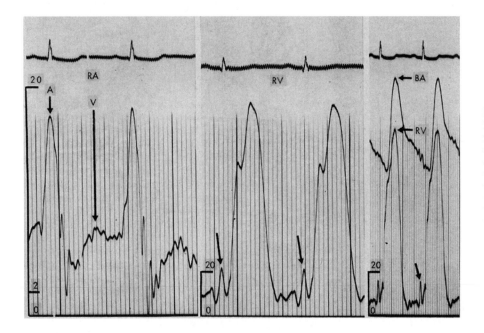

Figure 15–18

Pressure pulses from a cyanotic 34-year-old man with a nonrestrictive ostium secundum atrial septal defect and pulmonary vascular disease. Giant A waves in the right atrium (RA first panel) were transmitted into the right ventricle (RV) as presystolic distention (second panel, *arrows*). Elevated right ventricular systolic pressure is shown in the third panel. BA, brachial artery.

(see Fig. 15–27).[260] Wide fixed splitting is an auscultatory hallmark of atrial septal defect.[24,26,40,57,77,259,260] The aortic and pulmonary components are widely split during expiration, and the degree of splitting does not change during inspiration (Figs. 15–20, 15–22 and 15–23) or during the Valsalva maneuver (Fig 15–24). Wide splitting is caused by a delay in the pulmonary component associated with an increase in pulmonary vascular capacitance and an increase in *hangout interval* between the descending limbs of the pulmonary arterial and right ventricular pressure pulses.[103,252,326,386,387] As pulmonary artery pressure rises, the hangout interval decreases and the split then becomes a function of the relative durations of right and left ventricu-

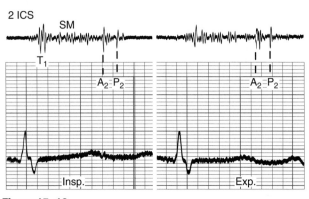

Figure 15–19

Phonocardiogram from a 13-year-old girl with a nonrestrictive ostium secundum atrial septal defect and a 2.5-to-1 left-to-right shunt. The loud second component of the split first heart sound (T_1) is tricuspid and is maximum at the lower left sternal edge (LSE). M_1, mitral component. A soft pulmonary midsystolic murmur (SM) in the second left intercostal space (2 ICS) is followed by wide fixed splitting of the second heart sound. A_2, aortic component; P_2, pulmonary component.

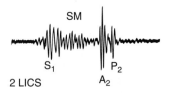

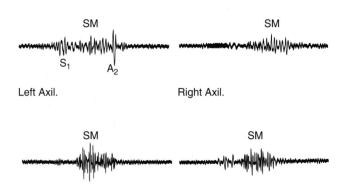

Figure 15–20

Phonocardiograms from a 21-year-old man with a nonrestrictive ostium secundum atrial septal defect. A grade 3/6 pulmonary midsystolic murmur (SM) in the second left intercostal space (2 LICS) is followed by wide splitting of second heart sound. A_2, aortic component; P_2, pulmonary component. Prominent systolic murmurs were present in the left axilla, right axilla and back because of rapid flow through peripheral pulmonary arteries. S_1, first heart sound.

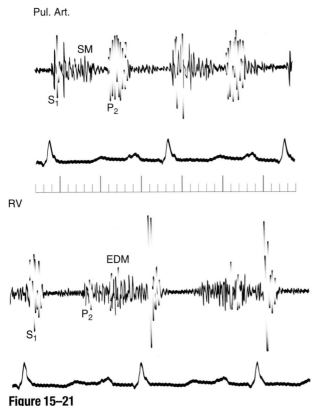

Figure 15–21

Intracardiac phonocardiograms from a 14-year-old boy with a nonrestrictive ostium secundum atrial septal defect and a 2.7-to-1 left-to-right shunt. A short midsystolic flow murmur (SM) was recorded in the main pulmonary artery (PUL ART). In the right ventricular outflow tract (RV), an early diastolic murmur of pulmonary regurgitation (EDM) was recorded despite normal pulmonary artery pressure.

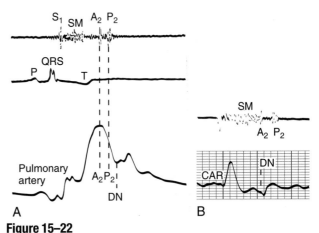

Figure 15–22

Tracings from a 28-year-old woman with a nonrestrictive ostium secundum atrial septal defect and a 2.3-to-1 left-to-right shunt. A, grade 2/6 pulmonary midsystolic murmur (SM) is followed by wide splitting of the second heart sound. The pulmonary component (P_2) coincides with the dicrotic notch of the pulmonary artery pressure pulse (DN). A_2, aortic component. B, The aortic component (A_2) coincides with the carotid dicrotic notch.

lar electromechanical systole, which is the same in both ventricles because a potential increase in duration of right ventricular systole due to volume overload is countered by accelerated ejection.[77,326] A healthy child examined in the *supine position* may exhibit relatively wide but not fixed splitting of the second heart sound. Reexamination in the sitting position confirms normal respiratory splitting.[78,335,386] Duration of diastole affects the degree of splitting by influencing the relative volumes of the right and left ventricles.[77,170] As diastole shortens, the split narrows, and as diastole lengthens, the split widens.[77,170] These patterns are evident in the beat-to-beat variations in cycle length with atrial fibrillation in which splitting tends to vary inversely with the duration of the preceding diastole.[77] *Absence of sinus arrhythmia* is a feature of atrial septal defect (see The Electrocardiogram, and Fig. 15–33B).

Fixed splitting means that the width of the split remains constant throughout active respiration and during the Valsalva maneuver. *Persistent splitting* means that the split widens during inspiration and narrows during expiration. Atrial septal defect is characterized by splitting of the second heart sound that is wide *and* fixed (Fig. 15–23). Wide fixed splitting is unlikely in neonates with atrial septal defect because there is little or no shunt in either direction.[248] During inspiration, the aortic and pulmonary components are equally delayed or do not move at all.[57,382] In the normal heart, inspiratory splitting is due chiefly to a delay in the

Figure 15–23

Phonocardiograms from a 26-year-old woman before and after surgical closure of a nonrestrictive ostium secundum atrial septal defect. *Before surgery* a grade 3/6 midsystolic pulmonary flow murmur (SM) was followed by wide fixed splitting of the second heart sound. A_2, aortic component; P_2, pulmonary component. *After surgery* the pulmonary systolic murmur virtually disappeared, and the second sound split normally. A pulmonary ejection sound (E) was present in the postoperative tracing.

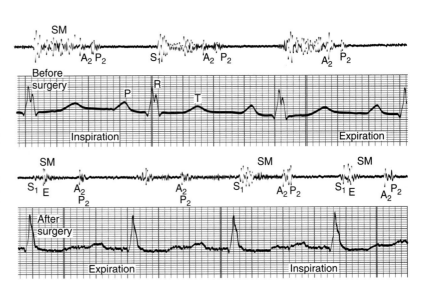

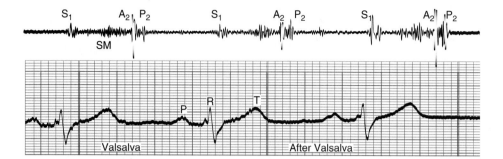

Figure 15–24

Phonocardiogram in the second left interspace during and after a Valsalva maneuver in a 17-year-old girl with a nonrestrictive ostium secundum atrial septal defect. Splitting of the second heart sound remained wide and fixed. S_1, first heart sound; SM, pulmonary midsystolic murmur.

pulmonary component of the second sound because the increase in pulmonary capacitance during inspiration is accompanied by an increase in the *hangout interval* (Fig. 15–25). The high pulmonary capacitance in atrial septal defect precludes an additional increase during inspiration, so there is no inspiratory delay in the hangout interval and no delay in the pulmonary component of the second sound. Phasic changes in systemic venous return during respiration are associated with reciprocal changes in volume of the left-to-right shunt, minimizing the respiratory variations in right and left ventricular filling.[24,40,171,259] Inspiration is accompanied by an increase in systemic venous return, so right ventricular filling is maintained or is increased while the left-to-right shunt decreases reciprocally, so left ventricular filling is maintained or is increased by the same amount. An inspiratory decrease in left-to-right shunt has been demonstrated in experimental animals[40] and in human subjects.[24,265]

These patterns of splitting do not prevail when partial anomalous pulmonary venous connection occurs with an *intact* atrial septum (Fig. 15–26).[259,311] Increased venous return during inspiration is not accompanied by a reciprocal decrease in left-to-right shunt because the atrial septum is intact. Accordingly, the aortic component of the second heart sound moves *toward* the first heart sound and the pulmonary

component moves *away*, so the split widens with inspiration and narrows with expiration (Figs. 15–26 and 15–27).

Rarely, an opening sound of the tricuspid valve follows the pulmonary component of the second heart sound.[15,260,352,417] Echocardiographic timing of the sound confirms that it coincides with abrupt arrest of the opening movement of the tricuspid valve in early diastole.[417] Mid-diastolic murmurs are due to augmented tricuspid flow.[156,245,260,315,358,368] Origin of the flow murmur at the tricuspid orifice has been demonstrated in experimental animals[358] and by intracardiac phonocardiography in human subjects (Fig. 15–28).[156,437] Tricuspid flow murmurs are medium frequency, impure, soft, short, presystolic or mid-diastolic, localized at the lower left sternal border, and do not increase with inspiration despite their right-sided origin. Intracardiac phonocardiograms identify low intensity inaudible diastolic murmurs within the atrial septal defect itself.[245,368,437] The combination of superficial impure presystolic and mid-diastolic murmurs together

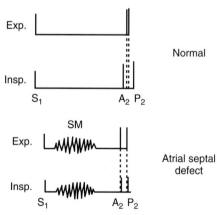

Figure 15–25

Illustration of respiratory behavior of the second heart sound in the normal heart and in the presence of a nonrestrictive atrial septal defect with a left-to-right shunt. *Normal inspiratory splitting* (INSP) is due chiefly to a delay in the pulmonary component (P_2) and less to movement of the aortic component (A_2) in the opposite direction. In *atrial septal defect*, the second sound is widely split during expiration (EXP) because the pulmonary component (P_2) is late. The split remains *fixed* during active inspiration and expiration because both components move equally and in the same direction or do not move at all. SM, systolic murmur.

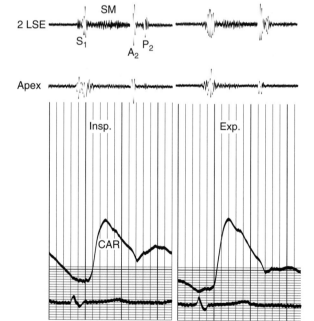

Figure 15–26

Phonocardiograms and carotid pulse (CAR) from a 16-year-old girl with anomalous pulmonary venous connection of the entire right lung to the inferior vena cava and an intact atrial septum (see Fig. 15–7). The second heart sound is *persistently* split, but the split is not *fixed*. A_2, aortic component; P_2, pulmonary component; SM, systolic murmur; 2 LSE, second intercostal space left sternal edge; INSP/EXP, inspiration and expiration.

RV

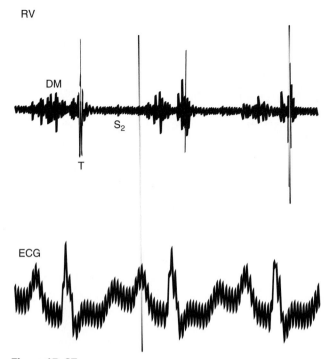

Figure 15–27
Intracardiac phonocardiogram from an 8-year-old female with a nonrestrictive ostium secundum atrial septal defect and 3 to 1 left-to-right shunt. The microphone in the *inflow* tract of the right ventricle just distal to the tricuspid valve recorded a middiastolic flow murmur (DM) and a loud tricuspid component of the first heart sound (T). S_2, second heart sound; RV, right ventricle.

with a superficial impure midsystolic murmur occasionally creates the impression of a pericardial rub. Occasionally, a rub in fact exists, and attention has been called to roughened pericardium and pericardial effusion in patients with atrial septal defect (Fig. 15–29).[5,243] A diastolic murmur of low- pressure pulmonary regurgitation is uncommon if not rare (Fig. 15–21) and is reserved for aneurysmal dilatation of the pulmonary trunk.[270] Atrial septal defects with pulmonary vascular disease and reversed shunts are accompanied by auscultatory signs of pulmonary hypertension (Figs. 15–30 and 15–31 and see Chapter 14).[207,260,333,408]

THE ELECTROCARDIOGRAM

Sinus node dysfunction has been identified as early as two to three years of age,[42,246,366,389] and accelerated atrial rhythms have been recorded on 24-hour ambulatory electrocardiograms in 35% of children with an atrial septal defect.[42] The incidence of atrial fibrillation, atrial flutter and supraventricular tachycardia increases in the fourth decade (Figs. 15–32 and 15–33).[109,181,254,366,369,422] *Sinus arrhythmia* is minimal or absent in children with atrial septal defect and does not occur in adults (Fig. 15–33B). Sinus arrhythmia depends on separation of the systemic and pulmonary venous returns, and with atrial septal defect, the two venous returns are not separated.[102]

Conduction defects are intrinsic parts of the anomaly and are usually age-related.[42,90,366,389] The PR interval tends to

be prolonged.[11,26,90] Atrioventricular node dysfunction begins in older children and is less frequent than sinus node dysfunction.[90,246,366,389] *Advanced* first-degree atrioventricular nodal block occurs with familial or less commonly nonfamilial atrial septal defect and occasionally culminates in complete heart block.[43,44,147,332] Some individuals in a family have an ostium secundum atrial septal defect and first-degree heart block, while others have PR prolongation with intact atrial septum.[43] In Holt-Oram syndrome (Figs. 15–15 and 15–16), PR interval prolongation, sinus bradycardia, and ectopic atrial rhythms are relatively common.[291,392]

Abnormal right atrial P waves are peaked rather than tall (see Fig. 15–35), but P wave configurations are usually normal (Fig. 15–34).[434] Prolonged P wave duration occurs when the terminal force is written by an enlarged right atrium.[282,372] The P wave axis with an *ostium secundum* atrial septal defect is inferior and to the left with upright P waves in leads 2, 3, and aVF (Figs. 15–34 and 15–35). The P wave axis with a *superior vena caval sinus venosus* atrial septal defect is leftward with inverted P waves in leads 2, 3, and aVF and an upright P wave in lead aVL (Fig. 15–36).[110,202]

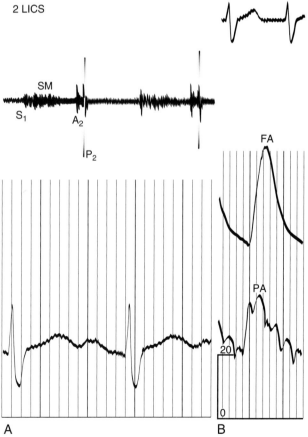

Figure 15–28
Tracings from a 4-year-old boy with a nonrestrictive ostium secundum atrial septal defect and a 2.3 to 1 left-to-right shunt. *A,* The pulmonary component of the split second sound is loud (P_2) even though the pulmonary arterial pressure was normal as shown in panel *b.* S_1, first heart sound; A_2, aortic component of the second sound; SM, systolic murmur; FA, femoral artery pulse; PA, pulmonary artery pulse.

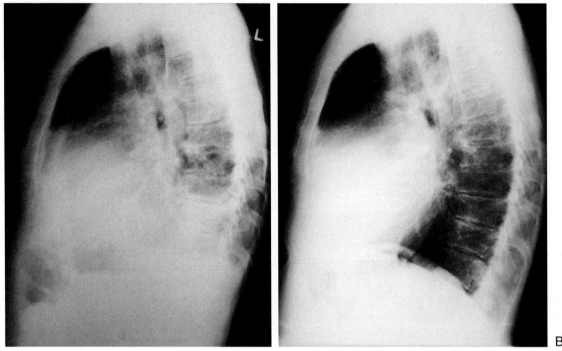

Figure 15–29

A, Lateral x-ray from a 65-year-old man with a nonrestrictive ostium secundum atrial septal defect and large pericardial and pleural effusions. *B,* The effusions were benign transudates that decreased appreciably after pericardiocentesis. Thickened pericardium was identified at surgery for closure of the atrial septal defect.

The atrial pacemaker is ectopic because the sinus venosus defect occupies the site of the sinoatrial node. Sinus venosus defects are occasionally accompanied by shifts from sinus rhythm with a normal P axis to an ectopic atrial rhythm with a leftward P axis.[110]

The QRS duration is slightly prolonged because of slurring of the terminal forces (Fig. 15–34). QRS duration increases with age, and may culminate in a pattern resembling complete right bundle branch block (Fig. 15–32). The QRS axis is vertical with clockwise depolarization that writes Q waves in leads 2, 3, and aVF (Figs. 15–34 and 15–35). Right axis deviation is reserved for symptomatic pulmonary hypertensive infants[125] or for young females with pulmonary vascular disease (Fig. 15–37). Left axis deviation is exceptional, and may represent acquired left anterior fascicular block in older adults (Fig. 15–32).[147,209]

An electrocardiographic hallmark of atrial septal defect is a QRS characterized by an rSr prime or an rsR prime in right precordial leads (Figs. 15–34 and 15–35).[26,36,47,271] The r prime wave in leads V_1 and aVR is slurred in contrast to thin terminal r waves in approximately 5% of normal electrocardiograms. Q waves are small or absent in left precordial leads because the shunt does not traverse the left ventricle (Figs. 15–34 to 15–36). The outflow tract of the right ventricle is the last portion of the heart to depolarize, and the enlargement and increased thickness caused by right ventricular volume overload are responsible for the rightward, superior, and anterior direction of the terminal force of the QRS as well as for the increased QRS dura-

tion.[49,257,308] The term *incomplete right bundle branch block* is a misnomer.[308]

A notch near the apex of the R waves in inferior leads of ostium secundum and sinus venosus atrial septal defects has been called *crochetage*[106] because the notch resembles the work of a crochet needle (Fig. 15–37). Crochetage is independent of the terminal force direction of the QRS, but when the rSr prime pattern occurs with crochetage in all inferior limb leads, the specificity of the electrocardiographic diagnosis of atrial septal defect is remarkably high.[106] Although crochetage has been correlated with shunt severity, the pattern has been reported with a patent foramen ovale and has been suggested as an electrocardiographic marker of a patent foramen ovale associated with ischemic embolic stroke.[46]

THE X-RAY

Increased pulmonary arterial vascularity extends to the periphery of the lung fields (Figs. 15–38 and 15–39). The pulmonary trunk and its proximal branches are dilated (Fig. 15–39). The left branch is usually obscured by an enlarged pulmonary trunk (Fig. 15–39), but the lateral view discloses dilatation of both branches (Figs. 15–39 and 15–40). The ascending aorta is seldom border-forming because the shunt does not traverse the aortic root (Figs. 15–38 and 15–39),[80,357] although angiographic and echocardiographic assessments indicate that the intrinsic caliber of the ascending aorta is not significantly reduced.[117] A sinus venosus atrial septal defect may be

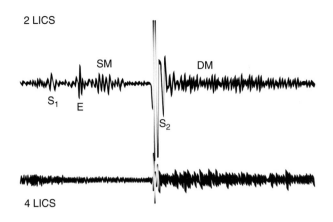

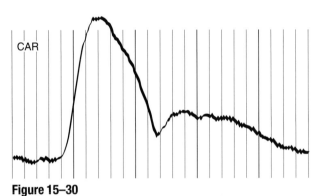

Figure 15–30

Tracings from a 28-year-old cyanotic woman with a nonrestrictive ostium secundum atrial septal defect and pulmonary vascular disease. A pulmonary ejection sound (E) introduced a soft short midsystolic murmur (SM) in the second left intercostal space (2 LICS). The second heart sound (S₂) is loud and single and introduced a decrescendo Graham Steell diastolic murmur (DM). S₁, first heart sound; 4 LICS, fourth left intercostal space; CAR, carotid pulse.

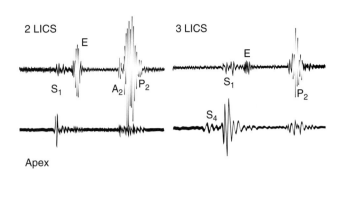

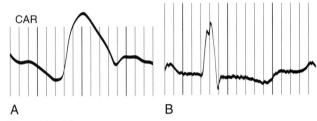

Figure 15–31

Tracings from a 32-year-old woman with a nonrestrictive ostium secundum atrial septal defect, pulmonary vascular disease, a 1.4 to 1 left-to-right shunt, and a small right-to-left shunt. Pulmonary artery systolic pressure was 90 mm Hg and systemic systolic pressure was 110 mm Hg. *A,* The first heart sound (S₁) is followed by a prominent pulmonary ejection sound (E) in the second left intercostal space (2 LICS). The second heart sound remained split, and the loud pulmonary component (P₂) was transmitted to the apex. A₂, aortic component. *B,* The ejection sound and the loud pulmonary component of the second sound were transmitted to the third left intercostal space (3 LICS). A fourth heart sound (S₄) was present at the lower left sternal border.

defect.[117,194,273] Left atrial enlargement is reserved for older adults after the advent of atrial fibrillation.[254,373] Volume elastic properties of the right and left atrium also play a role in determining relative atrial enlargement,

accompanied by localized enlargement or ampullary dilatation of the superior vena cava proximal to its attachment to the right atrium (Fig. 15–41).[34,110,128] Infants with large left-to-right shunts exhibit conspicuous pulmonary arterial and pulmonary venous vascularity with enlargement of all four cardiac chambers.[125,232,248] In older adults with moderate pulmonary hypertension and persistent left-to-right shunt, the pulmonary trunk and proximal branches are occasionally aneurysmal (Fig. 15–42). In young adults with pulmonary vascular disease and a balanced or reversed shunt, the pulmonary trunk and its branches are strikingly enlarged and calcified (Figs. 15–12 and 15–13).

Right atrial enlargement is characteristic (Figs. 15–39A and 15–43), but the left atrium is seldom enlarged despite a left-to-right shunt (Fig. 15–39B) because a major portion of pulmonary venous return is shunted directly into the right atrium owing to the proximity of the right pulmonary veins to the rim of the ostium secundum atrial septal

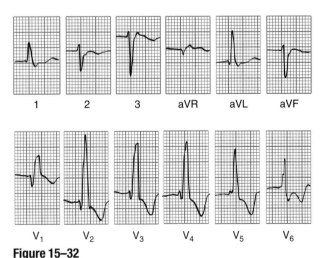

Figure 15–32

Electrocardiogram from an acyanotic man with a nonrestrictive ostium secundum atrial septal defect who died 3 months before his 95th birthday. The rhythm was atrial fibrillation. Left axis deviation was due to acquired left anterior fascicular block, and the right ventricular conduction defect was peripheral rather than central. The Q wave in lead V₁ reflected enlargement of the right atrium (see Fig. 15–43A).

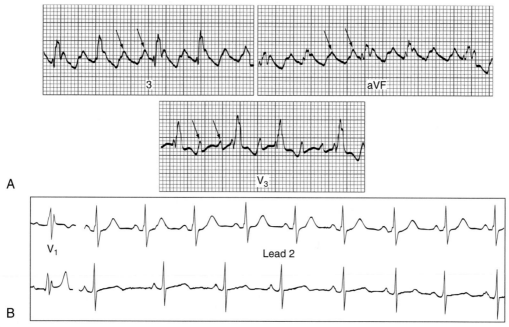

Figure 15–33

A, Leads 3, aVF, and V$_3$ from a 60-year-old woman with an ostium secundum atrial septal defect and a 2.6 to 1 left-to-right shunt. The rhythm is atrial flutter (*paired arrows*) with an irregular ventricular response. *B,* The upper rhythm strip (lead 2) illustrates *absence* of sinus arrhythmia in a 19-year-old female with a nonrestrictive ostium secundum atrial septal defect. The lower rhythm strip illustrates typical sinus arrhythmia that appeared after surgical closure of the atrial septal defect. The rsr′ in lead V$_1$ remained unchanged.

because for equal increments in volume the right atrium is more distensible than the left.[273]

An enlarged right ventricle occupies the apex and forms an acute angle with the left hemidiaphragm (Fig. 15–38). Dilatation of the outflow tract results in smooth continuity with the enlarged pulmonary trunk above (Fig. 15–38). In the lateral projection, the dilated right ventricle encroaches on the retrosternal space (Figs. 15–39B and 15–40) and displaces the left ventricle posteriorly. The size of the left ventricle is normal because its stroke volume is normal or

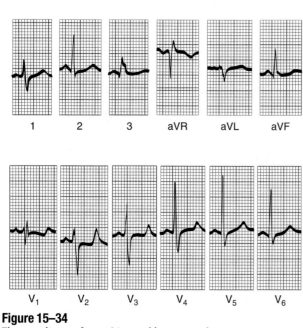

Figure 15–34

Electrocardiogram from a 24-year-old woman with a nonrestrictive ostium secundum atrial septal defect and a 2 to 1 left-to-right shunt. P waves are normal. The QRS axis is vertical with clockwise depolarization and Q waves in leads 2, 3, and aVF. The terminal QRS forces are directed upward, to the right and anterior and are slightly prolonged, so an rSr prime appears in lead V$_1$, a slurred terminal R wave appears in lead aVR, and slurred S waves appear in left precordial leads.

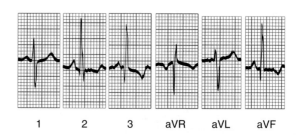

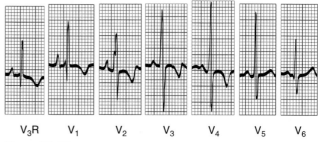

Figure 15–35

Electrocardiogram from a 5-year-old boy with a nonrestrictive ostium secundum atrial septal defect and a 3.5 to 1 shunt. P waves are peaked and tall in leads 2 and V$_3$R and in leads V$_{1-2}$. The QRS axis is vertical and depolarization is clockwise, so Q waves appear in leads 2, 3, and aVF. There is an rsR prime pattern in leads V$_1$ and V$_3$R.

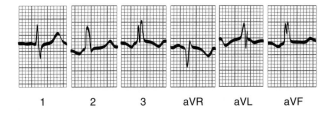

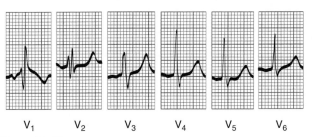

Figure 15–36

Electrocardiogram from a 25-year-old woman with a *superior vena caval sinus venosus* atrial septal defect. The P wave axis is leftward and markedly superior, so P waves are inverted in leads 2, 3 and aVF, are isoelectric in lead 1, and are slightly positive in lead aVR. Intracardiac electrophysiologic investigation identified an ectopic left atrial pacemaker. The QRS pattern is typical of a left-to-right shunt at atrial level, namely, a vertical QRS axis and prolonged terminal forces directed to the right, superior and anterior with an rSR prime in lead V$_1$ and S waves in left precordial leads.

reduced.[117] The relationship between the inferior vena caval shadow and the left ventricular shadow in the lateral projection distinguishes posterior displacement from intrinsic dilatation of the left ventricle (Fig. 15–44).[249] The lateral projection in adults often shows disproportionate anterior bowing of the upper third of the sternum (Fig. 15–39B). Atrial tachyarrhythmias, especially atrial fibrillation, initiate congestive heart failure with a progressive and often dramatic increase in heart size (Figs. 15–11 and 15–45).[373]

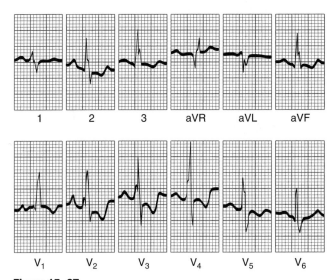

Figure 15–37

Electrocardiogram from a 32-year-old woman with a nonrestrictive ostium secundum atrial septal defect and a 2.6 to 1 left-to-right shunt. *Crochetage* is represented by notches on the R waves in leads 2, 3, and aVF.

In the *scimitar syndrome*, the confluence of right pulmonary veins forms a distinctive shadow parallel to or behind the right cardiac silhouette as the anomalous venous channels course downward to join the inferior vena cava (Figs. 15–6 to 15–8).[107,133,290,380,395] The heart is displaced into the right hemithorax because of hypoplasia of the right lung, but the anomalous venous channels may remain visible (Figs. 15–7 and 15–8).

THE ECHOCARDIOGRAM

Echocardiography with color flow imaging and Doppler interrogation establishes the location and size of an atrial septal defect and its physiologic consequences.[151] Transesophageal echocardiography is an important supplement to transthoracic imaging and has refined the anatomic assessment of the interatrial septum.[233,376] Transesophageal echocardiography identifies partial anomalous pulmonary venous connections,[16,33,50] and pulsed Doppler imaging identifies anomalous pulmonary venous connections in the fetus.[20] An ostium secundum atrial septal defect is represented by an echo-free space in the mid portion of the atrial septum (Fig. 15–9A). Color flow imaging confirms that the echo-free space is a true tissue defect, and pulsed Doppler imaging characterizes instantaneous flow patterns across the defect (Fig. 15–9B). A foramen ovale can be identified (Fig. 15–46C), color flow determines its patency,[13,75,336] and an in utero patent foramen ovale can be distinguished from an ostium secundum atrial septal defect.[185] Transthoracic and transesophageal echocardiography establish the diagnosis of atrial septal aneurysm (Fig. 15–47A), and

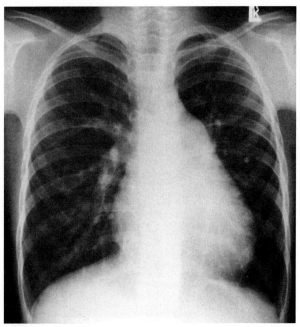

Figure 15–38

X-ray from a 5-year-old boy with a nonrestrictive ostium secundum atrial septal defect and a 2.5 to 1 left-to-right shunt. Pulmonary vascularity is increased, the pulmonary trunk and its right branch are prominent, but the ascending aorta is inconspicuous. The right atrium occupies the lower right cardiac border, and a dilated right ventricle occupies the apex.

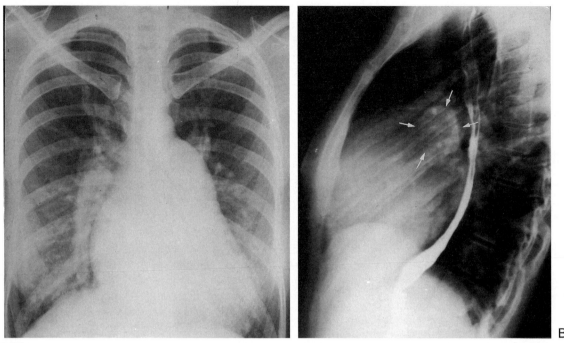

A   B

Figure 15–39

A and *B*, X-rays from a 31-year-old woman with a nonrestrictive ostium secundum atrial septal defect and a 3.2 to 1 left-to-right shunt. The frontal projection shows increased pulmonary arterial vascularity that extends to the periphery of the lung fields (enhanced by breast tissue). The pulmonary trunk and its right branch are dilated in contrast to the non border-forming ascending aorta. An enlarged right atrium occupies the lower right cardiac border, and an enlarged right ventricle occupies the apex. In the lateral projection, *arrows* bracket a dilated right pulmonary artery that was obscured in the frontal projection by the dilated pulmonary trunk. The retrosternal space is obliterated by enlargement of the right atrium and right ventricle despite an increase in anteroposterior chest dimension caused by bowing of the sternum. The left atrium is not enlarged in the barium esophagram.

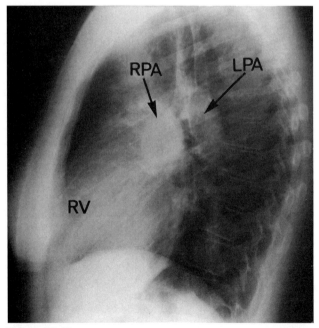

Figure 15–40

Lateral x-ray from a 48-year-old man with a nonrestrictive ostium secundum atrial septal defect and a 2.5 to 1 left-to-right shunt. The end-on right pulmonary artery (RPA) is dilated, and left pulmonary artery (LPA) appears as a large comma-like structure. The right ventricle (RV) encroaches on the retrosternal space. The left atrium is not enlarged.

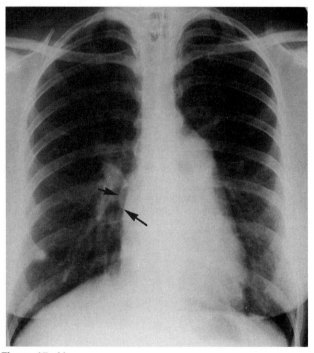

Figure 15–41

X-ray from a 26-year-old woman with a superior vena caval sinus venosus atrial septal defect and a 2 to 1 left-to-right shunt. *Arrows* bracket a subtle localized dilatation of the superior vena cava as it joins the right atrium. The x-ray otherwise resembles an ostium secundum atrial septal defect of equivalent size.

or young adults. Patients usually reach their fourth decade with little or no handicap. Preadolescents sometimes appear delicate and gracile. Dyspnea, fatigue, and recurrent lower respiratory infections are common. The left-to-right shunt in older adults is augmented by ischemic heart disease, systemic hypertension, and acquired calcific aortic stenosis that decrease left ventricular compliance. Atrial tachyarrhythmias, especially atrial fibrillation, precipitate congestive heart failure. The crests of the jugular venous A and V waves are equal (left atrialization). The right ventricular impulse is hyperdynamic, and a systolic pulsation is palpated over the dilated pulmonary trunk. The first heart sound is split with a loud tricuspid component. There is a grade 2/6 or 3/6 pulmonary midsystolic murmur, fixed splitting of the second heart sound, and a tricuspid mid-diastolic flow murmur. P waves are peaked but seldom tall. The QRS axis is vertical with clockwise depolarization and Q waves in leads 2, 3, and aVF. Terminal forces of the QRS are prolonged and point to the right and anterior, producing an rSr prime in lead V_1. Notching of the R waves in inferior leads results in a distinctive crochetage pattern. The x-ray shows increased pulmonary arterial vascularity, an inconspicuous ascending aorta, dilatation of the pulmonary trunk and its proximal branches, and enlargement of the right atrium and right ventricle. The scimitar syndrome is characterized by partial anomalous right pulmonary venous connection with infradiaphragmatic drainage and hypoplasia of the right lung. Echocardiography with color flow imaging and Doppler interrogation establishes the location and size of the atrial septal defect, its physiologic consequences, and the presence of partial anomalous pulmonary venous connections. A nonrestrictive ostium secundum atrial septal defect with pulmonary vascular disease is believed to represent the coexistence of primary pulmonary hypertension.

A superior vena caval sinus venosus atrial septal defect is clinically similar to an equivalent ostium secundum defect with two exceptions: 1) the atrial pacemaker is ectopic, the P wave axis is leftward, so inverted P waves appear in leads 2, 3, and aVF; and 2) the right hilus may show localized ampullary dilatation of the distal end of the superior vena cava as it joins the right atrium. Echocardiography confirms the location of the defect.

Ostium secundum atrial septal defects in young patients are among the most readily diagnosed congenital malformations of the heart, but these same defects sometimes defy clinical recognition in adults because of diagnostic ambiguities. The diagnosis of *mitral stenosis* is entertained (Table 15–1) because of dyspnea, orthopnea, atrial fibrillation, increased jugular venous V wave, a right ventricular impulse, a loud first heart sound, a delayed pulmonary component of the second heart sound mistaken for an opening snap, a tricuspid flow murmur mistaken for a mitral diastolic murmur, shunt vascularity mistaken for pulmonary venous congestion, and dilatation of the pulmonary trunk, the right atrium and occasionally the left atrium. *Mitral regurgitation* may be misdiagnosed as acquired (Table 15–2) because the holosystolic murmur of tricuspid regurgitation

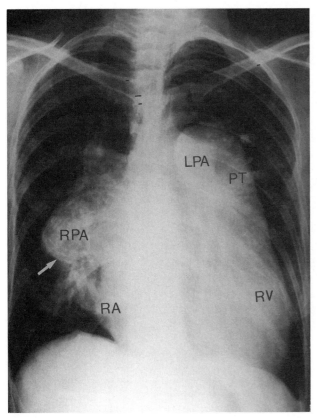

Figure 15–42
X-ray from a 64-year-old woman with a nonrestrictive ostium secundum atrial septal defect, pulmonary artery pressure of 60/38 mm Hg, and a 1.8 to 1 left-to-right shunt. Pulmonary vascularity is decreased. The pulmonary trunk (PT) and the right pulmonary artery (RPA) are aneurysmal, the right pulmonary artery contains a rim of calcium (*arrow*), and a dilated left pulmonary artery (LPA) is behind the pulmonary trunk. The ascending aorta is not seen. An enlarged right atrium occupies the lower right cardiac border, and an enlarged right ventricle (RV) occupies the apex.

color flow imaging or echocontrast determines whether an atrial septal defect coexists (Fig. 15–47B).*

Real time imaging identifies a dilated hyperkinetic right ventricle with paradoxical motion of the ventricular septum[127,269] and vigorous pulsations of the pulmonary trunk and its branches. The size, shape, and functional reserve of the left ventricle can be determined (Fig. 15–46B).[51,52]

A superior vena caval sinus venosus defect lies near the junction of the superior cava and the right atrium (Fig. 15–48A),[151,233] and an inferior vena caval sinus venosus defect lies just beyond the rim of the inferior vena cava (Fig. 15–48B).[336] An unroofed coronary sinus is identified by dilatation of the coronary sinus and by a defect between the sinus and left atrium.

SUMMARY

Ostium secundum atrial septal defects predominate in females and often come to light in asymptomatic children

*See references 13, 39, 56, 58, 96, 121, 131, 216, 331, 353, 390.

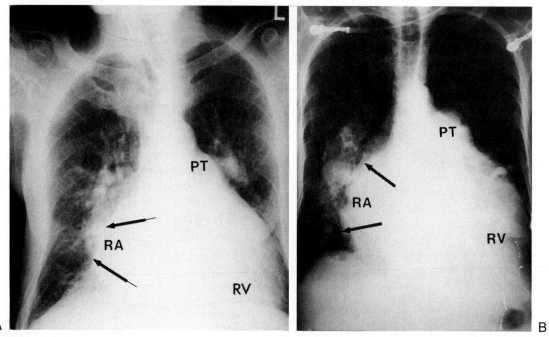

Figure 15–43

A, X-ray from the 95-year-old acyanotic man with a nonrestrictive ostium secundum atrial septal defect whose electrocardiogram in atrial fibrillation is shown in Figure 15–32. Pulmonary artery vascularity and pulmonary venous vascularity are increased. The pulmonary trunk (PT) is dilated, but the ascending aorta is not border-forming. The right atrium (RA) and the right ventricle (RV) are strikingly enlarged. *B,* X-ray from an 87-year-old acyanotic woman with a nonrestrictive ostium secundum atrial septal defect, severe tricuspid regurgitation, and atrial fibrillation. Pulmonary vascularity is decreased. The pulmonary trunk (PT) is dilated, its enlarged right branch contains eggshell calcification, but the ascending aorta is not border-forming. The right atrium (RA) and right ventricle (RV) are strikingly enlarged. At necropsy, a large thrombus resided in the dilated right pulmonary artery, and a smaller thrombus was found in the dilated left pulmonary artery.

is well heard at the apex, a delayed pulmonary component of the second sound followed by a tricuspid flow murmur is mistaken for an opening snap and the mid-diastolic murmur of coexisting mitral stenosis. Diagnostic ambiguity in older adults results from atrial arrhythmias, ischemic heart dis-

ease, systemic hypertension, and inverted left precordial T waves (Table 15–3).

Symptomatic infants with a large left-to-right shunt through an ostium secundum atrial septal defect pose a diagnostic problem to clinicians who are unaccustomed to

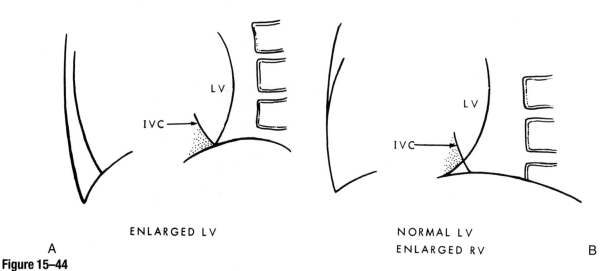

Figure 15–44

A, illustrates the relationship between the inferior vena cava (IVC) and the posterior silhouette of an enlarged left ventricle (LV) when the *right ventricle is normal.* The caval shadow at the level of the diaphragm lies *within* the left ventricular silhouette. *B,* illustrates the relationship between the inferior vena cava and the posterior silhouette of a normal left ventricle that is retrodisplaced by an *enlarged right ventricle.* The caval shadow at the level of the diaphragm lies *behind* the left ventricle. (Modified from Keats TE, Rudhe U, Foo GW: Inferior vena caval position in the differential diagnosis of atrial and ventricular septal defects. Radiology 83:616, 1964).

Figure 15–45
X-rays from an acyanotic woman with an ostium secundum atrial septal defect before and after the onset of atrial fibrillation. At age 49 years, the patient's x-ray shows increased pulmonary arterial vascularity, mild prominence of the pulmonary trunk and its right branch, and a moderate increase in right atrial size. At age 53 years, following the onset of atrial fibrillation, there is a considerable increase in size of the pulmonary trunk, right atrium, and right ventricle.

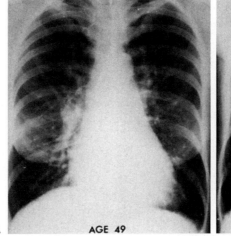
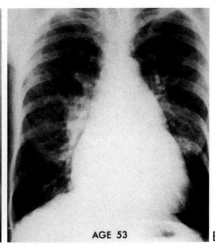

considering atrial septal defect as a diagnosis in neonates. Splitting of the second heart sound is variable and difficult to assess, the pulmonary component is increased, and a holosystolic murmur of tricuspid regurgitation and a tricuspid diastolic flow murmur are misinterpreted. The diagnosis is established by echocardiography. These infants often experience spontaneous closure of their atrial septal defect.

Lutembacher Syndrome

In 1811, Corvisart described the association of atrial septal defect with mitral stenosis,[97] and in 1916, Lutembacher* published the first comprehensive account of these two defects as a combination that has come to be called Lutembacher syndrome.[278] Opinion differs regarding what lesions the syndrome should include. Lutembacher believed that mitral stenosis was congenital even though his patient was 61 years old. The current consensus is that Lutembacher syndrome consists of a *congenital defect in the atrial septum* upon which *acquired mitral stenosis* is imposed.[98,150,188,196,242,370,403,427] The concept has been further broadened to include different anatomic types of congenital interatrial communications and different anatomic types of acquired mitral valve disease. What then constitutes an acceptable type of left-to-right shunt in Lutembacher syndrome?

When the interatrial communication is an ostium secundum atrial septal defect, the answer is clear.[150,242,296,403] However, a patent foramen ovale is not included in the definition even though Lutembacher stated that the high left atrial pressure of mitral stenosis might stretch the margins of a valve-incompetent foramen ovale and cause a left-to-right shunt.[188,289,403] There is an age-related

increase in mitral leaflet fibrosis and shortened fibrotic mitral chordae tendineae in ostium secundum atrial septal defects,[54,113,172,268,316] the functional consequence of which is mitral regurgitation, but it is debatable whether pure mitral regurgitation should be included in the definition of Lutembacher syndrome.[150,242] *Congenital* obstruction to left atrial flow that accompanies cor triatriatum or parachute mitral valve is occasionally associated with an atrial septal defect (see Chapter 9), but by convention the Lutembacher eponym is not applied. Partial anomalous pulmonary venous connection with intact atrial septum is a form of left-to-right shunt at atrial level, and cases have been reported with acquired mitral stenosis.† More

---

†See references 3, 6, 8, 63, 119, 166, 188, 196, 242, 393.

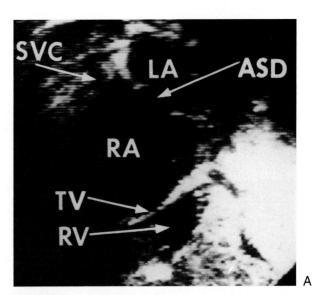

Figure 15–46
A, Echocardiogram (subcostal) from a 5-year-old girl with a nonrestrictive ostium secundum atrial septal defect (ASD) and an enlarged right atrium (RA). LA, left atrium; SVC, superior vena cava; TV, tricuspid valve; RV, right ventricle.

---

*Lutembacher is a German name, but Dr. Lutembacher spoke French, wrote in French, and preferred a French pronunciation of his name (Loo-tem-bah-share) because he was Alsatian, and Alsace-Lorraine was then a part of France. The pronunciation is now anglicized to Loo-tem-bah-ker.

Illustration continued on following page

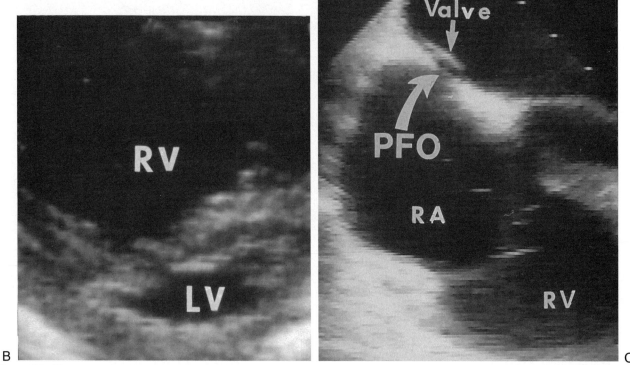

Figure 15–46

B, Echocardiogram (short axis) from a neonate with a nonrestrictive ostium secundum atrial septal defect, a large left-to-right shunt, and an enlarged right ventricle that flattened the ventricular septum and reduced the size of the left ventricle (LV). *C,* Transesophageal echocardiogram from a 30-year-old woman with transient ischemic attacks and a typical patent foramen ovale (PFO) guarded by a valve on its left atrial side. RA, right atrium; RV, right ventricle.

recently, *iatrogenic* Lutembacher syndrome has been applied to a defect in the atrial septal acquired during percutaneous transseptal mitral valvotomy for rheumatic mitral stenosis (see Fig. 15–52).[82] For the purposes of this chapter, Lutembacher syndrome is considered as the combination of *congenital* atrial septal defect and *acquired* rheumatic mitral stenosis.

When these disorders coexist, each modifies the hemodynamic and clinical expressions of the other.[30] Let us first examine the physiologic effects that mitral stenosis exerts

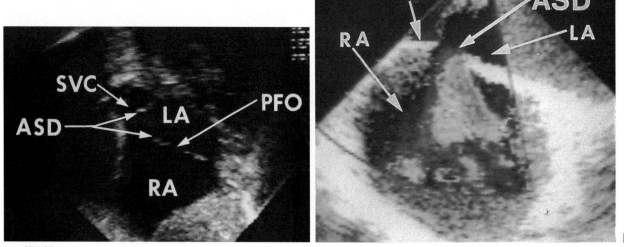

Figure 15–47

A, Echocardiogram from a 4-year-old male with a nonrestrictive sinus venosus atrial septal defect (ASD) of the superior vena caval type (SVC). The defect is at the junction of the superior vena cava and right atrium (RA) and is therefore remote from the midportion of the atrial septum as represented by the patent foramen ovale (PFO). LA, left atrium. *B,* Black-and-white print of a color flow image from a 34-year-old woman with a nonrestrictive inferior vena caval (IVC) sinus venosus atrial septal defect (ASD). LA, left atrium; RA, right atrium.

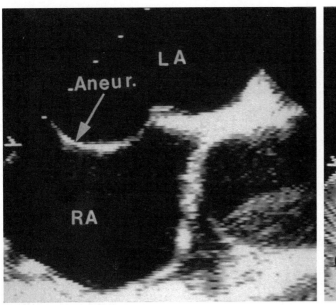 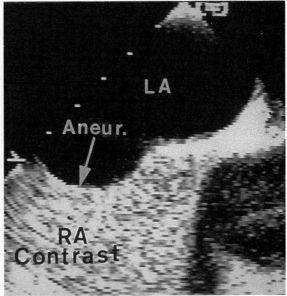

Figure 15–48

A, Transesophageal echocardiogram from a 29-year-old woman with transient ischemic attacks attributed to cerebral emboli from an atrial septal aneurysm (aneur) that oscillated vigorously from left to right and back again. RA, right atrium; LA, left atrium. B, Echo contrast in the right atrium outlined the aneurysm but identified no shunt.

on an atrial septal defect.[30] The left-to-right shunt across a nonrestrictive atrial septal defect is determined principally by the relative resistances to flow from left atrium into left ventricle, or from left atrium through the atrial septum into the right ventricle (see earlier). Mitral stenosis increases the resistance to flow from left atrium into the left ventricle, and in so doing augments the left-to-right shunt in proportion to the severity of mitral stenosis.[30,120,324,423] In the presence of a *restrictive* atrial septal defect, severe mitral stenosis generates a continuous left-to-right shunt because the pressure difference across the restrictive atrial septum exists throughout the cardiac cycle (see Fig. 15–52).[188,237,362]

Let us now examine the effects that an atrial septal defect exerts on mitral stenosis.[30] The idea that an interatrial communication might have a favorable hemodynamic effect was proposed in 1880 by Firkett[158] and in 1949 by Bland

and Sweet who surgically treated mitral stenosis by anastomosing a pulmonary vein to the azygos vein after which the left atrial pressure fell.[45] The mitral valve is normally the only exit from the left atrium. An atrial septal defect constitutes an alternative exit that decompresses the left atrium and in so doing, diminishes the mitral gradient.[188,370] Accordingly, mitral stenosis increases the shunt flow across an atrial septal defect, and an atrial septal defect decreases the gradient across a stenotic mitral valve. As the left-to-right shunt increases, left ventricular filling and stroke volume decline reciprocally. Conversely, an increase in pressure in the left atrium and pulmonary artery pressure causes right ventricular hypertrophy that decreases right

Table 15–2	ASD Secundum Diagnostic Ambiguities in Adults

Mitral Regurgitation

Atrial fibrillation

Apical holosystolic murmur

Wide splitting of second heart sound

Mid-diastolic murmur

Third heart sound

Table 15–3	ASD Secundum Diagnostic Ambiguities in Adults

Coexisting Acquired Heart Disease

Ischemic heart disease

Inverted left precordial T waves

Atrial tachyarrhythmias

Table 15–1	ASD Secundum Diagnostic Ambiguities in Adults

Mitral Stenosis

Dyspnea, orthopnea

Atrial fibrillation

Increased jugular venous V wave

Right ventricular impulse

Loud first heart sound

Delayed pulmonary component of a widely split second heart sound mistaken for mitral opening snap

Mid-diastolic tricuspid murmur

Increased pulmonary vascularity with dilatation of the pulmonary trunk, right ventricle, and left atrium

ASD, atrial septal defect.

ventricular distensibility, reduces the left-to-right shunt, and improves left ventricular filling.[370]

THE HISTORY

Lutembacher syndrome has a predilection for females because ostium secundum atrial septal defect and rheumatic mitral stenosis are both more prevalent in females.[30,403] The incidence of mitral stenosis in patients with atrial septal defect has been estimated at 4%.[30,100,403] The incidence of atrial septal defect in patients with mitral stenosis has been estimated at 0.6% to 0.7%.[30,100,403] Mitral stenosis is rheumatic even when Lutembacher syndrome is familial because it is the atrial septal defect that is transmitted.[98] Assuming a relatively uniform incidence of atrial septal defect, the incidence of coexisting rheumatic mitral stenosis depends on the geographic prevalence of rheumatic fever.[30] In underdeveloped countries, a history of rheumatic fever has been reported in 40% of patients with Lutembacher syndrome.[30,98,150,242]

The most important clinical consequence of a nonrestrictive atrial septal defect in Lutembacher syndrome is its ameliorating effect on the symptoms of mitral stenosis. Orthopnea, paroxysmal nocturnal dyspnea, pulmonary edema, and hemoptysis are infrequent and attenuated, and are replaced by fatigue due to reduced left ventricular filling and low cardiac output.[100,370] When Lutembacher syndrome consists of severe mitral stenosis with a *restrictive* atrial septal defect, the symptoms and clinical course resemble isolated mitral stenosis of equivalent severity.[30,242,403]

The ameliorating effects of an atrial septal defect were evident in Lutembacher's original patient, a 61 year old woman who had endured seven pregnancies.[278] Firkett's patient was a 74 year old woman who had endured 11 pregnancies.[158] An 81-year-old woman experienced no cardiac symptoms until her 75th year,[361] and survival to advanced age has been reaffirmed.[21,296,367,427] However, these reports should not obscure the unfavorable long-term outcome exerted by an atrial septal defect on mitral stenosis which increases the left-to-right shunt and predisposes to atrial fibrillation.[30,100,242,296] Susceptibility to infective endocarditis is increased by the presence of mitral stenosis in contrast to the negligible susceptibility of an uncomplicated ostium secundum atrial septal defect.

THE ARTERIAL PULSE

The arterial pulse is small because left ventricular stroke volume is small. Atrial fibrillation reduces the pulse still further (Fig. 15–49).[30,100]

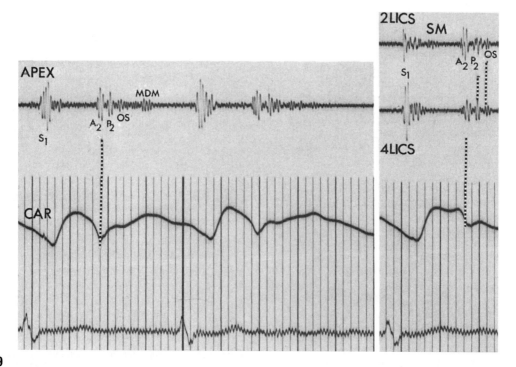

Figure 15–49

Tracings from a 42-year-old woman with Lutembacher syndrome that consisted of rheumatic mitral stenosis and a nonrestrictive superior vena caval sinus venosus atrial septal defect with a left-to-right shunt of 2.5 to 1, a mitral orifice of 1.1. cm², and pulmonary artery pressure of 38/18 mm Hg. The carotid pulse (CAR) was small because left ventricular stroke volume was reduced by atrial fibrillation shown in the rhythm strip below. Phonocardiogram at the apex recorded a prominent first heart sound (S_1), wide splitting of the second heart sound (A_2, aortic component; P_2, pulmonary component), an opening snap (OS), and a mid-diastolic murmur (MDM). The pulmonary component of the second sound was transmitted to the apex which was occupied by the right ventricle. In the second left intercostal space (2 LICS), the phonocardiogram shows a soft pulmonary midsystolic murmur (SM) and wide splitting of the second heart sound followed by an opening snap (OS). 4 LICS, fourth left intercostal space.

THE JUGULAR VENOUS PULSE

The right and left atrium function as a common chamber when the atrial septal defect is nonrestrictive, so the height and contour of the *left* atrial pressure pulse are transmitted into the *right* atrium and into the internal jugular vein.[120,423] Lutembacher syndrome is therefore responsible for an elevated mean jugular venous pressure in the absence of right ventricular failure, and for an elevated jugular venous A wave in the absence of pulmonary hypertension.

PRECORDIAL MOVEMENT AND PALPATION

The impulse of the right ventricle and pulmonary trunk are more prominent in Lutembacher syndrome with a nonrestrictive atrial septal defect than with an uncomplicated atrial septal defect of the same size, because mitral stenosis augments the left-to-right shunt. The underfilled left ventricle cannot be palpated. Diastolic thrill of mitral stenosis is exceptional because the velocity of mitral valve flow is comparatively low.

AUSCULTATION

The auscultatory signs of mitral stenosis are attenuated on two counts (Fig. 15–49).[150,403] First, flow is reduced across the stenotic mitral valve because left atrial blood has an alternative exit across the atrial septal defect, an explanation correctly offered by Lutembacher for the atypical characteristics of the mitral diastolic murmur.[278] Second, the auscultatory signs of uncomplicated mitral stenosis are heard best over the left ventricular impulse,[335] but in Lutembacher syndrome, the cardiac apex is occupied by the volume-overloaded right ventricle.

When a nonrestrictive atrial septal defect occurs with *mild* mitral stenosis, the auscultatory signs resemble those of the atrial septal defect.[403] Auscultatory yield is improved when the patient turns into a left lateral decubitus position and coughs briskly while the bell of the stethoscope is applied to the apex.[335] Mitral stenosis increases the left-to-right shunt and augments the mid-diastolic flow murmur across the pulmonary valve. Right ventricular dilatation is accompanied by the holosystolic murmur of tricuspid regurgitation that transmits to the apex inviting a mistaken diagnosis of mitral regurgitation.[30] Inspiratory augmentation of the tricuspid systolic murmur—Carvallo's sign—should prevent this error. When the atrial septal defect is restrictive, mitral stenosis produces a continuous shunt and a continuous murmur best heard at the lower *right* sternal border because the murmur is generated within the right atrial cavity.[188,237,362] The continuous murmur may increase with slow deep inspiration because of a delayed inspiratory increase in left atrial volume and pressure.[362] During the straining phase of the Valsalva maneuver, the interatrial gradient is reduced or abolished, and the continuous murmur diminishes.[362]

THE ELECTROCARDIOGRAM

When the atrial septal defect is restrictive, the electrocardiogram resembles mitral stenosis. When the atrial septal defect is nonrestrictive, the electrocardiogram resembles an atrial septal defect. Atrial fibrillation is frequent.[30] In the presence of sinus rhythm, P waves show left atrial abnormalities with a broad bifid configuration in lead 2 and a deep prolonged P terminal force in lead V_1 (Fig. 15–50).[403,415] Right ventricular hypertrophy is more common than with isolated atrial septal defect.

THE X-RAY

A *restrictive* atrial septal defect results in an x-ray that resembles mitral stenosis with pulmonary venous congestion and left atrial enlargement. When the atrial septal defect is *nonrestrictive*, the x-ray shows increased pulmonary arterial blood flow but little or no venous congestion because the left atrium decompresses (Fig. 15–51). Left atrial enlargement is less than expected for equivalent mitral stenosis but more than expected for an equivalent uncomplicated atrial septal defect (Fig. 15–51B).[30,150,415] Atrial fibrillation increases left atrial size.[30] Dilatation of the right atrium, right ventricle and pulmonary trunk exceeds expectations for an uncomplicated atrial septal defect because mitral stenosis augments the left-to-right shunt. It is unclear whether mitral valve calcification is actually infrequent or simply overlooked.

THE ECHOCARDIOGRAM

Echocardiography with color flow imaging and Doppler interrogation establishes the diagnosis of Lutembacher

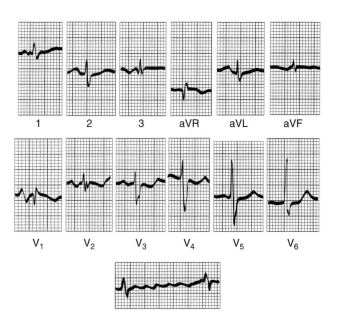

Figure 15–50
Electrocardiogram from the 42-year-old woman with Lutembacher syndrome whose phonocardiogram is shown in Figure 15–49. Broad notched left atrial P waves are present in lead 2 and aVL with a broad deep left atrial P terminal force in leads V_{1-2}. The leftward P wave axis with inverted P waves in leads 3 and aVF was due to an ectopic atrial pacemaker associated with the superior vena caval sinus venosus atrial septal defect. The QRS pattern resembles an ostium secundum atrial septal defect with a prolonged terminal force directed to the right, superior and anterior (rsr prime in lead V_1, r in aVR and a broad S wave in lead V_6). The rhythm strip below shows atrial fibrillation (see Fig. 15–49).

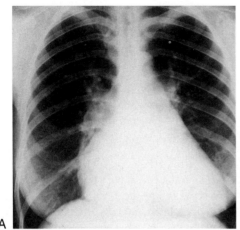
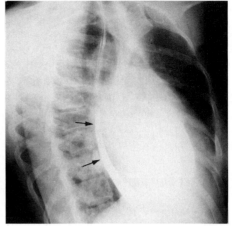

Figure 15–51

X-rays from the 42-year-old woman with Lutembacher syndrome referred to in Figures 15–49 and 15–50. The frontal projection shows no signs of pulmonary venous congestion. The pulmonary trunk is moderately prominent and merges with the shadow of the left atrial appendage resulting in a straight left cardiac border. The ascending aorta is not border forming. An enlarged right atrium occupies the lower right cardiac border, and an enlarged right ventricle occupies the apex. The right anterior oblique projection shows retrodisplacement of the barium esophagram by a moderately enlarged left atrium (*paired arrows*).

syndrome, identifies the location and size of the atrial septal defect and the degree of mitral stenosis (Fig. 15–52).[164,237] The continuous murmur at the right lower sternal border in the presence of a restrictive atrial septal defect coincides with Doppler flow patterns recorded by transesophageal echocardiography.[237]

SUMMARY

Lutembacher syndrome has a predilection for females because ostium secundum atrial septal defect and rheumatic mitral stenosis are both more prevalent in females. Despite rheumatic etiology of the mitral stenosis, a history of active rheumatic fever in childhood is obtained in less than half the cases.

When the atrial septal defect is *restrictive*, the clinical picture resembles isolated mitral stenosis. A continuous murmur is generated within the right atrial cavity and is heard at the right sternal border. The electrocardiogram shows left atrial P wave abnormalities, and the x-ray shows pulmonary venous congestion and left atrial enlargement.

A *nonrestrictive* atrial septal defect ameliorates the effects of mitral stenosis, and mitral stenosis augments the left-to-right interatrial shunt. Symptoms of pulmonary venous congestion are attenuated because the left atrium is decompressed. Mitral stenosis is a substrate for infective endocarditis. The arterial pulse is small especially with the advent of atrial fibrillation. The jugular venous pulse exhibits a prominent A wave in the absence of pulmonary hypertension because the left atrial pressure pulse is transmitted into the right atrium through the nonrestrictive atrial septal defect. Auscultatory signs of mitral stenosis are attenuated or absent. A pulmonary midsystolic flow murmur is prominent because right ventricular stroke volume is increased. The electrocardiogram in sinus rhythm shows left atrial P wave abnormalities. Right ventricular hypertrophy is more common than with an uncomplicated atrial septal defect. The x-ray shows increased pulmonary arterial blood flow with little or no pulmonary venous congestion. The right atrium, right ventricle, and pulmonary trunk

are considerably enlarged. Echocardiography with color flow imaging and Doppler interrogation establishes the presence and severity of mitral stenosis, identifies the location and size

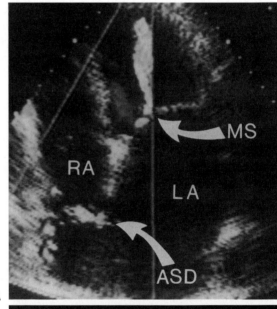
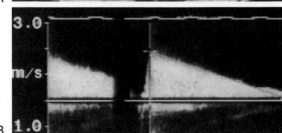

Figure 15–52

Echocardiogram from a 63-year-old woman with *iatrogenic* Lutembacher syndrome consisting of rheumatic mitral stenosis and an acquired interatrial communication produced during percutaneous transseptal mitral valvuloplasty. *A*, Black and white print of a color flow image shows a high-velocity diastolic jet from left atrium (LA) into right atrium (RA) through the acquired atrial septal defect (ASD). Mitral stenosis (MS) produced a high-velocity diastolic jet across the mitral valve. *B*, Continuous-wave Doppler across the stenotic mitral valve. The calculated orifice size was 1.8 cm^2.

of the atrial septal defect, and assesses the physiologic consequences of the combination.

When the atrial septal defect is *restrictive*, the clinical picture resembles isolated mitral stenosis. A continuous murmur is generated within the right atrial cavity and transmitted to the right sternal border. The electrocardiogram shows left atrial P wave abnormalities, and the x-ray shows pulmonary venous congestion and left atrial enlargement.

Common Atrium

Common atrium is a rare variety of interatrial communication characterized by absence or virtual absence of the atrial septum, vestigial remnants of which occasionally remain as diaphanous strands of tissue.[313] The right-sided portion of the common chamber has features of a morphologic *right* atrium (crista terminalis, pectinate muscles, right atrial appendage) and receives the superior and inferior vena cavae and the coronary sinus.[313] The left-sided portion of the common chamber has features of a morphologic *left* atrium (smooth nontrabeculated walls, left atrial appendage) and receives the pulmonary veins.[313] Common atrium therefore differs from atrial isomerism with a single atrial chamber that is either a bilateral morphologic right atrium or a bilateral morphologic left atrium (see Chapter 3). Absence of the atrial septum includes the ostium primum (atrioventricular septum) location, so there is a common atrioventricular valve (see Fig. 15–61) or a cleft anterior mitral leaflet (see Fig.15–59).[230,351] Partial anomalous pulmonary venous connections are frequent.[313] Systemic venous anomalies consist of superior vena caval connection to the left-sided portion of the common atrium, persistent left superior vena cava, and left hemiazygos vein.[116]

Physiologic consequences of common atrium resemble nonrestrictive atrial septal defect except for obligatory venoarterial mixing.[313] Common atrium is therefore a *cyanotic* malformation with *increased* pulmonary arterial blood flow.[351] Despite absence of the atrial septum, venoarterial mixing is usually no more than moderate with systemic arterial oxygen saturations that are often above 90%.[313,384] The relative magnitude of left-to-right and right-to-left components of interatrial mixing are determined chiefly by the distensibility characteristics of the right and left ventricles as in nonrestrictive atrial septal defect (see earlier).[384] At one end of the spectrum are patients with low pulmonary vascular resistance, distensible right ventricles, a large left-to-right shunt, and mild or absent cyanosis. At the other end of the spectrum are patients with high pulmonary vascular resistance, poorly distensible right ventricles, a significant right-to-left shunt, and conspicuous cyanosis.

THE HISTORY

Symptoms begin earlier and are more pronounced than with nonrestrictive atrial septal defects.[313] The majority of patients experience dyspnea, fatigue, respiratory infections, mild cyanosis, and physical underdevelopment in the first year of life. Occasional patients are relatively well into late childhood or early adolescence,[313,384] but rarely into adulthood (Fig. 15–59).

PHYSICAL APPEARANCE

Cyanosis occurs with insufficient evidence of pulmonary hypertension to account for its presence, and it may be insignificant at rest but induced by exercise or crying. Small or intermittent right-to-left shunts present in patients as highly colored cheeks or digital erythema. Down phenotype is not a feature of common atrium despite the presence of elements of an atrioventricular septal defect. Ellis-van Creveld syndrome—chondroectodermal dysplasia—is an important phenotype because 50% of patients with the syndrome have congenital heart disease and half of those have common atrium.[186,280,297,323] Ellis-van Creveld syndrome is autosomal recessive and is characterized by dwarfism with polydactyly of the hands that is invariable (Fig. 15–53A) and polydactyly of the feet in 10% of cases (Fig.15–53B).[323] *Polycarpaly* (a ninth or tenth carpal bone), *clinodactyly* (bent

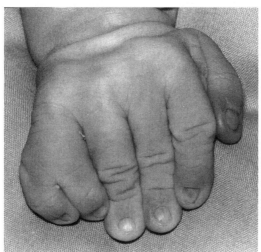
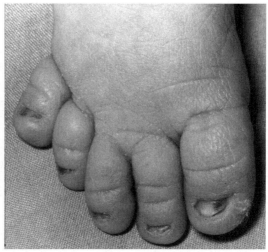

Figure 15–53
Photographs from a female neonate with Ellis-van Creveld syndrome and common atrium. *A*, The hand is characterized by a well-formed extra digit on its ulnar aspect (polydactyly), clinodactyly (bent fingers) and syndactyly (interdigital webbing). Hypoplasia of the nails is better seen in the foot (*B*) and in Figure 15–54.

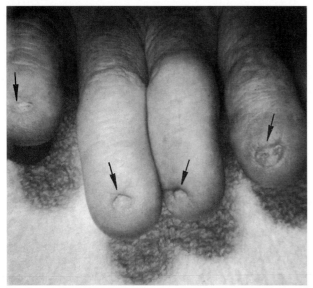

Figure 15–54
Close-up of the fingers of a 53-year-old female dwarf with Ellis-van Creveld syndrome and hypoplasia of the nails (*arrows*). (From Hearst JW: The Heart. 4th ed. New York, McGraw-Hill Book Company, 1978, with permission.)

finger), *syndactyly* (interdigital webbing), and *hypoplasia of the nails*[323,418] are common phenotypic features (Figs. 15–53 and 15–54). Premature eruption of malformed maxillary incisors, gingival hypertrophy, and multiple frenula are distinctive features (Fig. 15–55).

THE ARTERIAL PULSE, THE JUGULAR VENOUS PULSE, PRECORDIAL MOVEMENT AND PALPATION, AND AUSCULTATION

The arterial pulse, the jugular venous pulse, and precordial palpation are analogous to nonrestrictive ostium secundum atrial septal defect (see earlier). Auscultatory signs are also similar with the important exception of an apical holosystolic murmur of mitral regurgitation caused by the malformed left atrioventricular valve (Fig. 15–59B). An increase in the jugular A wave and a loud pulmonary component of the second heart sound reflect pulmonary hypertension that develops early.

THE ELECTROCARDIOGRAM

Absence of the atrial septum assumes deficiency of the superior vena caval sinus venosus location, the ostium primum or atrioventricular septal location, and the ostium secundum location. The electrocardiogram reflects deficiencies at all of these sites.[230] Leftward deviation of the P wave axis with inverted P waves in the inferior leads are analogous to the ectopic atrial pacemaker in a superior vena caval sinus venous atrial septal defect with an absent sinus node.[151,202,230,313,420] Left axis deviation of the QRS with counterclockwise depolarization (Figs. 15–56 and 15–57) and splintering of S waves in the inferior leads (Fig. 15–57) is analogous to the electrocardiogram of an atrioventricular septal defect.[230,313] The precordial leads are analogous to an ostium secundum atrial septal defect, but early development of pulmonary hypertension results in increased R wave amplitude in right precordial (Figs. 15–56 and 15–57). The electrocardiogram therefore reflects the combined absence of the superior, middle, and inferior portions of the atrial septum.

THE X-RAY

The chest x-ray is similar to nonrestrictive ostium secundum atrial septal defect (Figs. 15–58 and 15–59A).[313] Enlargement of the left atrial portion of the common atrium is seldom seen in the x-ray even in the presence of significant mitral regurgitation.

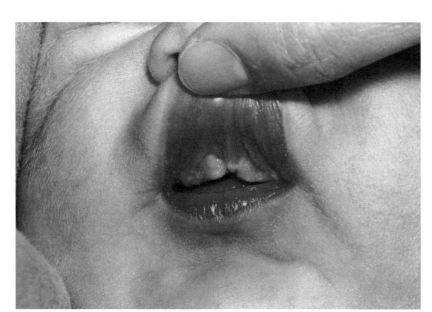

Figure 15–55
Female neonate with Ellis-van Creveld syndrome, premature eruption of malformed maxillary incisors, gingival hypertrophy, and multiple frenula.

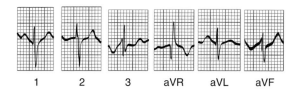

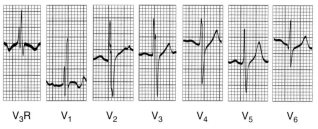

Figure 15–56

Electrocardiogram from a 5-year-old boy with common atrium, a cleft anterior mitral leaflet, and a 3.5 to 1 left-to-right shunt. The leftward shift of the P wave axis with inverted P waves in leads 2, 3, and aVF indicates an ectopic pacemaker because of an absent sinus node associated with a superior vena caval sinus venosus atrial septal defect. Left axis deviation with counterclockwise depolarization and splintered S waves in inferior leads indicates that the atrial septum was deficient in the ostium primum location. The terminal force of the QRS points to the right, superior and anterior as in an ostium secundum atrial septal defect.

THE ECHOCARDIOGRAM

Echocardiography with color flow imaging and Doppler interrogation identifies a common atrial chamber (Fig. 15–60), absence of the atrial septum, and a common atrioventricular valve or a cleft anterior mitral leaflet (Fig. 15–61). The right and left components of the common atrioventricular valve lie at the same level because the atrioventricular septum is absent (Fig. 15–61A). Color flow imaging identifies regurgitation across the left component of the common atrioventricular valve (Fig. 15–61B). The right ventricle is dilated (Fig.15–61A), the ventricular septum moves paradoxically, and the pulmonary trunk is dilated and pulsatile.

SUMMARY

The clinical features of common atrium resemble a nonrestrictive ostium secundum atrial septal defect with the following qualifications: 1) symptoms begin earlier and are more pronounced, 2) cyanosis occurs with *increased* pulmonary arterial blood flow and without sufficient pulmonary hypertension to account for its presence, 3) the P wave axis indicates absence of the sinus node with an ectopic atrial pacemaker because a superior vena caval sinus venosus atrial septal deficiency, 4) the QRS axis exhibits the left axis deviation and counterclockwise depolarization associated with an atrioventricular septal defect, and 5) echocardiography identifies absence of the atrial septum, a common atrioventricular valve, or a cleft anterior mitral leaflet.

Total Anomalous Pulmonary Venous Connection

In 1798, the Philosophical Transactions of the Royal Society in London published, "A description of a very unusual formation of the human heart,"[440] *total anomalous venous connection*. A 1942 review of 100 cases of anomalous pulmonary venous connections included 35 examples that were *total* anomalous.[61] The term applies when all four pulmonary veins connect anomalously to a systemic venous tributary of the right atrium or to the right atrium proper, but have no connection to the left atrium.[138,140] The malformation is isolated in approximately two thirds of patients so afflicted,[67,108,118,180] occurs in approximately four to six per 100,000 live births,[160] and accounts for about 2% of deaths from congenital heart disease in the first year of life. The association of total anomalous pulmonary venous connection with atrial isomerism is dealt with in Chapter 3.

Classifications take into account three features: 1) the pathway by which pulmonary venous blood reaches the right atrium, 2) the presence or absence of obstruction

Figure 15–57

Electrocardiogram from a 57-year-old cyanotic woman with common atrium, pulmonary hypertension, and moderate incompetence of the left-sided component of a common atrioventricular valve. The PR interval is prolonged. A normal P wave axis implies that the sinus node was intact despite a superior vena caval sinus venosus atrial septal defect. Peaked P waves in leads V$_{4-5}$ together with QS waves in leads V$_{1-3}$ are signs of right atrial enlargement, and broad bifid P waves in leads 3, aVL, aVF, and V$_6$ reflect a left atrial abnormality. Left axis deviation with counterclockwise depolarization and splintered S waves in leads 2, 3, and aVF imply an atrioventricular septal defect with a cleft anterior mitral leaflet. Right ventricular hypertrophy is manifested by tall R waves in right precordial leads and deep S waves in left precordial leads. QRS prolongation is due to increased duration of the terminal force that is directed to the right, superior and anterior.

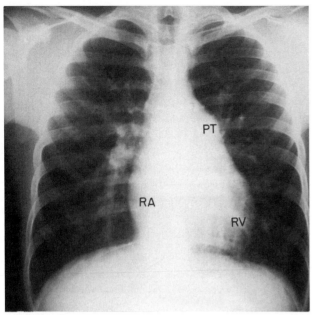

Figure 15–58

X-ray from a 5-year-old acyanotic boy with common atrium whose electrocardiogram is shown in Figure 15–56. The x-ray resembles an ostium secundum atrial septal defect. Pulmonary arterial vascularity is increased, the pulmonary trunk (PT) and its right branch are dilated, the right atrium (RA) is convex, and a prominent right ventricle (RV) occupies the apex.

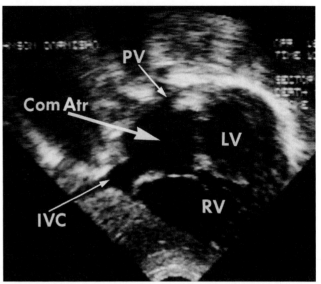

Figure 15–60

Echocardiogram (subcostal) from a female neonate with Ellis-van Creveld syndrome and common atrium (Com Atr). An atrial septum was absent. The inferior vena cava (IVC) entered the right sided portion of the common atrium, and the pulmonary veins (PV) entered the left sided portion of the common atrium. LV, left ventricle; RV, right ventricle.

along the course of the pathway, and 3) the nature of the interatrial communication.[108] The most widely used clinical classification recognizes *supradiaphragmatic* connections with or without obstruction, and *infradiaphrag-matic* or *infracardiac* connections that are always obstructed.[67,108,118,208,275,318] Supradiaphragmatic varieties constitute more than three fourths of cases.[108,118,180] Except for mixed connections and connections of all four pulmonary veins directly to the right atrium, all varieties of

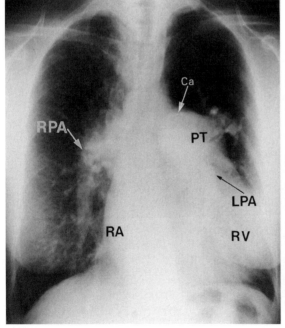

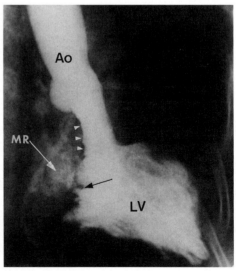

Figure 15–59

A, X-ray and left ventriculogram from the 57-year-old cyanotic woman with common atrium whose electrocardiogram is shown in Figure 15–57. The lung fields are oligemic. The ascending aorta is not border forming in contrast to the huge pulmonary trunk (PT) that contains a rim of calcium (Ca) in its upper margin. The right pulmonary artery (RPA) is dilated and tapers rapidly. A large left pulmonary artery (LPA) is behind the cardiac shadow. The right atrium (RA) is dilated, and an enlarged right ventricle (RV) occupies the apex. *B,* Left ventriculogram (LV) shows the typical gooseneck deformity (*small white arrowheads*) and the cleft anterior mitral leaflet (*black unmarked arrow*) of an atrioventricular septal defect. Mitral regurgitation (MR) was only moderate despite a malformed common atrioventricular valve.

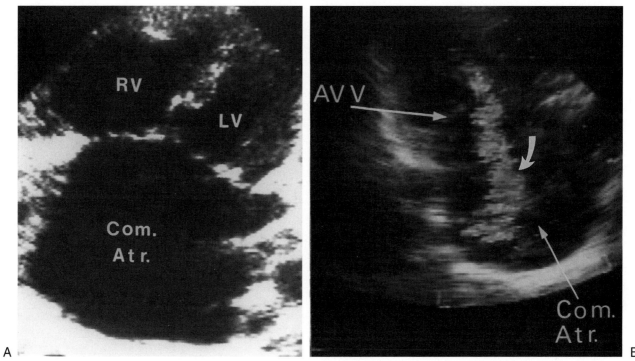

Figure 15–61

Echocardiogram with black and white print of a color flow image from the 57-year-old woman with common atrium referred to in Figures 15–57 and 15–59. *A,* Apical view shows the common atrium (Com. Atr.) and the common atrioventricular valve whose left and right components lie at the same level. LV, left ventricle; RV, right ventricle. *B,* Black and white print of a color flow image showing regurgitation (*unmarked curved arrow*) across the left component of the common atrioventricular valve (AVV). Com Atr, common atrium.

total anomalous pulmonary venous connections incorporate a *venous confluence* that receives the four pulmonary veins (Figs. 15–62 to 15–65). In the *supradiaphragmatic* varieties, the confluence joins the coronary sinus (Figs. 15–63 and 15–64) or a left vertical vein that ascends to join

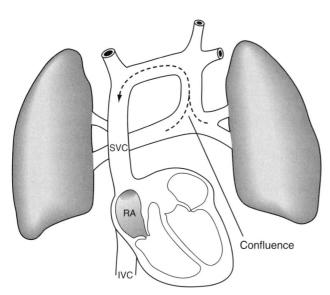

Figure 15–62

Illustration of total anomalous pulmonary venous connection in which blood from the confluence reaches the right atrium (RA) through an anomalous left vertical vein, an innominate bridge, and a right superior vena cava (SVC) (*dotted arrow*). IVC, inferior vena cava.

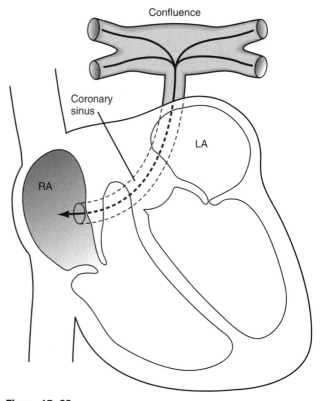

Figure 15–63

Illustration of total anomalous pulmonary venous connection in which the venous confluence joins the coronary sinus. RA, right atrium; LA, left atrium.

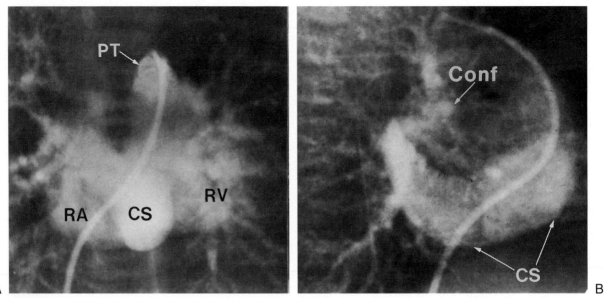

Figure 15–64
Angiocardiograms from a 2-month-old girl with total anomalous pulmonary venous connection to the coronary sinus. *A,* Levophase following injection of contrast material into the pulmonary trunk (PT) visualizes a dilated coronary sinus (CS) from which contrast enters the right atrium (RA) and right ventricle (RV). *B,* Lateral projection shows the confluence of pulmonary veins (Conf) entering a strikingly dilated coronary sinus (CS).

an innominate bridge to the right superior vena cava and right atrium (Figs. 15–62, 15–65, and 15–70). Obstruction of the vertical vein is caused by a *hemodynamic vise* formed posteriorly by the left bronchus and anteriorly by the pulmonary trunk (Figs. 15–65 and 15–66*B*).[118] Less commonly, the vertical vein is intrinsically obstructed.[277,388]

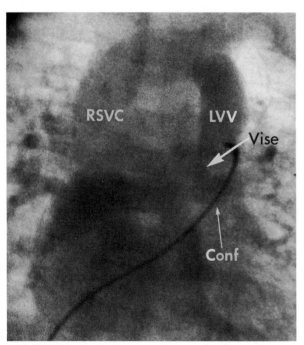

Figure 15–65
Levophase following injection of contrast material into the pulmonary trunk of a 3-month-old girl with total anomalous pulmonary venous connection and obstruction of the left vertical vein (LVV) by a *hemodynamic vise* that consisted of the dilated anterior pulmonary trunk and the posterior left bronchus (compare to Fig. 15–66 *B*). CONF, confluence; RSVC, right superior vena cava.

Obstruction is exceptional when the coronary sinus receives the venous confluence (Figs. 15–63 and 15–64) and results from stenosis of the right atrial ostium of the coronary sinus.[17,277,388] Rarely, the superior vena cava is obstructed at its junction with the right atrium. Uncommon connections include a venous confluence to the right superior vena cava via a right-sided anomalous venous channel (Fig. 15–67) or via the azygos venous system (Fig. 15–68).

Subdiaphragmatic or *infracardiac* total anomalous pulmonary venous connection refers to a venous confluence from which a vascular channel originates and descends anterior to the esophagus, penetrates the esophageal hiatus, and terminates in the portal vein or less commonly in the inferior vena cava or ductus venosus (Figs. 15–66*A* and 15–69).[118,168,180,275,318] Obstruction is almost invariable and is certain when the connection is to the portal vein because blood confronts resistance in the hepatic capillary bed. Alternatively, the descending venous channel is intrinsically obstructed or is compressed as it traverses the esophageal hiatus.[118]

An *interatrial communication* is the only exit from the right atrium and the only access to the left side of the heart. The communication varies from an obstructing patent foramen ovale to a nonrestrictive atrial septal defect.[118,180,183,388]

The *embryologic fault* responsible for total anomalous pulmonary venous connection is believed to be agenesis of the common pulmonary vein with persistence and enlargement of primitive communications between the pulmonary venous and the systemic venous beds.[32,67,118,183,276] The common pulmonary vein is a temporary outgrowth of the developing left atrium and joins the pulmonary veins as they arise from lung buds. When the common pulmonary vein fails to develop, the pulmonary venous plexus of lung buds does not join the left atrium but instead communicates with

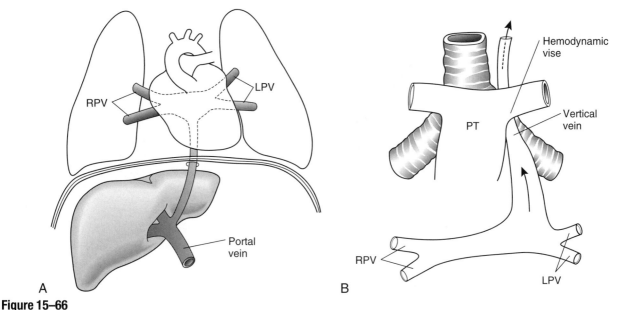

Figure 15–66

A, Illustration of the confluence of pulmonary veins giving rise to a vascular channel that enters the abdominal cavity through the diaphragmatic hiatus and terminates in the portal vein. RPV and LPV, right and left pulmonary veins. *B,* Illustration of the anomalous left vertical vein compressed in a *hemodynamic vise* consisting of the pulmonary trunk (PT) and the left bronchus.

systemic veins via anastomotic pathways that represent persistence and enlargement of embryonic vascular channels.

In fetal life, the *physiologic consequences* of total anomalous pulmonary venous connection are negligible because the amount of blood flowing through the lungs and through the pulmonary veins is negligible.[135] When the lungs expand at birth, an obligatory left-to-right shunt is established because pulmonary venous flow is necessarily into the right atrium where it mixes with systemic venous return.[135] Part of this mixture enters the right ventricle and part crosses the atrial septum to reach the left side of the heart.

Once the pulmonary and systemic venous returns converge in the right atrium, the response of the circulation depends on the size of the interatrial communication and the behavior of the pulmonary vascular bed.[67,118,135,180] A *restrictive patent foramen ovale* constitutes an obstruction that results in an increase in right atrial and pulmonary venous pressure, in pulmonary hypertension, and in a

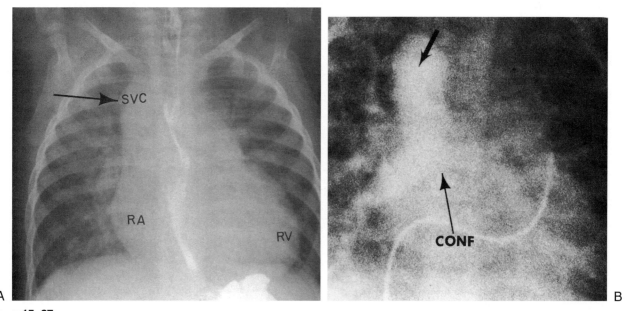

Figure 15–67

A, X-rays from a 10-month-old boy with total anomalous pulmonary venous connection into a right vertical vein that joined a right superior vena cava (SVC). *Arrow* points to the shadow formed by the superimposed right vertical vein and superior vena cava. Pulmonary arterial vascularity is increased. The right atrium (RA) is prominent, and an enlarged right ventricle (RV) occupies the apex. *B,* Levophase after contrast injection into the pulmonary trunk. The right and left pulmonary veins form a confluence (CONF) that rises as a right-sided anomalous pulmonary venous channel (*unmarked arrow*) and joins the right superior vena cava. Compare with right thoracic inlet in 15–67A.

decrease in flow to the left side of the heart. A *nonrestrictive atrial septal defect* provides free access to the left atrium, so the direction taken by right atrial blood becomes a function of the distensibility characteristics of the right and left ventricles.[67] Low pulmonary vascular resistance is accompanied by a dilated compliant right ventricle that receives a large volume of blood from the right atrium and ejects the large volume into the pulmonary circulation. Systemic flow is generally maintained despite a low left ventricular end-diastolic volume and ejection fraction and the small size of the left atrium and left ventricle. As pulmonary blood flow increases, pulmonary venous return to the right atrium increases, cyanosis is mild, and the oxygen saturation is high and equal in the right atrium, right ventricle, pulmonary trunk, left atrium and left ventricle. An increase in pulmonary vascular resistance induces right ventricular hypertrophy, so a smaller fraction of right atrial blood crosses the tricuspid valve into the hypertrophied noncompliant right ventricle. Pulmonary blood flow falls and cyanosis increases. Elevated pulmonary vascular resistance occurs more frequently with total anomalous pulmonary venous connection than with an isolated nonrestrictive atrial septal defect and an equilavent shunt.[118,180]

Pulmonary venous obstruction, whether supradiaphragmatic or infradiaphragmatic, results in pulmonary hypertension, reduced pulmonary blood flow,[118,180] and a decrease in the volume of pulmonary venous blood reaching the right atrium. Cyanosis increases as oxygen saturation of the right atrial mixture falls. Intrapulmonary and extrapulmonary veins exhibit intimal proliferation, abnormally thick walls and a reduction in size.[277] Even more malignant hemodynamic forces come into play when a

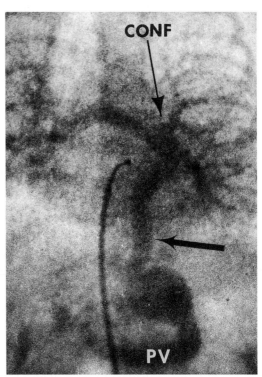

Figure 15–69

Levophase following injection of contrast material into the pulmonary trunk of a 4-day-old boy with infradiaphragmatic total anomalous pulmonary venous connection. Right and left pulmonary veins form a confluence (CONF) that gives rise to a vascular channel (*unmarked horizontal arrow*) that enters the abdominal cavity through the diaphragmatic hiatus and terminates in the portal vein (PV). Compare to Figure 15–66A. Obstruction was in the portal vein and hepatic bed rather than at the diaphragmatic hiatus, accounting for the subdiaphragmatic dilatation.

left vertical venous channel is compressed between the pulmonary trunk and the left bronchus (Figs. 15–65 and 15–66B). A rise in pulmonary venous pressure provokes pulmonary hypertension, pulmonary hypertension provokes further dilatation of the pulmonary trunk, the dilated hypertensive pulmonary trunk compresses the vertical venous channel still further, and the vicious cycle continues.

THE HISTORY

Sex ratio with supradiaphragmatic total anomalous pulmonary venous connections is about equal,[67,180,183] while infrahepatic connection to the portal vein strongly favors males.[108,180,208,275] These malformations have been reported in first cousins, siblings, monozygotic and dizygotic twins and in a father and his two children.[28,180,187,348,397] Total anomalous pulmonary venous connection with Holt-Oram syndrome has been described in a family with a history of atrial septal defect.[445]

The clinical course is abbreviated even in the absence of pulmonary venous obstruction. Seventy-five percent to ninety percent of symptomatic infants do not reach their first birthday, and most of those are dead within 3 to

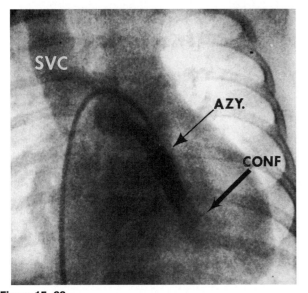

Figure 15–68

Angiogram from a 2-month-old boy with total anomalous pulmonary venous connection into a confluence (CONF) that joined a prominent right superior vena cava (SVC) via the azygos vein (AZY).

6 months.[118,180,356] Only 50% of patients who survive to age 3 months are alive at 1 year.[356] The malformation may not be suspected when pulmonary blood flow is increased and cyanosis is mild.[108] Before long, the infant becomes cyanotic and dyspneic with difficulty feeding and poor growth and development.[108,135] Those who survive their first year almost always have supradiaphragmatic connections, low pulmonary vascular resistance and a nonrestrictive atrial septal defect. A 10-year-old boy had *unobstructed infradiaphragmatic* connection to the inferior vena cava,[132] and a 17-year-old had *obstructed infradiaphragmatic* connection to the hepatic vein.[168] Exceptionally, patients reach their third, fourth, or fifth decade with relatively little disability and a clinical picture that resembles isolated ostium secundum atrial septal defect except for mild cyanosis.[62,67,83,108,183,299,301,329,398] A cyanotic woman with suprasystemic pulmonary vascular resistance was 54 years of age (Fig. 15–70), and a 62-year-old woman came to necropsy.[298] The oldest reported patient underwent surgical repair at age 66 years.[299]

In total anomalous pulmonary venous connection *with obstruction*, lifespan is brief and the clinical course is stormy. Tachypnea begins with expansion of the lungs because neonatal pulmonary blood flow is obstructed (Fig. 15–71).[67,118,180,275] Cyanosis is conspicuous because only a small portion of oxygenated pulmonary venous blood reaches the right atrium for mixing. When an infradiaphragmatic venous channel traverses the esophageal hiatus, feeding, crying and straining cause additional compression that aggravates the dyspnea and cyanosis.[275] Death from pulmonary edema and right ventricular failure comes within days, weeks or months after birth.[275]

Newborns with infradiaphragmatic connections and asplenia may have major esophageal varices.[167]

PHYSICAL APPEARANCE

Mild-to-moderate *cyanosis* occurs *with increased pulmonary blood flow* in total anomalous pulmonary venous connection without obstruction.[67] Infants with congestive heart failure are catabolic.[180] However, a relatively asymptomatic 46-year-old man had been cyanotic since childhood,[183] and an exceptional 39-year-old man was never overtly cyanotic.[67] Holt-Oram syndrome, Klippel-Feil syndrome,[180] and *cat eye* syndrome have been sporadically reported.[161,293,375]

THE ARTERIAL PULSE AND THE JUGULAR VENOUS PULSE

The arterial pulse is small because left ventricular stroke volume is reduced. The jugular venous pulse resembles the wave form of isolated ostium secundum atrial septal defect when the interatrial communication is nonrestrictive. At the inception of right ventricular failure, the right-to-left shunt increases while the jugular venous pressure remains relatively unchanged. Pulmonary hypertension with a restrictive interatrial communication results in a large even giant A wave.

PRECORDIAL MOVEMENT AND PALPATION

Precordial movement and palpation resemble a nonrestrictive ostium secundum atrial septal defect when the

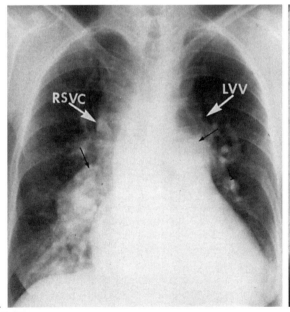 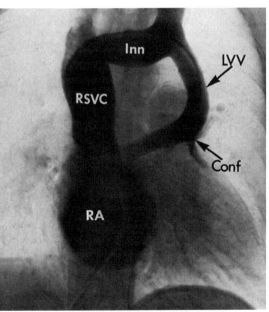

Figure 15–70

A, X-ray from a 54-year-old cyanotic woman with total anomalous pulmonary venous connection. The confluence of four pulmonary veins gave rise to a left vertical vein (LVV) that joined an innominate bridge and a right superior vena cava (RSVC). Pulmonary vascular resistance was above systemic level. The pulmonary trunk and right branch are dilated and contain calcium (*small black arrows*). *B,* Levophase following injection of contrast material into the pulmonary trunk showing the confluence (CONF), the left vertical vein (LVV), the innominate bridge (Inn), the right superior vena cava (RSVC), and the right atrium (RA).

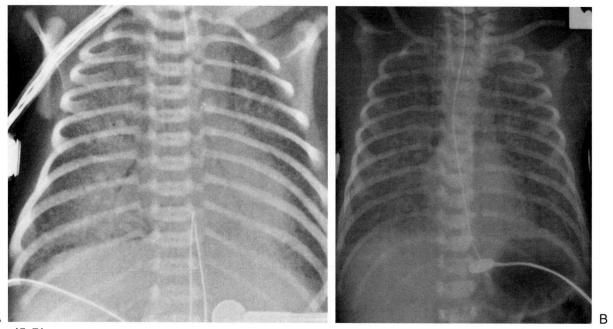

Figure 15–71

X-rays from two infants with total anomalous pulmonary venous connection and obstruction. The lungs in both x-rays show a striking stippled, reticular, ground glass appearance. *A,* Female neonate with infradiaphragmatic obstruction. The transverse liver and symmetric bronchi indicate right isomerism. *B,* Male neonate with atresia of a left vertical vein distal to the venous confluence. The dramatic appearance of the lungs is in marked contrast to the unimpressive cardiac silhouette.

interatrial communication is nonrestrictive, although these precordial signs begin earlier. A rise in pulmonary vascular resistance imposes afterload on the volume-loaded right ventricle, so its impulse becomes more striking (Fig. 15–72).[83,180] A hyperdynamic right ventricle is not a feature in neonates and infants with pulmonary vein obstruction because pulmonary blood flow is reduced.

AUSCULTATION

Auscultatory signs resemble an ostium secundum atrial septal defect when the interatrial communication is nonrestrictive. The tricuspid component of the first heart sound is loud, there is wide fixed splitting of the second heart sound (Figs. 15–73 and 15–74),[183] a pulmonary midsystolic murmur is generated by rapid ejection of a large right ventricular stroke volume into a dilated pulmonary trunk (Figs. 15–73 and 15–74), and a tricuspid diastolic flow murmur is common (Fig. 15–73).[180,439] The systolic murmur may have a wide thoracic distribution analogous to the peripheral pulmonary arterial murmurs with ostium secundum atrial septal defect and a hyperkinetic pulmonary circulation.[338] Pulmonary hypertension is accompanied by an ejection sound, attenuation of the pulmonary systolic flow murmur, loss of the tricuspid diastolic murmur, inspiratory splitting of the second heart sound (Fig. 15–72),[180] and a high-frequency early diastolic Graham Steell murmur (Fig. 15–75). An increased force of right atrial contraction generates a right ventricular fourth heart sound, and right ventricular failure is accompanied by a third heart sound and a holosystolic murmur of tricuspid regurgitation.[83,135,180]

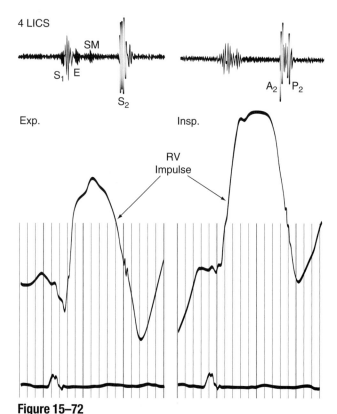

Figure 15–72

Tracings from a 13-year-old cyanotic girl with total anomalous pulmonary venous connection, systemic pulmonary artery pressure and a confluence of veins that joined the right superior vena cava. The right ventricular (RV) impulse is apparent. The second heart sound (S_2) splits normally during inspiration (INSP). The prominent pulmonary component (P_2) and the pulmonary ejection sound (E) were transmitted to the fourth left intercostal space (4 LICS). The pulmonary systolic murmur (SM) is attenuated. A_2, aortic component of the second sound.

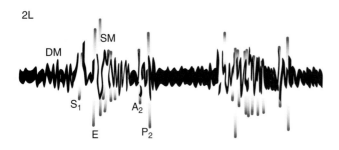

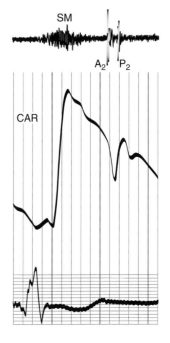

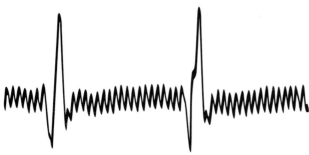

Figure 15–73

Phonocardiogram from a 9-month-old male with total anomalous pulmonary venous connection in which the four pulmonary veins joined the right atrium directly. A restrictive foramen ovale constituted a zone of pulmonary venous obstruction. The first heart sound (S_1) is preceded by a tricuspid diastolic flow murmur (DM) and followed by a pulmonary ejection sound (E) that introduced a prominent midsystolic flow murmur (SM). There is wide fixed splitting of the aortic (A_2) and pulmonary (P_2) components of the second heart sound. 2L, second left intercostal space.

Figure 15–74

Tracings from a 9-year-old boy with total anomalous pulmonary venous connection and low pulmonary vascular resistance. A prominent pulmonary systolic flow murmur (SM) ends before both components (A_2, P_2) of a widely split second heart sound. CAR, carotid pulse.

A continuous murmur is a noteworthy although uncommon auscultatory sign that originates in continuous flow through the venous confluence, the left vertical vein and left innominate vein (Fig. 15–62).[87,135] The continuous murmur has the quality of a soft venous hum and is maximum at the left upper sternal border. Less commonly, a continuous murmur is heard along the *right* upper sternal border where it is believed to originate from flow through a right-sided anomalous pulmonary venous channel into a right superior vena cava (Fig. 15–67).

In infants with pulmonary venous obstruction, auscultatory signs are governed by pulmonary hypertension rather than increased pulmonary blood flow.[208,275] Over half of these patients have no pulmonary systolic murmur because flow across the pulmonary valve is reduced, but an attenuated midsystolic murmur is generated by ejection into a dilated hypertensive pulmonary trunk. The second

Figure 15–75

Tracing from a moderately cyanotic 26-year-old man with total anomalous pulmonary venous connection to the right superior vena cava. Pulmonary artery systolic pressure was 87 mm Hg and the brachial arterial systolic pressure was 106 mm Hg. Phonocardiogram at the lower left sternal edge (LSE) shows a pulmonary ejection sound (E) and a Graham Steell diastolic murmur (DM) issuing from a loud single second heart sound (S_2). The ejection sound and diastolic murmur radiated to the apex because the apex was occupied by the right ventricle. CAR, carotid pulse.

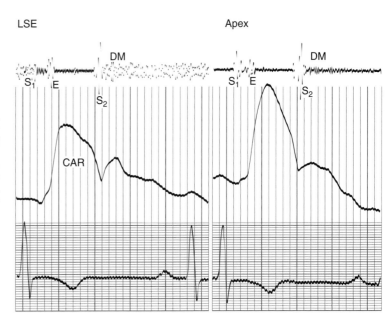

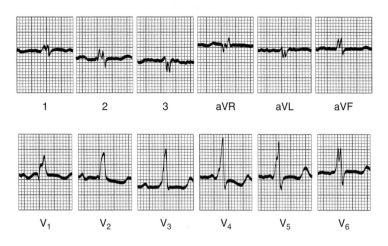

Figure 15–76

Electrocardiogram from a 49-year-old man with total anomalous pulmonary venous connection to a left vertical vein, a nonrestrictive ostium secundum atrial septal defect with a 2.5 to 1 shunt, and pulmonary artery pressure of 50/20 mm Hg. The PR interval is prolonged. The right ventricular conduction defect resembles the conduction defect in an adult with an ostium secundum atrial septal defect but the right precordial R waves are more prominent.

sound is single or closely split, and the pulmonary component is loud. A high frequency holosystolic murmur of tricuspid regurgitation accompanies pulmonary hypertensive right ventricular failure.

THE ELECTROCARDIOGRAM

The electrocardiogram resembles an ostium secundum atrial septal defect when the interatrial communication is nonrestrictive (Fig. 15–76). The PR interval tends to be prolonged (Fig. 15–76). Atrial fibrillation occurs in older patients as it does with ostium secundum atrial septal defect.[83] In the presence of pulmonary hypertension, the electrocardiogram exhibits peaked right atrial P waves, right axis deviation, tall right precordial R waves, inverted T waves and deep left precordial S waves of right ventricular hypertrophy (Figs.15–77 through 15–79).[135,180,183,197,275,394]

THE X-RAY

Cardiac enlargement begins within weeks.[135] Dilatation of the right ventricular outflow tract sometimes obscures an enlarged pulmonary trunk (Fig. 15–80). When the interatrial communication is nonrestrictive, the x-ray subsequently resembles an ostium secundum atrial septal defect with increased pulmonary blood flow, an enlarged pulmonary trunk and proximal branches, a small ascending aorta, a large right atrium, and a large right ventricle (Fig. 15–81).

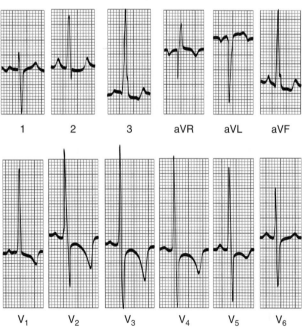

Figure 15–77

Electrocardiogram from a 13-year-old girl with total anomalous pulmonary venous connection to the right superior vena cava and systemic pulmonary artery pressure. Peaked right atrial P waves appear in leads 2 and aVF. There is right axis deviation and right ventricular hypertrophy reflected in the tall monophasic R waves and deeply inverted T waves in leads V_{1-4} and the deep S wave in lead V_6.

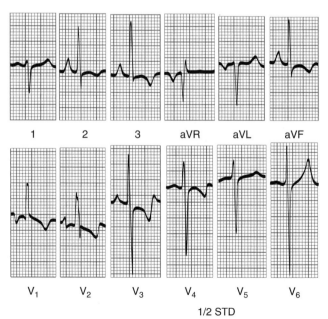

1/2 STD

Figure 15–78

Electrocardiogram from a 26-year-old man with total anomalous pulmonary venous connection to the right superior vena cava. Pulmonary artery systolic pressure was 87 mm Hg. Tall peaked right atrial P waves appear in leads 2, 3, and aVF. There is right axis deviation and right ventricular hypertrophy reflected in tall right precordial R waves, deeply inverted T waves, and deep left precordial S waves (half standardized).

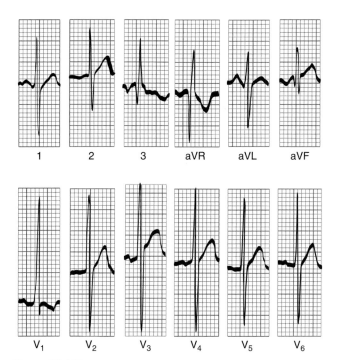

Figure 15–79

Electrocardiogram from a 9-month-old boy with total anomalous pulmonary venous connection of all four pulmonary veins directly into the right atrium. A restrictive foramen ovale caused pulmonary venous obstruction and severe pulmonary hypertension that promptly decreased after balloon atrial septostomy. The leftward and superior P wave axis indicates that the atrial pacemaker is ectopic. The QRS axis is vertical, and right ventricular hypertrophy is reflected in the tall monophasic R waves in right precordial leads and the deep S waves in left precordial leads.

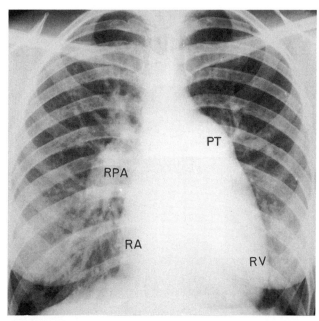

Figure 15–81

X-ray from a mildly cyanotic 21-year-old woman with total anomalous pulmonary venous connection to the the coronary sinus. The x-ray resembles an ostium secundum atrial septal defect with increased pulmonary arterial blood flow, dilatation of the pulmonary trunk (PT) and right pulmonary artery (RPA), an inconspicuous ascending aorta, and a dilated right ventricle (RV) and right atrium (RA).

Specific sites of anomalous pulmonary venous connections can be radiologically distinctive.[165] Prominence of the right upper cardiac border represents a right superior vena cava that receives the confluence of pulmonary veins via a right-sided anomalous venous channel (Figs. 15–67 and 15–80) or via the azygos vein (Fig. 15–68).[180] The coronary sinus dilates when it receives the confluence (Fig. 15–64) and may indent the esophagus.[183] Most distinctive is the figure of eight or snowman silhouette (Figs. 15–70 and 15–82A, B).[64,65,180,183,266,395,439] The upper portion of

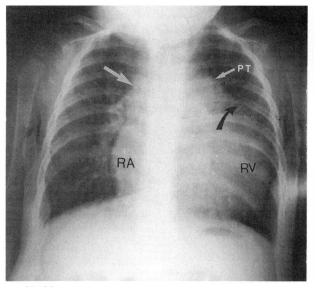

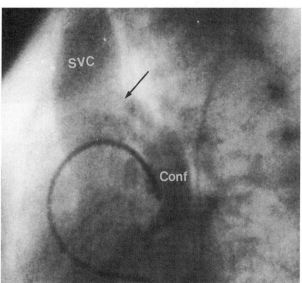

Figure 15–80

A, X-ray from a mildly cyanotic 5-month-old female with total anomalous pulmonary venous connection to a right superior vena cava which formed a prominent shadow at the right thoracic inlet (*large white arrow*). Pulmonary vascularity is increased. A dilated pulmonary trunk (PT) is obscured by the enlarged outflow tract (*curved black arrow*) of a dilated right ventricle (RV). *B,* Levophase of a pulmonary arteriogram showing the connection (*arrow*) of the confluence (Conf) to the right superior vena cava (SVC).

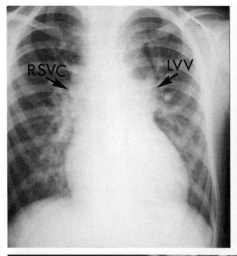

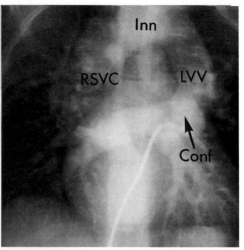

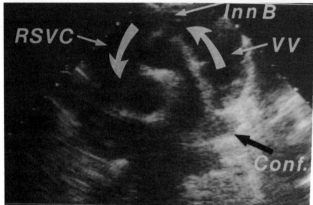

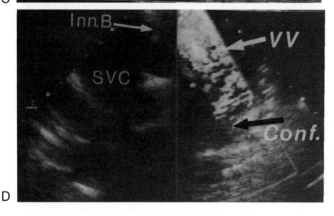

Figure 15–82

A, X-ray from a 6-year-old mildly cyanotic boy with total anomalous pulmonary venous connection. Pulmonary arterial vascularity is markedly increased. The cardiac silhouette has the distinctive *figure of eight* or *snowman* appearance. *B,* Levophase after injection of contrast material into the pulmonary trunk. Blood from the confluence of pulmonary veins (Conf) flows sequentially through a dilated left vertical vein (LVV), an innominate bridge (Inn), and a dilated right superior vena cava (RSVC), establishing the upper portion of the figure of eight. The lower portion of the figure of eight consists of the dilated right atrium and the dilated right ventricle. *C,* Echocardiogram from a 12-year-old girl with total anomalous pulmonary venous connection. The four pulmonary veins form a confluence (Conf) from which a dilated left vertical vein arises (VV, *upward curved arrow*) and continues as an innominate bridge (InnB) that joins a dilated right superior vena cava (RSVC, *downward curved arrow*). *D,* Black-and-white print of a color flow image showing unobstructed flow from the confluence into the vertical vein (VV).

the figure of eight is formed by the left vertical vein and the right superior vena cava. The lower portion is formed by the dilated right atrium and right ventricle. The snowman appearance does not reveal itself in the first few months of life because time must elapse before the distinctive venous channels develop sufficient size and radiodensity to be visible in the x-ray.[135,180,184]

Rarely, the communicating venous channel is formed within the substance of the lung rather than in the mediastinum where it bears a superficial resemblance to the *scimitar sign* of partial anomalous pulmonary venous connection (see earlier). However, agenesis of the right lung is rare with total anomalous pulmonary venous connection but is common in the scimitar syndrome.[178]

Total anomalous pulmonary venous connection with obstruction results in a very different radiologic picture (Fig. 15–71).[180,183,208,267,275,394] Pulmonary edema is striking with distention of the pulmonary veins and lymphatics and a reticular nodular ground glass appearance (Fig. 15–71).[180,183,355] The abnormal lung fields stand out in contrast to the comparatively unimpressive cardiac silhouette (Fig. 15–71B).[180,184,208]

THE ECHOCARDIOGRAM

Echocardiography with color flow imaging and Doppler interrogation locates the four pulmonary veins and their drainage sites, identifies the venous confluence and its connection(s), determines whether obstruction is present in the pulmonary venous pathways, identifies the location and the size of the interatrial communication and establishes the physiologic consequences (Figs. 15–82C, D and 15–83).[401] Color flow imaging establishes the direction and mean velocity of blood flow within the venous channels and permits assessment of the connections of individual pulmonary veins and of the venous confluence (Fig. 15–82D).[401] Doppler interrogation with color flow imaging identifies increased turbulence and velocity at sites of obstruction. When the venous connection is to the coronary sinus, all four pulmonary veins enter a confluence behind the left atrium (Figs. 15–64 and 15–83).

Color flow imaging identifies a confluence that joins a left vertical vein and an innominate bridge (Figs. 15–82C, D) or a confluence that joins a right vertical vein and right superior vena cava.[401] A restrictive interatrial communication causes obstruction to pulmonary venous flow when all four pulmonary veins connect to the right atrium directly.[401] With infradiaphragmatic connections, color flow imaging and Doppler interrogation identify the inferior vena cava and the anomalous venous channel adjacent to the aorta, and determine whether a localized site of obstruction is present in the anomalous channel as it descends below the diaphragm (Fig. 15–84).[401] Flow is pulsatile in the aorta but continuous in the anomalous venous channel.

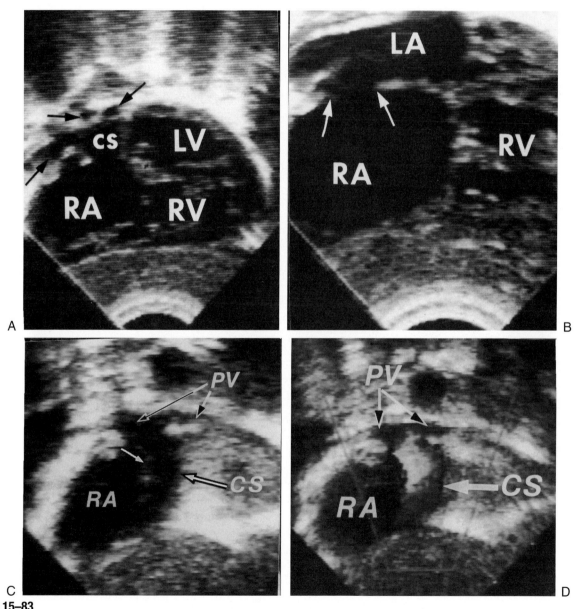

Figure 15–83

Echocardiograms (subcostal) from a 5-month-old girl with total anomalous pulmonary venous connection to the coronary sinus. *A*, Posterior angulation of the transducer visualized four pulmonary veins (*arrows*), the enlarged coronary sinus (cs), and its right atrial ostium (RA). LV, left ventricle; RV, right ventricle. *B*, A change in transducer angulation visualized a large ostium secundum atrial septal defect (*paired arrows*) and a dilated right atrium. LA, left atrium. *C, D*, Echocardiograms (subcostal) from a 3-week-old boy with total anomalous pulmonary venous connection to the coronary sinus. *C*, The pulmonary veins (PV) connect to a dilated coronary sinus (CS) that joins the right atrium (RA). *D*, Black and white print of a color flow image showing flow from pulmonary veins (PV) into the dilated coronary sinus (CS) and then into the right atrium (RA).

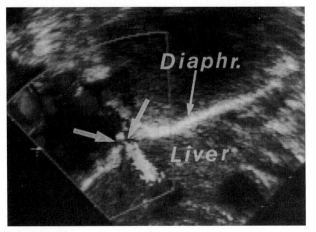

Figure 15–84
Black-and-white print of a color flow image from a 1-day-old girl with infra-diaphragmatic total anomalous pulmonary venous connection and obstruction at the diaphragmatic hiatus (*paired arrows*, Diaphr).

SUMMARY

A large left-to-right shunt is established shortly after birth when total anomalous pulmonary venous connection is accompanied by a nonrestrictive atrial septal defect, low pulmonary vascular resistance, and no obstruction. Dyspnea, cardiac failure, and physical underdevelopment begin shortly thereafter, and the majority of infants do not reach their first birthday. The clinical picture subsequently resembles a nonrestrictive ostium secundum atrial septal defect with the notable exception of mild-to-moderate cyanosis. Sex distribution is approximately equal in contrast to female preponderance in ostium secundum atrial septal defect. The right ventricular impulse is hyperdynamic. There is a prominent pulmonary midsystolic murmur, fixed splitting of the second heart sound, a prominent pulmonary component, and a tricuspid diastolic flow murmur. A soft humlike continuous murmur is occasionally heard along the upper left sternal border when a mildly compressed left vertical vein connects the venous confluence to the left innominate vein. The electrocardiogram shows right atrial P waves with right ventricular hypertrophy or may resemble an ostium secundum atrial septal defect. The distinctive x-ray features are the shadows caused by anomalous venous connections that emerge after the first few months of life. A prominent shadow at the right base represents the confluence of veins that joins the right superior vena cava via an anomalous right venous channel or via an azygos vein. The figure of eight or snowman appearance is caused by dilatation of the left vertical vein and right superior vena cava above and by dilatation of the right atrium and right ventricle below.

Total anomalous pulmonary venous connection with obstruction predominates in males especially when an infradiaphragmatic connection joins the portal vein. Lifespan is short and the clinical course is stormy with symptoms beginning at or shortly after birth. Death from pulmonary edema, congestive heart failure and hypoxia follows within weeks. Dyspnea and cyanosis are aggravated by crying, feeding or straining because the anomalous venous channel is further compressed at the esophageal hiatus. Cyanosis is conspicuous, the right ventricular impulse is relatively quiet, the pulmonary midsystolic murmur is attenuated or absent, and the second heart sound is closely split with a loud pulmonary component. The electrocardiogram shows right atrial P waves and right ventricular hypertrophy. The x-ray exhibits dramatic pulmonary venous congestion with a reticulated ground glass appearance in contrast to the unimpressive size of the cardiac silhouette.

Echocardiography with color flow imaging and Doppler interrogation locates the four pulmonary veins, identifies the venous confluence and its connection(s), determines whether there is obstruction in the pulmonary venous pathway, determines the location and size of the interatrial communication, and establishes the physiologic consequences of supradiaphragmatic or infradiaphragmatic total anomalous pulmonary venous connection.

Atrioventricular Septal Defects

The *atrioventricular septum* in the normal heart is a partition that separates the left ventricular outflow tract from the facing right atrium. The malformations discussed here are characterized by complete absence of the atrioventricular septum, and accordingly are called *atrioventricular septal defects*.[12,198,303,340,341,399,436] Additional features include a common atrioventricular ring, a five-leaflet valve that guards the common atrioventricular orifice, an unwedged left ventricular outflow tract, an aortic valve that is anterosuperior to the common atrioventricular junction, and disproportion of the left ventricular mass characterized by a longer distance from apex to aortic valve than from apex to the left atrioventricular valve.[12]

The different types of atrioventricular septal defects result from morphologic variations in the five-leaflet valve that guards the common atrioventricular orifice and from the relationship of the bridging leaflets to contiguous septal structures (Figs. 15–85 and 15–86).[12,436] In the normal heart, the two atrioventricular valves have *two separate* fibrous rings (annuli) that lie at *different levels* in the ventricular mass. In atrioventricular septal defects, a five-leaflet atrioventricular valve has a *single fibrous ring* (annulus) that lies at the *same horizontal level* in the ventricular mass (see Fig. 15–105).[12,303,340,350,436] The five-leaflet valve guards either a common atrioventricular orifice or separate right and left atrioventricular orifices (Fig. 15–86).[12] A left lateral leaflet is housed exclusively in the left ventricle, and a right inferior leaflet and a right anterosuperior leaflet are housed exclusively in the right ventricle (see Fig. 15–86). The other two leaflets are designated anterior and posterior bridging leaflets and have no counterparts in the normal heart.

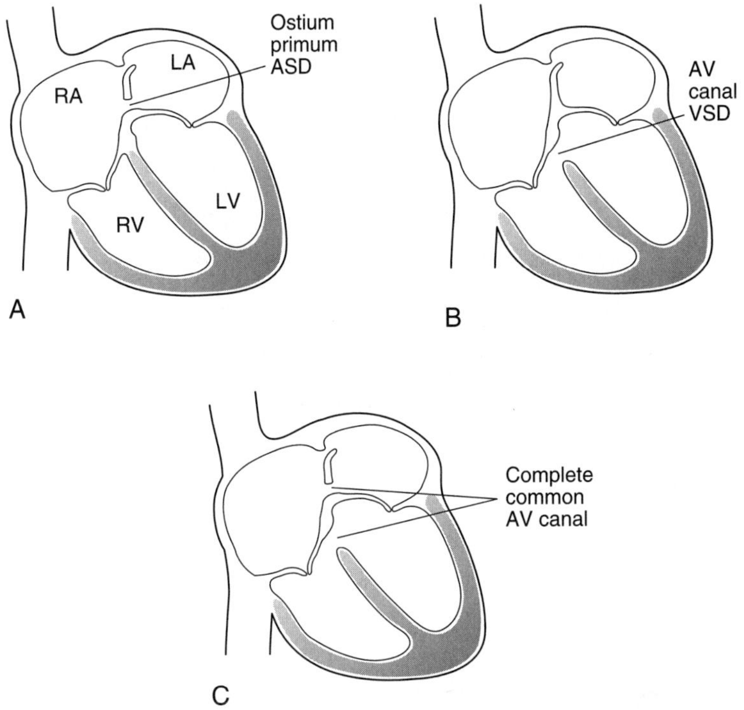

Figure 15–85

Schematic illustrations of the shunt levels in atrioventricular septal defects: *A*, an interatrial communication between the inferior atrial septum and the bridging leaflets, *B*, an interventricular communication between the bridging leaflets and crest of the ventricular septum, and *C*, interatrial *and* interventricular communications above and below a free-floating atrioventricular valve (complete common AV canal). RA, right atrium; LA, left atrium; RV, right ventricle; LV, left ventricle. (Modified from Anderson RH, Becker AE, Lucchese FE, et al: Morphology of Congenital Heart Disease. Baltimore, University Park Press, 1983.)

A common atrioventricular *orifice* lies within a common atrioventricular *annulus* when the anterior and posterior bridging leaflets are not divided by connecting leaflet tissue that runs in the ventricular septum (Fig. 15–86B). When the anterior and posterior bridging leaflets are divided by connecting leaflet tissue in the ventricular septum, separate left and right atrioventricular *orifices* lie within a common atrioventricular *annulus* (Fig. 15–86A). What has been called a *cleft* in the anterior *mitral* leaflet (Fig. 15–87) is a commissure between the left anterior and left posterior bridging leaflets (Fig. 15–86A). The margins of the left anterior and posterior bridging leaflets are supported by chordae tendineae that attach to the ventricular septum, an arrangement that is not represented in normal hearts.[139] The relationships of bridging leaflets to the adjacent ventricular septum and to the atrial septum determine the level of shunting through the atrioventricular septal defect (Fig. 15–85). When the bridging leaflets adhere to the crest of the ventricular septum, the shunt is at atrial level (Fig. 15–85A). The term *ostium primum* atrial septal defect does not properly characterize this interatrial communication which is not a defect in the atrial septum but instead represents absence of the atrioventricular septum.[198] When the bridging leaflets are attached to the distal end of the atrial septum, the shunt is ventricular level (Fig. 15–85B). When the bridging leaflets are free floating and unattached to either atrial or ventricular septum, shunts occur at both atrial and ventricular levels, an arrangement called *complete common atrioventricular canal* (Fig. 15–85C).

The unwedged position of the elongated left ventricular outflow tract together with the anterosuperior position of the aortic valve and the apical position of the deficient inlet septum results in a *gooseneck deformity* (Fig. 15–88). The left ventricular outflow tract is an elongated anteriorly displaced fibromuscular channel that lends itself to subaortic obstruction caused by an immobile ridge at the crest of the ventricular septum, by accessory chordal tissue arising from the left anterior atrioventricular valve leaflet which is fixed to the ventricular septum, by accessory papillary muscle tissue, by abnormally high insertion of the anterolateral papillary muscle, or by thickened tissue along the outflow septum and anterior left atrioventricular leaflet.[175,213,215] The papillary muscles are in an abnormal fore-aft arrangement that may result in a parachute valve or a double-orifice valve that reinforces left-to-right interatrial shunts.[93,130,213] Obstruction to left ventricular outflow augments the left-to-right shunts and augments regurgitation across the left atrioventricular valve.[162,175]

A common atrioventricular annulus is usually shared equally by the right and left ventricles, but the right-sided or the left-sided component of the annulus may be reduced in size. When the *right-sided* component is small, the right ventricle is hypoplastic, the tricuspid orifice overrides a malaligned inlet ventricular septum, and the right atrioventricular valve has attachments that straddle the ventricular septal defect.[218] When the *left-sided* component is small, the morphologic left ventricle is hypoplastic, but straddling does not occur despite atrioventricular malalignment because straddling is reserved for conoventricular malalignment.[212]

The *physiologic consequences* of an ostium primum atrial septal defect depend on its size and on the functional state of the left atrioventricular valve.[59,281] When the defect is nonrestrictive, the left atrium decompresses as it receives regurgitant flow from the left ventricle

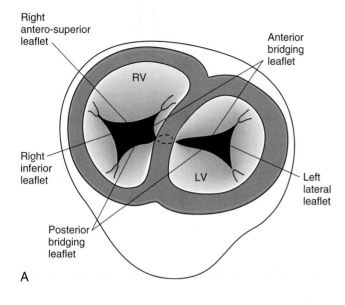

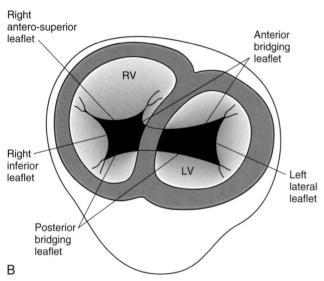

Figure 15–86

A, Illustration of the leaflet patterns in an atrioventricular septal defect with separate right and left atrioventricular orifices. Anterior and posterior bridging leaflets-now called by Anderson, et al, "superior" and "inferior" bridging leaflets-are connected by leaflet tissue that runs in the ventricular septum, an arrangement that results in a *cleft anterior mitral leaflet.* The cleft is more accurately characterized as the functional commissure between the anterior (superior) and posterior (inferior) bridging leaflets. *B*, Illustration of the leaflet patterns of a complete atrioventricular septal defect (complete common atrioventricular canal). The common valve consists of anterior (superior) and posterior (inferior) bridging leaflets that cross the septum, a small left lateral mural leaflet that is housed exclusively in the left ventricle, and small right inferior mural and anterosuperior leaflets that are housed exclusively in the right ventricle. (Modified from Anderson RH, Becker AE, Lucchese FE, et al: Morphology of Congenital Heart Disease. Baltimore, University Park Press, 1983.)

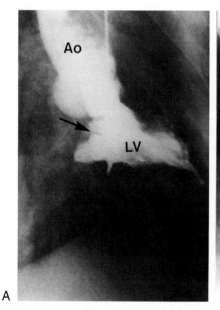

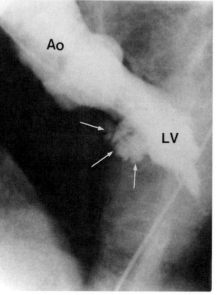

Figure 15–87

Left ventriculograms from a 71-year-old woman with a large left-to-right shunt through an ostium primum atrial septal defect. *A*, The left ventriculogram (LV) identifies a *cleft in the anterior mitral leaflet* (*unmarked arrow*) that represents the functional commissure between the anterior and posterior bridging leaflets. Ao, aorta. *B*, Long-axial view showing saccular herniation of atrioventricular valve tissue into the right ventricular inflow tract (*arrows*) effectively closing the inlet ventricular septal defect.

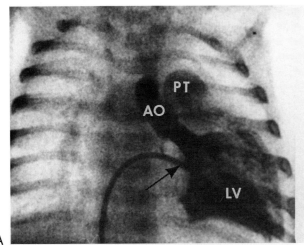

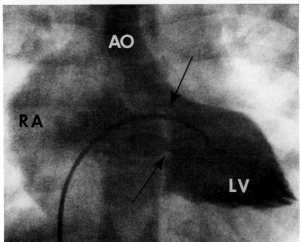

Figure 15–88

A, Left ventriculogram (LV) from an 8-week-old girl with a complete atrioventricular septal defect and a virtually competent common atrioventricular valve. *Arrow* points to the gooseneck deformity of the left ventricular outflow tract. A dilated pulmonary trunk (PT) visualized via the ventricular septal defect. *B,* Left ventriculogram from a 3-year-old female with a nonrestrictive ostium primum atrial septal defect and left atrioventricular valve regurgitation. A narrow jet (*lower arrow*) is received by a large right atrium (RA). The gooseneck deformity shown here (*upper arrow*) was better delineated during diastole. AO, aorta.

(Fig. 15–88*B*). When the atrial septal defect is restrictive, the clinical picture resembles isolated mitral regurgitation.[281,337] A nonrestrictive ventricular septal defect sets the stage for pulmonary vascular disease (see Chapter 17).[383] The physiologic consequences of complete atrioventricular septal defect are the sum of the nonrestrictive interatrial and interventricular communications and the degree of incompetence of the left and right components of the common atrioventricular valve (Figs. 15–88*A* and 15–89).

Down syndrome (see Physical Appearance) is an important independent variable in the proclivity for pulmonary vascular disease.[86,89,258,365,385] The proclivity does not depend on the size of the ventricular septal defect or even on the presence of congenital heart disease, but is coupled with Down syndrome per se.[86,258,365,400] Hypoventilation induced by upper airway abnormalities in Down patients causes pulmonary vascular disease.[89] The mid-facial region is small with short nasal passages, small oropharynx, small oral cavity, large tonsils and adenoids, and mandibular and maxillary hypoplasia. Another cause of pulmonary vascular disease is sleep apnea that results from retrodisplacement of an enlarged tongue (Fig. 15–90*A*) and from inspiratory collapse of the hypopharynx because of tracheomalacia.[9,89,365,400] More important causes of the proclivity for pulmonary vascular disease in Down syndrome are derived from morphometric studies of the lungs that disclose a reduction in the number of alveoli to approximately 35% of predicted and that disclose a reduction in the radial alveolar count which is an index of alveolar complexity.[9,201] These lung abnormalities are acquired postnatally because of faulty development.[220] The reduced internal surface area of the lungs implies a comparable reduction in cross-sectional area of the pulmonary vascular bed because the capillary surface area and the alveolar surface area are closely coupled.

Figure 15–89

A, X-ray of a 3-month-old boy with a complete atrioventricular septal defect. Pulmonary vascularity is increased. The dramatic increase in heart size reflects enlargement of the right atrium (RA) and right ventricle (RV). *B,* Left ventriculogram (LV) visualized the gooseneck deformity (*paired arrows*) of the outflow tract. Ao, aorta.

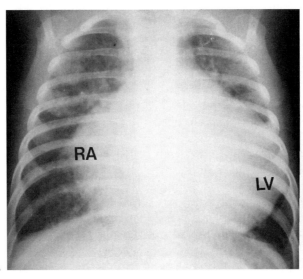

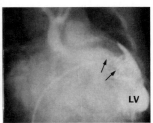

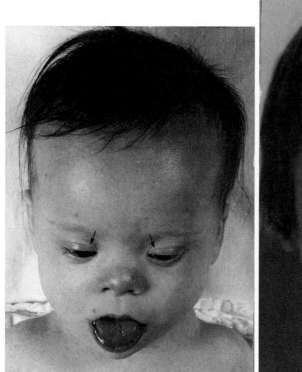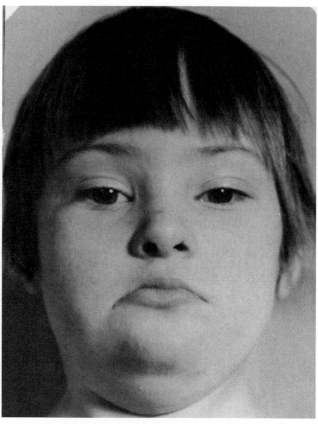

Figure 15–90

A, Facial appearance of a 6-month-old girl with Down syndrome, complete atrioventricular septal defect and a bidirectional shunt. The short flat nose is cyanotic, and the nasal bridge is depressed. The tongue is large and protuberant. *Two small arrows* point to oblique palpebral fissures. *B*, Nine year old female with Down syndrome. The corners of the mouth turn downward creating an expression of sadness. The nose is short and flat with a depressed nasal bridge. The inner epicanthic fold is subtle.

THE HISTORY

The male/female ratio in atrioventricular septal defects is approximately equal. An increased prevalence of trisomy 21 has been reported in the offspring of older gravida,[385] but the father rather than the mother has been incriminated as the source of extra chromosome 21.[223] The incidence of congenital heart disease in the offspring of females with atrioventricular septal defects has been estimated at 9.6% to 14.3%.[148] Families may have several affected members.[189,200]

The chief determinant of symptoms in a nonrestrictive ostium primum atrial septal defect is coexisting left AV valve regurgitation.[398] Severe regurgitation results in early congestive heart failure and a mortality of 33% in the first year.[398] Neonatal congestive heart failure is intractable when the left ventricle is hypoplastic.[162] Infants with complete atrioventricular septal defects develop congestive heart failure in the first six months of life (Fig. 15–89), and fetal hydrops has been reported.[217] Prolonged survival is exceptional, although one such patient lived to age 46 years[416] and another to age 73 years.[443] When a nonrestrictive ostium primum atrial septal defect exists with a functionally adequate left atrioventricular valve, adult survival is expected. Twelve percent of these patients reached or exceeded 60 years of age, but those beyond age 45 years

were symptomatic. The oldest reported patient was 79 years of age,[416] and the patient referred to in Figure 15–87 underwent cardiac surgery at age 71 years. Symptomatic deterioration is accelerated by atrial fibrillation or atrial flutter.[398] When a ventricular septal defect is the only component of an atrioventricular septal defect, the history resembles other forms of isolated ventricular septal defect of equivalent size (see Chapter 17).

Isolated left atrioventricular valve regurgitation generates a murmur that is mistaken for acquired mitral regurgitation, but detection at an early age should prevent this error. The risk of infective endocarditis coincides with regurgitation, not with abnormal structure of a functionally competent valve. Infective endocarditis is rare with complete atrioventricular septal defects.

Paradoxical emboli are rare with ostium primum atrial septal defects in contrast to ostium secundum defects because emboli that originate in the lower extremities are carried by inferior vena caval blood toward the *mid portion* of the atrial septum. *Superior* vena caval streaming targets the lower atrial septum, but emboli rarely originate in the upper extremities.

Spontaneous closure of the ventricular component of an atrioventricular septal defect is uncommon[234,327] and has been attributed to occlusion by tricuspid leaflet tissue derived from the bridging leaflets.[234] This mechanism is believed to have been operative in the 71 year old woman whose left ventriculogram is shown in Figure 15–87B.

Life expectancy for Down syndrome *without* congenital heart disease is significantly shorter than for comparable mentally retarded patients, suggesting an adverse effect on life expectancy that is unrelated either to congenital heart disease or to mental retardation.[25,73,89,287] Morbidity and mortality are adversely affected by respiratory tract infections, congenital anomalies of the gastrointestinal tract, increased risk of hepatitis B virus, hematologic, endocrinologic and immunologic disorders, and premature Alzheimer disease.[9] Hematologic disorders are unique, such as transient myelodysplasia in infancy, red cell macrocytosis, and increased susceptibility to acute megakaryocytic leukemia.[220] The gene for amyloid protein in Alzheimer disease has been cloned and localized to chromosome 21 proximal to the locus that delineates Down syndrome.[9,255,344,428] Virtually all Down patients over age 35 years have the characteristic central nervous system neuropathology and neurochemistry of Alzheimer syndrome.[115,255,304,344,428] Brain weights are lower in Down syndrome than in patients with senile Alzheimer disease, with differences most striking in the anterior frontal and anterior temporal regions.[115] Families with autosomal dominant Alzheimer disease produce a significantly higher than expected number of Down syndrome offspring.[115] Clinical dementia is uncommon, however, and must be distinguished from symptomatic hypothyroidism, which is common.[9] An association between autoimmune thyroid dysfunction and Down syndrome is widely recognized.[163]

PHYSICAL APPEARANCE

Down syndrome phenotype is the most distinctive physical appearance associated with an atrioventricular septal defect.[73,258,400,414] In 1866 Down wrote, "The face is flat and broad and destitute of prominence. The cheeks are round and extended laterally. The eyes are obliquely placed, and the internal canthi more than normally distant from one another. The palpebral fissure is very narrow. The lips are large and thick with transverse fissures. The tongue is long, thick, and is much roughened. The nose is small."[228] The incidence of trisomy 21 in the general population is approximately 1:800 live births, although the frequency is twice as great if based on *all* conceptuses because more than half of trisomy 21 fetuses are spontaneously aborted.[400] The association of congenital heart disease with Down syndrome was recognized in 1894 by Garrod[179] and in 1924 by Maude Abbott.[1] The incidence is about 50% compared with an incidence of 0.4% for infants with normal chromosomes. Complete atrioventricular septal defect accounts for two thirds of the congenital heart disease in Down syndrome.[73,400]

The phenotypic features of Down syndrome are numerous. The anteroposterior diameter of the skull is shortened. The inner epicanthic skin fold that inserts onto the lower lid may be prominent at birth (Fig. 15–91A). In Asian children with trisomy 21, the typical Down inner canthal fold is readily identified together with the normal Asian horizontal epicanthic fold above the outer canthus (Fig. 15–91B).[146] Brushfield spots (speckled iris) are distinctive ocular features that were described by Down[228] as

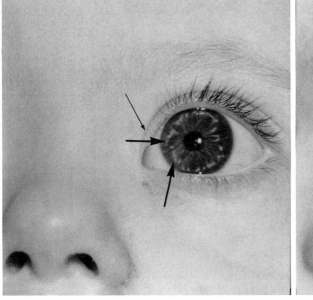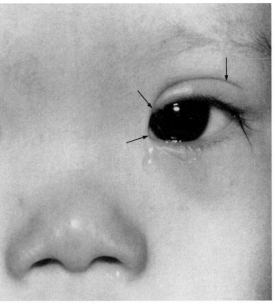

Figure 15–91

A, Brushfield spots (speckled iris, *large paired arrows*) readily seen in a blue-eyed female with Down syndrome. The typical inner epicanthic fold (*small upper left arrow*) inserts onto the lower lid. *B,* A 17-month-old Asian girl with Down syndrome. *Two arrows* on the left identify the typical inner epicanthic fold of Down syndrome. The *single vertical arrow* on the right identifies the normal horizontal Asian epicanthic fold above the outer canthus. Brushfield spots are not visible because the irises were dark brown.

fine white spots at the periphery of the iris readily seen in patients with blue-gray iris (Fig. 15–91A) but not in patients with dark brown iris.[146] The nose is small, the nasal bridge is depressed, and the nares are anteverted and narrow. The ears are low-set with overlapping or folding of the helix. The lips are prominent, thickened, and fissured, and the tongue is large and protuberant (Fig. 15–90A). The corners of the mouth turn down as a child's drawing of a sad face (Fig. 15–90B). The skin in infants is soft and velvety but in childhood the skin is dry, pale, and lax. Neonates have abundant skin and subcutaneous tissue in the posterior neck and exhibit absence of the Moro reflex. The hips can spontaneously dislocate between ages 2 and 10 years (Fig. 15–92B). The thoracic configuration reflects hyperinflation, and the abdomen tends to be protuberant because of reduced muscle tone and diastases recti. The hands are broad and stubby with a short curved fourth finger, a single transverse palmar crease (Fig. 15–92A) and a distal axial triradius. Short stubby feet are as common as short stubby hands.

THE ARTERIAL PULSE AND THE JUGULAR VENOUS PULSE

A small water-hammer pulse is due to rapid ejection of the large left ventricular stroke volume of severe left atrioventricular valve regurgitation. The arterial pulse is small in infants with an atrioventricular septal defect and congestive heart failure.

The V wave is dominant in the jugular venous pulse (Fig. 15–93) because the right atrium receives left ventricular systolic flow across an incompetent left AV valve *directly* through the atrioventricular septal defect or *indirectly* through an ostium primum atrial septal defect (Fig. 15–88B).[59] Congestive heart failure elevates the mean jugular venous pressure and elevates the A and V waves.

PRECORDIAL MOVEMENT AND PALPATION

An isolated nonrestrictive ostium primum atrial septal defect is associated with precordial movements analogous to an equivalent ostium secundum atrial septal defect. Coexisting left AV valve regurgitation is responsible for a left ventricular impulse and an apical systolic thrill that radiates toward the left sternal border because the right atrium receives the regurgitant flow (Fig. 15–88B). When regurgitation is severe and the interatrial communication is restrictive, systolic expansion of a large left atrium must be distinguished from an intrinsic right ventricular impulse of volume overload.

The right ventricular impulse is tumultuous with complete atrioventricular septal defect because of both volume and pressure overload. A dilated right ventricular outflow

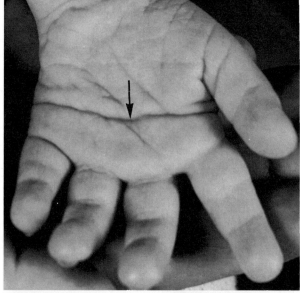

A

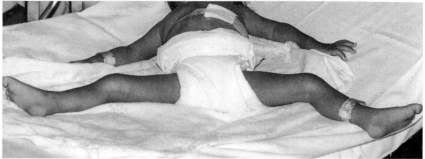

B

Figure 15–92

A, Transverse palmar crease in a 6-month-old infant with Down syndrome. *B*, Ninety degree external rotation of the hips in a 16-month-old child with Down syndrome. At age 3 years, the hips spontaneously dislocated.

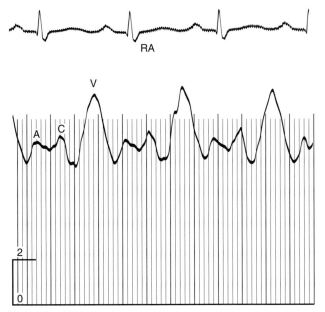

Figure 15–93

Right atrial pressure pulse (RA) from a 12-year-old girl with an ostium primum atrial septal defect and moderate left atrioventricular valve regurgitation. The V wave is prominent in the right atrium despite a competent right atrioventricular valve because left ventricular blood was ejected into the right atrium via the atrioventricular septal defect.

tract generates an impulse in the third left intercostal space, an enlarged pulmonary trunk generates an impulse in the second left intercostal space, and a volume overloaded left ventricle occupies the apex (Fig. 15–89B). The thrill of left AV valve regurgitation radiates toward the sternum where it is indistinguishable from thrills of ventricular septal defect and tricuspid regurgitation.

AUSCULTATION

An isolated nonrestrictive ostium primum atrial septal defect is accompanied by auscultatory signs analogous to a nonrestrictive ostium secundum atrial septal defect. Left atrioventricular valve regurgitation adds an apical holosystolic murmur that radiates toward the sternum (Figs. 15–94 and 15–95), sometimes as far as the right sternal edge because the right atrium receives regurgitant flow from the left ventricle (Fig. 15–88B). A systolic thrill has been identified over the right atrium at surgery. A pulmonary midsystolic flow murmur in the second left intercostal space is followed by wide fixed splitting of the second heart sound (Fig. 15–95). The delayed pulmonary component heard at the apex (Fig. 15–94B) can be mistaken for an opening snap which occasionally originates in the incompetent left AV valve. Mid-diastolic murmurs at the lower left sternal border are caused by augmented flow across the right atrioventricular valve (Figs. 15–94 through 15–96), and mid-diastolic murmurs at the apex are caused by augmented flow across the left atrioventricular valve.[337] An early to mid-diastolic murmur recorded within the right atrium has been ascribed to a tall left atrial V wave that generates a diastolic pressure gradient across a restrictive atrial septal defect.[399] When left

AV valve regurgitation is severe and the interatrial communication is restrictive or absent, auscultatory signs are analogous to isolated mitral regurgitation.[281,337] Wide persistent splitting of the second heart sound then reflects early closure of the aortic valve.[337]

The first heart sound is single and impure when a common atrioventricular orifice is equipped with a common atrioventricular valve. Early vibrations of a holosystolic murmur obscure the first heart sound that is soft because of prolongation of the PR interval. Wide fixed splitting of the second heart sound is difficult to identify because the aortic component is obscured by a holosystolic murmur, leaving an isolated loud pulmonary component. The high frequency murmur of left AV valve regurgitation preferentially radiates toward the sternum because the right atrium receives systolic flow from the left ventricle through the common atrioventricular canal. The regurgitant murmur radiates to the right of the sternum when the jet reaches the lateral wall of an enlarged right atrium. The ventricular septal defect murmur recorded with an intracardiac phonocardiogram coincides with the mid to lower left sternal border thoracic wall murmurs of left and right AV valve regurgitation.[156] Intracardiac phonocardiograms from within the right atrium cannot distinguish the murmurs of left and right AV valve regurgitation because the regurgitant stream from the left ventricle is directed into the right atrium. An increase in pulmonary vascular resistance diminishes the murmur of ventricular septal defect, reinforces the murmur across the right AV valve, and leaves the murmur across the

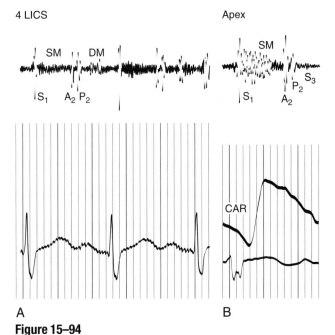

Figure 15–94

A, Phonocardiogram (4 LICS, fourth left intercostal space) of a 2-year-old boy with a nonrestrictive ostium primum atrial septal defect and severe left atrioventricular valve regurgitation. A holosystolic murmur (SM) radiates from the apex to the left sternal edge and is followed by fixed splitting of the second heart sound (A2/P2) and a tricuspid mid-diastolic flow murmur (DM). B, A prominent apical holosystolic decrescendo murmur ends at the split second heart sound which is followed by a left ventricular third heart sound (S₃).

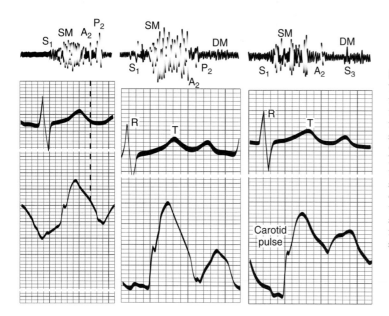

Figure 15–95

Tracings from a 13-year-old boy with a nonrestrictive ostium primum atrial septal defect and severe left atrioventricular valve regurgitation. In first panel (second left intercostal space), a prominent pulmonary midsystolic murmur (SM) ends before a second sound that is widely split with a prominent pulmonary component (P_2). The middle panel (lower left sternal border) shows the holosystolic murmur of left atrioventricular regurgitation that radiated from the apex and enveloped the aortic component of the second heart sound (A_2). P_2, pulmonary component, DM, mid-diastolic flow murmur across the right atrioventricular valve. In the third panel (apex), the systolic regurgitant murmur is softer, and a third heart sound (S_3) introduces a short mid-diastolic flow murmur (DM) across the left atrioventricular valve. S_1, first heart sound.

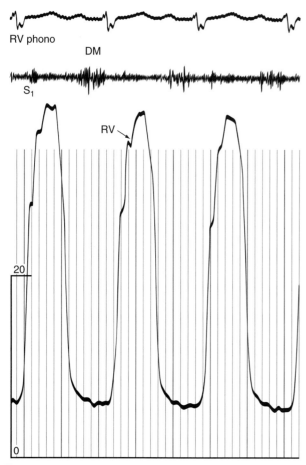

Figure 15–96

Recordings from a 5-year-old boy with a nonrestrictive ostium primum atrial septal defect and left atrioventricular valve regurgitation. The right ventricular intracardiac phonocardiogram (RV phono) recorded a mid-diastolic flow murmur (DM) across the right atrioventricular valve. The right ventricular pressure (RV) is slightly elevated.

left AV valve unchanged. A midsystolic murmur across the left ventricular outflow gooseneck (Fig. 15–88) is seldom recognized.

THE ELECTROCARDIOGRAM

In 1956, Toscano-Barbosa called attention to three electrocardiographic features of what came to be known as atrioventricular septal defects: the PR interval, the QRS axis, and the sequence of ventricular activation.[425] PR interval prolongation occurs in approximately 50% of cases because of delayed intraatrial and atrioventricular nodal conduction (see Fig. 15–99),[191,238,251,398,433] and complete atrioventricular block occasionally develops.[398] The incidence of atrial fibrillation and atrial flutter increases with age.

Toscano-Barbosa recognized that certain features of the QRS complex were distinct, stating that, "the similarity that may exist in the precordial leads may lead one astray from the differences that almost universally exist in the extremity leads which are of real discriminatory value."[425] These features are more clearly illustrated by vectorial analysis (Fig. 15–97).[425] Left axis deviation varies from moderate to extreme, and the QRS axis is either superior to the *left* or superior to the *right* with a mean that may reach minus 180 degrees.[48,134,154,271] Extreme left axis deviation is a feature of Down syndrome (Fig. 15–98). Counterclockwise depolarization results in Q waves in leads 1 and aVL (Fig. 15–99). The S waves in leads 2, 3 and aVF are characteristically notched on their upstrokes (Figs. 15–99 and 15–100) because of a change in direction of the terminal force of the QRS illustrated in the vector loop (Fig. 15–97). Occasional examples of *ostium secundum* atrial septal defects with left axis deviation represent acquired left anterior fascicular block (see Fig. 15–32).[209]

The mechanisms responsible for the characteristic QRS patterns in atrioventricular septal defects stem from congenital alterations of the excitation pathways into the ventri-

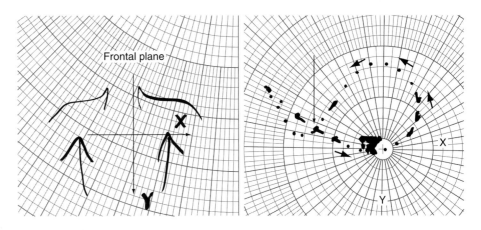

Figure 15–97

Vectorcardiogram from a 4-year-old girl with a complete atrioventricular septal defect. Depolarization is counterclockwise (*arrowheads*). The initial portion of QRS loop is superior and minus 90 degrees. The terminal portion of the loop abruptly changes direction (*long arrow*) and turns on itself.

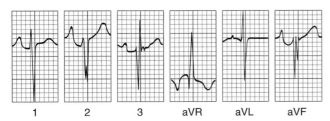

Figure 15–98

Limb leads from a symptomatic neonate with Down syndrome and a complete atrioventricular septal defect. Left axis deviation is extreme. Depolarization is counterclockwise with initial r waves in leads 2, 3, and aVF. The S waves in leads 2 and aVF are splintered.

cles[48,53,134,154,191,247,251,339] as Toscano-Barbosa originally proposed.[425] Anatomic studies of the atrioventricular conduction system in human and canine hearts have shed light on these distinctive QRS patterns.[48,53,154,263] Specialized conduction tissues in all types of atrioventricular septal defects have the same distribution. The AV node is positioned inferior and posterior to the coronary sinus. The atrioventricular conduction axis penetrates only at the crux, and the penetrating bundle is displaced posteriorly, lying on the posteroinferior rim of the ventricular component of the defect. The His bundle is shorter than normal and is posteriorly positioned. The left bundle branch is displaced posteriorly, and arises from the common bundle immediately after it enters the ventricular septum. The left anterior division of the left bundle branch has fewer fibers than normal and is increased in length. The left posterior division is shorter than normal and provides small branches to the posterobasal wall of the left ventricle. The right bundle branch is abnormally long.

These anatomic patterns correlate with electrophysiologic observations.[48,53,134,154,191,247] Short HV intervals are in accord with elaborate studies showing early activation of

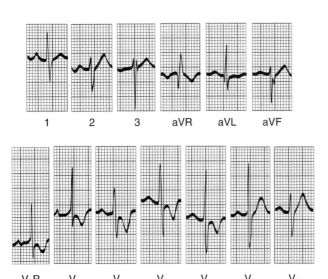

Figure 15–99

Electrocardiogram from a 5-year-old boy with a nonrestrictive ostium primum atrial septal defect and severe left atrioventricular valve regurgitation (see Fig. 15–96). The PR interval is prolonged. There is left axis deviation with counterclockwise depolarization and notching of the upstrokes of the S waves in leads 2, 3, and aVF. Right ventricular hypertrophy is indicated by the tall R waves in leads V_3R and V_1 and in the deep S waves in left precordial leads. The terminal tall R wave in lead aVR is slightly prolonged.

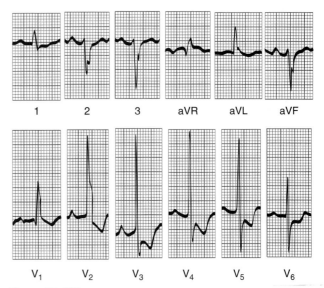

Figure 15–100

Electrocardiogram from a pulmonary hypertensive cyanotic 27-year-old man with a complete atrioventricular septal defect and a competent common atrioventricular valve. The PR interval is 200 msec. Peaked right atrial P waves appear in leads V_{2-3} and right atrial enlargement is indicated by the Q wave in lead V_1. There is left axis deviation with counterclockwise depolarization and notching of the upstrokes of the S waves in leads 2, 3, and aVF. The terminal r wave in lead aVR is prolonged. Right ventricular hypertrophy is indicated by tall monophasic R waves and ST-T wave changes in right precordial leads and by prominent S waves in left precordial leads.

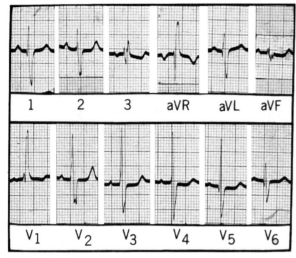

Figure 15–101

Electrocardiogram from a 12-year-old boy with a nonrestrictive ostium primum atrial septal defect, severe left atrioventricular valve regurgitation and pulmonary arterial systolic pressure of 45 mm Hg. P waves in leads 1 and 2 are peaked but not tall. Depolarization is counterclockwise with Q waves in leads 1 and aVL and a mean electrical axis of minus 90 degrees. The R wave in lead aVR is tall and slightly prolonged. Right ventricular hypertrophy is indicated by the tall R prime in lead V_1 and the deep prolonged S waves in leads V_{5-6}. Volume overload of the left ventricle is reflected in the lead V_5 Q wave and well-developed R wave.

the posterobasal left ventricular wall in human and canine atrioventricular septal defects.[48,53,134,154,247] Early posterobasal activation is consistent with posterior displacement of the left bundle branch and with a short posterior division that sends small branches to the posterobasal wall. Delayed activation of the anterior superior wall is appropriate for hypoplasia and increased length of the left anterior division of the left bundle branch.[48,53,154]

These anatomic and electrophysiologic observations provide acceptable explanations for the left axis deviation and for the depolarization pattern (Fig. 15–97). The delay in right ventricular activation results from increased length of the right bundle branch, not from slowed Purkinje conduction that is incorrectly implied by the terms *partial or complete right bundle branch block.*[48]

Right ventricular hypertrophy with an ostium primum atrial septal defect indicates pulmonary hypertension induced by left atrioventricular valve regurgitation (Figs. 15–99 and 15–101) or the pulmonary vascular disease of Down syndrome. Right ventricular hypertrophy with a complete atrioventricular septal defect reflects the pulmonary hypertension accompanying a nonrestrictive defect in the inlet septum (Fig. 15–100) whether or not pulmonary vascular disease coexists. Left precordial leads may exhibit Q waves and well-developed R waves of left ventricular volume overload.[251]

THE X-RAY

The x-ray in isolated *ostium primum atrial septal* defect has an x-ray analogous to an ostium secundum atrial septal

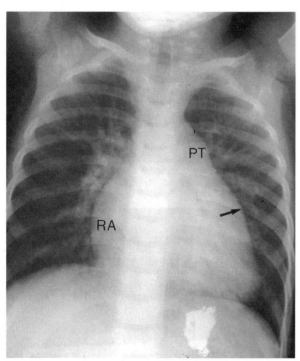

Figure 15–102

X-ray from a 3-year-old boy with a nonrestrictive ostium primum atrial septal defect and moderate regurgitation of the left atrioventricular valve. Pulmonary vascularity is increased, the pulmonary trunk (PT) is dilated, the right ventricular outflow tract is prominent (*arrow*), and the right atrium (RA) is enlarged. The ascending aorta is not seen. It is uncertain which ventricle occupies the apex.

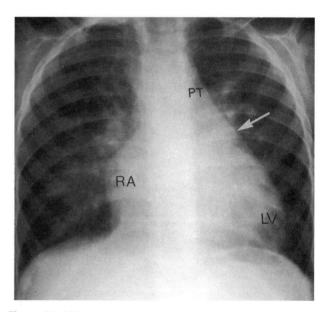

Figure 15–103

X-ray from a 19-month-old girl with a nonrestrictive ostium primum atrial septal defect, a restrictive inlet ventricular septal defect, a 2 to 1 left-to-right shunt and moderate to marked regurgitation of the left atrioventricular valve. An enlarged left atrial appendage (*arrow*) straightened the left cardiac border. A prominent right atrium (RA) occupies the right lower cardiac border, and a dilated left ventricle (LV) occupies the apex. Pulmonary vascularity is increased.

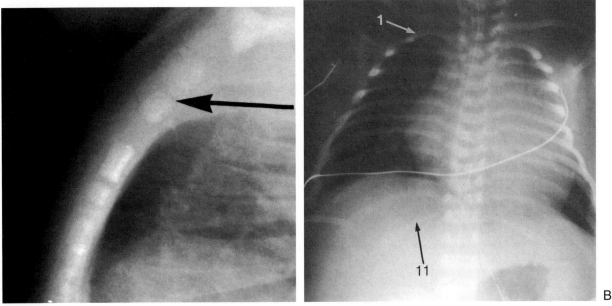

Figure 15–104

A, Double manubrial ossification center (*paired arrows*) in a 2-year-old boy with Down syndrome. *B*, Absence of the 12th rib in a neonate with Down syndrome. *Arrow* identifies the eleventh rib.

defect of equivalent size (Fig. 15–102). When *left AV valve regurgitation* coexists, the right atrium is especially enlarged because regurgitant flow is directed into the right atrial cavity (Fig. 15–88B). The left cardiac border is straightened by a prominent right ventricular outflow tract (Fig. 15–103). In infants and young children with a complete atrioventricular septal defect, pulmonary vascularity is increased and the enlarged cardiac silhouette may obscure all but a small portion of the lung fields (Fig. 15–89). A dilated right atrium occupies the right lower cardiac border, and the left ventricle may occupy the apex despite right ventricular enlargement (Fig. 15–89B). A dilated pulmonary trunk may be eclipsed by a prominent right ventricular outflow tract, and the ascending aorta is inconspicuous (Fig.15–89).

The lateral x-ray in Down syndrome may disclose a double manubrial ossification center (Fig. 15–104A),[225,262] and the posteroanterior projection consistently discloses an absent or rudimentary 12th rib (Fig.15–104B). Seckel syndrome is another phenotype in which there are 11 paired ribs.[244] Hyperinflation of the lungs caused by upper airway obstruction in Down syndrome flattens the hemidiaphragms.

THE ECHOCARDIOGRAM

Echocardiography with color flow imaging and Doppler interrogation establishes the type of atrioventricular septal defect and assesses the hemodynamic consequences. The diagnosis can be made in the fetus.[182,192] Cross sectional echocardiographic studies have characterized the pathognomonic morphologic features of atrioventricular septal defects

and have defined the relationships between septal structures and the atrioventricular junction.[204] Echocardiography identifies the atrioventricular valve attachments, identifies absence of the atrioventricular septum, and determines whether a common annulus is guarded by two separate atrioventricular valves or a common atrioventricular valve. Color flow imaging and Doppler interrogation establish atrial and ventricular level shunts and estimate the degree of atrioventricular valve regurgitation. The left ventricular outflow tract gooseneck can be recognized,[213] and the relative size of the left ventricular and right ventricular cavities can be defined.[195,303]

Absence of the atrioventricular septum is verified when the bridging leaflets cross at the same horizontal level above the crest of the ventricular septum (Figs. 15–105 and 15–108) and when fused chords are interposed between conjoined atrioventricular leaflets at the crest of the ventricular septum (Fig. 15–86B). An isolated atrial shunt exists when the bridging leaflets attach directly to the crest of the ventricular septum (Fig. 15–105) or attach indirectly by chordae tendineae (Fig. 15–108). Doppler interrogation and color flow imaging establish the level of the shunt (Fig. 15–106) and determine the competence of the right and left components of the atrioventricular valve. The left atrioventricular valve in the short axis assumes a triangular rather than a fish mouth appearance in diastole, and the *cleft* in the anterior leaflet is oriented toward the ventricular septum (Fig. 15–107) because the cleft is a functional commissure between the anterior and posterior bridging leaflets (Fig. 15–86A). Accessory chordae tendineae originate from the

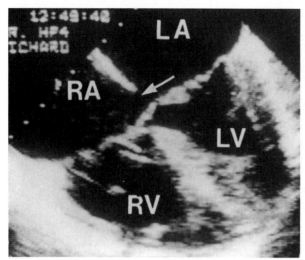

Figure 15–105

Transesophageal echocardiogram from a 54-year-old man with an isolated restrictive ostium primum atrial septal defect (*arrow*) at the distal end of an otherwise intact atrial septum. The right and left atrioventricular valves are at the same level because the atrioventricular septum was absent. LA and LV, left atrium and left ventricle; RA and RV, right atrium and right ventricle.

margins of the cleft and insert directly into the ventricular septum.

Continuity between the posterior aortic wall and the left atrioventricular valve is attenuated. Abnormal positions of the left ventricular papillary muscles can be identified, and a parachute or double orifice arrangement can be established. Interrogation of the left ventricular outflow tract is achieved from the subcostal view seeking the gooseneck deformity as shown in the angiocardiogram in Figure 15–88. Obstruction to left ventricular outflow is represented by a subaortic ridge, thick immobile chordal tissue, thin mobile chordal tissue, or an abnormally high or accessory papillary muscle.[213]

Complete atrioventricular septal defects are represented by bridging leaflets that float below the inferior margin of

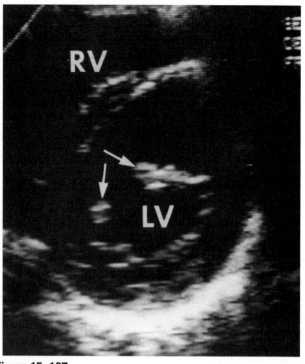

Figure 15–107

Echocardiogram (short axis) from a 6-year-old girl with a restrictive ostium primum atrial septal defect and a cleft anterior mitral leaflet (*paired arrows*) that points toward the right ventricle (RV). The cleft represents a functional commissure between the anterior and posterior bridging leaflets. The opened valve has a triangular shape.

the atrial septum and above the crest of the ventricular septum (Fig. 15–108*A*).

During diastole, the floating bridging leaflet moves away from the atrial septum into the ventricles, creating a *complete common atrioventricular canal* (Fig. 15–108*B*). The anterior bridging leaflet may contact the inferior margin of the atrial septum during systole, so the relationship between these structures should be examined in both phases of the cardiac cycle.

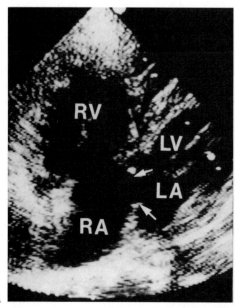

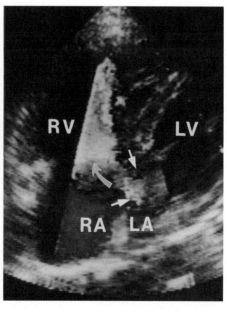

Figure 15–106

Echocardiogram from the 71-year-old woman whose angiocardiograms are shown in Figure 15–87. *A*, Apical four-chamber view showing a nonrestrictive ostium primum atrial septal defect (*paired arrows*). The right atrium (RA) and right ventricle (RV) are enlarged. *B*, Black-and-white print of a color flow image showing the left-to-right shunt across the ostium primum atrial septal defect (*paired arrows*) with flow continuing across the tricuspid valve (*curved arrow*) into the right ventricle (RV). LV, left ventricle; LA, left atrium.

A   B

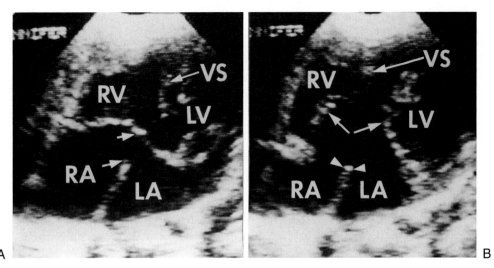

Figure 15–108
Echocardiograms (four-chamber) from a 2-year-old girl with a complete atrioventricular septal defect. *A*, The systolic frame shows a common atrioventricular valve whose bridging leaflets are at the same level because the atrioventricular septum is absent. The bridging leaflets float because they were unattached to either the distal atrial septum above (*unmarked paired arrows*) or to the crest of the ventricular septum (VS) below. The common atrioventricular canal lies between the crest of the ventricular septum and the distal atrial septum. RA and LA, right atrium and left atrium; RV and LV, right ventricle and left ventricle. *B*, The common AV valve as shown open in diastole (*paired oblique arrows*). *Paired arrowheads* identify the distal end of the atrial septum.

SUMMARY

An *ostium primum atrial septal defect* is clinically analogous to an ostium secundum atrial septal defect of equivalent size except for the QSR axis and the sequence of ventricular depolarization. When accompanied by left atrioventricular valve regurgitation, the clinical expressions are determined by the degree of regurgitation and the magnitude of the shunt. Congestive heart failure begins in childhood when the atrial septal defect is nonrestrictive and left AV valve regurgitation is severe. The incompetent left atrioventricular valve is susceptible to infective endocarditis. The jugular venous pulse displays a dominant V wave because the right atrium receives the regurgitant jet from the left ventricle. Precordial movement and palpitation are similar to ostium secundum atrial septal defect with the important addition of a left ventricular impulse and an apical systolic thrill. Auscultatory signs resemble those of ostium secundum atrial septal defect with the addition of the apical holosystolic murmur that radiates toward the sternum, occasionally as far as the right sternal border. A pulmonary midsystolic flow murmur is followed by fixed splitting of the second heart sound. The electrocardiogram shows left axis deviation with counterclockwise depolarization, splintered S waves in the inferior leads, and either an rsR prime pattern in right precordial leads or R waves of right ventricular hypertrophy. The x-ray resembles an ostium secundum atrial septal defect. Echocardiography with Doppler interrogation and color flow imaging establishes absence of the atrioventricular septum with the bridging leaflets at the same horizontal level. Color flow imaging identifies the left-to-right interatrial shunt and the degree of left AV valve regurgitation.

Complete atrioventricular septal defect becomes manifest in infancy because of congestive heart failure. Down phenotype is diagnostically important. The right ventricular impulse is hyperdynamic reflecting combined pressure and volume overload and eclipsing the left ventricular impulse. The murmur of left atrioventricular valve regurgitation preferentially radiates toward the sternum occasionally as far as the right anterior chest, and overlaps with the sites occupied by systolic murmurs of ventricular septal defect and right AV valve regurgitation. A mid-diastolic flow murmur is generated across the right atrioventricular valve. There is fixed splitting of the second heart sound with a prominent pulmonary component. The electrocardiogram shows left axis deviation, counterclockwise depolarization, splintering of the S waves in inferior leads and right ventricular hypertrophy in precordial leads. The x-ray shows increased pulmonary arterial vascularity and a considerable increase in heart size because of right atrial and right ventricular enlargement. Echocardiography identifies bridging leaflets of the common atrioventricular valve beneath the distal margin of the atrial septum and above the crest of the ventricular septum. Doppler interrogation and color flow imaging establish the levels of the interatrial and interventricular shunts and the degree of left and right AV regurgitation.

REFERENCES

1. Abbott ME: New accessions in cardiac anomalies. Int Am Museums Bull 10:111, 1924.
2. Adams CW: A reappraisal of life expectancy with atrial shunts of the secundum type. Dis Chest 48:357, 1965.
3. Adler LN, Berger RL, Starkey GWB, Abelmann WH: Anomalous pulmonary venous drainage associated with mitral stenosis. N Engl J Med 270:166, 1964.
4. Ainger LE, Pate JW: Ostium secundum atrial septal defects and congestive heart failure in infancy. Am J Cardiol 15:380, 1965.
5. Albers WH, Hugenholtz PG, Nadas AS: Constrictive pericarditis and atrial septal defect, secundum type. Am J Cardiol 23:850, 1969.
6. Aldridge HE, Wigle ED: Partial anomalous pulmonary venous drainage with intact interatrial septum associated with congenital mitral stenosis. Circulation 31:579, 1965.

7. Alexander JA, Rembert JC, Sealy WC, Greenfield JC: Shunt dynamics in experimental atrial septal defects. J Appl Physiol 39:281, 1975.

8. Alpert JS, Dexter L, Vieweg WVR, et al: Anomalous pulmonary venous return with intact atrial septum. Circulation 56:870, 1977.

9. Pueschel SM, Pueschel JK: Biomedical Concerns in Persons with Down Syndrome. Baltimore, Paul H Brooks Publishing, 1992.

10. Andersen M, Lyngborg K, Moller I, Wennevold A: The natural history of small atrial septal defect: Long-term follow-up with serial heart catheterizations. Am Heart J 92:302, 1976.

11. Anderson PAW, Rogers NC, Canent RV, Spach MS: Atrioventricular conduction in secundum atrial septal defects. Circulation 48:27, 1973.

12. Anderson, RH: New light on morphogenesis of atrioventricular septal defects. Int J Cardiol 18:79, 1988.

13. Mas J, Zuber M: Recurrent cerebrovascular events in patients with patent foramen ovale, atrial septal aneurysm, or both and cryptogenic stroke or transient ischemic attack. Am Heart J 130:1083, 1995.

14. Kimura K, Uemura S, Handa S, Terasaki M: Usefulness of saturation pulses in magnetic resonance imaging of partial anomalous pulmonary venous return. Angiology 52:331, 2001.

15. Aravanis, C.: Opening snap in relative tricuspid stenosis. Report of 2 cases of atrial septal defect. Am. J. Cardiol. 12:408, 1963.

16. Klecker RJ, Cristoforidis AJ, Sinclair DS. Vertical vein (partial anomalous pulmonary venous drainage). Am J Roentgenol. 175:867, 2000.

17. Arciniegas, E., Henry, J. G., and Green, E. W.: Stenosis of the coronary ostium. An unusual site of obstruction in total anomalous pulmonary venous drainage. J. Thorac. Cardiovasc. Surg. 79:303, 1980.

18. Arden, M. J., and Ferguson, M. J.: Interatrial septal defect in the elderly. A report on three patients. Geriatrics 17:745, 1962.

19. Arnfred, E.: Symptoms, signs, and hemodynamics in one hundred cases of atrial septal defect confirmed by operation. J. Cardiovasc. Surg. 7:349, 1966.

20. Feller PB, Allan LD. Abnormal pulmonary venous return diagnosed prenatally by pulsed Doppler flow imaging. Ultrasound Obstet Gynecol. 9:347, 1997.

21. Askey, J. M., and Kahler, J. E.: Longevity in extensive organic heart lesions: A case of Lutembacher's syndrome in a man aged 72. Ann. Intern. Med. 33:1031, 1950.

22. Assmann, H.: Die Klinische Roentgendiagnostik der Innern Erkrankungen. Leipzig, 1921.

23. Awan, I.H., Rice, R., and Moodie, D. S.: Spontaneous closure of atrial septal defect with interatrial aneurysm formation. Pediatr. Cardiol. 3:143, 1982.

24. Aygen, M. M., and Braunwald, E.: The splitting of the second heart sound in normal subjects and in patients with congenital heart disease. Circulation 25:328, 1962.

25. Baird, P. A., and Sadovnick, A. D.: Life expectancy in Down syndrome. J. Pediatr. 110:849, 1987.

26. Barber, J. M., Magidson, O., and Wood, P.: Atrial septal defect with special reference to electrocardiogram, pulmonary artery pressure and second heart sound Br. Heart J. 12:277, 1950.

27. Baron, M. G.: Abnormalities of the mitral valve in endocardial cushion defects. Circulation 45:672, 1972.

28. Baron, P., Gutgesell, H., Hawkins, E., and McNamara, D.: Infradiaphragmatic total anomalous pulmonary venous connection in siblings. Am. Heart J. 104:1107, 1982.

29. Barritt, S. W., Davies, D. H., and Jacob, G.: Heart sounds and pressures in atrial septal defect. Br. Heart J. 27:90, 1965.

30. Bashi, V. V., Ravikumar, E., Jairaj, P. S., Krishnaswami, S., and John, S.: Coexistent mitral valve disease with left-to-right shunt at atrial level: Clinical profile, hemodynamics, and surgical considerations in 67 consecutive patients. Am. Heart J. 114:406, 1987.

31. Bashour, T., Kabbani, S., Saalouke, M., and Cheng, T.O.: Persistent eustachian valve causing severe cyanosis in atrial septal defect with normal right heart pressures. Angiology 34:79, 1983.

32. Becher, M. W., Rockenmacher, S., Marin-Padilla, M.: Total anomalous pulmonary venous connection: persistence and atresia of the common pulmonary vein. Pediatr. Cardiol. 13:187, 1992.

33. Miller DS, Schwartz SL, Geggel RL, Smith JJ, Warner K, Pandian NG: Detection of partial anomalous right pulmonary venous return with an intact atrial septum by transesophageal echocardiography. J Am Soc Echocardiogr. 8:924, 1995.

34. Bedford, D. E.: The anatomical types of atrial septal defect. Their incidence and clinical diagnosis. Am. J. Cardiol. 6:568, 1960.

35. Bedford, D. E.: Atrial septal defect. Proc. R. Soc. Med. 54:779, 1961.

36. Bedford, D. E., Papp, C., and Parkinson, J.: Atrial septal defect. Br. Heart J. 3:37, 1941.

37. Posniak HV, Dudiak CM, Olson MC: Computed tomography diagnosis of partial anomalous pulmonary venous drainage. Cardiovasc Intervent Radiol 16:319, 1993.

38. Belkin, R. N., Hurwitz, D. J., and Kisslo, J.: Atrial septal aneurysm: Association with cerebrovascular and peripheral embolic events. Stroke 18:856, 1987.

39. Belkin, R.N., and Kisslo, J.: Atrial septal aneurysm: Recognition and clinical relevance. Am. Heart J. 120:948, 1990.

40. Berry, W. B., and Austen, W. G.: Respiratory variations in the magnitude of the left to right shunt in experimental interatrial communications. Am. J. Cardiol. 14:201, 1964.

41. Brili S, McClements B, Castellanos S, Apostolidou M, Barbetseas J, Pitsavos C: Significance of an atrial septal aneurysm in the presence of an ostium secundum atrial septal defect. Transesophageal echocardiographic study. Cardiology 86:421, 1995.

42. Bink-Boelkens, M. T. E., Bergstra, A., and Landsman, M. L. J.: Functional abnormalities of the conduction system in children with atrial septal defect. Int. J. Cardiol. 20:263, 1988.

43. Bizarro, R. O., Callahan, J. A., Feldt, R. H., Kurland, L. T., Gordon, H., and Brandenburg. R. O.: Familial atrial septal defect with prolonged atrioventricular conduction. Circulation 41:677, 1970.

44. Bjornstad, P. G.: Secundum type atrial septal defect with prolonged PR interval and autosomal dominant mode of inheritance. Br. Heart J. 36:1149, 1974.

45. Bland, E. F., and Sweet, R. H.: A venous shunt for advanced mitral stenosis. J. A. M. A. 140:1259, 1949.

46. Ay H, Buonanno FS, Abraham SA, Kistler JP, Koroshetz WJ: An electrocardiographic criterion for the diagnosis of patent foramen ovale associated with ischemic stroke. Stroke 29:1393, 1998.

47. Blumenschein, S. D., Barr, R. C., Spach, M. S., and Gentzler, R. C.: Quantitative frank vectorcardiograms of normal children and a comparison to those of patients with atrial defects. Am. Heart J. 83:332, 1972.

48. Boineau, J. P., Moore, E. N., and Patterson, D. F: Relationship between the ECG, ventricular activation, and the ventricular conduction system in ostium primum ASD. Circulation 48:556, 1973.

49. Boineau, J. P., Spach, M. S., and Ayers, C. R.: Genesis of the electrocardiogram in atrial septal defect. Am. Heart J. 68:637, 1964.

50. Ammash NM, Seward JB, Warnes CA, Commolly HM, O'Leary PW, Danielson GK: Partial anomalous pulmonary venous connection: diagnosis by transesophageal echocardiography. J Am Coll Cardiol. 29:1351, 1997.

51. Bonow, R. O., Borer, J. S., Rosing, D. R., Bacharach, S. L., Green, M. V., and Kent, K. M.: Left ventricular functional reserve in adult patients with atrial septal defect. Circulation 63:1315, 1981.

52. Booth, D. C., Wisenbaugh, T., Smith, M., and DeMaria, A. N.: Left ventricular distensibility and passive elastic stiffness in atrial septal defect. J. Am. Coll. Cardiol. 12:1231, 1988.

53. Borkon, A. M., Pieroni, D. R., Varghese, P. J., Ho, C. S., and Rowe, R. D.: The superior QRS axis in ostium primum ASD: A proposed mechanism. Am. Heart J. 90:215, 1975.

54. Boucher, C. A., Liberthson, R. R., and Buckley, M. J.: Secundum atrial septal defect and significant mitral regurgitation. Incidence, management and morphology basis. Chest 75:697, 1979.

55. Bourdillon, P. D., Foale, R. A., and Somerville, J.: Persistent left superior vena cava with coronary sinus and left atrial connections. Eur. J. Cardiol. 11:227, 1980.

56. Sadaniantz A: A jumping rope giant atrial septal aneurysm and territorial disputes. Clin Cardiol. 25:42, 2002.

57. Boyer, S. H., and Chisholm, A. W.: Second heart sound in atrial septal defect. Circulation 18:697, 1958.

58. Brand, A., Keren, A., Branski, D., Abrahamov, A., and Stern, S.: Natural course of atrial septal aneurysm in children and the potential for spontaneous closure of associated atrial septal defect. Am. J. Cardiol. 64:996, 1989.

59. Brandenberg, R. O., and DuShane, J. W.: Clinical features of persistent common atrioventricular canal. Proc. Staff Meet. Mayo Clin. 31:509, 1956.

60. Fuse S, Tomita H, Hatakeyama K, Kubu N, Abe N: Effect of size of a secundum atrial septal defect on shunt volume. Am J Cardiol. 88:1447, 2001.

61. Brody, H.: Drainage of pulmonary veins into the right side of the heart. Arch. Pathol. 33:221, 1942.

62. Bruce, R. A., and Hagen, J. M. V.: Anomaly of total pulmonary venous connection. Report of a case with survival for 31 years. Am. Heart. J. 47:785, 1954.

63. Bruschke, A. V. G., and Block, A.: Anomalous pulmonary venous drainage associated with mitral valve disease. Am. Heart J. 78:437, 1969.

64. Bruwer, A.: Roentgenologic findings in total anomalous pulmonary venous connection. Proc. Staff Meet. Mayo Clin. 31:171, 1956.

65. Bruwer, A. J.: Posteroanterior chest roentgenogram in two types of anomalous pulmonary venous connection. J. Thorac. Cardiovasc. Surg. 32:119, 1956.

66. Kerut EK, Norfleet WT, Plotnick GD, Giles TD: Patent foramen ovale: A review of associated conditions and the impact of physical size. J Am Coll Cardiol. 38:613, 2001.

67. Burroughs, J. T., and Edwards, J. E.: Total anomalous pulmonary venous connection. Am. Heart J. 59:913, 1960.

68. Campbell, M.: Natural history of atrial septal defect. Br. Heart J. 32:820, 1970.

69. Campbell, M., and Polani, P. E.: Factors in the aetiology of atrial septal defect. Br. Heart J. 23:477, 1961.

70. Campbell, M., Neill, C., and Suzmon, S.: The prognosis of atrial septal defect. Br. Med. J. 1:1375, 1957.

71. Canada, W. J., Goodale, F., and Currens, J. H.: Defect of the interatrial septum, with thrombosis of the pulmonary artery. N. Engl. J. Med. 248:309, 1953.

72. Canter, C.E., Martin, T.C., Spray, T.L., Weldon, C. S., and Strauss, A. W.: Scimitar syndrome in childhood. Am. J. Cardiol 58:652, 1986.

73. Carmi, R., Boughman, J. A., and Ferencz, C.: Endocardial cushion defect: Further studies of "isolated" versus "syndromic" occurrence. Am. J. Med. Genet. 43:569, 1992.

74. Medina A, de Lezo JS, Caballero E, Ortega RJ: Platypnea-orthodeoxia due to aortic elongation. Circulation 104:741, 2001.

75. Agmon Y, Khandheria BK, Meissner I, Gentile F, Sicks JD: Comparison of frequency of patent foramen ovale by transesophageal echocardiography in patients with cerebral ischemic events versus in subjects in the general population. Am J Cardiol. 88:330, 2001.

76. Cascos, A. S.: Holt-Oram syndrome. Acta Paediatr. Scand. 56:313, 1967.

77. Castle, R.F.: Variables affecting the splitting of the second heart sound in atrial septal defect. Am. Heart J. 73:468, 1967.

78. Castle, R. F., Hedden, C. A., and Davis, N. P.: Variables affecting splitting of second heart sound in normal children. Pediatrics 43:183, 1969.

79. Cayler, G. G.: Spontaneous functional closure of symptomatic atrial septal defects. New Engl. J. Med. 276:65, 1967.

80. Chait, A., and Zucker, M.: Superior vena cava in evaluation of atrial septal defect. Am. J. Roentgenol. 103:104, 1968.

81. Chassinat, R.: Observation d'anomalies anatomiques remarquables de l'appareil circulatoire avec hepatocele congénitale, n'ayant donné lieu pendant la vie à aucun symptôme particulier. Arch. Gen. Méd. Paris 11:80, 1836.

82. Chen, C., Lin, S., Hsu, T., Chen, C., Wang, S., and Chang, M.: Iatrogenic Lutembacher's syndrome after percutaneous transluminal mitral valvotomy. Am. Heart J. 119:209, 1990.

83. Chen, M., Chu, S., and Lee, Y.: Total anomalous pulmonary venous connexion in an adult: A rare anomaly. Int. J. Cardiol. 31:107, 1991.

84. Chen, S., Arcilla, R. A., Cassels, D. E., Thilenius, O. G., and Ranninger, K.: Abnormal initial QRS vectors in atrial septal defect. Am J Cardiol 24:346, 1969.

85. Basson CT, Cowley GS, Solomon SD, Weissman B, Poznanski AK: The clinical and genetic spectrum of the Holt-Oram syndrome (heart-hand syndrome). N Engl J Med. 330:885, 1994.

86. Chi, T., and Krovetz, J.: The pulmonary vascular bed in children with Down's syndrome. J. Pediatr. 86:533, 1975.

87. Chia, B., Tan, N., and Tan, L.: Total anomalous pulmonary venous drainage. Am. J. Cardiol. 34:850, 1974.

88. Basson CT, Solomon SD, Weissman B, MacRae CA, Poznanski AK Prieto F: Genetic heterogeneity of heart-hand syndromes. Circulation 91:1326, 1995.

89. Clapp, S., Perry, B. L., Farooki, Z. Q., Jackson, W. L., Karpawich, P. P., Hakini, M., Arciniegas, E., Green, E. W., and Pinsky, W. W.: Down's syndrome, complete atrioventricular canal, and pulmonary vascular obstructive disease. J. Thorac. Cardiovasc. Surg. 100:115, 1990.

90. Clark, E. B., and Kugler, J. D.: Preoperative secundum atrial septal defect with coexisting sinus node and atrioventricular node dysfunction. Circulation 65:976, 1982.

91. Cockerhan, J. T., Martin, T. C., Gutierrez, F. R., Hartman, A. F., Goldring, D., and Strauss, A. W.: Spontaneous closure of secundum atrial septal defect in infants and young children. Am. J. Cardiol. 52:1267, 1983.

92. Cohle, S. D., Titus, J. L., Kim, H., and Erickson, E.: Communication of the coronary sinus with both atria. Arch. Pathol. Lab. Med. 105:407, 1981.

93. Cooke, R. A., Chambers, J. B., and Curry, P. V. L.: Doppler echocardiography of double orifice of the left atrioventricular valve in atrioventricular septal defect. Int. J. Cardiol. 32:254, 1991.

94. Cooksey, J. D., Parker, B. M., and Weldon, C. S.: Atrial septal defect and calcification of the tricuspid valve. Br. Heart J. 32:409, 1970.

95. Ashida K, Itoh A, Naruko T, Otsuka M, Sakanoue Y: Familial scimitar syndrome. Circulation 103:126, 2001.

96. Burger AJ, Sherman HB, Charlamb NJ: Low incidence of embolic strokes with atrial septal aneurysms. Am Heart J. 139:149, 2000.

97. Corvisart, J. N.: Essai sur les Maladies et les Lésions Organiques du Coeur et des Gros Vaisseaux. 2nd ed Paris, 1811.

98. Courter, S. R., Felson, B., and McGuire, J.: Familial interauricular septal defect with mitral stenosis (Lutembacher's syndrome). Am. J. Med. Sci. 216:501, 1948.

99. Crafoord, C., and Senning, A.: Persistent atrioventricular canal. Am. J. Cardiol. 6:618, 1960.

100. Craig, R. J., and Selzer, A.: Natural history and prognosis of atrial septal defect. Circulation 37:805, 1968.

101. Cumming, G. R.: Functional closure of atrial septal defect. Am. J. Cardiol. 22:888, 1968.

102. Finley JP, Nugent ST, Hellenbrand W, Craig M, Gillis DA: Sinus arrhythmia in children with atrial septal defect. Br Heart J. 61: 280, 1989.

103. Curtiss, E. I., Matthews, R. G., and Shaver, J. A.: Mechanism of normal splitting of the second heart sound. Circulation 51:157, 1975.

104. Dalen, J. E., Bruce, R. A., and Cobb, L. A.: Interaction of chronic hypoxia of moderate altitude on pulmonary hypertension complicating defect of the atrial septum. New Engl. J. Med. 266:272, 1962.

105. Dalen, J. E., Haynes, F. W., and Dexter, L.: Life expectancy with atrial septal defect. J.A.M.A. 200:442, 1967.

106. Heller J, Hagege AA, Besse B, Desnos M, Marie F, Guerot C: "Crochetage" (notch) on R wave in inferior limb leads: A new independent electrocardiographic sign of atrial septal defect. J Am Coll Cardiol. 27:877, 1996.

107. Dalith, F., and Neufeld, H.: Radiological diagnosis of anomalous pulmonary venous connection. A tomographic study. Radiology 74:1, 1960.

108. Darling, R. C., Rothney, W. B., and Craig, J. M.: Total pulmonary venous drainage into the right side of the heart. Report of 17 autopsied cases not associated with other major cardiovascular anomalies. Lab. Invest. 6:44, 1957.

109. Dave, K. S., Parkrashi, B. C., Wooler, G. H., and Iones, C. U.: Atrial septal defects in adults. Am. J. Cardiol. 31:7, 1973.

110. Davia, J. E., Cheitlin, M.D., and Bedynek, J. L.: Sinus venosus atrial septal defect. Am. Heart J. 85:177, 1973.

111. Davidson, H. G.: Atrial septal defect in a mother and her children. Acta Med. Scand. 160:447, 1958.

112. Brockhoff CJ, Kober H, Tsilimngas N, Dapper F, Munzel T, Meinertz T: Holt-Oram syndrome. Circulation 99:1395, 1999.

113. Davies, M. J.: Mitral valve in atrial septal defect. Br. Heart J. 46:126, 1981.

114. D'Cruz, I. A., and Arcilla, R. A.: Anomalous venous drainage of the left lung into the inferior vena cava. Am. Heart J. 67:539, 1964.

115. de la Monte, S. M., and Hedley-Whyth, E. T.: Small cerebral hemispheres in adults with Down syndrome: Contributions of developmental arrest and lesions of Alzheimer's disease. J. Neuropathol. Exp. Neurol. 49:509, 1990.

116. De Leval, M. R., Ritter, D. G., McGoon, D. C., and Danielson, G. K.: Anomalous systemic venous connection. Proc. Mayo Clin. 50:599, 1975.

117. De Maria, A. N., Oliver, L. E., Borgren, H. G., George, L., and Mason, D. T.: Apparent reduction of aortic and left heart chamber size in atrial septal defect. Am. J. Cardiol. 42:545, 1978.

118. Delisle, G., Ando, M., Calder, A. L., Zuberbuhler, J. R., Rochenmacher, S., Alday, L. E., Mangini, O., van Praag, S., and van Praag, R.: Total anomalous pulmonary venous connection. Am. Heart J. 91:99, 1976.

119. Dev, V., Narula, J., Tandon, R., and Shrivastava, S.: Partial anomalous pulmonary venous drainage and intact atrial septum with mitral stenosis: The paradox of a small shunt. Clin. Cardiol. 11:780, 1988.

120. Dexter, L.: Atrial septal defect. Br. Heart J. 18:209, 1956.

121. DiPasquale, G., Andreoli, A., Grazi, P., Dominici, P., and Pinelli, G.: Cardioembolic stroke from atrial septal aneurysm. Stroke 19:640, 1988.

122. Agata AD, McGhie J, Taams MA, Cromme-Dijkhuis AH: Secundum atrial septal defect is a dynamic three-dimensional entity. Am Heart J. 137:1075, 1999.

123. Fransson S: The Botallo mystery. Clin Cardiol. 22:434, 1999.

124. Brassard M, Fouron J, van Doesburg NH, Mercier L, DeGuise P: Outcome of children with atrial septal defect considered too small for surgical closure. Am J Cardiol. 83:1552, 1999.

125. Dimich, I., Steinfeld, L., and Park, S. C.: Symptomatic atrial septal defect in infants. Am. Heart J. 85:601, 1973.

126. Dische, M. R., Teixeira, M. L., Winchester, P. H., and Engle, M. A.: Horseshoe lung associated with a variant of the scimitar syndrome. Br. Heart J. 36:617, 1974.

127. Iwasaki Y, Satomi G, Tasukochi S: Analysis of ventricular septal motion by Doppler tissue imaging in atrial septal defect and normal heart. Am J Cardiol. 83:206,1999

128. Dow, J. D.: The radiological diagnosis of the sinus venosus type of atrial septal defect. Guy's Hosp. Rep. 108:305, 1959.

129. Dow, J. W., and Dexter, L.: Circulatory dynamics in atrial septal defect. J. Clin. Invest. 29:809, 1950.

130. Draulans-Noë, H. A. Y., Wenink, A. C. G., and Quaegebeur, J: Single papillary muscle ("parachute valve") and double-orifice left ventricle in atrioventricular septal defect convergence of chordal attachment: Surgical anatomy and results of surgery. Pediatr. Cardiol. 11:29, 1990.

131. Raza M, Walters J, Soto H, Sharma M: Possible association of interatrial septal aneurysm with cerebral embolic episodes. Clin Cardiol. 22:814, 1999.

132. Duff, D. F., Nihill, M. R., Vargo, T. A., and Cooley, D. A.: Infradiaphragmatic total anomalous pulmonary venous return. Br. Heart J. 37:1093, 1975.

133. Dupuis, C., Charaf, L. A. C., Breviere, G., Apou, P., Remy-Jardin, M., and Helmius, G.: The "adult" form of scimitar syndrome. Am. J. Cardiol. 70:502, 1992.

134. Durrer, D., Roos, J. P., and van Dam, R. T.: The genesis of the electrocardiogram of patients with ostium primum defects (ventral atrial septal defects). Am. Heart J. 71:642, 1966.

135. DuShane, J. W.: Total anomalous pulmonary venous connection: Clinical aspects. Proc. Staff Meet. Mayo Clin. 31:167, 1956.

136. Eddleman, E. E., Jr., Holt, J. H., and Bancroft, W. H., Jr.: Computer analysis of the kinetocardiogram from patients with atrial septal defects. Am. Heart J. 71:435, 1966.

137. Edwards, J. E.: Functional pathology of the pulmonary vascular tree in congenital cardiac disease. Circulation 15:164, 1957.

138. Edwards, J. E.: Pathologic and developmental considerations in anomalous pulmonary venous connection. Proc. Staff Meet. Mayo Clin. 28:441, 1953.

139. Edwards, J. E.: The problem of mitral insufficiency caused by accessory chordae tendineae in persistent common atrioventricular canal. Proc. Staff Meet. Mayo Clin. 35:299, 1960.

140. Edwards, J. E., and Helmholz, H. F., Jr.: A classification of total anomalous pulmonary venous connection based on developmental considerations. Proc. Staff Meet. Mayo Clin. 31:151, 1956.

141. Ferrari VA, Reilly MP, Axel L, Sutton MGS: Scimitar syndrome Circulation 98:1583, 1998.

142. Otani H, Kagaya Y, Yamane Y, Chida M, Ito K, Namiuchi S: Long-term right ventricular volume overload increases myocardial fluorodeoxyglucose uptake in the interventricular septum in patients with atrial septal defect. Circulation 101:1686, 2000.

143. Bohm M: Holt-Oram syndrome. Circulation 98:2636, 1998.

144. Ellis. R. W. B., and van Creveld, S.: Syndrome characterized by ectodermal dysplasia, polydactyly, chondro-dysplasia and congenital morbus cordis; report of three cases. Arch. Dis. Child. 15:65, 1940.

145. O'Malley CD, Saunders JB de CM: Leonardo on the Human Body. New York, Dover Publications, Inc, 1952.

146. Emanuel, I., Huang, S., and Yeh, E.: Physical features of Chinese children with Down's syndrome. Am. J. Dis. Child. 115:398, 1968.

147. Emanuel, R., O'Brien, K., Somerville, J., Jefferson, K., and Hegde, M.: Association of secundum atrial septal defect with abnormalities of atrioventricular conduction or left axis deviation. Br. Heart J. 37:1085, 1975.

148. Emanuel, R., Somerville, J., Inns, A., and Withers, R.: Evidence of congenital heart disease in the offspring of parents with atrioventricular defects. Br. Heart J. 49:144, 1983.

149. Canada WJ, Goodale F, Currens JH: Defect in the atrial septum with thrombosis of the pulmonary artery. N Engl J Med. 248:309, 1953.

150. Espino-Vela, J.: Rheumatic heart disease associated with atrial septal defect; clinical and pathologic study of 12 cases of Lutembacher's syndrome. Am. Heart J. 57:185, 1959.

151. Ettedgui, J. A., Siewers, R. D., Anderson, R. H., Park, S. C., Pathl, E., and Zuberbuhler, J. R.: Diagnostic echocardiographic features of the sinus venosus defect. Br. Heart J. 64:329, 1990.

152. Niwa K, Perloff JK, Bhuta SM: Structural abnormalities of great arterial walls in congenital heart disease. Circulation 103:393, 2001.

153. Feldt, R. H., Avasthey, P., Yoshimasu, F., Kurland, L. T., and Titus, J. L.: Incidence of congenital heart disease in children born to residents of Olmsted County, Minnesota, 1950–1969. Mayo Clin. Proc. 46:794, 1971.

154. Feldt. R. H., DuShane, J. W., and Titus, J. L.: The atrioventricular conduction system in persistent common atrioventricular canal defect. Circulation 42:437, 1970.

155. Perloff JK, Koss B: Pregnancy in congenital heart disease. In Perloff JK and Child JS: Congenital Heart Disease in Adults. Philadelphia, WB Saunders Co, 1998.

156. Feruglio, G. A., and Sreenivasan, A.: Intracardiac phonocardiogram in thirty cases of atrial septal defect. Circulation 20:1087, 1959.

157. Agmon Y, Khandheria BK, Meissner I: Frequency of atrial septal aneurysm in patients with cerebral ischemic events. Circulation 99:1942, 1999.

158. Firkett, C. H.: Examen anatomique d'un cas de persistence du trou ovale de botal, avec lésions valvulaires considérables du coeur gauche, chez une femme de 74 ans. Ann. Soc. Méd. Chir. Liège 19:188, 1880.

159. Flamm, M. D., Cohn, K. E., and Hancock, E. W.: Ventricular function in atrial septal defect. Am. J. Med. 48:286, 1970.

160. Flyer, D. C., Buckley, L. P., Hellenbrand, W. E., Cohn, H. E., Kirklin, J. W., Nadas, A. S., Cartier, J. M., and Breibart, M. H.: Report of the New England Regional Infant Cardiac Program. Pediatrics 65 (Suppl):377, 1980.

161. Freedom, R. M., and Gerald, P. S.: Congenital cardiac disease and the "cat-eye" syndrome. Am. J. Dis. Child. 126:16, 1973.

162. Freedom, R. M., Bini, M., and Rowe, R. D.: Endocardial cushion defect and significant hypoplasia of the left ventricle. Eur. J. Cardiol. 74:263, 1978.

163. Friedman, D. L., Kastner, T., Pond, W. S., and O'Brien, D. R.: Thyroid dysfunction in individuals with Down syndrome. Arch. Int. Med. 149:1990, 1989.

164. Ananthasubramaniam K, Iyer G, Karthikeyan V: Giant left atrium secondary to tight mitral stenosis leading to acquired Lutembacher syndrome. J Am Soc Echocardiogr. 14:1033, 2001.

165. Krishnamoorthy KM: Radiological findings in total anomalous pulmonary venous connection. Heart 82:696, 1999.

166. Frye, R. L., Krebs, M., Rahimtoola, S. H., Ongley, P. A., Hallerman, F. J., and Wallace, R. B.: Partial anomalous pulmonary venous connection without atrial septal defect. Am. J. Cardiol. 22:242, 1968.

167. Chen HY, Chen SJ, Li YW, Wu MH, Wang JK, Tsai YF: Esophageal varices in congenital heart disease with total anomalous pulmonary venous connection. Int J Card Imaging 16:405, 2000.

168. Juneja R, Saxena A, Kothari SS, Taneja K: Obstructed infracardiac total anomalous pulmonary venous connection in an adult. Pediatr Cardiol 20:152, 1999.

169. Fukazawa, M., Fukushige, J., and Ueda, K.: Atrial septal defects in neonates with reference to spontaneous closure. Am. Heart J. 116:123, 1988.

170. Fukazawa, M., Fukushige, J., Ueda, Y., Ueda, K., and Sunagawa, K.: Effect of increase in heart rate on interatrial shunt in atrial septal defect. Pediatr. Cardiol. 13:146, 1992.

171. Furguson, J. J., Miller, M. J., Aroesty, J. M., Sahagian, P., Grossman, W., and McKay, R. G.: Assessment of right atrial pressure-volume relations in patients with and without an atrial septal defect. J. Am. Coll. Cardiol. 13:630, 1989.

172. Furuta, S., Wanibuchi, Y., Ino, T., and Aoki, K.: Etiology of mitral regurgitation in secundum atrial septal defect. Japanese Circulation J. 46:346, 1982.

173. Gall, J. C., Jr., Stern, A. M., Cohen, M. M., Adams, M. S., and Davidson, R. T.: Holt-Oram syndrome; clinical and genetic study of a large family. Am. J. Hum. Genet. 18:187, 1966.

174. Gallagher, M. E., Sperling, D. R., Gwinn, J. L., Meyer, B. W., and Flyer, D. C.: Functional drainage of the inferior vena cava into the left atrium. Am. J. Cardiol. 12:561, 1963.

175. Gallo, P., Formigari, R., Hokayem, N. J., D'Offizi, F., D'Alessandro, Francalanci, P., D'Amati, G., Colloridi, V., and Pizzuto, F.: Left ventricular outflow tract obstruction in atrioventricular septal defects: A pathologic and morphometric evaluation. Clin. Cardiol. 14:513, 1991.

176. Galve, E., Angel, J., Evangelista, A., Anivarro, I., Permanyer-Miralda, G., and Soler-Soler, J.: Bi-directional shunt in uncomplicated atrial septal defect. Br. Heart J. 51:480, 1984.

177. Garcia, R., and Taber, R. E.: Bacterial endocarditis of the pulmonic valve. Association with atrial septal defect of the ostium secundum type. Am. J. Cardiol. 18:275, 1966.

178. Saxena A, Sharma M, Shrivastava S: Right lung agenesis with total anomalous pulmonary venous drainage. Indian Heart J 46:177, 11994.

179. Garrod, A. E.: On the association of cardiac malformations with other congenital defects. St. Barth. Hosp. Rep. (London) 30:53, 1894.

180. Gatham, G. E., and Nadas, A. S.: Total anomalous pulmonary venous connection: Clinical and physiologic observations of 75 pediatric patients. Circulation 42:143, 1970.

181. Gault, J. H., Morrow, A. G., Gay, W. A., and Ross, J.: Atrial septal defect in patients over the age of 40 years. Circulation 37:261, 1968.

182. Delisle MF, Sandor GG, Tessier F, Farquharson DF: Outcome of fetuses diagnoses with atrioventricular septal defect. Obstet Gynecol. 94:763, 1999.

183. Gensen, J. B., and Blount, S. G.: Total anomalous pulmonary venous return. Am. Heart J. 82:387, 1971.

184. Genz, T., Locher, D., Genz, S., Schumacher, G., and Bühlmeyer, K.: Chest x-ray film patterns in children with isolated total anomalous pulmonary vein connection. Eur. J. Pediatr. 150:14, 1990.

185. Ghisla, R. P., Hannon, D. W., Meyer, R. A., and Kaplan, S.: Spontaneous closure of isolated ostium secundum atrial septal defects in infants: An echocardiographic study. Am. Heart J. 109:1327, 1985.

186. Giknis, F. L.: Single atrium and the Ellis-van Creveld syndrome. J. Pediatr. 62:558, 1963.

187. Gleason, M. M.: Concordant total anomalous pulmonary venous connection in dizygotic twins. Am. Heart J. 118:1338, 1989.

188. Goldfarb, B., and Wang, Y.: Mitral stenosis and left to right shunt at the atrial level. A broadened concept of the Lutembacher syndrome. Am. J. Cardiol 17:319, 1966.

189. Digilio MC, Marino B, Giannotti A, Dallapiccola J: Familiar atrioventricular septal defect: possible genetic mechanism. Br. Heart J. 72:301, 1994.

190. Goodman, D. J., and Hancock, E. W.: Secundum atrial septal defect associated with a cleft mitral valve. Br. Heart J. 35:1315, 1973.

191. Goodman, D. J., Harrison, D. C., and Cannom, D. S.: Atrioventricular conduction in patients with incomplete endocardial cushion defect. Circulation 49:631, 1974.

192. Allan LD: Atrioventricular septal defect in the fetus. Am J Obstet Gynecol 181:1250, 1999.

193. Gotsman, M. S., Astley, R., and Parsons, C. G.: Partial anomalous pulmonary venous drainage in association with atrial septal defect. Br. Heart J. 27:566, 1965.

194. Graham, T. P., Jarmakani, J.M., and Canent, R.V.: Left heart volume characteristics with a right ventricular volume overload: Total anomalous pulmonary venous connection and large atrial septal defect. Circulation 45:389, 1972.

195. Greene, A. C., Kotler, M. N., Mintz, G. S., Eshaphpour, E., and Segal, B. L.: Isolated cleft mitral valve. J. Cardiovasc. Ultrasonog. 1:13, 1982.

196. Gueron, M., and Gussarsky, J.: Lutembacher syndrome obsolete? A new modified concept of mitral valve disease and left to right shunt at atrial level. Am. Heart J. 91:535, 1976.

197. Guntheroth, W. G., Nadas, A. S., and Gross, R. E.: Transposition of the pulmonary veins. Circulation 18:117, 1958.

198. Gutgesell, H. P., and Huhta, J. C.: Cardiac septation in atrioventricular canal defect. J. Am. Coll. Cardiol. 8:1421, 1986.

199. Hagen, P. T., Scholz, D. G., and Edwards, W. D.: Incidence and size of patent foramen ovale during the first 10 decades of life. Mayo Clin. Proc. 59:17, 1984.

200. Kumar A, Williams CA, Victoria BE: Familial atrioventricular septal defect. Br. Heart J. 71:79, 1994.

201. Suzuki K, Yamaki S, Mimori S, Murakami Y, Mori K, Takahashi Y: Pulmonary vascular disease in Down syndrome with complete atrioventricular septal defect. Am J Cardiol 86:434, 2000.

202. Hancock, E. W.: Coronary sinus rhythm in sinus venosus defect and persistent left superior vena cava. Am. J. Cardiol. 14:608, 1964.

203. Hancock, E. W., Oliver, G. C., Swanson, M. J., and Hultgren, H. N.: Valsalva's maneuver in atrial septal defect. Am. Heart J. 65:50, 1963.

204. Falcao S, Daliento L, Ho SY, Rigby ML, Anderson RH: Cross sectional echocardiographic assessment of the extent of the atrial septum relative to the atrioventricular junction in atrioventricular septal defect. Heart 81:199, 1999.

205. Hanley, P. C., Tajik, A. J., Hynes, J. K., Edwards, W. D., Reeder, G. S., Haggler, D. J., and Seward, J. B.: Diagnosis and classification of atrial septal aneurysm by two-dimensional echocardiography: Report of 80 consecutive cases. J. Am. Coll. Cardiol. 6:1370, 1985.

206. Hara, M., and Char, F.: Partial cleft of septal mitral leaflet associated with atrial septal defect of the secundum type. Am. J. Cardiol. 17:282, 1966.

207. Harris, A.: The second heart sound in health and in pulmonary hypertension. Am. Heart J. 79:145, 1970.

208. Harris, G. B. C., Neuhauser, E. B. D., and Giedion, A.: Total anomalous pulmonary venous return below the diaphragm. The roentgen appearances in three patients diagnosed during life. Am. J. Roentgenol. 84:436, 1960.

209. Harrison, D. C., and Morrow, A. G.: Electrocardiographic evidence of left-axis deviation in patients with defects of the atrial septum of the secundum type. New Engl. J. Med. 269:743, 1963.

210. Hartmann, A. F., Jr., and Elliott, L. P.: Spontaneous physiologic closure of an atrial septal defect after infancy. Am. J. Cardiol. 19:290, 1967.

211. Harvey, J. R., Teague, S. M., Anderson, J. L., Voyles, W. F., and Thadani, U.: Clinically silent atrial septal defects with evidence for cerebral embolization. Ann. Int. Med. 105:695, 1986.

212. Fraisse A, del Nido PJ, Gaudart J, Geva T: Echocardiographic characteristics and outcome of straddling mitral valve. J Am Coll Cardiol. 38:819, 2001.

213. Sittiwangkul R, Ma RY, McCrindle BW, Coles JG, Smallhorn JF: Echocardiographic assessment of obstructive lesions in atrioventricular septal defects. J Am Coll Cardiol. 38:253, 2001

214. Hastreiter, A. R., Wennemark, J. R., Miller, R. A., and Paul, M. H.: Secundum atrial septal defects with congestive heart failure during infancy and early childhood. Am. Heart J. 64:467, 1962.

215. McElhinney DB, Reddy M, Silverman NH, Hanley FL: Accessory and anomalous atrioventricular valvar tissue causing outflow tract obstruction. J Am Coll Cardiol. 32:1741, 1998.

216. Haugland, H., and Vik-Mo, M.: Aneurysm of the atrial septum: Motion pattern in relation to respiratory and cardiac cycles. J. Clin. Ultrasound 14:52, 1986.

217. Huggon IA, Cook AC, Smeeton NC, Stat C, Magee AG, Sharma GK: Atrioventricular septal defects diagnosed during fetal life. J Am Coll Cardiol. 36:593, 2000.

218. Pessotto R, Padalino M, Rubino M, Kadoba K, Buchler JR, Van Praagh R: Straddling tricuspid valve as a sign of ventriculoatrial malalignment: A morphometric study of postmortem cases. Am Heart J. 138:1184, 1999

219. Heath, D., Helmholz, H. F., Jr., Burchell, H. B., DuShane, J. W., and Edwards, J. E.: Graded pulmonary vascular changes and hemodynamic findings in cases of atrial and ventricular septal defect and patent ductus arteriosus. Circulation 18:1155, 1958.

220. Pueschel SM and Pueschel JK.(eds). Biomedical Concerns in Persons with Down Syndrome. Baltimore, Paul H Brookes Publishing Co. 1992.

221. Hoffman, J. I. E., Rudolph, A. M., and Danilowicz, D.: Left to right atrial shunts in infants. Am. J. Cardiol. 30:868, 1972.

222. Holman, L. B.: Congenital heart disease and upper-extremity deformities. A report of two families. New Engl. J. Med. 272:437, 1965.

223. Holmes, L. B.: Decreasing age of mothers of infants with the Down syndrome. New Engl. J. Med. 298:1419, 1978.

224. Holt, M., and Oram, S.: Familial heart disease with skeletal malformation. Br. Heart J. 22:236, 1960.

225. Horns, J. W., and O'Loughlin, B. J.: Multiple manubrial ossification centers in mongolism. A.J.R. 93:395, 1965.

226. Howitt, G.: Atrial septal defect in three generations. Br. Heart J. 23:494, 1961.

227. Hudson, R.: Normal and abnormal interatrial septum. Br. Heart J. 17:489, 1955.

228. Down JL.: Observations on an ethnic classification of idiots. London Hospital Clinical Lectures and Reports, 3:259, 1866.

229. Hull, E.: Cause and effects of flow through defects of atrial septum. Am. Heart J. 38:350, 1949.

230. Hung, J., Ritter, D. G., Feldt, R. H., and Kincaid, O. W.: Electrocardiographic and angiographic features of common atrium. Chest 63:970, 1973.

231. Hung, J., Uren, R. F., Richmond, D. R., and Kelly, D. T.: The mechanism of abnormal septal motion in atrial septal defect. Circulation 63:142, 1981.

232. Hunt, C. E., and Lucas, R. V.: Symptomatic atrial septal defect in infancy. Circulation 47:1042, 1973.

233. Husmann., D., Daniel, W. G., Mugge, A., Ziemer, G., and Pearlman, A. S.: Value of transesophageal color Doppler echocardiography for detection of different types of atrial septal defect in adults. J. Am. Soc. Echo. 5:481, 1992.

234. Hwang, B., Hsieh, K., and Meng, C. C. L.: Importance of spontaneous closure of the ventricular part in atrioventricular septal defect. Jpn. Heart J. 33:205, 1992.

235. Brushfield T: Mongolism. Br J Children's Diseases. 21:241, 1924.

236. Hynes, K. M., Frye, R. L., Brandenburg, R. O., McGoon, D. C., Titus, J. L., and Giuliani, E. R.: Atrial septal defect (secundum) associated with mitral regurgitation. Am. J. Cardiol. 34:333, 1974.

237. Iga, K., Tomonaga, G., and Hori, K.: Continuous murmur in Lutembacher syndrome analyzed by Doppler echocardiography. Chest 101:565, 1992.

238. Jacobsen, J. R., Gillette, P. C., Corgett, B. N., Rabinovitch, M., and McNamara, D. G.: Intracardiac electrography in endocardial cushion defect. Circulation 54:599, 1976.

239. Jarmakani, J. M., George, B., and Wheller, J.: Ventricular volume characteristics in infants and children with endocardial cushion defects. Circulation 58:153, 1978.

240. Joffe, H.: Effect of age on pressure-flow dynamics in secundum atrial septal defect. Br. Heart J. 51:469, 1984.

241. Johansson, B., and Sievers, J.: Inheritance of atrial septal defect. Lancet 1:1224, 1967.

242. John, S., Munshi, S. C., Bhati, B. S., Gupta, R. P., Sukumar, I. P., and Cherian, G.: Coexistent mitral valve disease with left to right shunt at atrial level. J. Thorac. Cardiovasc. Surg. 60:174, 1970.

243. Just, H., and Mattingly, T. W.: Interatrial septal defect and pericardial disease. Am. Heart J. 76:157, 1968.

244. Seckel HPG: Bird-headed Dwarfs. Springfield Ill, Charles C Thomas, 1960.

245. Kambe, T., Hibi, N., Ito, H., Arakawa, T., Nishimura, K., Ishihara, H., Miwa, A., and Tada, H.: Clinical study of the flow murmurs at the defect area of atrial septal defect by means of intracardiac phonocardiography. Am. Heart J. 91:35, 1976.

246. Karpawich, P. P., Antillon, J. R., Cappola, P. R., and Agarwal, K. C.: Pre and postoperative electrophysiologic assessment of children with secundum atrial septal defect. Am. J. Cardiol. 55:519, 1985.

247. Karsh, R. B., Spach, M. S., and Barr, R. C.: Interpretation of isopotential surface maps in patients with ostium primum and secundum atrial septal defect. Circulation 41:913, 1970.

248. Kavanagh-Gray, D.: Atrial septal defect in infancy. Can. Med. Assoc. J. 89:491, 1963.

249. Keats, T. E., Rudhe, U., and Foo, G. W.: Inferior vena caval position in the differential diagnosis of atrial and ventricular septal defects. Radiology 83:616, 1964.

250. Khoury, G. H., and Hawes, C. R.: Atrial septal defect associated with pulmonary hypertension in children living at high altitudes. J. Pediatr. 70:432, 1967.

251. Kulbertius, H. E., Coyne, J. J., and Hallidie-Smith, K. A.: Electrocardiographic correlation of anatomical and haemodynamic data in ostium primum atrial septal defects. Br. Heart J. 30:464, 1968.

252. Kumar, S., and Luisada, A. A.: The second heart sound in atrial septal defect. Am. J. Cardiol. 28:168, 1971.

253. Kuzman, W. J.: Atrial septal defects in the older patient. Geriatrics 22:107, 1967.

254. Kuzman, W. J., and Yuskis, A. S.: Atrial septal defects in the older patient simulating acquired valvular heart disease. Am. J. Cardiol. 15:303, 1965.

255. Lai, F., and Williams, R. S.: A prospective study of Alzheimer disease in Down syndrome. Arch. Neurol. 46:849, 1989.

256. Landi, F., Cipriani, L., Cocchi, A., Zuccala, G., and Carbonin, P.: Ostium secundum atrial septal defect in the elderly. J. Am. Geriatr. Soc. 39:60, 1991.

257. Lasser, R. P., Borun, E. R., and Grishman, A.: Vectorcardiographic analysis of RSR complex of unipolar chest lead electrocardiogram. Am. Heart J. 41:667, 1951.

258. Laursen, H. B.: Congenital heart disease in Down's syndrome. Br. Heart J. 38:32, 1976.

259. Leatham, A.: The second heart sound-key to auscultation of the heart. Acta Cardiol. 19:395, 1964.

260. Leatham, A., and Gray, I. R.: Auscultatory and phonocardiographic signs of atrial septal defect. Br. Heart J. 18:193, 1956.

261. Lee, M. E., and Sade, R. M.: Coronary sinus septal defect. J. Thorac. Cardiovasc. Surg. 78:563, 1979.

262. Lees, R. F., and Caldicott, W. H. H.: Sternal anomalies and congenital heart disease. A.J.R. 124:423, 1975.

263. Lev, M.: The architecture of the conduction system in congenital heart disease. I. Common atrioventricular orifice. A.M.A. Arch Pathol. 65:174, 1958.

264. Lev, M., Paul, M. H., and Cassels, D. E.: Complete atrioventricular block associated with atrial septal defect of the fossa ovalis (secundum) type. A histopathologic study of the conduction systems. Am. J. Cardiol. 19:266, 1967.

265. Levin, A. R., Spach, M. S., Boineau, J. P., Canent, R. V., Jr., Capp, M. P., and Jewett, P. H.: Atrial pressure-flow dynamics in atrial septal defects (secundum type). Circulation 37:476, 1968.

266. Levin, B., and Borden, C. W.: Anomalous pulmonary venous drainage into left vertical vein. Radiology 63:317, 1954.

267. Levin, B., and White, H.: Total anomalous pulmonary venous drainage into the portal system. Radiology 76:894, 1961.

268. Liberthson, R. R., Boucher, C. A., Fallon, J. T., and Buckley, M. J.: Severe mitral regurgitation: A common occurrence in the aging patient with secundum atrial septal defect. Clin. Cardiol. 4:229, 1981.

269. Liberthson, R. R., Boucher, C. A., Strauss, H. W., Dinsmore, R. E., McKusick, K. A., and Pohst, G. M.: Right ventricular function in adult atrial septal defect. Am. J. Cardiol. 47:56, 1981.

270. Liberthson, R. R., Buckley, M. J., and Boucher, C. A.: Pulmonary regurgitation in large atrial shunts without pulmonary hypertension. Circulation 54:966, 1976.

271. Liebman, J., and Nadas, A. S.: The vectorcardiogram in the differential diagnosis of atrial septal defect in children. Circulation 22:956, 1960.

272. Lin, A. E., and Perloff, J. K.: Upper limb malformations associated with congenital heart disease. Am. J. Cardiol. 55:1576, 1985.

273. Little, R. C.: Volume elastic properties of right and left atrium. Am. J. Physiol. 158:237, 1949.

274. Lopez, J. F., Linn, H., and Shaffer, A. B.: The apical first heart sound as an aid in the diagnosis of atrial septal defect. Circulation 26:1296, 1962.

275. Lucas, R. V., Jr., Adams, P., Jr., Anderson, R. C., Varco, R. L., Edwards, J. E., and Lester, R. G.: Total anomalous pulmonary venous connection to the portal venous system: A cause of pulmonary venous obstruction. Am. J. Roentgenol. 86:561, 1961.

276. Lucas, R. V., Jr., Anderson, R. C., Amplatz, K., Adams, P., Jr., and Edwards, J. E.: Congenital causes of pulmonary venous obstruction. Pediatr. Clin. North Am. 10:781, 1963.

277. Lucas, R. V., Lock, J. E., Tandon, R., and Edwards, J. E.: Gross and histologic anatomy of total anomalous pulmonary venous connection. Am. J. Cardiol. 62:292, 1988.

278. Lutembacher, R.: De la stenose mitrale avec communication interauriculaire. Arch. Mal. Coeur 9:237, 1916.

279. Lynch, H. T., Brachenberg, K., Harris, R. E., and Becker, W.: Hereditary atrial septal defect. Am. J. Dis. Child. 132:600, 1978.

280. Lynch, J. I., Perry, L. W., Takakuwa, T., and Scott, L. P.: Congenital heart disease and chondroectodermal dysplasia. Am. J. Dis. Child. 115:80, 1968.

281. MacLeod, C. A.: Endocardial cushion defects with severe mitral insufficiency and small atrial septal defect. Circulation 26:755, 1962.

282. Macruz, R., Perloff, J. K., and Case, R. B.: A method for the electrocardiographic recognition of atrial enlargement. Circulation 17:882, 1958.

283. Magri, G., Jona, E., Messina, D., and Actisdato, A.: Direct recording of heart sounds and murmurs from the epicardial surface of the exposed human heart. Am. Heart J. 57:449, 1959.

284. Maillis, M. S., Cheng, T. O., Meyer, J. F., Crawley, I. S., and Lindsay, J.: Cyanosis in patients with atrial septal defect due to systemic venous drainage into the left atrium. Am. J. Cardiol. 33:674, 1974.

285. Mantini, E., Grondin, C. M., Lillehei, C. W., and Edwards, J. E.: Congenital anomalies involving the coronary sinus. Circulation 33:317, 1966.

286. Mardini, M. K., Sakati, N. A., Lewall, D. B., Christie, R., and Nyhan, W. L.: Scimitar syndrome. Clin. Pediatr. 21:350, 1982.

287. Marino, B., Vario, U., Corno, A., Nava, S., Guccione, P., Calabro, R., and Marcelletti, C.: Atrioventricular canal in Down syndrome: Prevalence of associated cardiac malformations compared with patients without Down syndrome. Am. J. Dis. Child. 144:1120, 1990.

288. Markman, P., Howitt, G., and Wade, E. G.: Atrial septal defect in the middle-aged and elderly. Quarterly J. Med. 34:409, 1965.

289. Marshall, R. J., and Warden, H. E.: Mitral valve disease complicated by left-to-right shunt at atrial level. Circulation 29:432, 1964.

290. Mascarenhas, E., Javier, R. P., and Samet, P.: Partial anomalous pulmonary venous connection and drainage. Am. J. Cardiol. 31:512, 1973.

291. Massumi, R. A., and Nutter, D. O.: The syndrome of familial defects of heart and upper extremities (Holt-Oram syndrome). Circulation 34:65, 1966.

292. Mathew, R., Thilenius, O. G., Arcilla, R. A.: Comparative response of right and left ventricles to volume overload. Am. J. Cardiol. 38:209, 1976.

293. McDermid, E. H., Duncan, A. M. V., Brach, K. R., Holden, J. J. A., Magenis, E., Sheehy, R., Burn, J., Kerdon, N., Noel, B., Schinzel, A., Teshima, I., and White, B. N.: Characterization of the supernumerary chromosomes in the cat eye syndrome. Science 232:646, 1986.

294. McDonald, I. L., McMurtry, T. J., and Dodek, A.: Atrial septal defect in adult identical twins. Clin. Cardiol. 6:507, 1983.

295. McDonald, L., Emanuel, R., and Towers, M.: Aspects of pulmonary blood flow in atrial septal defect. Br. Heart J. 21:279, 1959.

296. McGinn, S., and White, P. D.: Interauricular septal defect associated with mitral stenosis. Am. Heart J. 9:1, 1933.

297. McKusick, V. A., Egeland, J. A., Eldridge, R., and Krusen, D. E.: Dwarfism in the Amish. The Ellis-van Creveld syndrome. Johns Hopkins Med. J. 115:306, 1964.

298. McManus, B. M., Luetzeler, J., and Roberts, W. C.: Total anomalous pulmonary venous connection: Survival to age 62 years without surgical intervention. Am. Heart J. 103:298, 1982.

299. McMullan, M. H., and Fyke, F. E.: Total anomalous pulmonary venous connection: Surgical correction in a 66-year-old man. Ann. Thorac. Surg. 53:520, 1992.

300. Miao, C., Zuberbuhler, J. S., and Zuberbuhler, J. R.: Prevalence of congenital cardiac anomalies at high altitude. J. Am. Coll. Cardiol. 12:224, 1988.

301. Miller, G., and Pollock, B. E.: Total anomalous pulmonary venous drainage. Am. Heart J. 49:127, 1955.

302. Milnor, W. R., and Bertrand, C. A.: The electrocardiogram in atrial septal defect; a study of twenty-four cases, with observations on the RSR? V₁ pattern. Am. J. Med. 22:223, 1957.

303. Minich, L. A., Snider, A. R., Bove, E. L., Lupinetti, F. M., and Vermilion, R. P.: Echocardiographic evaluation of atrioventricular orifice anatomy in children with atrioventricular septal defect. J. Am. Coll. Cardiol. 19:149, 1992.

304. Mito, T., Pereyra, P. M., and Becker, L. E.: Neuropathology in patients with congenital heart disease and Down syndrome. Pediatr. Pathol. 11:867, 1991.

305. Mitsuoka, H., Chughtai, S., Cutarelli, R., Beg, R. A., Naraghipour, H., and Kay, E. B.: Holt-Oram syndrome associated with combined ostium primum and secundum atrial septal defects. Am. J. Cardiol. 36:967, 1975.

306. Mody, M. R.: Serial hemodynamic observations in secundum atrial septal defect with special reference to spontaneous closure. Am. J. Cardiol. 32:978, 1973.

307. Mody, M. R., Gallen, W. J., and Lepley, D.: Total anomalous pulmonary venous drainage below the diaphragm. Am. J. Cardiol. 24:575, 1969.

308. Moore, E. N., Boineau, J. P., and Patterson, D. F.: Incomplete right bundle branch block: An electrocardiographic enigma and possible misnomer. Circulation 44:678, 1971.

309. Morgan, B. C., Ricketts, H. J., and Winterscheid, L. C.: Inferior clockwise frontal plane forces in a child with endocardial cushion defect. Am. Heart J. 82:275, 1971.

310. Morgan, J. R., and Forker, A. D.: Syndrome of hypoplasia of the right lung and dextroposition of the heart: "Scimitar sign" with normal pulmonary venous drainage. Circulation 43:27, 1971.

311. Morrow, A. G., Arne, W. C., and Aygen, M. M.: Total unilateral anomalous pulmonary venous connection with intact atrial septum. Am. J. Cardiol. 9:933, 1962.

312. Movsowitz, C., Podolsky, L. A., Meyerowitz, C. B., Jacobs, L. E., and Kotler, M. N.: Patent foramen ovale: A nonfunctional embryological remnant or a potential cause of significant pathology? J. Am. Soc. Echocardio. 5:259, 1992.

313. Munoz-Armas, S., Gorrin, J. R. D., Anselmi, G., Hernandez, P. B., and Anselmi, A.: Single atrium. Am. J. Cardiol. 21:639, 1968.

314. Musewe, N. N., Alexander, D. J., Teshima, I., Smallhorn, J. F., and Freedom, R. M.: Echocardiographic evaluation of the spectrum of cardiac anomalies associated with trisomy 13 and trisomy 18. J. Am. Coll. Cardiol. 15:673, 1990.

315. Nadas, A. S., and Ellison, R. C.: Phonocardiographic analysis of diastolic flow murmur in secundum atrial septal defect and ventricular septal defect. Br. Heart J. 29:684, 1967.

316. Nagata, S., Nimura, Y., Sakakibara, H., Beppu, S., Park, Y., Kawazoe, K., and Fujita, T.: Mitral valve lesion associated with secundum atrial septal defect. Br. Heart J. 49:51, 1983.

317. Nagle, R. E., and Tamara, F. A.: Left parasternal impulse in pulmonary stenosis and atrial septal defect. Br. Heart J. 29:735, 1967.

318. Nakib, A., Moller, J. H., Kanjuh, V. I., and Edwards, J. E.: Anomalies of the pulmonary veins. Am. J. Cardiol. 20:77, 1967.

319. Nath, P. H., Delaney, D. J., Zollikofer, C., Ben-Sacher, G., Castaneda-Zuniga, W., Formanek, A., and Amplatz, K.: Coronary sinus-left atrial window. Radiology 135:319, 1980.

320. Neill, C. A., Ferencz, C., Sabiston, D. C., and Sheldon, H.: The familial occurrence of hypoplastic right lung with systemic arterial supply and venous drainage "scimitar syndrome." Bull. Johns Hopkins Hosp. 107:1, 1960.

321. Nora, J. J., McNamara, D. G., and Fraser, F. C.: Hereditary factors in atrial septal defect. Circulation 35:448, 1967.

322. Oakley, D., Naik, D., Verel, D., and Rajan, S.: Scimitar vein syndrome. Am. Heart J. 107:596, 1984.

323. Oliveira da Silva, E., Janovitz, D., and De Albuquerque, S. C.: Ellis-van Creveld syndrome: Report of 15 cases in an inbred kindred. J. Med. Genet. 17:349, 1980.

324. Opdyke, D. F., and Brecher, G. A.: Modifying effects of interatrial septal defect on the cardiodynamics of mitral stenosis. Am. J. Physiol. 164:573, 1951.

325. Opdyke, D. F., Duomarco, J., Dillon, W. H., Schreiber, H., Little, R. C., and Seely, R. D.: Study of simultaneous right and left atrial pressure pulses under normal and experimentally altered conditions. Am. J. Physiol. 154:258, 1946.

326. O'Toole, J. D., Reddy, P. S., Curtiss, E. I., and Shaver, J. A.: The mechanism of splitting of the second heart sound in atrial septal defect. Circulation 56:1047, 1977.

327. Pahl, E., Park, S. C., and Anderson, R. H.: Spontaneous closure of the ventricular component of an atrioventricular septal defect. Am. J. Cardiol. 60:1203, 1987.

328. Parikh, D. N., Fisher, J., Moses, J. W., Goldberg, H. L., Levin, A. R., Engle, M. A., and Borer, J. S.: Determinants and importance of atrial pressure morphology in atrial septal defect. Br. Heart J. 51:473, 1984.

329. Pastore, J. O., Akins, C. W., Zir, L. M., Buckley, M. J., and Dinsmore, R. E.: Total anomalous pulmonary venous connection and severe pulmonic stenosis in a 52 year old man. Circulation 55:206, 1977.

330. Patten, B. M.: The closure of the foramen ovale. Am. J. Anat. 48:19, 1931.

331. Pearson, A. C., Nagelhout, D., Castello, R., Gomez, C. R., and Labovitz, A. J.: Atrial septal aneurysm and stroke: Transesophageal echocardiographic study. J. Am. Coll. Cardiol. 18:1223, 1991.

332. Pease, W. E., Nordenberg, A., and Ladda, R. L.: Familial atrial septal defect with prolonged atrioventricular conduction. Circulation 53:759, 1976.

333. Perloff, J. K.: Auscultatory and phonocardiographic manifestations of pulmonary hypertension. Prog. Cardiovasc. Dis. 9:303, 1967.

334. Perloff, J. K.: Ostium secundum atrial septal defect-survival for 87 and 94 years. Am. J. Cardiol. 53:388, 1984.

335. Perloff, J. K.: Physical Examination of the Heart and Circulation. 3rd edition. Philadelphia, W. B. Saunders Company, 2000.

336. Perloff J. K., Koos B: Pregnancy in congenital heart disease. In Perloff, J. K., and Child, J. S.: Congenital Heart Disease in Adults. 2nd edition. Philadelphia, W. B. Saunders Company, 1998, p 91.

337. Perloff, J. K., and Harvey, W. P.: Auscultatory and phonocardiographic manifestations of pure mitral regurgitation. Prog. Cardiovasc. Dis. 5:172, 1962.

338. Perloff, J. K., Caulfield, W. H., and DeLeon, A. C.: Peripheral pulmonary artery murmur of atrial septal defect. Br. Heart J. 29:411, 1967.

339. Perloff, J. K., Roberts, N. K., and Cabeen, W. R.: Left axis deviation. Circulation 60:12, 1979.

340. Piccoli, G. P., Gerlis, L. M., Wilkinson, J. L., Lozadi, K., Macartney, F. J., and Anderson, R. H.: Morphology and classification of atrioventricular defects. Br. Heart J. 42:621, 1979.

341. Piccoli, G. P., Wilkinson, J. L., Macartney, F. J., Gerlis, L. M., and Anderson, R. H.: Morphology and classification of complete atrioventricular defects. Br. Heart J. 42:633, 1979.

342. Plass, R., Schmidt, K., and Guenther, K. H.: Intracardiac sounds and murmurs in atrial septal defect. Am. J. Cardiol. 28:173, 1971.

343. Popio, K. A., Gorlin, R., Teichholz, L. E., Cohn, P. F., Bechtel, D., and Herman, M. V.: Abnormalities of left ventricular function and geometry in adults with an atrial septal defect. Am. J. Cardiol. 36:302, 1975.

344. Potter, H.: Review and hypothesis: Alzheimer disease and Down syndrome-chromosome 21 nondysjunction may underlie both disorders. Am. J. Hum. Genet. 48:1192, 1991.

345. Pruzanski, W.: Familial congenital malformations of the heart and upper limbs. A syndrome of Holt-Oram. Cardiologia 45:21, 1964.

346. Pryor, R. E., Giannetto, L., and Bashore, T. M.: Surgical repair of atrial septal defect in an 89 year old man: Progressive shunt due to concomitant aortic stenosis. Am. Heart J. 118:423, 1989.

347. Raghib, G., Ruttenberg, H. D., Anderson, R. C., Amplatz, K., Adams, P., Jr., and Edwards, J. E.: Termination of left superior vena cava in left atrium, atrial septal defect, and absence of coronary sinus. A developmental complex. Circulation 31:906, 1965.

348. Raisher, B. D., Dowton, S. B., and Grant, J. W.: Father and two children with total anomalous pulmonary venous connection. Am. J. Med. Genet. 40:105, 1991.

349. Rasmussen, K.: Prediction of hemodynamic data in atrial septal defects of secundum type from simple and combined vectorcardiographic data. Am. Heart J. 87:413, 1974.

350. Rastelli, G. C., Kirklin, J. W., and Titus, J. L.: Anatomic observations on the complete form of persistent common atrioventricular canal with special reference to atrioventricular valves. Mayo Clin. Proc. 41:296, 1966.

351. Rastelli, G. C., Rahimtoola, S. H., Ongley, P. A., and McGoon, D. C.: Common atrium: Anatomy, hemodynamics, and surgery. J. Thorac. Cardiovasc. Surg. 55:834, 1968.

352. Rees, A., Farru, O., and Rodriguez, R.: Phonocardiographic, radiological and haemodynamic correlation in atrial septal defect. Br. Heart J. 34:781, 1972.

353. Rice, M. J., McDonald, R. W., and Reller, M. D.: Fetal atrial septal aneurysm: A cause of fetal atrial arrhythmias. J. Am. Coll. Cardiol. 12:1292, 1988.

354. Richer, T. J., Gallen, W. J., and Friedberg, D. Z.: Familial atrial septal defect in a single generation. Br. Heart J. 34:198, 1972.

355. Robinson, A. E., Chen, J. T. T., Bradford, W. D., and Lester, R. G.: Kerley B lines in total anomalous pulmonary venous connection below the diaphragm. Am. J. Cardiol. 24:436, 1969.

356. Rodriquez-Collado, J., Attie, F., Zabal, C., Troyo, P., Olvera, S., Vazquez, J., Gutierrez, B., and Vargas-Barron, J.: Total anomalous pulmonary venous connection in adults. J. Thorac. Cardiovasc. Surg. 103:877, 1992.

357. Roesler, H.: Interatrial septal defect. Arch. Intern. Med. 54:339, 1934.

358. Rogers, W. M., Harrison, J. S., Malm, J. R., Thomson, N., Simandl, E., al-Naaman, Y. D., Demetz, A., Deterling, R. A., Jr., Friend W., Andrews, W., and Donahoe, P.: Phonocardiographic criteria in the diagnosis of atrial and ventricular septal defects. An experimental and clinical study. J. Cardiovasc. Surg. 7:29, 1966.

359. Rokitansky, C.: Die Defecte der Scheidewande des Herzens. Vienne, 1875.

360. Romero, T., Covell, J., and Friedman, W. F.: A comparison of pressure-volume relations of the fetal newborn and adult heart. Am. J. Physiol. 222:1285, 1972.

361. Rosenthal, L.: Atrial septal defect with mitral stenosis (Lutembacher's syndrome) in a woman of 81. Br. Med. J. 2:1351, 1956.

362. Ross, J., Jr., Braunwald, E., Mason, D. T., Braunwald, N. S., and Morrow, A. G.: Interatrial communications and left atrial hypertension. A cause of continuous murmur. Circulation 28:853, 1963.

363. Rowe, E. D., and Uchida, I. A.: Cardiac malformation in Mongolism. A prospective study of 184 mongoloid children. Am. J. Med. 31:726, 1961.

364. Rowe, G. G., Castillo, C. A., Maxwell, G. M., Clifford, J. E., and Crumpton, C. W.: Atrial septal defect and the mechanism of shunt. Am. Heart J. 61:369, 1961.

365. Rowland, T. W., Nordstrom, L. G., Bean, M. S., and Burkhardt, H.: Chronic upper airway obstruction and pulmonary hypertension in Down's syndrome. Am. J. Dis. Child. 135:1050, 1981.

366. Ruschhaupt, D. G., Khoury, L., Thilenius, O. G., Replogle, R. L., and Arcilla, R. A.: Electrophysiologic abnormalities of children with ostium secundum atrial septal defect. Am. J. Cardiol. 53:1643, 1984.

367. Sailer, S.: Mitral stenosis with interauricular insufficiency. Am. J. Pathol. 12:259, 1936.

368. Sakamoto, T., Uozumi, Z., Change, S. Y., and Ueda, H.: Interatrial septal murmurs in secundum type atrial septal defect. Jpn. Heart J. 10:379, 1969.

369. Saksena, F. B., and Aldridge, H. E.: Atrial septal defect in the older patient. Circulation 42:1009, 1970.

370. Sambhi, M. P., and Zimmerman, H. A.: Pathologic physiology of Lutembacher syndrome. Am. J. Cardiol. 2:681, 1958.

371. Sanchez, J., Rodriquez-Torres, R., Lin, J., Goldstein, S., and Kavety, V.: Diagnostic value of the first heart sound in children with atrial septal defect. Am. J. Cardiol. 78:467, 1969.

372. Sanchez-Cascos, A., and Duechar, D.: The P wave in atrial septal defect. Br. Heart J. 25:202, 1963.

373. Sanders, C., Bittner, V., Nath, P. H., Breatnach, E. S., and Soto, B. S.: Atrial septal defect in older adults: Atypical radiologic appearances. Radiol. 167:123, 1988.

374. Schamroth, C. L., Sareli, P., Pocock, W. A., Davidoff, R., King, J., Reinach, G. S., and Barlow, J. B.: Pulmonary arterial thrombosis in secundum atrial septal defect. Am. J. Cardiol. 60:1152, 1987.

375. Schinzel, A., Schmid, W., Fracarro, M., Zuffardi, O., Opitz, J. M., Lindsten, J., Zetterqvist, P., Enell, H., Baccichetti, C., Tenconi, R., and Pagon, R. A.: The cat eye syndrome. Hum. Genet. 57:148, 1981.

376. Schwinger, M. E., Gindea, A. J., Freedberg, R. S., and Kronzon, I.: The anatomy of the interatrial septum: A transesophageal echocardiographic study. Am. Heart J. 119:1401, 1990.

377. Segall, H. N., and Spira, E. N.: A case of atrial septal defect observed during 25 years: Clinical and pathological data, with special reference to heart sounds and murmurs. Can. Med. Assoc. J. 90:636, 1964.

378. Seldon, W. A., Rubinstein, C., and Fraser, A. A.: The incidence of atrial septal defect in adults. Br. Heart J. 24:557, 1962.

379. Selzer, A., and Lewis, A. E.: The occurrence of chronic cyanosis in cases of atrial septal defect. Am. J. Med. Sciences 218:516, 1949.

380. Sepulveda, G., Lukas, D. S., and Steinberg, I.: Anomalous drainage of pulmonary veins; clinical, physiological and angiocardiographic features. Am. J. Med. 18:883, 1955.

381. Seward, J. B., Hayes, D. L., Smith, H. C., Williams, D. E., Rosenow, E. C., Reeder, G. S., Piehler, J. M., and Tajik, A. J.: Platypnea-orthodeoxia: Clinical profile, diagnostic work-up, management and report of 7 cases. Mayo Clin. Proc. 59:221, 1984.

382. Shafter, H. A.: Splitting of the second heart sound. Am. J. Cardiol. 6:1013, 1960.

383. Shah, C. V., Patel, M. K., and Hastreiter, A. R.: Hemodynamics of complete atrioventricular canal and its evolution with age. Am. J. Cardiol., 24:326, 1969.

384. Shaher, R. M., and Johnson, A. M.: The hemodynamics of common atrium. Guy's Hosp. Rep. 112:166, 1963.

385. Shaher, R. M., Farina, M. A., Porter, I., and Bishop, M.: Clinical aspects of congenital heart disease in mongolism. Am. J. Cardiol. 29:497, 1972.

386. Shaver, J. A., and O'Toole, J. D.: The second heart sound: Newer concepts. Mod. Concepts Cardiovasc. Dis. 46:7, 1976.

387. Shaver, J. A., Nadolny, R. A., O'Toole, J. D., Thompson, M. E., Reddy, P. S., Leon, D. F., and Curtiss, E. I.: Sound pressure correlates of the second heart sound. Circulation 49:316, 1974.

388. Sherman, F. E., and Bauersfeld, S. R.: Total, uncomplicated, anomalous pulmonary venous connection. Morphologic observations on 13 necropsy specimens from infants. Pediatrics 25:656, 1960.

389. Shiku, D. J., Stijns, M., Lintermans, J. P., and Vliers, A.: Influence of age on atrioventricular conduction intervals in children with and without atrial septal defect. J. Electrocardiol. 15:9, 1982.

390. Shiraishi, I., Hamaoka, K., Hayashi, S., Koh, E., Onouchi, Z., and Sawada, T.: Atrial septal aneurysm in infancy. Pediatr. Cardiol. 11:82, 1990.

391. Silver, M. D., and Dorsey, J. S.: Aneurysms of the septum primum in adults. Arch. Pathol. Lab. Med. 102:62, 1978.

392. Silverman, M. E., Copeland, A. J., and Hurst, J. W.: The Holt-Oram syndrome. Am. J. Cardiol. 25:11, 1970.

393. Singh, R., McGuire, L. B., Carpenter, M., and Dammann, J. F.: Mitral stenosis associated with partial anomalous pulmonary venous return (with intact atrial septum). Am. J. Cardiol. 28:226, 1971.

394. Smith, B., Frye, T. R., and Newtown, W. A., Jr.: Total anomalous pulmonary venous return. Am. J. Dis. Child. 101:41, 1961.

395. Snellen, H. A., and Albers, F. H.: The clinical diagnosis of anomalous pulmonary venous drainage. Circulation 6:801, 1952.

396. Snellen, H. A., and van Ingen, H. C., and Hoefsmit, E. C.: Patterns of anomalous pulmonary venous drainage. Circulation 38:45, 1968.

397. Solymar, L., Sabel, K., and Zetterqvist, P.: Total anomalous pulmonary venous connection in siblings: Report on three families. Acta. Paediatr. Scand. 76:124, 1987.

398. Somerville, J.: Ostium primum defect: Factors causing deterioration in the natural history. Br. Heart J. 27:413, 1965.

399. Somerville, J., and Resnekov, L.: The origin of an immediate diastolic murmur in atrioventricular defects. Circulation 32:797, 1965.

400. Spicer, R. L.: Cardiovascular disease in Down syndrome. Pediatr. Clin. North Am. 31:1331, 1984.

401. Sreeram, N., and Walsh, K.: Diagnosis of total anomalous pulmonary venous draining by Doppler color flow imaging. J. Am. Coll. Cardiol. 19:1577, 1992.

402. Starke, H., Schimke, R. N., and Dunn, M.: Upper-limb cardiovascular syndrome. A family study. Am. J. Cardiol. 19:588, 1967.

403. Steinbrunn, W., Cohn, K. E., and Selzer, A.: Atrial septal defect associated with mitral stenosis: The Lutembacher syndrome revisited. Am. J. Med. 48:295, 1970.

404. Stewart, J. R., Schaff, H. V., Fortuin, N. J., and Brawley, R. K.: Partial anomalous pulmonary venous return with intact atrial septum. Thorax 38:859, 1983.

405. Stollberger, C., Schneider, B., Abzieher, F., Wollner, T., Meinertz, T., and Slany, J.: Diagnosis of patent foramen ovale by transesophageal contrast echocardiography. Am. J. Cardiol. 71:604, 1993.

406. Storstein, O., and Tveten, H.: Anomalous drainage of pulmonary veins from right lung to superior vena cava with patent foramen ovale as cause of congestive heart failure in 68-year-old man. Acta Med. Scand. 148:77, 1954.

407. Sutherland, H. D.: A case with three atrial septal defects. Br. Heart J. 25:267, 1963.

408. Sutton, G., Harris, A., and Leatham, A.: Second heart sound in pulmonary hypertension. Br. Heart J. 39:743, 1968.

409. Swan, H. J. C., Burchell, H. B., and Wood, E. H.: Effect of oxygen on pulmonary vascular resistance in patients with pulmonary hypertension associated with atrial septal defect. Circulation 20:66, 1959.

410. Swan, H. J. C., Burchell, H. B., and Wood E. H.: A symposium on anomalous pulmonary venous connection. Proc. Staff Meet. Mayo Clin. 28:452, 1953.

411. Swan, H. J. C., Hetzel, P. S., Burchell, H. B., and Wood, E. H.: Relative contribution of blood from each lung to the left to right shunt in atrial septal defect. Circulation 14:200, 1956.

412. Swan, H. J. C., Kirklin, J. W., Becu, L. M., and Wood, E. H.: Anomalous connections of right pulmonary veins to superior vena cava with interatrial communications. Hemodynamic data in eight cases. Circulation 16:54, 1957.

413. Sweeney, L. J., and Rosenquist, G. C.: The normal anatomy of the atrial septum in the human heart. Am. Heart J. 98:194, 1979.

414. Tandon, R., and Edwards, J. E.: Cardiac malformations associated with Down's syndrome. Circulation 47:1349, 1973.

415. Tandon, R., Manchanda, S. C., and Roy, S. B.: Mitral stenosis with left to right shunt at atrial level. Br. Heart J. 33:773, 1971.

416. Tandon, R., Moller, J. H., and Edwards, J. E.: Unusual longevity in persistent common atrioventricular canal. Circulation 50:619, 1974.

417. Tavel, M. E., Baugh, D., Fisch, C., and Feigenbaum, H.: Opening snap of the tricuspid valve in atrial septal defect. Am. Heart J. 80:550, 1970.

418. Taylor, G. A., Jordan, C. E., Dorst, S. K., and Dorst, J. P.: Polycarpaly and other abnormalities of the wrist in chondroectodermal dysplasia. Radiology 151:393, 1984.

419. Thiron, J., Cribier, A., Cazor, J., and Letac, B.: Variations in height of jugular "a" wave in relation to heart rate in normal subjects and in patients with atrial septal defect. Br. Heart J. 44:37, 1984.

420. Thomas, H. M., Spicer, M. J., and Nelson, W. P.: Evaluation of P wave axis in distinguishing anatomical site of atrial septal defect. Br. Heart J. 35:738, 1973.

421. Thomas, J. D., Tabakin, B. S., and Ittleman, F. P.: Atrial septal defect with right-to-left shunt despite normal pulmonary artery pressure. J. Am. Coll. Cardiol. 9:221, 1987.

422. Tikoff, G., Schmidt, A. M., and Hecht, H. H.: Atrial fibrillation in atrial septal defect. Arch. Intern. Med. 121:402, 1968.

423. Tikoff, G., Schmidt, A. M., Kuida, H., and Hecht, H. H.: Heart failure in atrial septal defect. Am. J. Med. 39:533, 1965.

424. Timmis, G. C., Gordon, S., and Reed, J. O.: Spontaneous closure of an atrial septal defect. J.A.M.A. 176:17, 1966.

425. Toscano-Barbosa, E., Brandenburg, R. O., and Burchell, H. B.: Symposium on persistent common atrioventricular canal; electrocardiographic studies of cases with intracardiac malformations of the atrio-ventricular canal. Proc. Staff Meet. Mayo Clin. 31:513, 1956.

426. Ugarte, M., Salamanca, F. E., and Quero, M.: Endocardial cushion defects. An anatomical study of 54 specimens. Br. Heart J. 38:674, 1976.

427. Uhley, M. H.: Lutembacher's syndrome and a new concept of the dynamics of interatrial septal defect. Am. Heart J. 24:315, 1942.

428. VanCamp, G., Stinissen, P., Van Hul, W., Backhovens, H., Wehnert, A., VandenBerge, A., and VanBroeckhoven, C.: Selection of human chromosome 21-specific DNA probes for genetic analysis in Alzheimer's dementia and Down syndrome. Hum. Genet. 83:58, 1989.

429. von Rokitansky, C.: Die Defecte der Scheidewande des Herzens. Pathologischanatomische Abhandlung. Vienna, W. Braumuller, 1875.

430. Wagenvoort, C. A., Neufeld, H. N., DuShane, J. W., and Edwards, J. E.: The pulmonary arterial tree in atrial septal defect. A quantitative study of anatomic features in fetuses, infants, and children. Circulation 23:733, 1961.

431. Wagstaffee, W. W.: Two cases of free communication between the auricles, by deficiency of the upper part of the septum auricularum. Trans. Pathol. Soc. 19:96, 1868.

432. Waider, W., and Craige, E.: First heart sound and ejection sounds. Echocardiographic and phonocardiographic correlations with valvular events. Am. J. Cardiol. 35:346, 1975.

433. Waldo, A. L., Kaiser, G. A., Bowman, F. O., and Malm, J. R.: Etiology of prolongation of the PR interval in patients with an endocardial cushion defect. Circulation 48:19, 1973.

434. Walker, W. J., Mattingly, T. W., Pollock, B. E., Carmichael, D. B., Inmon, T. W., and Forrester, R. H.: Electrocardiographic and hemodynamic correlation in atrial septal defect. Am. Heart J. 52:547, 1956.

435. Welch, C. C., Gibson, D. C., and Fox, L. M.: Atrial septum secundum defects and mitral regurgitation. Am. J. Med. Sci. 252:45, 1966.

436. Wenink, A. C. G., and Zevallos, J.: Developmental aspects of atrioventricular septal defects. Int. J. Cardiol. 18:65, 1988.

437. Wennevold, A.: The diastolic murmur of atrial septal defects as detected by intracardiac phonocardiography. Circulation 34:132, 1966.

438. Weyman, A. E., Wann, S., Feigenbaum, H., and Dillon, J. C.: Mechanism of abnormal septal motion in patients with right ventricular volume overload. Circulation 54:179, 1976.

439. Whitaker, W.: Total pulmonary venous drainage through a persistent left superior vena cava. Br. Heart J. 16:177, 1954.

440. Wilson, J.: A description of a very unusual formation of the human heart. Philos. Trans. R. Soc. Lond. 88:346, 1798.

441. Winslow, M.: Mem. Acad. Roy. d. Sci. 1739. Cited by Otto, A. W.: Lehrbuch der pathologischen Anatomie der Menschen und der Tiere. Berlin, A. Rucker, 1830.

442. Winters, W. L., Jr., Cortes, F., McDonough, M., Tyson, R. R., Baier, H., Gimenez, J., and Davila, J. C.: Venoarterial shunting from inferior vena cava to left atrium in atrial septal defects with normal right heart pressures. Report of 2 cases. Am. J. Cardiol. 19:293, 1967.

443. Zion, M. M., Rosenman, D., Balkin, J., and Glaser, J.: Complete atrioventricular canal with survival to the eighth decade. Chest 85:437, 1984.

444. Inoue T, Ichihara M, Uchida T, Sakai Y, Hayashi T, Morrooka S: Three-dimensional computed tomography showing partial anomalous pulmonary venous connection complicated by the scimitar syndrome. Circulation 105:663, 2002.

445. Sanchez-Cascos A: Holt-Oram syndrome. Acta Paediatr Scand 56:313, 1967.

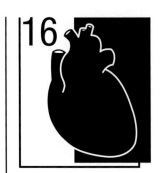

Pulmonary Stenosis with Interatrial Communication

In 1769, Giovanni Battista Morgagni described pulmonary stenosis with patent foramen ovale,[30] and in 1848 Thomas Peacock reported on *Contraction of the Orifice of the Pulmonary Artery and Communication Between the Cavities of the Auricles by a Foramen Ovale.*[34] The combination of pulmonary stenosis with reversed interatrial shunt has been called the *triologie de Fallot.*[23] Right ventricular outflow obstruction is usually represented by mobile dome pulmonary valve stenosis (Fig. 16–1), or much less commonly by stenosis of the pulmonary artery and its branches (Fig. 16–2).[7,12,13,16,18,20,29,35,38–40,42] Infundibular obstruction takes the form of secondary hypertrophic subpulmonary stenosis (Fig. 16–3).[7,8,12,21,25,44] Subinfundibular stenosis in a neonate was assigned to a right ventricular fibroma.[28] The interatrial communication is represented by either a patent foramen ovale or an ostium secundum atrial septal defect,[*] less commonly by an ostium primum[36] or sinus venosus atrial defect[19] or anomalous pulmonary venous connection.[32] This chapter deals principally with pulmonary valve stenosis and either a patent foramen ovale or a nonrestrictive ostium secundum atrial septal defect.[35]

When the interatrial communication is an atrial septal defect, coexisting pulmonary stenosis is almost always in a mobile dome valve, only occasionally in the branches.[3,8,29,35,38,39] The interatrial communication is almost always an ostium secundum defect. When severe pulmonary valve stenosis coexists with a right-to-left interatrial shunt, the shunt is almost always across a patent foramen ovale rather than an atrial septal defect.[10,12,35] The combination of severe pulmonary valve stenosis with a right-to-left shunt through a patent foramen ovale is more common than pulmonary valve stenosis with a nonrestric-

tive atrial septal defect irrespective of the direction of the shunt.[35]

The physiologic consequences of pulmonary stenosis with an interatrial communication depend on the degree of obstruction to right ventricular outflow and the size of the interatrial communication.[10,35] Patients with severe pulmonary stenosis and a right-to-left interatrial shunt (Fig. 16–4) almost always have pulmonary valve stenosis and a

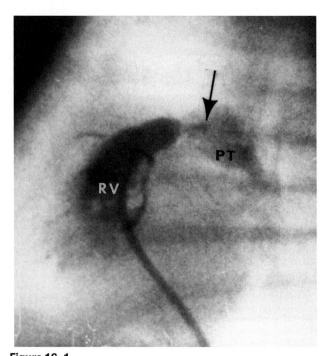

Figure 16–1
Lateral right ventricular angiocardiogram (RV) from a 2-day-old boy with pinpoint pulmonary valve stenosis, reversed shunt through a patent foramen ovale, and tricuspid regurgitation. *Arrow* identifies a tiny jet into the dilated pulmonary trunk (PT).

---

[*]3, 5, 8, 12, 14, 19, 31, 33, 35, 37, 39

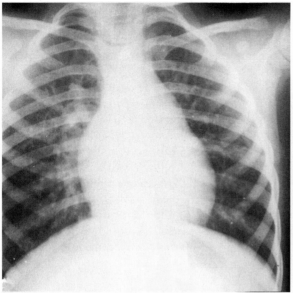
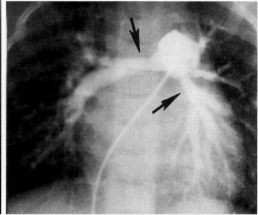

Figure 16–2

X-rays from a 5-year-old boy with stenosis of the pulmonary arterial branches (gradient 50 mm Hg) and a 2.2 to 1 left-to-right shunt through an ostium secundum atrial septal defect. *A,* Posteroanterior projection shows vascular lung fields, moderate dilatation of the pulmonary trunk, an inconspicuous ascending aorta, and a prominent right atrial convexity. *B,* Angiocardiogram with contrast material injected into the pulmonary trunk delineates stenoses of the right and left pulmonary arteries (*arrows*) with distal dilatation.

patent foramen ovale.[35] Patients with pulmonary stenosis and a left-to-right interatrial shunt almost always have mild to moderate pulmonary valve stenosis and a nonrestrictive ostium secundum atrial septal defect.[35] Severe pulmonary stenosis increases right atrial contraction that distends the right ventricle in presystole so it can achieve greater contractile force (Figs. 16–5 and 16–6). The large right atrial A wave is responsible for a presystolic right-to-left interatrial shunt. The high-pressure right atrium dilates, stretching the margins of the foramen ovale and increasing its patency. When right atrial blood escapes through the interatrial communication, pulmonary flow reciprocally falls.

A nonrestrictive atrial septal defect with mild to moderate pulmonary valve stenosis clinically resembles an isolated atrial septal defect (see Chapter 15). Small gradients should not be mistaken for mild pulmonary stenosis, because small gradients occur in isolated ostium secundum atrial septal defects with large left-to-right shunts and hyperkinetic right ventricular ejection across a normal pulmonary valve.

The History

Severe pulmonary stenosis with a right-to-left shunt across a patent foramen ovale is analogous to isolated severe pulmonary valve stenosis (see Chapter 11) except for cyanosis, which can date from birth[10,14] or can begin in childhood, puberty, or young adulthood.[1,7,8,14,22,39] Infants come to attention because of a murmur, but neonates with pinpoint pulmonary stenosis (see Fig. 16–1) have disarmingly soft murmurs. Symptoms can be appreciable when cyanosis is mild[14,41] because right ventricular pressure can exceed systemic before the right-to-left inter-

atrial shunt becomes manifest. However, one boy became cyanotic only when engaged in sports,[8] a woman with severe pulmonary stenosis and reversed interatrial shunt was in good health until age 40 years,[19] and a woman with a gradient of 120 mm Hg underwent surgical repair at age 58 years (see Fig. 16–5).

Giddiness, lightheadedness, or syncope may be experienced with exertion. Large jugular venous A waves (see Fig. 16–5) are sometimes subjectively sensed, especially after effort or excitement. Chest pain occasionally resembles angina pectoris attributed to ischemia in the high-pressure hypertrophied right ventricle. Death is due to right ventricular failure, or less commonly to hypoxia, cerebral abscess, or infective endocarditis.[12,38,39]

Nonrestrictive atrial septal defects with mild to moderate pulmonary stenosis are clinically analogous to isolated nonrestrictive ostium secundum atrial septal defects (see Chapter 15), although pulmonary stenosis attracts attention earlier because of the conspicuous murmur.[10,18] Cases of relatively asymptomatic survival into the sixth and seventh decades are on record, including a 59-year-old man with a large sinus venous defect and calcific pulmonary stenosis.[19] Familial pulmonary valve stenosis with atrial septal defect was reported in a mother and her two children.[9]

Physical Appearance

Pulmonary stenosis with a right-to-left shunt through a patent foramen ovale results in trivial to marked cyanosis that may be evident only during exercise.[2,8,15] Growth and development are poor when right ventricular failure begins in infancy or early childhood. Mild or intermittent

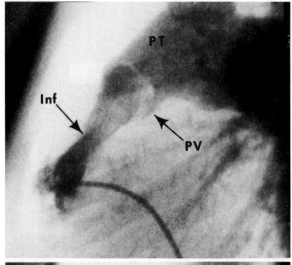

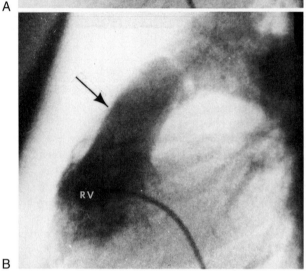

Figure 16–3

A, Lateral right ventricular angiocardiogram in a 5-year-old girl with severe mobile pulmonary valve stenosis (PV) and dynamic systolic narrowing of the infundibulum (Inf). There was a 1.4 to 1 left-to-right shunt through an atrial septal defect despite suprasystemic right ventricular pressure. The pulmonary trunk (PT) was dilated. *B,* Diastolic frame shows disappearance of infundibulum narrowing *(arrow).* RV, right ventricle.

right-to-left shunts are sometimes manifested by redness of the fingertips and toes rather than by cyanosis[41] (see Fig. 16–4) or by highly colored cheeks.[1,8] Central cyanosis of a right-to-left shunt must be distinguished from peripheral cyanosis of diminished skin blood flow caused by the low cardiac output of severe pulmonary stenosis. Peripheral cyanosis is accompanied by cold hands and feet and tends to be more pronounced in the lower extremities. When skin blood flow is improved by warmth, peripheral cyanosis diminishes and may vanish while central cyanosis becomes more evident. Children with a nonrestrictive atrial septal defect and mild to moderate pulmonary stenosis may have a delicate gracile body habitus with weight more affected than height (see Fig. 15–14). Noonan syndrome (see Fig. 11–7C) is associated with dysplastic pulmonary valve stenosis, which may coexist with an atrial septal defect.

The Arterial Pulse

In cases of severe pulmonary stenosis with right-to-left interatrial shunt, the systemic arterial pulse is small unless the reversed shunt is sufficient to maintain adequate left ventricular stroke volume. With the advent of right ventricular failure, the arterial pulse decreases despite increased flow of right atrial blood into the left side of the heart.

The Jugular Venous Pulse

When pulmonary stenosis coexists with a nonrestrictive atrial septal defect, the hypertrophied right ventricle is less distensible, and the right atrium contracts with greater force, so the A waves are prominent. The contour and height of the jugular pulse is determined by the presence and degree of pulmonary stenosis, not by the atrial defect. When pulmonary stenosis is severe enough to reverse the shunt, jugular venous A waves are large or even giant (see

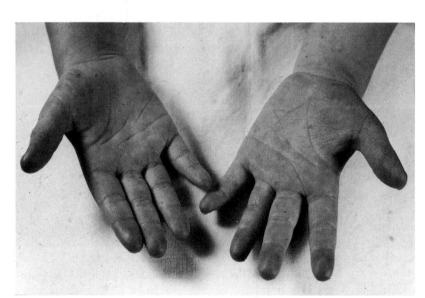

Figure 16–4

Red fingertips without cyanosis or clubbing in a 6-year-old boy with severe mobile pulmonary valve stenosis (gradient 108 mm Hg), a small intermittent right-to-left shunt across a patent foramen ovale, and a normal systemic arterial oxygen saturation.

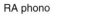

RA phono

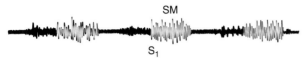

SM

S₁

RA pulse

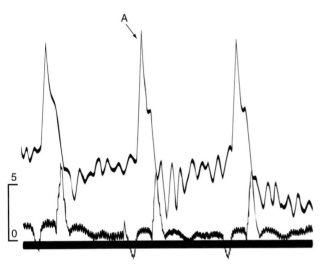

A

5

0

Figure 16–5

Tracings from a cyanotic woman who underwent surgical repair at 58 years of age for severe mobile pulmonary valve stenosis (gradient 120 mm Hg) that was associated with a reversed shunt through a patent foramen ovale. Large A waves (*arrow*) were present in the right atrial pressure pulse (RA). The right atrial intracardiac phonocardiogram (RA PHONO) recorded holosystolic murmur (SM) of tricuspid regurgitation. A soft presystolic murmur is represented by vibrations just before the first heart sound (S₁).

Figs. 16–5 and 16–6A). With the advent of right ventricular failure, the A wave remains dominant while the mean jugular venous pressure rises and with it the V wave, especially if tricuspid regurgitation coexists.

Precordial Movement and Palpation

Pulmonary stenosis with a right-to-left interatrial shunt is associated with precordial palpation similar to severe isolated pulmonary valve stenosis (see Chapter 11). A nonrestrictive atrial septal defect with mild to moderate pulmonary stenosis generates precordial signs similar to those of an isolated atrial septal defect of equivalent size, with the exception of a systolic thrill, which almost invariably means coexisting pulmonary valve stenosis.[15]

Auscultation

Severe pulmonary valve stenosis with a right-to-left interatrial shunt is accompanied by auscultatory signs analogous to those of isolated severe pulmonary stenosis (see Chapter

24). The stenotic murmur is maximum in the second left intercostal space (see Fig. 16–7) and radiates upward and to the left. The murmur is long, extending up to or beyond the aortic component of the second heart sound (Figs. 16–7 and 16–8C,D).[43] A grade 4/6 murmur peaks late in systole, assumes a kite-shaped configuration,[17,43] and obscures the aortic component of the second heart sound (see Figs. 16–7 and 16–8D). In the neonate with critical pulmonary valve stenosis and right ventricular failure, the pulmonary stenotic murmur is short and soft, and the pulmonary component of the second heart sound is delayed, soft, or absent (see Figs. 16–7 and 16–8D). The most prominent auscultatory sign may be the holosystolic murmur of tricuspid regurgitation (see Fig. 16–5).

Presystolic distention of the right ventricle (see Fig. 16–6B) is accompanied by a fourth heart sound that is occasionally long enough to qualify as a murmur (see Figs. 16–5 and 16–7). A short presystolic murmur can be generated as powerful right atrial contraction forces blood across a restrictive patent foramen ovale. Alternatively, a large right atrial A wave transmitted into the right ventricle (see Fig. 16–6) can exceed the pulmonary artery diastolic pressure, open the pulmonary valve, and generate presystolic flow and a presystolic murmur.

When a nonrestrictive atrial septal defect is associated with mild to moderate pulmonary stenosis, the auscultatory signs resemble an isolated nonrestrictive ostium

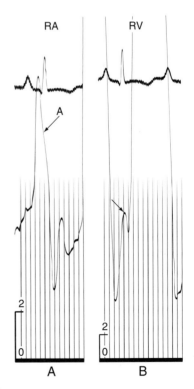

RA

RV

A

2

0

2

0

A

B

Figure 16–6

Right atrial (RA) and right ventricular (RV) pressure pulses from a 15-month-old cyanotic boy with severe mobile pulmonary valve stenosis (gradient 105 mm Hg) and a right-to-left shunt across a patent foramen ovale. A, There were large A waves (*arrow*) in the right atrial pressure pulse. B, The A wave was transmitted into the right ventricle (RV) as presystolic distention (*arrow*).

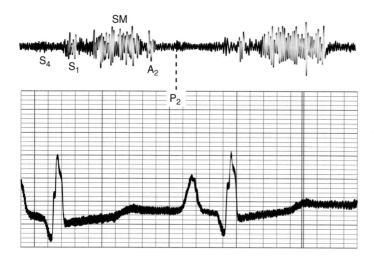

Figure 16–7

Phonocardiogram from the second left intercostal space of a 5-month-old cyanotic girl with severe mobile pulmonary valve stenosis, a right-to-left shunt across a patent foramen ovale, and suprasystolic right ventricular pressure. A fourth heart sound (S_4) in the first cycle became a short presystolic murmur in the next cycle. A long systolic murmur (SM) goes up to the aortic component on the second heart sound (A_2). The pulmonary component (P_2) is late and diminutive (*arrow*). Tall peaked right atrial P waves appear in lead 2 of the electrocardiogram.

secundum atrial septal defect, with three exceptions. First, an ejection sound is generated by the mobile stenotic pulmonary valve. Second, the pulmonary systolic murmur is loud and long (Figs. 16–9 and 16–10). Third, the second heart sound is more widely split owing to greater delay in the pulmonary component (see Figs. 16–8*B,C*, 16–9, and 16–10). The greater the degree of pulmonary stenosis, the later and softer the pulmonary component of the second heart sound (see Figs. 16–7 and 16–8).

Stenosis of the pulmonary artery and its branches with an ostium secundum atrial septal defect (Fig. 16–11) is accompanied by especially wide thoracic distribution of systolic murmurs that are reinforced by the hyperkinetic pulmonary blood flow of the atrial septal defect. The second heart sound is persistently split because of the atrial septal defect (see Fig. 16–11).

The Electrocardiogram

The electrocardiogram of pulmonary valve stenosis with right-to-left interatrial shunt is similar to that of severe iso-lated pulmonary valve stenosis (Figs. 16–12 and 16–13; see Chapter 11).[6,31] Peaked right atrial P waves appear in lead 2 and in right precordial leads (see Figs. 16–7, 16–12, and 16–13) and are occasionally exceptionally tall (see Figs. 16–7 and 16–12).[2,8] P wave duration in lead 2 is prolonged when a large right atrium writes the terminal inscription of the P wave.[26] Right axis deviation (see Fig. 16–12) is occasionally extreme (see Fig. 16–13). The terminal QRS forces may be prolonged and slurred (see Fig. 16–13). Severe right ventricular hypertrophy with suprasystemic right ventricular pressure is manifested by R waves of great amplitude in right and mid-precordial leads with upward convexity of ST segments and deeply inverted T waves, and by deep left precordial S waves (see Figs. 16–12 and 16–13).[6,7,31] The striking ST segment and T wave patterns sometimes extend to lead V_4.[31] Small q waves appear in lead V_1 (see Fig. 16–13) when the electrode topographically overlies a large right atrium (see Chapter 13).

The electrocardiogram of a nonrestrictive atrial septal defect with left-to-right shunt and mild to moderate pulmonary stenosis is similar to that of an isolated ostium

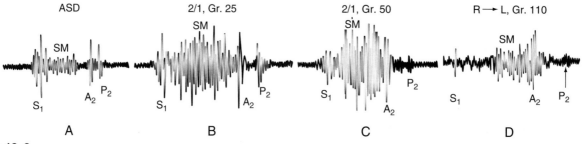

Figure 16–8

Phonocardiograms from the second left intercostal space of four patients whose congenital heart disease varied from isolated atrial septal defect (ASD) to atrial septal defect with mild, moderate, or severe pulmonary valve stenosis. *A,* Isolated atrial septal defect with 2.5 to 1 left-to-right shunt. A short soft systolic murmur (SM) ends well before both components of the split second heart sound. A_2, aortic component; P_2, pulmonary component. *B,* Atrial septal defect with a 2 to 1 left-to-right shunt and a 25 mm Hg gradient across a stenotic pulmonary valve. The systolic murmur is louder and longer and goes up to but does not obscure the aortic component of the second heart sound. The splitting is wider because pulmonary closure is later. *C,* Atrial septal defect with a 2 to 1 left-to-right shunt and 50 mm Hg gradient across a stenotic pulmonary valve. The loud long systolic murmur now extends beyond the aortic component of the second heart sound. The pulmonary component is soft and even later. *D,* Severe pulmonary valve stenosis (gradient 110 mm Hg) with right-to-left shunt through a patent foramen ovale. A kite-shaped systolic murmur envelopes the aortic component of the second sound. The pulmonary component is diminutive and delayed.

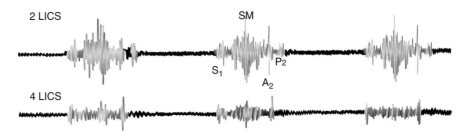

Figure 16–9

Phonocardiogram from a 23-year-old man with a 2.4 to 1 left-to-right shunt through an ostium secundum atrial septal defect and a 45 mm Hg gradient across a mobile stenotic pulmonary valve. The first heart sound (S_1) is normal. A prominent crescendo-decrescendo systolic murmur (SM) maximal in the second left intercostal space (2 LICS) goes up to but does not envelope the aortic component of the second heart sound (A_2). The pulmonary component (P_2) is delayed and soft. 4 LICS, fourth left intercostal space.

secundum atrial septal defect (see Chapter 15) except for right ventricular hypertrophy (Figs. 16–14 and 16–15). P waves may be peaked and moderately tall (see Fig. 16–14). The QRS axis is vertical or rightward (see Figs. 16–14 and 16–15). Terminal force prolongation widens the R wave in lead aVR and widens the S waves in leads 1, aVL, and V_6 (see Figs. 16–14 and 16–15). An rsR prime pattern in lead V_1 is represented by a smaller s wave and a taller R prime than in atrial septal defect without pulmonary stenosis (see Figs. 16–14 and 16–15).

The X-Ray

Severe pulmonary stenosis with a right-to-left interatrial shunt is associated with a chest x-ray analogous to isolated severe pulmonary valve stenosis (Fig. 16–16; see Chapter 11). Lung fields are oligemic because right atrial blood escapes across the atrial septum, reducing the right ventricular output, and decreased pulmonary blood flow becomes more apparent with the advent of right

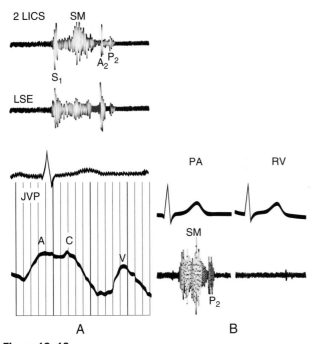

Figure 16–10

Phonocardiograms from a 6-year-old girl with a 2.3 to 1 left-to-right shunt across an ostium secundum atrial septal defect and a 25 mm Hg gradient across a mobile stenotic pulmonary valve. A, A prominent crescendo-decrescendo systolic murmur (SM) in the second left intercostal space (2 LICS) ends before the aortic component of the second heart sound (A_2). The pulmonary component (P_2) is moderately delayed and relatively soft. The systolic murmur is softer and shorter at the lower left sternal edge (LSE), where both components of the split second heart sound are recorded. The jugular venous pulse exhibits a small dominant A wave and a blunted X descent (lower tracing). B, Intracardiac phonocardiogram from within the main pulmonary artery (PA) recorded a prominent crescendo-decrescendo systolic murmur (SM) that ends before pulmonary valve closure (P_2). The murmur vanished when the microphone was withdrawn into the right ventricle (RV).

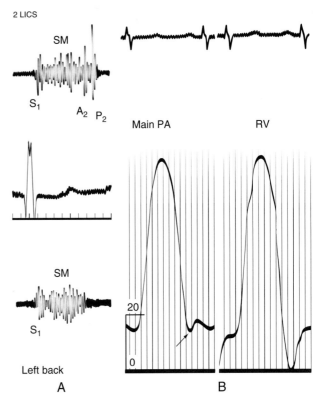

Figure 16–11

Tracings from a 5-year-old boy with bilateral pulmonary artery stenosis (gradient 50 mm Hg), an ostium secundum atrial septal defect, and a 2.2 to 1 left-to-right shunt. A, The phonocardiograms show systolic murmurs (SM) of approximately equal intensity in the second left intercostal space (2 LICS) and in the left back. Persistent splitting of the second heart sound (A_2/P_2) was due to the atrial septal defect. B, The pressure pulse in the main pulmonary artery (PA) shows the characteristic contour of bilateral stenosis of pulmonary artery branches with a steep rise and a rapid fall to a low dicrotic notch (arrow). The right ventricular pulse (RV) is shown for comparison.

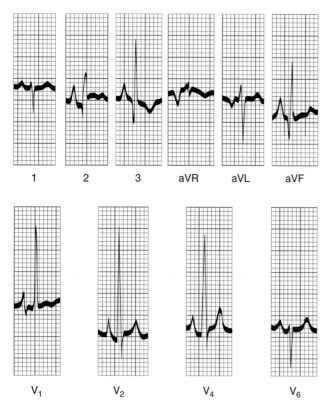

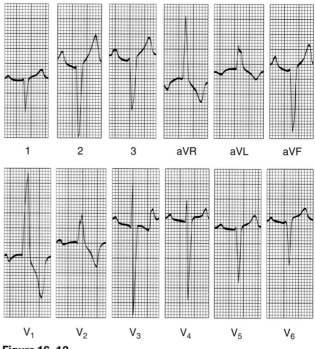

Figure 16–12

Electrocardiogram from the 5-month-old cyanotic girl with severe pulmonary valve stenosis and a right-to-left shunt across a patent foramen ovale referred to in Figure 16–7. Tall peaked right atrial P waves are present in leads 2, 3, aVF, and V_{1-4} appropriate for a 20 mm Hg A wave in the right atrial pressure pulse. There is right axis deviation and right ventricular hypertrophy manifested by tall monophasic R waves in leads V_{1-4} and a deep S wave in lead V_6 appropriate for suprasystemic right ventricular pressure.

Figure 16–13

Electrocardiogram from a 20-year-old man with severe mobile pulmonary valve stenosis (gradient 110 mm Hg) and a right-to-left shunt across a patent foramen ovale. A tall right atrial P wave is present in lead 2. Small q waves in right precordial leads are evidence of right atrial enlargement. The PR interval is prolonged. Right ventricular hypertrophy is reflected in the striking right axis deviation, the tall monophasic R wave and deeply inverted T wave in lead V_1, and the deep S wave in lead V_6.

ventricular failure. The pulmonary trunk is dilated (Fig. 16–17, and see Figs. 16–1, 16–3, and 16–16) for reasons analogous to the dilatation in cases of isolated mobile pulmonary valve stenosis (see Chapter 11).[7,8,12,38] Heart size is increased because of enlargement of the right atrium and right ventricle (see Figs. 16–16 and 16–17).[8,12,14,22] The right ventricular apex is not boot-shaped, because the size of the left ventricle is not reduced (see Fig. 16–16) (see Chapter 18).

The x-rays of a nonrestrictive atrial septal defect with mild to moderate pulmonary stenosis are indistinguishable from isolated ostium secundum atrial septal defect (Fig. 16–18).[27]

The Echocardiogram

The echocardiogram of severe mobile pulmonary valve stenosis with a right-to-left shunt through a patent foramen ovale is similar to isolated severe pulmonary valve stenosis (see Chapter 14). Color flow imaging records a high-velocity jet directed toward the left pulmonary artery (Fig. 16–19A) and the continuous wave Doppler signal

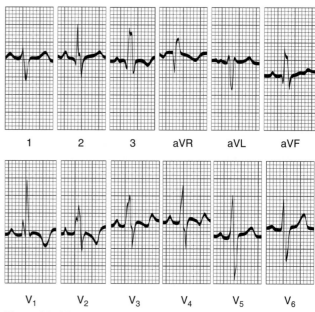

Figure 16–14

Electrocardiogram from an 18-year-old man with an ostium secundum atrial septal defect, a 2 to 1 left-to-right shunt, and a 25 mm Hg gradient across a mobile stenotic pulmonary valve. The P waves in lead 2 and in leads V_{2-4} are peaked but not tall. Right ventricular hypertrophy of pulmonary stenosis is manifested by right axis deviation, a tall R prime wave in lead V_1, and deep S waves in leads V_{5-6}. Prolongation of the terminal portion of the QRS axis in lead aVR is appropriate for the atrial septal defect.

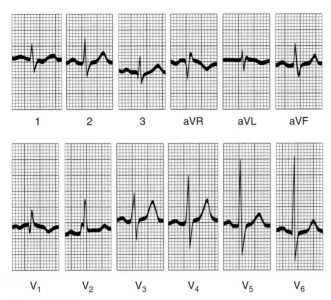

Figure 16–15

Electrocardiogram from the 23-year-old man with a 2.4 to 1 left-to-right shunt through an ostium secundum atrial septal defect and a 45 mm Hg gradient across a mobile stenotic pulmonary valve referred to in Figure 16–9. The normal P waves, the vertical QRS axis, the rsR prime in lead V_1, and the slightly prolonged terminal force in leads V_1 and aVR are appropriate for the atrial septal defect.

establishes the peak velocity and the gradient (Fig. 16–19B). Two-dimensional imaging identifies the patent foramen ovale with its valve (see Fig. 15–46), and color flow imaging defines the right-to-left shunt.

The echocardiogram of nonrestrictive ostium secundum atrial septal defect with mild to moderate pulmonary valve stenosis is analogous to an isolated atrial septal defect of the same location and size (see Chapter 15) except for coexisting pulmonary stenosis. Real-time imaging identifies the mobile stenotic pulmonary valve, and Doppler interrogation establishes the gradient (Fig. 16–20).

Summary

Severe pulmonary valve stenosis with a right-to-left interatrial shunt is accompanied by a conspicuous systolic murmur in a neonate except for the disarmingly soft murmur associated with pinpoint pulmonary valve stenosis and right ventricular failure. Mild or intermittent cyanosis or digital erythema precedes persistent cyanosis. Symptoms can be appreciable while cyanosis is mild. Giddiness, lightheadedness, and occasionally syncope occur, especially with effort. Physical underdevelopment coincides with right ventricular failure. Large A waves appear in the jugular venous pulse and are in contrast to the small systemic arterial pulse. The right ventricular impulse is strong and sustained and is accompanied by presystolic distention. There is a systolic thrill in the second left intercostal space. A pulmonary ejection sound precedes the pulmonary stenotic murmur, which is loud and long, extending up to or beyond the aortic component of the second heart sound. The pulmonary component of

Figure 16–16

X-rays from the 15-month-old cyanotic boy with severe mobile pulmonary valve stenosis, suprasystemic right ventricular pressure, and a right-to-left shunt across a patent foramen ovale. The jugular venous pulse is shown in Figure 16–6. *A,* The pulmonary trunk (PT) is dilated and an enlarged right ventricle (RV) occupies the apex. *B,* In the left anterior oblique, a dilated right ventricle (RV) displaces the left ventricle posteriorly. *C,* In the lateral projection, the normal location of the inferior vena cava *(arrow)* at the junction of the left ventricle and diaphragm indicates that the left ventricle is not enlarged.

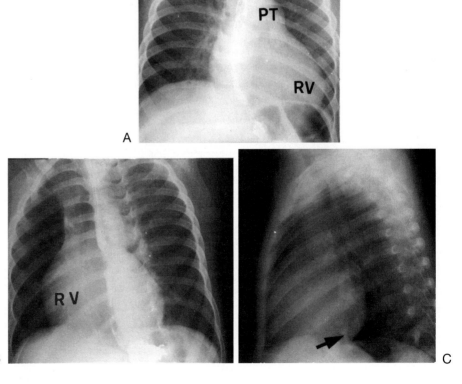

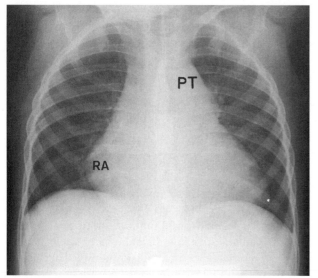

Figure 16–17

X-ray from a 30-month-old cyanotic boy with severe mobile pulmonary valve stenosis, a right ventricular systolic pressure of 130 mm Hg, and a right-to-left shunt across a patent foramen ovale. The pulmonary trunk (PT) is dilated. Right atrial enlargement (RA) was in response to severe tricuspid regurgitation.

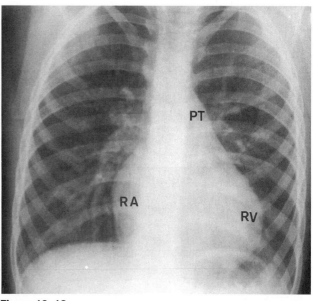

Figure 16–18

X-ray from a 10-year-old girl with an ostium secundum atrial septal defect, a 2.1 to 1 left to right shunt, and a 25 mm Hg gradient across a mobile stenotic pulmonary valve. The x-ray closely resembles an isolated ostium secundum atrial septal defect with increased pulmonary blood flow, a dilated pulmonary trunk (PT), an inconspicuous ascending aorta, a prominent right atrium (RA), and an enlarged right ventricle (RV) at the apex.

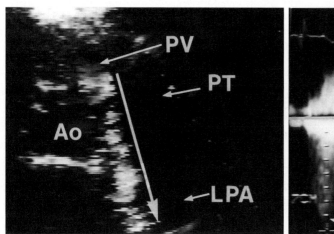

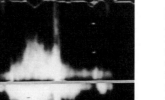

Figure 16–19

A, Black and white print of a color flow image from a 28-year-old woman with severe mobile pulmonary valve stenosis and a right-to-left shunt through a patent foramen ovale. A high-velocity jet across the pulmonary valve (PV) traverses the pulmonary trunk (PT) and enters the left pulmonary artery (LPA). Ao, aorta. *B,* Continuous wave Doppler across the pulmonary valve records a velocity of 7.0 m/sec, indicating a peak instantaneous gradient of 190 mm Hg.

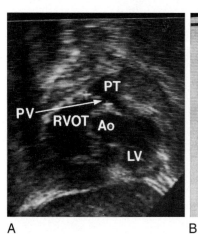

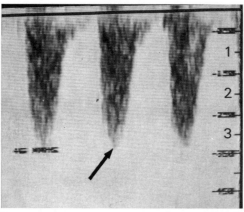

Figure 16–20

Echocardiogram with Doppler interrogation from a 7-year-old girl with mobile pulmonary valve stenosis and a left-to-right shunt through an ostium secundum atrial septal defect. *A,* Subcostal view shows the stenotic pulmonary valve (PV) above a well-formed right ventricular outflow tract (RVOT). The pulmonary trunk (PT) is dilated. Ao, aorta; LV, left ventricle. *B,* Continuous-wave Doppler across the stenotic pulmonary valve records a peak velocity (*arrow*) of 3.4 m/sec indicating a peak instantaneous gradient of 46 mm Hg.

the second heart sound is delayed, soft, or inaudible. Right atrial P waves can be strikingly tall, and right axis deviation is sometimes extreme. Right precordial leads show R waves of great amplitude followed by upward convexity of the ST segments and deep inversion of the T waves, while left precordial leads exhibit deep S waves and upright T waves. The lung fields are oligemic, the pulmonary trunk is dilated, the ascending aorta is inconspicuous, and the cardiac silhouette reflects enlargement of the right atrium and right ventricle. Real-time echocardiography identifies the mobile stenotic pulmonary valve, Doppler interrogation determines the gradient, and color flow imaging detects the right-to-left shunt across a patent foramen ovale.

Nonrestrictive atrial septal defect with left-to-right shunt and mild to moderate pulmonary stenosis clinically resembles an isolated ostium secundum atrial septal defect, but when pulmonary stenosis coexists, the malformation is discovered earlier because of the prominent pulmonary stenotic murmur. The jugular venous pulse shows dominant A waves rather than equal A and V crests. The right ventricular impulse is dynamic and a pulmonary stenotic thrill is consistently present. Auscultatory signs are similar to those of isolated ostium secundum atrial septal defect, but the pulmonary stenotic murmur is louder and longer, a pulmonary ejection sound is likely, and fixed splitting of the second heart sound is associated with a delayed and softer pulmonary component. The electrocardiogram shows right ventricular hypertrophy that would be inappropriate for an isolated atrial septal defect. The x-ray and echocardiogram resemble isolated ostium secundum atrial septal defect, except for the pulmonic stenotic Doppler gradient.

REFERENCES

1. Abrahams DG, Wood P: Pulmonary stenosis with normal aortic root. Br Heart J 13:519, 1951.
2. Allanby KD, Campbell M: Congenital pulmonary stenosis with closed ventricular septum. Guy's Hosp Rep 98:18, 1949.
3. Arnett EN, Aisner SC, Lewis KB, et al: Pulmonic stenosis, atrial septal defect and left-to-right shunting with intact ventricular septum. Chest 78:759, 1980.
4. Bierman FZ, Williams RG: Subxiphoid two-dimensional imaging of the interatrial septum in infants and neonates with congenital heart disease. Circulation 60:80, 1979.
5. Broadbent JC, Wood EH, Burchell HB: Left-to-right intracardiac shunts in the presence of pulmonary stenosis. Proc Staff Meet Mayo Clin 28:101, 1953.
6. Burch GE, DePasquale NP: The electrocardiogram, vectorcardiogram, and ventricular gradient in combined pulmonary stenosis and interatrial communication. Am J Cardiol 7:646, 1961.
7. Callahan JA, Brandenburg RO, Swan HJC: Pulmonary stenosis and interatrial communication with cyanosis: Hemodynamic and clinical study of ten patients. Am J Med 19:189, 1955.
8. Campbell M: Simple pulmonary stenosis: Pulmonary valvular stenosis with a closed ventricular septum. Br Heart J 16:273, 1954.
9. Ciuffo AA, Cunningham E, Traill TA: Familial pulmonary valve stenosis, atrial septal defect, and unique electrocardiogram abnormalities. J Med Genet 22:311, 1985.
10. deCastro CM, Nelson WP, Jones RC, et al: Pulmonary stenosis: Cyanosis, interatrial communication and inadequate right ventricu-

11. Dueghar DC, Zak GA: Cardiac catheterization in congenital heart disease. I. Four cases of pulmonary stenosis with increased pulmonary blood flow. Guy's Hosp Rep 101:1, 1952.
12. Edwards JE, Carey LS, Neufeld HN, Lester RG: Congenital Heart Disease. Philadelphia, W.B. Saunders, 1965.
13. Eldridge FL, Hultgren HN: Pulmonary stenosis and increased pulmonary blood flow. Am Heart J 49:838, 1955.
14. Engle MA, Taussig HB: Valvular pulmonic stenosis with intact ventricular septum and patent foramen ovale: Report of illustrative cases and analysis of clinical syndrome. Circulation 2:481, 1950.
15. Evans JR, Rowe RD, Keith JD: The clinical diagnosis of atrial septal defect in children. Am J Med 30:345, 1961.
16. Franchi RH, Gay BB Jr: Congenital stenosis of the pulmonary artery branches: A classification, with postmortem findings in two cases. Am J Med 35:512, 1963.
17. Gamboa R, Hugenholtz PG, Nadas AS: Accuracy of the phonocardiogram in assessing severity of aortic and pulmonic stenosis. Circulation 30:35, 1964.
18. Grissom RL, Campbell JA, Selverstone LA, et al: Clinical and physiologic studies of patients with pulmonic stenosis and auricular septal defects. J Lab Clin Med 36:831, 1950.
19. Hardy WE, Gnoj J, Ayers SM, et al: Pulmonic stenosis and associated atrial septal defects in older patients. Am J Cardiol 24:130, 1969.
20. Hubbard TF, Koszewski BJ: Pulmonary stenosis with increased pulmonary blood flow. Arch Intern Med 97:327, 1956.
21. Johnson AM: Hypertrophic infundibular stenosis complicating simple pulmonary valve stenosis. Br Heart J 21:429, 1959.
22. Johnson RP, Johnson EE: Congenital pulmonic stenosis with open foramen ovale in infancy. Report of five proved cases. Am Heart J 44:344, 1952.
23. Joly F, Carlotti J, Sicot JR, Piton A: Cardiopathies congénitales, les triologies de Fallot. Arch Mal Coeur 43:687, 1950.
24. Leatham A, Weitzman D: Auscultatory and phonocardiographic signs of pulmonary stenosis. Br Heart J 19:303, 1957.
25. Little JB, Lavender JP, DeSanctis RW: The narrow infundibulum in pulmonary valvular stenosis: Its preoperative diagnosis by angiocardiography. Circulation 28:182, 1963.
26. Macruz R, Perloff JK, Case RB: A method for the electrocardiographic recognition of atrial enlargement. Circulation 17:882, 1958.
27. Magidson O, Cosby RS, Dimitroff SP, et al: Pulmonary stenosis with left to right shunt. Am J Med 17:311, 1954.
28. Marin-Garcia J, Fitch CW, Shenefelt RE: Primary right ventricular tumor (fibroma) simulating cyanotic heart disease in a newborn. J Am Coll Cardiol 3:868, 1984.
29. Moffitt GR Jr, Zinsser HF Jr, Kuo PT, et al: Pulmonary stenosis with left to right intracardiac shunts. Am J Med 16:521, 1954.
30. Morgagni JB: Seats and Causes of Diseases. London, Millar & Cadell in the Strand and Johnson & Payne in Pater-Noster Row, 1769.
31. Munoz-Armas S, del Toro A, Sodi-Pollares D, de la Cruz MV: Tetralogy of Fallot and pulmonic stenosis with intact interventricular septum: Anatomic and electrocardiographic study. Am J Cardiol 21:773, 1968.
32. Neptune WB, Bailey CP, Goldberg H: The surgical correction of atrial septal defects associated with transposition of the pulmonary veins. J Thorac Cardiovasc Surg 25:623, 1953.
33. Ordway NK, Levy L II, Hyman AL, Bagnetto RL: Pulmonary stenosis with patent foramen ovale. Am Heart J 40:271, 1950.
34. Peacock TB: Contraction of the orifice of the pulmonary artery and communication between the cavities of the auricles by the foramen ovale. Trans Pathol Soc London 1:200, 1848.
35. Roberts WC, Shemin RJ, Kent KM: Frequency and direction of interatrial shunting in valvular pulmonic stenosis with intact ventricular septum and without left ventricular inflow or outflow obstruction. Am Heart J 99:142, 1980.
36. Rudolph AM, Nadas AS, Goodale WT: Intracardiac left-to-right shunt with pulmonic stenosis. Am Heart J 48:808, 1954.
37. Selzer A, Carnes WH: The role of pulmonary stenosis in the production of chronic cyanosis. Am Heart J 45:382, 1953.
38. Selzer A, Carnes WH: The types of pulmonary stenosis and their clinical recognition. Mod Concepts Cardiovasc Dis 18:45, 1949.
39. Selzer A, Carnes WH, Noble CA Jr, et al: The syndrome of pulmonary stenosis with patent foramen ovale. Am J Med 6:3, 1949.
40. Shafter HA, Bliss HA: Pulmonary artery stenosis. Am J Med 26:517, 1959.

41. Silverman BK, Nadas AS, Wittenborg MH, et al: Pulmonary stenosis with intact ventricular septum: Correlation of clinical and physiologic data, with review of operative results. Am J Med 20:53, 1956.

42. Vermillion MB, Leight L, Davis LA: Pulmonary artery stenosis. Circulation 17:55, 1958.

43. Vogelpoel L, Schrire V: Auscultatory and phonocardiographic assessment of pulmonary stenosis with intact ventricular septum. Circulation 22:55, 1960.

44. White PD, Hurst JW, Fennell RH: Survival to the age of seventy-five years with congenital pulmonary stenosis and patent foramen ovale. Circulation 2:558, 1950.

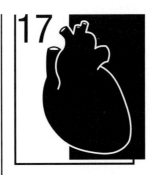

Ventricular Septal Defect

A developmental defect of the heart occurs from which cyanosis does not ensue in spite of the fact that a communication exists between the cavities of the two ventricles and in spite of the fact that admixture of venous blood and arterial blood occurs. This congenital defect, which is even compatible with a long life, is a simple one. It comprises a defect in the interventricular septum.[188]

Henri Roger, 1879

At necropsy, as described by Roger, "The ventricular walls [in ventricular septal defect] show no alteration, but in the upper portion of the interventricular septum beneath the mitral valve is an orifice that establishes a communication between the two ventricles."[188]

Roger also recognized the high incidence of this defect: "Among the congenital defects of the heart compatible with life and perhaps a long one, one of the most frequent which I have encountered . . . is the communication between the two ventricles because of failure of occlusion of the interventricular septum."[188]

Ventricular septal defects are the most common gross morphologic congenital malformations of the heart or circulation except for the bicuspid aortic valve (see Chapter 7), accounting for approximately 20% of all cases of congenital heart disease. Prevalence is reportedly as high as 3.3 to 3.8 per 1,000 live births,[64,74,100,135,268] an incidence that takes into account the frequency of spontaneous closure and the facility of echocardiographic diagnosis in the neonate especially the diagnosis of small defects in the muscular trabecular septum.[101,102,135,159,265]

Henri Roger believed that "this congenital defect . . . is a simple one,"[188] but more than a century later, there is still no uniform consensus on how best to characterize and classify the diverse types of defects to which the ventricular septum is subject. The ventricular septum is a complex nonplanar partition whose components are best defined according to anatomic landmarks on the right side of the septal surface (Fig. 17–1).[7,13,85,208] There are three major muscular components—the inlet septum (lightly trabeculated), the trabecular septum (heavily trabeculated), and the infundibular septum (non-trabeculated). Ventricular septal defects vary in size, shape and location, and are classified according to their relationship to the membranous, inlet, trabecular, and infundibular septum. The *membranous septum* is divided by

the tricuspid annulus into ventriculo-atrial and interventricular components and abuts the three major components of the muscular septum which radiate from it (see Fig. 17–1). The *inlet septum* is limited by the tensor attachments of the tricuspid valve. The location of the *infundibular* or *outlet septum* is defined by its name. The *trabecular septum* lies between the inlet septum and the infundibular septum.

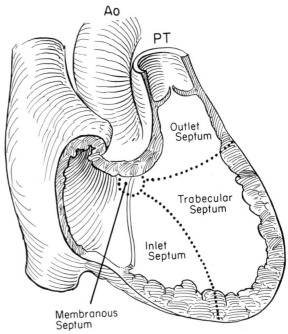

Figure 17–1

Four components of the ventricular septurn shown here from the right ventricular aspect are now described by Anderson, et al, as inlet and outlet components of the right ventricle because these areas do not correspond to septal structures as initially suggested. (Modified from Anderson RH, Becker AE, Lucchese E et al: Morphology of Congenital Heart Disease, Baltimore, University Park Press, 1983.)

Approximately 80% of ventricular septal defects are *perimembranous*, the prefix *peri* underscoring extension into adjacent portions of the inlet, trabecular, and infundubular septum (see Fig. 17–1). Large perimembranous defects encroach upon all three portions of the contiguous muscular septum (Fig. 17–2*A*). *Muscular ventricular septal defects* are prevalent in neonates with estimates as high as 53/1000 live births, but approximately 90% close spontaneously within 1 to 10 months of age.[274]

Atrioventricular conduction tissue penetrates the ventriculo-atrial portion of the membranous septum, with the His bundle and bundle branches running beneath the deficient interventricular component of the membranous septum close to the free edge of the ventricular septal defect.[7,8,225]

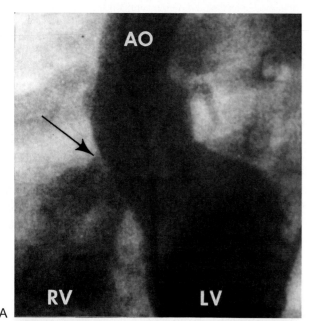

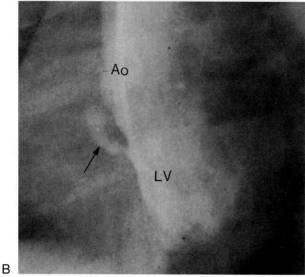

Figure 17–2

A, Left anterior oblique left ventriculogram (LV) from a 4-year-old boy with a moderately restrictive perimembranous ventricular septal defect (*arrow*). RV, right ventricle; AO, aorta. *B*, Left anterior oblique left ventriculogram (LV) from a 21 year old male with a tiny perimembranous ventricular septal defect (*arrow*).

The most common types of *muscular* defects are within the trabecular septum.[7,19,73,85,195,243] These malformations, which are more evident from the left septal surface, vary from small to large, from single to multiple (Fig. 17–3), to a honeycombed Swiss cheese structure with sieve-like fenestrations, to tortuous sinusoidal tracks threaded among septal trabeculae without through-and-through perforations.[7,17,73,85,195,243] Sieve-like fenestrations or multiple small muscular defects have the same net functional effect as a single large defect.

Isolated defects in the *inlet septum* represent approximately 8% of ventricular septal defects at surgery.[129] There is a difference between an inlet ventricular septal defect that is bordered entirely by myocardium and an inlet defect that involves the basal portion near the cardiac crux and is bordered in part by bridging atrioventricular valve tissue (see Chapter 15).[7,8,13,85,208,209]

The *infundibular septum* is represented by a small portion of muscle interposed between the outflow components of the left and right ventricles.[83] A sleeve of subpulmonary infundibulum supports the leaflets of the pulmonary valve and separates the right ventricular outflow tract from the surface of the heart rather than from the left ventricular outflow track. Ventricular septal defects in the infundibular septum are also called supracristal, subpulmonary, subarterial, or doubly committed, and account for approximately 5% to 7% of these defects in North America and Western Europe but for approximately 30% in Asian patients.[8,10,19,83,129] Infundibular septal defects can be entirely muscular or can be partially rimmed by semilunar valve tissue (subarterial).[85] The defect is considered *doubly committed subarterial* when there is little or no muscle interposed between the outflow components of the left and right ventricles together with absence of the septal component of the subpulmonary infundibulum, so the aortic and pulmonary leaflets are in fibrous continuity.[7,8,19,83,85,129,208] Because doubly committed subarterial defects lie immediately beneath the valves of both arterial trunks, the left and right coronary cusps of the aortic valve tend to prolapse into the outflow tract of the right ventricle (see section on *Ventricular Septal Defect with Aortic Regurgitation*). Much less commonly, a pulmonary cusp prolapses through the defect.[80]

Atrioventricular septal malalignment[85] involves an inlet ventricular septal defect and is usually accompanied by straddling of the tensor apparatus of an atrioventricular valve that inserts (straddles) onto both sides of the ventricular septum.[242] So-called *Eisenmenger malalignment* is represented by a perimembranous ventricular septal defect that occurs with anterior deviation of the infundibular septum.[253,269] Not relevant to this chapter is *malalignment between infundibular and trabecular septum* that is associated with Fallot's tetralogy (see Chapter 18) or much less commonly with coarctation of the aorta (see Chapter 8).

The tendency for ventricular septal defects—especially perimembranous and trabecular muscular defects—to decrease in size finds its ultimate expression in *complete*

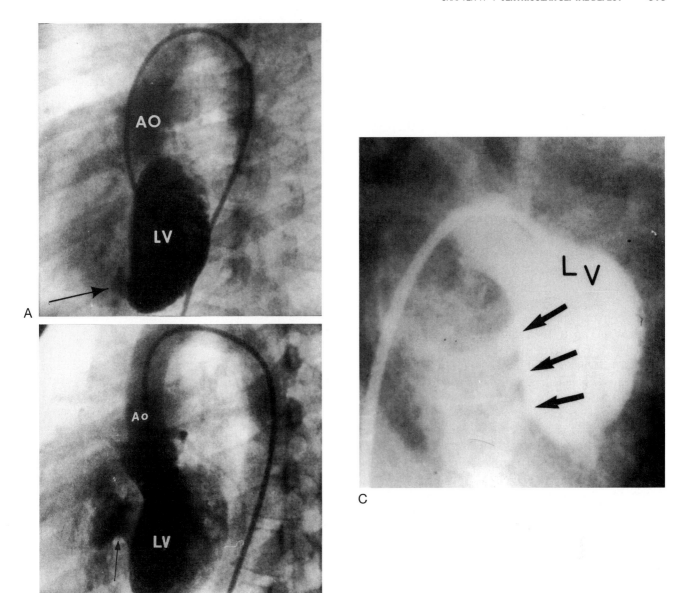

Figure 17–3
A, Left anterior oblique left ventriculogram (LV) from a 5-year-old girl with a restrictive ventricular septal defect in the low muscular/trabecular septum (*arrow*). AO, aorta. *B,* Left anterior oblique left ventriculogram from a 6-year-old girl with a nonrestrictive ventricular septal defect in the mid portion of the muscular/trabecular septum (*arrow*). *C,* Lateral left ventriculogram (LV) from a three week old male with three moderately restrictive defects in the muscular/trabecular septum.

spontaneous closure.[9,20,78,101,132,205] A ventricular septal defect may remain anatomically open but functionally closed with absent or negligible shunt (Figs. 17–2*B* and 17–4). Henri Roger did not anticipate spontaneous closure. "The pathologic state of the heart existing before birth and consisting of an arrest of development is not susceptible to favorable changes, either by spontaneous evolution or by medical or surgical intervention."[188] In 1918, two reports speculated that ventricular septal defects might undergo spontaneous closure.[71,240] One report was entitled "The Possibility of a Loud Congenital Heart Murmur Disappearing When a Child Grows Up."[71] The other report carried the title "Can the Clinical Manifestations of Congenital Heart Disease Disappear with

the General Growth and Development of the Patient?"[240] However, four decades elapsed before spontaneous closure was firmly documented.* In 1960, Paul Wood wrote, "In any large series of geriatric necropsies . . . atrial septal defect is always well represented, but where's the maladie de Roger? Assuming it does not provide immortality, it must either close spontaneously in middle life or have long since run its mortal course."

The *incidence of spontaneous closure* varies considerably depending on the population under consideration, the method of diagnostic investigation, the type of defect, and

---

*See references 3, 28, 33, 51, 60, 78, 101, 102, 127, 142, 145, 150, 151, 198, 204, 236, 265, 266, 274, 275.

whether the defect(s) are solitary or multiple.[146,265] Incidence is estimated at 50% to 75% for restrictive perimembranous and trabecular muscular defects observed from birth.* The incidence of spontaneous closure for trabecular muscular defects[146] is reportedly equal to or somewhat higher than the incidence for perimembranous defects.[227,261] Moderately restrictive and nonrestrictive defects can also close spontaneously, but the probability is comparatively low with an incidence estimated at 5% to 10%.[52,60,78,127,146,150,155] Most defects that are destined to close do so within the first year of life[146,227] with approximately 60% closing before age three years and 90% closing before age 8 years.[5,20,28,33,44,99,101,127,151] Spontaneous closure has been reported in older children and young adults[70,99,127,217] and has been documented at age 23 years,[198] between age 26 years and 33 years,[28,246] and at age 46 years.[33] *Multiple* ventricular septal defects have a strong tendency to close, a conclusion appropriate for the observation that multiple defects are three times more prevalent in neonates than after 1 year of age.[63] Ventricular septal defects in preterm infants are about twice as frequent as in full-term infants, but the rate of spontaneous closure is the same,[146] calling into question the notion that defects reflect incomplete ventricular septation.[145] A spontaneously closed defect in the muscular trabecular septum is funnel-shaped with a sealed orifice on its right ventricular aspect and a residual patent orifice on its left ventricular aspect, with endocardial proliferation in the lumen of the funnel and hypertrophy around the exit. Muscular defects represented by Swiss cheese fenestrations do not close spontaneously. Defects in the inlet septum seldom decrease in size[205,276] but occasionally become occluded by bridging atrioventricular valve tissue (see Fig.15–87B). A decrease in size of the malaligned ventricular septal defect of Fallot's tetralogy is exceptional (see Chapter 18).[153]

The mechanism(s) by which perimembranous ventricular septal defects close include adherence of septal tricuspid leaflet tissue to the margins of the defect, less commonly prolapse of an aortic cusp, and rarely intrusion of a sinus of Valsalva aneurysm.* A reduction in size of a perimembranous ventricular septal defect by adherence of tricuspid leaflet tissue is seldom accompanied by tricuspid regurgitation.[103]

Laennec described a *ventricular septal aneurysm* in 1826.[70] There is a strong tendency for perimembranous defects to close with formation of an aneurysm derived from the tricuspid valve (Figs. 17–4 and 17–31B).[20,70,87,112,144,182,218,233] Septal aneurysms are, as a rule, relatively small (Fig. 17–4), but exceptionally a septal aneurysm expands to considerable size,[105] and a giant aneurysm of the membranous septum revealed itself as a mediastinal mass.[200]

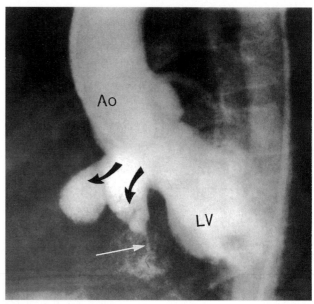

Figure 17–4

Left anterior oblique left ventriculogram (LV) from a 9-year-old girl with a perimembranous ventricular septal defect, a septal aneurysm (*arrow*), and a persistent small shunt. AO, aorta.

A *blind septal aneurysm* occasionally represents a *sui generis* congenital malformation of the interventricular portion of the membranous septum rather than a sequel to spontaneous closure of a perimembranous defect.* Familial congenital septal aneurysms have been reported, although rarely.[38] These aneurysms are, with notable exceptions, well-tolerated and have been discovered incidentally at necropsy in patients beyond the eighth decade.[98] Complications include infective endocarditis, conduction disturbances, intra-aneurysmal thrombosis with systemic embolism, aortic or tricuspid regurgitation, and obstruction to right ventricular outflow (see Fig. 18–11).[34,98,170,180,223] Blind congenital aneurysms may spontaneously perforate, establishing a left-to-right shunt into either the right ventricle or right atrium.[34,98,110,180,203,218,223,250]

The *hemodynamic classification* of ventricular septal defects is relatively straightforward because *physiologic consequences* depend essentially on the size of the defect and on the pulmonary vascular resistance.[193,194,261] These two variables often change with time, and the physiologic and clinical manifestations change accordingly. It has been postulated that a defect in the ventricular septum, whether open or spontaneously closed, might adversely affect left ventricular systolic function.[28,168] This postulation is relevant to impaired function or premature left ventricular failure in an occasional patient with a restrictive defect and a negligible shunt.[28,168]

When the resistance that limits or restricts the left-to-right shunt resides at the site of the ventricular septal defect, the term *restrictive* is applied, indicating that left

*See references 5, 28, 33, 44, 99, 101, 127, 151, 261, 265, 266, 275.
*See references 3, 9, 28, 39, 78, 127, 142, 187, 207, 218.

*See references 16, 34, 93, 98, 105, 110, 118, 180, 189, 203, 223.

ventricular systolic pressure is higher than right ventricular systolic pressure. Restrictive defects include those with normal right ventricular systolic pressure and those with right ventricular systolic pressure that is elevated but less than systemic (moderately restrictive). When the left-to-right shunt is not limited or restricted at the site of the ventricular septal pressures, the term *nonrestrictive* is applied. Right and left ventricular systolic pressure—and therefore pulmonary arterial and aortic systolic pressures—are identical, so the magnitude of the left-to-right shunt is governed by pulmonary vascular resistance.

Ventricular septal defects fall into four *anatomic physiologic categories* (Fig. 17–5): 1) *restrictive defects* with normal right ventricular and pulmonary artery systolic pressures and normal pulmonary vascular resistance; 2) *moderately restrictive defects* with higher than normal right ventricular and pulmonary artery systolic pressure and with low but variable pulmonary vascular resistance;

3) *nonrestrictive defects* with identical right ventricular and left ventricular systolic pressures and with elevated but variable subsystemic pulmonary vascular resistance; and 4) *nonrestrictive defects* with identical right and left ventricular systolic pressures and suprasystemic pulmonary vascular resistance—*Eisenmenger syndrome.*

Henri Roger's account of the physiology of a restrictive ventricular septal defect with normal pulmonary vascular resistance still applies.[188] "The mixture of arterial and venous blood which takes place is scarcely contestable when we recall the differences of pressure which exist, according to the experiments of Marey, between the two ventricles, the force of contraction of the left is equal to 128 mm Hg, that of the right only 25 mm Hg."

Restrictive ventricular septal defects—*maladie de Roger*—cause little or no functional derangement because the shunt is small and the pressures and resistances in the pulmonary circulation are normal (Fig. 17–5A).[194] A

Figure 17–5

Schematic illustrations of restrictive, moderately restrictive, and nonrestrictive ventricular septal defects (VSD). *A,* Restrictive VSD with normal pulmonary vascular resistance (PVR) and a small left-to-right shunt (*arrow*). *B,* Moderately restrictive VSD with low but variable pulmonary vascular resistance and a moderate left-to-right shunt. *C,* Nonrestrictive VSD with a large left-to-right shunt. *D,* Nonrestrictive VSD with suprasystemic pulmonary vascular resistance and reversed shunt (Eisenmenger syndrome). Ao, aorta; RA, right atrium; RV, right ventricle; LV, left ventricle; LA, left atrium; PT, pulmonary trunk.

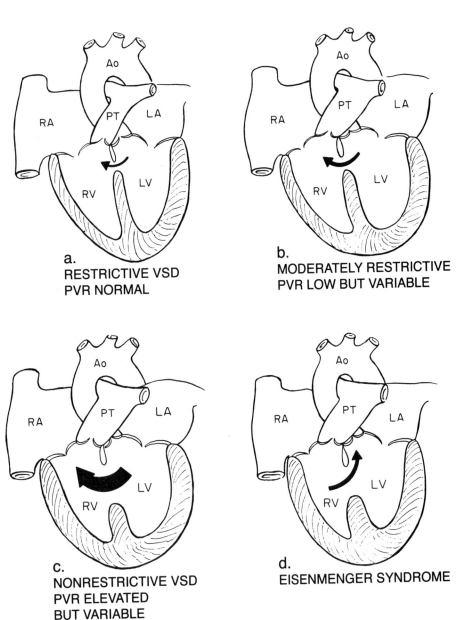

a.
RESTRICTIVE VSD
PVR NORMAL

b.
MODERATELY RESTRICTIVE
PVR LOW BUT VARIABLE

c.
NONRESTRICTIVE VSD
PVR ELEVATED
BUT VARIABLE

d.
EISENMENGER SYNDROME

restrictive defect represents a site of obligatory resistance between the left and right ventricles, thus limiting the magnitude of the left-to-right shunt and precluding delivery of left ventricular systolic pressure into the right ventricle and pulmonary trunk. Shunt flow is systolic with minor diastolic flow generated by the normal differences in left and right ventricular distensibility and end-diastolic pressure (see The Echocardiogram).[207]

A *moderately restrictive* ventricular septal defect is characterized by right ventricular systolic pressure that is above normal but less than systemic and by a low but variable pulmonary vascular resistance that rarely progresses.[114] The left ventricle adapts to a moderate increase in volume, and the right ventricle adapts to a moderate increase in pressure. Left ventricular systolic pressure *falls* more rapidly than right ventricular systolic pressure, favoring instant to instant right-to-left shunting. However, left ventricular *systolic* pressure *rises* more rapidly than right ventricular systolic pressure, favoring left-to-right shunting, so small right-to-left shunts are quantitatively returned to the right ventricle with the next systole. An increase in end-diastolic pressure in the volume loaded left ventricle is coupled to diastolic shunting.[66,81,207] Moderately restrictive defects in the trabecular muscular septum decrease in size during ventricular contraction, and in so doing decrease the systolic shunt, which is followed by shunting in diastole.[95] With isotonic exercise, systemic vascular resistance falls while pulmonary vascular resistance changes little if at all,[21] so a normal increment in systemic flow is achieved without a corresponding increase in left-to-right shunt.[21]

A *nonrestrictive ventricular septal defect* indicates that the right and left ventricles behave physiologically as a common chamber with identical peak systemic systolic pressures. The volume and direction of flow through the defect depend on the relative resistances in the pulmonary and systemic circulations. A nonrestrictive defect with elevated but variable pulmonary vascular resistance (Fig. 17–5C) imposes excessive volume overload on the left ventricle and imposes obligatory systemic systolic pressure afterloaded on the right ventricle. A persistently large left-to-right shunt culminates in depressed systolic function of the volume overloaded left ventricle.[106] A rise in pulmonary vascular resistance prompts a reciprocal fall in left-to-right shunt and a fall in volume overload of the left ventricle, while systolic pressure in the two ventricles necessarily remains identical as in the fetus. When pulmonary vascular resistance is suprasystemic, the architecture of the pulmonary vascular bed resembles primary pulmonary hypertension as described in Chapter 14, and the left-to-right shunt is replaced by a right-to left-shunt— Eisenmenger syndrome (Fig. 17–5D).* Right ventricle function is analogous to the function of the normal fetal right ventricle that is equipped to cope with systemic vascular resistance.[285]

In *neonates with a nonrestrictive ventricular septal defect*, the vasoreactive immature pulmonary resistance vessels play a pivotal role in regulating blood flow through the defect. The physiologic fall in neonatal pulmonary vascular resistance is delayed because of the interplay between shunt size and pulmonary vasoreactivity. In infants with a *moderately restrictive ventricular septal defect*, two additional mechanisms adjust the volume and direction of the shunt and the level of pulmonary arterial pressure. The most favorable mechanism is a decrease in size of the defect. A much less common mechanism is acquired obstruction to right ventricular outflow that reduces left ventricular volume overload and protects the pulmonary vascular bed (see Chapter 18).[228] When and to what extent these regulatory mechanisms exert their influence determines the hemodynamic and clinical course in patients with moderately restrictive and nonrestrictive ventricular septal defects.[27,28,44,131,132,157,211,238]

THE HISTORY

Ventricular septal defects occur in a wide range of mammals and birds with four-chambered hearts[159] with an incidence unrelated to sex, race, maternal age, or birth order[28,31,101,148,159,241] Ventricular septal defects are found in 3.3% of first-degree relatives of index patients.[47] Among first-degree relatives with congenital heart disease, one third have ventricular septal defects.[159] Between 30% and 60% of siblings of index patients have ventricular septal defects,[162] and siblings of patients with ventricular septal defects have three times the incidence of ventricular septal defects compared to the incidence in the general population.[159] Ventricular septal defects have been reported in identical twins[25,192] but with a high frequency of discordance.[159] Parents with a spontaneously closed ventricular septal defect can have offspring with a ventricular septal defect.[161] Birth weights are low in approximately 18% of full-term infants with ventricular septal defects,[126] and dysmaturity is in addition to and apart from the prevalence of ventricular septal defects in preterm infants. Heterotrisomy is a significant factor in ventricular septal defects with Down syndrome.[262]

Restrictive ventricular septal defects come to light because a systolic murmur is detected at the first well-baby examination but not at birth. A murmur that is present at birth is a feature of ventricular septal defect with a left ventricular to right atrial communication because the shunt exists *in utero* and therefore exists at birth (see later section).[185] *Very small defects* with trivial early systolic shunts escape detection because the accompanying early soft systolic murmurs are not detected or mistaken for a normal or innocent murmur (see Auscultation). The diagnosis is necessarily missed if the physical examination is performed after the ventricular septal defect has spontaneously closed. Spontaneous closure accounts for the striking age-related disparity in the incidence of ventricular septal defects from birth to maturity[9,31,45,84,99,109,146,227,238] and

---

*See references 44, 72, 91, 92, 97, 132, 157, 237, 248.

leaves the patient with no shunt and a functionally normal heart that still harbors a morphologic abnormality, especially if spontaneous closure is accompanied by a septal aneurysm (See Fig. 17–4).[103]

Infective endocarditis is a risk in restrictive ventricular septal defects but rarely occurs before eruption of the second teeth.[28,31,45,114,152,167,201,228,238,252] Roger aptly stated that, "Prevention of complications is by means of hygiene."[188] Infective endocarditis is usually on the septal tricuspid leaflet at site of the jet impact. Muscular defects have a low incidence of infective endocarditis because the jet dissipates within the right ventricular cavity without striking the septal tricuspid leaflet.[195]

Longevity is likely to be normal[33,114,270] as Roger stated:

I have observed several patients for 5, 12, and 15 years; these children have grown like others and not one has died prematurely. I have occasionally visited a woman whose children I attended from early ages. She had always been in excellent health and had never complained of cardiac difficulties. On auscultation I was greatly surprised to hear a murmur. I asked her if physicians had ever found anything wrong with her heart, and she told me that Guersant the Elder (the famous pediatrician who was my first master in infantile pathology) had recognized in her a few days after birth a cardiac malformation. This woman has now passed her fiftieth year; her health continues to be perfect and she is the mother of four children.

Despite the existence of an uncomplicated defect in the interventricular septum, patients may attain or even surpass the average span of human life.[188]

Moderately restrictive ventricular septal defects with low but variable pulmonary vascular resistance (See Fig. 17–5B) escape detection in the newborn nursery because the delayed fall in neonatal pulmonary vascular resistance results in delayed in onset of the shunt and delayed onset of the murmur. Congestive heart failure within the first few months of life is in response to a large left-to-right shunt that is established after the fall in pulmonary vascular resistance. Parents report that their infant fatigues or coughs while feeding, sweats excessively, is restless when recumbent, and sleeps poorly. Parents may detect a thrill when they touch their infant's chest and may detect a hyperactive precordium when holding the infant next to their chest. Spontaneous symptomatic improvement is related to a decrease in size of the defect, a favorable trend that may culminate in complete spontaneous closure (Fig. 17–6) (see earlier).

Patients with moderately restrictive defects and a moderate left-to-right shunt tolerate isotonic exercise because the exercise-induced increment in systemic blood flow is achieved without a corresponding increase in shunt (see earlier).[21] However, persistence of a significant shunt and protracted left ventricular volume overload incurs the risk of congestive heart failure.[114,228] Only occasional patients achieve adulthood (Fig. 17–7), one reaching age 65 years (Fig. 17–8B) and another reaching age 79 years.[67] Susceptibility to infective endocarditis is ongoing.[108,114,167]

Nonrestrictive ventricular septal defects with elevated but variable pulmonary vascular resistance (See Fig. 17–5C) present in infancy with congestive heart failure and little prospect that the defect will decrease in size. A minority of patients undergo relatively little fall in neonatal pulmonary vascular resistance, so the shunts are small and the early clinical course is deceptively benign. Most infants have large shunts and experience congestive heart failure with poor growth and development, labored breathing, frequent lower respiratory infections, difficulty feeding, and excessive diaphoresis.[6,44,73,141,228] Dyspnea and irritability are most pronounced when the infant is supine and improve when the baby is held upright or is placed in an infant seat. Feeding patterns are typical. A hungry infant awakens from a fretful sleep, feeds vigorously only to stop short of satisfaction because of dyspnea; falls asleep again, exhausted by the effort, only to awaken with renewed hunger and to repeat the

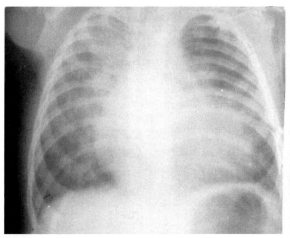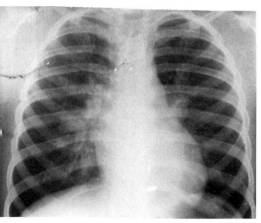

A B

Figure 17–6

X-rays at age 3 months (*A*) and 6 years (*B*) from the same patient with a moderately restrictive perimembranous ventricular septal defect that closed spontaneously. *A,* X-ray at 3 months with congestive heart failure, a 3.5 to 1 left-to-right shunt, and a pulmonary artery pressure of 68/22 mm Hg. Pulmonary venous congestion and cardiac enlargement are striking. *B,* At age 6 years, pulmonary vascularity was normal. There was mild residual enlargement of the pulmonary trunk and its proximal branches and a moderately convex left ventricle.

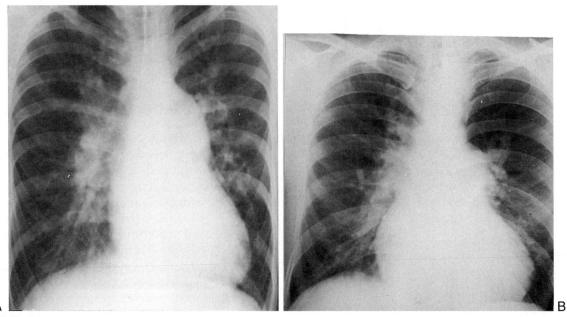

Figure 17–7
A, X-ray from a 17-year-old man with a moderately restrictive perimembranous ventricular septal defect, a 2.6 to 1 left-to-right shunt, and a pulmonary artery pressure of 75/23 mm Hg. Pulmonary arterial vascularity is increased, the pulmonary trunk and its proximal branches are markedly dilated, and a moderately enlarged convex left ventricle occupies the apex. *B*, X-ray from a 39-year-old man with a nonrestrictive perimembranous ventricular septal defect and a bidirectional shunt (arterial oxygen saturation 88%). Pulmonary arterial vascularity is increased, the pulmonary trunk and its proximal branches are markedly dilated, an enlarged convex left ventricle occupies the apex, and a prominent right atrium forms the right lower cardiac border.

frustrating cycle. Regulation of the large left-to-right shunt with amelioration of symptoms is almost always due to a rise in pulmonary vascular resistance.[27,52,101,150,238] When pulmonary resistance exceeds systemic resistance, the shunt is reversed, the patient is cyanotic,[44,91,114,167,248] and a condition that Maude Abbott called *Eisenmenger's complex* exists.[1]

Victor Eisenmenger published his account in 1897 in a paper entitled *Congenital Defects of the Ventricular Septum*.[56] Paul Wood, in his landmark publication of 1958, introduced the term *Eisenmenger syndrome* (Fig. 17–9), which he defined as "pulmonary hypertension with reversed shunt."[248] Wood quoted from Eisenmenger:

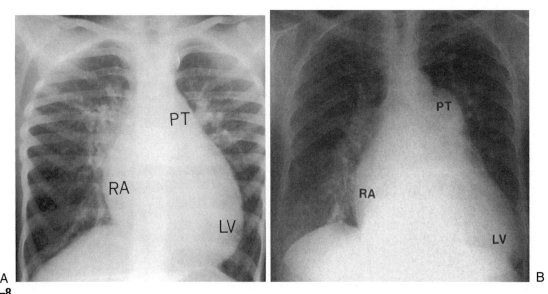

Figure 17–8
X-rays from two patients 60 years apart in age, both of whom had perimembranous ventricular septal defects. *A*, The 5-year-old boy had a moderately restrictive ventricular septal defect, a left-to-right shunt of 2.6 to 1, and a pulmonary artery pressure of 43/13 mm Hg. Pulmonary arterial vascularity is increased, the pulmonary trunk (PT) is moderately dilated, an enlarged left ventricle (LV) occupies the apex, and a prominent right atrium occupies the right lower cardiac border. *B*, This 65-year-old woman had a moderately restrictive perimembranous ventricular septal defect, a 2.7 to 1 left-to-right shunt, and pulmonary artery pressure of 55/32 mm Hg. Pulmonary arterial vascularity is increased, the pulmonary trunk (PT) is markedly dilated, an enlarged left ventricle (LV) occupies the apex, and a prominent right atrium (RA) occupies the lower right cardiac border.

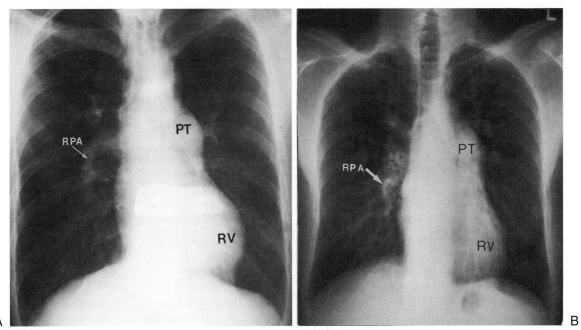

Figure 17–9
X-rays from two patients 42 years apart in age, both of whom had a nonrestrictive perimembranous ventricular septal defects and suprasystemic pulmonary vascular resistance (Eisenmenger syndrome). *A,* X-rays from the 25-year-old man shows clear lung fields, a markedly dilated pulmonary trunk (PT), an enlarged right pulmonary artery (RPA), and a nondilated convex right ventricle (RV) at the apex. *B,* X-ray from the 67-year-old man who died at age 69 years of legionnaires' disease. The lung fields are clear, the pulmonary trunk and the right pulmonary artery are markedly dilated, and a nondilated convex right ventricle (RV) occupies the apex.

"The patient was a powerfully built man of 32 who gave a history of cyanosis and moderate breathlessness since infancy. He managed well enough, until January, 1894 when dyspnea increased and edema set in. Seven months later (August) he was admitted to hospital in a state of heart failure. He improved with rest and digitalis, but collapsed and died more or less suddenly on November 13 following a large hemoptysis. At necropsy, a 2- to 2.5-cm defect was found in the perimembranous septum."

Cyanotic congenital heart disease represented here by Eisenmenger syndrome is a multisystem systemic disorder involving red blood cell mass and hemostasis, the central nervous system, bilirubin kinetics, the systemic vascular bed, the coronary circulation, the myocardium, uric acid metabolism and clearance, the kidneys, respiration, the digits, the long bones, and gynecologic endocrinology.[174,272] *Morbidity and mortality* in Eisenmenger syndrome are influenced by modern medical management of the multisystem disorders.[174,222,272] *Longevity* is approximately one to two decades longer than in early reports.[79,114,191,239,272] Right ventricular failure is uncommon[272,285] (Eisenmenger's original report[248] not withstanding), unless acquired systemic hypertension imposes disproportionate afterload.

Erythrocytosis is an adaptive response to the decrease in tissue oxygenation and arterial hypoxemia that stimulates renal release of erythropoietin, which in turn stimulates an increase in the number of red blood cells. Because erythrocytosis is an adaptive response designed to offset the hypoxemic deficit in tissue oxygenation, appropriate equi- librium conditions are established at elevated hematocrit levels. Erythrocytosis does not incur risk of stroke due to cerebral arterial thrombosis in older children, adolescents, and adults irrespective of hematocrit level, iron stores, or cerebral hyperviscosity symptoms.[281] However, cyanotic children younger than age 4 years with iron-deficient erythrocytosis experience thrombosis of intracranial venous sinuses but not of cerebral arteries.[281]

Hemostatic abnormalities have been recognized for over 50 years in patients with cyanotic congenital heart disease.[281] Platelet counts are usually in the low range of normal, and many clotting factor disorders have been identified, most recently acquired von Willebrand factor abnormalities.[280] The bleeding tendency is mucocutaneous and is characterized by easy bruising, gingival bleeding, epistaxis, menorrhagia, and increased risk of traumatic bleeding. Pulmonary hemorrhage—defined as hemoptysis (external) and/or intrapulmonary (internal)—is the most serious type of bleeding, and varies from mild and occasional to copious, recurrent, massive and fatal.[42,88,248,272,281] Victor Eisenmenger's patient "died more or less suddenly . . . following a large hemoptysis."[248] Massive intrapulmonary hemorrhage is a common cause of sudden death in Eisenmenger syndrome.[272] *Bilirubin* is formed from the breakdown of heme, a process that is excessive in the presence of cyanotic congenital heart disease and that coincides with a substantial increase in the amount of unconjugated bilirubin in the bile.[281] Calcium bilirubinate gallstones develop because unconjugated bilirubin is virtually water insoluble at physiologic pH.[281]

Systemic vascular dilatation is in response to endothelial-derived nitric oxide and prostaglandins that are released in response to the increase in endothelial shear stress inherent in the erythrocytotic perfusate. Increased arteriolar dilatation and tissue vascularity contribute to the bleeding tendency.[174] Paradoxical emboli announce themselves as transient ischemic attacks or strokes, or as renal or splenic infarcts (Fig. 17–10). Syncope can be caused by heat-induced vasodilatation of hot humid weather or a hot shower or bath.

The *extramural coronary arteries* are dilated, elongated, and tortuous, even aneurysmal (coronary ectasia).[174] Vasodilator nitric oxide and prostaglandins are released from coronary artery endothelium in response to the increased shear stress of erythrocytosis. Dilatation of the coronary arteries is accompanied by an increase in extramural coronary artery blood flow that does not encroach upon coronary vascular reserve because of remodeling of the myocardial microvascular circulation.[283]

Hyperuricemia results from decreased renal clearance and/or increased production of urate. Elevated plasma uric acid levels are common in cyanotic adults, and are secondary to enhanced urate reabsorption that results from renal hypoperfusion reinforced by a high filtration fraction.[174] Acute gouty arthritis is uncommon but not rare.

Renal involvement is represented by functional abnormalities and abnormalities of structure.[174,272,279] Decreased clearance of urate is a functional abnormality, but hyperuricemia in turn exerts little or no deleterious effect on renal function.[272,279] Proteinuria, another functional abnormality, is caused by increased glomerular hydraulic pressure in response to a combination of the high viscosity of erythrocytotic blood entering the afferent glomerular arteriole in concert with obligatory ultrafiltration from afferent to afferent arteriole. There are two distinct morphologic glomerular abnormalities in cyanotic adults.[272,279] The vascular abnormality is characterized by dilatation of hilar arterioles and glomerular capillaries in response to intraglomerular release of nitric oxide.[279] The non-vascular abnormality is characterized by an increase in glomerular cellularity in response to platelet derived growth factor and transforming growth factor-beta in the cytoplasm of systemic venous megakaryocytes that are shunted into the systemic arterial circulation and lodge in glomerular tufts.[279]

Cardiorespiratory responses to isotonic exercise in cyanotic congenital heart disease significantly influence the dynamics of oxygen uptake and ventilation.[256,281] Prolonged onset and recovery of oxygen uptake kinetics incur large oxygen deficits that result in hypoxemia even with low levels of exercise, suggesting that patients with left-to-right shunts rely heavily on anaerobic metabolism. Hyperventilation, which is subjectively perceived as dyspnea, is present at rest and increases excessively during

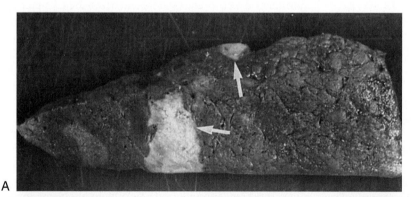

A

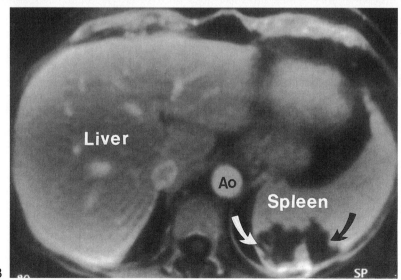

B

Figure 17–10

A shows splenic infarcts (*white arrows*) caused by paradoxical emboli in a 42-year-old woman with a nonrestrictive perimembranous ventricular septal defect and Eisenmenger syndrome. *B* is an abdominal computed tomographic scan that shows splenic infarcts (*curved arrows*) caused by paradoxical emboli in a 19-year-old man with a nonrestrictive perimembranous ventricular septal defect and Eisenmenger syndrome.

exercise because the augmentation in right-to-left shunt induced by exercise is accompanied by an increase in systemic arterial carbon dioxide and a decrease in pH that stimulate the respiratory center and carotid bodies.[256,281]

Clubbing of the digits and hypertrophic osteoarthropathy share a common pathogenesis.[281] Systemic venous megakaryocytes are shunted into the systemic arterial circulation (see comments on *renal involvement*) and impact in the digits and subperiosteum. Platelet-derived growth factor and transforming growth factor-beta are released from megakaryocytic cytoplasm and promote cell proliferation, protein synthesis, connective tissue formation, and deposition of extracellular matrix that are responsible for clubbing and hypertrophic osteoarthropathy.[281]

Pregnancy poses excessive risk in females with Eisenmenger syndrome. Maternal mortality exceeds 50%, and there is an independently high risk of fetal wastage because of uterine hypoxemia associated with cyanosis *per se*.[173,178,272]

Sudden death often results from massive intrapulmonary hemorrhage,[272] less commonly from rupture of a dilated hypertensive pulmonary trunk,[284] rarely from ventricular tachycardia.[114] A cerebral abscess in early life can result in a *seizure disorder* in adulthood, or the abscess can occur initially in adulthood.[28,248,281]

PHYSICAL APPEARANCE

The commonest abnormal physical appearances are poor growth and development, frailty and cachexia in infants with the catabolic effects of congestive heart failure caused by a large left-to-right shunt,[28,75,141,238] and cyanosis caused by a reversed shunt in Eisenmenger syndrome. Growth and development are also influenced by intrauterine and genetic factors and by low birth weight.[126] Young patients with nonrestrictive ventricular septal defects and balanced shunts may become cyanotic only after exercise or crying.[42] Harrison's grooves are due to thoracic retraction caused by chronic dyspnea (Fig. 17–11).

Asian patients are likely to have doubly committed subarterial ventricular septal defects (see earlier).[83] Ventricular septal defects also coincide with the physical appearance of trisomy 18 (see Figs. 19–5 and 20–11) and Down syndrome (see Figs. 15–90 and 15–91).[14,137,147,230] Additional relationships exist between physical appearance and ventricular septal defects in trisomy 13, trisomy 8 and 9 mosaic; rare aberrations such as 5p– (*cri du chat*), 13q–, and 18q–[128,161]; Holt Oram syndrome[267]; Cornelia de Lange syndrome[162]; Klippel-Feil syndrome[163]; cardiofacial syndrome[36]; and fetal alcohol syndrome.[212]

THE ARTERIAL PULSE

Moderately restrictive defects with relatively low pulmonary vascular resistance are associated with a brisk arterial pulse because of vigorous ejection from a volume loaded left ventricle. Nonrestrictive defects with large left-to-right shunts and congestive heart failure are associated with a diminished arterial pulse and pulsus alternans. The arterial pulse in Eisenmenger syndrome is normal because systemic stroke volume is maintained (Fig. 17–12).[248]

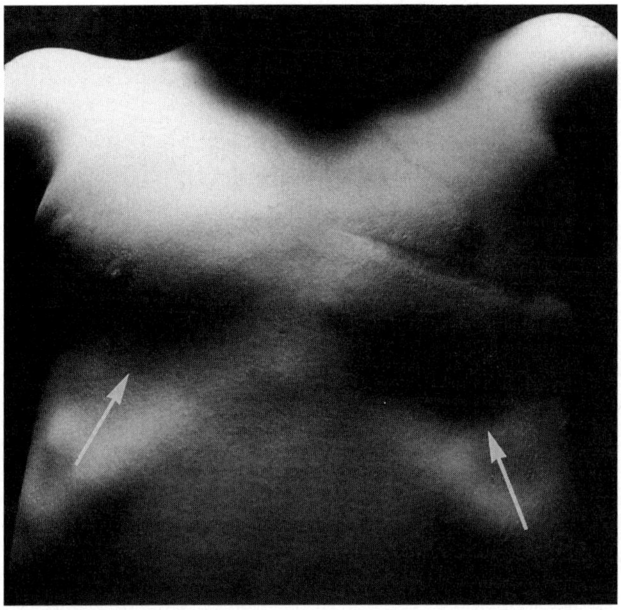

Figure 17–11
Photograph of the chest of an 8-year-old boy with a moderately restrictive perimembranous ventricular septal defect and a 2.7 to 1 left-to-right shunt. Lighting was adjusted to highlight prominent Harrison's grooves (*white arrows*) caused by chronic dyspnea. The left thoracotomy scar was from repair of coarctation of the aorta.

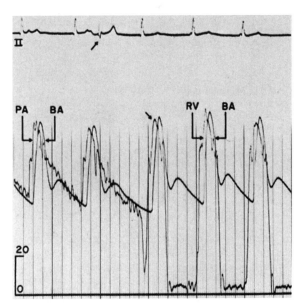

Figure 17–12
Pressure pulses from an 18- year-old man with a nonrestrictive perimembranous ventricular septal defect and Eisenmenger syndrome. The brachial artery pulse (BA) was identical with the pulmonary artery pulse (PA). The diastolic portions of the brachial and pulmonary artery pressure pulses were identical because pulmonary vascular resistance was the same as systemic vascular resistance. As the catheter was withdrawn into the right ventricle (RV), the peak systolic pressure remained the same as the brachial arterial systolic pressure (BA).

THE JUGULAR VENOUS PULSE

Moderately restrictive and nonrestrictive ventricular septal defects with congestive heart failure are associated with an elevated mean jugular venous pressure and an increase in A and V waves. The jugular venous pulse in Eisenmenger syndrome is normal or nearly so, with small dominant A waves (Fig. 17–13). Large A waves are exceptional because right ventricular systolic pressure does not exceed systemic level, so the right ventricle requires little extra help from its atrium because systemic afterload exists from birth.

PRECORDIAL MOVEMENT AND PALPATION

Roger stated that when a *ventricular septal defect is restrictive*, "it coincides with no other sign of organic disease with the exception of the harsh thrill which accompanies it."[188] The thrill is maximum in the third or fourth left intercostal space at the left sternal border. A subarterial ventricular septal defect directs the shunt into the pulmonary trunk, so the accompanying thrill is maximum in the second or first and second left intercostal space with radiation upward and to the left and into the neck.[61,183,213]

In a *moderately restrictive* ventricular septal defect with large left-to-right shunt, the volume overloaded left ventricle is dynamic, the dilated pulmonary trunk is palpable in the second left intercostal space, while the moderately afterloaded right ventricle is less impressive.

A *nonrestrictive* ventricular septal defect with low pulmonary vascular resistance and obligatory systemic pressure in the right ventricle and pulmonary trunk is associated with a dynamic volume overloaded left ventricle, a pressure overloaded systemic right ventricle, a palpable dilated hypertensive pulmonary trunk, and a palpable pulmonary closure sound. In Eisenmenger syndrome, the hypertensive right ventricular impulse displaces the left ventricle from the apex. The dilated hypertensive pulmonary trunk is palpable together with the loud pulmonary closure sound.

AUSCULTATION

A *very restrictive* ventricular septal defect in the perimembranous or trabecular septum (See Fig. 17–2B) is accompanied by a murmur that is a soft, highly localized, high frequency, early systolic decrescendo (Fig. 17–14) and that is easily overlooked in restless infants. The early systolic timing results from a shunt that is confined to early systole because small perimembranous or muscular defects decrease in size or obliterate in late systole.[149] An early systolic murmur lengthens *during* a premature ventricular beat because reduced left ventricular contractility cannot close the defect during late systole.[152] Conversely, more vigorous left ventricular contraction during the *post premature* beat closes the ventricular septal defect earlier in systole and further shortens the early systolic murmur. During the course of spontaneous closure, the holosystolic murmur of ventricular septal defect becomes early systolic before disappearing altogether (see Fig.17–18).[60,112]

The murmur of a moderately restrictive or restrictive perimembranous ventricular septal defect is typically holosystolic, high frequency, grade 4/6 or louder, and maximum in the third and fourth intercostal spaces at the left sternal border (Figs. 17–15 and 17–16), precordial sites that are topographically appropriate for the intracardiac location of the murmur (Fig. 17–15).[65] Muscular ventricu-

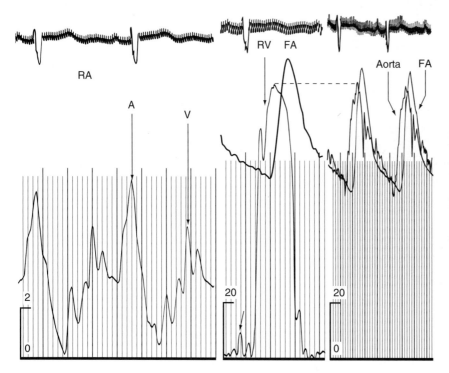

Figure 17–13

Tracings from an 11-year-old boy with a nonrestrictive perimembranous ventricular septal defect and Eisenmenger syndrome. A dominant wave is present in the right atrial (RA) pressure pulse. The *second panel* shows identical *diastolic* pressures in the aorta and femoral artery (FA). The femoral artery *systolic* pressure is slightly higher than the right ventricular and aortic systolic pressure because of peripheral amplification.

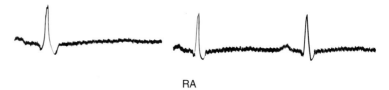

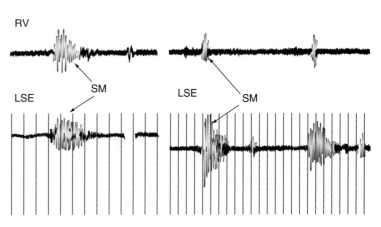

Figure 17–14

Phonocardiograms from a 4-year-old girl with a tiny perimembranous ventricular septal defect and a trivial left-to-right shunt. A soft pure high-frequency early systolic murmur (SM) was recorded within the cavity of the right ventricle (RV), and an identical precordial murmur was recorded externally at the lower left sternal edge (LSE). When the intracardiac microphone was withdrawn from right ventricle into right atrium (RA), the murmur vanished, establishing its origin within the right ventricular cavity.

lar septal defect murmurs are maximum at the same precordial sites as murmurs of perimembranous defects.[73,102] The typical murmur is holosystolic (Figs. 17–15 and 17–16) corresponding to the holosystolic pressure difference across the defect.[121] Roger recognized this mechanism when he wrote that the murmur "is so prolonged that it entirely occupies the period of the natural tic-tac of the normal heart sounds," and is "accompanied by no other physical signs save only the purring thrill."[188] When tricuspid chordae tendineae bridge the defect, the murmur has musical overtones assuming the pitch of an aeolian harp.

Moderately restrictive ventricular septal defects are accompanied by loud harsh holosystolic murmurs when pulmonary vascular resistance is below systemic level (Fig. 17–16). A plateau-shaped holosystolic murmur is sometimes accentuated in midsystole because of superimposition of a pulmonary flow murmur.[35,121]

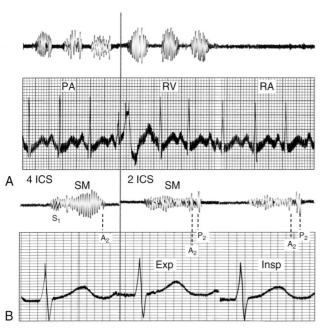

Figure 17–15

Phonocardiograms from a 4-year-old girl with a restrictive perimembranous ventricular septal defect, a 1.4 to 1 left-to-right shunt and normal pulmonary artery pressure. *A*, The intracardiac microphone recorded a prominent midsystolic systolic murmur (SM) in the main pulmonary artery (PA). When the microphone was withdrawn into the outflow tract of the right ventricle (RV), a holosystolic ventricular septal defect murmur was recorded. The holosystolic murmur vanished when the microphone was withdrawn into the right atrium (RA). *B*, Phonocardiogram on the thoracic wall at the fourth left intercostal space (4 ICS) recorded a holosystolic murmur identical with the holosystolic murmur recorded within the right ventricular outflow tract. The second heart sound in the second left intercostal space (2 ICS) exhibited persistent but not fixed splitting. S_1, first heart sound; A_2, aortic component; P_2, pulmonary component.

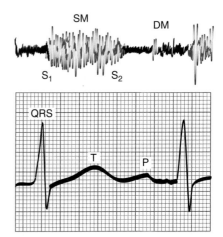

Figure 17–16

Phonocardiogram recorded over the left ventricular impulse of a 2-year-old girl with a moderately restrictive perimembranous ventricular septal defect and a 2.5 to 1 left-to-right shunt. A holosystolic murmur (SM) is followed by a mid-diastolic-presystolic murmur (DM) due to increased flow across the mitral valve. Note the bifid left atrial P wave abnormality. S_1, first heart sound; S_2, second heart sound.

The shunt in *subarterial ventricular septal defects* is directly into the pulmonary trunk, so the accompanying murmur like the thrill, is maximum in the second or first and second left intercostal space (Fig. 17–17) with radiation upward toward the left clavicle into the suprasternal notch and into the left side of the neck.[61,102,183,213] The shape of the murmur tends to be crescendo or crescendo-decrescendo (Fig. 17–17).[61,213]

A decrease in size or spontaneous closure of a perimembranous ventricular septal defect can be accompanied by a *septal aneurysm* that may harbor a small left-to-right shunt[70,180] (Fig. 17–4) but otherwise resembles a blind congenital membranous septal aneurysm (see earlier).[39,93,105,118,170,203] Septal aneurysms are usually occult, disclosing no evidence of their presence, but occasionally there are auscultatory clues.[93] The aneurysm may contain one or more small perforations (see Fig. 17–4) that generate a late systolic murmur or a holosystolic murmur with late systolic accentuation that results from stretching of the aneurysmal pouch, which enhances late systolic patency of small perforations.[70,130,176,177,180,203] Murmurs have also been attributed to entry of blood into a *sealed* blind aneurysmal pouch during ventricular systole.[34,170] Systolic tensing of the aneurysm sometimes produces a midsystolic click that may introduce a late systolic murmur.[176] The aneurysm occasionally protrudes into the outflow tract of the right ventricle (see Fig. 17–4), causing a midsystolic murmur in the second left intercostal space.[170,180] A septal aneurysm occasionally causes the murmur of tricuspid regurgitation[103,118,245] that can be identified during active respiration (Carvallo's sign).[172]

The prominent holosystolic murmur of a moderately restrictive ventricular septal defect often buries both components of the second sound, rendering the pulmonary component audible only during inspiration as it emerges from the murmur (Fig. 17–17). Analysis of the second heart sound benefits from exaggerated splitting (Fig. 17–15B).[90,121,122] Attention has been called to wide splitting with subarterial defects (Fig. 17–17).[61,213]

Moderately restrictive or nonrestrictive ventricular septal defects with large left-to-right shunts are associated with short mid-diastolic murmurs at the apex due to torrential flow across the mitral valve[75,102,121,154,199] (Fig.17–16) as originally described by Laubry and Pezzi in 1921.[119] These murmurs are often preceded by a third heart sound[75] especially in the presence of left ventricular failure. Intracardiac phonocardiograms confirm the presence of mid-diastolic murmurs within the inflow tract of the left ventricle just beyond the mitral valve.[65]

Nonrestrictive ventricular septal defects with elevated pulmonary vascular resistance reflect the effects of progressive pulmonary vascular disease on the length and loudness of the accompanying systolic murmur.[171] As pulmonary resistance approaches the systemic level, the holosystolic murmur shortens and softens (Figs. 17–18C, 17–18D and 17–19),[199] its shape becomes decrescendo (Figs. 17–18 and 17–19), and the murmur becomes early systolic (Fig. 17–18D) before disappearing altogether as the shunt is reversed (Fig. 17–18E).[171,248]

Auscultatory analysis of the *second heart sound* benefits from an increase in intensity of the pulmonary component and from an increase in pulmonary vascular resistance that

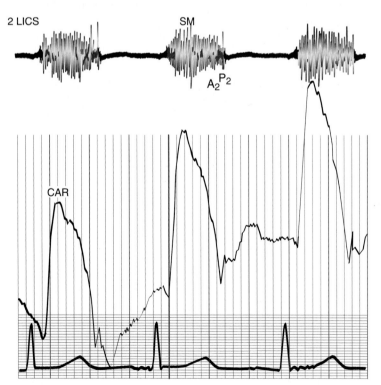

Figure 17–17

Phonocardiogram from a 5-year-old boy with a moderately restrictive subarterial ventricular septal defect, a 2 to 1 left-to-right shunt, and a pulmonary artery pressure of 80/36 mm Hg. The holosystolic systolic murmur (SM) was maximum in the second left intercostal costal space (2 LICS) because blood was shunted directly into the pulmonary trunk from the left ventricle through the subarterial ventricular septal defect. There is relatively wide splitting of the second heart sound due to delayed closure of the pulmonary valve. A_2/P_2, aortic and pulmonary components of the second heart sound; CAR, carotid pulse.

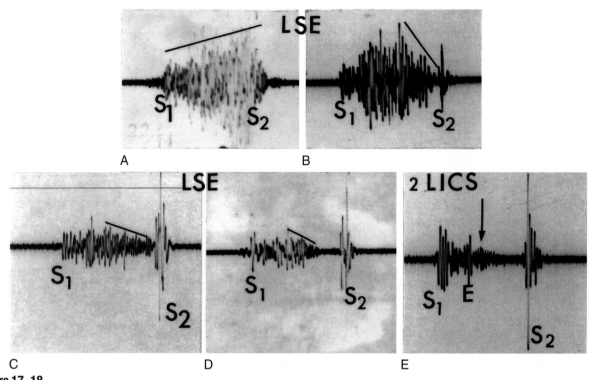

Figure 17–18

Phonocardiograms from five patients with perimembranous ventricular septal defects and pulmonary vascular resistance ranging from normal (*A*) to suprasystemic (*E*). The tracings show modifications of the murmur from a restrictive nonpulmonary hypertensive left-to-right shunt (*A*) to a pulmonary hypertensive right-to-left shunt (*E*). In Eisenmenger syndrome (*E*), a pulmonary ejection sound (E) introduces a short midsystolic murmur caused by flow into a dilated hypertensive pulmonary trunk. LSE, left sternal edge; PA, pulmonary artery; 2 LICS, second left intercostal space.

softens the murmur in later systole.[171] As pulmonary resistance rises, the degree of splitting decreases (Fig. 17–19),[102,171,199] and the second sound is single in Eisenmenger syndrome (Fig. 17–18*E*).[89,121,171,199,216,248] The two components fuse because the respective descending limbs of the left and right ventricular pressure pulses cross the aortic and pulmonary arterial pressure pulses at the same time. The aortic and pulmonary arterial dicrotic notches are synchronous, so the two components of the second sound are synchronous.[89]

When suprasystemic pulmonary vascular resistance abolishes the left-to-right shunt, the auscultatory signs are those of pure pulmonary hypertension (Fig. 17–18*E* and see Chapter 14).[171] Flow into the dilated hypertensive pulmonary trunk causes a pulmonary ejection sound that introduces a short soft midsystolic murmur.[171] A high-frequency Graham Steell murmur issues from a loud pulmonary component of the second heart sound. The Graham Steell murmur is the only diastolic murmur that is present when the shunt is reversed, because the mid-diastolic murmur across the mitral valve disappears as pulmonary blood flow decreases. Rarely, the murmur of pulmonary regurgitation is caused by prolapse of a pulmonary cusp through a subarterial ventricular septal defect.[80]

THE ELECTROCARDIOGRAM

The electrocardiogram is a useful reflection of the physiologic derangements but not the anatomic location of a ventricular septal defect. The tracing is influenced by the size of the defect, the size of the left-to-right shunt, and the pulmonary vascular resistance (see Fig. 17–5), that is, by the presence and degree of volume overload of the left ventricle and the presence and degree of pressure overload of the right ventricle.

A *restrictive* ventricular septal defect with normal pulmonary artery pressure is associated with a normal electrocardiogram,[169,199,226,235] but an RSR prime pattern is occasionally present in lead V_1. When a restrictive perimembranous defect is accompanied by a septal aneurysm, there is an increased incidence of rhythm and conduction disturbances, especially atrial fibrillation, paroxysmal atrial tachycardia, junctional rhythm, atrial flutter, and complete heart block.[11,34,93,105,114,118,180,189,223]

Moderately restrictive ventricular septal defects with large left-to-right shunts are associated with broad notched left atrial P waves in lead 1 and 2 and with a broad deep P terminal force in lead V_1 (Fig. 17–20).[75,169,226] The QRS axis is normal (Fig. 17–20), although left axis deviation occurs in about 5% of restrictive or moderately restrictive perimembranous defects (Fig. 17–21).[12,62,68,199,202,277] Inlet ventricular septal defects are associated with left axis deviation when they are a component of an atrioventricular septal defect (see Chapter 15).[75,158,169,199] The incidence of left axis deviation increases in the presence of ventricular septal aneurysms,[277] and left axis has been found in as many as

40% of patients with multiple ventricular septal defects, an observation unrelated to either the number of defects or their locations.[68] Volume overload of the left ventricle is reflected in tall R waves and tall peaked T waves in leads 2, 3, and aVF[54] and in prominent Q waves, tall R waves and tall peaked T waves in leads V_{5-6} (Fig. 17–20).[169,199,235,247]

A *nonrestrictive* ventricular septal defect with a large left-to-right shunt exhibits right atrial or combined atrial P wave abnormalities especially in lead 2 and in leads V_{1-2} (Fig. 17–22).[75] The QRS axis shifts moderately to the right (Figs. 17–22 and 17–23). Biventricular hypertrophy is reflected in the increased R wave amplitude in lead V_1, in

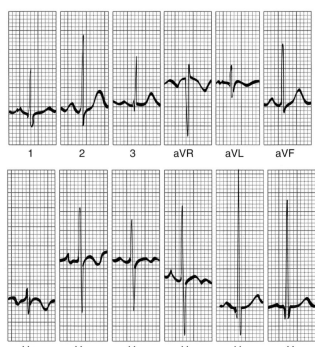

Figure 17–20

Electrocardiogram from a 14-month-old girl with a moderately restrictive perimembranous ventricular septal defect, a 2.5 to 1 left-to-right shunt and a pulmonary artery pressure of 38/16 mm Hg. A bifid left atrial P wave abnormality is present in lead 1, and the P wave in lead V_1 has a deep broad terminal left artial component. The QRS axis is normal. Deep Q waves, tall R waves and upright T waves in leads V_{5-6} are signs of left ventricular volume overload.

the deep Q waves, tall R waves, and tall peaked T waves in leads V_{5-6}, and in large equidiphasic RS complexes (the Katz-Wachtel phenomenon) in midprecordial leads (Figs. 17–22 and 17–23).[111,169,186,226] Infants with nonrestrictive ventricular septal defects and large left-to-right shunts

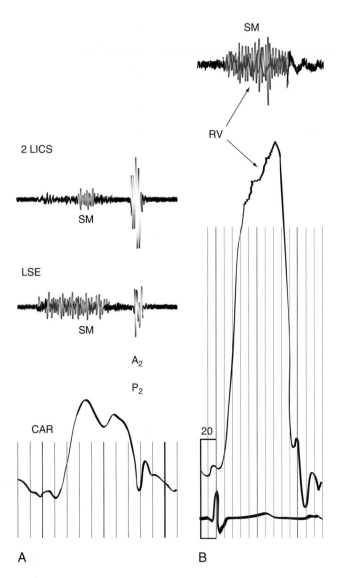

Figure 17–19

Tracings from a 6-year-old boy with a nonrestrictive perimembranous ventricular septal defect, elevated pulmonary vascular resistance, and a 1.8 to 1 left-to-right shunt. *A*, The thoracic wall systolic murmur (SM) at the left sternal edge (LSE) was early systolic, ending before the second heart sound (A2/P2) even though the same murmur recorded by an intracardiac microphone within the cavity of the right ventricle was holosystolic (*B*). RV, right ventricle; 2 LICS, second left intercostal space; A_2, aortic component; P_2, pulmonary component; CAR, carotid pulse.

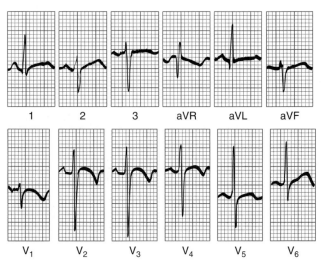

Figure 17–21

Electrocardiogram from a 3-year-old girl with a moderately restrictive perimembranous ventricular septal defect, a 2 to 1 left-to-right shunt, and a pulmonary artery pressure of 32/15 mm Hg. There is left axis deviation with counterclockwise depolarization.

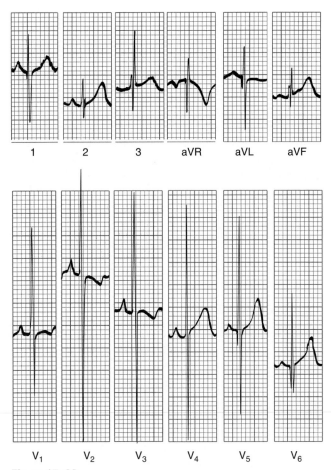

Figure 17–22

Electrocardiogram from a 3-month-old girl with a nonrestrictive perimembranous ventricular septal defect and a 3.5 to 1 left-to-right shunt. Peaked right atrial P waves appear in leads V_{1-4}. Right ventricular hypertrophy is manifested by prominent R waves in right precordial leads and prominent S waves in left precordial leads. Left ventricular volume overload is reflected in the deep Q waves, well-developed R waves, and tall peaked T waves in leads V_{5-6}. Combined ventricular hypertrophy is represented by the large RS complexes in leads V_{2-4}.

occasionally exhibit marked right axis deviation and pure or relatively pure right ventricular hypertrophy except for large equidiphasic complexes in one or more midprecordial leads (Fig. 17–24).

In Eisenmenger syndrome, P waves are often normal in younger patients (Fig. 17–25) and moderately peaked in older patients. Right axis deviation is moderate. Lead V_1 exhibits a tall monophasic R wave (Fig. 17–25) that is occasionally notched on its upstroke and followed by a small s wave. Prominent S waves appear in left precordial leads, but combined ventricular hypertrophy is lacking (Fig. 17–25).

THE X-RAY

Vaquez and Bordet described the radiologic signs of ventricular septal defect in 1913.[231] *Small defects* that were moderately restrictive at birth show residual signs of the initially larger left-to-right shunt, especially an increase in

size of the left ventricle and dilatation of the pulmonary trunk and its branches (Figs. 17–6B and 17–26).

Moderately restrictive ventricular septal defects with low but variable pulmonary vascular resistance (Fig. 17–5B) exhibit radiologic signs that correspond to the magnitude of the left-to-right shunt and the presence and degree of pulmonary hypertension. When pulmonary vascular resistance is relatively low, increased pulmonary arterial vascularity and pulmonary venous congestion coexist (Figs. 17–6A and 17–27).[234] Large shunts in infants may be accompanied by hyperinflated lungs with flat hemidiaphragms.[50] Right atrial dilatation accompanies congestive heart failure (Figs. 17–6A and 17–27). Enlargement of the left atrium is best recognized in the lateral projection (Fig. 17–27B) and may be more impressive than enlargement of the left ventricle.[75,199] An increase in size of the pulmonary trunk and its branches reflects the magnitude and chronicity of pulmonary arterial blood flow and the level of pulmonary arterial pressure (see Figs. 17–7 and 17–8).[107] The size of the ascending aorta is not increased because the left-to-right shunt is intracardiac and therefore does not traverse the aortic root (see Fig. 17–8).[199] In the lateral projection, the *lower* sternum is apt to protrude anteriorly whereas the *upper* sternum is relatively straight.

Nonrestrictive ventricular septal defects with elevated but variable pulmonary vascular resistance present in infancy with

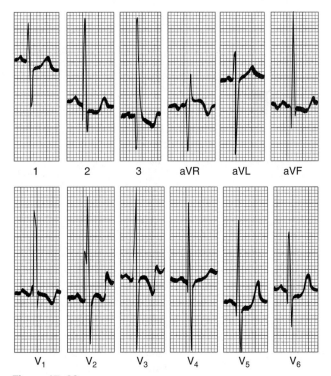

Figure 17–23

Electrocardiogram from a 6-year-old girl with a nonrestrictive perimembranous ventricular septal defect and a 3 to 1 left-to-right shunt. The QRS axis is plus 90°. Volume overload of the left ventricle is indicated by deep Q waves, prominent R waves and tall peaked T waves in leads V_{5-6}, and by deep Q waves and tall R waves in leads 2, 3 and aVF. Right ventricular hypertrophy is indicated by tall right precordial R waves and deep left precordial S waves. Biventricular hypertrophy is manifested by large RS complexes in mid precordial leads.

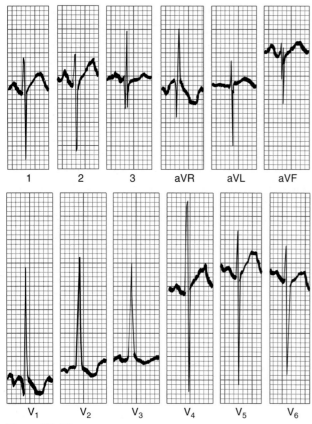

Figure 17–24

Electrocardiogram from a 3-month-old girl with a nonrestrictive muscular ventricular septal defect and a 3.4 to 1 left-to-right shunt. A right atrial abnormality is indicated by the peaked P wave in lead 2 and the q wave in lead V_1. Note the similarity of leads aVR and V_1. The QRS shows pure right ventricular hypertrophy with marked right axis deviation, a tall R wave in lead aVR, a 23-mm R wave in lead V_1 and deep left precordial S waves. A left ventricular contribution is confined to the large equidiphasic RS complex in V_4.

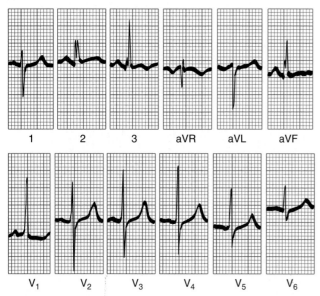

Figure 17–25

Electrocardiogram from a 19-year-old man with a nonrestrictive perimembranous ventricular septal defect and Eisenmenger syndrome. The shunt was balanced at age 5 years and reversed at age 9 years. The P waves are normal. Right axis deviation is mild. Right ventricular hypertrophy is manifested by the tall monophasic R wave in lead V_1. The tracing reflects pure pressure overload of the right ventricle.

congestive heart failure, pulmonary venous congestion, and radiologic enlargement of all four chambers. X-rays resemble those of moderately restrictive defects with large left-to-right shunts (see Figs. 17–6*A* and 17–7). In the exceptional adult, the pulmonary trunk and its branches are aneurysmal (Fig. 17–28). As pulmonary vascular resistance rises, the left-to-right shunt falls reciprocally, congestive heart failure is ameliorated, the heart size decreases, but enlargement of the pulmonary trunk and its branches persists (see Fig. 17–6*B*). When suprasystemic pulmonary vascular resistance reverses the shunt—*Eisenmenger syndrome* (see Fig. 17–5*D*)—the lung fields are oligemic; right atrial, left atrial, and left ventricular sizes are normal; and the hypertrophied but nondilated right ventricle occupies the apex (see Fig. 17–9). Except for enlargement of the pulmonary trunk and its branches and a convex apical right ventricle, the cardiac silhouette is deceptively unimpressive (see Fig. 17–9).

THE ECHOCARDIOGRAM

Transthoracic and transesophageal echocardiography with color flow imaging and Doppler interrogation establish the presence, location and physiologic consequences of ventricular septal defects (Fig. 17–29).[85,94,103,165,207,214,282] Three-dimensional echocardiography enhances assessment.[258,259] Shunt flow can be examined in the fetus by color Doppler M-mode.[260] Small multiple defects in the muscular septum,[215] spontaneous closure of perimembranous or muscular defects,[265] and septal aneurysms[257] can

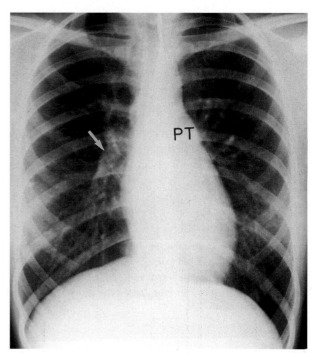

Figure 17–26

X-ray from a 15-year-old girl with a restrictive perimembranous ventricular septal defect, a left-to-right shunt of 1.4 to 1 and normal pulmonary artery pressure. The pulmonary trunk and its right branch are moderately prominent because the ventricular septal defect was previously larger. The x-ray is otherwise normal.

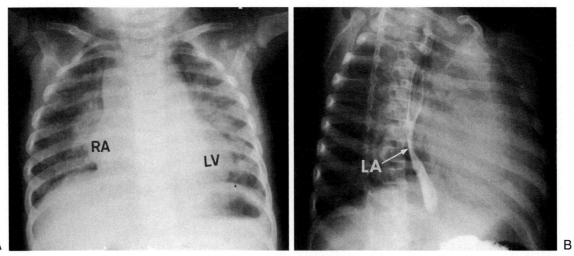

Figure 17–27

X-rays from a 7-month-old girl with a moderately restrictive perimembranous ventricular septal defect, a 3 to 1 left-to-right shunt, and a pulmonary artery pressure of 45/18 mm Hg. *A,* There is increased pulmonary arterial blood flow, increased pulmonary venous vascularity, a convex left ventricle at the apex, and a prominent right atrium at the right lower cardiac border. *B,* The right anterior oblique view shows retrodisplacement of the barium esophagram by an enlarged left atrium (LA).

be identified, and Swiss cheese defects in the trabecular muscular septum are recognized by color flow imaging. Right ventricular systolic pressure and pulmonary artery systolic and diastolic pressure can be estimated (Fig. 17–30).

Shunt flow across a ventricular septal defect is complex and was first characterized by angiocardiography[124,209] but

is now characterized with echocardiography.[207,215] Flow is bidirectional.[207,215] Isovolumetric contraction is accompanied by left-to-right shunting, with flow patterns during ventricular ejection depending in part on the size of the ventricular septal defect (Fig. 17–30). In nonrestrictive defects, the direction of flow is determined by the relative resistances in the pulmonary and systemic vascular

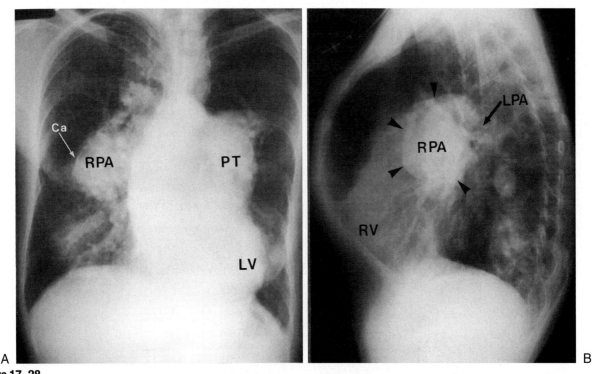

Figure 17–28

Remarkable x-rays from a 39-year-old woman with a nonrestrictive perimembranous ventricular septal defect and a 2.3 to 1 left-to-right shunt. *A,* There is aneurysmal dilatation of the pulmonary trunk (PT) and the right pulmonary artery (RPA) which contained a thin rim of calcium (Ca). Pulmonary arterial vascularity is increased, and a convex left ventricle (LV) occupied the apex. Rightward scoliosis is apparent. *B,* Lateral view shows the aneurysmal right pulmonary artery end-on, a dilated left pulmonary artery (LPA), an enlarged right ventricle (RV), and striking pectus carinatum.

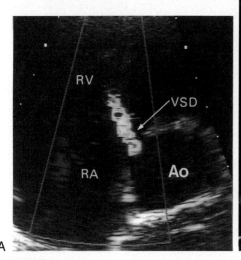

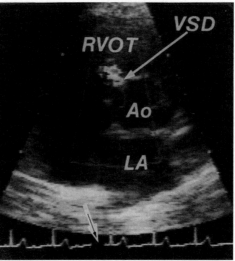

Figure 17–29

A, Black-and-white print of a color flow image in the short axis from a 41-year-old man with a restrictive perimembranous ventricular septal defect (VSD). *Arrow* points to the high-velocity systolic jet through the VSD. Ao, aorta; RA/RV, right atrium/right ventricle. *B*, Black-and-white print of a short axis color flow image from a 23-year-old woman with a restrictive perimembranous ventricular septal defect. *Arrow* points to *diastolic* flow into the right ventricular outflow tract (RVOT). See arrow in the electrocardiogram rhythm strip for timing.

beds.[207] Isovolumetric relaxation coincides with right-to-left flow. Two flow patterns have been identified during ventricular diastole.[207] Transient right-to-left flow occurs at the time of mitral valve opening followed by left-to-right flow from mid-diastole to the time of mitral valve closure.[207]

Echocardiography with color flow imaging locates the ventricular septal defect in the perimembranous septum (Fig. 17–31), in the muscular septum (Figs. 17–32 and 17–33), in the infundibular septum, or in the inlet septum (Fig. 17–34). Two-dimensional imaging identifies a septal aneurysm (Figs. 17–31B and 17–35A), and color flow imaging determines whether or not the aneurysm harbors a residual shunt (Fig. 17–35B). Aneurysm formation war-

rants color flow interrogation of the tricuspid valve for the presence of tricuspid regurgitation.[103,245] Inlet ventricular septal defects may be accompanied by atrioventricular valve straddling (Fig. 17–34). A subarterial defect is associated with color flow directed toward the pulmonary trunk (Fig. 17–36) with continuity of aortic and pulmonary valves in the roof of the defect[94,276] and with aortic regurgitation due to prolapse of the right or noncoronary cusp (see Fig. 17–45).

SUMMARY

Perimembranous and trabecular muscular ventricular septal defects that are trivial at birth go unrecognized unless the

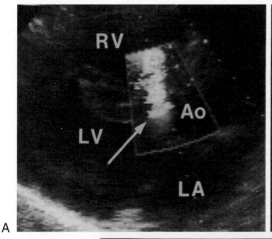

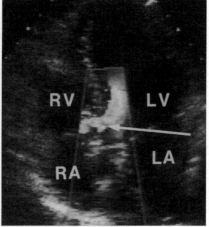

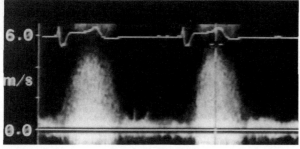

Figure 17–30

A, Black-and-white print of a short axis color flow image from a 40-year-old woman with a restrictive perimembranous ventricular septal defect. A high velocity jet (*arrow*) is directed into the outflow tract of the right ventricle (RV). LV/LA, left ventricle/left atrium; Ao, aorta. *B*, Apical four-chamber view shows the high-velocity jet traversing the perimembranous ventricular septal defect. *C*, Continuous wave Doppler across the ventricular septal defect recorded a left ventricular-to-right ventricular gradient of 130 mm Hg indicating a normal right ventricular systolic pressure.

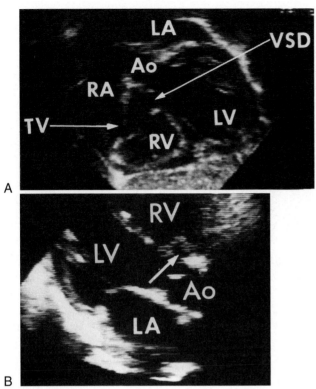

A

B

Figure 17–31
A, Subcostal four-chamber view shows a moderately restrictive perimembranous ventricular septal defect (VSD) and defines the relationship of the defect to the aorta (Ao) and tricuspid valve (TV). RV/LV, right ventricle/left ventricle; RA/LA, right atrium/left atrium. *B*, Echocardiogram from a 3-year-old girl with a restrictive perimembranous ventricular septal defect that closed spontaneously. Parasternal long-axis view shows a septal aneurysm (*arrow*) projecting into the outflow tract of the right ventricle (RV).

soft high frequency early systolic murmur is identified before the defect spontaneously closes. *A defect that is restrictive but not trivial* comes to light because of a left

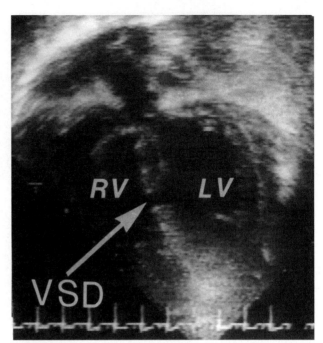

Figure 17–33
Echocardiogram (subcostal) from a 3-month-old boy with a restrictive ventricular septal defect (VSD) in the midportion of the trabecular muscular septum. RV/LV, right ventricle/left ventricle.

parasternal holosystolic murmur which is the only evidence of its presence. Restrictive defects in the perimembranous or muscular septum usually close spontaneously during the course of which the holosystolic murmur becomes early systolic before disappearing. Restrictive perimembranous defects are substrates for infective endocarditis.

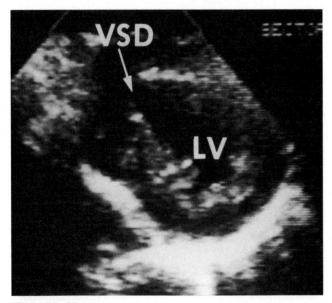

Figure 17–32
Echocardiogram in the short axis from a 1-year-old boy with a moderately restrictive ventricular septal defect (VSD) in the trabecular muscular septum. LV, left ventricle.

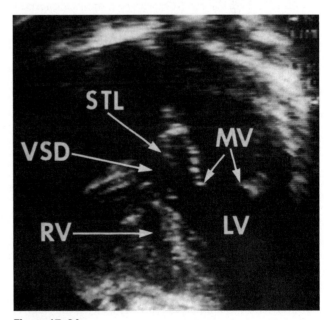

Figure 17–34
Echocardiogram (subcostal) from a 4-year-old girl with an inlet ventricular septal defect (VSD) and straddling of the septal tricuspid leaflet (STL). The right ventricle (RV) was significantly reduced in size. LV, left ventricle; MV, mitral valve.

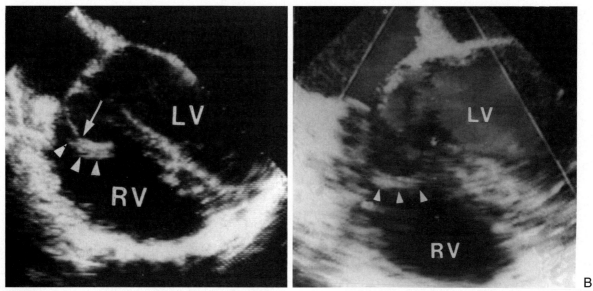

Figure 17–35

A, Echocardiograms from a 4-year-old boy with aneurysm formation (*arrowheads*) following spontaneous closure of a moderately restrictive perimembranous ventricular septal defect (*arrow*). LV/RV, left/right ventricle. B, Black-and-white print of a color flow image from the same patient showing the sealed aneurysm that filled during ventricular systole.

Moderately restrictive ventricular septal defects with low but variable pulmonary vascular resistance present with congestive heart failure in infancy. Holosystolic murmurs are absent at birth but obvious at the first well-baby examination. Infants with large shunts and congestive heart failure thrive poorly. The physical examination reveals retarded growth and development, a hyperdynamic left ventricular impulse, a variable right ventricular impulse, a left parasternal systolic thrill with a prominent holosystolic murmur, and an apical middiastolic flow murmur across the mitral valve. The electrocardiogram shows left atrial P wave abnormalities and volume overload of the left ventricle with variable degrees of right ventricular hypertrophy. X-rays reveal vascular lung fields that are a combination of increased pulmonary arterial blood flow and pulmonary venous congestion. All four cardiac chambers and the pulmonary trunk are dilated. Echocardiography with color flow imaging and Doppler interrogation establishes the presence and location of the ventricular septal defect and determines its physiologic consequences. Perimembranous and trabecular muscular defects tend to decrease in size and close spontaneously except for Swiss cheese defects. Reduction in size of the defect curtails excessive pulmonary arterial blood flow, curtails left ventricular volume overload, and ameliorates congestive heart failure.

Nonrestrictive ventricular septal defects with elevated but variable pulmonary vascular resistance present in infancy with congestive heart failure and its catabolic effects. If pulmonary vascular resistance remains sufficiently high to limit the shunt, the infant deceptively escapes the stage of heart failure with few ill effects, but goes on to confront a progressive rise in pulmonary vascular resistance. When the shunt is large, the physical examination reveals a dynamic precordium due to volume overload of the left ventricle and dilatation of the hypertensive right ventricle.

A systolic thrill and holosystolic murmur are accompanied by a loud pulmonary closure sound and an apical middiastolic flow murmur across the mitral valve. The electrocardiogram shows biatrial P waves and biventricular hypertrophy. The x-ray discloses shunt vascularity and pulmonary venous congestion with dilatation of the pulmonary trunk and all four cardiac chambers. A rise in pulmonary vascular resistance decreases pulmonary blood flow and ameliorates congestive heart failure. When pulmonary resistance is suprasystemic, the shunt is reversed and Eisenmenger syndrome exists. The physical examination then reveals symmetric cyanosis, a normal jugular

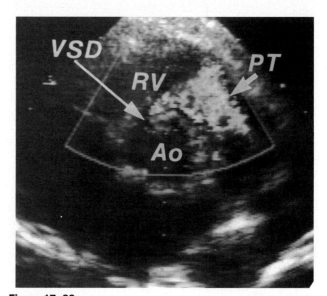

Figure 17–36

Black-and-white print of a color flow image in the short axis from a 10-year-old girl with a subarterial ventricular septal defect (VSD). The systolic jet (*arrow*) is directed into the pulmonary trunk (PT). There was no aortic regurgitation. Ao, aorta; RV, right ventricle.

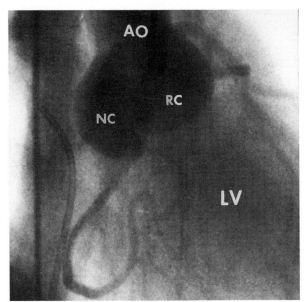

Figure 17–37

Right anterior oblique aortogram (AO) from a 19-year-old man with a restrictive perimembranous ventricular septal defect. Mild-to-moderate aortic regurgitation opacifies the left ventricle (LV). There is sagging of the noncoronary cusp (NC) and right coronary cusp (RC).

venous pulse with a small dominant A wave, a relatively modest right ventricular impulse, a palpable pulmonary trunk, and a palpable pulmonary component of the second heart sound. Auscultation discloses signs of pure pulmonary hypertension—a pulmonary ejection sound, a short pulmonary midsystolic murmur, a loud single second heart sound, and a Graham Steell murmur. The electrocardiogram shows right atrial P waves and relatively pure right ventricu-

lar hypertrophy. The x-ray reveals oligemic lung fields and an unimpressive cardiac silhouette except for a dilated pulmonary trunk and a convex right ventricle at the apex.

Ventricular Septal Defect with Aortic Regurgitation

In 1921 Laubry and Pezzi published a postmortem account of ventricular septal defect with an incompetent aortic valve.[119] Eleven years later Laubry, Routier and Soulie described two patients with ventricular septal defects, a loud aortic diastolic murmur, a wide pulse pressure, and at necropsy prolapsed aortic cusps.[120] The prevalence of aortic regurgitation with ventricular septal defect depends largely on the relative prevalence of perimembranous versus doubly committed subarterial defects.[*] *Perimembranous* defects are more common in Caucasians with an incidence of aortic regurgitation of approximately 5% to 8%.[45,53,156,184,219] *Subarterial* defects are more common in Asians with an incidence of aortic regurgitation of approximately 30%.[10,46,83,139,184,209]

Perimembranous defects are located immediately beneath the commissure between the right coronary cusp and the noncoronary cusp.[156,179,219] Aortic regurgitation is associated with sagging or herniation of the right coronary cusp or both the right coronary cusp and the noncoronary cusp (Figs. 17–37 and 17–38).[46,139,179,184,206,254,255] Herniation sometimes protrudes into the right ventricular outflow tract and causes obstruction[40,113,219,229] or

---

*See references 45, 46, 53, 83, 139, 156, 166, 184, 197, 219.

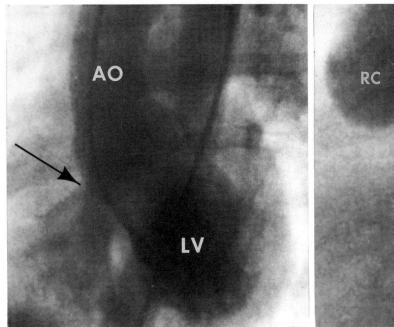

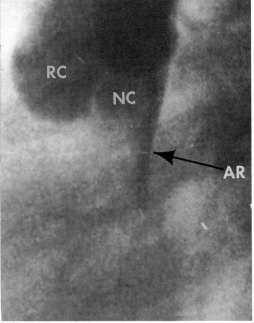

A   B

Figure 17–38

Angiograms from a 5-year-old boy with a moderately restrictive perimembranous ventricular septal defect and mild aortic regurgitation. *A,* Left anterior oblique left ventriculogram (LV) discloses the shunt (*arrow*). AO, aorta. *B,* Lateral aortogram shows sagging of the right coronary cusp (RC) and noncoronary (NC) cusp with mild aortic regurgitation (AR).

protrudes through the ventricular septal defect and reduces the left-to-right shunt.[156,179]

The morphologic basis for aortic regurgitation is ascribed to a structural abnormality at the right coronary-noncoronary commissure.[139,220,229] The abnormality is aggravated if not caused by the high-velocity jet accompanying the ventricular septal defect shunt which is in accordance with observations that aortic regurgitation develops years *after* birth[86,179] and that when the high velocity jet is absent as in Eisenmenger syndrome, aortic regurgitation is virtually unknown.[156,179]

The typical sequence begins with the structural abnormality responsible for faulty aortic leaflet apposition followed by sagging of the noncoronary cusp and right coronary cusp (Figs. 17–37 and 17–38).[113,179,206,220,229] Once the cusps fall below the normal closure line, the aortic valve becomes incompetent, and the impact of the regurgitant jet provokes leaflet elongation, thickening, distortion, and progression of the incompetence.[179,220]

Ventricular septal defects in the infundibular septum are located immediately beneath the aortic and pulmonary valves that constitute a contiguous roof over the defect which is therefore doubly committed and subarterial.[8,46,83,197] The aortic and pulmonary valves are in fibrous continuity with each other because the infundibular septum including the septal portion of the subpulmonary infundibulum are deficient.[83] The aortic valve lacks support, so the right and noncoronary sinuses move into the right ventricular outflow tract causing aortic regurgitation and occasionally causing a subpulmonary gradient.[156,179,208,229]

The *physiologic consequences* of aortic regurgitation with a ventricular septal defect are borne by the left ventricle, which receives the sum of the regurgitant volume from the aorta and the shunt volume from the ventricular septal defect. Aortic regurgitation begins insidiously and is gradually progressive unless infective endocarditis supervenes (see The History). The left-to-right shunt is larger for a given degree of regurgitation when regurgitation is associated with a *subarterial* defect which does not decrease in size unless partially occluded by the prolapsed right coronary cusp.[197] Aortic regurgitant volume and shunt volume both contribute significantly to left ventricular volume overload. Conversely, a *perimembranous* ventricular defect tends to get smaller as the degree of aortic regurgitation increases, so aortic regurgitant volume rather than shunt volume is the major contributor to left ventricular volume overload.[156,179] The shunt can be trivial or even absent in the presence of severe aortic regurgitation (Fig. 17–39).[156,179]

THE HISTORY

When aortic regurgitation coexists with ventricular septal defect, the male/female ratio is as high as 2:1 in contrast to the equal sex distribution when a ventricular septal defect occurs in isolation (see earlier).[40,113,148,156,166,179,184,206] Echocardiography and aortography in both perimembranous and subarterial ventricular septal defects detect herniation

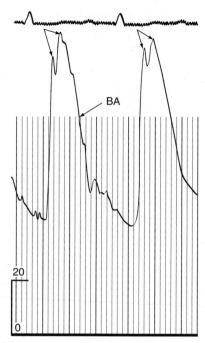

Figure 17–39
Brachial arterial pulse (BA) from a 21-year-old man with a restrictive perimembranous ventricular septal defect and severe aortic regurgitation. The left-to-right shunt was 1.5 to 1. The pulmonary artery pressure was normal. The brachial pulse shows a brisk rise, bisferiens (twin) peaks and a wide pulse pressure (115/55 mm Hg).

of the right and noncoronary cusps before the onset of aortic regurgitation,[46,83,139,197] which seldom begins before age 2 years or after age 10 years and peaks between 5 and 9 years of age.[45,86,113,148,156,166]

The diagnosis can sometimes be suspected based on the history. The typical murmur of ventricular septal defect is present for years, more commonly in a male. Between age 5 years and 9 years, an additional murmur is discovered. The patient becomes aware of neck pulsations, chest pain, diaphoresis, and vigorous precordial movement, especially at night when lying in the left lateral recumbent position. Infective endocarditis, to which the incompetent aortic valve is highly susceptible, accelerates regurgitant flow and left ventricular failure.[166,184]

THE ARTERIAL PULSE

The arterial pulse gradually becomes the bounding water-hammer pulse of severe aortic regurgitation with a wide pulse pressure, bisferiens peaks (Fig. 17–39), pistol shot sounds over the femoral arteries, and capillary pulsations in the nail beds (see Chapter 7).[53,156] Taussig said of one patient that "The head shook with each cardiac impulse and the pulsations of the dorsalis pedis were readily felt through the bed clothes."[221]

PRECORDIAL MOVEMENT AND PALPATION

The greater the degree of aortic regurgitation, the more dynamic the left ventricular impulse. A right ventricular impulse is inconspicuous or absent.

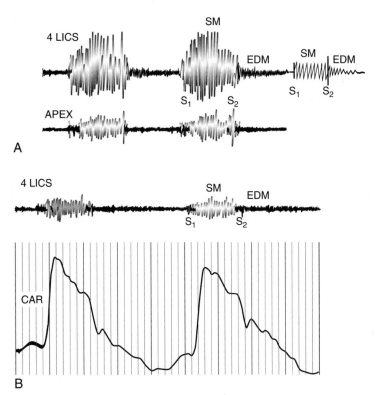

Figure 17–40

A, Tracings from an 8-year-old boy with a moderately restrictive perimembranous ventricular septal defect, a 2 to 1 left-to-right shunt, and mild aortic regurgitation. A prominent holosystolic murmur (SM) is followed by a soft high-frequency early diastolic murmur of aortic regurgitation (EDM). The holosystolic and early diastolic murmurs are schematically illustrated on the right (see Fig 17–41*A*). 4 LICS, fourth left intercostal space. At the apex, the holosystolic murmur remained prominent, but the aortic regurgitation murmur was absent. *B,* Tracings from a 17-year-old boy with a restrictive perimembranous ventricular septal defect, a 1.3 to 1 shunt, and moderate aortic regurgitation (brachial arterial pressure 135/50 mm Hg). In the fourth left intercostal space (4 LICS), there was the high- frequency holosystolic murmur of a restrictive ventricular septal defect and a soft early diastolic murmur of aortic regurgitation. CAR, carotid pulse.

AUSCULTATION

The murmurs of ventricular septal defect and aortic regurgitation are *not continuous* (see Fig. 17–41*B*) but are *holosystolic and early diastolic* (Figs. 17–40 and 17–41*A*).[156,172,179,206] The holosystolic portion of the murmur is typical of ventricular septal defect with intracardiac location in the right ventricular cavity and thoracic wall location at the overlying left sternal border site (Figs. 17–40 and 17–41*A*).[65] The diastolic portion of the murmur is characteristic of aortic regurgitation, that is, high-frequency decrescendo beginning with the aortic component of the second heart sound (Figs. 17–40 and 17–41*A*). The systolic/diastolic murmurs do not peak around the second heart sound and therefore differ from the murmur of patent ductus arteriosus which is continuous and envelopes the second heart sound, peaking around it (Fig. 17–41*B* and see Chapter 20). Eddy sounds that punctuate the ductus murmur in latter systole and early diastole are absent with ventricular septal defect and aortic regurgitation. Both the systolic and diastolic portions of the continuous murmur of patent ductus are maximum in the first or second left intercostal space. The *systolic* portion of the murmur of ventricular septal defect with aortic regurgitation is loudest in the third or fourth intercostal space, and the *diastolic* portion is heard at the mid to lower left sternal border (Fig. 17–40). Uncertainty arises in the *third* left intercostal space when the systolic and diastolic murmurs are both prominent and sometimes create the mistaken impression of a continuous murmur.

Distinction between an aortic regurgitation murmur and a Graham Steell murmur is difficult if not impossible on purely auscultatory grounds.[172] However, aortic regurgitation rarely occurs with Eisenmenger syndrome, so a high frequency early diastolic murmur is likely to be Graham Steell.[171] Conversely, in the presence of a restrictive ventricular septal defect, an early diastolic murmur is presumptively aortic regurgitation especially if the patient is male and certainly if the systemic arterial pulse is waterhammer. When the shunt is small and aortic regurgitation is severe, an apical mid-diastolic murmur is an Austin Flint rumble and not increased shunt flow across the mitral valve.[156]

THE ELECTROCARDIOGRAM

The electrocardiogram is useful in focusing attention on disproportionate left ventricular hypertrophy of aortic

Figure 17–41

Schematic illustrations of (*A*) a holosystolic murmur (SM) followed by an early diastolic murmur (EDM) in contrast to (*B*) a continuous murmur that envelops the second heart sound and peaks around it.

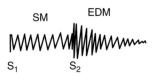

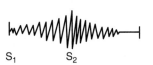

A

B

regurgitation in the presence of a restrictive ventricular septal defect (Fig. 17–42).When a restrictive defect occurs with severe aortic regurgitation, the tracing resembles aortic regurgitation rather than ventricular septal defect. Deep Q waves, tall R waves, deeply inverted T waves, and coved ST segments appear in left precordial leads (Fig. 17–42). Distinctions are less clear when a subarterial ventricular septal defect coexists with moderate aortic regurgitation and a moderate left-to-right shunt.

THE X-RAY

A key point in the x-ray is the combination of left ventricular enlargement that is disproportionate to the modest radiologic evidence of a left-to-right shunt (Fig. 17–43).[156] The x-ray resembles severe aortic regurgitation rather than ventricular septal defect (Fig. 17–43). The ascending aorta is prominent and pulsates vigorously on fluoroscopy or in real time echocardiography. When the ventricular septal defect is subarterial, the aortic root is inconspicuous despite appreciable regurgitant flow because the ventricular septal defect remains large enough to divert a sizable fraction of left ventricular stroke volume into the pulmonary circulation (Fig. 17–44). Whether the ventricular septal defect is perimembranous or subarterial, the onset of aortic regurgitation is mild and insidious, so the x-ray initially reflects the left-to-right shunt and not aortic regurgitation. As time goes on, the balance shifts as described previously.

THE ECHOCARDIOGRAM

Transthoracic and transesophageal echocardiography with Doppler interrogation and color flow imaging locate the ventricular septal defect as perimembranous or subarterial,

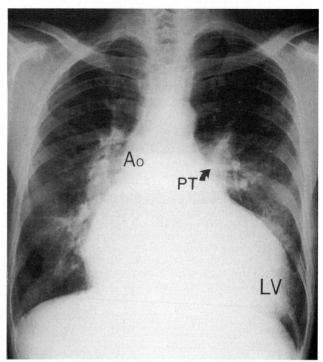

Figure 17–43

X-ray from a 21-year-old man with a restrictive perimembranous ventricular septal defect, a left-to-right shunt of 1.4 to 1 and severe aortic regurgitation. The electrocardiogram is shown in Figure 17–42. The pulmonary trunk (PT) is only mildly convex, but relatively prominent pulmonary vascularity implies that the shunt had previously been larger and the ventricular septal defect had decreased in size. The large left ventricle LV) and the dilated ascending aorta (Ao) are the result of aortic regurgitation not the left-to-right shunt.

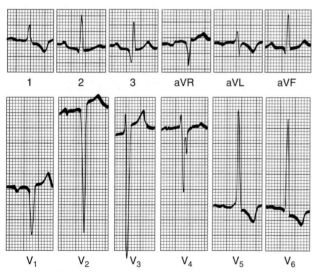

Figure 17–42

Electrocardiogram from a 21-year-old man with a restrictive perimembranous ventricular septal defect and severe aortic regurgitation. The tracing resembles isolated severe aortic regurgitation with PR interval prolongation, deep QS waves in right precordial leads and tall R waves with deeply inverted T waves and coved ST segments in left precordial leads typical of left ventricular volume overload.

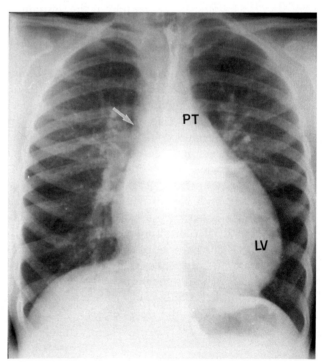

Figure 17–44

X-ray from a 14-year-old boy with moderately severe aortic regurgitation and a 2 to 1 left-to-right shunt through a subarterial ventricular septal defect. The left ventricle (LV) is considerably enlarged because of a combination of volume overload from moderately severe aortic regurgitation and a 2 to 1 left-to-right shunt. Pulmonary vascularity is increased, the pulmonary trunk (PT) is slightly convex, and the aortic root (Ao) is inconspicuous.

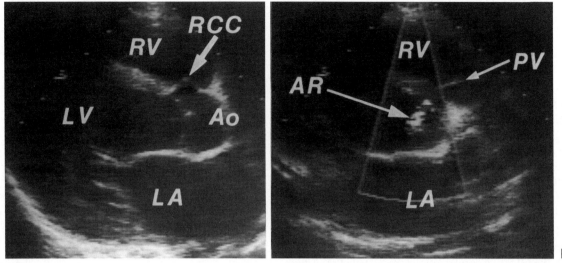

Figure 17–45

Echocardiograms from a 4-year-old boy with a moderately restrictive perimembranous ventricular septal defect and aortic regurgitation. *A*, The parasternal long-axis view shows prolapse of the right coronary cusp (RCC) into the ventricular septal defect. Ao, aorta; RV/LV, right ventricle/left ventricle; LA, left atrium. *B*, Black-and-white print of a color flow image in the short axis showing aortic regurgitation (AR). PV, pulmonary valve.

identify prolapse of the right and/or noncoronary cusps, and establish the presence and degree of aortic regurgitation.[46,83,160,197,255] Aortic regurgitation associated with prolapse of the right coronary cusp into a perimembranous ventricular septal defect is illustrated in Figure 17–45. Prolapse of the right coronary cusp can be distinguished from an aneurysm of the membranous septum.[46] Color flow imaging identifies flow across a perimembranous ventricular septal defect (Fig. 17–46*A*) and establishes the presence and degree of aortic regurgitation (Figs. 17–45*B* and 17–46*B*). A subarterial ventricular septal defect is recognized by its proximity to the pulmonary and aortic valves whose sinuses are contiguous without interposed infundibular septum.[197] The systolic jet through the subarterial ventricular septal defect is directed into the pulmonary trunk (see Fig. 17–36). Echocardiography with color flow imaging can identify prolapse of the right coro-

nary cusp or noncoronary aortic cusp before the onset of aortic regurgitation.[83,197] Doppler interrogation determines the presence and degree of right ventricular outflow obstruction caused by prolapse of an elongated right coronary cusp through the ventricular septal defect.[197]

SUMMARY

Patients with ventricular septal defect and aortic regurgitation are likely to be male. The ventricular septal defect murmur dates from infancy. Between 5 years and 9 years of age, the murmur of aortic regurgitation makes its appearance and is followed by insidious progression of regurgitant flow with gradual development of a bounding arterial pulse and a dynamic left ventricular impulse. The systolic/diastolic murmurs of ventricular septal defect and aortic regurgitation are not continuous but are holosystolic

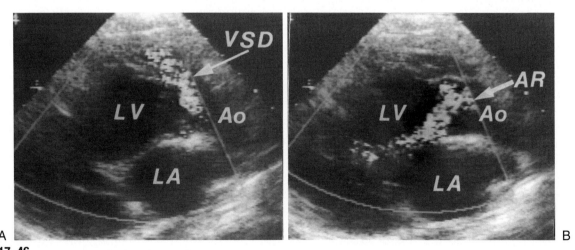

Figure 17–46

Black-and-white prints of color flow images in the parasternal long axis from an 8-year-old girl with a restrictive perimembranous ventricular septal defect and aortic regurgitation. *A*, There is a high-velocity jet across the ventricular septal defect (VSD). Ao, aorta; LV, left ventricle; LA, left atrium. *B*, Diastolic frame shows the high velocity jet of aortic regurgitation (AR).

and early diastolic, do not peak around the second heart sound, and do not contain eddy sounds. The electrocardiogram and x-ray disclose left ventricular hypertrophy and left ventricular enlargement out of proportion to the size of the left-to-right shunt. Echocardiography with color flow imaging and Doppler interrogation identifies the ventricular septal defect in the perimembranous septum or in the infundibular septum and establishes the presence and degree of aortic regurgitation.

Left Ventricular to Right Atrial Communication

In 1838, Thurnman described a left ventricular to right atrial communication in which a cleft tricuspid septal leaflet adhered to a ventricular septal defect.[224] Two decades later, Hillier described "Congenital malformation of the heart; perforation of the septum ventriculorum, establishing a communication between the left ventricle and the right atrium."[96] Similar if not identical reports appeared from Merkel in 1869[140] and from Preicz in 1890.[181] The publication of Gerbode and associates in 1958 stimulated renewed interest in the malformation that is sometimes called the Gerbode defect.[76]

A perimembranous ventricular septal defect is an obligatory component of the two varieties of left ventricular to right atrial communications illustrated in (Fig. 17–47).* The first and more common variety is characterized by a defect in the *intraventricular portion* of the membranous septum that opens into the right ventricle and then communicates with the right atrium through an anatomic deficiency in the septal tricuspid leaflet which is tethered to the crest of the ventricular septum (Fig. 17–47A). The deficiency in the septal tricuspid leaflet takes the form of perforations, clefts and widening, or absence of the commissure between the anterior and septal tricuspid leaflet.[190] A septal aneurysm is almost always present.[32,82] The ventriculoatrial communication originally described by Thurnman was this first variety.[224] In the second and much less common variety, the defect is in the *atrioventricular* portion of the membranous septum, so left ventricular blood enters the right atrium directly (Fig. 17–47E). This type of left ventricular to right atrial communication differs structurally from the atrioventricular septal defect discussed in Chapter 15.

The *physiologic consequences* of left ventricular to right atrial communications depend on the size of the defect and on the pulmonary vascular resistance as in other types of ventricular septal defects. However, the *chronology of the shunt* differs distinctively because shunt flow begins *in utero* in response to the obligatory differences in systolic pressure between the left ventricle and right atrium.[185] The right atrium accepts the shunt with little or no elevation of

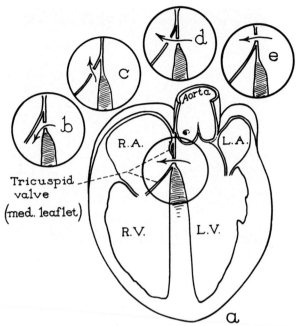

Figure 17–47
Schematic illustrations of the two varieties of left ventricular to right atrial communications originally proposed by Perry, Burchell, and Edwards in 1949.[175] The variety depicted in the large sketch (*a*) consists of a defect in the *intraventricular* portion of the membranous septum with tethering of the septal tricuspid leaflet to the crest of the ventricular septal defect. RA/LA, right atrium/left atrium; RV/LV, right ventricle/left ventricle. Insert *e* depicts the variety in which a defect in the *atrioventricular* portion of the membranous septum creates a direct communication from left ventricle into right atrium. Insets *b, c,* and *d* are variations of a *subanular* defect in the membranous septum. (With permission from Perry EL, Burchell HB, Edwards JE: Congenital communication between left ventricle and right atrium. Proc Staff Meet Mayo Clin 24:198, 1949.)

pressure because right atrial distensibility and volume increase appropriately, and because the ventricular septal defect is usually restrictive,[30,76,115,185] a feature that also accounts for normal or near normal pulmonary artery pressure. Left ventricular blood that is received by the right atrium during ventricular systole (Fig. 17–48) enters the right ventricle during the next diastole, establishing right ventricular volume overload. The shunt volume then finds its way through the pulmonary circulation, so volume overload of the left side of the heart coexists.

THE HISTORY

Sex distribution is equal or with slight female preponderance.[55,185] One patient with a left ventricular-to-right atrial communication had a sibling with an isolated perimembranous ventricular septal defect.[82] The clinical course is for all practical purposes, indistinguishable from that described earlier for restrictive or moderately restrictive perimembranous ventricular septal defects. However, an important difference is the *chronology* of the murmur, because onset of the shunt and therefore the onset of the murmur do not depend on the neonatal fall in pulmonary vascular resistance (see earlier). The shunt is present *in utero* because of the obligatory differences in systolic pressure between left ventricle and right atrium, so the mur-

---

*See references 15, 30, 58, 76, 77, 104, 115, 138, 175, 185, 190, 210.

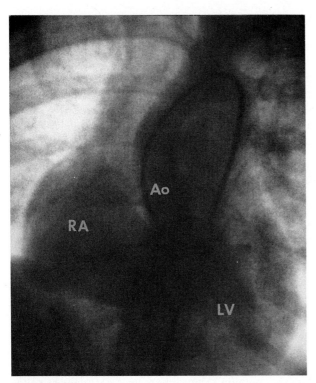

Figure 17–48
Angiocardiogram from a 4-year-old girl with a perimembranous ventricular septal defect and a left ventricular (LV) to right atrial (RA) shunt. Ao, ascending aorta.

mur that is generated by the shunt is present at birth.[185] The lesion is susceptible to infective endocarditis as in other perimembranous ventricular septal defects.[15,138,249]

THE JUGULAR VENOUS PULSE

Large V waves are seldom present and the mean jugular venous pressure is seldom elevated (Fig. 17–49) even though the left ventricle ejects into the right atrium,[76,115] because right atrial volume and distensibility increase in proportion to the shunt (see earlier).[30,76,115,185]

PRECORDIAL MOVEMENT AND PALPATION

The left-to-right shunt is received by the right atrium and then enters the right ventricle, which is volume overloaded. The right ventricular impulse is disproportionately prominent compared to ventricular septal defects of comparable size in other locations and is analogous to the volume overloaded right ventricular impulse of an ostium secundum atrial septal defect (see Chapter 15), but the apex is occupied by an equally volume overloaded *left* ventricle.

AUSCULTATION

The quality, configuration, and intensity of the systolic murmur generated by a left ventricular to right atrial communication are indistinguishable from murmurs of other ventricular septal defects of comparable size.[30,58,76,138] The *topographic location* of the murmur is its only distin-

guishing feature because the shunt is received by a right atrium that underlies the *right* lower sternal border (Fig. 17–49). The systolic murmur is recorded within the right atrial cavity[29] (Fig. 17–50) and is therefore located in a relatively rightward thoracic position (Fig. 17–49).[196] Because equal volumes of blood traverse the tricuspid and mitral valves, mid-diastolic murmurs can be generated across both of these valves depending on shunt volume.

The splitting, respiratory movement, and intensity of the second heart sound are the same as in a comparable isolated perimembranous ventricular septal defect. The split widens normally during inspiration because systemic venous return to the right side of the heart increases without a reciprocal decline in left-to-right shunt. The systolic shunt that is responsible for volume overload of the right ventricle traverses the left ventricle, so both ventricles handle equal volumes that are ejected against different resistances. Low pulmonary vascular resistance and increased pulmonary capacitance delay the pulmonary component of the second sound, but the persistent split moves normally with respiration because an intact atrial septum prevents a reciprocal decline in left-to-right shunt that

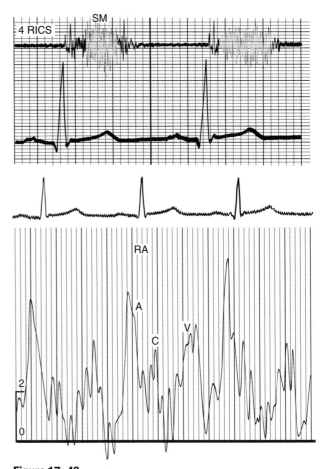

Figure 17–49
Tracings from a 17-year-old boy with a left ventricular to right atrial communication and a 2 to 1 left-to-right shunt. A prominent holosystolic murmur (SM) was present in the fourth right intercostal space (4 RICS). The right atrial (RA) pressure pulse did not show a large V wave even though the right atrium received shunt flow from the left ventricle.

RA phono

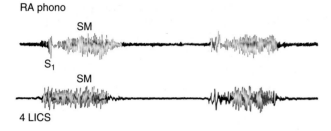

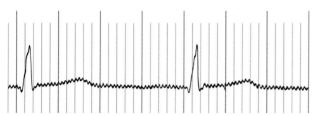

Figure 17–50

Tracings from the 17-year-old boy referred to in Figure 17–49. Intracardiac phonocardiogram within the right atrial cavity (RA PHONO) recorded a holosystolic murmur (SM), and the thoracic wall phonocardiogram in the fourth left intercostal space (4 LICS) recorded an identical murmur.

accompanies an ostium secundum atrial septal defect (see Chapter 15). *Normal intensity* of the pulmonary component of the second sound is a useful sign because it indicates that right ventricular enlargement is not due to pulmonary hypertension but instead to volume overload.

THE ELECTROCARDIOGRAM

There is an age-related increase in the incidence of supraventricular tachycardia, atrial flutter, and atrial fibrillation.[125,185] Tall peaked right atrial P waves date from infancy because the right atrium is the early recipient of the left-to-right shunt. PR interval prolongation reflects right atrial enlargement, and biatrial P wave abnormalities are common because both atria handle an equivalent volume (Fig. 17–51).[133,185]

An rSr' in lead V_1 and a terminal r wave in leads aVR and V_3R are electrocardiographic signs of right ventricular volume overload. Prominent left precordial Q waves, tall R waves and prominent upright T waves are signs of coexisting left ventricular volume overload (Fig. 17–51). A useful electrocardiographic pattern is the combination of tall peaked *right* atrial P waves with *left* ventricular hypertrophy.[76,115,138,185]

THE X-RAY

The most distinctive feature in the x-ray is enlargement of the right atrium that is out of proportion to the enlargement of the pulmonary trunk (Fig. 17–52).[55,58,76,115,125,138,164] The cardiac silhouette occasionally has a ball-like shape with the right side of the ball formed by the large right atrium and the left side of the ball formed by dilatation of the right ventricular infundibulum and the left ventricle (Fig. 17–52A).[125,185]

THE ECHOCARDIOGRAM

Echocardiography identifies the perimembranous location of the ventricular septal defect (Fig. 17–53A), and color flow imaging identifies the flow pattern from left ventricle into right atrium (Fig. 17–53B).[94,282] The relationship of the ventricular septal defect to the tricuspid valve can be established (Fig. 17–53A), and a ventricular septal aneurysm can be identified.

SUMMARY

The clinical features of a left ventricular to right atrial communication resemble those of a comparable isolated perimembranous ventricular septal defect but with a number of important variations. The systolic murmur is present *in utero* and therefore at birth, and the murmur occupies a relatively rightward thoracic position because it originates within the right atrium. Precordial palpation identifies both right and left ventricular impulses. The electrocardiogram shows tall peaked right atrial P waves without right ventricular hypertrophy but instead with evidence of left ventricular volume overload. Atrial arrhythmias are relatively common. The x-ray reveals enlargement of the right atrium that is disproportionate to the size of the pulmonary trunk. Echocardiography identifies the perimembranous ventricular septal defect, and color flow imaging records shunt flow from left ventricle into right atrium. The relationship of the ventricular septal defect to the tricuspid valve can be established, and a ventricular septal aneurysm can be identified.

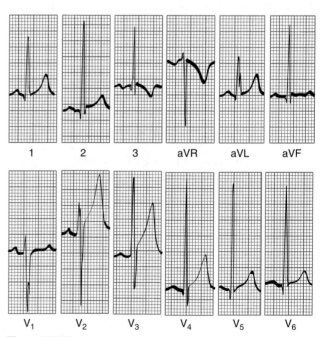

Figure 17–51

Electrocardiogram from the 17-year-old boy referred to in Figure 17–49. The tracing resembles an isolated ventricular septal defect. Volume overload of the left ventricle is represented by prominent Q waves, tall R waves and peaked T waves in leads V_{5-6}. Slight peaking of the P wave in lead V_2 is the only suggestion of a right atrial abnormality.

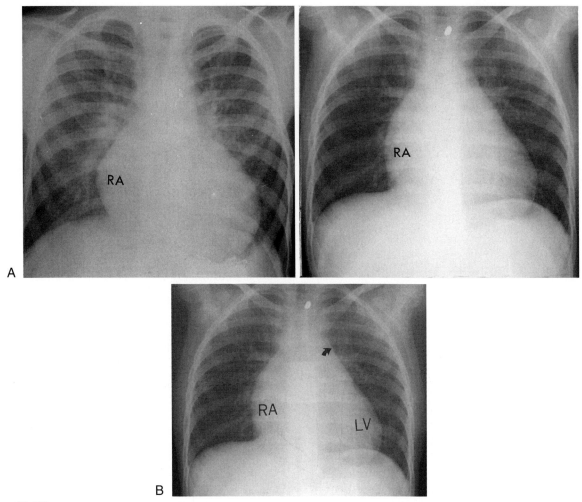

Figure 17–52

A, X-ray from a 4-year-old girl with a left ventricular to right atrial communication and a 2 to 1 left-to-right shunt. Pulmonary vascularity is increased. The right atrium (RA) is disproportionately enlarged compared to the inconspicuous pulmonary trunk. A dilated left ventricle occupies the apex and extends below the left hemidiaphragm. *B,* X-ray from a 10-year-old boy with a left ventricular to right atrial communication and a 2 to 1 left-to-right shunt. Pulmonary arterial vascularity is increased. The right atrium (RA) is disproportionately enlarged compared to the inconspicuous pulmonary trunk (*arrow*). A dilated left ventricle (LV) occupies the apex and extends below the left hemidiaphragm.

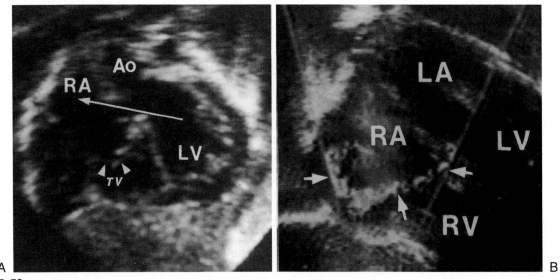

Figure 17–53

A, Echocardiogram from a 3-month-old boy with a left ventricular (LV) to right atrial communication (*arrow*, RA). The defect is in the *atrioventricular* portion of the membranous septum resulting in a direct communication from the left ventricle into the right atrium (see Fig. 17–47e). TV, tricuspid valve; Ao, aorta. *B,* Black-and-white print of a color flow image from the same patient. Three *arrows* identify jets that enter the right atrium through the left ventricular to right atrial communication. LA, left atrium; RV, right ventricle.

REFERENCES

1. Abbott ME: Congenital heart disease. In Nelson's Loose Leaf Medicine, vol 5. New York, Thomas Nelson and Sons, 1932.
2. Agustsson MH, Arcilla RA, Bicoff JP, et al: Spontaneous functional closure of ventricular septal defects in 14 children demonstrated by serial cardiac catheterizations and angiocardiography. Pediatrics 31:958, 1963.
3. Albers HJ, Carroll SE, Coles JC: Spontaneous closure of a membranous ventricular septal defect. Necropsy finding with clinical application. Br Med J 2:1162, 1962.
4. Allwork SP, Maladie du Roger: A new translation for the centenary. Am Heart J 98:307, 1979.
5. Alpert BS, Mellits ED, Rowe RD: Spontaneous closure of small ventricular septal defects. Am J Dis Child 125:194, 1973.
6. Alter BP, Czapek EE, Rowe RD: Sweating in congenital heart disease. Pediatrics 41:123, 1968.
7. Anderson RH, Wilcox BR: The surgical anatomy of ventricular septal defect. J Cardiac Surg 7:17, 1992.
8. Anderson RH, Becker AE, Lucchese FA, et al: Morphology of Congenital Heart Disease. Baltimore, University Park Press, 1983.
9. Anderson RH, Lenox CC, Zuberbuhler JR: Mechanisms of closure of perimembranous ventricular septal defect. Am J Cardiol 52:341, 1983.
10. Anzai T, Iijima T, Yoshiea I, et al: The natural history and timing of the radical operation for subpulmonic ventricular septal defects. Jpn J Surg 21:487, 1991.
11. Assad-Morell JL, Tajik AJ, Giuliani ER: Aneurysm of membranous interventricular septum: Echocardiographic features. Mayo Clin Proc 49:164, 1974.
12. Backman H: Influence of structural and functional features of ventricular septal defect on frontal plane QRS axis of the electrocardiogram. Br Heart J 34:274, 1972.
13. Baker EJ, Leung MP, Anderson RH, et al: The cross sectional anatomy of ventricular septal defects: A reappraisal. Br Heart J 59:339, 1988.
14. Balderston SM, Shaffer EM, Washington RL, Sondheimer HM: Congenital polyvalvular disease in trisomy 18: Echocardiographic diagnosis. Pediatr Cardiol 11:138, 1990.
15. Barclay RS, Reid JM, Coleman EN, et al: Communication between the left ventricle and the right atrium. Thorax 22:473, 1967.
16. Baron MG, Wolf BS, Grishman A, Van Mierop LHS: Aneurysm of the membranous septum. AJR 91:1303, 1964.
17. Baron MG, Wolf BS, Steinfeld L, Gordon A: Left ventricular angiocardiography in the study of ventricular septal defects. Radiology 81:223, 1963.
18. Barron JV, Sahn DJ, Valdez-Cruz LM, et al: Two-dimensional echocardiographic evaluation of overriding and straddling atrioventricular valves associated with complex congenital heart disease. Am Heart J 107:1006, 1983.
19. Becu LM, Fontana RS, DuShane JW, et al: Anatomic and pathologic studies in ventricular septal defect. Circulation 14:349, 1956.
20. Beerman LB, Park SC, Fischer DR, et al: Ventricular septal defect associated with aneurysm of the membranous septum. J Am Coll Cardiol 5:118, 1985.
21. Bendien C, Bossina KK, Buurma AE, et al: Hemodynamic effects of dynamic exercise in children and adolescents with moderate-to-small ventricular septal defects. Circulation 70:929, 1984.
22. Beregovich J, Bleifer S, Donoso E, Grishman A: The vectorcardiogram and electrocardiogram in ventricular septal defect, with special reference to the diagnosis of combined ventricular hypertrophy. Br Heart J 22:205, 1960.
23. Bharati S, McAllister HA, Lev M: Straddling and displaced atrioventricular orifices and valves. Circulation 60:673, 1979.
24. Bissett GS, Hirschfeld SS: Severe pulmonary hypertension associated with a small ventricular septal defect. Circulation 67:470, 1982.
25. Blair E, Herman R, Crowley RA: Interventricular septal defect in identical twins. J Thorac Cardiovasc Surg 50:197, 1965.
26. Blieden LC, Moller JH: Small ventricular septal defect associated with severe pulmonary hypertension. Br Heart J 52:117, 1984.
27. Bliss HA, Moffat JE: Hemodynamic events during the development of cyanosis and heart failure in a patient with large ventricular septal defect. Circulation 30:101, 1964.
28. Bloomfield DK: The natural history of ventricular septal defect in patients surviving infancy. Circulation 29:914, 1964.
29. Bouchard F, Wolff F, Kalmanson D: Left ventricle-right atrium communication: Diagnosed by catheterization and intracardiac phonocardiography. Arch Mal Coeur 54:1310, 1961.
30. Braunwald E, Morrow AG: Left ventricular-right atrial communication. Diagnosis by clinical, hemodynamic and angiographic methods. Am J Med 28:913, 1960.
31. Brotmacher L, Campbell M: The natural history of ventricular septal defect. Br Heart J 20:97, 1958.
32. Burrows PE, Fellows KE, Keane JF: Cineangiography of the perimembranous ventricular septum with left ventricular-right atrial shunt. J Am Coll Cardiol 1:1129, 1983.
33. Campbell M: Natural history of ventricular septal defect. Br Heart J 33:246, 1971.
34. Campbell RW, Steinmetz EF, Helmen CH: Congenital aneurysm of the membranous portion of the ventricular septum. A cause for holosystolic murmurs. Circulation 30:223, 1964.
35. Castle RF, Craige E: Auscultation of the heart in infants and children. Pediatrics 26:511, 1960.
36. Cayler GG: Cardiofacial syndrome: Congenital heart disease and facial weakness, a hitherto unrecognized association. Arch Dis Child 44:69, 1969.
37. Char F, Adams P Jr, Anderson RC: Electrocardiographic findings in one hundred verified cases of ventricular septal defect. Am J Dis Child 97:48, 1959.
38. Chen M, Rigby ML, Redington AN: Familial aneurysms of the interventricular septum. Br Heart J 65:104, 1991.
39. Chesler E, Korns ME, Edwards JE: Anomalies of the tricuspid valve, including pouches, resembling aneurysms of the membranous ventricular septum. Am J Cardiol 21:661, 1968.
40. Chung KJ, Manning JA: Ventricular septal defect associated with aortic insufficiency. Am Heart J 87:435, 1974.
41. Clark RJ, White PD: Congenital aneurysmal defect of membranous portion of ventricular septum associated with heart block, ventricular flutter, Adams-Stokes syndrome and death. Circulation 5:725, 1952.
42. Clarkson PM, Frye RL, DuShane JW, et al. Prognosis for patients with ventricular septal defect and severe pulmonary vascular obstructive disease. Circulation 38:129, 1968.
43. Claypool JG, Ruth W, Lin TK: Ventricular septal defect with aortic incompetence simulating patent ductus arteriosus. Am Heart J 54:788, 1957.
44. Collins G, Calder L, Rose V, et al: Ventricular septal defect: Clinical and hemodynamic changes in the first five years of life. Am Heart J 84:695, 1972.
45. Corone P, Doyon F, Gaudeau S, et al: Natural history of ventricular septal defect. Circulation 55:908, 1977.
46. Craig BG, Smallhorn JF, Burrows P, et al: Cross-sectional echocardiography in the evaluation of aortic valve prolapse associated with ventricular septal defect. Am Heart J 112:800, 1986.
47. Czeizel A, Meszaros M: Two family studies of children with ventricular septal defect. Eur J Pediatr 136:81, 1981.
48. Danaraj TJ: Ventricular septal defect simulating patent ductus arteriosus. Br Heart J 18:279, 1956.
49. Das SK, Jahnke EJ, Walker WJ: Aneurysm of the membranous septum with interventricular septal defect producing right ventricular outflow obstruction. Circulation 30:429, 1964.
50. Davies H, Williams J, Wood P: Lung stiffness in states of abnormal pulmonary blood flow and pressure. Br Heart J 24:129, 1962.
51. deCarvalho-Azevedo A, Toledo AN, deCarvalho AA, et al: Ventricular septal defect; an example of its relative diminution. Acta Cardiol 13:513, 1958.
52. Diehl AM, Kittle F, Crockett JE: Spontaneous complete closure of a high-flow, high-pressure ventricular septal defect. Lancet 81:572, 1961.
53. Dimich I, Steinfeld L, Litwak RS, et al: Subpulmonic ventricular septal defect associated with aortic insufficiency. Am J Cardiol 32:325, 1973.
54. DuShane JW, Weidman WH, Brandenberg RO, et al: The electrocardiogram in children with ventricular septal defect and severe pulmonary hypertension. Correlation with response of pulmonary arterial pressure to surgical repairs. Circulation 22:49, 1960.
55. Edwards JE, Carey, L.S., Neufeld, H.N., and Lester, R.G.: Congenital Heart Disease. Philadelphia, W.B. Saunders Company, 1965.
56. Eisenmenger, V.: Die angeborenen Defecte der Kammerscheidewand des Herzens. Z. Klin. Med. 32(Suppl. 1): 1897.

57. Elliott, L. P., and Schiebler, G. L.: X-ray Diagnosis of Congenital Heart Disease. Springfield, Illinois, Charles C Thomas, 1968.

58. Elliott, L. P., Gedgaudas, E., Levy, M. J., and Edwards, J. E.: The roentgenologic findings in left ventricular-right atrial communication. Am. J. Roentgenol. 93:304, 1965.

59. Ellis, J. H., Moodie, D. S., Sterba, R., and Gill, C. C.: Ventricular septal defect in the adult: Natural and unnatural history. Am. Heart J. 114:115, 1987.

60. Evans, J. R., Rowe, R. D., and Keith, J. D.: Spontaneous closure of ventricular septal defects. Circulation 22:1044, 1960.

61. Farru, O., Duffau, G., and Rodriguez, R.: Auscultatory and phonocardiographic characteristics of supracristal ventricular septal defect. Br. Heart J. 33:238, 1971.

62. Farru-Albohaire, O., Arcil, G., and Hernandez, I.: An association between axis deviation and an aneurysmal defect in children with a perimembranous ventricular septal defect. Br. Heart J. 64:146, 1990.

63. Fellows, K. E., Westerman, G. R., and Keane, J. F.: Angiography of multiple ventricular septal defects in infancy. Circulation 66:1094, 1982.

64. Ferencz, C., Rubin, J. D., Brenner, J. I., Neill, C. A., Perry, L. W., Hepner, S. I., Downing, J. W., and McCarter, R. J.: Congenital heart disease: Prevalence at livebirth. Am. J. Epidemiol. 121:31, 1985.

65. Feruglio, G. A., and Gunston, R. W.: Intracardiac phonocardiography in ventricular septal defect. Circulation 21:49, 1960.

66. Fisher, E. A., DuBrow, I. W., and Hastreiter, A. R.: Right ventricular volume in congenital heart disease. Am. J. Cardiol. 36:67, 1975.

67. Fontana, R. S., and Edwards, J. E.: Congenital Cardiac Disease. Philadelphia, W. B. Saunders Company, 1962.

68. Fox, K. M., Patel, R. G., Graham, G. R., Taylor, J. F. N., Stark, J., De Leval, M. R., and Macartney, F. J.: Multiple and single ventricular septal defect. Br. Heart J. 40:141, 1978.

69. Freedom, R. M., Bini, R., Dische, R., and Rowe, R. D.: The straddling mitral valve. Eur. J. Cardiol. 8:27, 1978.

70. Freedom, R. M., White, R. D., Pieroni, D. R., Varghese, P. J., Krovetz, L. J., and Rowe, R. D.: The natural history of the so-called aneurysm of the membranous ventricular septum in childhood. Circulation 49:375, 1974.

71. French, H.: The possibility of a loud congenital heart murmur disappearing when a child grows up. Guy's Hosp. Rep. 32:87, 1918.

72. Friedli, B., Kidd, B. S. L., Mustard, W. T., and Keith, J. D.: Ventricular septal defect with increased pulmonary vascular resistance. Am. J. Cardiol. 33:403, 1974.

73. Friedman, W. F., Mehrizi, A., and Pusch, A. L.: Multiple muscular ventricular septal defects. Circulation 32:35, 1965.

74. Fyler, D. C.: Report of the New England regional infant cardiac program. Pediatrics 65(Suppl.):375, 1980.

75. Fyler, D. C., Rudolph, A. M., Wittenborg, M. H., and Nadas, A. S.: Ventricular septal defect in infants and children; a correlation of clinical, physiologic, and autopsy data. Circulation 18:833, 1958.

76. Gerbode, F., Hultgren, H., Melrose, D., and Osborn, J.: Syndrome of left ventricular-right atrial shunt. Successful surgical repair of defect in five cases, with observation of bradycardia on closure. Ann. Surg. 148:433, 1958.

77. Gibson, R.: The syndrome of the left ventricular to right atrial shunt. Br. Heart J. 22:589, 1960.

78. Glancy, D. L., and Roberts, W. C.: Complete spontaneous closure of ventricular septal defect. Am. J. Med. 43:846, 1967.

79. Gould, L., and Gopalaswamy, C.: Late survival of a patient with ventricular septal defect and Eisenmenger's syndrome. Angiology 33:769, 1982.

80. Gould, L., and Lyon, A. F.: Prolapse of the pulmonic valve through a ventricular septal defect. Am. J. Cardiol. 18:127, 1966.

81. Graham, T. P., Atwood, G. F., Boucek, R. J., Cordell, D., and Boerth, R. D.: Right ventricular volume characteristics in ventricular septal defect. Circulation 54:800, 1976.

82. Grenadier, E., Shem-Tov, A., Motro, M., and Palant, A.: Echocardiographic diagnosis of left ventricular-right atrial communication. Am. Heart J. 106:407, 1983.

83. Griffin, M. L., Sullivan, I. D., Anderson, R. H., and Macartney, F. J.: Doubly committed subarterial ventricular septal defect: New morphological criteria with echocardiographic and angiographic correlation. Br. Heart J. 59:474, 1988.

84. Griffiths, S. P., Blumenthal, S., Jameson, A. G., Ellis, K., Morgan, B. C., and Malm, J. R.: Ventricular septal defect. Survival in adult life. Am. J. Med. 37:23, 1964.

85. Hagler, D. J., Edwards, W. D., Seward, J. B., and Tajik, A. J.: Standardized nomenclature of the ventricular septum and ventricular septal defects, with applications for two-dimensional echocardiography. Mayo Clin. Proc. 60:741, 1985.

86. Halloran, K. H., Talner, N. S., and Browne, M. J.: A study of ventricular septal defect associated with aortic insufficiency. Am. Heart J. 69:320, 1965.

87. Hamby, R. I., Raia, F., and Apiado, O.: Aneurysm of the pars membranacea. Report of three adult cases and a review of the literature. Am. Heart J. 79:688, 1970.

88. Haroutunian, L. M., and Neill, C. A.: Pulmonary complications of congenital heart disease: Hemoptysis. Am. Heart J. 84:540, 1972.

89. Harris, A.: The second heart sound in health and in pulmonary hypertension. Am. Heart J. 79:145, 1970.

90. Harris, C., Wise, J., and Oakley, C. M.: Fixed splitting of the second heart sound in ventricular septal defect. Br. Heart J. 33:428, 1971.

91. Haworth, S. G.: Pulmonary vascular disease in ventricular septal defect: Structural and functional correlations in lung biopsies from 85 patients, with outcome of intracardiac repair. J. Pathol. 152:157, 1987.

92. Heath, D., Helmholz, H. F., Jr., Burchell, H. B., DuShane, J. W., and Edwards, J. E.: Graded pulmonary vascular changes and hemodynamic findings in case of atrial and ventricular septal defect and patent ductus arteriosus. Circulation 18:1155, 1958.

93. Heggtveit, H. A.: Congenital aneurysm of the membranous septum associated with bundle branch block. Am. J. Cardiol. 14:112, 1964.

94. Helmcke, F., de Souza, A., Nanda, N. C., Villacosta, I., Gatewood, R., Colvin, E, and Soto, B.: Two-dimensional and color Doppler assessment of ventricular septal defect of congenital origin. Am. J. Cardiol. 63:1112, 1989.

95. Herbert, W. H.: Hydrogen-detected ventricular septal defects. Br. Heart J. 31:766, 1969.

96. Hillier, T.: Congenital malformation of the heart; perforation of the septum ventriculorum, establishing a communication between the left ventricle and the right atrium. Trans. Pathol. Soc. Lond. 10:110, 1859.

97. Hislop, A., Haworth, S. G., Shinebourne, E. A., and Reid, L.: Quantitative structural analysis of pulmonary vessels in isolated ventricular septal defect in infancy. Br. Heart J. 37:1014, 1975.

98. Hoeffel, J. C., Henry, M., Flizot, M., Luceri, R., and Pernot, C.: Radiologic patterns of aneurysms of the membranous septum. Am. Heart J. 91:450, 1976.

99. Hoffman, J. I. E.: Natural history of congenital heart disease. Problems in its assessment with special reference to ventricular septal defects. Circulation 37:97, 1968.

100. Hoffman, J. I. E., and Christianson, R.: Congenital heart disease in a cohort of 19,502 births with long-term follow-up. Am. J. Cardiol. 42:641, 1978.

101. Hoffman, J. I. E., and Rudolph, A. M.: The natural history of ventricular septal defects in infancy. Am. J. Cardiol. 16:634, 1965.

102. Hollman, A., Morgan, J. J., Goodwin, J. F., and Fields, H.: Auscultatory and phonocardiographic findings in ventricular septal defect. A study of 93 surgically treated patients. Circulation 28:94, 1963.

103. Hornberger, L. K., Sahn, D. J., Krabill, K. A., Sherman, F. S., Swensson, R. E., Pesonen, E., Hagen-Ansert, S., and Chung, K. J.: Elucidation of the natural history of ventricular septal defects by serial Doppler color flow mapping studies. J. Am. Coll. Cardiol. 13:1111, 1989.

104. Hutchin, P., and Peters, R. M.: Left ventricular-right atrial communication with aortic insufficiency. Ann. Thorac. Surg. 4:344, 1967.

105. Jain, A. C., and Rosenthal, R.: Aneurysm of the membranous ventricular septum. Br. Heart J. 29:60, 1967.

106. Jarmakani, J. M., Graham, T. P., and Canent, R. V.: Left ventricular contractile state in children with successfully corrected ventricular septal defect. Circulation 45:I-102, 1972.

107. Jarmakani, J. M. M., Graham, T. P., Benson, D. W., Canent, R. V., and Greenfield, J. C.: In vivo pressure-radius relationships of the pulmonary artery in children with congenital heart disease. Circulation 43:585, 1971.

108. Johnson, D. H., Rosenthal, A., and Nadas, A. S.: A forty year review of bacterial endocarditis in infancy and childhood. Circulation, 51:581, 1975.

109. Kaplan, S., Dauod, G. I., Benzing, G., III, Devine, F. J., Glass, I. H., and McGuire, J.: Natural history of ventricular septal defect. Am. J. Dis. Child. 105:581, 1963.

110. Kasparian, H., Brest, A. M., and Novack, P.: Congenital aneurysm of the membranous ventricular septum. Arch. Intern. Med. 116:753, 1965.

111. Katz, L. N., and Wachtel, H.: Diphasic QRS type of electrocardiogram in congenital heart disease. Am. Heart J. 13:202, 1937.

112. Kavanagh-Gray, D.: Spontaneous closure of a ventricular septal defect. Can. Med. Assoc. J. 87:868, 1962.

113. Kawashima, Y., Danno, M., Shimizu, Y., Matsuda, H., Miyamoto, T., Fujita, T., Kozuka, T., and Manabe, H.: Ventricular septal defect associated with aortic insufficiency: Anatomic classification and method of operation. Circulation 47:1057, 1973.

114. Kidd, L., Driscoll, D. J., Gersony, W. M., Hayes, C. J., Keane, J. F., O'Fallon, W. M., Pieroni, D. R., Wolfe, R. R., and Weidman, W. H.: Second natural history study of congenital heart defects: Results of treatment of patients with ventricular septal defects. Circulation 87(Suppl. 1):38, 1993.

115. Kramer, R. A., and Abrams, H. L.: Radiologic aspects of operable heart disease. VII. Left ventricular-right atrial shunts. Radiology 78:171, 1962.

116. Lambert, E. C., Kelsch, J. V., and Vlad, P.: Differential diagnosis of ventricular septal defect in infancy. Am. J. Cardiol. 11:447, 1963.

117. Lambert, M. E., Widlansky, S., Franken, E. A., Hurwitz, R., Nielson, R., and Nasser, W. K.: Natural history of ventricular septal defects associated with ventricular septal aneurysms. Am. Heart J. 88:566, 1974.

118. Larsen, K. A., and Noer, T.: Cardiac aneurysm of the membranous portion of the interventricular septum. Acta Med. Scand. 166:401, 1960.

119. Laubry, C., and Pezzi, C.: Traité des Maladies Congénitales du Coeur. Paris, J. B. Baillière et Fils, 1921.

120. Laubry, C., Routier, D., and Soulie, P.: Les souffles de la maladie de Roger. Rev. Méd. Paris 50:439, 1933.

121. Leatham, A., and Segal, B.: Auscultatory and phono-cardiographic signs of ventricular septal defect with left-to-right shunt. Circulation 25:318, 1962.

122. Lessof, M.: Heart sounds and murmurs in ventricular septal defect. Guy's Hosp. Rep. 108:361, 1959.

123. Lev, M., and Saphir, O.: Congenital aneurysm of the membranous septum. Arch. Pathol. 25:819, 1938.

124. Levin, A. R., Spach, M. S., and Canent, R. V.: Intracardiac pressure-flow dynamics in isolated ventricular septal defects. Circulation 35:430, 1967.

125. Levy, M., and Lillehei, C. W.: Left ventricular-right atrial canal. Ten cases surgically. Am. J. Cardiol. 10:623, 1962.

126. Levy, R. J., Rosenthal, A., Miettenen, O. S., and Nadas, A. S.: Determinants of growth in patients with ventricular septal defect. Circulation 57:793, 1978.

127. Lim, D., and Keith, J. D.: Spontaneous closure of ventricular septal defect. Am. Heart J. 80:432, 1970.

128. Lin, A. E., and Perloff, J. K.: Upper limb malformations associated with congenital heart disease. Am. J. Cardiol. 55:1576, 1985.

129. Lincoln, C., Jamieson, S., Shinebourne, E., and Anderson, R. H.: Transatrial repair of ventricular septal defects with reference to their anatomic classification. J. Thorac. Cardiovasc. Surg. 74:183, 1977.

130. Linhart, J. W., and Razi, B.: Late systolic murmur. A clue to the diagnosis of aneurysm of the membranous septum. Chest 60:283, 1971.

131. Lucas, R. V., Jr., Adams, P., Jr., Anderson, R. C., Meyne, N. G., Lillehei, C. W., and Varco, R. L.: The natural history of isolated ventricular septal defect. A serial physiologic study. Circulation 24:1372, 1961.

132. Lynfield, J., Gasul, B. M., Arcilla, R., and Luan, L. L.: The natural history of ventricular septal defects in infancy and childhood. Based on serial cardiac catheterization studies. Am. J. Cardiol. 5:357, 1961.

133. Macruz, R., Perloff, J. K., and Case, R. B.: A method for the electrocardiographic recognition of atrial enlargement. Circulation 17:882, 1958.

134. Marino, B., Papa, M., Guccione, P., Corno, A., Marasini, M., and Calabro, R.: Ventricular septal defect in Down syndrome. Am. J. Dis. Child. 144:544, 1990.

135. Martin, G. R., Perry, L. W., and Ferencz, C.: Increased prevalence of ventricular septal defect: Epidemic or improved diagnosis. Pediatrics 83:200, 1989.

136. Mason, D., and Hunter, W. C.: Localized congenital defects of cardiac interventricular septum; study of three cases. Am. J. Pathol. 13:835, 1937.

137. Matsuoka, R., Misugi, K., Goto, A., Gilbert, E. F., and Ando, M.: Congenital heart anomalies in the trisomy 18 syndrome, with reference to congenital polyvalvular disease. Am. J. Med. Genet. 14:657, 1983.

138. Mellins, R. B., Cheng, G., Ellis, K., Jameson, A. G., Malm, J. R., and Blumenthal, S.: Ventricular septal defect with shunt from left ventricle to right atrium. Bacterial endocarditis as a complication. Br. Heart J. 26:584, 1964.

139. Menahem, S., Johns, J. A., Del Torso, S., Goh, T. H., and Venables, A. W.: Evaluation of aortic valve prolapse in ventricular septal defect. Br. Heart J. 56:242, 1986.

140. Merkel, G.: Zur Kasuistik der totalen Herzerkrankungen. Virchows Arch. Pathol. Anat. 48:488, 1869.

141. Miller, R. H., Schiebler, G. L., Grumbar, P., and Krovetz, L. J.: Relation of hemodynamics to height and weight percentiles in children with ventricular septal defects. Am. Heart J. 78:523, 1969.

142. Miller, W. L., and Kovachevich, R.: Self-sealing ventricular septal defects of the heart. Report of two cases. Am. Heart J. 66:798, 1963.

143. Milo, S., Ho, S. W., Macartney, F. J., Wilkinson, J. L., Becker, A. E., Wenink, A. C. G., Gittenberger de Groot, A. C., and Anderson, R. H.: Straddling and overriding atrioventricular valves. Am. J. Cardiol. 44:1122, 1979.

144. Misra, K. P., Hildner, F. J., Cohen, L. S., Narula, O. S., and Samet, P.: Aneurysm of the membranous ventricular septum: A mechanism for spontaneous closure of ventricular septal defect. New Engl. J. Med. 283:58, 1970.

145. Mitchell, S. C., Berendes, H. W., and Clark, W. M., Jr.: The normal closure of the ventricular septum. Am. Heart J. 73:334, 1967.

146. Moe, D. G., and Guntheroth, W. G.: Spontaneous closure of uncomplicated ventricular septal defect. Am. J. Cardiol. 60:674, 1987.

147. Moene, R. J., Sobotka-Plojhar, M., Oppenheimer-Dekker, A., and Lindhout, D.: Ventricular septal defect with overriding aorta in trisomy-18. Eur. J. Pediatr. 147:556, 1988.

148. Momma, K., Toyama, K., Takao, A., Ando, M., Nakazawa, M., Hirosawa, K., and Amai, Y.: Natural history of subarterial infundibular ventricular septal defect. Am. Heart J., 108:1312, 1984.

149. Moncada, R., Bicoff, J. P., Arcilla, R. A., Agustsson, M. H., Lendrum, B. L., and Gasul, B. M.: Retrograde left ventricular angiocardiography in ventricular septal defect. Am. J. Cardiol. 11:436, 1963.

150. Moore, D., Vlad, P., and Lambert, E. C.: Spontaneous closure of ventricular septal defect following cardiac failure in infancy. J. Pediatr. 66:712, 1965.

151. Moss, A. J.: Conquest of the ventricular septal defect—a period of uncertainty. Am. J. Cardiol. 25:457, 1970.

152. Mudd, J. G., Aykent, Y., Williams, V. L., Hanlon, C. R., and Fagan, L. F.: The natural history of 252 patients with proved ventricular septal defects. Am. J. Med. 39:946, 1965.

153. Musewe, N. N., Smallhorn, J. E., Moes, C. A. F., Freedom, R. M., and Trusler, G. A.: Echocardiographic evaluation of obstructive mechanism of tetralogy of Fallot with restrictive ventricular septal defect. Am. J. Cardiol. 61:664, 1988.

154. Nadas, A. S., and Ellison, R. C.: Phonocardiographic analysis of diastolic flow murmurs in secundum atrial septal defect and ventricular septal defect. Br. Heart J. 29:684, 1967.

155. Nadas, A. S., Scott, L. P., Hauck, A. J., and Rudolph, A. M.: Spontaneous functional closing of ventricular septal defects. New Engl. J. Med. 264:309, 1961.

156. Nadas, A. S., Thilenius, O. G., LaFarge, C. G., and Hauck, A. J.: Ventricular septal defect with aortic regurgitation. Medical and pathologic aspects. Circulation 29:862, 1964.

157. Naeye, R. L.: The pulmonary arterial bed in ventricular septal defect. Anatomic features in childhood. Circulation 34:962, 1966.

158. Neufeld, H. N., Titus, J. L., DuShane, J. W., Burchell, H. B., and Edwards, J. E.: Isolated ventricular septal defect of the persistent common atrioventricular canal type. Circulation 23:685, 1961.

159. Newman, T. B.: Etiology of ventricular septal defects: An epidemiologic approach. Pediatrics 76:741, 1985.

160. Nishimura, R. A., Miller, F. A., Callahan, M. J., Benassi, R. C., Seward, J. B., and Tajik, A. J.: Doppler echocardiography: Theory, instrumentation, technique, and application. Mayo Clin. Proc. 60:321, 1985.

161. Nora, J. J.: Update on the etiology of congenital heart disease and genetic counseling. In Van Praagh, R., and Takao, A. (eds.): Etiology and Morphogenesis of Congenital Heart Disease. Mount Kisco, New York, Futura Publishing Company, 1980.

162. Nora, J. J., and Nora, A. H.: The genetic contribution to congenital heart disease. *In* Nora, J. J., and Takao, A. (eds.): Congenital Heart Disease. Mount Kisco, New York, Futura Publishing Company, 1984.

163. Nora, J. J., Cohen, M., and Maxwell, G. M.: Klippel-Feil syndrome with congenital heart disease. Am. J. Dis. Child. 102:110, 1961.

164. Nordenstrom, B., and Ovenfors, C. O.: Septal defect between the left ventricle and the right atrium diagnosed by cardioangiography. Acta. Radiol. 54:393, 1960.

165. Orita, Y., Hirata, T., Kikuchi, Y., Takeshita, A., and Nakamura, M.: Two-dimensional echocardiographic demonstration of so-called aneurysm of the membranous ventricular septum in adults. J. Cardiovasc. Ultrasonog. 3:261, 1984.

166. Otterstad, J. E., Ihlen, H., and Vatne, K.: Aortic regurgitation associated with ventricular septal defects in adults. Acta Med. Scand. 218:85, 1985.

167. Otterstad, J. E., Nitter-Hauge, S., and Myhre, E.: Isolated ventricular septal defects in adults: Clinical and haemodynamic findings. Br. Heart J. 50:343, 1983.

168. Otterstad, J. E., Simonsen, S., and Erikssen, J.: Hemodynamic findings at rest and during mild supine exercise in adults with isolated uncomplicated ventricular septal defects. Circulation 71:650, 1985.

169. Papadopoulos, C., Lee, Y. C., and Scherlin, L.: Isolated ventricular septal defect. Electrocardiographic, vectorcardiographic and catheterization data. Am. J. Cardiol. 16:359, 1965.

170. Perasalo, O., Halonen, P. I., Pyorala, K., and Telivuo, L.: Aneurysm of the membranous ventricular septum causing obstruction of the right ventricular outflow tract in a case of ventricular septal defect. Acta Chir. Scand. 383(Suppl.):123, 1961.

171. Perloff, J. K.: Auscultatory and phonocardiographic manifestations of pulmonary hypertension. Prog. Cardiovasc. Dis 9:303, 1967.

172. Perloff, J. K.: Physical Examination of the Heart and Circulation. 3rd ed, Philadelphia, W. B. Saunders Company, 2000

173. Perloff, J. K.: Pregnancy in congenital heart disease: The mother and the fetus. *In* Perloff, J. K., and Child, JS: Congenital Heart Disease in Adults 2nd ed. Philadelphia, W. B. Saunders Company, 1998.

174. Perloff JK, Rosove MH, Sietsema KE, Territo MC. Cyanotic congenital heart disease: A multisystem systemic disorder. In Perloff JK and Child JS. Congenital Heart Disease in Adults 2nd ed. WB Saunders Co Philadelphia, 1998, p. 199.

175. Perry, E. L., Burchell, H. B., and Edwards, J. E.: Cardiac clinics; congenital communication between left ventricle and right atrium; co-existing ventricular septal defect and double tricuspid orifice. Proc. Staff Meet. Mayo Clin. 24:198, 1949.

176. Pickering, D., and Keith, J. D.: Systolic clicks with ventricular septal defects. A sign of aneurysm of ventricular septum? Br. Heart J. 33:538, 1971.

177. Pieroni, D. R., Bell, B. B., Krovetz, L. J., Varghese, P. J., and Rowe, R. D.: Auscultatory recognition of aneurysm of the membranous ventricular septum associated with small ventricular septal defect. Circulation 44:733, 1971.

178. Pitts, J. A., Crosby, W. M., and Basta, L. L.: Eisenmenger's syndrome in pregnancy. Am. Heart J. 93:321, 1977.

179. Plauth, W. H., Jr., Braunwald, E., Rockoff, S. D., Mason, D. T., and Morrow, A. G.: Ventricular septal defect and aortic regurgitation. Clinical, hemodynamic and surgical considerations. Am. J. Med. 39:552, 1965.

180. Pombo, E., Pilapil, V. R., Lehan, P. H.: Aneurysm of the membranous ventricular septum. Am. Heart J. 79:188, 1970.

181. Preicz, H.: Beitrage zur Lehre von den angeborenen Herzanomalien. Beitr. Pathol. Anat. 7:234, 1890.

182. Ramaciotti, C., Keren, A., and Silverman, N. H.: Importance of (perimembranous) ventricular septal aneurysm in the natural history of isolated perimembranous ventricular septal defect. Am. J. Cardiol. 57:268, 1986.

183. Reynolds, J. L.: Supracristal ventricular septal defect. Am. J. Cardiol. 18:610, 1966.

184. Rhodes, L. A., Keane, J. F., Keane, J. P., Fellows, K. E., Jonas, R. A., Castaneda, A. R., and Nadas, A. S.: Long follow-up (to 43 years) of ventricular septal defect with audible aortic regurgitation. Am. J. Cardiol. 66:340, 1990.

185. Riemenschneider, T. A., and Moss, A. J.: Left ventricular-right atrial communication. Am. J. Cardiol. 19:710, 1967.

186. Riggs, T., Mehta, S., Hirschfeld, S., Borkat, G., and Liebman, J.: Ventricular septal defect in infancy: A combined vectorcardiographic and echocardiographic study. Circulation 59:385, 1979.

187. Roberts, W. C., Morrow, A. G., Mason, D. T., and Braunwald, E.: Spontaneous closure of ventricular septal defect. Anatomic proof in an adult with tricuspid atresia. Circulation 27:90, 1963.

188. Roger, H.: Clinical researches on the congenital communication of the two sides of the heart by failure of occlusion of the interventricular septum. Bull. de l'Acad. de Méd. 8:1074, 1879. (*In* Willius, F. A., and Keys, T. E.: Classics of Cardiology. Malabar, Florida, Robert E. Krieger Publishing Company, 1983.)

189. Rogers, H. M., Evans, I. C., and Domeier, L. H.: Congenital aneurysm of the membranous portion of the ventricular septum. Am. Heart J. 43:781, 1952.

190. Rosenquist, G. C., and Sweeney, L. J.: Normal variations in tricuspid valve attachments to the membranous ventricular septum: A clue to the etiology of left ventricular to right atrial communication. Am. Heart J. 89:186, 1975.

191. Rosove, M. H., Perloff, J. K., Hocking, W. G., Child, J. S., Canobbio, M. M., and Skorton, D. J.: Chronic hypoxaemia and decompensated erythrocytosis in cyanotic congenital heart disease. Lancet 2:313, 1986.

192. Rubenstein, H. J., and Weaver, K. H.: Monozygotic twins concordant for ventricular septal defects. Case report and review of the literature of congenital heart disease in monozygotic twins. Am. J. Cardiol. 15:386, 1965.

193. Rudolph, A. M.: The changes in the circulation after birth: Their importance in congenital heart disease. Circulation 41:343, 1970.

194. Rudolph, A. M., and Nadas, A. S.: The pulmonary circulation and congenital heart disease. New Engl. J. Med. 267:968, 1962.

195. Saab, N. G., Burchell, H. B., DuShane, J. W., and Titus, J. L.: Muscular ventricular septal defects. Am. J. Cardiol. 18:713, 1966.

196. Sakakibara, S., and Konno, S.: Left ventricular-right atrial communication. Ann. Surg. 158:93, 1963.

197. Schmidt, K. G., Cassidy, S. C., Silverman, N. H., and Stanger, P.: Doubly committed subarterial ventricular septal defects: Echocardiographic features and surgical implications. J. Am. Coll. Cardiol. 12:1538, 1988.

198. Schott, G. D.: Documentation of spontaneous functional closure of a ventricular septal defect during adult life. Br. Heart J. 35:1214, 1973.

199. Schrire, V., Vogelpoel, L., Beck, W., Nellen, M., and Swanepoel, A.: Ventricular septal defect: The clinical spectrum. Br. Heart J. 27:813, 1965.

200. Sethia, B., and Cotter, L.: Giant aneurysm of the membranous septum. Br. Heart J. 46:107, 1981.

201. Shah, P., Singh, W. S. A., Rose, V., and Keith, J. D.: Incidence of bacterial endocarditis in ventricular septal defects. Circulation 34:127, 1966.

202. Shaw, N. J., Godman, M. J., Hawes, A., and Sutherland, G. R.: Superior QRS axis in ventricular septal defect. Br. Heart J. 62:281, 1989.

203. Shumacker, H. B., Jr., and Glover, J.: Congenital aneurysms of the ventricular septum. Am. Heart J. 66:405, 1963.

204. Simmons, R. F., Moller, J. H., and Edwards, J. E.: Anatomic evidence for spontaneous closure of ventricular septal defect. Circulation 34:38, 1966.

205. Somerville, J.: Congenital heart disease—changes in form and function. Br. Heart J. 41:1, 1979.

206. Somerville, J., Brandao, A., and Ross, D. N.: Aortic regurgitation with ventricular septal defect. Circulation 41:317, 1970.

207. Sommer, R. J., Golinko, R. J., and Ritter, S. B.: Intracardiac shunting in children with ventricular septal defect: Evaluation with Doppler color flow mapping. J. Am. Coll. Cardiol. 16:1437, 1990.

208. Soto, B., Becker, A. E., Moulaert, A. J., Lie, J. T., and Anderson, R. H.: Classification of ventricular septal defects. Br. Heart J. 43:332, 1980.

209. Soto, B., Ceballos, R., and Kirklin, J. W.: Ventricular septal defects: A surgical viewpoint. J. Am. Coll. Cardiol. 14:1291, 1989.

210. Stahlman, M., Kaplan, S., Helmsworth, J. A., Clark, L. C., and Scott, H. W., Jr.: Syndrome of left ventricular-right atrial shunt resulting from high interventricular septal defect associated with defective septal leaflet of tricuspid valve. Circulation 12:813, 1955.

211. Stanton, R. E., and Fyler, D. C.: The natural history of pulmonary hypertension in children with ventricular septal defects assessed by serial right-heart catheterization. Pediatrics 27:621, 1961.

212. Steeg, C. N., and Woolf, P.: Cardiovascular malformations in the fetal alcohol syndrome. Am. Heart J. 98:635, 1979.

213. Steinfeld, L., Dimich, I., Park, S. C., and Baron, M. G.: Clinical diagnosis of isolated subpulmonic (supracristal) ventricular septal defect. Am. J. Cardiol. 30:19, 1972.

214. Sutherland, G. R., Godman, M. J., Smallhorn, J. F., Guiterras, P., Anderson, R. H., and Hunter, S.: Ventricular septal defects. Two dimensional echocardiographic and morphological correlations. Br. Heart J. 47:316, 1982.

215. Sutherland, G. R., Snyllie, J. H., Ogilvie, B. C., and Keeton, B. R.: Colour flow imaging in the diagnosis of multiple ventricular septal defects. Br. Heart J. 62:43, 1989.

216. Sutton, G., Harris, A., and Leatham, A.: Second heart sound in pulmonary hypertension. Br. Heart J. 30:743, 1968.

217. Suzuki, H., and Lucas, R. V., Jr.: Spontaneous closure of ventricular septal defects. Anatomic evidence in three patients. Arch. Pathol. 84:31, 1967.

218. Tandon, R., and Edwards, J. E.: Aneurysmlike formations in relation to membranous ventricular septum. Circulation 47:1089, 1973.

219. Tatsuno, K., Konno, S., and Sakakibara, S.: Ventricular septal defect with aortic insufficiency. Am. Heart J. 85:13, 1973.

220. Tatsuno, K., Konno, S., Ando, M., and Sakakibara, S.: Pathogenetic mechanisms of prolapsing aortic valve and aortic regurgitation associated with ventricular septal defect. Circulation 48:1028, 1973.

221. Taussig, H. B., and Semans, J. H.: Severe aortic insufficiency in association with a congenital malformation of the heart of the Eisenmenger type. Bull. Johns Hopkins Hosp. 66:157, 1940.

222. Territo, M. C., Rosove, M. H., and Perloff, J. K.: Cyanotic congenital heart disease: Hematologic management, renal function, and urate metabolism. *In* Perloff, J. K., and Child, J. S. (eds.): Congenital Heart Disease in Adults. Philadelphia, W. B. Saunders Company, 1991.

223. Thery, C., Lekieffre, J., and Dupuis, C.: Atrioventricular block secondary to a congenital aneurysm of the membranous septum. Br. Heart J. 37:1097, 1975.

224. Thurnman, J.: On aneurysms of the heart. Med. Chir. Trans. R. Med. Chir. Soc. London 21:187, 1838.

225. Titus, J. L., Daugherty, G. W., and Edwards, J. E.: Anatomy of the atrioventricular conduction system in ventricular septal defect. Circulation 28:72, 1963.

226. Toscano-Barboza, E., and DuShane, J. W.: Ventricular septal defect. Correlation of electrocardiographic and hemodynamic findings in 60 proved cases. Am. J. Cardiol. 3:721, 1959.

227. Trowitzsch, E., Braun, W., Stute, M., and Pielemeier, W.: Diagnosis, therapy, and outcome of ventricular septal defects in the first year of life: A two-dimensional colour-Doppler echocardiography study. Eur. J. Pediatr. 149:758, 1990.

228. Van-Hare, G. F., Soffer, L. J., Sivakoff, M. C., and Liebman, J.: Twenty-five-year experience with ventricular septal defect in infants and children. Am. Heart J. 114:606, 1987.

229. Van Praagh, R., and McNamara, J. J.: Anatomic types of ventricular septal defects with aortic insufficiency. Am. Heart J. 75:604, 1968.

230. Van Praagh, S., Truman, T., Firpo, A., Bano-Rodrigo, A., Fried, R., McManus, B., Engle, M. A., and Van Praagh, R.: Cardiac malformations in trisomy 18: A study of 41 postmortem cases. J. Am. Coll. Cardiol. 13:1586, 1989.

231. Vaquez, H., and Bordet, E.: Le Coeur et l'Aorte, Études Radiographiques. Paris. J. B. Baillière et Fils, 1913.

232. Varghese, P. J., Allen, J. R., Rosenquist, G. C., and Rowe, R. D.: Natural history of ventricular septal defect with right-sided aortic arch. Br. Heart J. 32:537, 1970.

233. Varghese, P. J., Izukawa, T., Celermajer, J., Simon, A., and Rowe, R. D.: Aneurysm of the membranous ventricular septum. A method of spontaneous closure of small ventricular septal defect. Am. J. Cardiol. 24:531, 1969.

234. Vickers, C. W., Kincaid, O. W., DuShane, J. W., and Kirklin, J. W.: Ventricular septal defect and severe pulmonary hypertension: Radiologic considerations in selection of patients for surgery. Radiology 75:69, 1960.

235. Vince, D. J., and Keith, J. D.: The electrocardiogram in ventricular septal defect. Circulation 24:225, 1961.

236. Wade, G., and Wright, J. P.: Spontaneous closure of ventricular septal defects. Lancet 1:737, 1963.

237. Wagenvoort, C. A., Neufeld, H. N., DuShane, J. W., and Edwards, J. E.: The pulmonary arterial tree in ventricular septal defect. A quantitative study of anatomic features in fetuses, infants and children. Circulation 23:740, 1961.

238. Walker, W. J., Garcia-Gonzalez, E., Hall, R. J., Czarnecki, S. W., Franklin, R. B., Das, S. K., and Cheitlin, M. D.: Interventricular septal defect: Analysis of 415 catheterized cases, 90 with serial hemodynamic studies. Circulation 31:54, 1965.

239. Warnes, C. A., Boger, J. E., and Roberts, W. C.: Eisenmenger ventricular septal defect with prolonged survival. Am. J. Cardiol. 54:460, 1984.

240. Weber, F. P.: Can the clinical manifestations of congenital heart disease disappear with the general growth and development of the patient? Br. J. Child. 15:113, 1918.

241. Weidman, W. H., Blount, S. G., DuShane, J. W., Gersony, W. M., Hayes, C. J., and Nadas, A. S.: Clinical course in ventricular septal defect: Natural history study. Circulation (Suppl. 1), 1, 1977.

242. Wenink, A. C. G., and Gittenberger de Groot, A. C.: Straddling mitral and tricuspid valves. Am. J. Cardiol. 49:1959, 1982.

243. Wenink, A. C. G., Oppenheimer-Dekker, A., and Moulaert, A. J.: Muscular ventricular septal defects. Am. J. Cardiol. 43:259, 1979.

244. Winchell, P., and Bashour, F.: Ventricular septal defect with aortic incompetence simulating patent ductus arteriosus. Am. J. Med. 20:361, 1956.

245. Winslow, T. M., Redberg, R. F., Foster, E., and Schiller, N. B.: Transesophageal echocardiographic detection of abnormalities of the tricuspid valve in adults associated with spontaneous closure of perimembranous ventricular septal defect. Am. J. Cardiol. 70:967, 1992.

246. Wise, J. R., and Wilson, W. S.: Angiographic documentation of spontaneous closure of ventricular septal defect in an adult. Chest 75:90, 1979.

247. Witham, A. C., and McDaniel, J. S.: Electrocardiogram, vectorcardiogram and hemodynamics in ventricular septal defect. Am. Heart J. 79:335, 1970.

248. Wood, P.: The Eisenmenger syndrome, or pulmonary hypertension with reversed central shunt. Br. Med. J. 2:701, 755, 1958.

249. Yacoub, M. H., Mansur, A., Towers, M., and Westbury, H.: Bacterial endocarditis complicating left ventricle to right atrium communication. Br. J. Dis. Chest 66:78, 1972.

250. Yang, S. S., Maranhao, V., Ablaza, S. G. G., Morse, D. P., and Goldberg, H.: Aneurysm of the membranous portion of the ventricular septum. Am. J. Cardiol. 23:83, 1969.

251. Young, D., and Mark, H.: Fate of the patient with the Eisenmenger syndrome. Am. J. Cardiol. 28:658, 1971.

252. Zakrzewski, T., and Keith, J. D.: Bacterial endocarditis in infants and children. J. Pediatr. 67:1179, 1965.

253. Zielinsky, P., Rossi, M., Haertel, J. C., Vitola, D., Lucchese, F. A., and Rodrigues, R.: Subaortic fibrous ridge and ventricular septal defect: Role of septal malalignment. Circulation 75:1124, 1987.

254. Butter A, Duncan W, Weather DD, Hosking M, Cornel G: Aortic peolapse in ventricular septal defect and its association with aortic regurgitation. Can J Cardiol 14:833, 1998.

255. Leung MP, Chau KT, Chiu C, Yung TC, Mok CK: Intraoperative TEE assessment of ventricular septal defect with aortic regurgitation. Ann Thorac Surg 61:854, 1996.

256. Sietsema KE, Cooper DM, Perloff JK, Rosove MH, Child JS, Cannobio MM, Whipp BJ, Wasserman K: Dynamics of oxygen uptake during exercise in adults with cyanotic congenital heart disease. Circulation 73:1137, 1986.

257. Dipchand AI, Boutin C: Left ventricular septal aneurysm. Circulation 98:1697, 1998.
Ammash N, Warnes CA: Cerebrovascular events in adult patients with cyanotic congenital heart disease. J Am Coll Cardiol 28:768, 1996.

258. Ishii M, Hashino K, Eto G, Tsutsumi T, Himeno W, Sugahara Y, Muta H, Kato H: Qualitative assessment of severity of ventricular septal defect by three-dimensional reconstruction of color Doppler-imaged vena contracta and flow convergence region. Circulation 103:664, 2001.

259. Dall'Agata A, Cromme-Dijkhuis AH, Meijboom FJ, Bogers AJJC: Three-dimensional echocardiography enhances the assessment of ventricular septal defect. Am J Cardiol 83:1578, 1999.

260. Lethor JP, Marcon F, de Moor M, King MEE: Physiology of ventricular septal defect shunt flow in the fetus examined by color Doppler M-mode. Circulation 101:93, 2000.

261. Ahunbay G, Onat T, Celebi A, Batmaz G: Regression of right ventricular pressure in ventricular septal defect in infancy. Pediatr Cardiol 20:336,1999.

262. Baptista MJ, Fairbrother UL, Howard CM, Farrer MJ, Davies GE: Heterotrisomy, a significant contributing factor to ventricular septal defect associated with Down syndrome? Hum Genet 107:476, 2000.

263. Diglio MC, Marino B, Grazioli S, Agostino D, Giamnotti A, Dallapiccola B: Comparison of occurrence of genetic syndromes in ventricular septal defect with pulmonic stenosis (classic tetralogy of Fallot) versus ventricular septal defect with pulmonic stenosis. Am J Cardiol 77:1375, 1996.

264. Du ZD, Roguin N, Barak M, Bihari SG, Ben EM: High prevalence of muscular ventricular septal defects in preterm neonates. Am J Cardiol 78:1183, 1996.

265. Du ZD, Roguin N, Wu XJ: Spontaneous closure of muscular ventricular septal defect identified by echocardiography in neonates. Cardiol Young 8:500, 1998.

266. Krovetz LJ: Spontaneous closure of ventricular septal defect Am J Cardiol 81:100, 1998.

267. Kumar A, Van Mierop LH, Epstein ML: Pathogenetic implications of muscular ventricular septal defect in Holt-Oram syndrome. Am J Cardiol 73:993, 1994.

268. Grech V: Epidemiology and diagnosis of ventricular septal defect in Malta. Cardiol Young 8:329, 1998.

269. Fukuda T, Suzuki T, Ito T: Clinical and morphologic features of per-imembranous ventricular septal defect with overriding of the aorta—the so-called Eisenmenger ventricular septal defect. Cardiol Young 10:343, 2000.

270. Magee AG, Fenn L, Vellekoop J, Godman MJ: Left ventricular function in adolescents and adults with restrictive ventricular septal defect and moderate left-to-right shunting. Cardiol Young 10:126, 2000.

271. Liberman L, Kaufman s, Alfayyadh M, Hordof AJ, Apfel HD: Noninvasive prediction of pulmonary artery pressure in patients with isolated ventricular septal defect. Pediatr Cardiol 21:197, 2000.

272. Niwa K, Perloff JK, Kaplan S, Child JC, Miner PD: Eisenmenger syndrome in adults: ventricular septal defect, truncus arteriosus, univentricular heart. J Am Coll Cardiol 34:223, 1999.

273. Mori K, Matsuoka S, Tatara K, Hayabuchi Y, Nii M, Kuroda Y. Echocardiographic evaluation of the development of aortic valve prolapse in supracristal ventricular septal defect. Eur L Pediatr 154:176, 1995.

274. Onat T, Ahunbay G, Batmaz G, Celebi A: Natural course of isolated ventricular septal defect during adolescence. Pediatr Cardiol 19:230, 1998.

275. Wang JK, Wu MH, Chiu IS, Chu SH, Hung CR: Malalignment type of ventricular septal defect in double-chambered right ventricle. Am J Cardiol 77:839, 1996.

276. Shirali GS, Smith EO, Geva T: Quantitation of echocardiographic predictors of outcome in infants with isolated ventricular septal defect. Am Heart J 130:1228, 1995.

277. Tomita H, Arakaki Y, Yagihara T, Echigo S: Incidence of spontaneous closure of outlet ventricular septal defect. Jpn Circ J 65:364, 2001.

278. Tutar HE, Atalay S, Turkay S, Imamoglu A: QRS axis in isolated perimembranous ventricular septal defect and influences of morphological factors on QRS axis. J Electrocardiol 34:197, 2001.

279. Perloff JK, Latta H, Barsotti P: Pathogenesis of the glomerular abnormality in cyanotic congenital heart disease. Am J Cardiol 86:1198, 2000.

280. Territo MC, Perloff JK, Rosove MH, Moake JL, Runge A: Acquired von Willebrand factor abnormalities in adults with congenital heart disease. Clin Appl Thrombosis/ Hemostasis 4:257, 1998.

281. Perloff JK: Cyanotic congenital heart disease: A multisystem disorder. In Perloff JK and Child JS: Congenital Heart Disease in Adults, 2nd ed. Philadelphia, WB Saunders Co, 1998, p 199.

282. Child JS: Transthoracic and transesophageal echocardiographic imaging: Anatomic and homodynamic assessment. In Perloff JK and Child JS: Congenital Heart Disease in Adults, 2nd ed. Phialdelphia, WB Saunders Co, 1998.

283. Brunken RC, Perloff JK, Czernin J, Huang S, Campisi R, Purcell, Miner PD, Child JS, Schelbert HR: Coronary blood flow and myocardial perfusion reserve in adults with cyanotic congenital heart disease. In press.

284. Niwa K, Perloff JK, Bhuta S, Laks H, Drinkwater DC, Child JS, Miner PD.Structural abnormalities of great atrerial walls in congenital heart disease. Circulation 103:393, 2001.

285. Hopkins WE, Waggoner AD: Severe pulmonary hypertension without right ventricular failure: The unique hearts of patients with Eisenmenger syndrome. Am J Cardiol 89:34, 2002.

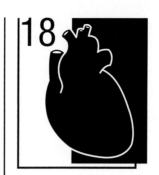

Ventricular Septal Defect with Pulmonary Stenosis

Ventricular septal defects with obstruction to right ventricular outflow encompass a wide range of anatomic, physiologic and clinical disorders. *Nonrestrictive* ventricular septal defects occur with pulmonary stenosis that varies from *mild* to *severe* to *complete* (pulmonary atresia). *Restrictive* ventricular septal defects occur with pulmonary stenosis that varies from *mild* to *severe*. The central concern of this chapter is *Fallot's tetralogy*, which is the most familiar and prevalent combination of these two defects.

The classic paper by Etienne-Louis Arthur Fallot—"L'Anatomie Pathologique de la Maladie Bleue" (Fig 18–1A)—appeared in 1888 in an obscure journal published in Marseille where Fallot lived throughout his life.[11,79] The malformation reported by Fallot was originally described in 1671 by Niels Stensen,[6] better known by his Latinized name, Nicholas Steno, who was equally distinguished as anatomist, geologist, and theologian.[142,148,220] Steno wrote:

"When I opened the right ventricle . . . the probe that was passed forward and upward along the interventricular septum entered directly into the aorta just as readily as the probe passed from left ventricle into aorta. The same aortic canal . . . was common to both ventricles. Thus, the aorta receives blood from both ventricles at the same time . . . as it partly straddles the right ventricle" (Fig. 18–1B).[220]

One hundred years later, the clinical and anatomical features of Fallot's tetralogy were described by Eduard Sandifort of Leyden[148,189,220] followed by William Hunter (1784),[123] James Hope (1839)[121] and Thomas Peacock (1866).[169] In 1872, Sir Thomas Watson wrote, "The septum between the ventricles was imperfect in its upper part; and the aorta belonged as much to one ventricle as to the other. The pulmonary artery would not admit a goosequill; the walls of the right ventricle were as thick as those of the left."[217] Fallot made an anatomic diagnosis at the bedside, was proved right at postmortem, and coined

the term *tetralogy*.[79] "This malformation consists of a true anatomopathologic type represented by the following tetralogy: 1) stenosis of the pulmonary artery; 2) interventricular communication; 3) deviation of the origin of the aorta to the right; 4) hypertrophy, almost always concentric, of the right ventricle."[79] Fallot requested that no eulogy be published after his death, but the tetralogy that bears his name remains one of the most familiar eponyms in cardiovascular medicine.[11]

The four salient anatomic components of Fallot's tetralogy result from a specific morphogenetic abnormality—*malalignment of the infundibular septum*.[198] In the normal heart, division of the fetal conotruncal segment culminates in alignment of the infundibular septum with the muscular trabecular septum. In Fallot's tetralogy, the infundibular septum deviates anteriorly and cephalad and is therefore not aligned with the trabecular septum, creating a ventricular septal defect at the site of malalignment. The deviation of the infundibular septum encroaches on the right ventricular outflow tract causing infundibular stenosis and a biventricular overriding aorta (Fig. 18–2).[198] The degree of override and the size of the biventricular aorta are determined chiefly by the degree of malalignment,[198] but the size of the aorta is also determined by an inherent medial abnormality.[5] The nonrestrictive malaligned ventricular septal defect results in systemic systolic pressure in the right ventricle and in concentric right ventricular hypertrophy.

The malaligned ventricular septal defect is located in the perimembranous septum with extension into the infundibular septum.[198] The crest of the muscular trabecular septum forms the floor of the defect which is roofed by the valve of the overriding aorta setting the stage for aortic regurgitation.[42,200] Rarely, the ventricular septal defect is part of an atrioventricular septal defect (see Chapter

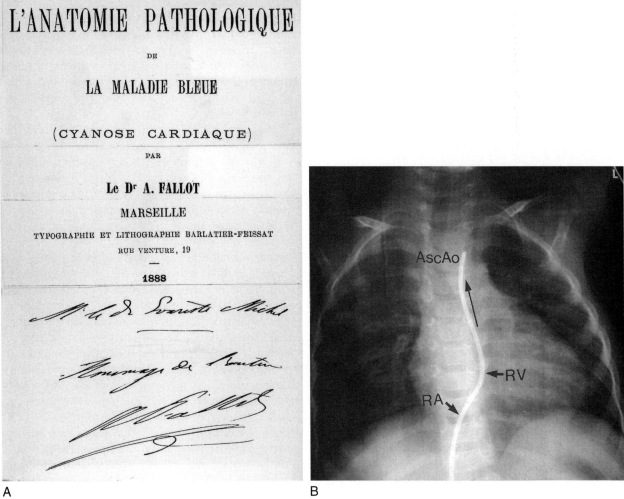

Figure 18–1

A, Cover of Fallot's 1888 publication inscribed to Messieur le Docteur S. Michel, "Homage from the author," and signed "E Fallot." *B,* Catheter following the path of Nicholas Steno's probe, "When I opened the right ventricle...the probe that was passed forward and upward along the interventricular septum entered directly into aorta...." RA, right atrium; RV, right ventricle; AscAo, ascending aorta.

15).[201,207] Muscular ventricular septal defects occasionally coexist with the malaligned defect, but usually close spontaneously in the first year of life. The nonrestrictive malaligned ventricular septal defect of Fallot's tetralogy *remains* nonrestrictive. Only occasionally does accessory or excessive tricuspid valve tissue reduce the size of the defect (see Fig. 18–18).[76,89,102,119] The occluding accessory or excessive tricuspid valve tissue is fixed to the edges of the defect by short chordae tendineae or is tethered by long chordae that permit wide excursions through the defect. The malaligned ventricular septal defect of Fallot's tetralogy is associated with normal atrioventricular conduction.

Malalignment of the infundibular septum is the essential if not the only cause of obstruction to right ventricular outflow[198] which also results from hypertrophy of the septoparietal trabeculations, the trabecula septomarginalis, and the infundibular septum (Fig. 18–3A). Anterior and cephalad malalignment of the infundibular septum can narrow the entire right ventricular outflow tract (Fig.

18–3A, B).[58,198] The greater the malalignment, the greater the aortic override and the more severe the obstruction. The pulmonary valve is frequently stenotic and bicuspid Fig. 18–3B), less commonly unicommissural unicuspid.[4] A hypoplastic pulmonary annulus or stenosis of the ostium of the infundibulum is occasionally the main site of obstruction (Fig. 18–4). The pulmonary trunk, its bifurcation, and its right and left branches tend to be segmentally or diffusely hypoplastic (Fig. 18–5B).[191]

Pulmonary atresia with a nonrestrictive malaligned ventricular septal defect is the ultimate expression of severity in Fallot's tetralogy. The right ventricle terminates blindly against an atretic pulmonary valve or against imperforate muscle (Figs. 18–6A and 18–7B).[71] The pulmonary trunk is either a vestigial cord or a hypoplastic funnel-shaped channel that widens as it approaches the bifurcation. The proximal pulmonary arteries are hypoplastic (Fig. 18–7D) and may be discontinuous.[71] The entire right ventricular output enters the systemic circulation via the nonrestrictive malaligned ventricular septal defect (Figs. 18–6A and

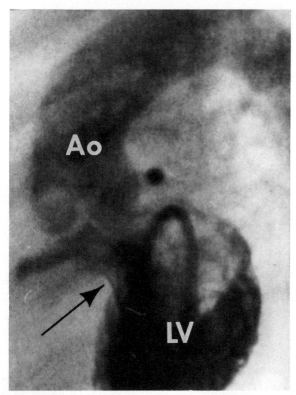

Figure 18–2
Left anterior oblique left ventriculogram (LV) from an 8-month-old girl with cyanotic Fallot's tetralogy. The enlarged aorta (Ao) significantly overrides the ventricular septum (*arrow*).

18–7B). The biventricular aorta is dilated (Figs. 18–6A and 18–7A,B) and often continues as a right aortic arch (Fig. 18–8A). The lungs are perfused by systemic to pulmonary arterial collaterals (Figs 18–6B and 18–7C,D)

upon which survival depends.[77,112,113,127,139,151,180,205] Exceptionally, the pulmonary circulation is supplied primarily if not exclusively by a long, narrow sigmoid-shaped ductus arteriosus (see Fig. 18–38B) that is structurally a muscular systemic artery similar to a systemic arterial collateral. This ductal structure is appropriate for intrauterine flow, which is directed *from* the aorta *into* the pulmonary artery.

One of the most characteristic features of Fallot's tetralogy with pulmonary atresia is a pulmonary circulation supplied entirely by collateral arteries that serve both a nutritive function and the respiratory function of gas exchange.[205] The three types of arterial blood supply to the lungs include major systemic arterial collaterals, the distinctive ductus arteriosus that is a muscular systemic artery structurally similar to a collateral artery, and small diffuse pleural arterial plexuses.[139] *Systemic arterial collaterals* are classified according to their origins, namely: 1) *bronchial arterial collaterals* that originate as their name indicates and anastomose to pulmonary arteries within the lung (Fig. 18–6B)[66,180]; 2) *direct systemic arterial collaterals* that originate from the descending aorta, enter the hilum, and then assume the structure and distribution of intrapulmonary arteries (Figs. 18–7C,D)[180]; and 3) *indirect systemic arterial collaterals* that originate from major aortic branches other than bronchial arteries (internal mammary, innominate, subclavian) and anastomose to proximal pulmonary arteries outside the lung (Fig.18–8B).[77,151,180] All three major types of systemic arterial collaterals are present when Fallot's tetralogy occurs with *pulmonary atresia*, but only bronchial collaterals are present when the tetralogy occurs with *pulmonary stenosis*.[180] Approximately 10% of arterial collaterals originate from coronary arteries.[25,62,100,166]

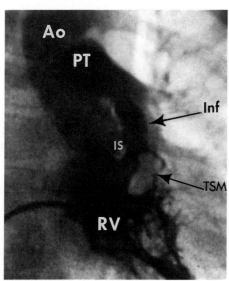

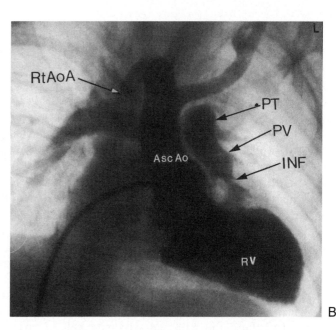

Figure 18–3
A, Right ventriculogram (RV) from a 5-year-old boy with Fallot's tetralogy. The infundibular septum (IS) and the trabecula septomarginalis (TSM) are hypertrophied. The aorta (Ao) visualizes from the right ventricle and is larger than the pulmonary trunk (PT). INF, infundibulum. *B,* Right ventriculogram (RV) from a 15-month-old boy with Fallot's tetralogy. There is hourglass narrowing of the hypertrophied infundibulum (INF), a dome-shaped stenotic pulmonary valve (PV), and a well-formed annulus and pulmonary trunk (PT). The dilated ascending aorta (AscAo) visualizes from the right ventricle and continues as a right aortic arch (RtAoA).

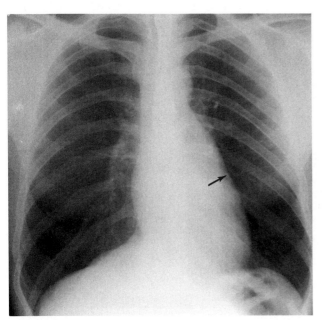

Figure 18–4

X-ray from a mildly cyanotic 37-year-old man with Fallot's tetralogy. *Arrow* points to a localized indentation at the site of stenosis of the ostium of the infundibulum above which the infundibular chamber is mildly convex. The x-ray is otherwise normal.

Direct aortic to pulmonary collaterals originate from intersegmental branches of the dorsal aorta during the third and fourth weeks of gestation.[66,180] *Bronchial arterial collaterals* develop in the ninth gestational week after the paired intersegmental arteries have been resorbed[66,180] and do not coexist with direct aortic collaterals.[180] *Indirect collaterals* arise later in gestation, and therefore coexist with bronchial collateral vessels but not with direct aortic *collaterals*.[180] A particular collateral artery supplies a particular

segment of lung, but duplicate blood supplies occasionally occur.[77] A single type of collateral blood supply usually predominates in a given patient.[180] Lung growth and survival depend on the size and patency of the collateral arteries.[112] Diminished pulmonary blood flow has an adverse effect on the growth of peripheral pulmonary arteries.[180]

Bronchial arterial *collaterals* are characterized by *intrapulmonary* anastomoses, direct arterial *collaterals* by *hilar* anatomoses, and indirect arterial *collaterals* by *extrapulmonary* anatomoses.[180] Thus, systemic arterial *collaterals* anastomose with pulmonary arteries in one of three locations: 1) intrapulmonary, 2) extrapulmonary, and 3) hilar.[180]

Systemic arterial collaterals have a strong tendency to harbor intimal cushions (proliferations) that serve as sites of potential segmental stenosis (Fig.18–8B).[112,113,180] In the absence of segmental stenoses, large collateral arteries transmit systemic arterial pressure into the pulmonary vascular bed resulting in morphologic changes analogous to pulmonary vascular disease (see Chapter 14).[7,180] Stenotic sites protect the intrapulmonary resistance vessels from systemic pressure but at the price of compromising regional pulmonary blood flow. The pulmonary circulation is effective in gas exchange regardless of the type of systemic arterial collateral. A reduction in lung volume coincides with a reduction in the total number of alveoli despite an increase in alveolar density.[127]

In 1947, Taussig observed that the ductus arteriosus was seldom structurally normal in Fallot's tetralogy with pulmonary atresia.[202] The *normal* fetal ductus serves as a conduit for right ventricular flow from pulmonary trunk into aorta. This function cannot be served when pulmonary atresia diverts the entire right ventricular output into the aorta via the nonrestrictive malaligned ventricular septal defect. Not surprisingly, the ductus is malformed or

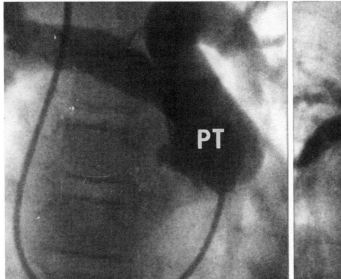
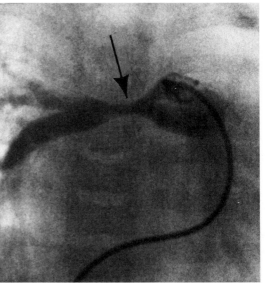

Figure 18–5

A, Pulmonary arteriogram from a 12-year-old boy with Fallot's tetralogy and a normally formed pulmonary trunk (PT) and proximal branches. *B,* Pulmonary arteriogram from a 9-month-old female with Fallot's tetralogy and tubular hypoplasia of the right pulmonary artery (*arrow*). Similar obstruction was present in the left pulmonary artery.

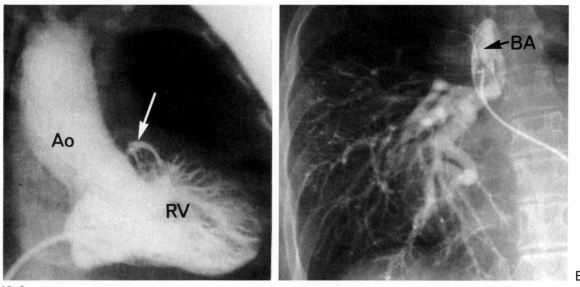

Figure 18–6

A, Right ventriculogram (RV) from a 5-year-old boy with Fallot's tetralogy and pulmonary atresia. *Arrow* points to the blind infundibulum. The aortic root (Ao) is conspicuously dilated, and continues as a right aortic arch. *B*, Selective opacification of a large right bronchial arterial collateral (BA) that connects to intrapulmonary arteries.

absent when pulmonary atresia exists from early fetal life. Absence of a ductus indicates that normal intrauterine ductal function was usurped, rendering the ductus superfluous. If a ductus is present, it serves as a long narrow branch of the aorta that carries systemic arterial blood *from* the aorta *into* the pulmonary trunk.[112,139] The ductus is narrow because it delivers blood only to the lungs which represents no more than 5% to 10% of the combined ventricular output. The ductus is long because it first runs distally, diverging from the aortic arch, and then turns back to join the proximal left pulmonary artery (see Fig. 18–38B).

Aortic regurgitation occurs in Fallot's tetralogy because the malaligned ventricular septal defect is partially roofed by the aortic valve.[42,101,138,150,198,200] Herniation of aortic cusps occurs less frequently with Fallot's tetralogy than with isolated subarterial ventricular septal defects,[150] a difference that has been ascribed to the dissimilar flow patterns that impact on the aortic valve.[150] In cyanotic Fallot's tetralogy, the aortic valve is not subjected to turbulent flow because the left ventricle ejects directly into the aorta without generating a left-to-right jet.[150] Nevertheless, there is an age-related increase in aortic regurgitation[42,146] related in part to progressive aortic root dilatation associated with an inherent medial abnormality.[5] Aortic regurgitation causes volume overload of *both* ventricles because the aorta is biventricular,[146] and an incompetent aortic valve is susceptible to infective endocarditis, which can suddenly and catastrophically augment the degree of biventricular regurgitation (see The History).[146]

A right aortic arch is a feature of Fallot's tetralogy.[111,138,184] The incidence increases as the severity of right ventricular outflow obstruction increases (Fig. 18–3B) and reaches approximately 25% with pulmonary atresia (Figs.18–6A and 18–8A).

Anomalous origin and distribution of *coronary arteries* are common (see Chapter 32).[56,57,83,88,91,124] The incidence of coronary artery anomalies is influenced by aortopulmonary rotation and is higher when the aortic root is anterior to or side-by-side with the pulmonary trunk.[88] Anomalous coronary arteries are of no *functional* importance but are of considerable *surgical* importance. The commonest anomalies are origin of a conus artery or the left anterior descending artery from either the right coronary artery or the right sinus of Valsalva (Fig. 18–9).[57,83,124] Less common is origin of a single coronary artery from the right sinus of Valsalva.[57] Relatively frequent are fistulous communications between coronary arteries and the pulmonary artery or right atrium, and collateral communications between coronary arteries and bronchial arteries.[25,56,57,62,166] Rarely, the left anterior descending coronary artery originates from the pulmonary artery.[226]

Fallot recognized that, "... at times, there is an additional entirely accessory defect, namely, patency of the foramen ovale."[79] An atrial septal defect occasionally coexists with Fallot's tetralogy,[138,184] but the term *pentalogy* is longer used.

Obstruction to right ventricular outflow with ventricular septal defect is not necessarily represented by Fallot's tetralogy. *Pulmonary valve stenosis* occasionally occurs with an isolated *perimembranous* ventricular septal defect (Fig. 18–10). The degree of stenosis varies from trivial to severe, the size of the ventricular septal defect varies from small to nonrestrictive, and right ventricular systolic pressure varies from normal to suprasystemic.[16] Other examples of the combination include pulmonary valve stenosis with a *muscular* ventricular septal defect,[190] obstruction to right ventricular outflow caused by protrusion of a large *ventricular*

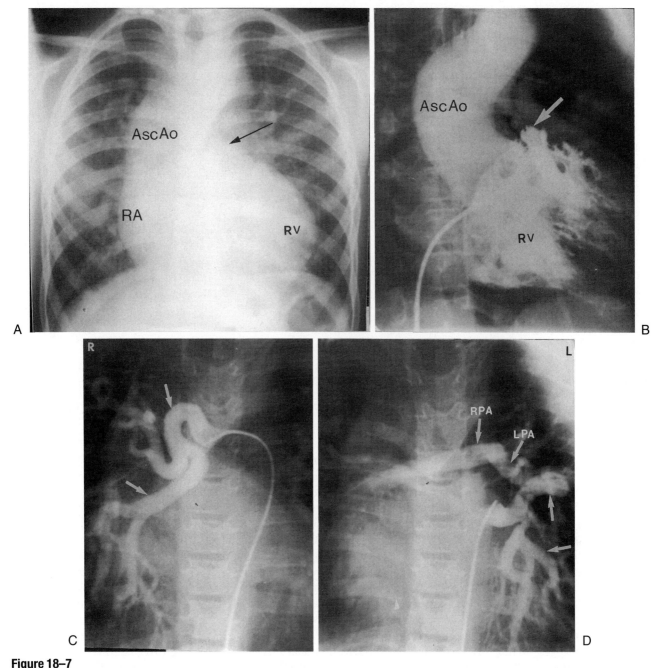

Figure 18–7

A, X-ray from a 3-year-old boy with Fallot's tetralogy and pulmonary atresia. The ascending aorta (AscAo) is conspicuously dilated, the main pulmonary artery segment (*arrow*) is not border-forming, the right lower cardiac border is occupied by a convex right atrium (RA), and the apex is occupied by a convex right ventricle (RV). *B*, Right ventriculogram showing the blind outflow tract of pulmonary atresia (*arrow*) and a conspicuously dilated ascending aorta (AscAo). *C*, Selective visualization of a direct right arterial collateral (*arrows*) that arose from the descending thoracic aorta and had a hilar anastomosis. *D*, The right pulmonary artery (RPA) and left pulmonary artery (LPA) are hypoplastic but continuous. A direct systemic arterial collateral (*two unmarked arrows*) arose from the descending aorta and had a hilar anastomosis. A vestigial pulmonary trunk was not visualized.

septal aneurysm into the right ventricular outflow tract (Fig. 18–11), and double-chambered right ventricle with a *perimembranous*[60,92,103,109,110,173,185] or a *malaligned* ventricular septal defect (Fig. 18–12).[55,58] Sir Arthur Keith in his 1909 Hunterian lecture focused on obstructing right ventricular muscular bundles[128] that may consist of a hypertrophied moderator band,[185] a hypertrophied trabecula septomarginalis, or a fibromuscular diaphragm,[14] with obstruction that varies from nil to severe to complete.[92,110,115,185] A ventricular septal defect that commu-

nicates with the proximal high-pressure compartment results in a right-to-left shunt.[110]

Taussig described two infants with a loud holosystolic murmur at the lower left sternal border and increased pulmonary blood flow, prompting the diagnosis of ventricular septal defect.[204] Several years later, both patients were cyanotic with pulmonary midsystolic murmurs and decreased pulmonary blood flow, prompting a change in the diagnosis to Fallot's tetralogy. Gasul formalized the notion that progressive infundibular obstruction

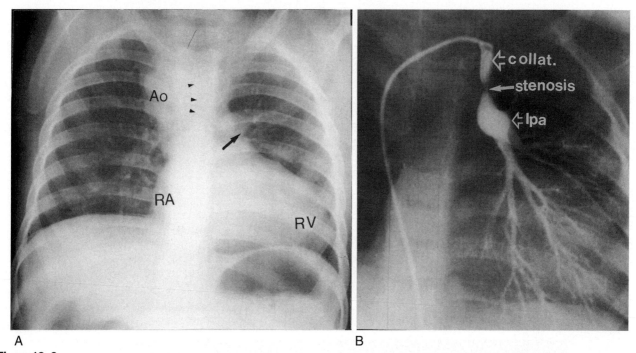

Figure 18–8

A, X-ray from a 2-year-old girl with Fallot's tetralogy and pulmonary atresia. The lung fields have the lacy appearance of systemic arterial collateral circulation. The ascending aorta (Ao) continues as a prominent right aortic arch and displaces the trachea to the left (*three unmarked arrowheads*). An enlarged boot-shaped right ventricle (RV) occupies the apex, and a convex right atrium (RA) occupies the lower right cardiac border. *B*, Selective opacification of an indirect systemic arterial collateral (collat) that originated from the left subclavian artery. There was a zone of stenosis in the collateral artery before the left pulmonary artery (lpa) visualized.

sometimes occurred with ventricular septal defect (Fig. 18–13),[99] and confirmatory reports soon appeared.[16,104,147, 176,193,208] The acquired obstruction usually results from hypertrophy of right ventricular muscle bundles and only rarely from a malaligned infundibular septum.[176]

The *physiologic consequences* of Fallot's tetralogy depend essentially on two variables—the degree of obstruction to right ventricular outflow and to a lesser extent systemic vascular resistance. The magnitude and direction of the shunt are determined by the resistance at the site(s) of pulmonary stenosis compared to systemic vascular resistance. When pulmonary stenosis offers the lesser resistance, the shunt is left-to-right. When the resistances are equal, the shunt is balanced. When right ventricular outflow resistance exceeds systemic resistance, the shunt is right-to-left. The amount of aortic override is not the issue, although the degree of override tends to coincide with the degree of obstruction to right ventricular outflow, which is the issue. When right ventricular blood preferentially flows into the aorta, pulmonary blood flow is reciprocally reduced, so the left side of the heart is underfilled.[95,126] The ultimate expression of right ventricular outflow obstruction is *pulmonary atresia*, which commits the entire right ventricular output to the aorta. Pulmonary blood flow then depends on systemic arterial collaterals, which provide the lungs with normal or increased flow, so cyanosis can be mild or even absent.[61] Unobstructed flow through arterial collaterals sets the stage for pulmonary vascular disease. Stenoses in arterial collaterals protect the

pulmonary vascular bed but at the price of reduced pulmonary blood flow. Irrespective of the degree of right ventricular outflow obstruction in Fallot's tetralogy, right ventricular systolic pressure cannot exceed systemic pressure because the ventricular septal defect is nonrestrictive. Accordingly, a ceiling is placed on the degree of pressure overload that pulmonary stenosis can impose on the right ventricle. When pulmonary stenosis is severe, right ventricular pressure overload is determined by systemic vascular resistance. Increased systemic resistance associated with systemic hypertension or less commonly acquired calcific aortic stenosis (see Fig. 18–33*B*) improves pulmonary blood flow but increases right ventricular afterload. Aortic regurgitation imposes volume load on the already pressure-overloaded right ventricle.

Morphologic changes may be *secondary* to the physiologic derangements of Fallot's tetralogy. Tricuspid leaflets develop fibrous thickening because right ventricular systolic pressure is systemic, but the leaflets seldom become incompetent. The right ventricle ejects against systemic resistance without an increase in filling pressure, so right atrial pressure remains normal, and systolic function of the hypertrophied right ventricle remains normal (Fig.18–14*B*, *C*).[126] The underfilled left ventricle is reduced in size with reduced stroke volume.[95,126] Low pressure and low flow in the pulmonary circulation alter the small muscular arteries and arterioles and cause thinning of the media with interruption of elastic tissue and widespread thromboses.[24,84,182]

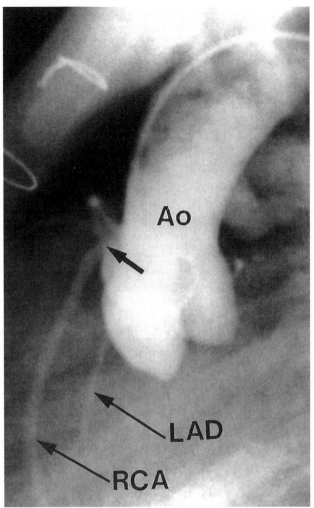

Figure 18–9
Aortogram (Ao) from a 6-year- old boy with Fallot's tetralogy. The left anterior descending coronary artery (LAD) and the right coronary artery (RCA) arose from a single ostium (*arrow*). A branch of the left anterior descending artery crossed the right ventricular outflow tract. The circumflex coronary (not shown) originated from the right coronary artery.

When *severe* pulmonary stenosis occurs with a *restrictive* ventricular septal defect, right ventricular systolic pressure exceeds systemic, and the hypertrophied right ventricle dilates and fails. A physiologically analogous state exists when accessory tricuspid leaflet tissue partially occludes the malaligned ventricular septal defect of Fallot's tetralogy (see Fig. 18–18).[76,89,102] A *restrictive* ventricular septal defect with *mild* pulmonary stenosis produces few or no physiologic derangements.

THE HISTORY

Sex distribution in Fallot's tetralogy is approximately equal. The malformation recurs in families and has been reported in siblings[65,167,225,228] including triplets,[45] and in parents and offspring.[67,228] Two brothers with DiGeorge syndrome had Fallot's tetralogy. Birth weight tends to be lower than normal, and growth and development are generally retarded.[184] Hereditary cardiovascular defects in Keeshond dogs include typical Fallot's tetralogy and isolated ventricular septal defect with pulmonary stenosis.[168]

The tetralogy usually comes to light in neonates and infants.[26,184] When the shunt is left-to-right, initial suspicion is a prominent systolic murmur in an acyanotic patient. When the shunt is balanced, the murmur persists in addition to mild, intermittent, or stress-induced cyanosis. When the shunt is reversed, the prominence of the systolic murmur is inversely proportional to the prominence of cyanosis (see Auscultation).

The clinical course in early infancy is often benign. Mild to moderate neonatal cyanosis tends to increase, but cyanosis may be delayed for months. Its appearance is related to increased oxygen requirements of the growing infant rather than to progressive obstruction to right ventricular outflow.[26,136,184] Infants with Fallot's tetralogy and pulmonary atresia can be mildly cyanotic or acyanotic

Figure 18–10
Right ventriculograms (RV) from a 23-month-old boy with pulmonary valve stenosis, a nonrestrictive perimembranous ventricular septal defect, and a balanced shunt. The plane of the ventricular septum is relatively vertical (*A*) because a well-developed left ventricle occupied the apex. A normal-sized aorta (Ao) and pulmonary trunk (PT) fill simultaneously. In the lateral projection (*B*), pulmonary stenosis is seen to originate in a slightly thickened valve (*arrow*). The pulmonary trunk is mildly dilated. The infundibulum is normal.

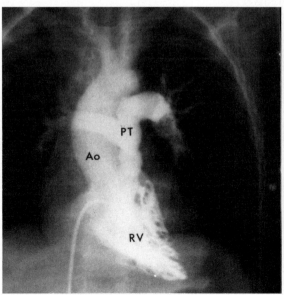

A

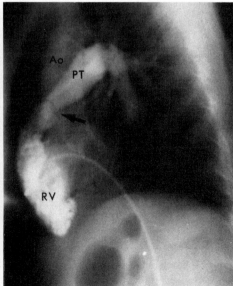

B

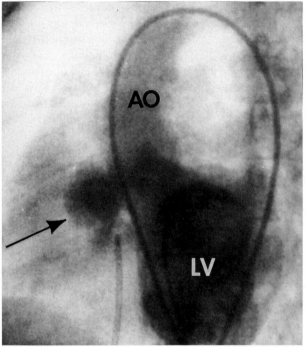

Figure 18–11
Lateral left ventriculogram (LV) from an 8-year-old boy with a large ventricular septal aneurysm (*arrow*) that obstructed the right ventricular outflow tract. A restrictive perimembranous ventricular septal defect had spontaneously closed. Systolic pressure proximal to the obstructing aneurysm was 70 mm Hg and distal to the aneurysm was 30 mm Hg. (Ao = aorta).

because of abundant collateral circulation.[61] Few patients remain acyanotic after the first several years of life, and by 5 to 8 years of age, the majority of children are conspicuously cyanotic and symptomatic with cyanosis closely coupled to the severity of pulmonary stenosis.

In an analysis of survival patterns based on 566 necropsy cases of Fallot's tetralogy, two thirds of patients reached their first birthday, approximately half reached age 3 years and approximately one fourth completed the first decade of life.[23,188] The rate of attrition was then 6.4% per year with 11% alive at age 20 years, 6% at age 30 years, and 3% at age 40 years.[23,188] Nevertheless, Fallot's tetralogy remains the most common type of congenital heart disease in cyanotic children after 4 years of age, and represents the a large proportion of adults with cyanotic congenital heart disease.[114,148] Fallot recognized this tendency when he wrote, "We have seen from our observations that cyanosis, especially in the adult, is the result of a small number of cardiac malformations well determined. One of these cardiac malformations is much more frequent than others . . ." namely, the tetralogy of which he spoke.[79] Fallot's oldest patient was 36 years of age,[79] and survivals between the fifth and seventh decades are uncommon but not rare.[*] A 64-year-old woman had the tetralogy, which was diagnosed in 1895 by G.A. Gibson, best known for his description of the continuous murmur of patent ductus arteriosus.[148] In 1929, White and Sprague published an account of the American composer Henry F. Gilbert who lived a productive life to age 60 years.[219] Another patient played cricket and football as a schoolboy and survived to age 62 years.[153] Fallot's tetralogy with *pulmonary atresia* has a life expectancy without surgery as low as 50% in 1 year and 8% in 10 years,[23] but a satisfactory amount of collateral blood flow occasionally permits survival into

---

[*]See references 1, 8, 10, 18, 27, 29, 36, 50, 114, 125, 148, 153, 183, 197, 215, 219.

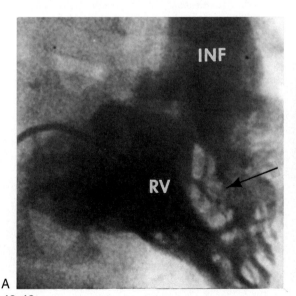

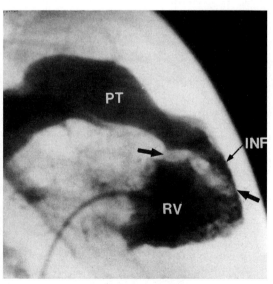

Figure 18–12
A, Right ventriculogram (RV) from an acyanotic 8-year-old boy with a *double-chambered right ventricle* caused by an hypertrophied trabecula septomarginalis (*arrow*). A restrictive perimembranous ventricular septal defect coexisted. Systolic pressure in the inflow tract of the right ventricle was 50 mm Hg higher than systolic pressure in the pulmonary trunk and infundibulum (INF). *B*, Lateral right ventriculogram showing the prominent muscular partition (*arrows*) that separated the high-pressure inflow portion of the right ventricle from the low-pressure infundibular portion creating a *two-chambered right ventricle*.

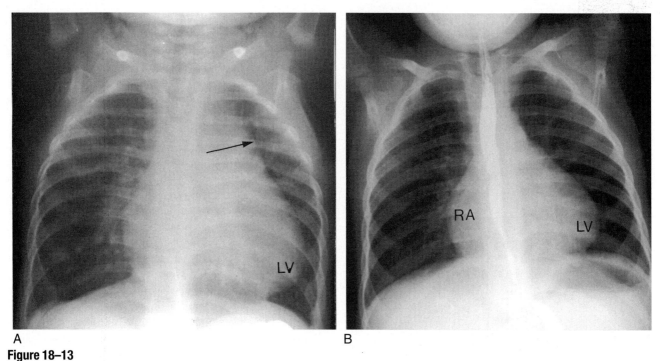

Figure 18–13

A, X-ray from an acyanotic 7-month-old girl with a large left-to-right shunt through a moderately restrictive perimembranous ventricular septal defect. Pulmonary arterial vascularity is increased, an enlarged convex left ventricle (LV) occupies the apex, the right atrium occupies the right lower cardiac border, and the left thoracic inlet is obscured by thymus (*arrow*). *B*, X-ray at 2 years of age after progressive acquired obstruction to right ventricular outflow had reversed the shunt. Pulmonary arterial vascularity is reduced, the left ventricle LV) is no longer dilated, but the right atrium (RA) remains prominent. Thymus has disappeared.

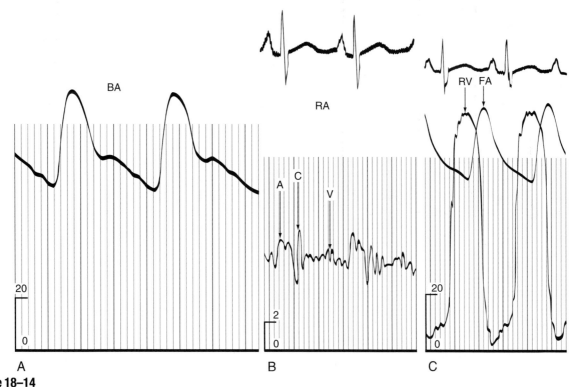

Figure 18–14

A, Normal brachial arterial (BA) pulse in a 9-year-old girl with Fallot's tetralogy. *B*, Normal right atrial pressure pulse (RA) from a 5-year-old boy with Fallot's tetralogy. *C*, Right ventricular (RV) systolic pressure is virtually identical with femoral arterial (FA) systolic pressure. Right ventricular end-diastolic pressure is normal.

Illustration continued on following page

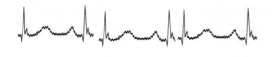

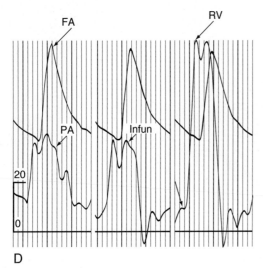

Figure 18–14, *Continued*

D, Catheter withdrawal tracings from a 3-year-old mildly cyanotic girl with Fallot's tetralogy. Identical systolic pressure of 40 mm Hg in the pulmonary artery (PA) and infundibulum (INFUN) abruptly increases to systemic level in the right ventricle (RV) where the end diastolic pressure was normal (*lower left arrow*).

adolescence and adulthood.[3,27,77,98,118,133,146,197,200] One such patient lived to age 54 years,[197] and another lived to age 55 years despite acquired calcific aortic stenosis and regurgitation (see Fig. 18–33B).

Pregnancy is poorly tolerated.[170] The gestational decrease in systemic vascular resistance increases the right-to-left shunt, and the labile systemic vascular resistance during labor and delivery results in abrupt oscillations in hypoxemia. Fetal wastage is high,[170] and live born offspring are dysmature.

Right ventricular function is good in Fallot's tetralogy. The neonatal right ventricle is well equipped to eject against systemic vascular resistance and is seldom called on to do more because the nonrestrictive ventricular septal defect permits decompression into the aorta.[114,126] Right ventricular failure is uncommon with the following exceptions.[48,114,184,203] *Pulmonary atresia with large systemic arterial collaterals* causes biventricular failure in the first few weeks of life.[61] *Accessory tricuspid leaflet tissue* that partially occludes the ventricular septal defect causes suprasystemic right ventricular systolic pressure and the right ventricular failure.[48,76,89,102] *Absence of the pulmonary valve* (see later section) imposes volume overload on the pressure-overloaded right ventricle, which may fail.[155,187] *Systemic hypertension* results in an increase in left *and* right ventricular afterload and in right ventricular or biventricular failure.[20,48,120] *Acquired calcific stenosis* of the biventricular aortic valve is physiologically analogous

to systemic hypertension because it imposes increased afterload on both the right and left ventricles (see Fig. 18–33B). *Acquired regurgitation* of the biventricular aortic valve may induce right ventricular failure by imposing volume overload on the pressure overloaded right ventricle.[42,146] *Infective endocarditis* on the incompetent aortic valve can result in catastrophic acute severe biventricular aortic regurgitation.

Isotonic exercise is accompanied by a decrease in systemic vascular resistance in the face of fixed obstruction to right ventricular outflow, significantly increasing venoarterial mixing and significantly influencing the dynamics of oxygen uptake and ventilation.[195,196] Exercise-induced hypoxemia and increased carbon dioxide content stimulate the respiratory center and the carotid body, provoking hyperventilation that is subjectively perceived as dyspnea.[195,196]

Hypoxic spells that are variously called paroxysmal hyperpnea, syncopal attacks, or hypoxic, anoxic, or hypercyanotic spells, are dramatic and alarming features of Fallot's tetralogy.[26,30,106,129,159,194,199,223] A typical spell begins with a progressive increase in the rate and depth of respiration and culminates in paroxysmal hyperpnea; deepening cyanosis; limpness; syncope; and occasionally in convulsions, cerebrovascular accidents, and death.[30,159,223] Electroencephalographic abnormalities during an hypoxic spell are similar to those of acute hypoxic episodes of other causes.[59] Peak incidence is between the second and sixth month of life with an occasional spell as early as the first month but comparatively few spells after age 2 years. Spells are typically initiated by the stress of feeding, crying, or a bowel movement, particularly after an infant awakens from a long deep sleep.[106,159] Attacks sometimes occur without an apparent precipitating cause, especially in deeply cyanotic infants although spells do not necessarily coincide with the degree of cyanosis.[30,159] The spells were originally attributed to infundibular contraction caused by sympathetic stimulation which was believed to divert right ventricular blood into the aorta,[194,223] but the occurrence of spells in the presence of pulmonary *atresia* argued against this theory.[194] It is now believed that vulnerable respiratory control mechanisms, which are especially sensitive after prolonged deep sleep, react to the sudden increase in cardiac output provoked by feeding, crying, or straining and initiate the following vicious circle.[106,159] As heart rate and cardiac output increase, venous return increases in the face of fixed obstruction to right ventricular outflow, so the right-to-left shunt increases. Infundibular contraction may reinforce this pattern but does not initiate it.[194,199] The increased right-to-left shunt causes in a fall in systemic arterial pO_2 and pH and in a rise in pCO_2, a blood gas composition to which a sleep-sensitive respiratory center and carotid body overreact, provoking hyperpnea, which in turn further increases the cardiac output and perpetuates the cycle. *Supraventricular tachycardia* and *rapid atrial pacing* initiate spells by inducing infundibular narrowing which increases the right-to-left shunt[129,194,199,227] and sheds light on the pathogenesis of *spontaneous* spells. Five mechanisms are therefore involved in the pathogenesis of Fallot spells: 1) an acceleration in heart rate, 2) an increase in cardiac output and venous return, 3) an increase in right-to-left shunt, 4) vulnerable respiratory control centers, and 5) infundibular contraction. Manual compression of the abdominal aorta can abort a spell by decreasing cardiac output and decreasing venous return.[68]

Squatting for relief of dyspnea is a time-honored hallmark of Fallot's tetralogy (Fig. 18–15).[31,32,140,162,203] William Hunter made the following observations on the effects of posture in 1784:

"Any hurry upon his spirits or brisk motion of his body would generally occasion a fit. And for some of the last years of his life he found out by his own observations that when the fit was coming upon him, he would escape it altogether, or at least take considerably from its violence or duration by instantly lying down upon the carpet on his left side, and remaining immovable in that position for about 10 minutes. I saw the experiments made with success."[123]

Taussig described the preference for certain postures other than squatting, namely, the knee-chest position, lying down, or sitting with legs drawn underneath (Fig. 18–16).[203] Parents may hold their breathless infant upright with its legs flexed upon its abdomen (Fig. 18–16, no. 4). Young adults cross their legs during quiet standing or sitting, a variation that is relatively ineffective. Habitual squatters assume the position effortlessly (Fig. 18–15). The mechanisms by which squatting exerts its beneficial effects are as follows[31,32,107,141,162]: 1) Quiet standing after exercise-induced peripheral vasodilatation predisposes to orthostatic hypotension and faintness, a tendency that is exaggerated in hypoxemic patients. Squatting counteracts orthostatic hypotension and diminishes or prevents post-exertion orthostatic faintness.[107,162] 2) Squatting increases systemic vascular resistance, diverts right ventricular blood into the pulmonary circulation, and increases the amount of oxygenated blood entering the left side of the heart.[107,162,192] The left ventricle delivers the larger volume of oxygenated blood into the systemic circulation, so systemic arterial pO_2 and pH increase and pCO_2 decreases, blunting the stimulus to the respiratory center and carotid body and relieving the hyperventilatory dyspnea.[107] 3) The effect of squatting on *systemic venous return* is an even more effective means by which hyperventilatory dyspnea is relieved.[107] Isotonic leg exercise reduces the oxygen saturation of venous effluent returning to the heart from the lower extremities. Squatting mechanically curtails lower extremity venous return, decreases the volume of

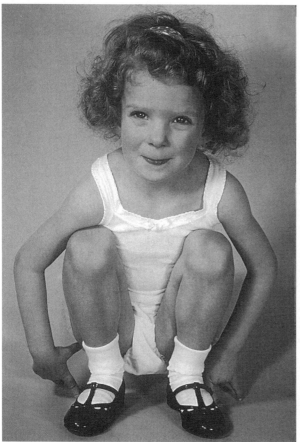
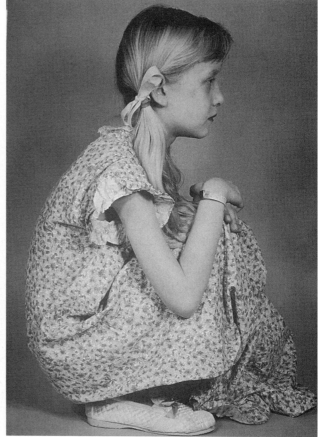

A   B

Figure 18–15

A and *B*, Photographs showing typical squatting postures assumed effortlessly in two children with Fallot's tetralogy.

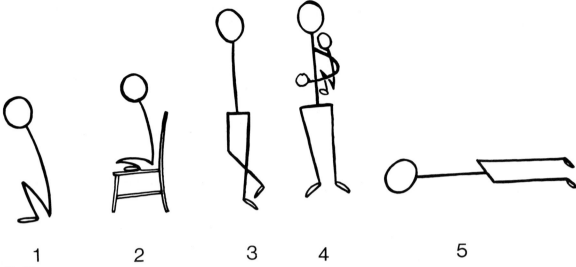

Figure 18–16
Line drawings illustrating various postures assumed for relief of dyspnea in Fallot's tetralogy: 1) squatting, 2) sitting with legs drawn underneath (squatting equivalent), 3) legs crossed while standing, 4) infant held with legs flexed on its abdomen, and 5) lying down. (Modified from Lurie PR: Postural effects in tetralogy of Fallot. Am J Med 15:297, 1953.)

unsaturated venous blood delivered to the heart, and increases the oxygen saturation of right ventricular blood. 4) Right ventricular blood shunted into the systemic circulation has a higher oxygen content and pH and a lower pCO_2 content.[107] 5) The higher pO_2 and pH and the lower pCO_2 reduce the stimulus to the respiratory center and carotid body and reduce the hyperventilatory dyspnea.

Recurrent hypoxic spells can lead to brain damage and mental retardation.[120] Cerebral venous sinus thromboses and small occult thromboses may become manifest after prolonged hypoxic spells.[184] Hypernasal resonance or nasal speech (velopharyngeal insufficiency) may develop after repeated or prolonged spells because nasal resonance is compromised by improper approximation of the velum (soft palate) and the pharyngeal walls, a disturbance that has been ascribed in part to central nervous system damage caused by hypoxic spells.[135]

Pulmonary stenosis and aortic regurgitation[42,74] are substrates for infective endocarditis. Wheezing and stridor have been attributed to tracheal compression by an enlarged aorta.[43] Iron-deficient erythrocytosis in patients less than four years of age increases the risk of cerebral venous sinus thrombosis.[172] Brain abscess and cerebral embolism add to the list of central nervous system complications.[22,86,149,172,184]

The *physiologic consequences and clinical course* of a nonrestrictive ventricular septal defect are favorably influenced by mild to moderate *acquired* obstruction to right ventricular outflow (see earlier[176] and see Chapter 17). The clinical picture initially resembles an isolated nonrestrictive ventricular septal defect with large left-to-right shunt (see Fig. 18–13A). With the development of right ventricular outflow obstruction, excessive pulmonary blood flow and volume overload of the left ventricle are curtailed,[99,136,147,193,208] symptoms related to the left-to-right shunt diminish, and physical development improves.

Obstruction to right ventricular outflow may progress enough to reverse the shunt, resulting in late onset cyanosis (see Fig. 18–13B).

When a *restrictive* ventricular septal defect is accompanied by *severe* pulmonary valve stenosis, the clinical picture resembles isolated pulmonary stenosis with intact ventricular septum (see Chapter 11). A *restrictive* ventricular septal defect with *mild* pulmonary stenosis is associated with a conspicuous murmur and few or no symptoms, but with the risk of infective endocarditis.

PHYSICAL APPEARANCE

Patients with cyanotic Fallot's tetralogy are as a rule physically underdeveloped.[15,184] Excessive collateral arterial blood flow accompanying pulmonary atresia can cause congestive heart failure and poor physical development in infants. Cyanosis in Fallot's tetralogy varies from absent to severe and is symmetrically distributed. John Hunter described such a patient: "I was consulted about a young gentleman's health. From his infancy, every considerable exertion produced a seeming tendency to suffocation and a change from the scarlet tinge to the modena or purple."[178] Cyanosis may become manifest only after crying, feeding, or exercise because stress increases venous return to the obstructed right ventricle and augments the right-to-left shunt. When there is a history of squatting or an analogous posture, it is useful to have the patient or parent illustrate the posture so that it can be witnessed (see Figs.18–15 and 18–16).

Fallot's tetralogy is associated with a number of distinctive phenotypes[130]: CATCH 22 (monosomy 22q11.2),[72,78,87] Down trisomy 21,[201,207] velocardiofacial (Shprintzen) syndrome, CHARGE, and Goldenhar syndrome[105] (oculoauriculovertebral dysplasia). Poland syndrome, correctly described by Author Fallot as congenital pectoral dysplasia,[11] is characterized by absence of a pectoralis major muscle (Fig. 18–17), syndactyly, brachydactyly, and hypoplasia of the ipsilateral hand.[144]

THE ARTERIAL PULSE

The arterial pulse is normal irrespective of the severity of pulmonary stenosis (see Fig.18–14C, D). When the shunt is balanced, the left ventricle maintains a normal stroke volume, and when there is severe pulmonary stenosis or atresia, a reduced left ventricular stroke volume is supplemented by right ventricular blood ejected directly into the aorta.[126] A *brisk* arterial pulse with wide pulse pressure is a feature of large systemic arterial collateral flow[61] or aortic regurgitation.[42]

An accurate estimate of the right ventricular outflow gradient requires little more than bedside determination of the blood pressure. Right ventricular systolic pressure is the same as systemic systolic pressure (see Fig. 18–14C, D), so the stenotic gradient is the difference between the cuff brachial arterial systolic pressure and an estimated pulmonary arterial systolic pressure, 15 to 25 mm Hg depending on age and severity of pulmonary stenosis. The estimate is refined by considering that pulmonary arterial pressure is lowest when cyanosis is severe and normal when cyanosis is mild.

THE JUGULAR VENOUS PULSE

The jugular pulse is normal (see Fig. 18–14B). A neonatal right ventricle has an inherent capacity to eject against systemic resistance without extra help from its atrium. In Fallot's tetralogy, resistance to right ventricular discharge is at but not above systemic because the nonrestrictive ventricular septal defect permits decompression into the aorta (see Fig. 18–14C, D). The right ventricle maintains its neonatal capacity to eject at systemic level without increasing its filling pressure. Accordingly, the right atrium is not required to increase its contractile force, so the jugular venous pulse remains normal in height and waveform. If accessory tricuspid leaflet tissue partially occludes the ventricular septal defect, right ventricular systolic pressure exceeds systemic (Fig. 18–18) and the A wave becomes prominent.[119] In the presence of systemic hypertension, the right ventricle contracts from an increased end-diastolic fiber length induced by forceful right atrial contraction which is reflected in the jugular venous pulse as an increase in the A wave.[120] Acquired stenosis of the biventricular aortic valve has a similar effect on the right ventricle and right atrium. A minor feature of the jugular venous pulse is related to a persistent left superior vena cava[122,138] in the presence of which the *left* jugular pulse is more prominent than the right.[54,122]

PRECORDIAL MOVEMENT AND PALPATION

James Hope in 1839 described an "increase of pulsation at the inferior part of the sternum, indicative of right ventricular hypertrophy."[121] The right ventricle in Fallot's tetralogy ejects at systemic pressure without dilating and with little or no increase in the force of contraction. Accordingly, the accompanying precordial impulse is gentle and is analogous to a normal neonatal right ventricular impulse. In Fallot's tetralogy, however, the impulse persists as the neonate matures because right ventricular systolic pressure remains at systemic level. The right ventricular impulse is relegated to the fourth and fifth left intercostal spaces and subxiphoid area because the stenosis is infundibular (see Fig. 18–14D). A *left* ventricular impulse is conspicuous by its absence because the left ventricle is underfilled. Abundant flow through large systemic arterial collaterals augments left ventricular filling, but even then a left ventricular impulse is seldom palpated. *Subinfundibular* stenosis or double-chambered right ventricle (see Fig. 18–12) relegates the right ventricular impulse to the *fifth* left intercostal space and subxiphoid area.

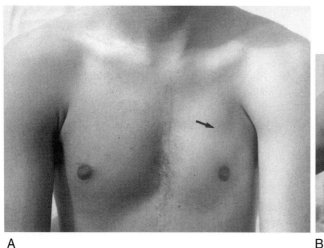

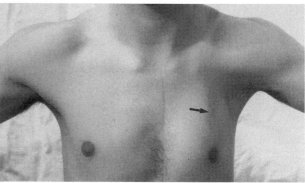

A   **B**

Figure 18–17

Photographs of a 16-year-old boy with Fallot's tetralogy and Poland syndrome. *A*, The left chest is mildly flattened (*arrow*). *B*, Raising the arms exaggerates the appearance of agenesis of the left pectoralis major muscle (*arrow*) with lateral displacement of the nipple. Compare with the normal right chest.

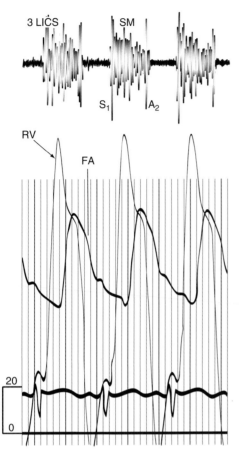

Figure 18–18

Tracings from a 3-year-old girl with Fallot's tetralogy. Right ventricular (RV) systolic pressure exceeded femoral arterial systolic pressure (FA) because accessory tricuspid leaflet tissue partially occluded the ventricular septal defect. As a result, a long loud pulmonary stenotic murmur (SM) went up to the aortic component of the second heart sound (A_2). Right ventricular end-diastolic pressure was 28 mm Hg (see calibration below). S_1, first heart sound; 3LICS, third left intercostal space.

A dilated *right aortic arch* (see Fig. 18–6) may reveal itself by an impulse at the right sternoclavicular junction. The aortic component of the second heart sound is often palpable in the second left intercostal space because a hypoplastic or atretic anterior pulmonary trunk is all that guards the enlarged aortic root. Systolic thrills do not originate at sites of severe stenosis because right ventricular blood flow is diverted from the pulmonary trunk into the aorta. Lesser degrees of obstruction as in acyanotic Fallot's tetralogy are accompanied by thrills because of sufficient flow across the site of stenosis.

AUSCULTATION

The physiology of Fallot's tetralogy is nicely reflected in the accompanying auscultatory signs. Ejection sounds originate in a dilated *aorta* (see Figs. 18–6A and 18–7A) and are therefore important auscultatory signs of severe pulmonary stenosis or pulmonary atresia (Fig. 18–19; (see

Figs. 18–21 and 18–23 thru 18–25).[133,136,211,212] The aortic ejection sound is maximum at the upper *right* sternal border but when loud, is heard along the left sternal border and toward the apex. The ejection sound may selectively decrease with inspiration (Fig. 18–19) even though it originates in a dilated aortic root rather than in the pulmonary valve (see Chapter 11). *Pulmonary* ejection sounds are absent because the stenotic bicuspid pulmonary valve is not sufficiently mobile (see Fig. 18–3).

Nearly 50 years before Fallot's report, James Hope wrote:

"A loud superficial murmur with the first heart sound in the third left intercostal space may proceed from a contraction of the pulmonary orifice or from an opening out of the right ventricle into the left ventricle, or from both these lesions conjoined. When these lesions coincide with cyanosis, the double lesion is almost positive and an increase of pulsation at the inferior part of the sternum, indicative of right ventricular hypertrophy is a corroborative circumstance."[121]

The systolic murmur that Hope described referred to cyanotic Fallot's tetralogy and originated at the sites of stenosis rather than across the ventricular septal defect (Fig. 18–20).[85] The murmur is maximum in the third left intercostal space because the stenosis is infundibular. *Subinfundibular* stenosis results in a lower murmur site.[173]

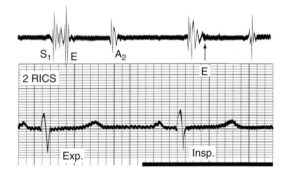

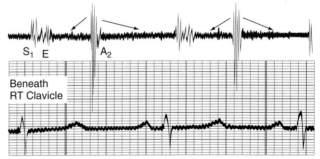

Figure 18–19

Phonocardiograms from an 11-year-old girl with Fallot's tetralogy and pulmonary atresia. Tracing from the second right intercostal space (2 RICS) shows an aortic ejection sound (E) that was prominent during expiration (EXP) but absent during inspiration (INSP). Phonocardiogram from beneath the right clavicle shows a soft continuous murmur (*paired arrows*). S_1, first heart sound; A_2, aortic component of the second sound.

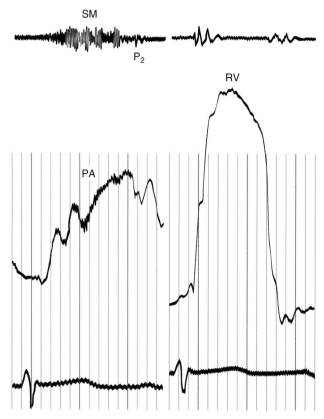

Figure 18–20

Intracardiac phonocardiogram, pulmonary arterial (PA) pressure pulse and right ventricular (RV) pressure pulse in a 10-year-old girl with severe Fallot's tetralogy. A soft systolic stenotic murmur (SM) was recorded in the main pulmonary artery (PA) but not in the right ventricle (RV). The faint pulmonary component of the second heart sound (P_2) was recorded by the intracardiac microphone but was neither heard nor recorded on the chest wall. Pressure pulses not calibrated.

The duration and configuration of the systolic murmur are determined by the balance between the resistance at the site of stenosis and the resistance in the systemic vascular bed. Transient changes in this balance are reflected in transient changes in the length and loudness of the murmur. These auscultatory signs are closely coupled to the severity of pulmonary stenosis (Fig. 18–21).[211,212] A holosystolic murmur extending up to the aortic component of the second heart sound reflects a *left-to-right* shunt across the ventricular septal defect (Fig. 18–21B). As pulmonary stenosis increases, the shunt murmur becomes decrescendo, diminishing and ending before the aortic component of the second sound (Fig. 18–21C). When the shunt is balanced, the ventricular septal defect is silent, and the previously obscured pulmonary stenotic murmur emerges (Fig. 18–21D). A further increase in the degree of pulmonary stenosis diverts right ventricular blood into the aorta and away from the pulmonary trunk, so the pulmonary stenotic murmur becomes shorter and softer (Fig. 18–21E). Severe pulmonary stenosis is reflected in an even shorter and softer systolic murmur and by an ejection sound that is generated in the dilated aortic root (Fig. 18–21F). Pulmonary atresia abolishes right ventricular to pulmonary arterial flow and

abolishes the pulmonary stenotic murmur. An aortic ejection sound may be followed by no murmur (Fig. 18–21G) or a trivial midsystolic murmur into the dilated aortic root.

During hypoxic spells, pulmonary arterial blood flow sharply declines, the pulmonary stenotic murmur shortens and softens, and with loss of consciousness, the murmur disappears.[211,223] Vasoactive drugs induce analogous changes by altering systemic vascular resistance.[211,213,214] Pressor agents increase systemic vascular resistance and increase the resistance to right ventricular discharge into the aorta.[20,120] The right-to-left shunt decreases, right ventricular blood is diverted into the pulmonary artery, and the pulmonary stenotic murmur becomes louder and longer. Amyl nitrite has the opposite effect, inducing a decrease in systemic vascular resistance, a decrease in resistance to right ventricular discharge into the aorta, a decrease in flow into the pulmonary trunk, with softening and shortening of the stenotic murmur (Fig. 18–22).

Continuous murmurs are auscultatory signs of pulmonary *atresia* and occur in over 80% of such patients (Figs. 18–19 and 18–23 through 18–25). Continuous murmurs originate in direct and indirect systemic arterial collaterals, and therefore do not occur in Fallot's tetralogy with pulmonary stenosis because the collaterals are confined to bronchial arteries (see Fig. 18–6B).[180] Intensity of continuous murmurs ranges from grade 3/6 to soft humming murmurs that are easily overlooked especially at nonprecordial sites. Continuous murmurs are heard beneath the clavicles, in the back, to the right and left of the sternum, and in the right and left axillae (Figs. 18–23 through 18–25). Thoracic locations vary from patient to patient and from time to time in the same patient.[38,133] Continuous murmur may peak before and after the second heart sound (Figs. 18–23 and 18–25) or may peak in systolic as with other arterial continuous murmurs (Fig 18–24), creating the mistaken impression of a long intracardiac systolic murmur, especially if the murmur is located at the left sternal edge.

The murmur of tricuspid regurgitation occurs in the occasional adult with right ventricular failure caused by systemic hypertension or acquired aortic stenosis, or in the occasional patient with suprasystemic right ventricular pressure due to partial occlusion of the ventricular septal defect by tricuspid leaflet tissue.

Diastolic murmurs are caused by aortic regurgitation or much less frequently by absent pulmonary valve (see later section).[42,150,211] The aortic regurgitant murmur is high frequency decrescendo, beginning with the prominent single aortic component of the second heart sound (Fig. 18–24A). Continuous murmurs from collateral circulation preclude detection of the murmur of aortic regurgitation, and a brisk arterial pulse may indicate abundant collateral flow rather than aortic regurgitant flow. However, conspicuous cyanosis with a brisk arterial pulse favors aortic regurgitation because arterial collaterals that are large enough to cause bounding pulses are also large enough to increase pulmonary arterial blood flow and minimize

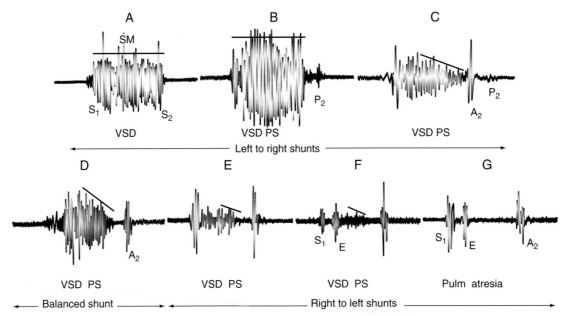

Figure 18–21

Series of phonocardiograms showing auscultatory modifications incurred when varying degrees of pulmonary stenosis (PS) are imposed on a nonrestrictive ventricular septal defect (VSD). *A,* Holosystolic murmur of isolated ventricular septal defect. *B,* Holosystolic murmur of ventricular septal defect with mild pulmonary stenosis. The pulmonary component of the second heart sound (P_2) is delayed but readily identified. *C,* The ventricular septal defect murmur decreases in latter systole because moderately severe pulmonary stenosis decreased the left-to-right shunt in latter systole. The pulmonary component of the second heart sound is softer and further delayed. *D,* The ventricular septal defect murmur is replaced by a relatively long pulmonary stenotic murmur because right ventricular outflow resistance equals systemic vascular resistance, so the shunt is balanced and the ventricular septal defect is silent. The second sound is the single aortic component (A_2) because the pulmonary component is inaudible. *E,* The pulmonary stenotic murmur shortens and softens when right ventricular outflow resistance exceeds systemic vascular resistance because right ventricular blood is diverted into the aorta. The single second sound is the aortic component. *F,* The systolic murmur is shorter and softer because severe pulmonary stenosis diverts still more right ventricular blood into the aorta and away from the pulmonary artery. An *aortic* ejection (E) originates in the dilated ascending aorta. The single second sound is the aortic component. *G,* The pulmonary stenotic murmur vanishes in the presence of pulmonary atresia. An aortic ejection sound (E) originates in the dilated ascending aorta. The single second sound is the aortic component (A_2).

cyanosis. Large collateral arteries that deliver abundant pulmonary blood flow occasionally cause mitral middiastolic murmurs (Fig. 18–24*A*). Rarely, a bicuspid stenotic pulmonary valve is incompetent, generating a delayed medium frequency diastolic murmur of low-pressure pulmonary regurgitation (Fig. 18–24*B*).

A soft delayed pulmonary component of the second heart sound is often detected when cyanosis is mild or absent (see Figs. 18–20 and 18–21*C*).[28,85,206,211,212,214] When cyanosis is marked, the pulmonary closure sound is usually inaudible, and with pulmonary atresia, there is no pulmonary component because there is no functional pulmonary valve. The pulmonary component is soft or absent because right ventricular blood preferentially enters the aorta, so pulmonary blood flow and pulmonary artery pressure are abnormally low. Amyl nitrite inhalation reduces pulmonary arterial flow still further, and makes an audible pulmonary second sound disappear (see Fig. 18–22).[171,213] Inaudibility is also related to pulmonary valve leaflets that are thickened and bicuspid, so that brisk closing excursions are precluded. The aortic component of the second heart sound behaves differently as Thomas Peacock wrote in 1866. "The aorta is unusually large and from the powerful reaction on the valves during diastole of the heart, a loud ringing second sound is heard on listening at the upper part of the sternum."[169] Peacock's loud ringing

second sound referred to the single loud aortic component (Figs. 18–25 and 18–26). A *delay* in the pulmonary component is due to two variables.[211] First, a relatively long interval is required for high right ventricular systolic pressure to fall below the pulmonary arterial incisura. Second, delayed relaxation of the infundibulum contributes to late pulmonary valve closure by supporting the column of blood in the pulmonary trunk after the right ventricle has begun to relax.[28]

Fourth heart sounds are exceptional because the force of right atrial contraction is seldom increased. Third heart sounds rarely occur on either side of the heart because right ventricular failure is uncommon and left ventricular filling is reduced. With systemic hypertension, right ventricular or biventricular failure may be accompanied by third and fourth heart sounds. With pulmonary atresia and large systemic to pulmonary arterial collaterals, increased blood flow across the mitral valve sometimes generates a left ventricular third sound and a short middiastolic murmur (see Fig. 18–24).

Severe pulmonary valve stenosis with a *restrictive* perimembranous ventricular septal defect results in auscultatory signs similar if not identical to the auscultatory signs of severe *isolated* pulmonary stenosis. Suprasystemic right ventricular systolic pressure abolishes the left-to-right shunt, so a long pulmonary stenotic murmur exists

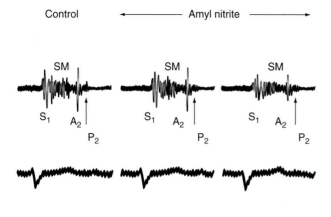

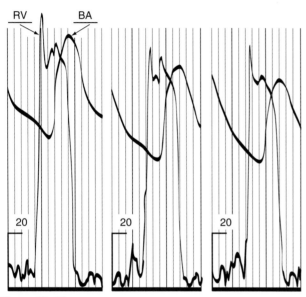

Figure 18–22

Tracings from a mildly cyanotic 3-year-old girl with Fallot's tetralogy and a balanced shunt. Amyl nitrite inhalation induced a fall in systemic vascular resistance and a parallel fall in right ventricular (RV) and brachial arterial (BA) pressures. Blood from the right ventricle preferentially entered the aorta, pulmonary blood flow reciprocally decreased, the pulmonary stenotic murmur (SM) shortened and softened, and the faint pulmonary component of the second sound (P₂) disappeared.

alone.[119,165] An analogous loud long pulmonary stenotic murmur is generated when accessory tricuspid leaflet tissue partially occludes the malaligned ventricular septal defect (see Fig. 18–18).[165]

Mild pulmonary valve stenosis with a *restrictive* ventricular septal defect results in auscultatory signs dominated by the holosystolic murmur of the ventricular septal defect. Suspicion of coexisting pulmonary valve stenosis depends on the presence of a pulmonary ejection sound and a right ventricular impulse.

THE ELECTROCARDIOGRAM

The electrocardiogram is a relatively reliable reflection of the physiology of Fallot's tetralogy.[19,37,64,114] Because the force of right atrial contraction is not increased and the right atrium is not enlarged, P waves may be peaked but are seldom increased in amplitude (Figs. 18–27 and 18–28), and are often normal in young patients. P wave duration may be short (Fig. 18–27) because the left atrium is under-filled and relatively small.[145] The PR interval is normal because the conduction system is normal.[53,137]

The QRS axis is the same as the axis of a normal newborn[64,174] (Fig. 18–27). The important point is that the QRS axis and the direction of ventricular depolarization do not change as the neonate matures because the functional demands on the right ventricle do not change (Figs. 18–27 and 18–28).[64,174] The QRS duration is normal without notching or slurring,[19,64] but in an occasional adult, there is a peripheral conduction delay.[2,114] Left axis deviation with counterclockwise depolarization is reserved for Fallot's tetralogy with an atrioventricular septal defect (see Chapter 15).[82]

Right ventricular hypertrophy is characterized by a tall monophasic R wave confined to lead V_1 with an abrupt change to an rS pattern in lead V_2 (Figs. 18–27, 18–28 and 18–29).[19,53,64,174] The presence and depth of Q waves and the amplitude of R waves in leads V_{5-6} are sensitive signs of the magnitude of pulmonary blood flow and left ventricular filling. Reduced pulmonary flow with an underfilled left ventricle is accompanied by rS patterns in leads V_{2-6} (Fig. 18–27). A balanced shunt is accompanied by small q waves and well-developed R waves in lead V_{5-6} (Fig. 18–28).

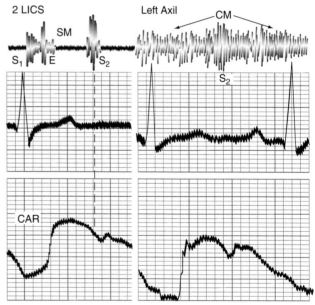

Figure 18–23

Phonocardiograms from an 11-year-old girl with Fallot's tetralogy and pulmonary atresia. In the second left intercostal space (2LICS), an aortic ejection sound (E) follows the first heart sound (S₁) by a delay appropriate for the isometric contraction time incurred by systemic vascular resistance. The ejection sound introduces a soft short systolic murmur that originated in the dilated ascending aorta. The aortic component of the second sound (A₂) is loud because the aorta was dilated and guarded anteriorly by a hypoplastic pulmonary trunk. In the left axilla (LT. AXIL.), a continuous murmur (CM) peaked before and after the second heart sound.

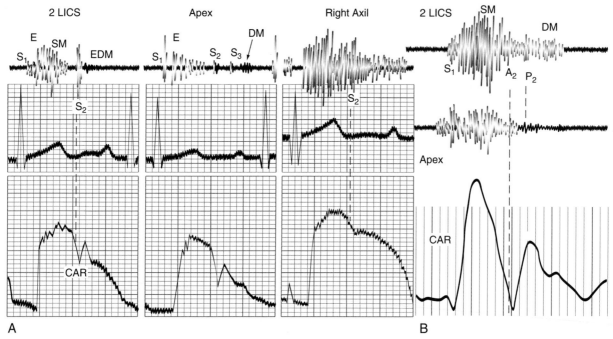

Figure 18–24

A, Phonocardiograms from a 15-year-old boy with Fallot's tetralogy and pulmonary atresia. In the second left intercostal space (2 LICS), an aortic ejection sound (E) merges with a prominent short midsystolic murmur (SM). The single second sound (S₂) is the aortic component that introduces an early diastolic murmur of aortic regurgitation (EDM). The aortic ejection sound is more obvious at the apex where the systolic murmur is softer. A third heart sound (S₃) is followed by a soft short mid-diastolic murmur (DM) across the mitral valve. A continuous murmur in the right axilla (RT AXIL) is louder in systole. CAR, carotid pulse. *B,* Tracings from a mildly cyanotic 12-year-old male with Fallot's tetralogy and a stenotic and incompetent bicuspid pulmonary valve. A long loud midsystolic murmur of pulmonary stenosis envelopes the aortic component of the second heart sound (A₂). A medium pitched low pressure mid-diastolic murmur (DM) begins with the delayed pulmonary component of the second sound (P₂).

A left-to-right shunt is accompanied by deeper left precordial Q waves and relatively tall R waves (Fig. 18–29).

Right precordial T waves are upright or inverted with almost equal frequency (Figs. 18–27 thru 18–29). The deeply inverted right precordial T waves that characterize severe pulmonary stenosis with intact ventricular septum seldom occur because right ventricular systolic pressure does not exceed systemic pressure.

With pulmonary atresia and an abundant collateral arterial circulation, P waves are broad and bifid because of increased flow into the left atrium. Q waves with well-developed R waves appear in leads V_{5-6} because of increased flow into the left ventricle, and ST segment and T wave abnormalities may be present in mid-precordial leads (Fig. 18–30).

Acquired obstruction to right ventricular outflow with a nonrestrictive ventricular septal defect results in an electrocardiogram that initially resembles isolated ventricular septal defect of equivalent size. As outflow obstruction increases, right ventricular systolic pressure remains unchanged, but pulmonary blood flow and left ventricular volume decrease. Left precordial qR complexes become less prominent, while tall right precordial R waves persist.[136]

In *double-chambered right ventricle,* the increase in right ventricular pressure and mass are confined to the proximal hypertensive compartment. Precordial leads display a normal QRS progression from V_{1-6} (Fig. 18–31).[34,60,92,97,103,185]

An upright T wave in lead V_3R may be the only electrocardiographic sign of right ventricular hypertrophy.[103]

Restrictive ventricular septal defects with *severe* pulmonary valve stenosis have electrocardiograms indistinguishable from isolated pulmonary stenosis with intact ventricular septum.[165] *Restrictive* ventricular septal defects with *mild* pulmonary stenosis are associated with modest signs of right ventricular hypertrophy manifested by a relatively vertical QRS axis, an rSr′ pattern in lead V_1, and persistent upright right precordial T waves.

THE X-RAY

In cyanotic Fallot's tetralogy, pulmonary vascularity is reduced and the middle and outer thirds of the lung fields show a paucity of vascular markings because of a reduction in size of intrapulmonary arteries and veins (Fig. 18–32).[117,184,203] The right lung is occasionally less vascular than the left lung.[221] In the presence of pulmonary atresia, systemic arterial collaterals that anastomose with *segmental* or *lobar intrapulmonary* arteries produce a lacy reticular pattern without the normal diminution in vessel caliber toward the periphery (Fig. 18–33A).[39,133] Systemic arterial collaterals or bronchial collaterals that anastomose with *hilar* or *extrapulmonary* arteries result in normal intrapulmonary branching (see Figs.18–6B, 18–7C,D and 18–8B). The patterns of collateral arterial circulation are not uniform, with some areas oligemic and other areas

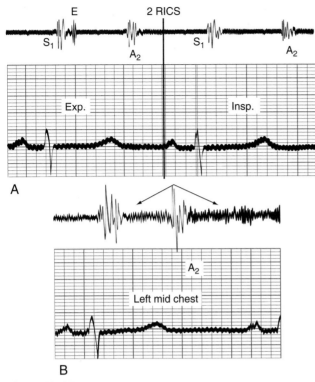

Figure 18–25

Phonocardiograms from a 4-year-old child with Fallot's tetralogy and pulmonary atresia. *A,* In the second right intercostal space (2 RICS), an aortic ejection sound (E) is prominent during expiration (EXP) and absent during inspiration (INSP). *B,* In the left midchest, a soft continuous murmur is of equal intensity in systole and diastole (*paired arrows*). S_1, first heart sound; A_2, aortic component of the second heart sound.

normal or hypervascular (Fig. 18–34). Systemic collateral arteries rarely cause rib notching because they do not run in intercostal grooves.[222]

The concave main pulmonary artery segment of pulmonary atresia stands out in bold relief, especially in the presence of a dilated right aortic arch (Figs. 18–32 and 18–33A).[120,133,184] The size of the ascending aorta tends to vary inversely with the size of the pulmonary trunk (see Fig. 18–3), culminating in the conspicuously dilated ascending aorta of pulmonary atresia (Fig. 18–33). However, dilatation of the ascending aorta is also determined by inherent medial abnormalities.[5] A *right aortic arch* occurs in 20% to 30% of patients with Fallot's tetralogy with the highest incidence in pulmonary atresia (Figs. 18–6A and 18–33A).[111,120,133,138,184] A right arch is usually accompanied by a right descending aorta that runs as a fine line parallel to the vertebral column (Fig. 18–33; see Fig. 18–36). A right aortic arch indents the *right side* of the trachea (see Fig. 18–8A), and a left aortic arch indents the *left side* of the trachea (Fig. 18–33B). A dilated anomalous left subclavian artery may pass behind the esophagus and cause a localized posterior indentation (Fig. 18–35).[209] A left superior vena cava is common and may cast its shadow at the left thoracic inlet.[94]

The *size* of the heart in cyanotic Fallot's tetralogy is normal (see Fig. 18–32).[120,184,203] The right atrium and right

ventricle cope with systemic resistance without dilating, and the left atrium and left ventricle are underfilled and are therefore small. Cardiac size in pulmonary atresia tends to be larger in response to flow through systemic arterial collaterals (Figs. 18–33 and 18–34).[114,133,184]

The *configuration* of the heart has long been a subject of interest in Fallot's tetralogy because of the distinctive bootshaped or *coeur en sabot* appearance (see Fig. 18–32).[17,120,184,203] The configuration has also been likened to a golf club wood or driver, especially when a right aortic arch and a concave main pulmonary artery segment accentuate the configuration of the left cardiac border (see Figs. 18–6A and 18–8A). The boot shape results from the combination of a small underfilled left ventricle that lies above a horizontal ventricular septum, inferior to which is a concentrically hypertrophied but nondilated right ventricle (see

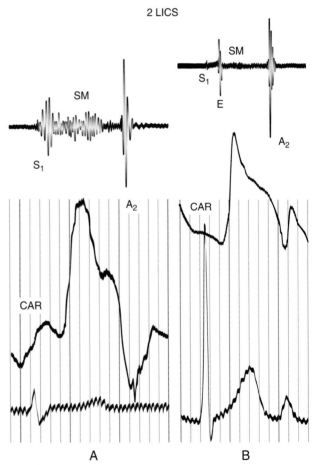

Figure 18–26

A, Tracings from a 2-year-old moderately cyanotic girl with Fallot's tetralogy. A grade 3/6 pulmonary stenotic murmur (SM) ends before the aortic component of the second sound (A_2), which was loud because a dilated aorta was guarded by a small anterior pulmonary trunk. *B,* Tracings from an 18-month-old girl with Fallot's tetralogy and pulmonary atresia. A prominent aortic ejection sound (E) introduces a soft short systolic murmur (SM) that originated in the dilated aortic root. The interval between the first heart sound and ejection sound is appropriate for the isovolumetric contraction time incurred by systemic vascular resistance. The aortic component of the second sound (A_2) was loud because a dilated aorta was guarded by a hypoplastic anterior pulmonary trunk. 2 LICS, second left intercostal space; CAR, carotid pulse.

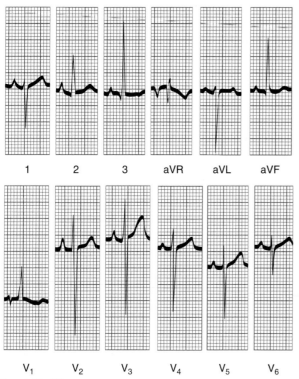

Figure 18–27

Electrocardiogram from a 2-year-old girl with cyanotic Fallot's tetralogy. P waves in leads 1, 2, 3 and V$_{2-3}$ are distinctly peaked. There is moderate right axis deviation with clockwise depolarization. Right ventricular hypertrophy is represented by a notched monophasic R wave in lead V$_1$. Right precordial T waves were normal because right ventricular systolic pressure did not exceed systemic systolic pressure. There is the typical abrupt change from an R wave in lead V$_1$ to an rS in lead V$_2$. Q waves are absent in left precordial leads because the left ventricle was underfilled.

Fig. 18–32A). The *coeur en sabot* is uncommon in neonates because intrauterine left ventricular volume is normal. In pulmonary atresia, the boot-shape may be present at birth (see Fig. 18–33A). In *acyanotic* Fallot's tetralogy or in pulmonary atresia with *large systemic arterial collaterals*, a well-formed convex apex is the result of normal if not increased left ventricular filling (Fig. 18–34). When right ventricular outflow obstruction is represented by stenosis of the *ostium of the infundibulum,* a localized indentation marks the site of obstruction above which the infundibular chamber is slightly convex (Figs. 18–4 and 18–36).

A nonrestrictive ventricular septal defect with *acquired* obstruction to right ventricular outflow initially exhibits increased pulmonary vascularity with enlargement of the left ventricle, left atrium, and pulmonary trunk (see Fig. 18–13A). Progressive obstruction results in a decline in pulmonary arterial blood flow and in normalization of the size of the left atrium and left ventricle (see Fig. 18–13B).[104,136] When a nonrestrictive *perimembranous* ventricular septal defect occurs with *pulmonary valve stenosis*, the radiologic picture is determined by the degree of pulmonary stenosis. The size of the ascending aorta is normal, the pulmonary trunk is dilated, and the ventricular septum is vertical rather than horizontal (see Fig. 18–10). When a malaligned

ventricular septal defect is partially occluded by tricuspid leaflet tissue, the right ventricle may dilate and fail. When a restrictive perimembranous ventricular septal defect occurs with mild pulmonary valve stenosis, the x-ray resembles isolated pulmonary valve stenosis.

THE ECHOCARDIOGRAM

Echocardiography with color flow imaging and Doppler interrogation provides morphologic and physiologic assessment of Fallot's tetralogy and its variations.[89] Thymic aplasia or hypoplasia can be identified in patients with DiGeorge syndrome.[51] Continuous wave Doppler establishes the outflow gradient and identifies the combination of valvular and infundibular pulmonary stenosis (Fig. 18–37). The malaligned ventricular septal defect is recognized with anterior and cephalic deviation of the infundibular septum and a biventricular aorta (Figs. 18–38 and

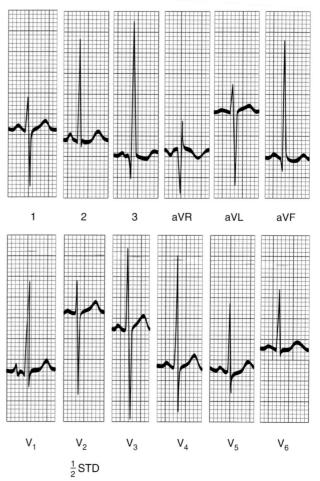

Figure 18–28

Electrocardiogram from a mildly cyanotic 3-year-old girl with Fallot's tetralogy. P waves are normal. There is moderate right axis deviation with clockwise depolarization. Right ventricular hypertrophy is represented by a tall monophasic R wave in lead V$_1$ with the typical abrupt change to an rS complex in lead V$_2$. Right precordial T waves remain upright because right ventricular systolic pressure did not exceed systemic systolic pressure. Prominent R waves in left precordial leads reflect an adequately filled and well-developed left ventricle. The large equidiphasic in RS complex in lead V$_3$ suggests biventricular hypertrophy. Leads V$_{2-3}$ are half standardized.

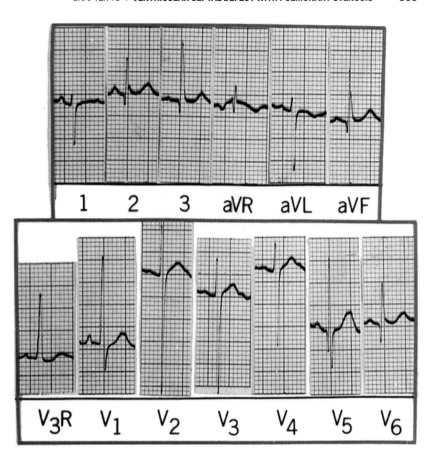

Figure 18–29

Electrocardiogram from a 2-year-old girl with acyanotic Fallot's tetralogy and a left-to-right shunt of 1.4/1. P waves in leads 1 and V_1 are slightly peaked. There is moderate right axis deviation with clockwise depolarization. Right ventricular hypertrophy is represented by tall monophasic R waves in leads V_3R and V_1 with the typical abrupt change to an rS complex in lead V_2. T waves are upright in right precordial leads because right ventricular systolic pressure did not exceed systemic systolic pressure. The well-developed R waves and prominent Q waves in leads V_{5-6} indicate adequate filling of a well-developed left ventricle.

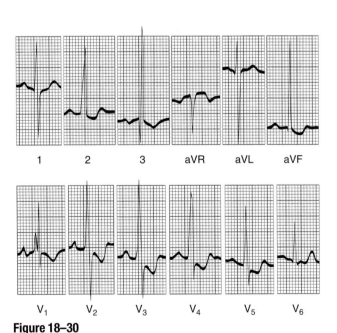

Figure 18–30

Electrocardiogram from a 15-year-old boy with Fallot's tetralogy and pulmonary atresia. P waves are slightly peaked in leads V_{1-2}. Right axis deviation is moderate. Right ventricular hypertrophy is represented by a tall, notched R wave in lead V_1 with atypical extension of the tall R wave to midprecordial leads together with inverted T waves and ST segment depressions. Prominent R waves in left precordial leads and the q wave in lead V_6 indicate an adequately filled well-developed left ventricle due to abundant aortopulmonary collateral flow.

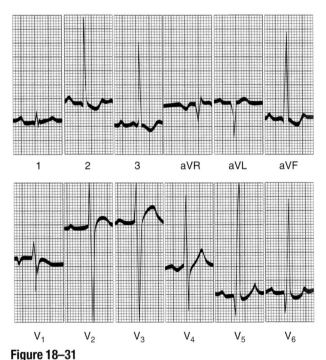

Figure 18–31

Electrocardiogram from a 23-year-old man with a nonrestrictive perimembranous ventricular septal defect and a *double-chambered* right ventricle. Right ventricular hypertrophy is conspicuously absent in both limb leads and precordial leads because only the most proximal portion of the right ventricle was hypertensive. The left ventricular volume overload pattern in leads V_{5-6} was due to a surgical shunt.

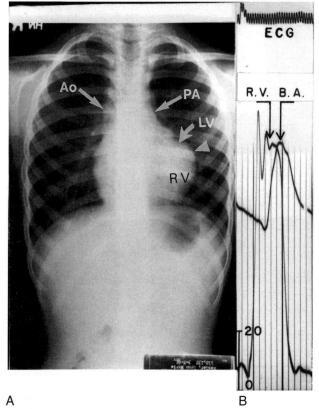

A

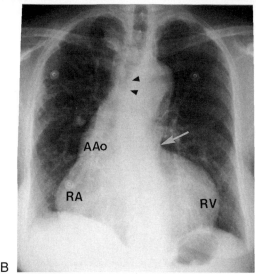

B

Figure 18–32

A, X-ray from a 4-year-old girl with classic cyanotic Fallot's tetralogy. The heart is typically boot-shaped because a small underfilled left ventricle (LV) lies superior to a relatively horizontal ventricular septum and an elevated interventricular sulcus (*unmarked arrowhead*) inferior to which lies the concentrically hypertrophied apex forming right ventricle (RV). The ascending aorta (Ao) is prominent, the main pulmonary artery segment (PA) is concave, and the lungs are oligemic. *B,* Systolic pressures are identical in the right ventricular (RV) and brachial artery (BA) because the ventricular septal defect was nonrestrictive.

18–39). The pulmonary trunk and its proximal branches can be assessed (Fig. 18–39). A right aortic arch is imaged from suprasternal notch and subclavicular windows, and the presence and degree of aortic regurgitation can be established with color flow. Echocardiography identifies excessive tricuspid leaflet tissue partially occluding the malaligned ventricular septal defect, and color flow imaging with continuous-wave Doppler interrogation establishes the degree of restriction across the partially occluded defect.[89] Pulmonary atresia is diagnosed when pulmonary valve echoes are absent and when color flow imaging and continuous wave Doppler detect no flow across the right ventricular outflow tract (Fig. 18–38A). The distinctive narrow serpentine elongated arterialized ductus arteriosus can be identified (Fig. 18–38B).

Obstructing or nonobstructing subinfundibular muscle bundles of a double-chambered right ventricle can be imaged, the degree of obstruction can be established with color flow and Doppler interrogation (Fig. 18–40), and a coexisting perimembranous ventricular septal defect can be detected.[216]

Fallot's Tetralogy with Absent Pulmonary Valve

In 1847, Cheevers described the combination of absent pulmonary valve, ventricular septal defect, annular stenosis, and dilatation of the pulmonary trunk and its branches.[47] The malformation was confirmed in 1908 by Royer and Wilson[186] and reconfirmed in 1927 by Kurtz, Sprague, and White.[132] The incidence of absent pulmonary valve

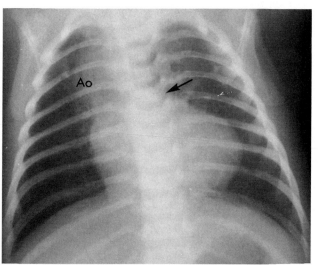

A

B

Figure 18–33

X-rays from two patients who were 55 years apart in age. *A,* Twenty-day-old boy with Fallot's tetralogy and pulmonary atresia. The boot-shaped apex is emphasized by the concave main pulmonary artery segment (*arrow*) and the right aortic arch (Ao). The lung fields show the lacy appearance of systemic arterial collateral circulation. *B,* X-ray from a 55-year-old woman with Fallot's tetralogy, pulmonary atresia, and acquired calcific stenosis and regurgitation of a biventricular aortic valve. Death was due to biventricular failure. The lung fields show the lacy appearance of systemic arterial collaterals. The dilated ascending aorta (AAo) continues as a left aortic arch that deviates the trachea to the right (*arrowheads*) and descends along the left side of the vertebral column. The main pulmonary artery segment is concave (*arrow*). An enlarged right atrium (RA) occupies the lower right cardiac border. The apex-forming right ventricle (RV) is convex and not boot-shaped because the left ventricle was well-developed owing to adequate filling from systemic arterial collateral circulation.

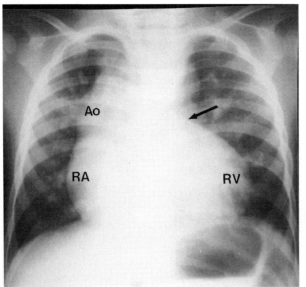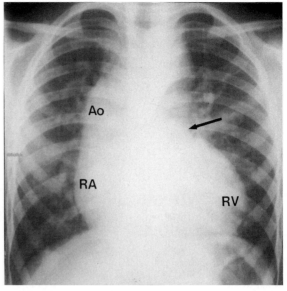

Figure 18–34

X-rays from the 3-year-old boy with Fallot's tetralogy and pulmonary atresia whose angiograms are shown in Figure 18–7. There is nonhomogeneous pulmonary vascularity reflecting nonuniform distribution of systemic arterial collateral flow (see Fig. 18–7). The ascending aorta (Ao) is dilated and the main pulmonary artery segment is concave (*arrow*). A prominent right atrium (RA) occupies the lower right cardiac border. The apex forming right ventricle (RV) is convex and not boot-shaped because the left ventricle was well-developed owing to adequate filling from systemic arterial collateral circulation.

in patients with Fallot's tetralogy ranges from 2.4% to 6.3%.[35,138,181] Pulmonary valve tissue is completely lacking or consists of rudimentary remnants of avascular myxomatous connective tissue.[75] Rarely, absence of the pulmonary valve occurs with absence of a pulmonary artery[12,33] (see later section) and with systemic to pulmonary artery collat-

erals.[44] Obstruction to right ventricular outflow resides at the narrow pulmonary annulus, not at the malaligned infundibular septum.[33] Stenosis of the infundibulum or narrowing of the pulmonary trunk above the annulus is exceptional.[33] The pulmonary trunk and especially its proximal branches dilate massively (Fig. 18–41) together with the infundibulum (Fig.18–41C).[33,75,134,143,155,175,187]

The malformation can be recognized in the fetus.[93] Regurgitant volume *in utero* is returned to the pulmonary

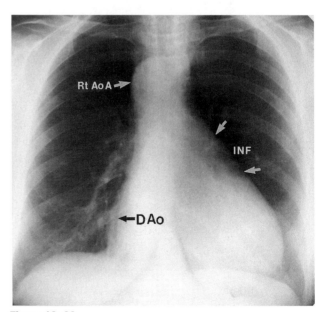

Figure 18–35

Lateral x-ray from a 5-year-old girl with Fallot's tetralogy, pulmonary atresia, a right aortic arch, and an aberrant left subclavian artery (LSA) that indents the posterior aspect of the barium-filled esophagus.

Figure 18–36

X-ray from a 62-year-old woman with stenosis of the ostium of the infundibulum (INF) and a restrictive perimembranous ventricular septal defect. *Paired arrows* bracket the slightly convex infundibulum. A right aortic arch (RtAoA) continued as a right descending aorta (DAo).

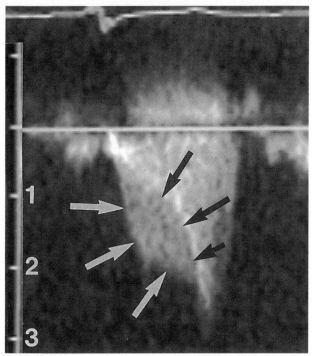

Figure 18–37
Continuous wave Doppler from an 18-month-old girl with Fallot's tetralogy, a stenotic bicuspid pulmonary valve, and a stenotic infundibulum. The Doppler signal across the pulmonary valve (*white arrows*) contains within it the profile of coexisting infundibular stenosis (*black arrows*).

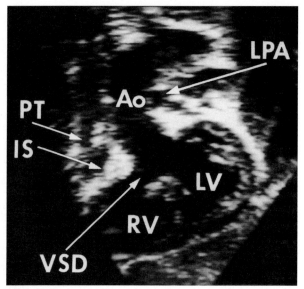

Figure 18–39
Echocardiogram (subcostal view) from an 18-month-old girl with cyanotic Fallot's tetralogy, a malaligned infundibular septum (IS), a narrow right ventricular outflow tract and a hypoplastic pulmonary trunk (PT). The large ventricular septal defect (VSD) lies beneath the biventricular aorta (Ao). RV, right ventricle; LV, left ventricle; LPA, left pulmonary artery.

trunk during each right ventricular systole, distending the pulmonary trunk and its branches, more so when egress is curtailed by agenesis of the ductus arteriosus[75,93,179] even though decompression is achieved via the nonrestrictive ventricular septal defect.[93] *Diastolic collapse* of the central pulmonary arteries occurs after each systole, with diastolic flow accelerated by elastic recoil of the proximal pulmonary arteries.[93] Medial abnormalities in the walls of the dilated proximal pulmonary arteries have been attributed to *in utero* flow patterns, but the medial abnormalities *per se* contribute materially to the massive dilatation (Fig. 18–41

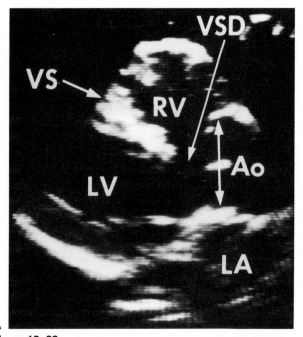

Figure 18–38
A, Echocardiogram (parasternal long axis) from a 22-year-old male with Fallot's tetralogy and pulmonary atresia. A nonrestrictive malaligned ventricular septal defect (VSD) lies beneath a dilated biventricular aorta (Ao). VS, ventricular septum; LA, left atrium; RV, right ventricle; LV, left ventricle. B, Black-and-white print of a color flow image from a neonate with Fallot's tetralogy and pulmonary atresia. The arterialized ductus is typically narrow, serpentine, and elongated. Ao, aorta; Dao, descending aorta.

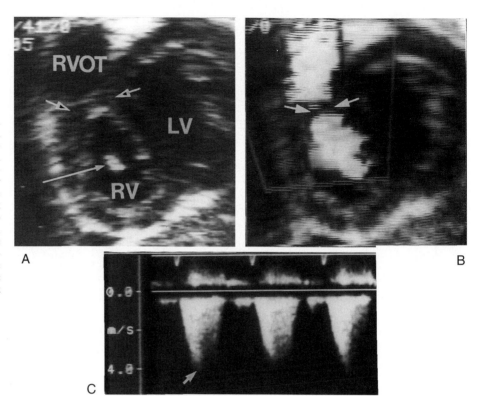

Figure 18–40
A, Echocardiogram (subcostal view) from a 2-year-old girl with double-chambered right ventricle and a restrictive perimembranous ventricular septal defect. Paired arrows identify the anomalous muscle bundles that separate the hypertensive inflow portion of the right ventricle (RV) from the low pressure right ventricular outflow tract (RVOT). The *long unmarked arrow* points to a large right ventricular papillary muscle. *B*, Black-and-white print of a color flow image shows the site of subinfundibular obstruction (*paired arrows*). *C*, Continuous wave Doppler recorded a peak velocity of 4m/sec across the obstruction (64 mm Hg peak instantaneous gradient).

and 18–42).[5,179] Morphometric studies have revealed a bizarre pattern of abnormal hilar branching in addition to the proximal pulmonary artery abnormalities.[154,179] Tufts of pulmonary arteries are entwined among compressed intrapulmonary bronchi.[179] Compression of small bronchi by abnormal branching patterns of intrapulmonary arteries together with compression of the trachea and bronchi by dilated *proximal* pulmonary arteries are major complications of the malformation.[33,69,116,175,179,181] An important feature of the experimental fetal rat model of congenitally absent pulmonary valve is the degree of bronchial deformity, which suggests that an inherent bronchial abnormality is an essential part of the syndrome.[158]

The *physiologic consequences* of Fallot's tetralogy with absent pulmonary valve are borne by the right ventricle which is subjected to the massive volume overload of severe pulmonary regurgitation in addition to the combined resistance to discharge incurred by annular obstruction and the nonrestrictive ventricular septal defect.[12] The doubly beset right ventricle dilates and fails, its filling pressure rises and equilibrates with pulmonary arterial diastolic pressure, and right atrial pressure rises in parallel. Right ventricular failure and tracheobronchial compression are responsible for the high morbidity and mortality.[46]

THE HISTORY

The malformation usually causes respiratory distress (tracheobronchial obstruction) and right ventricular failure soon after birth, but an occasional patient experiences infancy with surprisingly few symptoms.[33,69,75,134,164,175,181]

The symptoms related to bronchial obstruction occasionally improve during the course of tracheobronchial maturation, although emphysema, atelectasis, and pulmonary infection are common.[33,134,175] It is often uncertain whether early cyanosis is due to respiratory distress or to a right-to-left shunt. However, the degree of cyanosis typically diminishes with age[134,143,175] because a decrease in pulmonary vascular resistance decreases pulmonary regurgitant flow, decreases volume overload of the pressure-overloaded right ventricle, and decreases the right-to-left shunt.[134,143]

THE ARTERIAL PULSE, THE JUGULAR VENOUS PULSE, AND PRECORDIAL PALPATION

Right ventricular failure curtails aortic flow and reduces the systemic arterial pulse. The jugular venous pulse is elevated in parallel with the elevated right ventricular filling pressure. The A wave remains dominant until tricuspid regurgitation obliterates the X descent and increases the crest of the V wave. The right ventricular impulse is especially dynamic because of the combined effects of volume and pressure overload. A dilated infundibulum[75,143] (Fig. 18–41C) can palpated in the third left intercostal space, and a dilated pulsatile pulmonary trunk is palpated in the *second left* intercostal space (Fig. 18–41A). A systolic thrill is common because augmented right ventricular stroke volume is rapidly ejected across a hypoplastic pulmonary annulus. The diastolic thrill of pulmonary regurgitation is common because flow is accelerated by diastolic recoil of the dilated proximal pulmonary arteries.

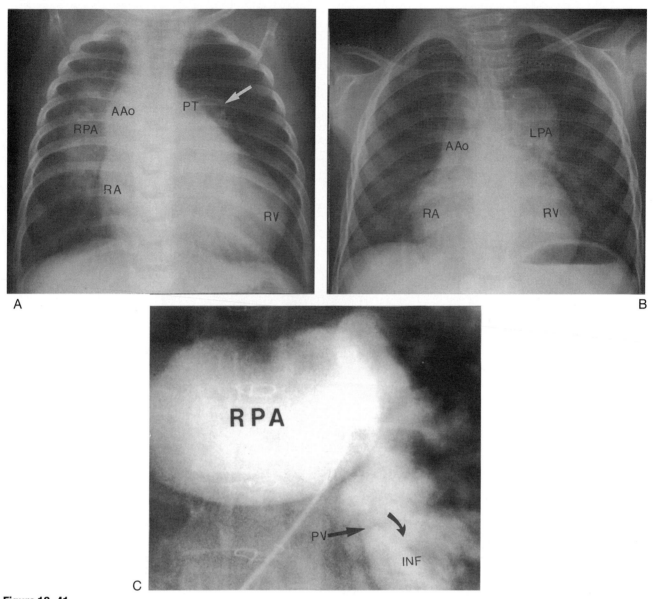

Figure 18–41

A, X-ray from a 6-month-old boy with Fallot's tetralogy and absent pulmonary valve. The *right* pulmonary artery (RPA) is aneurysmal. A dilated left pulmonary artery (*arrow*) is partially obscured by the large pulmonary trunk (PT). The ascending aorta (AAo) is dilated. A large right atrium (RA) occupies the right lower cardiac border, and an enlarged right ventricle (RV) occupies the apex. *B,* X-ray from an 8-month-old boy with Fallot's tetralogy and absent pulmonary valve. The *left* pulmonary artery (LPA) is aneurysmal. The ascending aorta (AAo) is dilated. An enlarged right atrium occupies the right lower cardiac border, and an enlarged right ventricle (RV) occupies the apex and extends below the left hemidiaphragm. *C,* Pulmonary arteriogram from a 26-year-old man with Fallot's tetralogy and absent pulmonary valve. The right pulmonary artery (RPA) is aneurysmal. The site of the absent pulmonary valve (PV) is identified by the straight *arrow*. The *curved arrow* identifies regurgitant flow into the dilated infundibulum (INF).

AUSCULTATION

Wheezing and stertorous breathing of tracheobronchial compression interfere with auscultation. A pulmonary ejection sound is absent despite dilatation of the pulmonary trunk because the pulmonary valve is absent.[108] The pulmonary component of the second heart sound is categorically absent because there is no valve mechanism.[108,143,155,187] The aortic component of the second sound is muted by interposition of the dilated anterior pulmonary trunk.[143] A midsystolic murmur is maximum in the second left intercostal space and is loud, harsh, and long because a large right ventricular stroke volume is ejected across a narrow annulus into a dilated pul-

monary trunk (Fig. 18–42).[75,90,143] The regurgitant murmur is analogous to the diastolic murmur of isolated severe congenital pulmonary valve regurgitation (see Chapter 12).[40,90,108,143,155,156,187,211] A distinct gap exists between the aortic component of the second heart sound and the onset of the diastolic murmur that coincides with the expected delayed timing of the absent pulmonary closure sound. The diastolic murmur is usually grade 3/6 and is impure and often harsh, ending well before the subsequent first heart sound (Fig. 18–42). The crescendo portion of the diastolic murmur may be comparatively long because of a delayed fall in pressure associated with impaired infundibular relaxation and increased diastolic stiffness.[90] The combi-

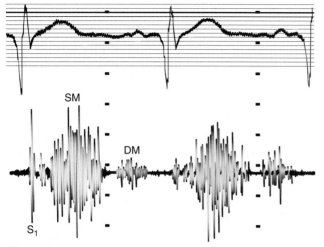

Figure 18–42

Phonocardiogram from the third left intercostal space of a 2-month-old girl with Fallot's tetralogy and absent pulmonary valve. A long loud midsystolic murmur (SM) is followed by a murmur-free interval before the onset of a mid-diastolic murmur (DM). The pulmonary component of the second heart sound is absent because the pulmonary valve is absent. The aortic component of the second heart sound is obscured by the long systolic murmur.

nation of a long, loud, harsh systolic murmur followed by a shorter harsh diastolic murmur creates the distinctive auscultatory impression of *sawing wood*.

THE ELECTROCARDIOGRAM

The P wave is usually both peaked *and* tall (Fig. 18–43). The QRS axis is rightward. However, the chief electro-cardiographic difference between Fallot's tetralogy with

absent pulmonary valve and classic cyanotic Fallot's tetralogy is the precordial lead pattern of right ventricular hypertrophy. When the pulmonary valve is absent, the tall monophasic R wave in lead V_1 extends into adjacent precordial leads (Fig. 18–43) in contrast to Fallot's tetralogy in which the tall right precordial R wave is characteristically confined to lead V_1 (see Fig. 18–27).

THE X-RAY

Radiologic features of Fallot's tetralogy with absent pulmonary valve are striking.[40,63,69,108,156,187] The pulmonary trunk and proximal branches dilate, often massively (see Fig. 18–41). Infundibular dilatation (Fig. 18–41C) may project leftward as a hump-shaped shadow.[187] A conspicuously dilated right ventricle occupies the apex, and an enlarged right atrium forms the right lower cardiac silhouette (Fig. 18–41A,B). Pulmonary vascularity is normal rather than decreased, although assessment is compromised by emphysema, hyperinflation, and atelectasis.[75,134,175] Rarely the right or left pulmonary artery arises directly from the aorta and lung vascularity is greater on the ipsilateral side.[35]

THE ECHOCARDIOGRAM

Echocardiography with color flow imaging and Doppler interrogation establishes the diagnosis and hemodynamic consequences of Fallot's tetralogy with absent pulmonary valve.[93] The malaligned ventricular septal defect is nonrestrictive (Figs. 18–44 and 18–45). An echodense ridge

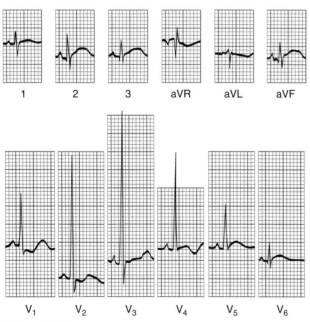

Figure 18–43

Electrocardiogram from a female neonate with Fallot's tetralogy and absent pulmonary valve. P waves are peaked and tall in leads 2 and aVF and in the midprecordium. The QRS axis is plus 90 degrees. Tall monophasic R waves of right ventricular hypertrophy are present in lead V_1 and extend into contiguous midprecordial leads.

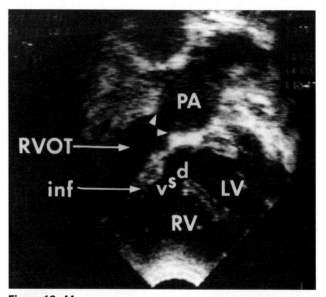

Figure 18–44

Echocardiogram (subcostal view) from a 23-month-old boy with Fallot's tetralogy and an absent pulmonary valve. The main pulmonary artery (PA) and right ventricular outflow tract (RVOT) are dilated. Echogenic ridges project into the lumen at the expected site of the pulmonary valve (*paired arrowheads*). The infundibular septum (inf) is malaligned, and the ventricular septal defect (vsd) is nonrestrictive. RV, right ventricle; LV, left ventricle.

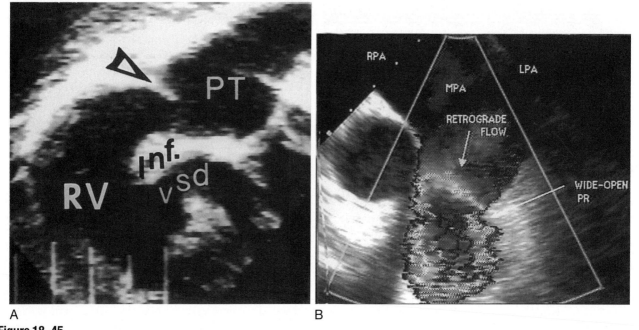

Figure 18–45

A, Echocardiogram (subcostal view) from a 4-year-old boy with Fallot's tetralogy and absent pulmonary valve. The *large arrowhead* points to an echogenic ridge at the site of the absent pulmonary valve. The pulmonary trunk (PT) is dilated. inf, infundibulum; vsd, ventricular septal defect. *B*, Echocardiogram from a 26-year-old man with Fallot's tetralogy and absent pulmonary valve. Black-and-white print of a color flow image shows retrograde flow and wide open pulmonary regurgitation (PR). MPA, main pulmonary artery; RPA/LPA, right/left pulmonary artery.

projects into the lumen at the expected site of the absent pulmonary valve (Figs. 18–44 and 18–45*A*). The infundibulum, pulmonary trunk, and proximal branches are dilated (Figs. 18–44 and 18–45*A*). Color flow imaging characterizes the pulmonary regurgitation (Fig. 18–45*B*), and Doppler interrogation characterizes flow patterns across the absent pulmonary valve and the pulmonary annulus (Fig. 18–46).

Fallot's Tetralogy with Absence of a Pulmonary Artery

Congenital absence of a pulmonary artery is usually associated with Fallot's tetralogy[73,152,161,221] and only rarely occurs in isolation.[2,3] It is almost always the *left* pulmonary artery that is absent (Figs. 18–47 and 18–48). When the

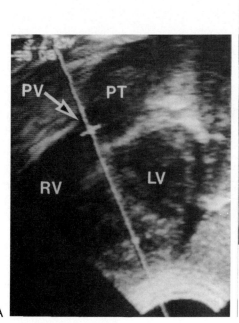

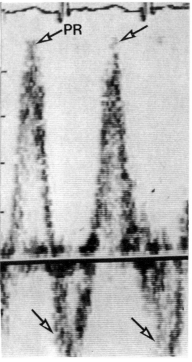

Figure 18–46

A, Echocardiogram (subcostal view) from a 4-year-old girl with Fallot's tetralogy and absent pulmonary valve. The Doppler sample volume is at the site of the absent pulmonary valve (PV). The pulmonary trunk (PT) and right ventricular outflow tract (RV) are dilated. LV, left ventricle. *B*, The Doppler signal is systolic/diastolic and not continuous, appropriate for the to-and-fro murmur which was systolic/diastolic and not continuous (see Fig 18–42). The larger signal is pulmonary regurgitation (PR).

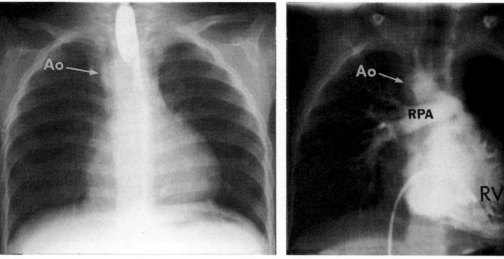

Figure 18–47

A, X-ray from an infant with Fallot's tetralogy and absent left pulmonary artery. The left hemithorax is smaller than the right hemithorax (posterior ribs are closer), but lung vascularity is not diminished. The aortic arch (Ao) and descending aorta are right-sided. *B*, The right ventriculogram (RV) from the same patient opacifies the right pulmonary artery (RPA), but not the left pulmonary artery, which is absent. The right aortic arch (Ao) visualized simultaneously.

right pulmonary artery is absent, the blood supply to the ipsilateral lung is often derived solely from the coronary arteries.[96] Congenital *absence* of a pulmonary artery differs from *anomalous origin* of a pulmonary artery from the ascending aorta, a malformation that also occurs with the tetralogy.[160] When the *left* pulmonary artery is absent, the murmur of pulmonary stenosis radiates into the *right* pulmonary artery and into the *right* upper chest.[161] The x-ray is diagnostically useful when the left hemithorax is small, the left hemidiaphragm is elevated, and left lung is hypovascular (Fig. 18–47*A*).[73,152,161,218,221] The aortic arch is usually on the *right* when the *left* pulmonary artery is congenitally absent (Fig. 18–47).[13,73,152,177] When the left pulmonary artery originates from the ascending aorta, the *ipsilateral* lung is relatively *hypervascular*.

SUMMARY

In *classic Fallot's tetralogy*, cyanosis is usually detected a few weeks after birth. The majority of patients are cyanotic by 6 months of age. Pulmonary atresia is accompanied by mild or absent neonatal cyanosis when pulmonary blood flow is appreciably increased by large systemic to pulmonary artery collaterals. Physical underdevelopment is common. Distinctive attacks of hyperpnea, deepening cyanosis, and syncope occur especially in the first 6 months of life and are provoked by feeding, straining, or crying. Squatting is the characteristic posture assumed for relief of dyspnea. Right ventricular failure is conspicuous by its absence, with few exceptions. The arterial pulse and the jugular venous pulse are normal. Precordial palpation detects a gentle right ventricular impulse that is confined to the lower left sternal border and subxiphoid area. A right sternoclavicular impulse indicates a right aortic arch with a dilated ascending aorta. The length and loudness of the pulmonary stenotic murmur vary inversely with the sever-

ity of right ventricular outflow obstruction. An aortic ejection sound is anticipated when the aortic root is dilated, and is consistently present in the dilated ascending aorta of pulmonary atresia. Pulmonary ejection sounds are absent because a bicuspid pulmonary valve is not sufficiently mobile. A single second heart sound is the aortic component. A soft delayed pulmonary component is reserved for the occasional patient with adequate flow into a well-formed pulmonary trunk. Continuous murmurs originate in the aortopulmonary collaterals that accompany Fallot's tetralogy with pulmonary atresia. P waves are normal or peaked but not tall. The QRS axis retains a normal neonatal direction. Right ventricular hypertrophy is characterized

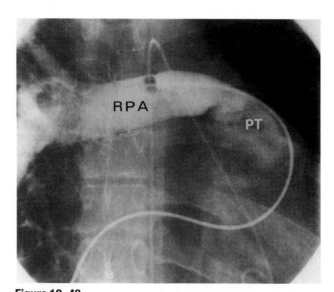

Figure 18–48

Selective pulmonary arteriogram from a 28-year-old man with Fallot's tetralogy and absent left pulmonary artery. The pulmonary trunk (PT) continues as the right pulmonary artery (RPA). The aortic arch was atypically left-sided.

by a tall monophasic R wave confined to lead V_1 with the abrupt transition to an rS complex in lead V_2. Q waves and well-developed R waves in left precordial leads reflect adequate pulmonary arterial blood flow and adequate left ventricular filling. The x-ray shows reduced pulmonary vascularity except for increased aortopulmonary collateral blood flow with pulmonary atresia. The ascending aorta is enlarged and often right-sided. The main pulmonary artery segment is distinctively concave. Cardiac size is normal, but the contour is characteristically boot-shaped. The echocardiogram reveals a biventricular aorta, a malaligned ventricular septal defect, and a narrow right ventricular outflow tract.

Fallot's tetralogy with absent pulmonary valve announces itself shortly after birth by symptoms of tracheobronchial compression and right ventricular failure. Neonatal cyanosis improves with age. The jugular venous pulse is elevated because of an increase in right ventricular filling pressure. A systolic impulse is palpated over the volume-overloaded right ventricle, over the dilated infundibulum, and over an aneurysmal pulmonary trunk. A systolic thrill is present in the second left intercostal space. The mid-diastolic murmur of pulmonary regurgitation begins at an interval after the aortic component of the second heart sound at the expected timing of the absent pulmonary component, or after the end of the long harsh systolic murmur. The systolic/diastolic murmurs are to and fro and not continuous. The x-ray discloses massive, often aneurysmal dilation of the pulmonary trunk and its proximal branches. The right atrium and especially the right ventricle are appreciably enlarged. The electrocardiogram is characterized by P waves that are peaked and tall, a rightward QRS axis and tall monophasic R waves of right ventricular hypertrophy that extend beyond lead V_1. Echocardiography identifies a dense band of echoes at the expected site of the absent pulmonary valve, and identifies the malaligned ventricular septal defect and the biventricular aorta. Color flow imaging establishes severe pulmonary regurgitation, and Doppler interrogation records the systolic/diastolic flow patterns across the right ventricular outflow tract.

Fallot's tetralogy with absent left pulmonary artery is characterized by a relatively small left hemithorax, an elevated left hemidiaphragm, and an ipsilateral decrease in pulmonary vascularity. The murmur of pulmonary stenosis radiates preferentially into the right pulmonary artery and the right upper chest because the left pulmonary artery is absent.

REFERENCES

1. Abraham AS, Atkinson M, Mitchell WM: Fallot's tetralogy with some features of Marfan's syndrome and survival to fifty-eight years. Br Heart J 23:110, 1961.
2. Abraham KA, Cherian G, Rao YD, et al: Tetralogy of Fallot in adults. A report of 147 patients. Am J Med 66:811, 1979.
3. Al-Attar AS: Pulmonary atresia in young adults. Int Surg 46:443, 1966.
4. Altrichter PM, Olson LJ, Edwards WD, et al: Surgical pathology of the pulmonary valve: A study of 116 cases spanning 15 years. Mayo Clin Proc 64:1352, 1989.
5. Niwa K, Perloff JK, Bhuta SM, et al: Structural abnormalities of great arterial walls in congenital heart disease. Light and electron microscopic analyses. Circulation 103:393, 2001.
6. Steno N: Anatomicus regij hafniensis embryo monstro affinis parisiis dissectus. Acta Med et Philosophia, Hafminsia 1:200, 1671.
7. Andriko J, Robinowitz M, Moore J, Virmani R: Necrotizing arteritis in uncorrected tetralogy of Fallot with pulmonary atresia. Pediatr Cardiol 13:233, 1992.
8. Anonymous: A case of long survival with Fallot's tetralogy. Demonstrated at the Post-Graduate Medical School of London. BMJ 2:748, 1966.
9. Bahler RC, Carson P, Traks E, et al: Absent right pulmonary artery. Am J Med 46:64, 1969.
10. Bain GO: Tetralogy of Fallot: Survival to seventieth year. Report of a case. AMA Arch Pathol 58:176, 1954.
11. Acierno LJ.: Etienne-Louis Fallot: Is it his tetralogy? Profiles in Cardiology. Clin Cardiol 22:321, 1999.
12. Jekel L, Benatar A, Bennink GB, et al: Tetralogy of Fallot with absent pulmonary valve. Scand Cardiovasc J 32:213, 1998.
13. Barrett O Jr, Walker WJ: Tetralogy of Fallot with absent left pulmonary artery: Report of a case with anomalous development of the right hilar vasculature and non-functioning right lung. Am Heart J 55:357, 1958.
14. Bashour TT, Kabbani S, Sandouk A, Cheng TO: Double-chambered right ventricle due to fibromuscular diaphragm. Am Heart J 107:792, 1984.
15. Baum D, Stern MP: Adipose hypocellularity in cyanotic congenital heart disease. Circulation 55:916, 1977.
16. Becu L, Ikkos D, Ljundqvist A, Rudhe U: Evolution of ventricular septal defect and pulmonary stenosis with left to right shunt into classic tetralogy of Fallot. A case report with clinical, angiocardiographic and anatomic correlations. Am J Cardiol 7:598, 1961.
17. Bedford DE: Three cases of congenital heart disease with cyanosis in adults. Proc R Soc Med 23:130, 1929.
18. Bedford, D. E.: Two cases of Fallot's tetralogy, shown at the section in 1929, exhibiting unusual longevity. Proc. R. Soc. Med. 49:314, 1956.
19. Bender, S. R., Dreifus, L. S., and Downing, D.: Anatomic and electrocardiographic correlation of Fallot's tetralogy. A study of 100 proved cases. Am. J. Cardiol. 7:475, 1961.
20. Benge, W., and White, C. W.: Systemic hypertension complicating tetralogy of Fallot. Am. J. Cardiol. 42:295, 1978.
21. Berry, T. E., Muster, A. J., and Paul, M. H.: Transient neonatal tricuspid regurgitation: Possible relation with premature closure of the ductus arteriosus. J. Am. Coll. Cardiol. 2:1178, 1983.
22. Berthrong, M., and Sabiston, D. C., Jr.: Cerebral lesions in congenital heart disease. A review of autopsies on 162 cases. Bull. Johns Hopkins Hosp. 89:384, 1951.
23. Bertranou, E. G., Blackstone, E. H., Hazelrig, J. B., Turner, M. E., and Kirklin, J. W.: Life expectancy without surgery in tetralogy of Fallot. Am. J. Cardiol. 42:458, 1978.
24. Best, P. V., and Heath, D.: Pulmonary thrombosis in cyanotic congenital heart disease without pulmonary hypertension. J. Pathol. Bacteriol. 75:281, 1958.
25. Bogers, A. J. J. C., Rohmer, J., Wolsky, S. A. E., Quaegebeur, J. M., and Huysmans, H. A.: Coronary artery fistula as source of pulmonary circulation in pulmonary atresia with ventricular septal defect. Thor. Cardiovasc. Surg. 38:30, 1990.
26. Bonchek, L. I., Starr, A., Sunderland, C. O., and Menashe, V. D.: Natural history of tetralogy of Fallot in infancy. Circulation 48:392, 1973.
27. Bopp, P., Rost, J., and Duchosal, P. W.: Unusual longevity in Fallot's tetralogy and pseudotruncus arteriosus. Br. Heart J. 25:735, 1963.
28. Bousvaros, G. A.: Pulmonary second sound in the tetralogy of Fallot. Am. Heart J. 61:570, 1961.
29. Bowie, E. A.: Longevity in tetralogy and trilogy of Fallot. Discussion of cases in patients surviving 40 years and presentation of two further cases. Am. Heart J. 62:125, 1961.
30. Braudo, J. L., and Zion, M. M.: The cyanotic (syncopal) attack in Fallot's tetralogy. Br. Med. J. 1:1323, 1959.
31. Brotmacher, L.: Hemodynamic effects of squatting during recovery from exertion. Br. Heart J. 19:567, 1957.
32. Brotmacher, L.: Hemodynamic effects of squatting during repose. Br. Heart J. 19:559, 1957.

33. Buendia, A., Attie, F., Ovseyevitz, J., Zghaib, A., Zamora, C., Zavaleta, D., Vargas-Barron, J., and Richheimer, R.: Congenital absence of pulmonary valve leaflets. Br. Heart J. 50:31, 1983.

34. Byrum, C. J., Dick, M., Behrendt, D. M., Hees, P., and Rosenthal, A.: Excitation of the double chambered right ventricle. Am. J. Cardiol. 49:1254, 1982.

35. Calder, A. L., Brandt, P. W. T., Barratt-Boyes, B. G., and Neutze, J. M.: Variant of tetralogy of Fallot with absent pulmonary valve leaflets and origin of one pulmonary artery from the ascending aorta. Am. J. Cardiol. 46:106, 1980.

36. Campbell, M.: Natural history of cyanotic malformations and comparison of all common cardiac malformations. Br. Heart J. 34:3, 1972.

37. Campbell, M.: Simple pulmonary stenosis; pulmonary valvular stenosis with closed ventricular septum. Br. Heart J. 16:273, 1954.

38. Campbell, M., and Deuchar, D. C.: Continuous murmurs in cyanotic congenital heart disease. Br. Heart J. 23:173, 1961.

39. Campbell, M., and Gardner, F. E.: Radiological features of enlarged bronchial arteries. Br. Heart J. 12:183, 1950.

40. Campeau, L., Gilbert, G., and Aerichide, N.: Absence of the pulmonary valve. Report of two cases associated with other congenital lesions. Am. J. Cardiol. 8:113, 1961.

41. Campeau, L. A., Ruble, P. E., and Cooksey, W. B.: Congenital absence of the pulmonary valve. Circulation:15:397, 1957.

42. Capelli, H., Ross, D., and Somerville, J.: Aortic regurgitation in tetralogy of Fallot and pulmonary atresia. Am. J. Cardiol. 49:1979, 1982.

43. Capitanio, M. A., Wolfson, B. J., Faerber, E. N., Williams, J. L., and Balsara, R. K.: Obstruction of the airway by the aorta. A.J.R. 140:675, 1983.

44. Siwik ES, Preminger TJ, Patel CR. Association of systemic to pulmonary collateral arteries with tetralogy of Fallot and absent pulmonary valve. Am J Cardiol. 77:547, 1996.

45. Cassidy, S. C., and Allen, H. D.: Tetralogy of Fallot in triplet siblings. Am. J. Cardiol. 67:1442, 1991.

46. Donofrio MT, Jacobs ML, Rychik J. Tetralogy of Fallot with absent pulmonary valve: echocardiographic morphometric features of the right-sided structures and their relationship to presentation and outcome. J Am Soc Echocardiogr. 10:556,1997.

47. Cheevers, N.: Retrecissement congenital de l'orfice pulmonaire. Arch. Med. Fourth Series 15:488, 1847.

48. Chesler, E., Joffe, H. S., Beck, W., and Schrire, V.: Tetralogy of Fallot and heart failure. Am. Heart J. 81:321, 1971.

49. Lee W, Smith RS, Comstock CH, Kirk JS, Riggs T, Weinhouse E. Tetralogy of Fallot: prenatal diagnosis and postnatal survival. Obstet Gynecol. 86:583, 1995.

50. Chin, J., Bashour, T., and Kabbani, S.: Tetralogy of Fallot in the elderly. Clin. Cardiol. 7:453, 1984.

51. Moran AM, Colan SD, Mayer JE, van der Velde ME. Echocardiographic identification of thymic hypoplasia in tetralogy of Fallot/tetralogy pulmonary atresia. AmJ Cardiol. 84:1268, 1999.

52. Coelho, E., de Paiva, E., and Nunes, A.: Malformations of the pulmonary artery and its branches, including two cases of absence of the right pulmonary artery. Am. J. Cardiol. 13:462, 1964.

53. Coelho, E., de Paiva, E., de Padua, F., Nunes, A., Amram, S., Bordalo, E., and Luis, S.: Tetralogy of Fallot. Angiocardiographic, electrocardiographic, vectorcardiographic, and hemodynamic studies of the Fallot-type complex. Am. J. Cardiol. 7:538, 1961.

54. Colman, A. L.: Diagnosis of left superior vena cava by clinical inspection, a new physical sign. Am. Heart J. 73:115, 1967.

55. Wang JK, Wu MH, Chang CI, Chiu IS, Chu SH, Hung CR. Malignant-type ventricular septal defect in double-chambered right ventricle. Am J Cardiol. 77:839, 1996.

56. Dabizzi, R. P., Caprioli, G., Aiazzi, L., Castelli, C., Baldrighi, G., Parenzan, L., and Baldright, V.: Distribution and anomalies of coronary arteries in tetralogy of Fallot. Circulation 61:95, 1980.

57. Dabizzi, R. P., Teodori, G., Barletta, G. A, Caprioli, G., Baldrighi, G., and Baldrichi, V.: Associated coronary and cardiac anomalies in the tetralogy of Fallot. An angiographic study. Eur. Heart J. 11:692, 1990.

58. Daliento, L., Grisolia, E. F., Frescura, C., and Thiene, G.: Anomalous muscle bundle of the sub-pulmonary outflow in tetralogy of Fallot. Int. J. Cardiol. 6:547, 1984.

59. Daniels, S. R., Bates, S. R., and Kaplan, S.: EEG monitoring during paroxysmal hyperpnea of tetralogy of Fallot: An epileptic or hypoxic phenomenon? J. Child. Neurol. 2:98, 1987.

60. Danilowicz, D., and Ishmael, R.: Anomalous right ventricular muscle bundle. Clin. Cardiol. 4:146, 1981.

61. Danilowicz, D., and Ross, J.: Pulmonary atresia without cyanosis. Report of two cases with ventricular septal defect and increased pulmonary blood flow. Br. Heart J. 33:138, 1971.

62. Dark, J. H., and Pollock, J. C. S.: Coronary artery-pulmonary artery fistula in tetralogy of Fallot with pulmonary atresia. Eur. Heart J. 6:714, 1985.

63. D'Cruz, I. A., Lendrum, B. L., and Novak, G.: Congenital absence of the pulmonary valve. Am. Heart J. 68:728, 1964.

64. DePasquale, N. P., and Burch, G. E.: The electrocardiogram, vectrocardiogram, and ventricular gradient in the tetralogy of Fallot. Circulation 24:94, 1961.

65. Der Kaloustian, V. M., Ratl, H., Malouf, J., Hatem, J., Slim, M., Tomeh, A., Khouri, J., and Kutayli, F.: Tetralogy of Fallot with pulmonary atresia in siblings. Am. J. Med. Genet. 21:119, 1985.

66. DeRuiter, M. C., Gittenberger-de Groot, A. C., Poelmann, R. E., Van Iperen, L., and Mentink, M. M. T.: Development of the pharyngeal arch system related to the pulmonary and bronchial vessels in the ovian embryo. Circulation. 87:1306, 1993.

67. Di Chiara, J. A., Pieroni, D. R., Gingell, R. L., and Bannerman, R. M.: Familial pulmonary atresia. Am. J. Dis. Child. 134:506, 1980.

68. Van Roekins CN, Zukergerg AL. Emergency management of hypercyanotic crises in tetralogy of Fallot. Ann Emer Med. 25:256, 1995.

69. Dunnigan, A., Oldham, H. N., and Benson, D. W.: Absent pulmonary valve syndrome in infancy. Am. J. Cardiol. 48:117, 1981.

70. East, T., and Barnard, W. G.: Pulmonary atresia and hypertrophy of bronchial arteries. Lancet 1:834, 1938.

71. Edwards, J. E., and McGoon, D. C.: Absence of anatomic origin from heart of pulmonary arterial supply. Circulation 47:393, 1973.

72. Hofbeck M, Rauch A, Buheitel G, Leipold G, von der EJ, Pfeiffer R. Monosomy 22q11 in patients with pulmonary atresis, ventricular septal defect, and major aortopulmonary collateral arteries. Heart 79:180, 1998.

73. Emanuel, R. W., and Pattinson, J. N.: Absence of left pulmonary artery in Fallot's tetrad. Br. Heart J. 18:289, 1956.

74. Emanuel, R., Somerville, J., Prusty, S., and Ross, D.: Aortic regurgitation from infective endocarditis in Fallot's tetralogy and pulmonary atresia. Br. Heart J. 37:365, 1975.

75. Emmanouilides, G. C., Thanopoulos, B., Siassi, B., and Fishbein, M.: Agenesis of ductus arteriosus associated with the syndrome of tetralogy of Fallot and absent pulmonary valve. Am. J. Cardiol. 37:403, 1976.

76. Faggian, G., Frescura, C., Thiene, G., Bortolotti, U., Mazzucco, A., and Anderson, R. H.: Accessory tricuspid valve tissue causing obstruction of the ventricular septal defect in tetralogy of Fallot. Br. Heart J. 49:324, 1983.

77. Faller, K., Haworth, S. G., Taylor, J. F. N., and Macartney, F. J.: Duplicate sources of pulmonary blood supply in pulmonary atresia with ventricular septal defect. Br. Heart J. 46:263, 1981.

78. Hofbeck M, Leipold G, Rauch A, Buheitel G, Singer H. Clinical relevance of monosomy 22q11.2 in children with pulmonary atresia and ventricular septal defect. Eur J Pediatr 158:302, 1999.

79. Fallot, A.: Contribution à l'anatomie pathologique de la maladie bleue (cyanose cardiaque). Marseille Medical. 25:418, 1888.

80. Digilio MC, Marino B, Grazioli S, Agostino D, Gianotti A, Dallapiccola B. Comparison of occurrence of genetic syndromes in ventricular septal defect with pulmonic stenosis (classic tetralogy of Fallot) versus ventricular septal defect with pulmonic atresia. Am J Cardiol. 77:1375, 1996.

81. Feigin, I., and Rosenthal, J.: The tetralogy of Fallot. Am. Heart J. 26:302, 1943.

82. Feldt, R. H., DuShane, J. W., and Titus, J. L.: The anatomy of the atrioventricular conduction system in ventricular septal defect and tetralogy of Fallot: Correlations with the electrocardiogram and vectorcardiogram. Circulation 34:774, 1966.

83. Fellows, K. E., Freed, M. D., Keane, J. F., Van Praagh, R., Bernhard, W. F., and Castenada, A. C.: Results of routine preoperative coronary angiography in tetralogy of Fallot. Circulation 51:561, 1975.

84. Ferencz, C.: The pulmonary vascular bed in tetralogy of Fallot. I. Changes associated with pulmonic stenosis. Bull. Johns Hopkins Hosp. 106:81, 1960.

85. Feruglio, G. A., and Gunton, R. W.: Intracardiac phonocardiography in ventricular septal defect. Circulation 21:49, 1960.

86. Fischbein, C. A., Rosenthal, A., Fischer, E. G., Nadas, A. S., and Welch, K.: Risk factors for brain abscess in patients with congenital heart disease. Am. J. Cardiol. 34:97, 1974.

87. Momma K, Kondo C, Ando M, Matsuoka R, Takao A. Tetralogy of Fallot associated with chromosome 22q11 deletion. Am J Cardiol. 76:618, 1995.

88. Chiu I, Wu C, Wang J, Wu M, Chu S, Hung C, Lue H. Influence of aortopulmonary rotation on the anomalous coronary artery pattern in tetralogy of Fallot. Am J Cardiol. 85:780, 2000.

89. Flanagan, M. F., Foran, R. B., Van Praagh, R., Jonas, R., and Sanders, S. P.: Tetralogy of Fallot with obstruction of the ventricular septal defect: Spectrum of echocardiographic findings. J. Am. Coll. Cardiol. 11:386, 1988.

90. Fontana, M. E., and Wooley, C. F.: The murmur of pulmonic regurgitation in tetralogy of Fallot with absent pulmonary valve. Circulation 57:986, 1978.

91. Gupta D, Saxena A, Kothari S, Jueneja M, Sharma S, VenuGopal P. Detection of coronary artery anomalies in tetralogy of Fallot using a specific angiographic protocol. Am J Cardiol. 87:241, 2001.

92. Forster, J. W., and Humphries, J. O.: Right ventricular anomalous muscle bundle. Circulation 43:115, 1971.

93. Fouron, J. C., Sahn, D. J., Bender, R., Block, R., Schneider, H., Fromberger, H., Fromberger, P., Hagen-Ansert, S., and Daily, P.: Prenatal diagnosis and circulatory characteristics in tetralogy of Fallot with absent pulmonary valve. Am. J. Cardiol. 64:547, 1989.

94. Fraser, R. S., Dvorkin, J., Rossall, R. E., and Eidem, R.: Left superior vena cava: A review of associated congenital heart lesions, catheterization data and roentgenologic findings. Am. J. Med. 31:711, 1961.

95. Fukuda, J., Izumi, T., Matsukawa, T., and Eguchi, S.: Development of left ventricular muscle in tetralogy of Fallot. Jpn. Circ. J. 48:465, 1984.

96. Gupta K, Livesay JJ, Lufschanowski R. Absent right pulmonary artery with coronary collaterals supplying the affected lung. Circulation 104:12, 2001.

97. Gale, G. E., Heimann, K. W., and Barlow, J. B.: Double-chambered right ventricle. Br. Heart J. 31:291, 1969.

98. Garcia, R., Cargill, J. W., and Drake, E. H.: Pseudotruncus arteriosus, Report of the oldest surviving patient. Am. Heart J. 78:537, 1969.

99. Gasul, B. M., Dillon, R. F., Vrla, V., and Hait, G.: Ventricular septal defects. Their natural transformation into those with infundibular stenosis or into the cyanotic or noncyanotic type of tetralogy of Fallot. J.A.M.A. 164:847, 1957.

100. Amin Z, McElhinney DB, Reddy VM, Moore P, Hanley FL, Teitel DF. Coronary to pulmonary artery collaterals in patients with pulmonary atresia and ventricular septal defect. Ann Thorac Surg. 70:119, 2000.

101. Glancy, D. L., Morrow, A. G., and Roberts, W. C.: Malformations of the aortic valve in patients with the tetralogy of Fallot. Am. Heart J. 76:755, 1968.

102. Glaser, J., Rosenmann, D., Balkin, J., and Zion, M. M.: Acquired obstruction of the ventricular septal defect in tetralogy of Fallot. Cardiol. 76:309, 1989.

103. Goitein, K. J., Neches, W. H., Park, S. C., Mathews, R. A., Lenox, C. C., and Zuberbuhler, J. R.: Electrocardiogram in double chamber right ventricle. Am. J. Cardiol. 45:604, 1980.

104. Gotsman, M. S.: Increasing obstruction to the outflow tract in Fallot's tetralogy. Br. Heart J. 28:615, 1966.

105. Greenwood, R. D., Rosenthal, A., Sommer, A., Wolff, G., and Craenen, J.: Cardiovascular malformations in oculoauriculovertebral dysplasia (Goldenhar syndrome). J. Pediatr. 85:816, 1974.

106. Guntheroth, W. G., Morgan, B. C., and Mullins, G. L.: Physiologic studies of paroxysmal hyperpnea in cyanotic congenital heart disease. Circulation 31:70, 1965.

107. Guntheroth, W. G., Morgan, B. C., Mullins, G. L., and Baum, D.: Venous return with knee-chest position and squatting in tetralogy of Fallot. Am. Heart J. 75:313, 1968.

108. Harris, B. C., Shaver, J. A., Kroetz, F. W., and Leonard, J. J.: Congenital pulmonary valvular insufficiency complicating tetralogy of Fallot. Am. J. Cardiol. 23:864, 1969.

109. Hartmann, A. F., Jr., Goldring, D., and Carlsson, E.: Development of right ventricular obstruction by aberrant muscular bands. Circulation 30:679, 1964.

110. Hartmann, A. F., Jr., Tsifutis, A. A., Arvidsson, H., and Goldring, D.: The two-chambered right ventricle. Report of nine cases. Circulation 26:279, 1962.

111. Hastreiter, A. R., D'Cruz, I. A., and Cantez, T.: Right-sided aorta. Br. Heart J. 28:722, 1966.

112. Haworth, S. G.: Collateral arteries in pulmonary atresia with ventricular septal defect. Br. Heart J. 44:5, 1980.

113. Haworth, S. G., and Macartney, F. J.: Growth and development of pulmonary circulation in pulmonary atresia with ventricular septal defect and major aortopulmonary collaterals. Br. Heart J. 44:14, 1980.

114. Higgins, C. B., and Mulder, D. G.: Tetralogy of Fallot in the adult. Am. J. Cardiol. 29:837, 1972.

115. Hindle, W. V., Jr., Engle, M. A., and Hagstrom, J. W. C.: Anomalous right ventricular muscles: A clinicopathologic study. Am. J. Cardiol. 21:487, 1968.

116. Hiraishi, S., Bargeron, L. B., Isabel-Jones, J. B., Emmanouilides, G. C., Friedman, W. F., and Jarmakani, J. M.: Ventricular and pulmonary artery volumes in patients with absent pulmonary valve. Circulation 67:183, 1983.

117. Hislop, A., and Reid, L.: Structural changes in the pulmonary arteries and veins in Tetralogy of Fallot. Br. Heart J. 35:1178, 1973.

118. Hofbeck, M., Sunnegardh, J. T., Burrows, P. E., Moes, C. A. F., Lightfoot, N., Williams, W. G., Trusler, G. A., and Freedom, R. M.: Analysis of survival in patients with pulmonic valve atresia and ventricular septal defect. Am. J. Cardiol. 67:737, 1991.

119. Hoffman, J. I. E., Rudolph, A. M., Nadas, A. A., and Gross, R. E.: Pulmonic stenosis, ventricular septal defect, and right ventricular pressure above systemic level. Circulation 22:405, 1960.

120. Holladay, W. E., Jr., and Witham, A. C.: The tetralogy of Fallot; the variability of its clinical manifestations. Arch. Intern. Med. 100:400, 1957.

121. Hope, J.: Diseases of the Heart. London, J. Churchill & Sons, 1839.

122. Horitz, S., Esquivel, J., Attie, F., Lupi, E., and Espino-Vela, J.: Clinical diagnosis of persistent left superior vena cava by observation of jugular pulses. Am. Heart J. 86:759, 1973.

123. Hunter, W.: Three cases of malformation of the heart, case II. Medical Observations and Inquiries by a Society of Physicians in London 6:291, 1784.

124. Hurwitz, R. A., Smith, W., King, H., Girod, D. A., and Caldwell, R. L.: Tetralogy of Fallot with abnormal coronary artery: 1967 to 1977. J. Thorac. Cardiovasc. Surg. 80:129, 1980.

125. Iga, K., Hori, K., Matsumura, T., Gen, H., Kitaguchi, S., Tomonaga, G., and Tamamura, T.: A case of unusual longevity of tetralogy of Fallot confirmed by cardiac catheterization. Jpn. Circ. J. 55:962, 1991.

126. Jarmakani, J. M. M., Graham, T. T., Canent, R. V., and Jewett, T. H.: Left heart function in children with tetralogy of Fallot before and after palliative or corrective surgery. Circulation 46:478, 1972.

127. Johnson, R. J., and Haworth, S. G.: Pulmonary vascular and alveolar development in tetralogy of Fallot. Thorax 37:893, 1982.

128. Keith, A.: The Hunterian lectures on malformations of the heart. Lancet 2:359, 1909.

129. King, S. B., and Franch, R. H.: Production of increased right to left shunting by rapid heart rates in patients with tetralogy of Fallot. Circulation 44:265, 1971.

130. Kinouchi, A., Mori, K., Ando, M., and Takao, A.: Facial appearance of patients with conotruncal anomalies. Pediatr. Jpn. 17:84, 1976.

131. Krongrad, E., Ritter, D. B., Hawe, A., Kincaid, O. W., and McGoon, D. C.: Pulmonary atresia or severe pulmonic stenosis and coronary artery-to-pulmonary artery fistula. Circulation 46:1005, 1972.

132. Kurtz, C. M., Sprague, H. B., and White, P. D.: Congenital heart disease; interventricular septal defects with associated anomalies in series of three cases examined post mortem, and living patient 58 years old with cyanosis and clubbing of fingers. Am. Heart J. 3:77, 1927.

133. LaFargue, R. T., Vogel, J. H. K., Pryor, R., and Blount, S. G., Jr.: Pseudotruncus arteriosus. A review of twenty-one cases with observations on oldest reported case. Am. J. Cardiol. 19:239, 1967.

134. Lakier, J. B., Stanger, P., Heymann, M. A., Hoffman, J. I. E., and Rudolph, A. M.: Tetralogy of Fallot with absent pulmonary valve: Natural history and hemodynamic considerations. Circulation 50:167, 1974.

135. Laskin, R. L., Salazar, R., Witzel, M. A., and Rose, V.: Velopharyngeal insufficiency in tetralogy of Fallot. Pediatr. Cardiol. 4:41, 1983.

136. Lendrum, B. L., Agustsson, M. H., Arcilla, R. A., Gasul, B. M., and Mercado, H. G.: Natural history of patients with "acyanotic" tetralogy of Fallot. Circulation 24:979, 1961.

137. Lev, M.: The architecture of the conduction system in congenital heart disease. II. Tetralogy of Fallot. A.M.A. Arch. Pathol. 67:572, 1959.

138. Lev, M., and Eckner, F. A.: The pathologic anatomy of tetralogy of Fallot and its variations. Dis. Chest 45:251, 1964.

139. Liao, P., Edwards, W. D., Julsrud, P. R., Puga, F. J., Danielson, G. K., and Feldt, R. H.: Pulmonary blood supply in patients with pulmonary atresia and ventricular septal defect. J. Am. Coll. Cardiol. 6:1343, 1985.

140. Lund, G. W.: Growth study of children with tetralogy of Fallot. J. Pediatr. 41:572, 1952.

141. Lurie, P. R.: Postural effects in tetralogy of Fallot. Am. J. Med. 15:297, 1953.

142. Maas, V.: Nicolai Steno: Opera Philosophica 2:49, 1910.

143. Macartney, F. J., and Miller, G. A. H.: Congenital absence of the pulmonary valve. Br. Heart J. 32:483, 1970.

144. Mace, J. W., Kaplan, J. M., Schanberger, J. E., and Gotlin, R. W.: Poland's syndrome. Clin. Pediatr. 11:98, 1972.

145. Macruz, R., Perloff, J. K., and Case, R. B.: A method for the electrocardiographic recognition of atrial enlargement. Circulation 17:882, 1958.

146. Marelli, A. J., Perloff, J. K., Child, J. S., and Laks, H.: Pulmonary atresia with ventricular septal defect in adults. Circulation 89:243, 1994.

147. Maron, B. J., Ferrans, V. J., and White, R. I.: Unusual evolution of acquired infundibular stenosis in patients with ventricular septal defect. Circulation 48:1092, 1973.

148. Marquis, R. M.: Longevity and the early history of tetralogy of Fallot. Br. Med. J. 1:819, 1956.

149. Martelle, R. R., and Linde, L. M.: Cerebrovascular accidents with tetralogy of Fallot. Am. J. Dis. Child. 101:206, 1961.

150. Matsuda, H., Ihara, K., Mori, T., Kitamura, S., and Kawashima, Y.: Tetralogy of Fallot with aortic insufficiency. Ann. Thorac. Surg. 29:529, 1980.

151. McGoon, M. D., Fulton, R. E., Davis, G. D., Ritter, D. G., Neill, C. A., and White, R. I.: Systemic collateral and pulmonary stenosis in patients with congenital pulmonary valve atresia and ventricular septal defect. Circulation 56:473, 1977.

152. McKim, J. S., and Wiglesworth, F. W.: Absence of left pulmonary artery; report of six cases with autopsy findings in three. Am. Heart J. 47:845, 1954.

153. Meindok, H.: Longevity in the tetralogy of Fallot. Thorax 19:12, 1964.

154. Milanesi, O., Talenti, E., Pellegrino, P. A., and Thiene, G.: Abnormal pulmonary artery branching in tetralogy of Fallot with "absent" pulmonary valve. Int. J. Cardiol. 6:375, 1984.

155. Miller, R. A., Lev, M., and Paul, M. H.: Congenital absence of the pulmonary valve. The clinical syndrome of tetralogy of Fallot with pulmonary regurgitation. Circulation 26:266, 1962.

156. Miller, R. A., White, H., and Lev, M.: Congenital absence of the pulmonary valve: Clinical and pathological syndrome. Circulation 18:759, 1958.

157. Miller, S. J.: Tetralogy of Fallot: Report of a case that survived to his fifty-seventh year and died following surgical relief of gallstone ileus. Ann. Intern. Med. 36:901, 1952.

158. Momma, K., Ando, M., Takao, A.: Fetal cardiac morphology of tetralogy of Fallot with absent pulmonary valve in the rat. Circulation 82:1343, 1990.

159. Morgan, B. C., Guntheroth, W. G., Bloom, R. S., and Fyler, D. C.: A clinical profile of paroxysmal hyperpnea in cyanotic congenital heart disease. Circulation 31:66, 1965.

160. Morgan, J. R.: Left pulmonary artery from ascending aorta in tetralogy of Fallot. Circulation 45:653, 1972.

161. Nadas, A. S., Rosenbaum, H. D., Wittenborg, M. H., and Rudolph, A. M.: Tetralogy of Fallot with unilateral pulmonary atresia; clinically diagnosable and surgically significant variant. Circulation 8:328, 1953.

162. O'Donnell, T. V., and McIlroy, M. B.: The circulatory effects of squatting. Am. Heart J. 64:347, 1962.

163. Onesti, S. J., Jr., and Harned, H. S. Jr.: Absence of the pulmonary valve associated with ventricular septal defect. Am. J. Cardiol. 2:496, 1958.

164. Osman, M. Z., Meng, C. C. L., and Girdany, B. R.: Congenital absence of the pulmonary valve. Am. J. Roentgenol. 106:58, 1969.

165. Padmanabhan, J., Varghese, P. J., Lloyd, S., and Haller, J. A.: Tetralogy of Fallot with suprasystemic pressure in the right ventricle. Am. Heart J. 82:805, 1971.

166. Pahl, E., Fong, L., Anderson, R. H., Park, S. C., and Zuberbuhler, J. R.: Fistulous communications between a solitary coronary artery and the pulmonary arteries as the primary source of pulmonary blood supply in tetralogy of Fallot with pulmonary valve atresia. Am. J. Cardiol. 63:140, 1989.

167. Pankau, R., Siekmeyer, W., and Stoffregen, R.: Tetralogy of Fallot in three sibs. Am. J. Med Genet. 37:532, 1990.

168. Patterson, D. F., Pyle, R. L., Van Mierop, L., Melbin, J., and Olson, M.: Hereditary defects of the conotruncal septum in Keeshond dogs: Pathologic and genetic studies. Am. J. Cardiol. 34:187, 1974.

169. Peacock, T. B.: On Malformations of the Human Heart. London, J. Churchill & Sons, 1866.

170. Perloff, J. K.: Pregnancy in congenital heart disease. *In* Perloff, J. K., and Child, J. S. 2nd edition. Congenital Heart Disease in Adults. Philadelphia, W. B. Saunders Company, 1998.

171. Perloff, J. K., Calvin, J., DeLeon, A. C., and Bowen, P.: Systemic hemodynamic effects of amyl nitrite in normal man. Am. Heart J. 66:460, 1963.

172. Perloff, J. K., and Marelli, A.: Neurologic and psychosocial disorders in adults with congenital heart disease. Heart Dis. Stroke 1:218, 1992.

173. Perloff, J. K., Ronan, J. A., DeLeon, A. C.: Ventricular septal defect with the "two-chambered right ventricle." Am. J. Cardiol. 16:894, 1965.

174. Pileggi, F., Bocanegra, J., Tranchisi, J., Macruz, R., Borges, S., Portugal, O., Villarinho, M. G., Barbato, E., and Descourt, L. V.: The electrocardiogram in tetralogy of Fallot: A study of 142 cases. Am. Heart J. 59:667, 1960.

175. Pinsky, W. W., Nihill, M. R., Mullins, C. E., Harrison, G., and McNamara, D. G.: The absent pulmonary valve syndrome. Circulation 57:159, 1978.

176. Pongiglione, G., Freedom, R. M., Cook, D., and Rowe, R. D.: Mechanism of acquired right ventricular outflow tract obstruction in patients with ventricular septal defect. Am. J. Cardiol. 50:776, 1982.

177. Pool, P. E., Vogel, J. H. K., and Blount, S. G.: Congenital unilateral absence of a pulmonary artery. Am. J. Cardiol. 10:706, 1962.

178. Qvist, G.: John Hunter 1728–1793. London, William Heinemann Medical Books Limited, 1981.

179. Rabinovitch, M., Grady, S., David, I., Van Praagh, R., Sauer, V., Buhlmeyer, K., Casteneda, A. R., and Reid, L.: Compression of intrapulmonary bronchi by abnormally branching pulmonary arteries associated with absent pulmonary valves. Am. J. Cardiol. 50:804, 1982.

180. Rabinovitch, M., Herrera-de Leon, V., Castenada, A., and Reid, L.: Growth and development of the pulmonary vascular bed in patients with tetralogy of Fallot with or without pulmonary atresia. Circulation 64:1234, 1981.

181. Rao, P. S., and Lawrie, G. M.: Absent pulmonary valve syndrome. Br. Heart J. 50:586, 1983.

182. Rich, A. R.: A hitherto unrecognized tendency to the development of widespread pulmonary vascular obstruction in patients with congenital pulmonary stenosis (tetralogy of Fallot). Bull. Johns Hopkins Hosp. 82:389, 1948.

183. Rosenthal, L.: Longevity and the tetralogy of Fallot. Br. Med. J. 1:1107, 1956.

184. Rowe, R. D., Vlad, P., and Keith, J. D.: Experiences with 180 cases of tetralogy of Fallot in infants and children. Can. Med. Assoc. J. 73:23, 1955.

185. Rowland, T. W., Rosenthal, A., and Castenada, A. R.: Double-chamber right ventricle. Am. Heart J. 89:455, 1975.

186. Royer, B. F., and Wilson, J. D.: Incomplete heterotaxy with unusual heart malformations. Arch. Pediatr. 25:881, 1908.

187. Ruttenberg, H. D., Carey, L. S., Adams, P., and Edwards, J. E.: Absence of the pulmonary valve in the tetralogy of Fallot. Am. J. Roentgenol. 91:500, 1964.

188. Rygg, I. H., Oelsen, K., and Boesen, I.: Life history of tetralogy of Fallot. Dan. Med. Bull. 18 (Suppl. II): 25, 1971.

189. Sandifort, E.: Observationes Anatomico-Pathological. Lugduni Batavorum, Eyk and D. Vygh, 1777.

190. Sautter, R. D., Emanuel, D. A., and Doege, K. H.: Association of pulmonary valvular stenosis and muscular ventricular septal defect. Report of a case in a patient aged seventy-five years. Am. J. Cardiol. 16:743, 1965.

191. Sharma, S. N., Sharma, S., Shrivastava, S., Rajani, M., and Tandon, R.: Pulmonary arterial anatomy in tetralogy of Fallot. Int. J. Cardiol. 25:33, 1989.

192. Sharpey-Shafer, E. P.: Effects of squatting on the normal and failing circulation. Br. Med. J. 1:1072, 1956.

193. Shepherd, R. L., Glancy, D. L., Jaffe, R. B., Perloff, J. K., and Epstein, S. E.: Acquired subvalvular right ventricular outflow obstruction in patients with ventricular septal defect. Am. J. Med. 53:444, 1972.
194. Shinebourne, E. A., Anderson, R. H., and Bowyer, J. J.: Variations in clinical presentation of Fallot's tetralogy in infancy. Br. Heart J. 37:946, 1975.
195. Sietsema, K. E., Cooper, D. M., Perloff, J. K., Rosove, M. H., Child, J. S., Canobbio, M. M., Whipp, B. J., and Wassermann, K.: Dynamics of oxygen uptake during exercise in adults with cyanotic congenital heart disease. Circulation 73:1137, 1986.
196. Sietsema, K. E., Cooper, D. M., Perloff, J. K., Child J. S., Rosove, M. H., Wasserman, K., and Whipp, B. J.: Control of ventilation during exercise in patients with central venous-to-systemic arterial shunts. J. Appl. Physiol. 64:234, 1988.
197. Smitherton, T. C., Nimetz, A. A., and Friedlich, A. L.: Pulmonary atresia with ventricular septal defect: Report of the oldest surviving case. Chest 67:603, 1975.
198. Soto, B., Pacifico, A. D., Ceballos, R., and Bargeron, L. M.: Tetralogy of Fallot: An angiographic-pathologic correlative study. Circulation 64:558, 1981.
199. Steeg, C. N., and Hordof, A.: The hemodynamic effects of supraventricular tachycardia in ventricular septal defect with pulmonary outflow tract obstruction. Am. Heart J. 90:245, 1975.
200. Sudhir, K., Gupta, K., Abraham, A. K., Cherian, M. P., Reddy, N. K., and Cherian, M. K., Pulmonary atresia with ventricular septal defect in adult patients. Clin. Cardiol. 10:350, 1987.
201. Tandon, R., Moller, J. H., and Edwards, J. E.: Tetralogy of Fallot associated with persistent common atrioventricular canal (endocardial cushion defect). Br. Heart J. 36:197, 1974.
202. Taussig, H. B.: Clinical and pathological findings in cases of truncus arteriosus in infancy. Am. J. Med. 2:26, 1947.
203. Taussig, H. B.: Congenital Malformations of the Heart. New York, The Commonwealth Fund, 1947.
204. Taussig, H. B.: Left to right shunts in infancy. In Lam, C. R. (ed.): Henry Ford Hospital International Symposium on Cardiovascular Surgery. Philadelphia, W. B. Saunders Company, 1955.
205. Thiene, G., Frescura, C., Bini, R. M., Valente, M., and Gallucci, V.: Histology of pulmonary arterial supply in pulmonary atresia with ventricular septal defect. Circulation 60:1066, 1979.
206. Toffler, O. B.: The pulmonary component of the second heart sound in Fallot's tetralogy. Br. Heart J. 25:509, 1963.
207. Uretzky, G., Puga, F. J., Danielson, G. K., Feldt, R. H., Julsrud, P. R., Seward, J. B., Edwards, W. D., and McGoon, D. C.: Complete atrioventricular canal associated with tetralogy of Fallot. J. Thorac. Cardiovasc. Surg. 87:756, 1984.
208. Varghese, P. J., Allen, J. R., Rosenquist, G. C., and Rowe, R. D.: Natural history of ventricular septal defect with right-sided aortic arch. Br. Heart J. 32:537, 1970.
209. Velasquez, G., Nath, P. H., Castaneda-Zuniga, W. R., Amplatz, K., and Formanck, A.: Aberrant left subclavian artery in tetralogy of Fallot. Am. J. Cardiol. 45:811, 1980.
210. Venables, A. W.: Absence of the pulmonary valve with ventricular septal defect. Br. Heart J. 24:293, 1962.
211. Vogelpoel, L., and Schrire, V.: Auscultatory and phonocardiographic assessment of Fallot's tetralogy. Circulation 22:73, 1960.
212. Vogelpoel, L., and Schrire, V.: Role of auscultation in differentiation of Fallot's tetralogy from severe pulmonary stenosis with intact ventricular septum and right-to-left interatrial shunt. Circulation 11:714, 1955.
213. Vogelpoel, L., Schrire, V., Nellen, M., and Swanepoel, A.: The use of amyl nitrite in the differentiation of Fallot's tetralogy and pulmonary stenosis with intact ventricular septum. Am. Heart J. 57:803, 1959.
214. Vogelpoel, L., Schrire, V., Nellen, M., and Swanepoel, A.: The use of phenylephrine in the differentiation of Fallot's tetralogy from pulmonary stenosis with intact ventricular septum. Am. Heart J. 59:489, 1960.
215. Volini, I. F., and Flaxman, N.: Tetralogy of Fallot; report of a case in man who lived to his forty-first year. J.A.M.A. 111:2000, 1938.
216. Von Doenhoff, L. J., and Nanda, N. C.: Obstruction within the right ventricular body. Two-dimensional echocardiographic features. Am. J. Cardiol. 51:1498, 1983.
217. Watson, T.: Lectures on the Principles and Practice of Physic. Vol II. Philadelphia, Henry C. Lea, 1872.
218. Werber, J., Ramilo, J. L., London, R., and Harris, V. J.: Unilateral absence of a pulmonary artery. Chest 84:729, 1983.
219. White, P. D., and Sprague, H. B.: Tetralogy of Fallot; report of a case of a noted musician, who lived to his 60th year. J.A.M.A. 92:787, 1929.
220. Willius, F. A.: An unusually early description of the tetralogy of Fallot. Proc. Staff Meet. Mayo Clin. 23:316, 1948.
221. Wilson, W. J., and Amplatz, K.: Unequal vascularity in tetralogy of Fallot. Am. J. Roentgenol. 100:318, 1967.
222. Wong, H. O., and Ang, A. H.: Unilateral rib notching in Fallot's tetralogy due to systemic-pulmonary collateral vessels. Br. Heart J. 35:226, 1973.
223. Wood, P.: Attacks of deeper cyanosis and loss of consciousness (syncope) in Fallot's tetralogy. Br. Heart J. 20:282, 1958.
224. Wood, P., Magidson, O., and Wilson, P. A. O.: Ventricular septal defect with a note on acyanotic Fallot's tetralogy. Br. Heart J. 16:387, 1954.
225. Wulfsberg, E. A., Zintz, E. J., and Moore, J. W.: The inheritance of conotruncal malformations: A review and report of two siblings with tetralogy of Fallot with pulmonary atresia. Clin. Genet. 40:12, 1991.
226. Yamaguchi, M., Tsukube, T., Hosokawa, Y., Ohashi, H., and Oshima, Y.: Pulmonary origin of left anterior descending coronary artery in tetralogy of Fallot. Ann. Thorac. Surg. 52:310, 1991.
227. Young, D., and Elbl, F.: Supraventricular tachycardia as cause of cyanotic syncopal spells in tetralogy of Fallot. New Engl. J. Med. 284:1359, 1971.
228. Zellers, T. M., Driscoll, D. J., and Michels, V. V.: Prevalence of significant congenital heart defects in children of parents with Fallot's tetralogy. Am. J. Cardiol. 65:523, 1990.

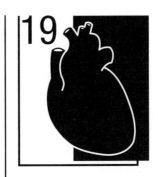

Double Outlet Ventricle

Double outlet ventricle refers to abnormal ventriculoarterial alignments in which both great arteries originate exclusively or predominantly from either a morphologic right ventricle or a morphologic left ventricle in hearts equipped with two ventricles.[13,14,17,26,59-61,69,76,80] This chapter is concerned with double outlet ventricles in hearts with concordant atrioventricular connections to each of two morphologically distinct ventricles (biventricular atrioventricular connections). The incidence of *double outlet right ventricle* has been estimated at 0.09 per 1000 live births or 4.5% of necropsy cases of congenital heart disease.[80] *Double outlet left ventricle* is among the rarest of the ventriculoarterial malalignments, representing less than 5% of double outlet ventricles.

The earliest report of *double outlet right ventricle* was published in French in 1703.[80] Ninety years elapsed before an English language publication appeared.[2] Double outlet right ventricle was known to Peacock in 1866,[65] and was called *partial transposition* by Vierordt in 1898[81] to signify that the aorta was transposed but the pulmonary trunk was normally aligned. In 1949, Taussig and Bing published a case of *complete transposition of the aorta* and *levoposition of the pulmonary artery* which originated chiefly from the right ventricle.[77] Three years later a case was described in which the right ventricle gave rise to both great arteries,[16] and in 1957 Witham formalized the term *double outlet right ventricle*[83] which is now preferred to the synonymous term *right ventricular origin of both great arteries*.[59-61]

It has been argued that double outlet right ventricle is virtually unclassifiable because of its complex and diverse anatomy.[80] However, certain features are sufficiently recurrent to serve as the basis for the classification in this chapter. Three essential gross morphologic features include: 1) the connections of the great arteries to the ventricles; 2) the location, size, and relationship of the ventricular septal defect to the great arteries; and 3) the absence, presence and degree of pulmonary stenosis (Table 19–1).

A double outlet morphologic right ventricle gives rise to both great arteries which are separated from each other by an outlet septum housed exclusively in the right ventricle.[69] An conus resides beneath each of the two great arterial valves (double conuses), although either conus may be attenuated. The position of the outlet septum determines two types of infundibular relationships, namely, anterior/posterior and side-by-side.[26,63,69] In the anterior/posterior relationship which is more common, the aorta arises from the posterior infundibulum and the ventricular septal defect is subaortic. In the side-by-side relationship, which is less common, the pulmonary trunk arises from the medial infundibulum and the ventricular septal defect is subpulmonary.

Table 19–1 | Double Outlet Right Ventricle: *Clinical Classification*

Common Types

Subaortic ventricular septal defect without pulmonary stenosis:

　Low pulmonary vascular resistance

　High pulmonary vascular resistance

Subpulmonary ventricular septal defect without pulmonary stenosis:

　Low pulmonary vascular resistance

　High pulmonary vascular resistance

Less Common Types

Doubly committed ventricular septal defect

Uncommitted ventricular septal defect

Intact ventricular septum

Connections of the Great Arteries to the Ventricles

The aorta is either to the right of and anterior to the pulmonary trunk or side-by-side with the aorta to the right.[20,69,75,76] Each great artery arises above a conus which prevents fibrous continuity with atrioventricular valve tissue,[17,63] but conal attenuation occasionally permits fibrous continuity.[12,17,26,37,48,63,74,75,79] When each great artery is equipped with a separate conus and both great arteries arise exclusively from the right ventricle, the term *double outlet right ventricle* is not questioned. Unresolved is the appropriate terminology for hearts with a biventricular great arterial valve.[17] Double outlet right ventricle with a *subaortic* ventricular septal defect, pulmonary stenosis, and greater than 50 % aortic override resembles Fallot's tetralogy (Table 19–2, see Chapter 18). Double outlet right ventricle with a *subpulmonary* ventricular septal defect and a biventricular pulmonary trunk that is posterior and therefore not border forming resembles complete transposition of the great arteries (Table 19–2, see Chapter 27). It has been proposed that double outlet right ventricle, Fallot's tetralogy, and complete transposition of the great arteries may represent a spectrum of anomalies that result from variable embryonic arrest of the normal rotation of the junction of the outflow tract and the great arteries.[14]

Relationship of the Ventricular Septal Defect to the Great Arteries

A ventricular septal defect provides the left ventricle with its only exit (Fig. 19–1). The ventricular septal defect is usually subaortic or subpulmonary, but less commonly the defect is committed to both great arteries or to neither great artery, or the ventricular septum is intact (Table 19–1).[35,51,59,60,61,75,76,80] The major determinant of intracardiac streaming is the location of the ventricular septal defect. When the defect is committed to the aorta, blood flow is selectively channeled into the aorta (Fig. 19–1A). Rarely, the ventricular septal defect is in the muscular or

Table 19–2 | **Double Outlet Right Ventricle: Major Clinical Patterns**

A. *Subaortic* ventricular septal defect, no pulmonary stenosis, low pulmonary vascular resistance—resembles nonrestrictive perimembranous ventricular septal defect.

B. *Subaortic* ventricular septal defect, no pulmonary stenosis, high pulmonary vascular resistance—Eisenmenger syndrome.

C. *Subaortic* ventricular septal defect with pulmonary stenosis—resembles Fallot's tetralogy.

D. *Subpulmonary* ventricular septal defect with no pulmonary stenosis—resembles complete transposition of the great arteries with nonrestrictive ventricular septal defect.

inlet septum and is therefore committed to neither great artery. Streaming is secondarily influenced by obstruction to ventricular outflow, especially pulmonary, and by pulmonary vascular resistance.

In 1949, Taussig and Bing described a malformation referred to as "complete transposition of the aorta and levoposition of the pulmonary artery" (see earlier).[77] The aorta arose completely from the right ventricle, a nonrestrictive ventricular septal defect was subpulmonary, and the pulmonary trunk was biventricular although it arose principally from the right ventricle.[49,77] Left ventricular blood selectively entered the pulmonary artery through the subpulmonary ventricular septal defect (Figs. 19–1D and 19–2).[37,74,76,77,79,82] The Taussig-Bing anomaly constitutes less than 10% of cases of double outlet right ventricle.[48,49]

Obstruction to Ventricular Outflow

Pulmonary stenosis is present in 40% to 70% of cases of double outlet right ventricle with subaortic ventricular septal defect[7,25,57,59,74,76] (see Fig. 19–1C) and is represented by an underdeveloped subpulmonary conus or by a stenotic bicuspid pulmonary valve.[25,59,75,80] In the presence of pulmonary artesia (Fig. 19–3), the right ventricle has a single functional outlet—the aorta—so *double outlet* then refers to ventriculoarterial *alignment*.[80] Pulmonary stenosis is exceptional when the ventricular septal is subpulmonary.[2,25,56]

A nonrestrictive ventricular septal defect is physiologically advantageous because it provides the left ventricle with an unobstructed exit. A restrictive subaortic ventricular septal defect or a spontaneous decrease in size is a form of subaortic stenosis.[46,55,61,66] The decrease in size may culminate in complete closure,[51,66] or rarely the ventricular septum is congenitally intact and the left ventricle is hypoplastic.[24,51,76] Aortic stenosis is also caused by underdevelopment of the subaortic infundibulum which occurs in about 50% of cases with a subaortic ventricular septal defect.[49,80]

Nearly a third of patients with *straddling atrioventricular valves* (biventricular insertion of chordae tendineae) have double outlet right ventricle (see Fig. 19–10).[68] The straddle can involve the right-sided or left-sided atrioventricular valve.[68] *Overriding* refers to biventricular commitment of the atrioventricular annulus which is not a feature of double outlet right ventricle.

The *atrioventricular node* is in its normal location, and the conduction system penetrates the right side of the central fibrous body (see The Electrocardiogram).[12,78] The location of the atrioventricular bundle is related to the ventricular septal defect as in isolated ventricular septal defect (see Chapter 17).

The classification of double outlet right ventricle in Table 19–1 is based on the anatomic faults that are principally responsible for the physiologic derangements and

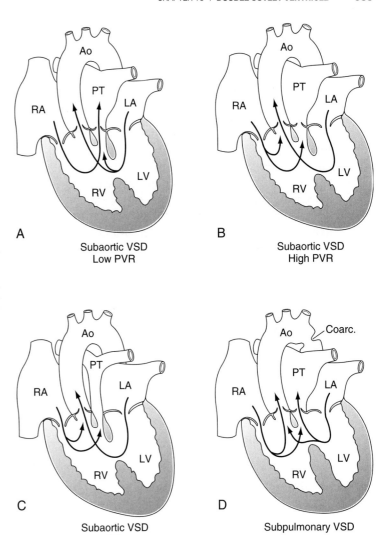

Figure 19–1

Illustrations of four major clinical patterns of double outlet right ventricle (see Tables 19–1 and 19–2). *A, Subaortic* ventricular septal defect (VSD), low pulmonary vascular resistance, no pulmonary stenosis. *B, Subaortic* ventricular septal defect, high pulmonary vascular resistance. *C, Subaortic* ventricular septal defect with pulmonary stenosis. *D, Subpulmonary* ventricular septal defect. Ao, aorta; RA, right atrium; PT, pulmonary trunk; LA, left atrium; LV, left ventricle; RV, right ventricle.

clinical manifestations that result from a subaortic or subpulmonary ventricular septal defect and from the absence or presence of pulmonary stenosis or pulmonary vascular disease.

The *physiologic consequences* of double outlet right ventricle with a *subaortic* ventricular septal defect and *no pulmonary stenosis* resemble an isolated nonrestrictive perimembranous ventricular septal defect (Table 19–2; see Chapter 17). Because the defect is committed to the aorta, left ventricular blood selectively enters the aorta. Low pulmonary vascular resistance permits a substantial portion of left ventricular blood to stream into the pulmonary circulation, and permits right ventricular blood to stream almost exclusively into the pulmonary trunk (see Fig. 19–1A). Pulmonary blood flow is increased, and aortic oxygen saturation is virtually normal. As pulmonary vascular resistance rises, right ventricular blood is diverted into the aorta, and left ventricular blood is diverted away from the pulmonary trunk (see Fig. 19–1B). Pulmonary blood flow declines, and aortic oxygen saturation declines in parallel.

When *pulmonary stenosis* coexists with double outlet right ventricle, the ventricular septal defect is almost always *subaortic*.[7,25,57,59] Pulmonary stenosis may initially be absent or mild and then develop and progress.[31] Pulmonary stenosis diverts right ventricular and left ventricular blood away from the pulmonary artery and into the aorta (see Fig. 19–1C), so pulmonary blood flow and aortic oxygen saturation fall. The more severe the pulmonary stenosis, the more blood from the right and left ventricles enters the aorta, and in the presence of pulmonary atresia, all blood from both ventricles enters the aorta (Fig. 19–3).[71] Double outlet right ventricle with a nonrestrictive subaortic ventricular septal defect and severe pulmonary stenosis or atresia physiologically resembles Fallot's tetralogy (Table 19–2; see Chapter 18).[2,7,25,59,71,74]

When the ventricular septal defect is *subpulmonary*, left ventricular blood preferentially enters into the pulmonary trunk and right ventricular blood preferentially enters the aorta (see Figs. 19–1D and 19–2), so pulmonary artery oxygen saturation exceeds aortic oxygen saturation. When pulmonary vascular resistance is low, pulmonary blood flow is increased, systemic arterial oxygen saturation is high, cyanosis is relatively mild, and the

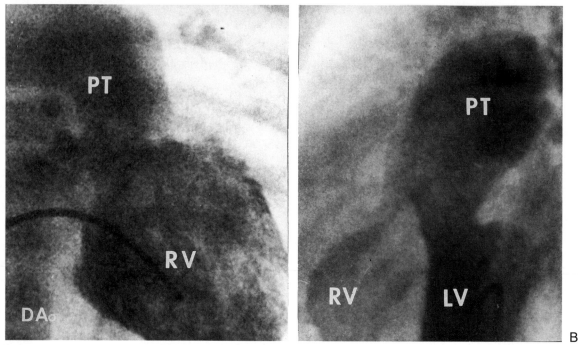

Figure 19–2
Angiocardiograms from a 20-month-old boy with double outlet right ventricle and a subpulmonary ventricular septal defect. *A*, The right ventriculogram (RV) shows a large pulmonary trunk (PT) arising from a dilated right ventricle. DA, descending aorta. *B*, Left oblique left ventriculogram showing selective flow from left ventricle (LV) into a dilated biventricular pulmonary trunk (PT). The right ventricle (RV) faintly visualizes.

left ventricle is volume overloaded as in complete transposition of the great arteries (see Chapter 27). A rise in pulmonary vascular resistance diverts right ventricular blood away from the pulmonary artery into the aorta. Pulmonary blood flow declines, systemic arterial oxygen saturation falls, and left ventricular volume overload is curtailed (see Fig. 19–1*D*).

Double Outlet Right Ventricle and Subaortic Ventricular Septal Defect without Pulmonary Stenosis

The clinical manifestations closely resemble isolated non-restrictive perimembranous ventricular septal defect (see

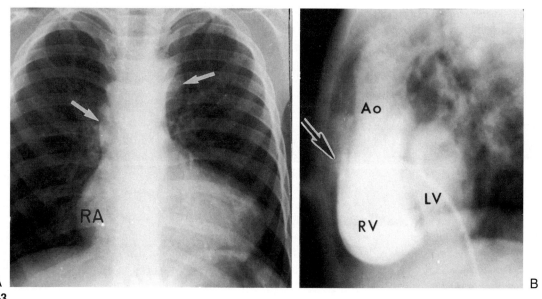

Figure 19–3
A, X-ray from a 3-year-old boy with double outlet right ventricle, subaortic ventricular septal defect, and pulmonary atresia. Lung fields show the lacy appearance of systemic-to-pulmonary arterial collaterals. The pulmonary trunk is conspicuously absent, and the ascending and transverse aorta are correspondingly large. The apex is boot-shaped and prominent. The right atrium (RA) is moderately convex. *B*, Lateral right ventriculogram (RV) showing the blind outflow tract (*arrow*) and the dilated aorta (Ao) that arises anterior to the ventricular septum. LV, left ventricle.

Figs. 19–1*A* and 19–1*B* and Table 19–2). Male/female ratio is estimated at 1.7 to 1.[27,80] A large kindred included a second cousin with double outlet right ventricle, a first cousin with complete transposition of the great arteries, and two siblings with truncus arteriosus.[67]

THE HISTORY

The murmur of ventricular septal defect dates from birth because flow from the left ventricle through the defect is obligatory and does not await the neonatal fall in pulmonary vascular resistance. However, the intensity of the systolic murmur increases as neonatal pulmonary resistance falls and as the increased left ventricular stroke volume is ejected through the ventricular septal defect into both great arteries. Increased pulmonary blood flow results in volume overload of the left ventricle, congestive heart failure, and poor growth and development.[31,60,61] Cyanosis is mild or absent because left ventricular blood preferentially enters the aorta and right ventricular blood preferentially enters the pulmonary artery (see Fig. 19–1*A*). A rise in pulmonary vascular resistance curtails pulmonary blood flow and relieves the left ventricle of volume overload. Patients occasionally reach young adulthood (Fig. 19–4*A*)[31,61]; one underwent intracardiac repair

at age 53 years (Fig. 19–4*B*), and one survived to age 65 years.[36]

PHYSICAL APPEARANCE

Transient neonatal cyanosis coincides with the transient elevation in neonatal pulmonary vascular resistance. The subsequent fall in pulmonary vascular resistance is accompanied by an increase in pulmonary blood flow, volume overload of the left ventricle and the catabolic appearance associated with congestive heart failure. A subsequent rise in pulmonary resistance diverts left ventricular blood away from the pulmonary trunk and diverts right ventricular blood into the aorta (see Fig. 19–1*B*)—Eisenmenger syndrome—with the appearance of cyanosis and clubbing (Table 19–2*B*). Double outlet right ventricle is occasionally associated with trisomy 18 and the distinctive overlapping fingers (clinodactyly), rocker bottom feet, and lax skin (Fig. 19–5).[18,38,70,72,73]

THE ARTERIAL PULSE

The arterial pulse is brisk when pulmonary blood flow is increased and the volume-overloaded left ventricle is functionally normal. A rise in pulmonary vascular resistance curtails left ventricular volume overload and normalizes the arterial pulse.

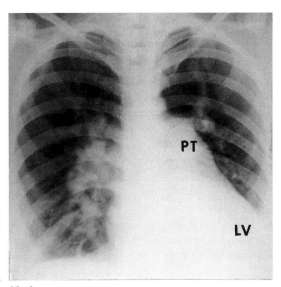

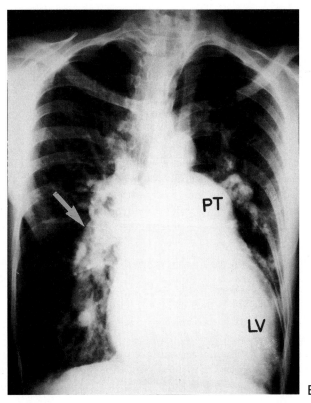

A

B

Figure 19–4

A, X-ray from an acyanotic 24-year-old woman with double outlet right ventricle, a subaortic ventricular septal defect and a pulmonary to systemic flow ratio of 2 to 1. Pulmonary vascularity is increased, the pulmonary trunk (PT) and its proximal branches are dilated, the ascending aorta is not border-forming, and a large left ventricle (LV) occupies the apex. The x-ray resembles a nonrestrictive perimembranous ventricular septal defect. *B,* X-ray from a 53-year-old man with double outlet right ventricle, subaortic ventricular septal defect, and a pulmonary to systemic flow ratio of 1.7 to 1. The pulmonary trunk and its right branch are markedly dilated, and an enlarged left ventricle occupies the apex. Distortion of the clavicles is due to scoliosis.

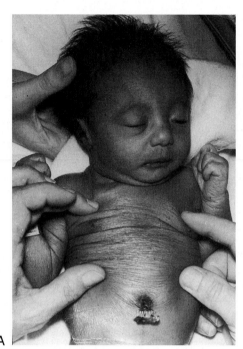

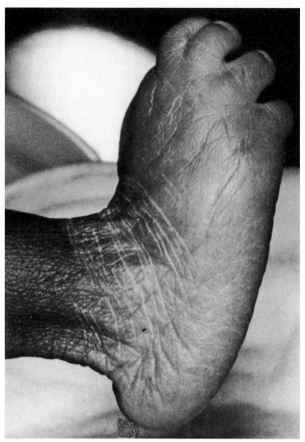

Figure 19–5
Photographs of a 6-week-old boy with (*A*) the characteristic clenched fists, overlapping fingers (clinodactyly), lax skin, and (*B*) rocker bottom feet of trisomy 18. The infant had double outlet right ventricle with a subaortic ventricular septal defect.

THE JUGULAR VENOUS PULSE

The jugular venous A wave, V wave, and mean pressure are elevated when biventricular failure results from increased pulmonary blood flow. The height and waveform of the jugular venous pulse normalize when pulmonary vascular resistance increases. The right ventricle then ejects at systemic resistance with little extra help from the right atrium, as in Eisenmenger syndrome (see Chapter 17).

PRECORDIAL MOVEMENT AND PALPATION

Harrison's grooves result from chronic dyspnea. A right ventricular impulse is accompanied by the impulse of a dilated hypertensive pulmonary trunk and a palpable pulmonary valve closure sound. The thrill generated by the ventricular septal defect is maximum in the third and fourth intercostal spaces at the left sternal border (see Auscultation).

A rise in pulmonary vascular resistance curtails pulmonary blood flow and decreases left ventricular volume overload, so the left ventricular impulse is inconspicuous or absent as in Eisenmenger syndrome. The right ventricular impulse, the palpable pulmonary trunk, and the palpable pulmonary closure sound persist.

AUSCULTATION

The first heart sound is soft because the PR interval tends to be prolonged (see The Electrocardiogram).[44,60] *Low pulmonary vascular resistance* results in a holosystolic murmur of ventricular septal defect that is maximum in the third and fourth intercostal spaces at the left sternal border. The pulmonary component of the second heart sound is loud because the hypertensive dilated pulmonary trunk is anterior. The aortic component of the second sound is prominent because the aortic valve lies side by side and to the right of the pulmonary trunk rather than posterior. Inspiratory splitting of the second is preserved as long as pulmonary vascular resistance is less than systemic. Increased flow across the mitral valve generates an apical mid-diastolic murmur.

Elevated pulmonary vascular resistance induces a fall in pulmonary blood flow and in left ventricular volume overload (see Fig. 19–1*B*). The murmur of ventricular septal defect becomes decrescendo and softer (Fig. 19–6) but does not disappear because flow from left ventricle into aorta is obligatory. Except for the soft decrescendo murmur, the auscultatory signs are analogous to Eisenmenger syndrome with an isolated nonrestrictive ventricular septal defect, namely, a pulmonary ejection sound, a loud single second

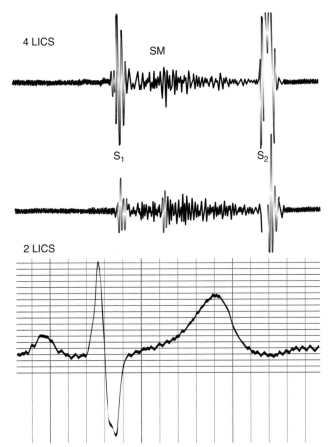

Figure 19–6

Phonocardiogram from a 10-year-old boy with double outlet right ventricle, subaortic ventricular septal defect, elevated pulmonary vascular resistance and a pulmonary to systemic flow ratio of 1.2 to 1. There is a relatively soft decrescendo systolic murmur (SM) in the fourth left intercostal space (4 LICS). The second heart sound (S_2) is loud and single. Lead 2 of electrocardiogram shows left axis deviation. 2 LICS, second left intercostal space; S_1, first heart sound.

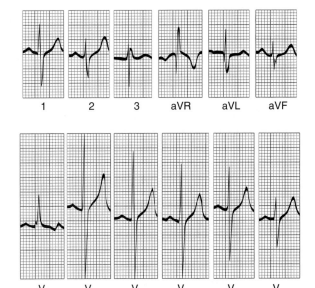

Figure 19–7

Electrocardiogram from an acyanotic 24-year-old woman with double outlet right ventricle, subaortic ventricular septal defect and a pulmonary to systemic flow ratio of 2 to 1. The PR interval is 200 msec. There is left axis deviation with counterclockwise depolarization. The qR in lead V_1 indicates right atrial enlargement, and the deep S waves in V_{5-6} indicate right ventricular hypertrophy. Biventricular hypertrophy is manifested by large RS complexes in leads V_{3-5} (V_{3-6} are half standardized).

heart sound, and a Graham Steell murmur of pulmonary hypertensive pulmonary regurgitation (see Chapter 17).

THE ELECTROCARDIOGRAM

PR interval prolongation is common[60] (Fig. 19–7) because of the unusually long course of the common atrioventricular bundle.[44] Peaked right atrial P waves are associated with bifid broad left atrial P waves when pulmonary blood flow is increased. (Fig. 19–8). Left axis deviation with counterclockwise depolarization is an important feature of double outlet right ventricle with a subaortic ventricular septal defect, no pulmonary stenosis, and increased pulmonary blood flow.[31,44,60,78] (Fig. 19–7). The mechanism of left axis deviation is unknown but cannot be related to an abnormality of the conduction system which is structurally the same when pulmonary vascular resistance is elevated and there is right axis deviation (Fig. 19–8) or when double outlet right ventricle coexists with pulmonary stenosis and right axis deviation.[78] The QRS duration is normal, but right ventricular conduction defects

sometimes occur including right bundle branch block.[44] Right ventricular hypertrophy is obligatory and is manifested by tall R waves in leads V_1 and aVR with deep S waves in left precordial leads (Figs. 19–7 and 19–8). Left

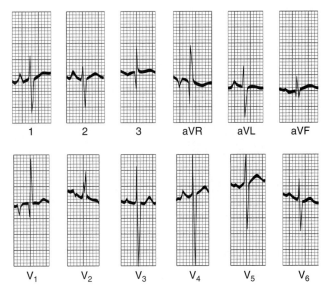

Figure 19–8

Electrocardiogram from a 6-week-old boy with double outlet right ventricle, subaortic ventricular septal defect, moderately elevated pulmonary vascular resistance, and trisomy 18 (see Fig. 19–5). Peaked right atrial P waves are present in leads 1 and 2, and a broad bifid left atrial P wave is present in lead V_2. There is moderate right axis deviation with clockwise depolarization. The q wave in lead V_1 indicates right atrial enlargement. Right ventricular hypertrophy is manifested by tall R waves in leads V_1 and aVR and by deep S waves in left precordial leads.

ventricular volume overload is indicated by large RS complexes in mid-precordial leads and by tall R waves in left precordial leads (Fig. 19–7). Elevated pulmonary vascular resistance is associated with right axis deviation and pure right ventricular hypertrophy (Fig. 19–8).

THE X-RAY

The x-ray with double outlet right ventricle, nonrestrictive subaortic ventricular septal defect, and low pulmonary vascular resistance is analogous to isolated nonrestrictive perimembranous ventricular septal defect with increased pulmonary blood flow (Figs. 19–4 and 19–9 A).[20,27,31,60,61] Thymus is present even though there is transposition of the aorta (Fig. 19–9B) in contrast to complete transposition of both great arteries in which thymus is typically absent (see Chapter 27). The pulmonary trunk is prominent because it is not posterior to the aorta and it carries increased volume at systemic pressure (see Fig.19–4). Left atrial and left ventricular enlargement reflect the volume overload of increased pulmonary blood flow (see Fig. 19–4). Dilatation of the right atrium and right ventricle become conspicuous with the advent of congestive heart failure.

The lung fields are oligemic when *pulmonary vascular resistance is elevated* either before the neonatal fall in resistance (Fig. 19–9B) or after the development of pulmonary vascular disease which curtails left ventricular volume overload. The right ventricle copes with systemic resistance without significant enlargement. The x-ray is indistinguishable from Eisenmenger syndrome with a nonrestrictive ventricular septal defect (see Fig. 17–9 in Chapter 17).[20]

THE ECHOCARDIOGRAM

Echocardiography with color flow imaging and Doppler interrogation provides diagnostic information on: 1) right ventricular origin and spatial relationships of the great arteries, 2) the presence and position of the infundibular septum, 3) the size of the ventricular septal defect and its relationship to the aortic and pulmonary valves, 4) mitral/semilunar valve discontinuity (see Figs. 19–19 and 19–20),[54] and straddling atrioventricular valve tensor apparatus (Fig. 19–10). The aortic root and pulmonary trunk are parallel to each other and are separated by a prominent outlet septum. The aorta arises entirely from the right ventricle and the pulmonary trunk arises predominantly if not entirely from the right ventricle (see Fig. 19–19). The great arteries appear as double circles in the short axis, with the aorta to the right of the pulmonary trunk as in complete transposition of the great arteries (see Chapter 27). The pulmonary trunk is identified by its bifurcation into right and left branches, and the aorta is identified by its brachiocephalic branches. Bilateral subarterial conuses separate the aortic and pulmonary valves from the atrioventricular valves. The course of the outlet septum establishes the alignment of the ventricular septal defect with the aortic or the pulmonary valve. If the outlet septum curves leftward toward the ventriculo/infundibular fold, the ventricular septal defect becomes subaortic. If the outlet septum is straight and parallel to the trabecular septum, the ventricular septal defect becomes subpulmonary. The echocardiogram identifies a single coronary artery which is estimated to occur in 11% of cases of double outlet right ventricle(see Chapter 32).[43]

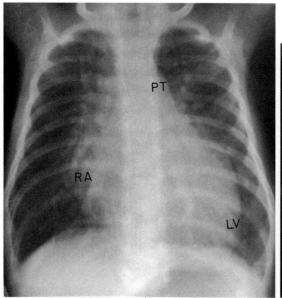 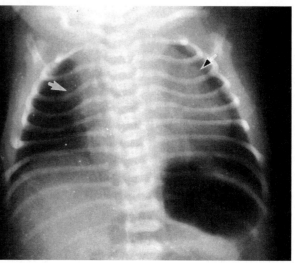

Figure 19–9

A, X-ray from an acyanotic 8-week-old boy with double outlet right ventricle, a subaortic ventricular septal defect, and a pulmonary to systemic flow ratio of 2.4 to 1. The film is over-penetrated, but pulmonary vascularity is increased. The pulmonary trunk (PT) is moderately convex, a dilated left ventricle (LV) occupies the apex, and a prominent right atrium (RA) forms the right lower cardiac border. *B,* X-ray from a one day old male with double outlet right ventricle and a subaortic ventricular septal defect. A large thymus alters the cardiac silhouette which is otherwise normal for age.

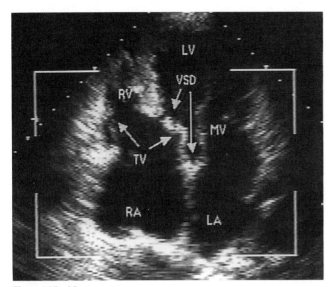

Figure 19–10
Echocardiogram (apical four-chamber) from a 7-year-old boy with double outlet right ventricle and a subaortic ventricular septal defect. The septal leaflet of the tricuspid valve (TV) straddles the ventricular septal defect (VSD) and inserts on both sides of the septum. RA/LA, right and left atrium; RV/LV, right and left ventricle; MV, mitral valve.

SUMMARY

Double outlet right ventricle with subaortic ventricular septal defect and no pulmonary stenosis may first come to light because of *transient neonatal cyanosis*. The subsequent fall in pulmonary vascular resistance with increased pulmonary blood flow results in congestive heart failure with poor growth and development. Physical examination reveals a hyperactive precordium with right and left ventricular impulses, a left parasternal systolic thrill and murmur of ventricular septal defect, a loud pulmonary component of the second sound with close splitting, and an apical mid-diastolic murmur of augmented flow across the mitral valve. The electrocardiogram is of special diagnostic importance because of left axis deviation with counterclockwise depolarization. The x-ray is indistinguishable from a nonrestrictive perimembranous ventricular septal defect with increased pulmonary blood flow.

Pulmonary vascular disease results in a clinical picture resembling Eisenmenger syndrome with a nonrestrictive ventricular septal defect, but double outlet right ventricle is suspected when pulmonary blood flow remains increased in the presence of cyanosis, and when a soft decrescendo left parasternal systolic murmur persists because of obligatory flow from left ventricle through the subaortic ventricular septal defect into the aorta. The echocardiogram with color flow imaging and Doppler interrogation identifies right ventricular origin of both great arteries and establishes the location, size, and great arterial commitments of the ventricular septal defect.

Double Outlet Right Ventricle with Subaortic Ventricular Septal Defect and Pulmonary Stenosis

Pulmonary stenosis occurs in over 50% of patients with double outlet right ventricle and a subaortic ventricular septal defect (see Table 19–2 C and Figs. 19–1B and 19–11). The clinical manifestations closely resemble Fallot's tetralogy (see Chapter 18).

THE HISTORY AND PHYSICAL APPEARANCE

Pulmonary stenosis varies from mild to severe to atresia and can be present at birth or delayed in onset with a progressive increase in severity (Fig. 19–11).[25] Cyanotic patients squat as in Fallot's tetralogy.[25] The clinical course and longevity are better than in double outlet right ventricle *without* pulmonary stenosis because pulmonary blood flow is more effectively regulated. (see earlier).[41,74]

THE JUGULAR VENOUS PULSE AND THE ARTERIAL PULSE

The A wave is normal because the right ventricle ejects at but not above systemic vascular resistance and does so without increased contractile force of the right atrium,

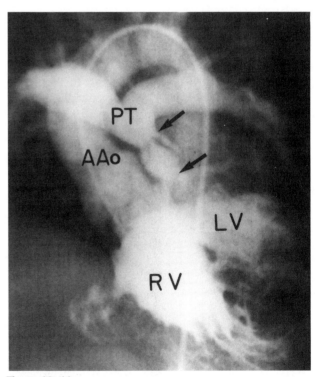

Figure 19–11
Angiocardiogram from a 15-month-old boy with double outlet right ventricle, a nonrestrictive subaortic ventricular septal defect, and pulmonary stenosis caused by the combination of an underdeveloped subpulmonary conus (*lower unmarked arrow*) and a bicuspid pulmonary valve (*upper unmarked arrow*). The ascending aorta (AAo) and the pulmonary trunk (PT) arise from the right ventricle (RV). LV, left ventricle.

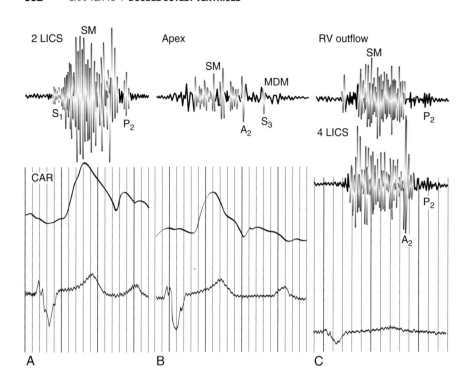

A   B   C

Figure 19–12

Phonocardiograms from an 18-year-old man with double outlet right ventricle, subaortic ventricular septal defect, and a 45-mm Hg subpulmonary gradient. *A*, In the second left intercostal space (2 LICS), a loud crescendo-decrescendo systolic murmur (SM) obscures the aortic component of the second heart sound. The pulmonary component (P_2) is delayed and prominent. *B*, The systolic murmur (SM) radiated to the apex where there was a prominent third heart sound (S_3) that introduced a mid-diastolic murmur (MDM) due to increased flow across the mitral valve. *C*, Intracardiac phonocardiogram from within the right ventricular outflow tract recorded a systolic murmur (SM) similar to the murmur in the second left intercostal space together with a delayed pulmonary closure sound (P_2). The simultaneous chest wall phonocardiogram in the fourth left intercostal space (4 LICS) recorded a decrescendo holosystolic murmur and the delayed P_2. A_2, aortic component of the second sound; CAR, carotid pulse.

analogous to Fallot's tetralogy (see Chapter 18). The arterial pulse is normal because biventricular ejection into the aorta maintains a normal stroke volume.

PRECORDIAL MOVEMENT AND PALPATION

The right ventricular impulse is analogous to the gentle impulse of a normal neonatal heart and is assigned to the fourth and fifth left intercostal spaces and subxiphoid area because the stenosis is subpulmonary (Fig. 19–11). A systolic thrill is maximum in the third left intercostal space for the same reason. A left ventricular impulse is not palpable in cyanotic patients because pulmonary blood flow is reduced and the left ventricle is underfilled.

AUSCULTATION

Acyanotic patients with mild pulmonary stenosis have a holosystolic murmur of ventricular septal defect at the lower left sternal border and a midsystolic murmur of pulmonary stenosis in the second and third left intercostal spaces (Fig. 19–12 *A,C*). The pulmonary component of the second heart sound is appropriately delayed (Fig. 19–12*A*). An apical third heart sound introduces a mid-diastolic murmur generated across the mitral valve when pulmonary blood flow is increased (Fig. 19–12*B*).

Patients with severe pulmonary stenosis or pulmonary atresia have auscultatory signs indistinguishable from cyanotic Fallot's tetralogy (see Chapter 18). The duration of the pulmonary stenotic murmur varies inversely with the severity of stenosis. Pulmonary atresia is accompanied by an ejection sound and a soft midsystolic murmur into the dilated aorta and a loud single second heart sound due

to aortic valve closure (Fig. 19–13). Exceptionally, there is a long decrescendo systolic murmur at the left sternal border because of obligatory flow from left ventricle into aorta through a restrictive ventricular septal defect that constitutes a zone of subaortic stenosis.[25] A left ventricular

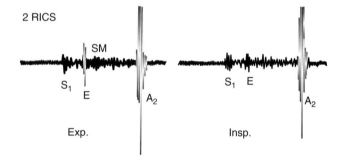

Exp.   Insp.

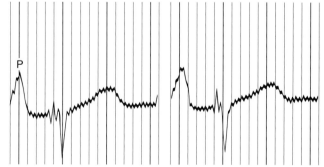

Figure 19–13

Phonocardiogram in the second right intercostal space (2 RICS) of a 3-year-old cyanotic boy with double outlet right ventricle, a subaortic ventricular septal defect, and pulmonary atresia. An aortic ejection sound (E) introduces a soft midsystolic murmur (SM) that ends before a loud single second heart sound that was the aortic component (A_2). The ejection sound decreased during inspiration (Insp.) despite aortic origin.

fourth heart sound may then be heard because an increased force of left atrial contraction is associated with the left ventricular hypertrophy of subaortic stenosis.[25] Audibility of the fourth heart sound is enhanced by prolongation of the PR interval.[57] An early diastolic murmur of aortic regurgitation is occasionally present in double outlet right ventricle with pulmonary stenosis as in Fallot's tetralogy.[31,41]

THE ELECTROCARDIOGRAM

Peaked right atrial P waves may occur even with mild pulmonary stenosis because the right ventricle is systemic, and may be accompanied by left atrial P waves because pulmonary blood flow is increased (Fig. 19–14). Severe pulmonary stenosis is accompanied by P waves that are either normal or peaked and low amplitude (Fig. 19–15) or occasionally peaked and tall (Fig. 19–16). P waves resemble Fallot's tetralogy, but in double outlet right ventricle the PR interval is likely to be prolonged (Figs. 19–14, 19–15 and 19–16).[57]

When pulmonary stenosis is *mild*, the electrocardiogram retains the left axis deviation and counterclockwise depolarization that occur in the absence of pulmonary stenosis (Fig. 19–14). As stenosis increases, the QRS axis becomes vertical or rightward. It is here that distinctive albeit subtle features arouse suspicion of double outlet right ventricle with pulmonary stenosis.[25,44,48,57] What is

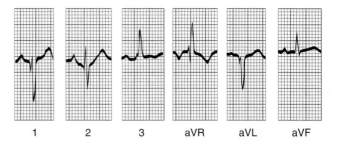

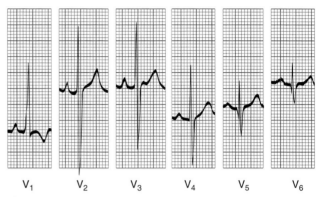

Figure 19–15

Electrocardiogram from a 13-year-old cyanotic girl with double outlet right ventricle, subaortic ventricular septal defect, and severe subpulmonary stenosis. Peaked right atrial P waves appear in leads 2 and V_{1-3}. The PR interval is 190 msec. Distinct q waves persist in leads 1 and aVL despite right axis deviation. Right ventricular hypertrophy is manifested by tall R waves in leads V_1 and aVR. The qR pattern in leads V_{5-6} indicates a moderately well-developed left ventricle.

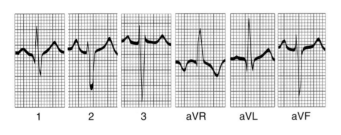

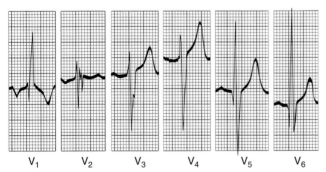

Figure 19–14

Electrocardiogram from an 18-year-old man with double outlet right ventricle, subaortic ventricular septal defect and a 45 mm Hg subpulmonary gradient. The PR interval is 210 msec. The right atrial P wave in lead 2 is tall peaked, and a deep broad left atrial P terminal force appears in lead V_1. There is left axis deviation with counterclockwise depolarization. Right ventricular hypertrophy is manifested by the tall R wave in lead V_1 and by the deep S waves in left precordial leads. Left ventricular volume overload is manifested in leads V_{5-6} by deep Q waves, tall R waves and tall peaked T waves. Terminal forces are prolonged with slurred S waves in inferior leads and a slurred R wave in lead aVR.

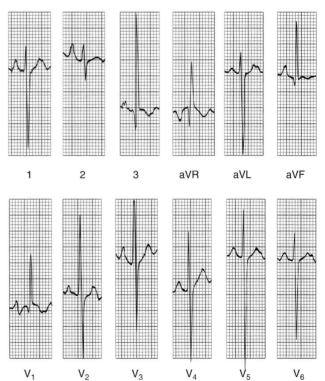

Figure 19–16

Electrocardiogram from a 3-year-old boy with double outlet right ventricle, subaortic ventricular septal defect, and pulmonary atresia. Tall peaked P waves appear in leads 1 and 2 and in midprecordial leads. The PR interval is 190 msec. There is marked right axis deviation. The q wave in lead V_1 reflects right atrial enlargement. Right ventricular hypertrophy is manifested by the tall R wave in lead V_1 and by the deep S waves in left precordial leads.

distinctive is the persistence of *counterclockwise* initial forces that generate q waves in leads 1 and aVL even when the axis is vertical or rightward (Fig. 19–15). Q waves in leads 1 and aVL are rare in neonates and young children[5] and are virtually unknown in Fallot's tetralogy (see Chapter 18).[57] The terminal forces are deep and prolonged with a tendency for broad slurred S waves in leads 1, aVL and V_{5-6} and a broad R wave in lead aVR (Figs. 19–14 and 19–15).[44,57] The electrocardiogram with pulmonary atresia is similar if not indistinguishable from Fallot's tetralogy with pulmonary atresia (Fig. 19–16).[57] A restrictive subaortic ventricular septal defect is functionally subaortic stenosis which can cause left ventricular hypertrophy.

THE X-RAY

The pulmonary trunk is not dilated because the stenosis is subpulmonary (Figs. 19–11 and 19–17). When pulmonary stenosis is mild, pulmonary vascularity is increased and the left ventricle is dilated (Fig. 19–17). When pulmonary stenosis is severe, pulmonary vascularity is reduced, the heart size is normal, and the apex is convex (Fig. 19–18A).[27] In the presence of pulmonary atresia, the ascending aorta is enlarged, the main pulmonary artery segment is concave, and the apex is boot-shaped (Figs. 19–3 *A, B* and 19–18*B*).

THE ECHOCARDIOGRAM

Echocardiography with color flow imaging and Doppler interrogation establishes the subaortic location of the ven-

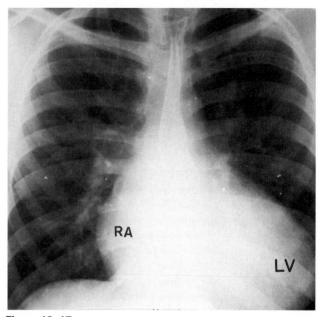

Figure 19–17

X-ray from an 18-year-old man with double outlet right ventricle, a subaortic ventricular septal defect, a 40 mm Hg subpulmonary gradient, and a pulmonary to systemic flow ratio of 2.2 to 1. The pulmonary trunk is not dilated even though pulmonary blood flow is increased. An enlarged left ventricle (LV) occupies the apex, and a prominent right atrium (RA) occupies the right lower cardiac border.

tricular septal defect and the presence, type, and degree of pulmonary stenosis (Figs. 19–19 and 19–20). Both great arteries are imaged above the right ventricle, and subpulmonary stenosis with a nondilated pulmonary trunk is identified (Fig. 19–19). Continuous wave Doppler estab-

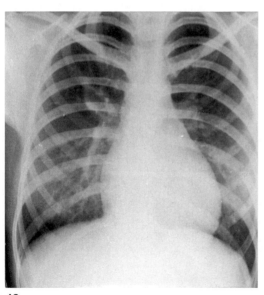

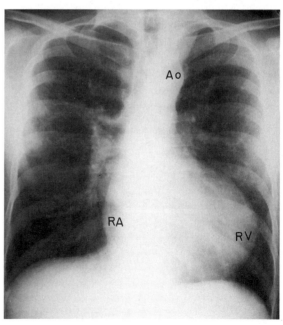

Figure 19–18

A, X-ray from a 13-year-old girl with double outlet right ventricle, subaortic ventricular septal defect, and severe subpulmonary stenosis. Pulmonary vascularity is normal. The heart size is normal with a slightly rounded apex. *B,* X-ray from a 29-year-old man with double outlet right ventricle, a subaortic ventricular septal defect, and pulmonary atresia (compare to Fig. 19–3 *A*). The lung fields have the lacy appearance of systemic to pulmonary artery collaterals. The pulmonary trunk is conspicuously absent, but the right and left branches are well-formed. The aortic knuckle (Ao) is prominent and continues as a left descending aorta. The boot-shaped apex is occupied by the right ventricle (RV). The right atrium (RA) is moderately convex.

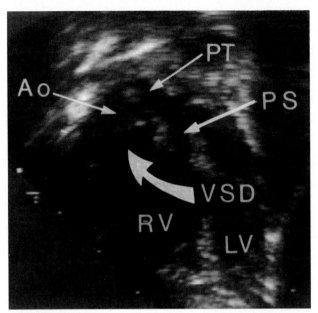

Figure 19–19

Echocardiogram (subcostal view) from a 2-month-old boy with double outlet right ventricle (RV), a subaortic ventricular septal defect (VSD), valvular and infundibular pulmonary stenosis (PS), and a hypoplastic pulmonary trunk (PT). The *large curved arrow* indicates the direction of blood flow from left ventricle (LV) through the ventricular septal defect into the aorta (Ao).

lishes the pulmonary stenotic gradient (Fig. 19–20B). Double-circle great arteries are seen in the short axis, and a bicuspid stenotic pulmonary valve is occasionally identified at the origin of the pulmonary trunk which is to the left of the aorta.

SUMMARY

Cyanosis coexists with increased pulmonary blood flow when pulmonary stenosis is mild. When pulmonary stenosis is severe, the electrocardiogram arouses suspicion especially because of q waves in leads 1 and aVL despite a vertical or rightward QRS axis. The PR interval tends to be prolonged. Terminal forces are slurred in leads 1, aVL, avR, and in leads V$_{5-6}$. A decrescendo systolic murmur may persist at the lower left sternal border because of obligatory flow from left ventricle across the ventricular septal defect into the right ventricular aorta. Echocardiography establishes the diagnosis of double outlet right ventricle with subaortic ventricular septal defect and subpulmonary or pulmonary valve stenosis.

Double Outlet Right Ventricle with Subpulmonary Ventricular Septal Defect: The Taussig-Bing Anomaly

Clinical manifestations of the Taussig-Bing anomaly resemble complete transposition of the great arteries with a

nonrestrictive ventricular septal defect (see Table 19–2 and Chapter 27). However, about 50% of patients have congenital malformations of the aortic arch including coarctation, isthmic hypoplasia, interruption, patent ductus arteriosus, and subaortic stenosis.[42,49,62,80,82]

THE HISTORY

Cyanosis dates from birth or early infancy because flow from right ventricle into aorta is obligatory (see Fig. 19–1D).[11,20,61,77,82] As neonatal pulmonary vascular resistance falls, left ventricular blood selectively enters the pulmonary trunk across the subpulmonary ventricular septal defect (see Fig. 19–2). Systemic arterial oxygen saturation is relatively high but at the price of increased pulmonary blood flow, left ventricular volume overload, and congestive heart failure.[74,82] The clinical course is especially poor when coarctation of the aorta elevates systemic systolic pressure and augments already abundant pulmonary blood flow by diverting still more right ventricular blood into the pulmonary trunk (see Fig. 19–1D).[62,74] A rise in pulmonary vascular resistance serves to regulate pulmonary blood flow and ameliorate congestive heart failure. Cyanosis increases but longevity improves and an occasional patient reaches the second, third, or fourth decade (Fig. 19–21).[11,19,20]

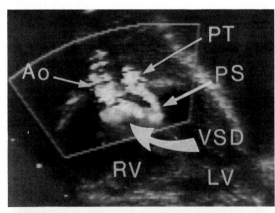

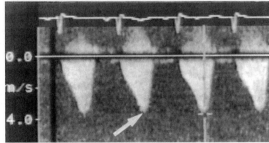

Figure 19–20

A, Black-and-white print of a color flow image from the 2-month-old boy with double outlet right ventricle, subaortic ventricular septal defect, and pulmonary stenosis whose two dimensional echocardiogram appears in Figure 19–19. Both great arteries arise from the right ventricle (RV). Blood flow through the ventricular septal defect (VSD) selectively enters the aorta, and the high velocity jet of pulmonary stenosis enters the pulmonary trunk. B, Continuous wave Doppler records a peak instantaneous gradient of 64 mm Hg from right ventricle to pulmonary trunk (peak velocity 4 m/sec).

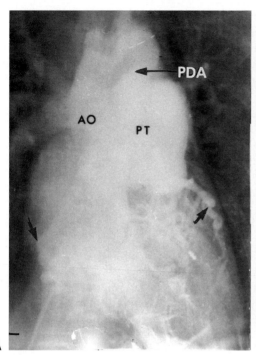

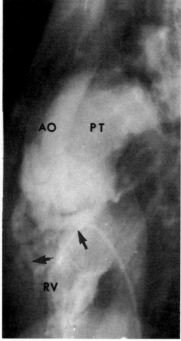

A

B

Figure 19–21

Right ventriculograms (RV) from a 40-year-old woman with the Taussig-Bing anomaly characterized by double outlet right ventricle, a subpulmonary ventricular septal defect, a biventricular pulmonary trunk, and pulmonary vascular disease. *A,* The ascending aorta (AO) and the pulmonary trunk (PT) are side by side with the aorta to the right. The large patent ductus arteriosus (PDA) was distal to coarctation of the aorta. *B,* Lateral projection shows the aorta (AO) anterior to the pulmonary trunk (PT). *Unmarked arrows* point to dilated ectatic coronary arteries (see Chapter 32). RV, right ventricle.

PHYSICAL APPEARANCE

Infants with increased pulmonary blood flow suffer the catabolic effects of congestive heart failure with poor growth and development. When a moderate elevation in pulmonary vascular resistance curtails pulmonary blood flow, congestive heart failure is relieved and growth and development improve. Suprasystemic pulmonary vascular resistance results in *reversed differential cyanosis,* a distinctive physical appearance that becomes manifest because ductal flow is right to left (Fig. 19–22).[82] The toes are *less* cyanotic and clubbed than the fingers because *oxygenated* blood from the left ventricle flows through the subpulmonary ventricular septal defect into the pulmonary trunk and through the patent ductus into the descending aorta, whereas *unoxygenated* blood from the right ventricle flows into the aorta and to the upper extremities. Trisomy 18 is another distinctive physical appearance that occurs with either a subpulmonary or a subaortic ventricular septal defect (see Fig. 19–5).[18,38,70,72,73]

THE ARTERIAL PULSE

Upper and lower extremity arterial pulses are diagnostically important because of the frequency of coarctation of the aorta.[60,61,74,82] The femoral pulses are preserved, however, when a nonrestrictive patent ductus is distal to the coarctation (Fig. 19–21).

THE JUGULAR VENOUS PULSE

The right atrial A wave, V wave, and mean pressure are elevated in the presence of biventricular failure. Increased pulmonary vascular resistance curtails pulmonary blood

flow and alleviates congestive heart failure, so the jugular venous pulse normalizes (Fig. 19–23, second panel).

PRECORDIAL MOVEMENT AND PALPATION

An obligatory right ventricular impulse becomes more conspicuous in the presence of biventricular failure. The dilated

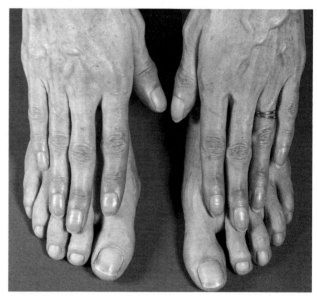

Figure 19–22

Photograph of the hands and feet of the 40-year-old woman with Taussig-Bing anomaly referred to in Figure 19–21. There is *reversed* differential cyanosis with fingers more cyanotic than toes because *unoxygenated* blood from the right ventricle entered the ascending aorta and the bracheocephalic arteries while *oxygenated* blood from the left ventricle entered the pulmonary trunk through the subpulmonary ventricular septal defect and preferentially flowed through the large patent ductus arteriosus into the descending thoracic aorta. Compare with Figure 20–12 in Chapter 20 that illustrates conventional differential cyanosis that characterizes a reversed shunt through an isolated patent ductus arteriosus.

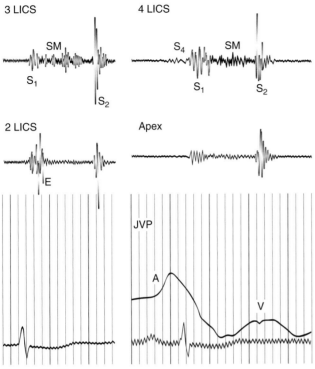

Figure 19–23

Phonocardiograms from the 40-year-old woman with the Taussig Bing anomaly referred to in Figures 19–21 and 19–22. A soft systolic murmur (SM) is maximum in the third left intercostal space (3 LICS) and ends before a loud single second heart sound (S_2). A pulmonary ejection sound (E) originated in the dilated hypertensive pulmonary trunk and was recorded in the second left intercostal space (2 LICS). A soft fourth heart sound (S_4) was recorded at the fourth left intercostal space (4 LICS). The jugular venous pulse (JVP) shows a small dominant A wave.

hypertensive pulmonary trunk (see Figs. 19–2 and 19–21) and the loud pulmonary second heart sound are palpated in the second left intercostal space. Volume overload of the left ventricle is responsible for a left ventricular impulse. A thrill is located as high as the second left intercostal space because the ventricular septal defect is subpulmonary. As pulmonary vascular resistance rises, pulmonary blood flow falls, left ventricular volume overload is curtailed, the left ventricular impulse may disappear, the right ventricular impulse decreases, and the ventricular septal defect thrill vanishes.

AUSCULTATION

A systolic murmur that originates at the ventricular septal defect may be located as high as second left intercostal space because the left ventricle ejects directly into the pulmonary trunk through the subpulmonary ventricular septal defect (see Fig. 19–1D).[11,82] The pulmonary component of the second heart sound is loud with splitting preserved as long as pulmonary resistance is lower than systemic. An apical middiastolic murmur signifies increased pulmonary blood flow with increased flow across the mitral valve. As pulmonary resistance rises, pulmonary blood flow and left ventricular volume overload decline, the murmur through the subpulmonary ventricular septal defect is attenuated (Fig. 19–23),

and the mitral flow murmur disappears. A pulmonary ejection sound, a soft short midsystolic murmur, and a Graham Steell murmur originate in the dilated hypertensive pulmonary trunk. The second heart sound is loud and single because of synchronous closure of aortic and pulmonary valves.

THE ELECTROCARDIOGRAM

PR interval prolongation is not as frequent as in double outlet right ventricle with subaortic ventricular septal defect (Fig. 19–24).[19] Biatrial P wave abnormalities reflect the combination of volume overload of the left atrium and right atrial enlargement caused by right ventricular failure. The QRS axis is vertical or rightward with clockwise depolarization[61] (Fig. 19–24) resembling the QRS axis of complete transposition of the great arteries with nonrestrictive ventricular septal defect (see Chapter 27). Right ventricular hypertrophy is reflected in tall R waves in lead V_1 and aVR and deep S waves in left precordial leads (Fig. 19–24). Volume overload of the left ventricle is represented by well-developed R waves in leads V_{5-6} (Fig. 19–24). Elevated pulmonary vascular resistance curtails pulmonary blood flow and reduces volume overload of the left ventricle, but right ventricular pressure overload is unchanged. Accordingly, tall peaked right atrial P waves persist with residual evidence of a left atrial abnormality, and with biventricular hypertrophy in midprecordial leads (Fig. 19–25).

THE X-RAY

An increase in pulmonary arterial and pulmonary venous vascularity results from low pulmonary vascular resistance

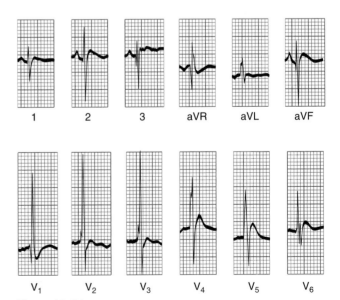

Figure 19–24

Electrocardiogram from a 3-month-old boy with double outlet right ventricle and a subpulmonary ventricular septal defect. The PR interval is normal. Peaked right atrial P waves appear in leads 2, 3, and aVF. The QRS axis is rightward with clockwise depolarization. Right ventricular hypertrophy is reflected in the tall R waves in leads V_{1-2} and in lead aVR and by prominent S waves in left precordial leads.

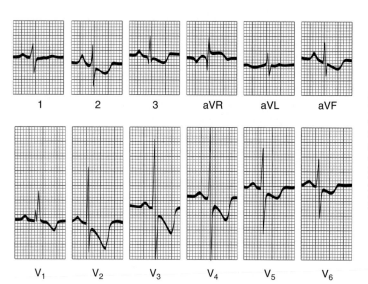

Figure 19–25

Electrocardiogram from the 40-year-old woman with the Taussig Bing anomaly referred to in Figures 19–21 and 19–22. The P wave in lead 2 is tall and peaked (right atrial abnormality) and broad (left atrial abnormality). The PR interval is 180 msec. The QRS axis is plus 90 degrees. Right ventricular hypertrophy is manifested by the rR pattern in lead V_1, the R wave in lead aVR, the deep S waves in left precordial leads, and the inverted T waves in right and midprecordial leads. Biventricular hypertrophy from a well-developed left ventricle is implied by the large RS complexes in midprecordial leads.

and congestive heart failure (Fig. 19–26). The left atrium and the left ventricle are enlarged because of volume overload, and the right atrium and right ventricle are enlarged because of congestive heart failure (Figs. 19–26 and 19–27). The dilated pulmonary trunk projects prominently to the left when the great arteries are side-by-side, and the x-ray resembles a nonrestrictive perimembranous ventricular septal defect (Fig. 19–28). When the dilated pulmonary trunk is posterior and therefore not border forming, the

x-ray then resembles complete transposition of the great arteries[11,19,77] (Fig. 19–26) except for the presence of a thymus (Fig.19–27). With the advent of pulmonary vascular disease, pulmonary arterial blood flow decreases, pulmonary venous vascularity disappears, volume overload of the left ventricle is curtailed, dilatation of the pulmonary trunk persists, and the x-ray resembles a nonrestrictive ventricular septal defect with Eisenmenger syndrome (Figs. 19–28 and 19–29).

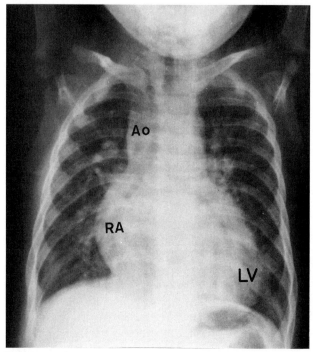

Figure 19–26

X-ray from a 4-month-old girl with Taussig Bing anomaly characterized by double outlet right ventricle, a subpulmonary ventricular septal defect, and a pulmonary to systemic flow ratio of 3 to 1. The dilated pulmonary trunk was not border-forming because it was posterior. The rightward and anterior ascending aorta is seen at the right thoracic inlet. Pulmonary vascularity is increased, a convex left ventricle (LV) occupies the apex, and a prominent right atrium (RA) occupies the right lower cardiac border.

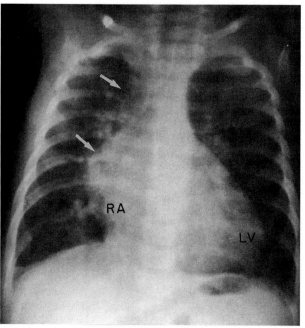

Figure 19–27

X-ray from a 3-month-old girl with the Taussig-Bing anomaly and coarctation of the aorta proximal to a ductus arteriosus. Pulmonary vascularity is increased, but the vascular pedicle is narrow because the posterior pulmonary trunk is not border forming. An enlarged left ventricle (LV) occupies the apex, and an enlarged right atrium (RA) occupies the right lower cardiac border. The x-ray resembles complete transposition of the great arteries except for the thymus (*arrow* and right hilus).

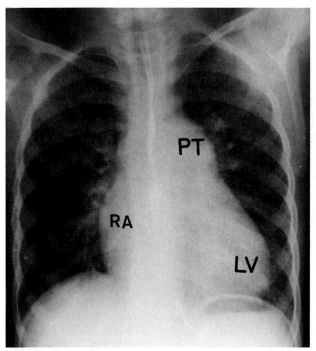

Figure 19–28
X-ray from a 10-year-old girl with the Taussig Bing anomaly, pulmonary vascular disease, and reversed shunt through a large patent ductus arteriosus. Pulmonary vascularity is normal, the pulmonary trunk (PT) is dilated, a moderately prominent right atrium (RA) forms the lower right cardiac border, and an enlarged left ventricle (LV) occupies the apex. Death followed a brain abscess.

THE ECHOCARDIOGRAM

The following points are relevant in addition to the echocardiographic features described in the section on double outlet right ventricle with *subaortic* ventricular septal defect: 1) the ventricular septal defect is subpulmonary (Figs. 19–30 and 19–31), 2) the pulmonary trunk overrides the subpulmonary ventricular septal defect (Fig. 19–30), 3) pulmonary stenosis is absent, and 4) subaortic stenosis, coarctation of the aorta, and patent ductus arteriosus often coexist.

SUMMARY

Double outlet right ventricle with subpulmonary ventricular septal defect—the Taussig Bing anomaly— resembles com-

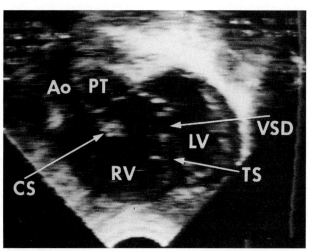

Figure 19–30
Echocardiogram (subcostal) from a 4-month-old girl with double outlet right ventricle and a subpulmonary ventricular septal defect (VSD). The ascending aorta (Ao) and the pulmonary trunk (PT) are parallel to each other, are separated by the conal septum (CS), and are positioned entirely above the right ventricle (RV). The conal septum is straight and parallel to the trabecular septum (TS), thus committing the ventricular septal defect to the pulmonary trunk. LV, left ventricle.

plete transposition of the great arteries with nonrestrictive ventricular septal defect. Both malformations are characterized by cyanosis with increased pulmonary blood flow. However, birth weights are not large in the Taussig-Bing anomaly, as they are in complete transposition, and there is a high incidence of aortic arch anomalies, especially coarctation of the aorta and patent ductus arteriosus. Pulmonary vascular disease with right-to-left shunt through a nonrestrictive patent ductus arteriosus results in distinctive reversed differential cyanosis with fingers more cyanotic than toes. A soft early systolic murmur persists at the left sternal border because of obligatory flow through the subpulmonary ventricular septal defect. The QRS axis is rightward as with complete transposition rather than the left axis deviation of double outlet right ventricle with subaortic ventricular septal defect. When the dilated pulmonary trunk is posterior and not border forming, the x-ray resembles complete transposition of the great arteries except for a thymic shadow. The x-ray, the physical signs, and the electrocardiogram otherwise resemble a nonrestrictive ventricular septal

Figure 19–29
X-rays from the 40-year-old woman with the Taussig Bing anomaly referred to in Figures 19–21 and 19–22. *A,* Pulmonary soft tissue densities are enhanced by breast tissue, but pulmonary vascularity is otherwise normal. The cardiac silhouette is normal except for the mildly convex pulmonary trunk (PT) that was dilated but posterior. *B,* The left anterior oblique projection confirms the normal size of the right atrium and of both ventricles.

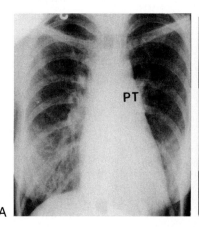

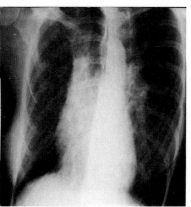

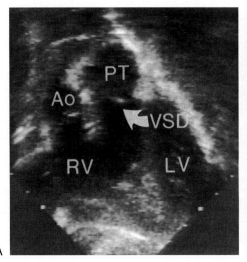
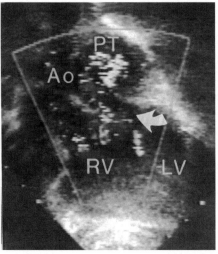

A   B

Figure 19–31

A, Echocardiogram from a 3-year-old boy with double outlet right ventricle and a nonrestrictive subpulmonary ventricular septal defect. The aorta (Ao) and the dilated pulmonary trunk (PT) arise entirely from the right ventricle (RV), and the ventricular septal defect (VSD) is committed to the pulmonary trunk. LV, left ventricle. *B,* Black-and-white print of a color flow image showing flow from left ventricle through the ventricular septal defect (*unmarked curved arrow*) into the dilated pulmonary trunk.

defect with Eisenmenger syndrome, but the early onset of cyanosis with increased pulmonary arterial blood flow should prevent error. The echocardiogram with color flow imaging and Doppler interrogation establishes the diagnosis of double outlet right ventricle, identifies the subpulmonary location of the ventricular septal defect, and identifies coexisting coarctation of the aorta and patent ductus arteriosus.

Double Outlet Left Ventricle

Origin of both great arteries from the morphologic *left* ventricle in biventricular hearts is among the rarest of ventriculo-great arterial malalignments.[4,13,21,23,39,52,80] The malformation was described in the early 19th century, was rediscovered in 1967, and was defined clinically and at necropsy in 1970.[64] Morphogenesis has been assigned to misalignment of the septal anlagen of the embryonic conus and the conal ridges.[34] Double outlet left ventricle is the

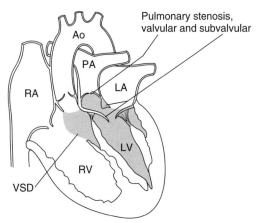

Figure 19–32

Drawing of double outlet left ventricle with a subaortic ventricular septal defect (VSD) and pulmonary stenosis that was valvular and subvalvular. The aorta (Ao) and pulmonary artery (PA) both arise from the *left* ventricle (LV). RV, right ventricle; RA, right atrium. (From Dadourian BJ, Perloff JK, Drinkwater DC, et al: Double outlet left ventricle: long survival after surgical correction. Ann Thorac Surg 51:159, 1991, with permission.)

converse of double outlet right ventricle because both great arteries arise entirely or predominantly from the morphologic *left* ventricle (Fig. 19–32).[34] The only exit for the right ventricle is a subaortic or subpulmonary ventricular septal defect.[13] Rarely, the ventricular septum is intact.[9]

The commoner type of this malformation in *situs solitus* with two well-formed noninverted ventricles is characterized by double outlet left ventricle with a *subaortic* ventricular septal defect that tends to occur with pulmonary stenosis (Fig. 19–32).[10] Less commonly, the ventricular septal defect is subpulmonary, and *aortic* stenosis is the outflow obstruction.[13,52]

Double outlet left ventricle with subaortic ventricular septal defect and pulmonary stenosis (Fig. 19–32) resembles cyanotic Fallot's tetralogy including a right aortic arch, hypoxic spells, and a pulmonary stenotic murmur whose length varies inversely with the severity of obstruction. The electrocardiogram shows right ventricular hypertrophy, and the x-ray shows little or no increase in cardiac size with normal or reduced pulmonary vascularity.[52] The echocardiogram with Doppler interrogation identifies two noninverted ventricles with left ventricular origin of both great arteries and establishes the location of the ventricular septal defect, and the presence and degree of pulmonary stenosis.[10,45] Double outlet *left* ventricle is distinguished from origin of both great arteries from an *inverted morphologic right ventricle* (Fig. 19–33).[8]

Double outlet left ventricle with *subaortic ventricular septal defect* and *no pulmonary stenosis* resembles complete transposition of the great arteries with a subaortic ventricular septal defect and a posterior aorta. The two circulations are in parallel, with blood from the left ventricle recirculating within the pulmonary circulation, and blood from the right ventricle recirculating within the systemic circulation (see Chapter 27). Cyanosis varies inversely with pulmonary arterial blood flow. When pulmonary vascular resistance is low, cyanosis exists with *increased* pulmonary blood flow as in complete transposition of the great arteries.

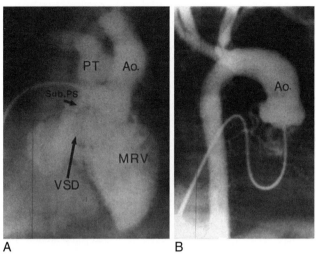

Figure 19–33

Angiocardiograms from a 3-year-old boy with congenitally corrected transposition of the great arteries, a ventricular septal defect (VSD), and subpulmonary stenosis (Sub PS). *A,* The aorta (Ao) and pulmonary trunk (PT) both arise from the morphologic right ventricle (MRV). The ascending aorta (Ao) is convex to the left, a feature confirmed in panel *B.*

Double outlet left ventricle with a nonrestrictive *subpulmonary* ventricular septal defect and no pulmonary stenosis resembles isolated nonrestrictive ventricular septal defect.[52] As neonatal pulmonary vascular resistance falls, left ventricular blood is increasingly diverted into the pulmonary artery, and right ventricular blood preferentially flows into the pulmonary artery because of the subpulmonary location of the ventricular septal defect. Pulmonary blood flow increases, the electrocardiogram reveals biventricular hypertrophy, cyanosis is minimal, and congestive heart failure results in poor growth and development.[52] Echocardiography identifies two noninverted ventricles, establishes left ventricular origin of both great arteries, and identifies the subpulmonary ventricular septal defect.[52]

REFERENCES

1. Abernathy J: Surgical and Physiological Essays. Part II. London, James Evans, 1793.
2. Agarwala B, Doyle EF, Danilowicz D, et al: Double-outlet right ventricle with pulmonic stenosis and anteriorly positioned aorta (Taussig-Bing variant). Am J Cardiol 32:850, 1973.
3. Ainger LE: Double outlet right ventricle: Intact ventricular septum, mitral stenosis, and blind left ventricle. Am Heart J 70:521, 1965.
4. Anderson R, Galbraith R, Gibson R, Miller G: Double outlet left ventricle. Br Heart J 36:554, 1974.
5. Robinson BW, Anisman PC, Sandhu S, et al: Significance of a Q wave in lead 1 in the newborn. Am J Cardiol 84:615, 1999.
6. Azevedo A, Toledo AN, deCarvalho AA, Roubach R: Transposition of aorta and levoposition of the pulmonary artery (Taussig-Bing syndrome). Am Heart J 52:249, 1956.
7. Baron MG: Angiographic differentiation between tetralogy of Fallot and double outlet right ventricle. Circulation 43:451, 1971.
8. Battistessa S, Soto B: Double outlet right ventricle with discordant atrioventricular connection: An angiographic analysis of 19 cases. Int J Cardiol 27:253, 1990.
9. Beitzke A, Suppan C: Double outlet left ventricle with intact ventricular septum. Int J Cardiol 5:175, 1984.
10. Bengur AR, Snider AR, Peters J, Merida-Asnus L: Two-dimensional echocardiographic features of double outlet left ventricle. Am Soc Echo 3:320, 1990.
11. Beuren, A: Differential diagnosis of the Taussig-Bing heart from complete transposition of the great vessels with a posteriorly overriding pulmonary artery. Circulation 21:1071, 1960.
12. Bharati, S., and Lev, M.: The conduction system in double outlet right ventricle with subpulmonic ventricular septal defect and related hearts (the Taussig-Bing group). Circulation 54:459, 1976.
13. Bharati, S., Lev, M., Steward, R., McAllister, H. A., and Kirklin, J. W.: The morphologic spectrum of double outlet left ventricle and its surgical significance. Circulation 58:558, 1978.
14. Bostrom, M. P. G., and Hutchins, G. M.: Arrested rotation of the outflow tract may explain double-outlet right ventricle. Circulation 77:1258, 1988.
15. Brandt, P. W. T., Calder, A. L., Barrat-Boyes, B. G., and Neutz, J. M.: Double outlet left ventricle. Morphology, cineangiocardiographic diagnosis and surgical treatment. Am. J. Cardiol. 38:897, 1976.
16. Braun, K., DeVries, A., Feingold, D. S., Ehrenfeld, N. E., Feldman, J., and Schorr, S.: Complete dextroposition of the aorta, pulmonary stenosis, interventricular septal defect, and patent foramen ovale. Am. Heart J. 43:773, 1952.
17. Walters HL, Mavroudis C, Tchervenkov CI, Jacobs JP, Lacour-Gayet F, Jacobs ML. Congenital heart surgery nomenclature and database: double outlet right ventricle. Ann Thorac Surg 69:S249, 2000
18. Butler, L. J., Snodgrass, G. J. A. I., France, N. E., Sinclair, L., and Russell, A.: E(16–18) trisomy syndrome: Analysis of 13 cases. Arch. Dis. Child. 40:600, 1965.
19. Campbell, M., and Hudson, R. E. B.: A case of Taussig-Bing transposition with survival for 34 years. Guy's Hosp. Rep. 107:14, 1958.
20. Carey, L. S., and Edwards, J. E.: Roentgenographic features in cases with origin of both great vessels from the right ventricle without pulmonary stenosis, Am. J. Roentgenol. 93:269, 1965.
21. Conti, V., Adams, F., and Mulder, D. G.: Double-outlet left ventricle. Ann. Thorac. Surg. 18:402, 1974.
22. Uemura H, Yagihara T, Kawashima Y, Nishigaki K, Kamiya T, Sy H, Anderson RH. Coronary arterial anatomy in double outlet right ventricle with subpulmonary stenosis. Ann Thorac Surg 59:591, 1995.
23. Dadourian, B. J., Perloff, J. K., Drinkwater, D. C., Child, J. S., and Mulder, D. G.: Double outlet left ventricle-long survival after surgical correction. Ann. Thorac. Surg. 51:159, 1991.
24. Davachi, F., Moller, J. H. and Edwards, J. E.: Origin of both great vessels from the right ventricle with intact ventricular septum. Am. Heart J. 75:790, 1968.
25. Dayem, M. K., Prager, L., Goodwin, J. F., and Steiner, R. E.: Double outlet right ventricle with pulmonary stenosis. Br. Heart J. 29:64, 1967.
26. de la Cruz, M. V., Cayre, R., Martinez, O. A., Sadowinski, S., and Serrano, A.: The infundibular interrelationships and the ventriculoarterial connection in double outlet right ventricle. Clinical and surgical implications. Int. J. Cardiol. 35:153, 1992.
27. De-wen, G., Mei-lin, L., Zhen-qiong, G., and Cheng, T. O.: Double outlet right ventricle: A clinical-roentgenologic-pathologic study of 28 consecutive patients. Chest 85:527, 1984.
28. Edwards, W. D.: Double outlet right ventricle and tetralogy of Fallot. Two distinct but not mutually exclusive entities. J. Thorac. Cardiovasc. Surg. 82:418, 1981.
29. Elliott, L. P., Amplatz, K., and Edwards, J. E.: Coronary arterial patterns in transposition complexes. Am. J. Cardiol. 17:362, 1966.
30. Elliott L. P., Adams, P., Jr., Levy, M. J., and Edwards, J. E.: Right ventricular aorta and biventricular pulmonary trunk, an uncommon form of transposition. Am. Heart J. 66:478, 1963.
31. Engle, M. A., Steinberg, I., Lukas, D. S., and Goldberg, H. P.: Acyanotic ventricular septal defect with both great vessels from the right ventricle. Am. Heart J. 66:755, 1963.
32. Ettinger, P. O., Weisse, A. B., Khan, M. J., and Levinson, G. E.: Double outlet right ventricle in an adult with aortic regurgitation. Am. J. Cardiol. 47:818, 1969.
33. Falholt, W., and Pedersen, A.: Complete transposition of aorta and levoposition of pulmonary artery; report of case diagnosed by cardiac catheterization. Acta Med. Scand. *142* (Suppl 266):393, 1952.
34. Manner J, Seidl W, Steding G. Embryological observations on the formal pathogenesis of double outlet left ventricle with a right ventricular infundibulum. Thorac Cardiovasc Surg 45:172, 1997.
35. Hagler, D. J., Edwards, W. D., Seward, J. B., and Tajik, A. J.: Standardized nomenclature of the ventricular septum and ventricular

septal defects, with applications for two- dimensional echocardiography. Mayo. Clin. Proc. 60:741, 1985.

36. Dikinson C, Walker S, Wilmshurst P. Double outlet right ventricle with unprotected pulmonary vasculature presenting in a woman of 65. Heart 76:187, 1996.

37. Hinkes, E., Rosenquist, G. C., and White, R. I.: Roentgenographic reexamination of the internal anatomy of the Taussig-Bing heart. Am. Heart J. 81:335, 1971.

38. James, A. E., Belcourt, C. L., Atkins, L., and Janower, M. L.: Trisomy 18. Radiology 92:37, 1969.

39. Kerr, A. R., Barcia, A., Bargeron, L. M., and Karklin, J. W.: Double outlet left ventricle with ventricular septal defect and pulmonary atresia. Am. Heart J. 81:688, 1971.

40. Khanolkar, U. B., and Kinare, S. G.: Taussig-Bing complex-a pathologic study of eight cases. Indian Heart J. 42:157, 1990.

41. Khattri, H. N., Misra, K. P., and Dutta, B. N.: Double outlet right ventricle with long survival. Br. Heart J. 30:569, 1968.

42. Khoury, G. H., and Gilbert, E. F.: Taussig-Bing malformation with coarctation of aorta. Angiology 21:143, 1970.

43. Ewing S, Silverman NH. Echocardiographic diagnosis of single coronary artery in double outlet right ventricle. Am J Cardiol. 77:535, 1996.

44. Krongrad, E., Ritter, D. G., Weidman, W. H., and DuShane, J. W.: Hemodynamic and anatomic correlation of electrocardiogram in double outlet right ventricle. Circulation 46:995, 1972.

45. Galal O, Hatle L, Al Halees Z. Changes of management in a patient with double outlet left ventricle. Cardiol Young. 9:602, 1999.

46. Lavoie, R., Sestier, F., Gilbert, G., Chameides, L., Van Praagh, R., and Grondin, P.: Double outlet right ventricle with left ventricular outflow tract obstruction due to small ventricular septal defect. Am. Heart J. 82:290, 1971.

47. Manner J, Seidl, Steding G. Embryological observations on the morphogenesis of double outlet right ventricle with subaortic ventricular septal defect and normal arrangement of the great arteries. Thorac Cardiovasc Surg. 43:307, 1995.

48. Lev, M., Bharati, S., Meng, L., Liberthson, R. R., Paul, M. H., and Idriss, F. A.: A concept of double outlet right ventricle. J. Thorac. Cardiovasc. Surg. 64:271, 1972.

49. Lev, M., Rimoldi, H. J., Eckner, F. O., Melhuish, P. B., Meng, L., and Paul, M. H.: The Taussig-Bing heart: Qualitative and quantitative anatomy. Arch. Pathol. 81:24, 1966.

50. Macartney, F. J., Rigby, M. L., Anderson, R. H., Stark, J., and Silverman, N. H.: Double outlet right ventricle. Cross sectional echocardiographic findings, their anatomical explanation and surgical relevance. Br. Heart J. 52:164, 1984.

51. MacMahon, H. E., and Lepa, M.: Double outlet right ventricle with intact interventricular septum. Circulation 30:745, 1964.

52. Marino, B., and Bevilacqua, M.: Double-outlet left ventricle: Two-dimensional echocardiographic diagnosis. Am. Heart J. 123:1075, 1992.

53. Marino, B., Loperfido, F., and Sardi, C. S.: Spontaneous closure of ventricular septal defect in a case of double outlet right ventricle. Br. Heart J. 49:608, 1983.

54. Child JS: Transthoracic and transesophageal echocardiographic imaging: Anatomiv and hemodynamic assessment. In Perloff JK and Child JS. Congenital Heart Disease in Adults 2nd edition, Philadelphia, WB Saunders Co, 1998, p91.

55. Mason, D. T., Morrow, A. G., Elkins, R. C., and Friedman, W. F.: Origin of both great vessels from the right ventricle associated with severe obstruction to left ventricular outflow. Am. J. Cardiol. 24:118, 1969.

56. Michaelsson, M., and Tuvemo, T.: Double outlet right ventricle with spontaneously developing pulmonary outflow obstruction. Br. Heart J. 36:937, 1974.

57. Mirowski, M., Mehrizi, A., and Taussig, H. B.: The electrocardiogram in patients with both great vessels arising from the right ventricle combined with pulmonary stenosis. An analysis of 22 cases with special reference to the differential diagnosis from the tetralogy of Fallot. Circulation 28:1116, 1963.

58. Mitchell, S. C., Korones, S. B., and Berendes, H. W.: Congenital heart disease in 56,109 births; incidence and natural history. Circulation 43:323, 1971.

59. Neufeld, H. N., DuShane, J. W., and Edwards, J. E.: Origin of the great vessels from the right ventricle. II. With pulmonary stenosis. Circulation 23:603, 1961.

60. Neufeld, H. N., DuShane, J. W., Wood, E. H., Kirklin, J. W., and Edwards, J. E.: Origin of both great vessels from the right ventricle. I. Without pulmonary stenosis. Circulation 23:399, 1961.

61. Neufeld, H. N., Lucas, R. V., Jr., Lester, R. G., Adams, P., Jr., Anderson, R. C., and Edwards, J. E.: Origin of both great vessels from the right ventricle without pulmonary stenosis. Br. Heart J. 24:393, 1962.

62. Parr, G. V. S., Waldhausen, J. A., Bharati, S., Lev, M., Fripp, R., and Whitman, V.: Coarctation in Taussig-Bing malformation of the heart. J. Thorac. Cardiovasc. Surg. 86:280, 1983.

63. Parsons, J. M., Baker, E. J., Anderson, R. H., Ladusans, E. J., Hayes, A., Fagg, N., Cook, A., Qureshi, S. A., Deverall, P. B., Maisey, M. N., and Tynan, M.: Double-outlet right ventricle: Morphologic demonstration using nuclear resonance imaging. J. Am. Coll. Cardiol. 18:168, 1991.

64. Paul, M. H., Muster, A. J., Sinha, S. N., Cole, R. B., and Van Praagh, R.: Double-outlet left ventricle. Circulation 41:129, 1970.

65. Peacock, T. B.: On Malformations of the Human Heart. 2nd ed. London, J. Churchill and Sons, 1866.

66. Rao, P. S., and Sissman, N. J.: Spontaneous closure of physiologically advantageous ventricular septal defects. Circulation 43:83, 1971.

67. Rein, A. J. J. T., Dollberg, S., and Gale, R.: Genetics of conotruncal malformations: Review of the literature and reports of a consanguineous kindred with various conotruncal malformations. Am. J. Med. Genet. 36:353, 1990.

68. Rice, M. J., Seward, J. B., Edwards, W. D., Hagler, D. J., Danielson, G. K., Puga, F. J., and Tajik, A. J.: Straddling atrioventricular valve: Two-dimensional echocardiographic diagnosis, classification and surgical implications. Am. J. Cardiol. 55:505, 1985.

69. Roberson, D. A., and Silverman, N. H.: Malaligned outlet septum with subpulmonary ventricular septal defect and abnormal ventriculoarterial connection: A morphologic spectrum defined echocardiographically. J. Am. Coll. Cardiol. 16:459, 1990.

70. Rogers, T. R., Hagstrom, J. W., and Engle, M. A.: Origin of both great vessels from the right ventricle associated with the trisomy-18 syndrome. Circulation 32:802, 1965.

71. Rogoff, J. H., and Anthony, W.: Double outlet right ventricle with pulmonary valve atresia. Am. Heart J. 72:259, 1966.

72. Rohde, R. A., Hodgeman, J. E., and Cleland, R. S.: Multiple congenital anomalies in the E-trisomy (group 16–18) syndrome. Pediatrics 33:258, 1964.

73. Smith, D. W.: The number 18 trisomy and D1 trisomy syndromes. Pediatr. Clin. North Am. 10.389, 1963.

74. Sondheimer, H. M., Freedom, R. M., and Olley, P. M.: Double-outlet right ventricle: Clinical spectrum and prognosis. Am. J. Cardiol. 39:709, 1977.

75. Sridaromont, S., Feldt, R. H., Ritter, D. G., Davis, G. D., and Edwards, J. E.: Double-outlet right ventricle: Hemodynamic and anatomic correlations. Am. J. Cardiol. 38:85, 1976.

76. Sridaromont, S., Ritter, D. G., Feldt, R. H., Davis, G. D., and Edwards, J. E.: Double outlet right ventricle: Anatomic and angiocardiographic correlations. Mayo Clin. Proc. 53:555, 1978.

77. Taussig, H. B., and Bing, R. J.: Complete transposition of aorta and levoposition of pulmonary artery; clinical, physiological, and pathological findings. Am. Heart J. 37:551, 1949.

78. Titus, J. H., Neufeld, H. N., and Edwards, J. E.: The atrioventricular system in hearts with both great vessels originating from the right ventricle. Am. Heart J. 67:588, 1964.

79. Van Praagh, R.: What is the Taussig-Bing malformation? Circulation 38:445, 1968.

80. Van Praagh, S., Davidoff, A., Chin, A., Shiel, F. S., Reynolds, J., and Van Praagh, R.: Double outlet right ventricle: Anatomic types and developmental implications based on a study of 101 autopsied cases. Coeur 8:389, 1982.

81. Vierordt, H.: Die angeborenen Herzkrankheiten. Spez. Pathol. Ther. 15:244, 1898.

82. Wedemeyer, A. L., Lucas, R. V., and Castenada, A. R.: Taussig-Bing malformation, coarctation of the aorta, and reversed patent ductus arteriosus. Circulation 42:1021, 1970.

83. Witham, A. C.: Double outlet right ventricle. A partial transposition complex. Am. Heart J. 53:928, 1957.

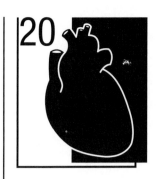

Patent Ductus
Arteriosus

In 1593, Giambattista Carcano described the ductus arteriosus in his book on the great cardiac vessels of the fetus.[39] However, Leo Bottali came to be associated with the arterial duct even though Bottali had misapplied the term *ductus* to the foramen ovale.[39] It was not until Rokitansky's handbook of 1844 followed by his beautifully illustrated monograph of 1852 that patent ductus arteriosus was recognized as a specific congenital malformation.[133] The incidence of isolated persistent patency of the ductus arteriosus has been estimated at 1:2000 to 1:5000 births or approximately 10% to 12% of all varieties of congenital heart disease.[8,37]

The pulmonary orifice of the ductus is located immediately to the left of the bifurcation of the pulmonary trunk near the origin of the left branch (Figs. 20–1 and 20–2). The aortic orifice of the ductus is located immediately distal to the origin of the left subclavian artery (Figs. 20–1 and 20–2). The patent ductus can be long and narrow or short and wide with all gradations in between (Figs. 20–3 through 20–5).[48,62,101,151] Closure begins at the pulmonary arterial end, so the ductus is larger at its aortic end and is shaped as a truncated cone (Figs. 20–3 and 20–4).[48,62,80,108] A widely patent aortic end with a sealed pulmonary end sets the stage for a ductal aneurysm (Fig. 20–6).[*] Patency confined to the pulmonary end is exceptional.[161] Anatomic variations include bilateral patent ductus,[67,87,111,112,114] left-sided patent ductus with right aortic arch,[185] right-sided patent ductus with right aortic arch,[69] and a patent ductus or ligamentum arteriosum as a component of a vascular ring (Fig. 20–7).[71]

Despite its seeming anatomic simplicity, the ductus arteriosus is as fascinating as it is complex. The *fetal patent ductus* is a major anatomic component of an intrauterine great artery consisting of pulmonary trunk/ductus/aortic continuity that delivers 85% of right ventricular output into the descending aorta.[16,206] *Persistent fetal circulation* applies when the intrauterine right-to-left ductal shunt persists after birth (see Chapter 14).[72] Persistent patency of the ductus arteriosus after birth is abnormal and therefore undesirable, although with certain forms of congenital heart disease survival depends on neonatal ductal patency. These *ductal dependent circulations* include malformations in which a patent ductus is the only source of pulmonary arterial blood flow (pulmonary atresia with intact ventricular septum), the only source of systemic arterial blood flow (aortic atresia or complete interruption of the aortic arch), or patent ductus as the only source of bidirectional blood flow (simple complete transposition of the great arteries).

The ductus arteriosus is derived from the sixth aortic arch. By the fourth month of gestation, ductal tissue is distinctive and differs histologically from pulmonary arterial and aortic tissue.[78,182] At 16 weeks gestation, the ductus consists of a muscular arterial channel and an endothelium separated by an internal elastic lamina and a thin subendothelial layer.[78,182] Ductal media can be aortic, pulmonary, and mixed because medial tissue differs at the aortic and pulmonary ends of the ductus.[80] As gestation proceeds, the intima thickens, and the subendothelial layer is invaded by cells from the media that disrupt the internal elastic lamina.[78] In the mature ductus at term, conspicuous intimal cushions protrude into the lumen of the ductus,[78] which is capable of contraction (functional closure) followed by anatomic closure that begins at the pulmonary arterial end.[80] Anatomic closure has been examined at the immunohistochemical level and ultrastructural level,[80,182] and a sequence of changes have been identified, namely: 1) separation of endothelium from the internal elastic lamina resulting in subendothelial edema; 2) enfolding and ingrowth of endothelial cells, migration of undifferentiated

---

[*]See references 26, 48, 62, 70, 76, 85, 90, 95, 101, 126, 150, 151.

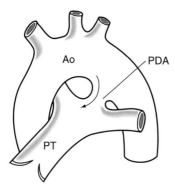

Patent ductus

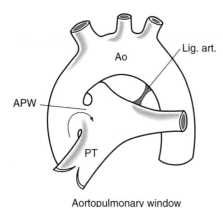

Aortopulmonary window

Figure 20–1

Illustrations of patent ductus arteriosus (PDA) and aortopulmonary window (APW). The aortic orifice of a *patent ductus arteriosus* inserts immediately beyond the origin of the left subclavian artery, and the pulmonary orifice inserts immediately to the left of the bifurcation of the pulmonary trunk (PT). An *aortopulmonary window* is a communication between adjacent walls of the ascending aorta (Ao) and the pulmonary trunk (PT) proximal to its bifurcation. LIG ART, ligamentum arteriosum.

medial smooth muscle cells into the subendothelium and fragmentation of the internal elastic lamina; 3) sealing of the lumen by endothelial cell apposition; and 4) accumulation of lipid droplets followed by intimal and outer subendothelial degenerative changes that spread centrally and peripherally and result in disappearance of endothelial cells at luminal apposition lines.[80] The normal process of functional closure begins within 10 to 15 hours after birth, is virtually complete (probe patent) by the second week of extrauterine life, and the ductus is anatomically closed (ligamentum arteriosum) 2 to 3 weeks after birth.[108,201,206] When a ductus is destined to remain patent, the intrauterine subendothelial internal elastic lamina lies adjacent to the intimal cushions, endothelial cells adhere closely to the elastic lamina, and subendothelial edema with enfolding of endothelial cells does not occur.[78,80,182] A ductus arteriosus that remains patent in full-term infants after 3 months of extrauterine life harbors these histologic features of persistent patency. Spontaneous closure is then unlikely.[77,79,182]

Ductal wall tone *in utero* is determined by an interplay between the constricting effects of oxygen (relatively weak because of low fetal pO_2) and the dilating effects of endoge-

nous prostaglandin E$_2$.[41,42,96,122,130,160,192] Prostaglandin synthetase inhibitors administered to mammalian fetuses or to pregnant ewes constrict the fetal ductus.[41,42,122,160] Intrauterine constriction deprives the fetal right ventricle of its only outlet.[16,122] As term approaches, the ductus becomes less responsive to prostaglandin E$_2$ and more responsive to oxygen, setting the stage for constriction that begins within a few hours after birth in full term infants.[41,43,144] Functional closure is closely coupled to the increase in extrauterine ambient oxygen tension, which exerts a direct constricting effect on the ductal wall. Constriction induced by oxygen has been related to inhibition of voltage-gated potassium channels.[169] Flow through the closing ductus is transiently bidirectional, followed by left-to-right flow[144] that rapidly decreases during the next 12 hours and cannot be detected at 48 hours.[57,98] Anatomic closure is the culmination of morphologic changes accrued during intrauterine ductal maturation.[41,43,78,80,81,138,182] Apoptosis and smooth muscle cell proliferation have been assigned a role in postnatal anatomical closure.[45]

Delayed closure of the ductus arteriosus is common in normal preterm infants.[13,53,57,110,130,163-165,195,204] Premature

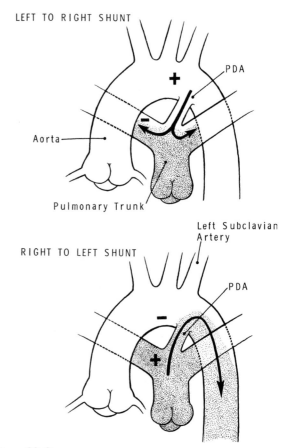

Figure 20–2

Illustrations of two major flow patterns in patent ductus arteriosus (PDA). The *upper* drawing illustrates a left-to-right shunt through a patent ductus in which pulmonary vascular resistance is lower than systemic vascular resistance. Shunt flow is from aorta into the pulmonary trunk. The *lower* drawing illustrates a right-to-left shunt through a patent ductus in which pulmonary vascular resistance is suprasystemic. Shunt flow is from pulmonary trunk into the aorta distal to the left subclavian artery.

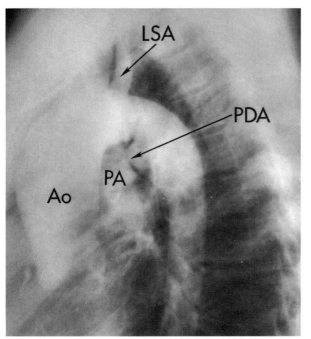

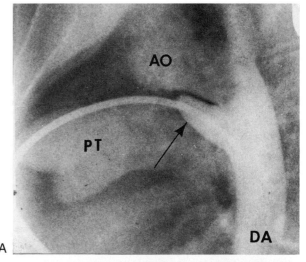

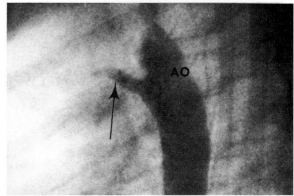

Figure 20–3

Lateral aortogram from a 14-year-old girl whose x-ray is shown in Fig. 20–28*A*. The conical shape of the ductus (PDA) is larger at its aortic end (Ao) and smaller at its pulmonary arterial end (PA). LSA, left subclavian artery.

neonates with a gestational age of 30 weeks or more usually experience spontaneous ductal closure within a time frame that corresponds to the timing of closure in full-term infants (Figs. 20–8 and 20–9).[164,165] Spontaneous closure in full-term infants is unlikely after 3 months of age,[77,79] and spontaneous closure in premature infants is unlikely after 1 year of age.[79]

Persistent patency of the ductus in premature infants coincides with respiratory distress, but subsequent ductal

Figure 20–4

A, Lateral angiogram from a 16-year-old girl. A catheter passed from the pulmonary trunk (PT) through a ductus arteriosus (*arrow*) which is distinctly larger at its aortic end than at its pulmonary end. AO, aortic arch; DA, descending aorta. *B*, Lateral angiogram from an 8-year-old boy with a restrictive tubular ductus arteriosus (*arrow*) that fills from the aorta (AO) and tapers markedly at its pulmonary end.

Figure 20–5

Angiocardiograms from a 3-year-old boy with a nonrestrictive patent ductus arteriosus (PDA), low pulmonary vascular resistance and a 3 to 1 left-to right shunt. *A*, The ascending aorta (Ao) is relatively small, but the pulmonary trunk (PT) and left ventricle (LV) are dilated. *B*, The patent ductus arteriosus (PDA) joins the relatively small ascending aorta (Ao) to the dilated pulmonary trunk (PT).

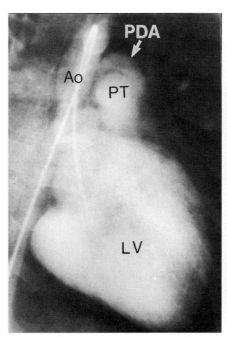

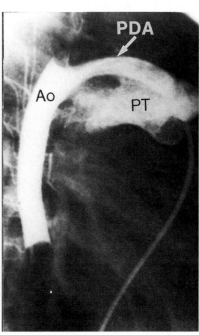

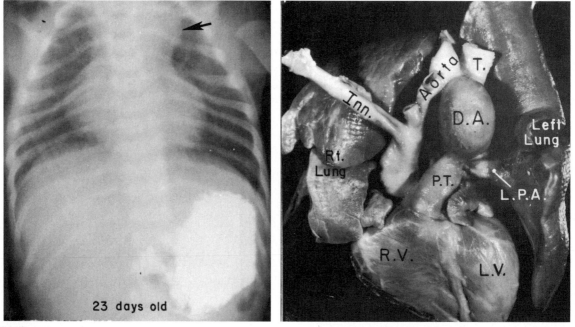

Figure 20–6

A, X-ray showing the striking convexity of a large ductal aneurysm (*arrow*) in a 23-day-old infant. (Pyloric stenosis accounted for retention of barium in the stomach.) *B*, Necropsy specimen shows the ductal aneurysm (DA) which was sealed at its pulmonary arterial end but open at its aortic end. Inn, innominate artery; T, trachea; PT, pulmonary trunk; LPA, left pulmonary artery; RV/LV, right and left ventricle.

closure may not improve respiratory distress.[51,164,165] Patent ductus in preterm infants can be associated with reduced cerebral blood flow due to a steal effect caused by

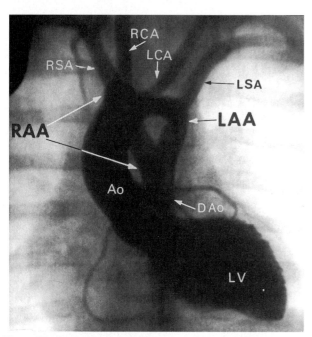

Figure 20–7

Angiocardiogram with contrast material injected into the left ventricle (LV) of a 15-year-old boy with a vascular ring. The ascending aorta (Ao) bifurcates into a right aortic arch (RAA) that passes anterior to the trachea and a left aortic arch (LAA) that passes posterior to the esophagus. The two aortic arches join to form the descending aorta (DAo). The esophagus and trachea were compressed within the vascular ring. All anatomic components of the vascular ring are visualized except the ligamentum arteriosum which was surgically divided. RSA/LSA, right subclavian and left subclavian artery; RCA/LCA, right carotid and left carotid artery.

the aortic-to-pulmonary shunt rather than to a limited capacity of the preterm left ventricle to achieve adequate cardiac output.[5,13,61,136]

First trimester maternal rubella with rash carries an 80% incidence of intrauterine viral infection[139] and results in deafness and cataracts (Fig. 20–10) and congenital malformations of the heart in two thirds of offspring. Patent ductus arteriosus accounts for one third of these malformations[79] and is characterized by maturational arrest and an immature wall of the type found at 16 weeks' gestation (see earlier).[79]

The *physiologic consequences* of persistent patency of the ductus arteriosus depend on five variables: 1) the size of the ductus, 2) the pulmonary vascular resistance, 3) the adaptive response of the left ventricle to volume overload, 4) prematurity, and 5) respiratory distress. When the ductus is *restrictive*, pulmonary vascular resistance is normal, right ventricular afterload is normal, a continuous gradient results in continuous flow from aorta to pulmonary artery, and the hemodynamic consequences are negligible. When the ductus is *moderately restrictive*, pulmonary vascular resistance is normal or nearly so, right ventricular afterload is not significantly increased, and continuous flow from aorta to pulmonary artery imposes moderate volume overload on the left ventricle. About 95% of isolated patent ductuses are restrictive or moderately restrictive. When the ductus is *nonrestrictive*, systolic pressure in the aorta and pulmonary trunk are at systemic level, and the direction of blood flow through the ductus depends on the relative resistances in the systemic and pulmonary vascular beds.[172] If pulmonary resistance is lower than systemic, a

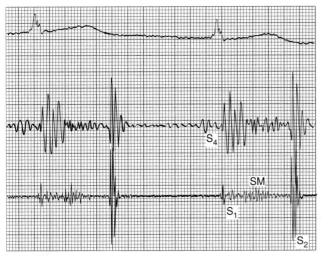

Figure 20–8
Phonocardiograms in the second left intercostal space of a 21-day-old premature boy with a nonrestrictive patent ductus arteriosus (see x-ray in Fig. 20–9). The low-frequency filter *upper* tracing shows a fourth heart sound (S$_4$). The high-frequency filter *lower* tracing shows a normal first heart sound (S$_1$) and an unimpressive early to midsystolic ductal murmur (SM) that fades before a loud single second heart sound (S$_2$).

left-to-right shunt is established and imposes volume overload on the left ventricle while right ventricular afterload remains at systemic level (see Fig. 20–2, *upper*). When pulmonary vascular resistance exceeds systemic resistance, the shunt is reversed (see Fig. 20–2, *lower*), volume overload of the left ventricle is curtailed, pressure overload of the right ventricle remains at systemic level, and the pulmonary vascular bed exhibits histologi-

cal changes analogous to primary pulmonary hypertension (see Chapter 14).[8,34,35,36,54,93,94,101,198]

The first section of this chapter is concerned with isolated persistent patency of the ductus arteriosus. The second section is devoted to aortopulmonary window, an anomaly that is embryologically unrelated to patent ductus but is physiologically and clinically similar.

The History

A newborn is typically pronounced normal and discharged as a well baby. Neonatal pulmonary vascular resistance falls, a left-to-right shunt is established, the ductus murmur emerges, and the diagnosis becomes apparent. Less commonly, a low-birth-weight neonate comes to attention because of systemic hypoperfusion or congestive heart failure without an incriminating ductus murmur (Fig. 20–8).[89,195,204] Absence of a murmur does not confirm ductal closure.[206] Doppler echocardiography occasionally detects a tiny patent ductus in infants without auscultatory signs of its presence,[105] or detects a tiny ductus in adults in whom the diagnosis had been missed (see Fig. 20–40).[192] Exceptional examples of spontaneous closure have been documented between 5 and 6 years of age, between 7 and 14 years,[18] after 17 years,[34] and at age 19 years.[27] Ductal closure occasionally results from healed infective endocarditis[40,73] or from occlusion by a thrombus.[66,107]

Vesalius described a valve or membrane of the ductus arteriosus in 1561.[64] A valvelike structure was subsequently found in stillborn human fetuses and in newborn

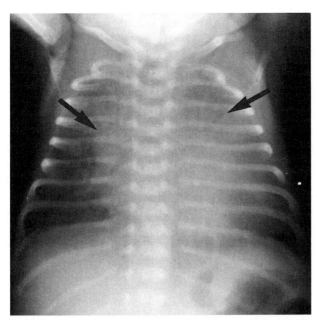

Figure 20–9
X-ray from the 21-day-old premature boy with a widely patent ductus arteriosus whose phonocardiogram is shown in Fig. 20–8. Pulmonary blood flow is increased, the heart is considerably enlarged, and a thymus obscures the base. By age 4 months, the ductus had spontaneously closed, the thymus had disappeared, and the x-ray was virtually normal.

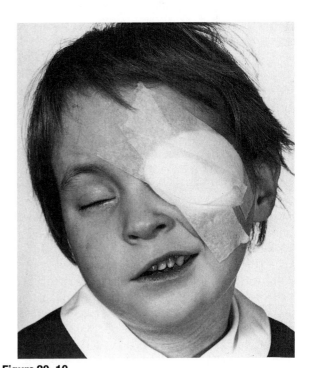

Figure 20–10
A 5-year-old girl whose mother had first trimester rubella. The bandage followed ophthalmic surgery for cataract. The child had a patent ductus arteriosus.

rabbits,[64] and a necropsy report in 1903 called attention to a perforated ductal valve.[197] Taussig confirmed the presence of a membranous valve at the pulmonary end of a ductus arteriosus and theorized that rupture of the valve might account for the sudden appearance of a ductus murmur, an event occasionally witnessed in children or young adults.[190] A continuous murmur intermittently appeared and disappeared in a patient with a veil-like valve at the pulmonary end of a ductus,[113] and the abrupt appearance of a loud continuous murmur was described in a 55-year-old man with a ductal membrane.[193] Rarely, a closed lumen is reopened by spontaneous intramural dissection of a ductal aneurysm.[21]

Patent ductus arteriosus predominates in females with a sex ratio of 2 or 3 to 1,[34] and female prevalence is even greater in older patients.[11,32,65,134,149] Canine patent ductus is also more common in females and can be hereditary.[154] There is a tendency for recurrence in siblings[3,8,23,27,32,120,128] and in offspring of parents with patent ductus.[3] Familial recurrence has been reported in three generations of a single family.[135] Identical twins may both have a patent ductus or the ductus may be patent in only one twin.[60,159]

In offspring of gravida with *maternal* rubella, patent ductus arteriosus and pulmonary artery stenosis are the anticipated coexisting congenital cardiac malformations (see Chapter 11).[33,59,84,173] Maternal rubella resulted in patent ductus arteriosus in one of a twin pair while the other twin had pulmonary artery stenosis. Low birth weight is a feature of the rubella syndrome, and infants fail to thrive even if the ductus is restrictive. A seasonal incidence of patent ductus in late winter and early spring coincided with the peak incidence of rubella.[173]

Persistent patency of the ductus arteriosus is about six times as frequent in high altitude residents as in sea level residents.[6] A predilection for increased pulmonary vascular resistance is a feature of high altitude births with patent ductus, and the predilection exists even when the ductus is restrictive.[6]

Congestive heart failure is the commonest cause of death related to patent ductus *per se*.[15,34,47,65] Rarely, death is due to a dissecting aneurysm of the ductus, to rupture of a ductal aneurysm,[92,150] or to rupture of a hypertensive aneurysmal pulmonary trunk.[48,109,175] Aneurysm of a *nonpatent* ductus (see Fig. 20–6) may be complicated by rupture, by spontaneous intramural dissection, by systemic embolism or infection, by recurrent laryngeal nerve paralysis, by compression of the pulmonary trunk, or by hemorrhagic erosion into the esophagus or tracheobronchial tree.[21,126]

Infective endarteritis occurs with a restrictive patent ductus because of the high velocity left-to-right shunt but does not occur with a nonrestrictive patent ductus and reversed shunt.[34,47,65] The infection is located at the narrow pulmonary arterial end of the ductus or at the site of an intimal jet lesion in the pulmonary artery opposite the ductus. Susceptibility has not been established for a tiny clinically silent ductus detected only by Doppler echocardiography (see Fig. 20–40).[103]

Abnormal patterns of cerebral arterial blood flow in infants, especially preterm neonates with a nonrestrictive patent ductus, predispose to central nervous system ischemia and to hemorrhage into the germinal matrix.[14,61,125,136] A sharp decrease in diastolic arterial flow velocity appears to act as a *steal* from the cerebral circulation. Increased pulse pressure and major fluctuations of blood flow velocity caused by opening and closing of the ductus may rupture capillaries of the germinal matrix and cause intraventricular hemorrhage.

After the first year of life, most patients with patent ductus arteriosus are asymptomatic. Beginning at the second decade, the risk of infective endarteritis exceeds the risk of congestive heart failure,[4,34,91,149] but in the third decade, more and more patients with moderately restrictive left-to-right shunts experience heart failure[32,34,65,134,142,149] while those with a restrictive patent ductus remain asymptomatic. A 20-year-old man with a patent ductus had been a cross-country runner,[32] and a woman led an active life as a schoolmistress and died at the age of 85 years because of gastrointestinal bleeding.[11] A number of reports have called attention to survival beyond age 60 years (see Fig. 20–16),[2,20,34,102,134,147,203,205] and one patient died at 90 years of age.[199]

A nonrestrictive patent ductus with *Eisenmenger syndrome* is complicated by the multisystem systemic disorders of cyanotic congenital heart disease (see Chapter 17).[142,180,191,202] Isotonic exercise with an Eisenmenger ductus tends to cause leg fatigue without dyspnea because the exercise-induced increase in right-to-left shunt is channeled into the descending aorta (see Figs. 20–2 and 20–12), precluding hypoxia-induced stimulation of the respiratory center and the carotid body.[9,54,142,179,191,202] Hypertrophic osteoarthropathy is confined to the lower extremities.[52,137,180,200] Left ventricular failure is absent because volume overload is curtailed. A dilated hypertensive pulmonary trunk may cause hoarseness by compressing the recurrent laryngeal nerve. Angina and syncope are not features of nonrestrictive patent ductus arteriosus and reserved shunt because right ventricular pressure cannot exceed systemic.[202] Cyanosis escapes attention when the cyanotic feet are not examined (see Physical Appearance). A young girl came to attention because she noticed that when she sat in a warm bath, her toes were blue but her fingers were pink.

Constriction or closure of the fetal ductus deprives the right ventricle of its only outlet, so neonates present with massive tricuspid regurgitation and right-to-left interatrial shunts.[16,122,192] Because salicylates cause constriction of the fetal ductus, the history should include inquiries about maternal aspirin ingestion followed up by salicylate levels on umbilical cord blood.[10]

Physical Appearance

Maternal rubella is associated with low birth weight and failure to thrive irrespective of ductal patency or ductal size.[47,60,159] An underdeveloped child with a patent ductus should be examined for cataracts, deafness, and mental retardation (Fig. 20–10).[118] Another distinctive phenotype is the overlapping fingers (clinodactyly), rocker bottom feet, and lax skin of *trisomy 18* (Fig. 20–11).[29,124,168] *Char syndrome* is an inherited disorder that maps to chromosome 6p12-p21 and is characterized by patent ductus arteriosus, facial dysmorphism, and abnormalities of the hand.[158,162,170]

Differential cyanosis and clubbing are important physical signs of patent ductus with reversed shunt (Figs. 20–2 and 20–12).[157,202] The toes are cyanosed and clubbed because unsaturated blood is delivered selectively to the lower extremities. When a small amount of unsaturated blood enters the left subclavian artery, the fingers of the left hand are mildly cyanosed and slightly clubbed, especially the thumb (Fig. 20–12A). The fingers of the right hand are normal because unsaturated blood does not reach the right subclavian artery. In the presence of *bilateral* patent ductus with reversed shunt, the *right* arm is cyanosed because the right subclavian artery receives desaturated blood from the pulmonary artery via the right ductus arteriosus.[112]

Older patients should be instructed to sit or squat with their hands placed alongside their feet or on the dorsum of the feet to facilitate comparison of fingers and toes (Fig. 20–12A). The right and left thumbs should be compared (Fig. 20–12A). Differential cyanosis is exaggerated by isotonic exercise or by warming the hands and feet, maneuvers that increase skin blood flow and exaggerate the color differences. In neonates with persistent fetal circulation, the right-to-left ductal shunt may cause distinctive differential cyanosis confined to the head, right shoulder, and right arm with a line of demarcation that runs obliquely from above the left shoulder to below the right axilla.[72]

Normal individuals, especially young women, may have *peripheral* cyanosis of the feet because of vasoconstriction,

Figure 20–11
Photographs of a female infant with patent ductus arteriosus, ventricular septal defect, and the physical appearance of trisomy 18 with lax skin and overlapping fingers (clinodactyly) (*B*). Rocker bottom feet (in *A*) are not well shown.

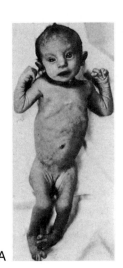

A

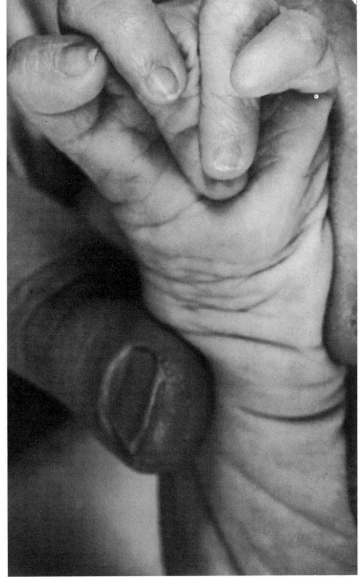

B

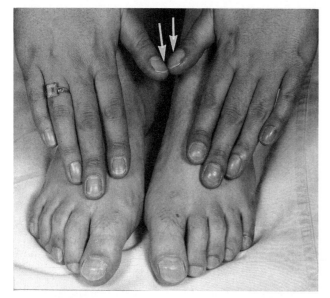

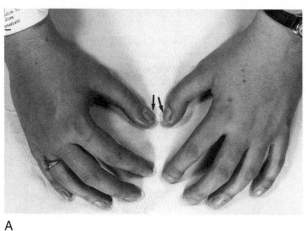

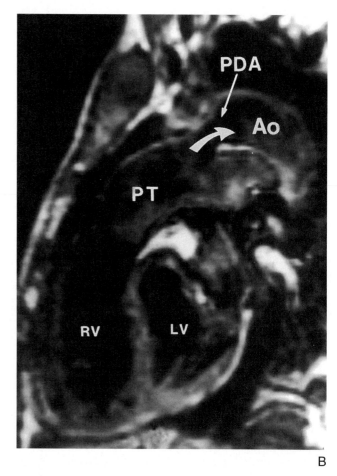

A B

Figure 20–12
A, Photographs of a 28-year-old woman with patent ductus arteriosus, suprasystemic pulmonary vascular resistance, and reversed shunt. The *upper photograph* shows the patient sitting with her hands placed on the dorsum of her feet. The right hand is acyanotic and the digits are not clubbed. The left hand is mildly cyanotic and the thumb is clubbed. The toes are cyanotic and clubbed. In the close-up (*lower photograph*), the right hand is acyanotic and the thumb is not clubbed (*arrow*). The left hand is mildly cyanotic and the thumb is clubbed (*arrow*). B, Magnetic resonance image from a 29-year-old woman with a nonrestrictive patent ductus and reversed shunt (*curved arrow*) from the pulmonary trunk (PT) through a nonrestrictive patent ductus arteriosus (PDA) into the aorta (Ao). (RV/LV = right and left ventricle.)

a mechanism that is suspected when the feet are cold. Diagnostic error is prevented by warming the extremities, which abolishes peripheral cyanosis but exaggerates central cyanosis.

The Arterial Pulse

Wide systemic arterial pulse pressure is an important physical sign of patent ductus arteriosus with a large left-to-right shunt.[157,172] The sign is especially useful in symptomatic neonates without a ductus murmur. However, the arterial pulse may be weak in preterm infants in whom systemic flow is reduced by the *steal* effect associated with aortopulmonary shunting (see earlier).[5,13,136] The typical pulse has a brisk rise, a single or bisferiens peak and a rapid collapse (Fig. 20–13). Diastolic flow from aortic root into

pulmonary trunk lowers the aortic *diastolic* pressure, and a large left ventricular stroke volume with forceful left ventricular contraction maintains or elevates aortic *systolic* pressure. The carotid, brachial, femoral, and even dorsalis pedis pulses can be bounding.[157] The superficial palmar arch as it crosses the heads of the metacarpals is sometimes evident as a strong pulsation.[187] An erythematous wheal cased by a mosquito bite blushed and blanched synchronously with the pulse in a child with a large patent ductus.[100]

The arterial pulse is usually normal when pulmonary vascular disease reverses the shunt. However, in the presence of pulmonary hypertensive pulmonary regurgitation, diastolic blood flow from the aorta through the ductus into the pulmonary artery and across the incompetent pulmonary valve into the right ventricle lowers the aortic diastolic pressure, so the pulse pressure widens.

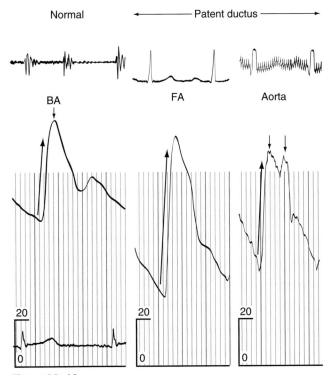

Figure 20–13
Femoral artery (FA) and central aortic pulses in two patients aged 18 months and 22 months with nonrestrictive patent ductus arteriosus and large left-to-right shunts. Pulse pressures are wide with a brisk rate of rise, a single or bisferiens (twin) peak and a rapid collapse. A normal brachial arterial pulse in the left panel is shown for comparison.

The Jugular Venous Pulse

Congestive heart failure results in an increase in mean jugular venous pressure and in the A and V waves. When suprasystemic pulmonary vascular resistance reverses the shunt, the A wave is relatively unimpressive because the right ventricle adapts to systemic vascular resistance without augmented right atrial contraction.

Precordial Movement and Palpation

A *moderately restrictive* patent ductus causes volume overload of the left ventricle with moderate pressure overload of the right ventricle. The left ventricular impulse is dynamic and the right ventricular impulse is unimpressive. George A. Gibson wrote, "When the ductus arteriosus is permanently patent, a very distinct thrill is to be felt—a thrill which distinctly follows the systole of the heart and persists until the diastolic phase has existed for some time."[74,133]

A *nonrestrictive ductus* with low pulmonary vascular resistance results in volume overload of the left ventricle and systemic systolic pressure in the right ventricle. The left ventricular impulse is hyperdynamic and the right ventricular impulse is sustained. A dilated pulmonary trunk is palpable together with a loud pulmonary closure sound. If a thrill is present, it is likely to be confined to systole (see Auscultation). When flow through the ductus is reversed, pulmonary hypertension exists without volume overload

of the left ventricle, so palpation detects only a right ventricular impulse. Symptomatic infants with a nonrestrictive patent ductus and low pulmonary vascular resistance have a hyperdynamic volume-overloaded left ventricular impulse accompanied by the conspicuous impulse of a hypertensive failing right ventricle.

Auscultation

Gibson characterized the murmur of patent ductus arteriosus[74]:

It persists through the second sound and dies away gradually during the long pause. The murmur is rough and thrilling. It begins softly and increases in intensity so as to reach its acme just about, or immediately after the incidence of the second sound, and from that point gradually wanes until its termination.

The description cannot be improved. Although Gibson was not the first to describe the continuous murmur of a patent ductus, he precisely characterized the murmur and confidently established the clinical diagnosis based on that characterization.[133] The classic murmur of uncomplicated patent ductus arteriosus rises to a peak in latter systole, continues without interruption through the second sound which it envelops, then declines in intensity during the course of diastole (Figs. 20–14 through 20–16). The murmur may be present during the entire cardiac cycle (Fig. 20–14) or there may be a

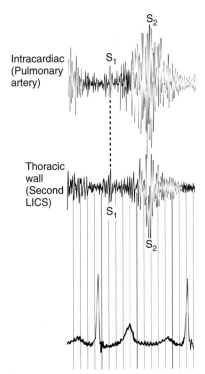

Figure 20–14
Phonocardiograms recorded simultaneously from within the pulmonary artery (PUL ART) and on the thoracic wall at the second left intercostal space (2nd LICS) of a 7-year-old girl with a moderately restrictive patent ductus arteriosus and a 2 to 1 left-to-right shunt. In Gibson's words, the murmur "begins softly and increases in intensity so as to reach its acme just about, or immediately after the incidence of the second heart sound, and from that point gradually wanes until its termination."[74]

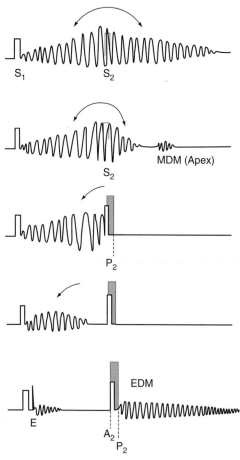

Figure 20–15

Illustrations of sequential modifications of the murmur of patent ductus from a nonpulmonary hypertensive left-to-right shunt (*above*) to a pulmonary hypertensive right-to-left shunt (*below*). MDM, mid-diastolic murmur; EDM, early diastolic murmur; A₂/P₂, aortic and pulmonary components of the second heart sound.

silent interval toward the end of diastole or immediately after the first heart sound (Fig. 20–15). The term *continuous* is best applied to the *uninterrupted* progression of a murmur through the second heart sound rather than to the presence of murmur throughout the cardiac cycle.[157] The ductus murmur is therefore continuous even when late diastole and early systole are murmur free.

High-velocity flow through a restrictive ductus generates a relatively soft high frequency continuous murmur. A moderately restrictive ductus generates a loud coarse *machinery* murmur punctuated by *eddy sounds* that are randomly distributed in the second half of systole and in the first half of diastole (Fig. 20–17A).[105,157] Intracardiac phonocardiography records the maximum intensity of the ductus murmur in the pulmonary artery at the pulmonary ostium of the ductus (see Fig. 20–14). Intraoperative phonocardiograms recorded from the surface of the pulmonary trunk show a similar localization.[129] These observations are in accord with the chest wall position of the ductus murmur, which is loudest in the first or second

intercostal space or beneath the left clavicle as Gibson originally stated.[133]

A relatively rare auscultatory variation is the intermittent disappearance and reappearance of an otherwise typical continuous ductal murmur.[113,117,177] Interruption of flow has been ascribed to acute angulations of an elongated ductus[117,177] or to a valve or veil-like structure within the ductal lumen (see earlier).[113] A similar mechanism has been proposed for the transient diastolic ductal murmur of the neonate.[152] Reappearance of a continuous murmur long after ductal closure has been ascribed to reopening caused by a tear in the valve of the ductus[197] or to spontaneous intramural dissection.[21]

The shape, length, and timing of the murmur of patent ductus arteriosus depend on instantaneous differences in pressure and flow between the aorta and pulmonary trunk (see Fig. 20–15).[97,123] At the beginning of systole, flow into the pulmonary artery is derived from the right ventricle rather than through the ductus. During the course of systole, the ductus contribution progressively increases, and during diastole flow into the pulmonary artery is from the ductus

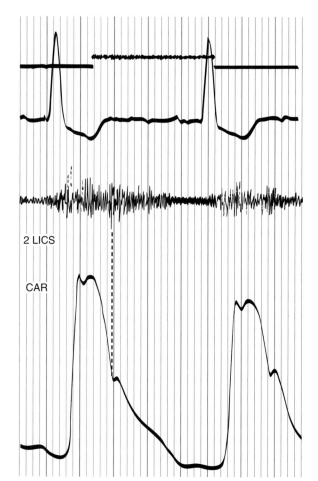

Figure 20–16

Tracings from an 84-year-old woman with a moderately restrictive patent ductus arteriosus (see x-ray in Fig. 20–38). The murmur in the second left intercostal space (2 LICS) continues through the second heart sound, which is timed by the dicrotic notch of the carotid pulse (CAR). The continuous murmur then faded, rendering late diastole murmur-free.

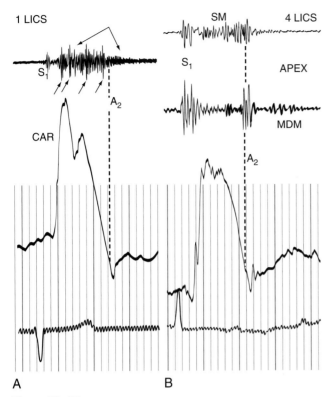

Figure 20–17

Tracings from an 18-year-old woman with a nonrestrictive patent ductus arteriosus, increased pulmonary vascular resistance, but a 2.3 to 1 left-to-right shunt. *A*, The ductus murmur in the first left intercostal space (1 LICS) continued (*paired arrows*) for a short distance after the aortic component of the second heart sound (A_2). Eddy sounds (*lower arrows*) punctuate the murmur. CAR, carotid pulse. *B*, In the fourth left intercostal space (4 LICS), the ductus murmur is holosystolic (SM) and devoid of eddy sounds. At the apex, the short low-frequency mid-diastolic murmur (MDM) was caused by augmented flow across the mitral valve.

alone.[156,157] *Systolic reinforcement* of the ductus murmur described by Skoda occurs because flow from aorta into pulmonary trunk is greater in systole, especially when the systemic pulse pressure is wide, and because systolic flow from right ventricle into pulmonary artery is reinforced by simultaneous flow from the ductus, whereas diastolic flow is derived from the ductus alone. As pulmonary vascular resistance rises, the pulmonary arterial and aortic diastolic pressures equilibrate (Fig. 20–18), diastolic ductal flow diminishes and finally vanishes, and the diastolic portion of the continuous murmur disappears, leaving a holosystolic murmur (Figs. 20–15, 20–19, and 20–20). With a further increase in pulmonary vascular resistance, the systolic portion of the ductus murmur shortens (Figs. 20–15 and 20–20) and ultimately disappears (Fig. 20–15), leaving the ductus murmur-free because right-to-left ductal flow does not generate a murmur.[156] The classic Gibson murmur is replaced by auscultatory signs of pulmonary hypertension, namely, a pulmonary ejection sound, a short pulmonary midsystolic murmur, a single or closely split second heart sound with a loud pulmonary component, and a Graham Steell murmur of hypertensive pulmonary regurgitation (Figs. 20–15 and 20–21).[156] The diagnosis of patent ductus

arteriosus cannot be based on auscultatory signs, but is confidently based on differential cyanosis (Fig. 20–12).

In the newborn, a transient systolic murmur due to left-to-right ductal flow is sometimes detected before physiologic closure.[25,28,86] The soft crescendo systolic murmur ends with the second sound or continues just beyond it.[25] These harmless transient preclosure neonatal murmurs are physiologically analogous to the not so harmless murmurs that appear when patent ductus arteriosus is accompanied by a subsequent increase in pulmonary vascular resistance. Even when a ductus is destined to remain patent, the

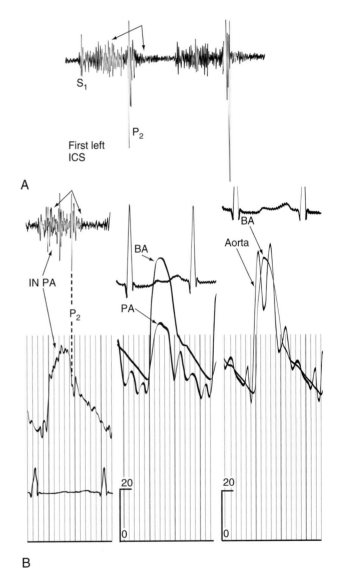

Figure 20–18

Tracings from a 15-year-old boy with a nonrestrictive patent ductus arteriosus, increased pulmonary vascular resistance, but a 2 to 1 left-to-right shunt. *A*, The ductus murmur in the first left intercostal space (ICS) continued through the timing of the second heart sound (*paired arrows*) but faded well before the subsequent first heart sound (S_1). *B*, An identical murmur was recorded within the pulmonary trunk at its bifurcation (*left panel*). The brachial arterial (BA) and pulmonary arterial (PA) pulses diverge in systole but converge in diastole (*center panel*), so the ductus murmur is maximum in systole and minimal in diastole (*left panel*). The right panel shows relatively low diastolic pressures in the brachial artery and in the aorta with a bisferiens (twin-peaked) pulse in the central aorta.

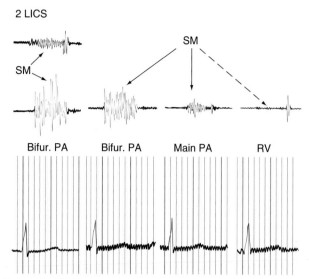

Figure 20–19

Tracings from an 11-year-old girl with a nonrestrictive patent ductus arteriosus, increased pulmonary vascular resistance, but a 2 to 1 left-to-right shunt. The first panel shows a holosystolic ductal murmur (SM) in the second left intercostal space (2 LICS) and a louder holosystolic ductal murmur recorded from within the pulmonary artery (PA) at its bifurcation. The remaining panels show the intracardiac murmur fading then vanishing as the catheter tip microphone was withdrawn from the bifurcation of the pulmonary artery to the main pulmonary artery and into the right ventricle (RV).

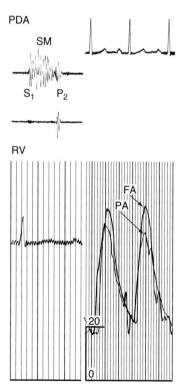

Figure 20–20

Tracings from a 3-year-old girl with a nonrestrictive patent ductus, increased pulmonary vascular resistance, but a 2.7 to 1 left-to-right shunt. The intracardiac microphone recorded a decrescendo holosystolic murmur *within the lumen* of the patent ductus arteriosus (PDA). The right ventricle (RV) was silent except for the pulmonary component of the second heart sound (P_2). The femoral arterial (FA) and pulmonary arterial (PA) pulses diverge in systole but are identical in diastole, so the ductus murmur that was confined to systole.

neonatal ductal murmur is initially systolic and becomes continuous only after pulmonary vascular resistance has fallen sufficiently to permit both systolic *and* diastolic ductal flow.

Shunt murmurs are often absent in infants with a nonrestrictive patent ductus and congestive heart failure (Fig. 20–8). Ductus murmurs are also absent in a significant number of preterm infants with respiratory distress and ductal patency.[12,145] Occasionally, a very large short ductus is devoid of murmur despite a large left-to-right shunt (Fig. 20–22).

Apical mid-diastolic murmurs are generated by increased flow across the mitral valve when the left-to-right shunt is large,[156] but these murmurs cannot not heard unless the diastolic portion of the continuous murmur is attenuated by an increase in pulmonary vascular resistance (Figs. 20–15, 20–17, and 20–23).[156] In patent ductus arteriosus with reversed shunt, a mid-diastolic murmur has been attributed to a *right-sided Austin Flint* mechanism associated with *pulmonary* regurgitation.[83] *To-and-fro murmurs* over the cranium of infants with a nonrestrictive patent ductus arteriosus have been ascribed to accelerated forward flow followed by rapid diastolic runoff.

The second heart sound is occasionally split paradoxically in the presence of a large left-to-right shunt.[82] Prolonged left ventricular ejection and short right ventricular ejection are held responsible.[82,172] The second sound is impossible to analyze because it is obscured by the continuous murmur and the eddy sounds, but an increase in pulmonary vascular resistance renders the second sound audible because the diastolic portion of the continuous murmur softens or disappears and the pulmonary component becomes louder (see Figs. 20–15, 20–17, and 20–18). When the shunt is reversed, the second sound is single or closely split, and the pulmonary component is loud (see Fig. 20–15). The second sound is widely split when depressed right ventricular contractility and prolonged right ventricular ejection delay the pulmonary component (see Figs. 20–21 and 20–22).

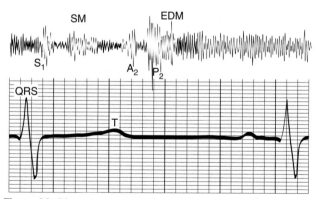

Figure 20–21

Phonocardiogram from the second left intercostal space of a 26-year-old woman with a nonrestrictive patent ductus arteriosus, suprasystemic pulmonary vascular resistance, and reversed shunt. The midsystolic murmur (SM) originated in the dilated hypertensive pulmonary trunk. The Graham Steell murmur (DM) issues from a loud delayed pulmonary component of the second heart sound (P_2). S_1, first heart sound; A_2, aortic component of the second sound.

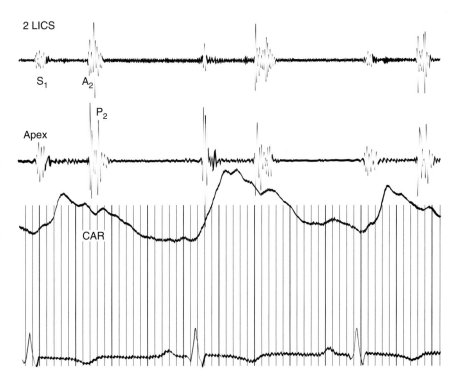

Figure 20–22

Tracings from a 30-year-old man with an unusually large short patent ductus arteriosus. Despite a 2 to 1 left-to-right shunt, a ductus murmur was neither heard nor recorded. 2 LICS, second left intercostal space. Relatively wide expiratory splitting of the second heart sound was caused by delay in the loud pulmonary component (P_2) that was transmitted to the apex. S_1, first heart sound; A_2, aortic component of the second sound; CAR, carotid pulse.

The Electrocardiogram

A *moderately restrictive* patent ductus arteriosus with increased pulmonary blood flow generates a bifid prolonged left atrial P wave in one or more limb leads and in right precordial leads (Figs. 20–24 and 20–25). Atrial fibrillation sometimes occurs in older patients.[47,134] The PR interval is prolonged in 10% to 20% of cases (Fig. 20–24).[140] The QRS axis is usually normal, but an occasional infant has right axis deviation, especially neonates with respiratory distress. Rare examples of left axis deviation have been reported,[49] and the rubella syndrome may be associated with an unusually superior QRS axis that points upward and to the left or right.[88] Volume overload of the left ventricle results in tall R waves with prominent q waves and tall peaked T waves in leads V_{5-6} (Figs. 20–25 and 20–26).

A *nonrestrictive* patent ductus with low pulmonary vascular resistance is associated with biatrial P waves and combined ventricular hypertrophy. Large equidiphasic RS complexes appear in most if not all precordial leads with tall R waves and prominent S waves in leads V_{5-6} (Figs. 20–25 and 20–26).

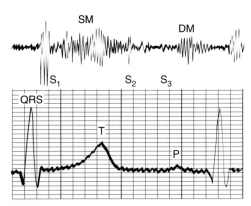

Figure 20–23

Phonocardiogram at the apex of a 5-year-old girl with a nonrestrictive patent ductus arteriosus and a 3 to 1 left-to-right shunt. The systolic portion of the ductus murmur (SM) was transmitted to the apex where a prominent mid-diastolic murmur (DM) was caused by augmented flow across the mitral valve.

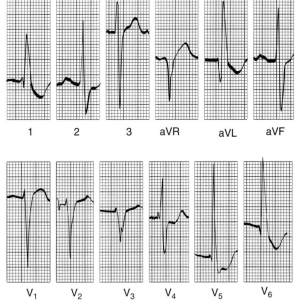

Figure 20–24

Electrocardiogram from a 37-year-old woman with a moderately restrictive patent ductus arteriosus, a 2.8 to 1 left-to-right shunt, and a pulmonary artery pressure of 48/18 mm Hg. (see x-ray in Fig. 20–32). A broad bifid left atrial P wave is present in lead 2. The PR interval is 200 msec. The QRS is prolonged and the axis is horizontal. Left ventricular volume overload is manifested by prominent q waves in leads aVL and V_6 and by tall R waves and ST-T wave changes in lead aVL and in leads V_{5-6}.

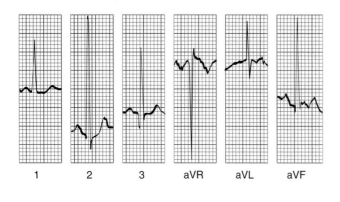

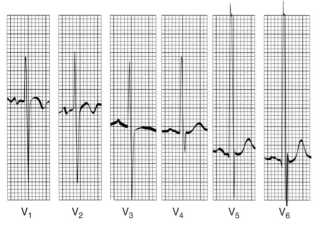

Figure 20–25

Electrocardiogram from a 19-month-old boy with a moderately restrictive patent ductus arteriosus, a 3 to 1 left-to-right shunt, and a pulmonary arterial pressure of 45/22 mm Hg. (see x-ray in Fig. 20–31). Biphasic left atrial P waves appear in leads V_{1-2}. The QRS axis is normal, so tall R waves of left ventricular volume overload appear in leads 2 and aVF. Volume overload of the left ventricle is also manifested by tall R waves and upright T waves in leads V_{5-6}. Right ventricular hypertrophy is manifested by prominent S waves in leads V_{5-6} and a prominent R wave in lead V_1. Leads V_{2-3} are half standardized and exhibit large RS complexes of biventricular hypertrophy.

Patent ductus with *pulmonary vascular disease and reversed shunt* is accompanied by peaked right atrial P waves in leads 2, 3, and V_1 (Fig. 20–27), and right ventricular hypertrophy manifested by right axis deviation, tall R waves in lead V_1 with inverted right precordial T waves, and prominent S waves in left precordial leads (see Fig. 20–27). R waves in leads V_{5-6} imply that a left-to-right shunt previously existed (see Fig. 20–27).

The X-Ray

The ductus itself is sometimes seen in the frontal projection as an inconspicuous soft convexity between the aortic knob and the pulmonary artery segment (Figs. 20–5*A* and 20–28).[186] A striking exaggeration of this inconspicuous shadow is an aneurysm of a nonpatent ductus (see Fig. 20–6).[62] Calcium appears in the ductus of older patients (Figs. 20–29 and 20–38*A*).[31,47,50]

A *moderately restrictive* patent ductus with low pulmonary vascular resistance results in increased pulmonary arterial vascularity, enlargement of the pulmonary trunk

and its proximal branches, and enlargement of the left atrium and left ventricle (Figs. 20–30, 20–31, and 20–32).[186] Asymmetric pulmonary vascularity is occasionally associated with a hyperlucent left lung.[174] The ascending aorta in infants is inconspicuous because intrauterine ductal flow excludes the aorta (see Figs. 20–5 and 20–30). After birth, left-to-right ductal flow recirculates through the aortic root, so the ascending aorta becomes prominent (see Fig. 20–3).[38] The x-ray of a *nonrestrictive* patent ductus in infants and children with low pulmonary vascular resistance exhibits a marked increase in pulmonary arterial vascularity with enlargement of all four cardiac chambers (Fig. 20–33).

The x-ray with a *nonrestrictive patent ductus and reversed shunt* exhibits reduced pulmonary vascularity, dilatation of the pulmonary trunk and its proximal branches, a normal or near normal left ventricle and left atrium, and an hypertrophied right ventricle that is not significantly dilated (Fig. 20–34).

The Echocardiogram

Echocardiography with color flow imaging and Doppler interrogation establishes the size of the patent ductus

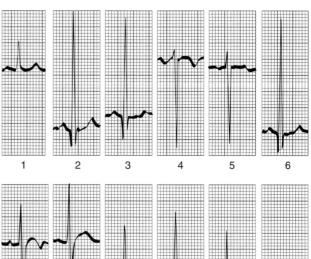

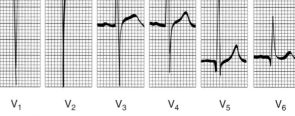

Figure 20–26

Electrocardiogram from a 16-year-old boy with a moderately restrictive patent ductus arteriosus, pulmonary artery pressure of 80/50 mm Hg, and a 2 to 1 left-to-right shunt. The QRS axis is normal and depolarization is clockwise, so prominent q waves and tall R waves of left ventricular volume overload appear in leads 2, 3, and aVF. Volume overload of the left ventricle is also manifested by the deep S wave in lead V_1 and by prominent q waves, tall R waves, and peaked upright T waves in leads V_{5-6}. Biventricular hypertrophy is reflected in the large RS complexes in leads V_{2-4}, which are half standardized.

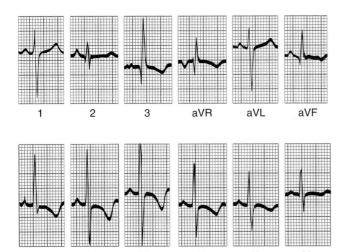

Figure 20–27

Electrocardiogram from a 28-year-old woman with a nonrestrictive patent ductus, suprasystemic pulmonary vascular resistance, and reversed shunt. Peaked right atrial P waves are present in lead 2 and leads V_{1-2}. Isolated right ventricular hypertrophy is manifested by right axis deviation, tall monophasic R waves and inverted T waves in leads V_{1-4} and prominent S waves in left precordial leads.

(Fig. 20–35), the flow dynamics through the ductus, and the physiologic consequences of persistent ductal patency.[97,104,106,110,123,183,192,196,204] Transesophageal echocardiography improves diagnostic accuracy.[127] When the shunt is entirely left-to-right, the flow disturbance within the ductus is continuous with peak velocity reinforced in latter systole because forward flow from the right ventricle coincides with shunt flow through the ductus (Fig. 20–36).[97,104,123] Systolic forward flow in the aorta distal to the orifice of the ductus is followed by reversed diastolic flow (Fig. 20–37). Velocities across the aortic isthmus and in the descending aorta are substantially increased in the presence of large ductal flow.[17] The color flow pattern in the pulmonary trunk consists of a ductal jet that adheres to the lateral wall, travels toward the pulmonary valve, and then reverses itself to travel up the medial wall (Fig. 20–38). Alternatively, a jet directed toward the pulmonary valve adheres to the medial wall of the pulmonary trunk (Fig. 20–39).

Color flow imaging with Doppler interrogation identifies the clinically silent nonrestrictive patent ductus in premature infants,[89,195,204] and identifies the tiny clinically silent ductus in older patients (Fig. 20–40).[103] *In utero* ductal closure is recognized by fetal echocardiography.[121,141] The reversed shunt in a nonrestrictive patent ductus with suprasystemic pulmonary vascular resistance can be identified with Doppler interrogation[97,104] and contrast echocardiography.[146] Right ventricular systolic pressure and pulmonary artery diastolic pressure can be estimated by continuous-wave Doppler interrogation of the jets of tricuspid and pulmonary regurgitation and by Doppler velocities across the ductus.

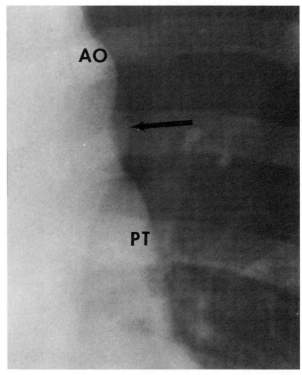

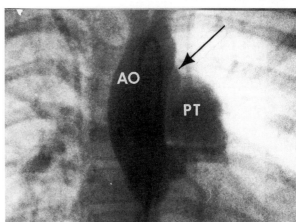

Figure 20–28

A, Close-up of a portion of the chest x-ray in the 14-year-old girl whose aortogram is shown in Figure 20–3. The soft convex shadow of the patent ductus (*black arrow*) is located between the aortic knuckle (AO) and pulmonary trunk (PT). The convex shadow represents the dilated aortic end of the conical ductus shown in the aortogram of Fig. 20–3. *B,* Aortogram in a 5-year-old girl with the convex shadow of a conical ductus (*arrow*) located between the aortic knuckle (AO) and the pulmonary trunk (PT). Compare with Figure 20–4.

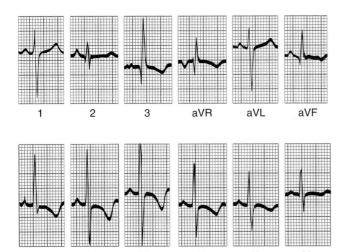

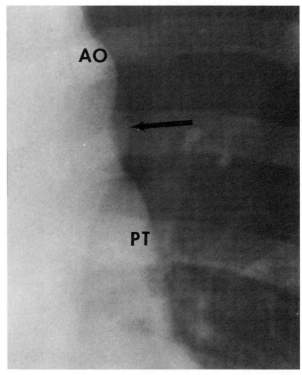

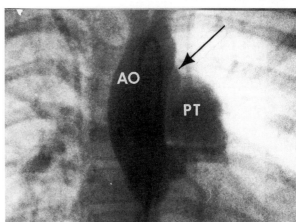

Summary

Clinical suspicion of patent ductus arteriosus is heightened by premature birth, maternal rubella, or birth at high altitude. The clinical signs are unmistakable in the majority of patients with a *moderately restrictive* patent ductus. The arterial pulse is brisk, the pulse pressure is wide, the left ventricular impulse is dynamic, and auscultation detects the distinctive continuous murmur that peaks around the second heart sound and is punctuated by eddy sounds. The electrocardiogram shows volume overload of

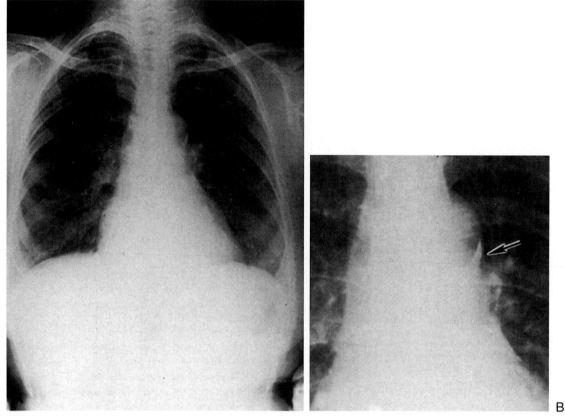

Figure 20–29

X-ray from a 63-year-old woman with a restrictive patent ductus and a left-to-right shunt of 1.3 to 1. Ductal calcification is represented by the comma-like density between the aortic knuckle and the main pulmonary artery segment. The right panel is a close-up of ductal calcification (*arrow*). The x-ray is otherwise normal.

the left ventricle, and the x-ray shows increased pulmonary arterial vascularity with enlargement of the left ventricle, left atrium, ascending aorta, and pulmonary trunk. Echocardiography with color flow imaging and Doppler interrogation establishes the size of the ductus, the flow dynamics

within the ductus and within the contiguous aorta and pulmonary trunk, and establishes the hemodynamic consequences of ductal patency.

A *nonrestrictive* patent ductus with low pulmonary vascular resistance presents in infancy with con-

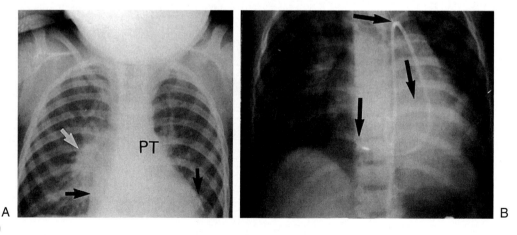

Figure 20–30

X-rays from a 13-month-old girl with a moderately restrictive patent ductus arteriosus, pulmonary artery pressure of 39/15 mm Hg, and a 2.3 to 1 left-to-right shunt. *A*, Pulmonary vascularity is increased, the pulmonary trunk (PT) and its right branch (*white arrow*) are prominent, but the ascending aorta is inconspicuous. The left cardiac border formed by a dilated left ventricle (*vertical black arrow*) and the right cardiac border is formed by a dilated right atrium (*horizontal black arrow*). *B*, A femoral artery catheter passed through the ductus at first acute bend (*upper horizontal arrow*), then into the pulmonary trunk across the pulmonary valve into the right ventricle (*right vertical arrow*), and finally across the tricuspid valve into the right atrium where the tip lies (*left vertical arrow*).

Figure 20–31

X-rays from the 19-month-old boy with a nonrestrictive patent ductus arteriosus and a 3 to 1 left-to-right shunt. The electrocardiogram is shown in Figure 20–25. *A,* The increased pulmonary vascularity is both arterial and venous. The pulmonary trunk (PT) and its right branch (*arrow*) are dilated. The apex is formed by an enlarged left ventricle (LV), and the right cardiac border is formed by a dilated right atrium (RA). *B,* The lateral barium esophagram shows a moderately enlarged left atrium (LA).

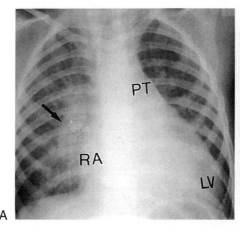
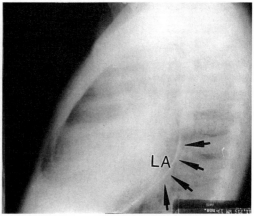

gestive heart failure. An incriminating ductus murmur is often absent, but the arterial pulses are bounding and the left and right ventricular impulses are hyperdynamic. Echocardiography establishes the diagnosis.

A *nonrestrictive* patent ductus with suprasystemic pulmonary vascular resistance and *reversed* shunt is recognized by distinctive differential cyanosis even though the ductus murmur is absent. The toes are cyanosed and clubbed, but the fingers are spared. The physical signs are those of pure pulmonary hypertension. The electrocardiogram shows right ventricular hypertrophy with little or no volume overload of the left ventricle. The x-ray exhibits normal or reduced pulmonary vascularity, dilatation of the pulmonary trunk, and an otherwise unimpressive cardiac silhouette. Echocardiography with color flow and contrast imaging confirms the diagnosis.

Aortopulmonary Window

In 1830, Professor John Elliotson in a lecture delivered at St. Thomas Hospital, London, described the first known case of aortopulmonary window.[58] This uncommon malformation consists of a communication, usually nonrestrictive, between adjacent walls of the ascending aorta and pulmonary trunk.[19,22,148,167] During early embryogenesis, two opposing proximal truncal cushions rapidly enlarge and fuse to form the *truncal septum* that separates the truncus arteriosus into aortic and pulmonary channels.[119,194] The more distal truncoaortic sac is then divided by the *aortopulmonary septum*. Maldevelopment of the truncal and aortopulmonary septum defines three morphologic types of aortopulmonary windows.[119] *First,* nonfusion of the embryonic aortopulmonary septum and the truncal septum results

Figure 20–32

A, X-rays from a 37-year-old woman with a moderately restrictive patent ductus and a 2.8 to 1 left-to-right shunt. The electrocardiogram is shown in Figure 20–24. Pulmonary vascularity is increased, the pulmonary trunk (PT) is prominent, the apex is occupied by a dilated convex left ventricle (LV), and the right cardiac border is formed by a dilated right atrium (RA). *B,* Lateral barium esophagram shows enlargement of the left atrium.

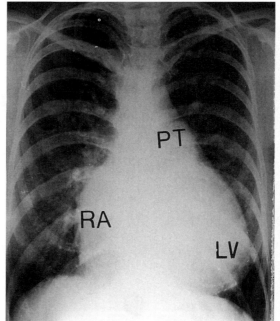
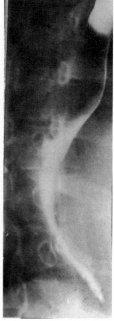

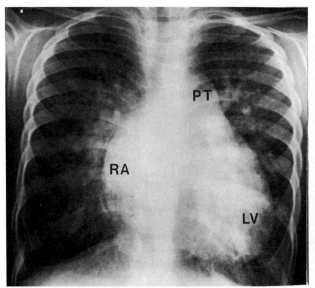

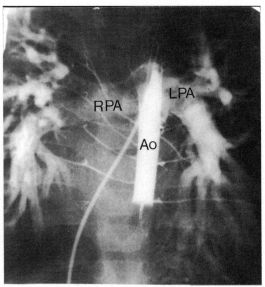

Figure 20–33

A, X-ray from a 3-year-old boy with a nonrestrictive patent ductus arteriosus, low pulmonary vascular resistance, and a 3 to 1 left-to-right shunt. Angiocardiograms are shown in Figure 20–5. Pulmonary blood flow is increased, the pulmonary trunk (PT) is dilated, an enlarged left ventricle (LV) occupies the apex, and an enlarged right atrium (RA) forms the right cardiac border. *B,* Right pulmonary artery (RPA) and left pulmonary artery (LPA) visualized through the patent ductus after contrast material was injected into the balloon-occluded descending aorta (Ao). The size of the intrapulmonary arteries was appreciably increased. Compare to the increased pulmonary vascularity in *panel A.*

in a circular moderate-sized defect located about midway between the great arterial valves and the bifurcation of the pulmonary trunk. *Second,* malalignment of the embryonic aortopulmonary septum and the truncal septum results in a defect that is similarly located but is helical rather than circular. *Third,* complete absence of the embryonic aortopulmonary septum results in a nonrestrictive defect. Although the morphogenesis of an aortopulmonary window is unrelated to the morphogenesis of a patent ductus arteriosus, the clinical manifestations and physiologic consequences of the two malformations are similar if not identical,[22,143,148,166] so inclusion of aortopulmonary window in this chapter is appropriate.

Coexisting anomalies are rare, with patent ductus arteriosus the most common, estimated at 12% (see Fig.

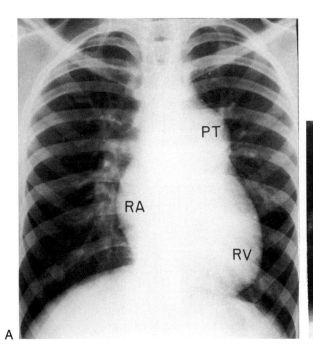

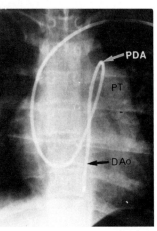

Figure 20–34

X-rays from a 14-year-old boy with a nonrestrictive patent ductus arteriosus, suprasystemic pulmonary vascular resistance, and reversed shunt. *A,* Pulmonary vascularity is decreased. The pulmonary trunk (PT) and its proximal branches are dilated, the hypertrophied right ventricle (RV) forms an acute angle with the left hemidiaphragm, and the right atrium (RA) is prominent. *B,* A catheter from the left median basilic vein entered the pulmonary trunk (PT), crossed the ductus (PDA), and came to rest in the descending aorta (DAo). The course of the catheter represents the pathway taken by unoxygenated blood through a reversed ductal shunt (see Figs. 20–2 *lower* and 20–12A).

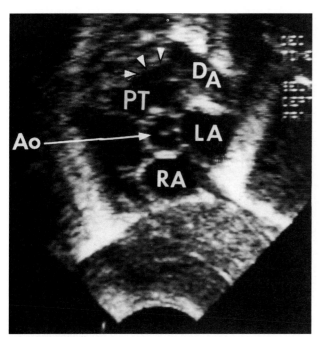

Figure 20–35
Echocardiogram showing a moderately restrictive patent ductus arteriosus (*three arrowheads*) in a 2-month-old infant. Ao, aortic valve; PT, pulmonary trunk; DA, descending aorta; RA/LA, right atrium and left atrium.

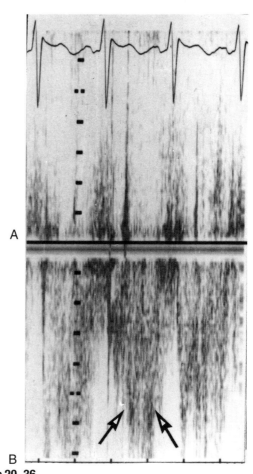

Figure 20–36
Continuous-wave Doppler from a 7-month-old girl with a moderately restrictive patent ductus arteriosus and a 3 to 1 left-to-right shunt. Peak ductal flow is in mid to late systole and then continues throughout diastole (*lower paired arrows*).

20–45).[44,148,166] Because an aortopulmonary window tends to be nonrestrictive, it is most often mistaken for a nonrestrictive ductus. When pulmonary vascular resistance is suprasystemic and the shunt is reversed, the clinical picture is indistinguishable from a nonrestrictive ventricular septal defect with Eisenmenger syndrome (see Chapter 17).[202] Aortopulmonary window and ventricular septal defect rarely coexist.[19,189]

Aortopulmonary window is somewhat more frequent in males in contrast to patent ductus.[143] Infective endocarditis is rare.[22,143] An appreciable percentage of infants with a nonrestrictive aortopulmonary window die of congestive heart failure in infancy or early childhood.[22,143,148,181,184] Although only a minority reach teenage or young adulthood, occasional survivals have been reported in the fourth or fifth decade[56,143,148] with survival favored by a rise in pulmonary vascular resistance or by a restrictive defect. The patient referred to in Figure 20–45 lived to age 58 years with an aortopulmonary window and Eisenmenger syndrome.

A bounding arterial pulse and wide pulse pressure are analogous to the arterial pulse in a nonrestrictive patent ductus with low pulmonary vascular resistance (Fig. 20–41).[19,44,148] When an aortopulmonary window exists with suprasystemic pulmonary vascular resistance and reversed shunt, unoxygenated blood enters the ascending aorta, so differential cyanosis does not occur. The clinical picture is then indistinguishable from nonrestrictive ventricular septal defect with Eisenmenger syndrome (see Chapter 17).

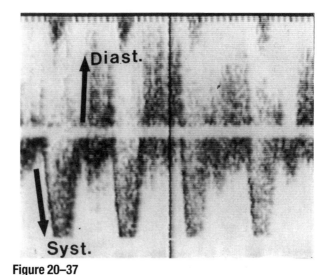

Figure 20–37
Pulsed Doppler from a 6-month-old girl with a moderately restrictive patent ductus arteriosus and a 2.8 to 1 left-to-right shunt. Sample volume in the descending aorta distal to the ductus recorded systolic flow (Syst) *down* the aorta and diastolic flow (Diast) in the opposite direction.

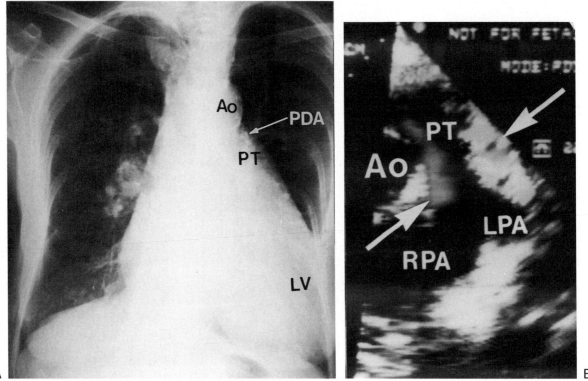

Figure 20–38

A, X-ray from the 84-year-old woman with a moderately restrictive patent ductus arteriosus (PDA) whose phonocardiogram is shown in Figure 20–16. The pulmonary trunk (PT) and its right branch are dilated. A thin rim of calcium appears in the transverse aorta (Ao). An enlarged left ventricle (LV) is at the apex, and an enlarged right atrium occupies the lower right cardiac border. *B,* Black-and-white print of a color flow image in the short axis. Ductal flow adheres to the lateral wall of the pulmonary trunk (*PT right arrow*), travels downward toward the pulmonary valve, and then upward along the medial wall of the pulmonary trunk (*left arrow*). RPA/LPA, right and left pulmonary artery; Ao, aorta.

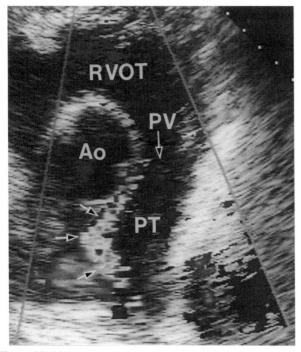

Figure 20–39

Black-and-white print of a color flow image from a 64-year-old man with a restrictive patent ductus arteriosus. Ductal flow (*three left arrows*) tracks along the medial wall of the pulmonary trunk (PT) downward toward the pulmonary valve (PV). RVOT, right ventricular outflow tract; Ao, aorta.

The physiologic mechanisms responsible for variations in the murmur of a nonrestrictive aortopulmonary window are analogous to the mechanisms that apply to nonrestrictive patent ductus arteriosus (see Fig. 20–15).[19] In 80% of patients, the murmur is systolic rather than continuous[143,148] (see Fig. 20–41) and is punctuated by eddy sounds (see Fig. 20–41). When a continuous murmur is present it is likely to be shortened (Fig. 20–42). A *moderately restrictive* aortopulmonary window generates a continuous murmur indistinguishable from the continuous murmur of a moderately restrictive patent ductus arteriosus.[19,44,75,143,148,178]

A nonrestrictive aortopulmonary window with *suprasystemic pulmonary vascular resistance and reversed shunt* is accompanied by auscultatory signs of pulmonary hypertension. No murmur is generated across the defect, but a Graham Steell murmur may appear before the shunt is reversed because of the considerable dilatation of the hypertensive pulmonary trunk.[19,75,148,181]

Systolic or continuous murmurs generated by an aortopulmonary window are typically maximum in the third left intercostal space.[22,44,56] A prominent *systolic* murmur at the mid to lower left sternal border invites the

Figure 20–40

A, Black-and-white print of a color flow image from a 35-year-old man with a tiny clinically silent patent ductus arteriosus. His daughter had a moderately restrictive patent ductus. *Paired arrows* identify ductal flow entering the pulmonary trunk (PT) immediately distal to the left pulmonary artery (LPA) and tracking along the medial wall of the pulmonary trunk toward the right ventricular outflow tract (RVOT). Ao, aorta. *B*, Lateral aortogram showing a conical ductus arteriosus (PDA) that was patent at its aortic end (Ao *paired white arrows*) but was a virtual thread at its pulmonary arterial end. LSA, left subclavian artery.

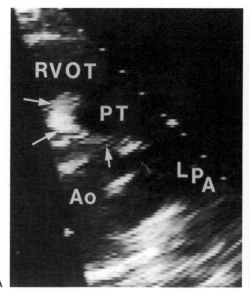
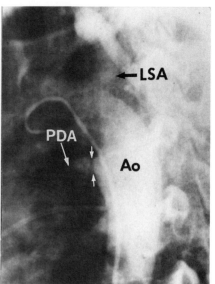

mistaken diagnosis of ventricular septal defect, but eddy sounds and a bounding arterial pulse should prevent this error (see Fig. 20–41). Apical mid-diastolic murmurs represent increased flow across the mitral valve (see Fig. 20–42).

The *electrocardiogram* of a nonrestrictive aortopulmonary window with low pulmonary vascular resistance reflects combined ventricular hypertrophy with volume overload of the left ventricle and pressure overload of the right ventricle analogous to a nonrestrictive patent ductus

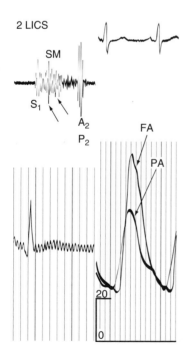

Figure 20–41

Tracings from a 2-year-old boy with an aortopulmonary window and a 3.4 to 1 left-to-right shunt. The phonocardiogram in the second left intercostal space (2 LICS) shows a decrescendo holosystolic murmur (SM) punctuated by eddy sounds (*paired arrows*). The single second heart sound is loud because the pulmonary component (P_2) was increased. The femoral (FA) and pulmonary arterial (PA) pressure pulses diverge in systole but are identical in diastole, so the murmur is confined to systole. S_1, first heart sound; A_2, aortic component of the second sound.

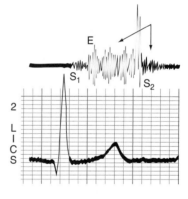
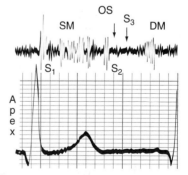

Figure 20–42

Phonocardiograms from a 14-year-old boy with an aortopulmonary window and a 3 to 1 left-to-right shunt. The systolic murmur (SM) in the second left intercostal space (2 LICS) continues (see *paired arrows*) just beyond the second heart sound (S_2). E, pulmonary ejection sound. At the apex, a soft third heart sound (S_3) and a mid-diastolic murmur (DM) were due to increased flow across the mitral valve, and there was a faint mitral opening sound (OS).

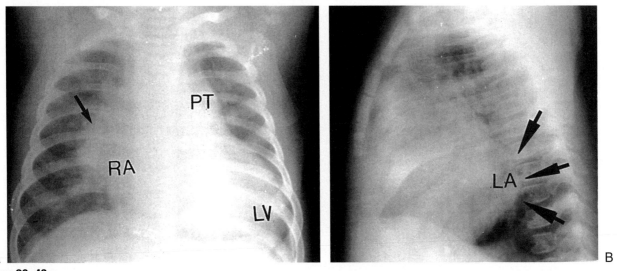

Figure 20–43

X-rays from a 5-month-old girl with an aortopulmonary window and a 3.5 to 1 left-to-right shunt. *A,* Pulmonary vascularity is increased, pulmonary venous congestion is evident at the right hilus (*arrow*), the pulmonary trunk (PT) is prominent, and a dilated left ventricle LV) occupies the apex. *B,* Lateral view shows an enlarged left atrium (LA).

with low pulmonary vascular resistance (see Fig. 20–25). When pulmonary vascular resistance is suprasystemic with reversed shunt, the electrocardiogram is analogous to nonrestrictive patent ductus with Eisenmenger syndrome (see Fig. 20–27).

The x-ray does not distinguish a nonrestrictive aortopulmonary window with low pulmonary vascular resistance from a nonrestrictive patent ductus with large left-to-right shunt (Figs. 20–43 and 20–44).[19] When the shunt is reversed (Fig. 20–45), the x-ray resembles a non-

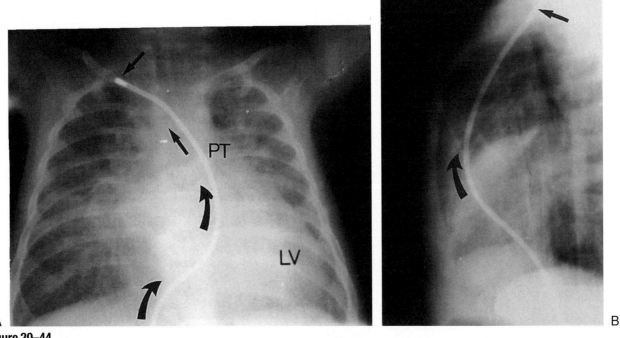

Figure 20–44

X rays from a 6-month-old boy with an aortopulmonary window and a 3.5 to 1 left-to-right shunt. *A,* Pulmonary arterial and pulmonary venous vascularity are markedly increased. A dilated left ventricle (LV) occupies the apex. The course of the femoral venous catheter is into the right atrium (*lower left arrow*), across the right ventricular outflow tract into the pulmonary trunk (PT), through the aortopulmonary window into the ascending aorta (*smaller oblique arrow*), and into the right subclavian artery (*upper arrow*). *B,* The lateral projection shows the catheter passing from pulmonary trunk (*curved arrow*) across the aortopulmonary window into the aorta and into the right subclavian artery (*upper arrow*).

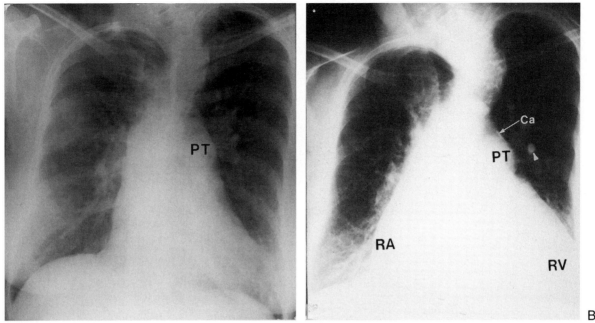

Figure 20–45

A, X-ray from a 51-year-old cyanotic woman with an aortopulmonary window, suprasystemic pulmonary vascular resistance, and reversed shunt. Pulmonary vascularity is normal. The pulmonary trunk (PT) and its proximal branches are moderately enlarged, but the cardiac size and configuration are virtually normal. *B,* X-ray 5 years later after the advent of atrial fibrillation. The right ventricle (RV) and right atrium (RA) are markedly dilated. The rim of calcium (Ca) above the dilated pulmonary trunk (PT) proved to lie in a restrictive patent ductus. The *unmarked arrowhead* adjacent to the pulmonary trunk identifies the cross section of a dilated intrapulmonary artery. The patient died in her 58th year.

restrictive patent ductus with right-to-left shunt (see Fig. 20–34).

Echocardiography localizes the aortopulmonary window between the ascending aorta and the pulmonary trunk just proximal to the bifurcation[7,166,176] (Fig. 20–46) and determines whether a patent ductus coexists. Color flow imaging identifies the shunt as left-to-right, right-to-left (Fig. 20–47), or bidirectional.

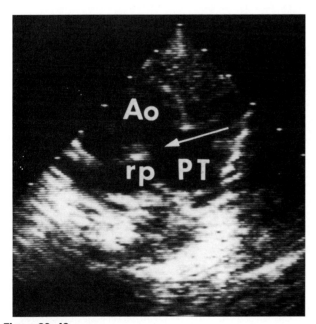

Figure 20–46

Echocardiogram (parasternal short-axis) from a 5-month-old girl with an aortopulmonary window (*arrow*) between the ascending aorta (Ao) and the pulmonary trunk (PT). rp, right pulmonary artery.

SUMMARY

Aortopulmonary window is an uncommon malformation that should be considered in acyanotic patients with clinical evidence of a nonrestrictive patent ductus arteriosus and a large left-to-right shunt. The murmur is usually systolic rather than continuous and is maximum in the third left intercostal space. The relatively low location of the murmur arouses suspicion of ventricular septal defect, but eddy sounds and a bounding arterial pulse prevent this error. A restrictive aortopulmonary window exhibits a continuous murmur and clinical signs indistinguishable from a restrictive patent ductus arteriosus except for the relatively low precordial location of the murmur. An aortopulmonary window with suprasystemic pulmonary vascular resistance and reversed shunt is clinically indistinguishable from a nonrestrictive ventricular septal defect with Eisenmenger syndrome. Echocardiography with color flow imaging and Doppler interrogation make the distinction.

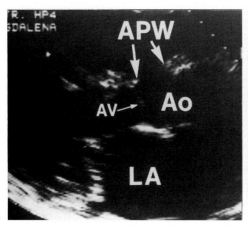
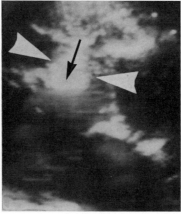

A
B

Figure 20–47

A, Echocardiogram (parasternal long-axis) from the 51-year-old patient whose x-rays are shown in Figure 20–45. *A*, *Paired arrows* identify the aortopulmonary window (APW). Ao, aorta; AV, aortic valve; LA, left atrium. *B*, Black-and-white print of a parasternal long-axis color flow image. Large arrowheads bracket a right-to-left shunt (*black arrow*) through the aortopulmonary window.

REFERENCES

1. Adams FH, Diehl A, Jorgens J, Veasy LG: Right heart catheterization in patent ductus arteriosus and aortic-pulmonary septal defect. J. Pediatr. 40:49, 1952.
2. Aiken JE, Bifulco E, Sullivan JJ Jr: Patent ductus arteriosus in the aged. Report of this disease in a 74 year old female. JAMA 177:330, 1961.
3. Wilkins JL: Risks to offspring of patients with patent ductus arteriosus. J. Med. Genet. 6:1, 1969.
4. Alter BP, Czapek EE, Rowe RD: Sweating in congenital heart disease. Pediatrics 41:123, 1968.
5. Alverson DC, Eldridge MW, Johnson JD, et al: Effect of patent ductus arteriosus on left ventricular output in premature infants. J. Pediatr. 102:754, 1983.
6. Alzamora-Castro V, Battilana G, Abugattas R, Sialer S: Patent ductus arteriosus and high altitude. Am. J. Cardiol. 5:761, 1960.
7. Garver KA, Hernandez RJ, Vermillion RP, Martin GM: Correlative imaging of aortopulmonary window: Demonstration with echocardiography, angiography, and MRI. Circulation 96:1036, 1997.
8. Anderson RC: Causative factors of congenital malformations. Patent ductus arteriosus. Pediatrics 14:143, 1954.
9. Anderson RC, Adams P, Jr, Varco RL: Patent ductus arteriosus with reversal of flow. Clinical study of ten children. Pediatrics 18:410, 1956.
10. Arcilla RA, Thilenius OG, Ranninger K: Congestive heart failure from suspected ductal closure in utero. J. Pediatr. 75:74, 1969.
11. Bain CWC: Longevity in patent ductus arteriosus. Br. Heart J. 19:574, 1957.
12. Baylen BG, Meyer RA, Korfhagen J, et al: Left ventricular performance in the critically ill premature infant with patent ductus arteriosus and pulmonary disease. Circulation 55:182, 1977.
13. Baylen BG, Ogata H, Ikegami M, et al: Left ventricular performance and regional blood flows before and after ductus arteriosus occlusion in premature lambs treated with surfactant. Circulation 67:837, 1983.
14. Bejar R, Merritt TA, Coen RW, et al: Pulsatility index, patent ductus arteriosus and brain damage. Pediatrics 69:818, 1982.
15. Benn J: The prognosis of patent ductus arteriosus. Br. Heart J. 9:283, 1947.
16. Berry TE, Muster AJ, Paul MH: Transient neonatal tricuspid regurgitation: Possible relation with premature closure of the ductus arteriosus. J. Am. Coll. Cardiol. 2:1178, 1983.
17. Guntheroth WG, Forster FK. Large ductal flow may cause high velocity in the descending aorta without coarctation. Am. J. Cardiol. 87:493, 2001.
18. Bishop, R. C.: Delayed closure of ductus arteriosus. Am. Heart J. 44:639, 1952.
19. Blieden, L. C., and Moller, J. H.: Aorticopulmonary septal defect. Br. Heart J. 36:630, 1974.
20. Boe, J., and Humerfelt, S.: Patent ductus arteriosus Botalli in an octogenarian followed for fifty years. Acta Med. Scand. 167:73, 1960.
21. Borow, K. M., Hessel, S. J., and Sloss, L. J.: Fistulous aneurysm of ductus arteriosus. Br. Heart J. 45:467, 1981.
22. Bosher, L. H., Jr., and McCue, C. M.: Diagnosis and surgical treatment of aortopulmonary fenestration. Circulation 25:456, 1962.
23. Boulay, R. J.: Patent ductus arteriosus in identical twins. Am. J. Cardiol. 7:270, 1961.
24. Glancy D.L., Wegman M., Dhurandhar R.W.: Aortic dissection and patent ductus arteriosus in three generations. Am J Cardiol 87:813, 2001.
25. Braudo, M., and Rowe, R. D.: Auscultation of the heart-early neonatal period. Am. J. Dis. Child. 101:67, 1961.
26. Dyamenahalli U, Smallhorn JF, Geva T, Fouron J, Cairns P, Jutras L, Hughes V, Rabinovitch M. Isolated ductus arteriosus aneurysm in the fetus and infant: A multi-institutional experience. J. Am. Coll. Cardiol. 36:262, 2000.
27. Burman, D.: Familial patent ductus arteriosus. Br. Heart J. 23:603, 1961.
28. Burnard, E. D.: A murmur from the ductus arteriosus in the newborn baby. Br. Med. J. 1:806, 1958.
29. Butler, L. J., Snodgrass, G. J., France, N. E., Sinclair, L., and Russell, A.: Trisomy syndrome: Analysis of thirteen cases. Arch. Dis. Child. 40:600, 1965.
30. Calder, L., Van Praagh, R., Van Praagh, S., Sears, W. P., Corwin, R., Levy, A., Keith, J. D., and Paul, M. H.: Truncus arteriosus communis. Am. Heart J., 92:23, 1976.
31. Calne, D. B., and Raftery, E. B.: Patent ductus arteriosus in an elderly man. Br. Heart J. 28:716, 1966.
32. Campbell, M.: Patent ductus arteriosus. Some notes on prognosis and on pulmonary hypertension. Br. Heart J. 17:511, 1955.
33. Campbell, M.: Place of maternal rubella in the aetiology of congenital heart disease. Br. Med. J. 1:691, 1961.
34. Campbell, M.: Natural history of patent ductus arteriosus. Br. Heart J. 30:4, 1968.
35. Campbell, M., and Hudson, R.: Patent ductus arteriosus with reversed shunt due to pulmonary hypertension. Guy's Hosp. Rep. 100:26, 1951.
36. Campbell, M., and Hudson, R.: The disappearance of the continuous murmur of patent ductus arteriosus. Guy's Hosp. Rep. 101:32, 1952.
37. Cargren, L. E.: The incidence of congenital heart disease in children born in Gothenburg 1941–1950. Br. Heart J. 21:40, 1959.
38. Castellanos, A., and Hernandez, F. A.: Size of ascending aorta in congenital cardiac lesions. Acta Radiol. 6:49, 1967.
39. Castiglioni, A.: A History of Medicine. New York, Alfred A. Knopf, 1947.
40. Chiles, N. H., Smith, H. L., Christensen, N. A., and Geraci, J. E.: Spontaneous healing of subacute bacterial endarteritis with closure of patent ductus arteriosus. Proc. Staff Meet. Mayo Clin. 28:520, 1953.
41. Clyman, R. I., and Heymann, M. A.: Pharmacology of the ductus arteriosus. Pediatr. Clin. North Am. 28:77, 1981.
42. Clyman, R. I., Campbell, D., Heymann, M. A., and Mauray, F.: Persistent responsiveness of the neonatal ductus arteriosus in immature lambs. Circulation 71:141, 1985.
43. Clyman, R. I., Mauray, F., Roman, C., Heymann, M. A., and Payne, B.: Factors determining the loss of ductus arteriosus responsiveness to prostaglandin E. Circulation 68:433, 1983.
44. Coleman, E. N., Barclay, R. S., Reid, J. M., and Stevenson, J. G.: Congenital aorto-pulmonary fistula combined with patent ductus arteriosus. Br. Heart J. 29:571, 1967.
45. Tananari Y, Maeno Y, Takagishi T, Sagaguri Y, Morimatsu M, Kato H. Role of apoptosis in the closure of neonatal ductus arteriosus. Jpn Circ J 64, 684, 2000.
46. Collett, R. W., and Edwards, J. E.: Persistent truncus arteriosus: Classification according to anatomic types. Surg. Clin. North Am. 29:1245, 1949.

47. Cosh, J. A.: Patent ductus arteriosus. A follow-up study of 73 cases. Br. Heart J. 19:13, 1957.

48. Cruikshank, B., and Marquis, R. M.: Spontaneous aneurysm of the ductus arteriosus. A review and report of the tenth adult case. Am. J. Med. 25:140, 1958.

49. Cruze, K., Elliott, L. P., Schiebler, G. L., and Wheat, M. W.: Unusual manifestations of patent ductus arteriosus in infancy. Dis. Chest 43:563, 1963.

50. Currarino, G., and Jackson, J. H.: Calcification of ductus arteriosus and ligamentum Botalli. Radiology 94:139, 1970.

51. Carboni MP, Ringel RE. Ductus arteriosus in premature infants beyond the second week of life. Pediatr Cardiol. 18:372, 1997.

52. Dailey, F. H., Genovese, P. D., and Behnke, R. H.: Patent ductus arteriosus with reversal of flow in adults. Ann. Intern. Med. 56:865, 1962.

53. Danilowicz, D., Rudolph, A. M., and Hoffman, J. I. E.: Delayed closure of the ductus arteriosus in premature infants. Pediatrics 37:74, 1966.

54. Davies, D. H., and Gazetopoulos, N.: Dyspnoea and differential hypercapnia in the "Eisenmenger ductus." Guy's Hosp. Rep. 115:175, 1966.

55. D'Heer, H. A. H., and van Nieuwenhuizen, C. L. C.: Diagnosis of congenital aortic septal defects. Description of two cases and special emphasis on a new method which allows an accurate diagnosis by means of cardiac catheterization. Circulation 12:58, 1956.

56. Downing, D. F.: Congenital aortic septal defect. Am. Heart J. 40:285, 1950.

57. Drayton, M. R., and Skidmore, R.: Ductus arteriosus blood flow during the first 48 hours of life. Archives Dis. Child. 62:1030, 1987.

58. Elliotson, J.: Case of malformation of the pulmonary artery and aorta. Lancet 1:247, 1830.

59. Emmanouilides, G. C., Linde, L. M., and Crittenden, I. H.: Pulmonary artery stenosis associated with patent ductus following maternal rubella. Circulation 29:514, 1964.

60. Engle, M. A., Holswade, G. R., Goldberg, H. P., and Glenn, F.: Present problems pertaining to the patency of the ductus artery. I. Persistence of growth retardation after successful surgery. Pediatrics 21:70, 1958.

61. Kurtis PS, Rosenkrantz TS, Zalneraitis EL. Cerebral blood flow and EEG changes in preterm infants with patent ductus arteriosus. Pediatr Neurol. 12:114, 1995.

62. Falcone, M. W., Perloff, J. K., and Roberts, W. C.: Aneurysm of the non-patent ductus arteriosus. Am. J. Cardiol. 29:422, 1972.

63. Farahmand, F., White, T. E., and Lucas, R. V., Jr.: Cranial bruit in patent ductus arteriosus. J. Pediatr. 64:441, 1964.

64. Fay, J. E., and Travill, M. B.: The "valve" of the ductus arteriosus—an enigma. Can. Med. Assoc. J. 97:78, 1967.

65. Fisher, R. G., Moodie, D. S., Sterba, R., and Gill, C. C.: Patent ductus arteriosus in adults-long-term follow-up: Nonsurgical versus surgical treatment. J. Am. Coll. Cardiol. 8:280, 1986.

66. Foulis, J.: On a case of patent ductus arteriosus with aneurysm of the pulmonary artery. Edinburgh Med. J. 29:1117, 1884.

67. Freedom, R. M., Moes, C. A. F., Pelech, A., Smallhorn, J., Rabinovitch, M., Olley, P. M., Williams, W. G., Trusler, G. A., and Rowe, R. D.: Bilateral ductus arteriosus. Am. J. Cardiol. 53:884, 1984.

68. Fripp, R. R., Whitman, V., Waldhausen, J. A., and Boal, D. K.: Ductus arteriosus aneurysm presenting as pulmonary artery obstruction. J. Am. Coll. Cardiol. 6:234, 1985.

69. Fu, M., Hung, J., Liao, P., and Chang, C.: Isolated right-sided patent ductus arteriosus in right-sided aortic arch. Chest 91:623, 1987.

70. Acherman RJ, Siassi B, Wells W, Goodwin M, DeVore G. Aneurysm of the ductus arteriosus. Am J Perinatol. 15:653, 1998.

71. Garti, I. J., Aygen, M. M., Vidne, B., and Levy, M. J.: Right aortic arch with mirror-image branching causing vascular ring. A new classification of the right aortic arch patterns. Br. J. Radiol. 46:115, 1973.

72. Gersony, W. M.: Persistence of the fetal circulation. J. Pediatr. 82:1103, 1973.

73. Gibb, W. T., Jr.: Acute bacterial endarteritis of a patent ductus arteriosus. New York J. Med. 41:1861, 1941.

74. Gibson, G. A.: Persistence of the arterial duct and its diagnosis. Edinburgh Med. J. 8:1, 1900.

75. Gibson, S., Potts, W. J., and Langewisch, W. H.: Aortic-pulmonary communication due to localized congenital defect of aortic septum. Pediatrics 6:357, 1950.

76. Ayabe T, Nakamura K, Nakajima S, Yano Y: Surgical management of ductus arteriosus aneurysm in adults. Jpn J Thorac Cardiovasc Surg. 48:304, 2000.

77. Gittenberger-de Groot, A. C.: Persistent ductus arteriosus: Most probably a primary congenital malformation. Br. Heart J. 39:610, 1977.

78. Gittenberger-de Groot, A. C., and Strengers, J. L. M.: Histopathology of the arterial duct (ductus arteriosus) with and without treatment with prostaglandin E1. Int. J. Cardiol. 19:153, 1988.

79. Gittenberger-de Groot, A. C., Moulaert, A. J. M., and Hitchcock, J. F.: Histology of the persistent ductus arteriosus in cases of congenital rubella. Circulation 62:183, 1980.

80. Gittenberger-de Groot, A. C., Strengers. J. L. M., Mentink, M., Poelmann, R. E., and Patterson, D. F.: Histologic studies on normal and persistent ductus arteriosus in the dog. J. Am. Coll. Cardiol. 6:394, 1985.

81. Gittenberger-de Groot, A. C., van Ertbruggen, I., Moulaert, A. J. M. G., and Harinck, E.: The ductus arteriosus in the preterm infant: Histologic and clinical observations. J. Pediatr. 96:88, 1980.

82. Gray, I. R.: Paradoxical splitting of the second heart sound. Br. Heart J. 18:21, 1956.

83. Green, E. W., Agruss, N. S., and Adolph, R. D.: Right sided Austin-Flint murmur. Am. J. Cardiol. 32:370, 1973.

84. Gregg, N. M.: Congenital cataract following German measles in the mother. Trans. Ophthalmol. Soc. Aust. 3:35, 1941.

85. Kopuz C, Erik MK. Gigantic patent ductus arteriosus-report of a newborn cadaver dissection and review of the literature. Surg Radiol Anat 18:343 1996.

86. Hallidie-Smith, K. A.: Murmur of persistent ductus arteriosus in premature infants. Arch. Dis. Child. 47:725, 1972.

87. Hallman, G. L., and Rosenberg, H. S.: Bilateral patent ductus arteriosus: Case report. Angiology 15:140, 1964.

88. Halloran, K. H., Sanyal, S. K., and Gardner, T. H.: Superiorly oriented electrocardiographic axis in infants with the rubella syndrome. Am. Heart J. 72:600, 1966.

89. Hammerman, C., Strates, E., and Valaitis, S.: The silent ductus: Its precursors and its aftermath. Pediatr. Cardiol. 7:121, 1986.

90. Taneja K, Gulati M, Jain M, Saxena A: Ductus arteriosus aneurysm in the adult. Clin Radiol. 52:231, 1997.

91. Hay, J. D.: Population and clinic studies of congenital heart disease in Liverpool. Br. Med. J. 2:661, 1966.

92. Hays, J. T.: Spontaneous aneurysm of a patent ductus arteriosus in an elderly patient. Chest 5:88, 1985.

93. Heath, D., and Whitaker, W.: The pulmonary vessels in patent ductus arteriosus. J. Pathol. Bacteriol. 70:285, 1955.

94. Heath, D., Helmholz, H. F., Jr., Burchell, H. B., DuShane, J. W., and Edwards, J. E.: Graded pulmonary vascular changes and hemodynamic findings in cases of atrial and ventricular septal defects and patent ductus arteriosus. Circulation 18:1155, 1958.

95. Maisel P, Brenner J. Spontaneous closure and thrombosis of a ductal aneurysm in a neonate. Cardiol Young. 9:503, 1999.

96. Heymann, M. A., Berman, W., Rudolph, A. R., and Whitman, V.: Dilatation of the ductus arteriosus by prostaglandin E1 in aortic arch abnormalities. Circulation 59:169, 1979.

97. Hiraishi, S., Horiguchi, Y., Misawa, H., Oguchi, K., Kadoi, N., Fujino, N., and Yashiro, K.: Noninvasive Doppler echocardiographic evaluation of shunt flow dynamics of the ductus arteriosus. Circulation 75:1146, 1987.

98. Hirsimaki, H., Jero, P., Saraste, M., Ekblad, H., Korvenranta, H., and Wanne, O.: Grading of the left-to-right shunting ductus arteriosus in neonates with bedside pulsed Doppler ultrasound. Am. J. Perinatol. 8:247, 1991.

99. Hochhaus, H.: Ueber das Offenbleiben des Ductus Botalli. Deutsch. Arch. Klin. Med. 51:1, 1893.

100. Holden, J. D., Jones, R. C., and Akers, W. A.: Patent ductus arteriosus diagnosed by a mosquito bite or the cutis Quincke. Arch. Dermatol. 94:742, 1966.

101. Holman, E., Gerbode, F., and Purdy, A.: The patent ductus. A review of 75 cases with surgical treatment including an aneurysm of the ductus and one of the pulmonary arteries. J. Thorac. Cardiovasc. Surg. 25:111, 1953.

102. Hornstein, T. R., Hellerstein, H. K., and Ankeney, J. L.: Patent ductus arteriosus in a 72-year-old woman. J.A.M.A. 199:580, 1967.

103. Houston, A. B., Gnanapragasam, J. P., Lim, M. K., Doig, W. B., and Coleman, E. N.: Doppler ultrasound and the silent ductus arteriosus. Br. Heart J. 65:97, 1991.

104. Houston, A. B., Lim, M. K., Doig, W. B., Gnanapragasam, J., Coleman, E. N., Jamieson, M. P. G., and Pollock, J. C. S.: Doppler flow characteristics in the assessment of pulmonary artery pressure in ductus arteriosus. Br. Heart J. 62:284, 1989.

105. Hubbard, T. F., and Neis, D. D.: The sounds at the base of the heart in cases of patent ductus arteriosus. Am. Heart J. 59:807, 1960.

106. Huhta, J. C., Cohen, M., and Gutgesell, H. P.: Patency of the ductus arteriosus in normal neonates. J. Am. Coll. Cardiol. 4:561, 1984.

107. Jager, B. V.: Noninfectious thrombosis of a patent ductus arteriosus. Report of a case, with autopsy. Am. Heart J. 20:236, 1940.

108. Jager, B. V., and Wollenman, O. J., Jr.: An anatomical study of the closure of the ductus arteriosus. Am. J. Pathol. 18:595, 1942.

109. Jayakrishnan, A. G., Loftus, D., Kelly, P., and Luke, D. A.: Spontaneous post-partum rupture of a patent ductus arteriosus. Histopathology 21:383, 1992.

110. Johnson, G. L., Breart, G. L., Gewitz, M. H., Brenner, J. I., Lang, P., Dooley, K. J., and Elleson, R. C.: Echocardiographic characteristics of premature infants with patent ductus arteriosus. Pediatrics 72:864, 1983.

111. Park IS, Kim YH, Ko JK. Bilateral patent ductus arteriosus and non-confluent pulmonary arteries in neonates as shown by radial artery angiography. Tex Heart Inst J. 24:384, 1997.

112. Keagy, K. S., Schall, S. A., and Herrington, R. T.: Selective cyanosis of the right arm. Pediatr. Cardiol. 3:301, 1982.

113. Keith, T. R., and Sagarminaga, J.: Spontaneously disappearing murmur of patent ductus arteriosus. A case report. Circulation 24:1235, 1961.

114. Kelsey, J. R., Jr., Gilmore, C. E., and Edwards, J. E.: Bilateral ductus arteriosus representing persistence of each sixth aortic arch. Report of a case in which there were associated isolated dextrocardia and ventricular septal defects. A.M.A. Arch. Pathol. 55:154, 1953.

115. King, D. H., Smith, E.O., Huhta, J. C., and Gutgesell, H. P.: Mitral and tricuspid annular diameter in normal children determind by two dimensional echocardiography. Am J Cardiol 55: 787, 1985.

116. Kitterman, J. A., et al.: Patent ductus arteriosus in premature infants. New Engl. J. Med. 287:473, 1972.

117. Kohler, C. M., and McNamara, D. G.: Elongated patent ductus arteriosus with intermittent shunting. Pediatrics 39:446, 1967.

118. Kornes, S. B., Ainger, L. E., Monif, G. R. G., Roane, J., Sever, J., and Fuste, F.: Congenital rubella syndrome: Study of 22 infants. Am. J. Dis. Child. 110:434, 1965.

119. Kutsche, L. M., and Van Mierop, L. H. S.: Anatomy and pathogenesis of aorticopulmonary septal defect. Am. J. Cardiol. 59:443, 1987.

120. Lamy, M., Degrouchy, J., and Schweisguth, O.: Genetic and nongenetic factors in the etiology of congenital heart disease: A study of 1188 cases. Am. J. Hum. Genet. 9:17, 1957.

121. Mielke G, Steil E, Breuer J, Goelz R: Circulatory changes following intrauterine closure of the ductus arteriosus in the human fetus and newborn. Prenatal Diagnosis 18:139, 1998.

122. Levin, D. L., Mills, L. J., and Weinberg, A. G.: Hemodynamic, pulmonary vascular, and myocardial abnormalities secondary to pharmacologic constriction of the fetal ductus arteriosus. Circulation 60:360, 1979.

123. Liao, P., Su, W., and Hung, J.: Doppler echocardiographic flow characteristics of isolated patent ductus arteriosus: Better delineation by Doppler color flow mapping. J. Am. Coll. Cardiol. 12:1285, 1988.

124. Lin, A., and Perloff, J. K.: Upper limb malformations and congenital heart disease. Am. J. Cardiol. 55:1576, 1985.

125. Lipman, B., Serwer, G. A., and Brazy, J. E.: Abnormal cerebral hemodynamics in preterm infants with patent ductus. Pediatrics 69:778, 1982.

126. Lund, J. T., Hansen, D., Brocks, V., Jensen, M. B., and Jacobsen, J. R.: Aneurysm of the ductus arteriosus in the neonate: Three case reports with a review of the literature. Pediatr. Cardiol. 13:222, 1992.

127. Shyu KG, Lai LP, Lin SC, Chang H, Chen JJ: Diagnostic accuracy of transesophageal echocardiography for detecting patent ductus arteriosus in adolescents and adults. Chest 108:1201, 1995.

128. Lynch, H. T., Grissom, R. L., Magnuson, C. R., and Krush, A.: Patent ductus arteriosus. Study of two families. J.A.M.A. 194:135, 1965.

129. Magri, G., Jona, E., Messina, D., and Actis-Dato, A.: Direct recording of heart sounds and murmurs from the epicardial surface of the exposed human heart. Am. Heart J. 57:449, 1959.

130. Mahoney, L., Clyman, R. I., and Heymann, M. A.: Decreased contractility of the ductus arteriosus in experimental pulmonic stenosis. Circulation 70:695, 1984.

131. Mark, H., and Young, D.: Spontaneous closure of the ductus arteriosus in a young adult. New Engl. J. Med. 269:416, 1963.

132. Marquis, R. M.: Congenital heart disease: The ductus arteriosus as pathfinder. Br. Heart 58:429, 1987.

133. Marquis, R. M.: The continuous murmur of persistence of the ductus arteriosus—an historical review. Eur. Heart J. 1:465, 1980.

134. Marquis, R. M., Miller, H. C., McCormack, R. J. M., Matthews, M. B., and Kitchin, A. H.: Persistence of ductus arteriosus with left to right shunt in the older patient. Br. Heart J. 48:469, 1982.

135. Martin, R. P., Banner, N. R., and Radley-Smith, R.: Familial persistent ductus arteriosus. Arch. Dis. Child. 61:906, 1986.

136. Martin, C. G., Snider, A. R., Katz, S. M., Peabody, J. L., and Brady, J. P.: Abnormal cerebral blood flow patterns in preterm infants with a large patent ductus arteriosus. J. Pediatr. 101:587, 1982.

137. Martinez-Lavin, M., Bobadilla, M., Casanova, J., Attie, F., and Martinez, M.: Hypertrophic osteoarthropathy in cyanotic congenital heart disease. Arthritis Rheum. 25:1186, 1982.

138. McMurphy, D. M., Heymann, M. A., Rudolph, A. M., and Melman, K. L.: Developmental change in construction of the ductus arteriosus. Pediatr. Res. 6:231, 1972.

139. Miller, E., Cradock-Watson, J. E., and Pollock, T. M.: Consequences of confirmed maternal rubella at successive stages of pregnancy. Lancet 2:781, 1982.

140. Mirowski, M., Arevalo, F., Medrano, G. A., and Cisneros, F. A.: Conduction disturbances in patent ductus arteriosus. A study of 200 cases before and after surgery with determination of the P-R index. Circulation 25:807, 1962.

141. Leal SD, Cavalle-Garrido T, Ryan G, Farine D. Isolated ductal closure in utero diagnosed by fetal echocardiography. Am J Perinatal 14:205, 1997.

142. Morgan, J. M., Gray, H. H., Miller, G. A. H., and Oldershaw, P. J.: The clinical features, management and outcome of persistence of the arterial duct presenting in adult life. Int. J. Cardiol. 27:193, 1990.

143. Morrow, A. G., Greenfield, L. J., and Braunwald, E.: Congenital aortopulmonary septal defect. Clincal and hemodynamic findings, surgical technic, and results of operative correction. Circulation 25:463, 1962.

144. Moss, A. J., Emmanouilides, G., and Duffie, E. R., Jr.: Closure of the ductus arteriosus in the newborn infant. Pediatrics 32:25, 1963.

145. Murphy, D. J., Vick, G. W., Ramsay, J. M., Danford, D. A., and Huhta, J. C.: Continuous wave Doppler echocardiography in patent ductus arteriosus. J. Cardiovasc. Ultrasonogr. 6:273, 1987.

146. Sohn DW, Kim YJ, Zo JH, Lee MM Paek YB. The value of contrast echocardiography in the diagnosis of patent ductus arteriosus with Eisenmenger's syndrome. L Am Soc Echocardiogr 14:57, 2001.

147. Ong K, Madan R, Patent ductus arteriosus diagnosed in old age. Am J Geriatr Cardiol 7:14, 1998.

148. Neufeld, H. N., Lester, R. G., Adams, P., Jr., Anderson, R. C., Lillehei, C. W., and Edwards, J. E.: Aorticopulmonary septal defect. Am. J. Cardiol. 9:12, 1962.

149. Ng, A. S., Vlietstra, R. E., Danielson, G. K., Smith, H. C., and Puga, F. J.: Patent ductus arteriosus in patients more than 50 years old. Int. J. Cardiol. 11:277, 1986.

150. Ohtsuka, S., Kahihana, M., Ishikawa, T., Noguchi, Y., Kuga, K., Ishimitsu, T., Sugishita, Y., Ito, I., Ijima, H., Hori, M., and Kimura, Y.: Aneurysm of patent ductus arteriosus in an adult case: Findings of cardiac catheterization, angiography, and pathology. Clin. Cardiol. 10:537, 1987.

151. Oldham, H. N., Jr., Collins, N. P., Pierce, G. E., Sabiston, D. C., Jr., and Blalock, A.: Giant patent ductus arteriosus. J. Thorac. Cardiovasc. Surg. 47:331, 1964.

152. Papadopoulos, G. S., and Folger, G. M.: Diastolic murmurs in the newborn of benign nature. Int. J. Cardiol. 3:107, 1983.

153. Ananthasubramaniam K Patent ductus arteriosus in the elderly. J Am Soc Echocardiogr 14:321,200Sietten LJ, Pierpont ME. Familial occurrence of patent ductus arteriosus. Am J Med Genet 57:27, 1995.

154. Patterson, D. F: Hereditary transmission of patent ductus arteriosus in the dog. Am. Heart J. 74:289, 1967.

155. Perlman, J. M., Hill, A., and Volpe, J. J.: The effect of patent ductus arteriosus on flow velocity in the anterior cerebral arteries: Ductal steal in the premature newborn infant. J. Pediatr. 99:767, 1981.

156. Perloff, J. K.: Auscultatory and phonocardiographic manifestations of pulmonary hypertension. Progr. Cardiovasc. Dis. 9:303, 1967.

157. Perloff, J. K. The Physical Examination of the Heart and Circulation.3ʳᵈ edition, Philadelphia, W. B. Saunders Company, 2000.

158. Satoda M, Pierpont ME, Diaz GA, Bornemeier RA, Gelb BD. Char syndrome, an inherited disorder with patent ductus maps to chromosome 6p12-p21. Circulation 99:3036, 1999.

159. Porter, W. B.: The effect of patent ductus arteriosus on body growth. Am. J. Med. Sci. 213:178, 1947.

160. Printz, M. P., Skidgel, R. A., and Friedman, W. F.: Studies of pulmonary prostaglandin biosynthetic and catabolic enzymes as factors in ductus arteriosus patency and closure. Pediatr. Res. 18:19, 1984.

161. Quiroga, C.: Partial persistence of the ductus arteriosus. Acta Radiol. 55:103, 1961.

162. Bertola DR, Kim CA, Sugayama SM, Utagawa CY, Albano LM, Gonzolez CH. Further delineation of Char syndrome. Pediatr Int 42:85, 2000.

163. Reller, M. D., Buffkin, D. C., Colasurdo, M. A., Rice, M. J., and McDonald, R. W.: Ductal patency in neonates with respiratory distress syndrome. A randomized surfactant trial. Am. J. Dis. Child. 145:1017, 1991.

164. Reller, M. D., Colasurdo, M. A., Rice, M. J., and McDonald, R. W.: The timing of spontaneous closure of the ductus arteriosus in infants with respiratory distress syndrome. Am. J. Cardiol. 66:75, 1990.

165. Reller, M. D., Ziegler, M. L., Rice, M. J., Salin, R. C., and McDonald, R. W.: Duration of ductal shunting in healthy preterm infants: An echocardiographic color flow Doppler study. J. Pediatr. 112:441, 1988.

166. Rice, M. J., Seward, J. B., Hagler, D. J., Mair, D. D., and Tajik, A. J.: Visualization of aortopulmonary window by two-dimensional echocardiography. Mayo Clin. Proc. 57:482, 1982.

167. Richardson, J., Doty, D., Rossi, N., and Ehrenhaft, J.: The spectrum of anomalies of aortopulmonary septation. J. Thorac. Cardiovasc. Surg. 78:21, 1979.

168. Rohde, R. A., Hodgmann, J. E., and Cleland, R. S.: Multiple congenital anomalies in the trisomy (group 16–18) syndrome. Pediatrics 33:258, 1964.

169. Michelakis E, Rebeyka I, Bateson J, Olley P, Puttagunta L, Archer S. Voltage-gated potassium channels in human ductus arteriosus. Lancet 356:134. 2000.

170. Satoda M, Zhao F, Diaz GA, Burn J, Goodship J, Davidson HR, Pierpont ME, Gelb BD. Mutations in TFAP2B cause Char syndrome, a familial form of patent ductus arteriosus. Nat Genet 25:42, 2000.

171. Rudolph, A. M., Mayer, F. E., Nadas, A. S., and Gross, R. E.: Patent ductus arteriosus. A clinical and hemodynamic study of 23 patients in the first year of life. Pediatrics 22:892, 1958.

172. Rudolph, A. M., Scarpelli, E. M., Golinko, R. J., and Gootman, N. L.: Hemodynamic basis for clinical manifestations of patent ductus arteriosus. Am. Heart J. 68:447, 1964.

173. Rutstein, D. B., Nickerson, R. J., and Heald, F. P.: Seasonal incidence of patent ductus arteriosus and maternal rubella. Am. J. Dis. Child. 84:199, 1952.

174. Sang, K., Bowen, A., Park, S. C., Galvis, A. G., and Young, L. W.: Patent ductus arteriosus. Its occurrence with unequal pulmonary vascularity and hyperlucent left lung. Am. J. Dis. Child. 135:637, 1981.

175. Sardesai, S. H., Marshall, R. J., Farrow, R., and Mourant, A. J.: Dissecting aneurysm of the pulmonary artery in a case of unoperated patent ductus arteriosus. Eur. Heart J. 11:670, 1990.

176. Satomi, G., Nakamura, K., Imai, Y., and Takao, A.: Two-dimensional echocardiographic diagnosis of aorticopulmonary window. Br. Heart J. 43:351, 1980.

177. Shapiro, W., Said, S. I., and Nova, P. L.: Intermittent disappearance of the murmur of patent ductus arteriosus. Circulation 22:226, 1960.

178. Shepherd, S. G., Park, F. R., and Kitchell, J. R.: Case of aorto-pulmonic communication incident to congenital aortic septal defect; discussion of embryologic changes involved. Am. Heart J. 27:733, 1944.

179. Sietsema, K. E., and Perloff, J. K.: Cyanotic congenital heart disease: Dynamics of oxygen uptake and control of ventilation during exercise. In Perloff, J. K., and Child, J. S.: Congenital Heart Disease in Adults. 2nd edition, Philadelphia, W. B. Saunders Company, 1998.

180. Perloff JK, Rosove MH, Sietsema KE, Territo MC. Cyanotic congenital heart disease: A multisystem systemic disorder. In Perloff JK and Child JS. Congenital Heart Disease in Adults. 2nd edition, Philadelphia, WB Saunders Co, 1998.

181. Skall-Jensen, J.: Congenital aortico-pulmonary fistula; a review of the literature and report of two cases. Acta Med. Scand. 160:221, 1958.

182. Slomp, J., van Munsteren, J. C., Polmann, R. E., de Reeder, E. G., Bogers, A. J. J. C., and Gittenberger-de Groot, A. C.: Formation of intimal cushions in the ductus arteriosus as a model for vascular intimal thickening. An immunohistochemical study of changes in extracellular matrix components. Atherosclerosis. 93:25, 1992.

183. Smallhorn, J. F., Gow, R., Olley, P. M., Freedom, R. M., Swyer, P. R., Perlman, M., and Rowe, R. D.: Combined non-invasive assessment of the patent ductus arteriosus in the preterm infant before and after indomethacin treatment. Am. J. Cardiol. 54:1300, 1984.

184. Spencer, H., and Dworken, H. J.: Congenital aortic septal defect with communication between aorta and pulmonary artery; case report and review of the literature. Circulation 2:880, 1950.

185. Steinberg, I.: Left-sided patent ductus arteriosus and right-sided aortic arch. Angiocardiographic findings in three cases. Circulation 28:1138, 1963.

186. Steinberg, I.: Roentgenography of patent ductus arteriosus. Am. J. Cardiol. 13:698, 1964.

187. Stuckey, D.: Pulmonary pulsation: A physical sign of patent ductus arteriosus in infancy. Med. J. Aust. 2:681, 1957.

188. Takenaka, K., Sakamoto, T., Shiota, T., Amano, W., Igarashi, T., and Sugimoto, T.: Diagnosis of patent ductus arteriosus in adults by biplane transesophageal color Doppler flow mapping. Am. J. Cardiol. 68:691, 1991.

189. Tandon, R., Silva, C. L., Moller, J. H., and Edwards, J. E.: Aorticopulmonary septal defect coexisting with ventricular septal defect. Circulation 50:188, 1974.

190. Taussig, H. B.: Congenital Malformations of the Heart. New York, The Commonwealth Fund, 1947.

191. Territo, M. C., Rosove, M., and Perloff, J. K.: Cyanotic congenital heart disease: Hematologic management, renal function, and urate metabolism. In Perloff, J. K., and Child, J. S: Congenital Heart Disease in Adults. Philadelphia, 2nd ed,W. B. Saunders Company, 1998.

192. Tulzer, G., Gudmundsson, S., Sharkey, A. M., Wood, D. C., Cohen, A. W., and Huhta, J. C.: Doppler echocardiography of fetal ductus arteriosus constriction versus increased right ventricular output. J. Am. Coll. Cardiol. 18:532, 1991.

193. Umebayashi, Y., Taira, A., Morishita, Y., and Arikawa, K.: Abrupt onset of patent ductus arteriosus in a 55-year-old man. Am. Heart J. 118:1067, 1989.

194. Van Praagh, R., and Van Praagh, S.: The anatomy of common aorticopulmonary trunk (truncus arteriosus communis) and its embryologic implications. A study of 57 necropsy cases. Am. J. Cardiol. 16:406, 1965.

195. van de Bor, M., Verloove-Vanhorick, S. P., Brand, R., and Ruys, J. H.: Patent ductus arteriosus in a cohort of 1338 preterm infants: A collaborative study. Pediatr. Perinatol. Epidemiol. 2:328, 1988.

196. Vick, G. W., Huhta, J. C., and Gutgesell, H. P.: Assessment of the ductus arteriosus in preterm infants utilizing suprasternal two-dimensional/Doppler echocardiography. J. Am. Coll. Cardiol. 5:973, 1985.

197. Wagner, O.: Beitrag zur pathologie des ductus arteriosus (Botalli). Deutsch Arch. Klin. Med. 79:90, 1903.

198. Whitaker, W., Heath, D., and Brown, J. W.: Patent ductus arteriosus with pulmonary hypertension. Br. Heart J. 17:121, 1955.

199. White, P. D., Mazurkie, S. J., and Boschetti, A. E.: Patency of the ductus arteriosus at 90. New Engl. J. Med. 280:146, 1969.

200. Williams, B., Ling, J., Leight, L., and McGaff, C. J.: Patent ductus arteriosus and osteoarthropathy. Arch. Intern. Med. 111:346, 1963.

201. Wilson, R. R.: Post-mortem observations on contraction of the human ductus arteriosus. Br. Med. J. 1:811, 1958.

202. Wood, P.: Eisenmenger's syndrome. Br. Med. J. 2:701, 755, 1958.

203. Woodruff, W. W., Gabliani, G., and Grant, A. O.: Patent ductus arteriosus in the elderly. Southern Med. J. 76:1436, 1983.

204. Zanardo, V., Milanesi, O., Trevisanuto, D., Rizzo, M., Ronconi, M., Stellin, G., and Cantarutti, F: Early screening and treatment of "silent" patent ductus arteriosus in prematures with RDS. J. Perinat. Med. 19:291, 1991.

205. Zarich, S., Leonardi, H., Pippin, J., Tuthill, J., and Lewis, S.: Patent ductus arteriosus in the elderly. Chest 94:1103, 1988.

206. Mahoney LT, Coryell KG, Lauer RM: The newborn transitional circulation: Two-dimensional Doppler echocardiographic study. J. Am. Coll. Cardiol. 6:623, 1985.

Anomalous Origin of the Left Coronary Artery from the Pulmonary Trunk

In 1886, H. St. John Brooks described two cases of "an abnormal coronary artery arising from the pulmonary artery."[14] The diagnosis was subsequently called into question, and the abnormal communication was attributed to a coronary arterial fistula.[95] The seminal report of Bland, White, and Garland in 1933[12] referred to Maude Abbott's case of a 60-year-old woman with anomalous origin of the left coronary artery from the pulmonary trunk (Fig. 21–1B). The names of Bland, White, and Garland remain as eponyms.[44] Anomalous origin of the left coronary artery from the pulmonary trunk is the most common *major* congenital malformation of the coronary circulation with an incidence of 1/300,000 live births.[62] More rarely, the *right* coronary artery (see Fig. 21–4),[47,88,106,109,116,121] the *left anterior descending* or *circumflex* coronary artery,[25,34,36,37,42,88,115] *both* coronary arteries,[11,28,48,109] or a *single* coronary artery[87] arise from the pulmonary trunk, or the left coronary artery or a coronary arterial branch originates from the right or left pulmonary artery.[10,42]

The anomalous left coronary artery is small and thin-walled, resembling a venous channel (Figs. 21–1 to 21–3).[15,21,62] The right coronary artery originates normally from its aortic sinus, is dilated and tortuous[8,26,30,62] (see Figs. 21–1 and 21–3), and rarely is aneurysmal.[7] The portion of left ventricle supplied by the anomalous left coronary artery becomes thin, scarred, and dilated[21,62] and is occasionally aneurysmal.[59,93] This aneurysm is acquired and not congenital.[107] The hypoperfused but viable portion of left ventricle *increases* its mass often appreciably[13,15] because of replication of immature cardiomyocytes in response to the hypoxemic stimulus.[90] The left ventricular endocardium exhibits fibroelastosis[62,86,93] and rarely focal calcification.[8,61,122] In adults with ischemic heart disease, newly formed elastic fibers appear within 3 or 4 weeks after a myocardial infarction and culminate in endocardial fibroelastosis in the vicinity of the infarct.[53]

Three theories have been proposed to explain the origin of a coronary artery from the pulmonary trunk.[48] The first two theories relate to division of the embryonic truncus arteriosus.[65] In the early embryo, two opposing truncal cushions enlarge and fuse to form the truncal septum, which divides the truncus arteriosus into aortic and pulmonary channels.[65] Assuming that the coronary arteries originate as two endothelial buds (see Chapter 32), displacement of the origin of one or both of these buds could assign either or both coronary arteries to the portion of the truncus arteriosus destined to become the pulmonary artery. Alternatively, faulty division of the truncus could incorporate one or both coronary artery buds into the pulmonary artery. The higher incidence of anomalous origin of the *left* coronary artery rather than the *right* coronary artery from the pulmonary trunk has been attributed to the proximity of the left aortic sinus to the truncal septum, so a relatively small displacement of the left coronary artery anlage would suffice to cause the left coronary artery ostium to lie within the pulmonary artery.[48] These theories presuppose that human coronary arteries originate as two endothelial buds that develop simultaneously with or before division of the truncus arteriosus (see Chapter 32). However, the coronary arteries may not appear until *after* the division of the truncus.[48] Nor do these theories explain the presence of a third (accessory) coronary artery or anomalous origin of one branch of the left coronary artery from the pulmonary trunk, and do not explain why the relative size of the pulmonary artery, the aorta, and their valves are not altered by the presumed displacement of the truncal septum.[48] The *involution and persistence* theory postulates that there are originally *six* coronary artery anlagen, three from the aorta and three from the pulmonary artery (see Chapter 32).[48] The two coronary arteries that are destined to be normal are believed to arise from two persistent anlagen in two separate aortic sinuses, whereas the anlagen in the third aortic sinus in addition to

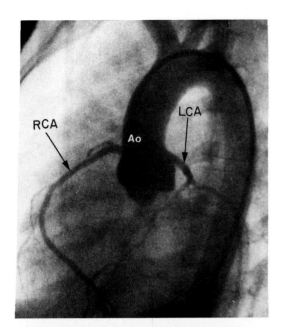

Figure 21–1

A, Aortogram (left anterior oblique) from a normal 5-year-old girl with a normal right coronary artery (RCA) and a normal left (LCA) coronary artery. AO, aorta. *B,* Right coronary arteriogram (lateral projection) from a 4-year-old girl with anomalous origin of the left coronary artery (LCA) from the pulmonary trunk (PT). A dilated right coronary artery originates from the aorta, and abundant intercoronary anastomoses communicate with the left coronary artery that originates from the pulmonary trunk. The direction of flow is from the right coronary artery through intercoronary anastomoses into the left coronary artery and into the pulmonary trunk.

all three anlagen in the pulmonary sinuses undergo involution.[48] By the same theory, anomalous origin of one or both coronary arteries could result from persistence of pulmonary artery coronary anlagen together with involution of the normally persistent aortic coronary anlagen.[48] Anomalous origin of the left coronary artery from the pulmonary trunk with a bicuspid aortic valve is believed to be the expression of a single morphogenic defect.[18,19] In the

Syrian hamster, a relationship has been proposed between anomalous origin of the left coronary artery and the developmental morphology of the semilunar valves.[18,19]

Myocardial ischemia is a serious sequel of anomalous origin of the left coronary artery from the pulmonary trunk. Ischemia does not stem from the fact that only *one* coronary artery originates from the aorta, because the functional consequences of a single coronary artery are benign[33,80,108] with few exceptions (see Chapter 32).[84,89] Nor is perfusion of the anomalous coronary artery by unoxygenated blood from the pulmonary trunk a satisfactory explanation, because in *cyanotic* congenital heart disease the oxygen content of coronary arterial blood can be exceedingly low without producing myocardial ischemia.[62] Why then does cardiac muscle become ischemic when the left coronary artery arises from the pulmonary trunk? The answer lies in the *direction* of blood flow through the coronary bed[8,9,35,98,125] as illustrated in the circulatory patterns of Figure 21–5. In fetal and early neonatal life, high pulmonary arterial pressure results in *antegrade* blood flow *into* the anomalous left coronary artery[83] (Fig. 21–5A). The subsequent decrease in pulmonary arterial pressure is accompanied by a parallel decrease in blood flow into the anomalous left coronary artery (Fig. 21–5B). During this crucial transition, myocardial perfusion depends almost entirely on perfusion from the right coronary artery (see Fig. 21–2).[6,35] Myocardial ischemia is a necessary sequel unless adequate circulation from right to left coronary artery is established via intercoronary anastomoses on which survival largely depends (see Fig. 21–2C).[21,35,93,101,118] Intercoronary anastomoses represent low-resistance pathways between the aorta and pulmonary trunk—*arteriovenous fistulae*[9,30]—that have two opposing effects: 1) the desirable effect of reestablishing left coronary arterial perfusion,[93] and 2) the undesirable effect of a coronary steal that bypasses the capillary bed and deprives the myocardium of oxygen.[9,35,69,81,98,99,118,119] The idea of retrograde flow through an anomalous left coronary artery was originally proposed by 1886 by St. John Brooks[14]: "Here are two arteries belonging to the different circulations—the pulmonary and the systemic—anastomosing with each other. In these circulations, as is well known, the arterial pressure is very much greater in the systemic than in the pulmonary; how then did the blood flow in the anomalous coronary artery? There cannot be a doubt that it acted very much after the manner of a vein, and that blood flowed through it towards the pulmonary artery, and from thence into the lungs."

Physiologic, pathologic, and clinical derangements arise from ischemic consequences of the transition from decreased antegrade perfusion of the anomalous left coronary artery to flow from the right coronary artery through the low-resistance intercoronary anastomoses into the left coronary artery then retrograde flow into the pulmonary trunk (see Fig. 21–5). Ischemia causes the left ventricle to labor under three handicaps: *first*, contractility is depressed because viable myocardium is compromised,[76] *second*, mitral regurgitation, which is a consequence of ischemic papillary muscle dysfunction,[31] adds to the hemodynamic burden

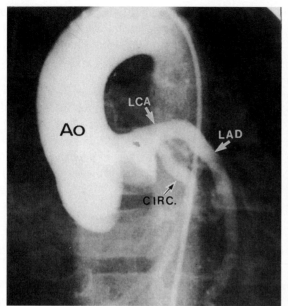

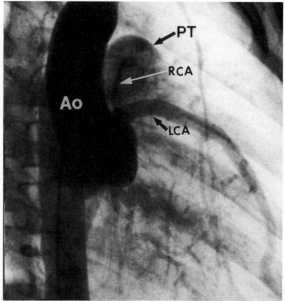

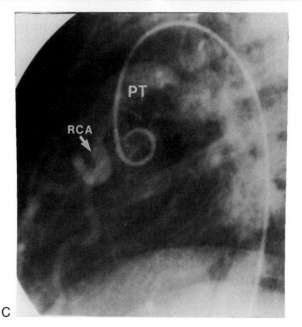

Figure 21–2

Aortograms with coronary artery visualization in a four-year-male with anomalous origin of the *right* coronary artery from the pulmonary trunk *A,* The left main coronary artery (LCA) originates from its aortic sinus and divides into the left anterior descending (LAD) and circumflex (CIRC) branches. (Ao = aorta) *B,* Intercoronary anastomoses from the left coronary (LCA) fill the right coronary artery (RCA) whose flow is *into* the pulmonary trunk (PT). *C,* The lateral projection shows the right coronary artery (RCA) entering the pulmonary trunk (PT).

(Fig. 21–6), and *third,* flow via the intercoronary anastomoses constitutes a left-to-right shunt that is occasionally sufficient to volume overload the left ventricle.[100] *Regional* abnormalities of wall motion characterize anomalous origin of the left coronary artery from the pulmonary trunk,[20,96] but infants tend to exhibit global hypokinesis.[20,96]

The History

Eighty-five percent of patients present in infancy. The outlook is most grave when *both* coronary arteries originate from the pulmonary trunk[11,28,48,109] and the outlook is

most favorable when the right coronary artery[47,73,88,103, 106,109,116,121] or a left anterior descending or circumflex coronary artery originates anomalously.[25,34,37,42,88,115] The clinical course is a continuum ranging from death in infancy to asymptomatic adult survival with all gradations in between.[*] Nevertheless, three general patterns emerge: 1) serious symptoms in early infancy with death before age 1 year, 2) early symptoms followed by gradual attenuation or disappearance of symptoms, and 3) absence or virtual absence of early symptoms with asymptomatic survival to

---

[*]See references 24, 35, 52, 56, 68, 70, 74, 75, 81, 86, 95, 111, 112, 114, 119, 124.

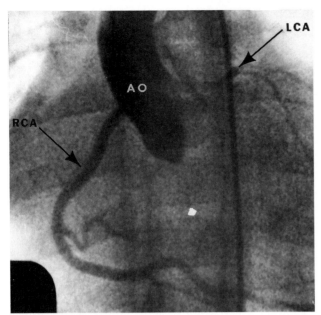

Figure 21–3
Anteroposterior aortogram from a four-month-old female showing a normal right coronary artery (RCA) arisng from the aorta (AO) and poorly developed intercoronary anastomoses faintly visualizing the left coronary artery (LCA).

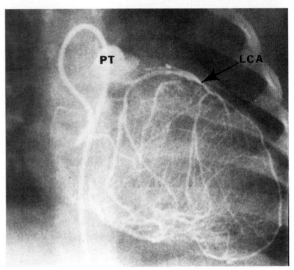

Figure 21–4
A, Anteroposterior semiselective right coronary arteriogram from the four-year-old female referred to in Figure 21–1B. The right coronary artery (RCA) arises from the aorta (AO) and communicates via abundant intercoronary anastomoses with the left coronary artery (LCA) that originates from the pulmonary trunk (PT). Flow is from the LCA into the PT. *B,* Later frame showing the proximal LCA and PT more clearly.

adulthood. Adult survival even to age 90 years[29] is much more likely with anomalous origin of the *right* coronary artery from the pulmonary trunk, which, however, is not necessarily benign.[73,103,106,116,121]

Eighty percent to 90% of patients with anomalous origin of the left coronary artery from the pulmonary trunk die in their first year.[*] Infants appear normal at birth and often remain so for about two months after which symptoms characteristically begin.[62,69,72,82,114,122] Irritability, dyspnea, wheezing, cough, diaphoresis, and ashen gray pallor are precipitated or aggravated by feeding, crying, or a bowel movement.[22,62,114,122] Growth and development are poor.[13,70,86] Death generally results from heart failure.[13,70,86] Symptomatic infants occasionally improve[55] only to die suddenly during a relatively asymptomatic childhood or adolescence.[70,86,122] Angina may be deferred until the teens,[26] or the anomaly may be discovered in asymptomatic children because of mitral regurgitation (Figs. 21–6 and 21–7).[30,40,93] About 15% of individuals with anomalous origin of the left coronary artery survive to adulthood,[13,62,66,79,111,124] some reaching the seventh or eighth decade.[7,38,64,77] One of the first known patients with the anomaly was the 60-year-old woman described by Maude Abbott in 1908.[1] The malformation reveals itself in adults because of the murmur of mitral regurgitation,[7,38,63,86,117] because of a continuous murmur mis-

taken for a patent ductus (see Fig. 21–7), or because of angina pectoris, myocardial infarction, congestive heart failure, atrial fibrillation, ventricular tachyarrhythmias, cardiac arrest, or sudden death.[*]

Physical Appearance

Acutely ill infants with rapid labored breathing, weak cry, cough, and diaphoresis present a dramatic clinical picture. Pallor and diaphoresis accompany episodes of myocardial ischemia (angina). Infants with chronic congestive heart failure are catabolic.[13,70,86,93]

---

[*]See references 8, 21, 24, 52, 59, 62, 69, 72, 93, 114, 122.

[*]See references 2, 3, 5, 9, 26, 40, 41, 43, 45, 46, 54, 62, 64, 68, 85, 95, 97, 112, 119, 122.

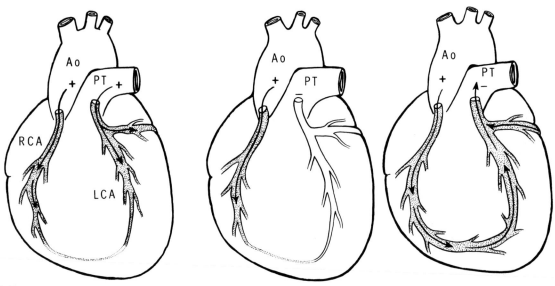

Figure 21–5

Flow patterns through the coronary bed in anomalous origin of the left coronary artery from the pulmonary trunk. *A,* In the fetus and early neonate, high pressure in the pulmonary trunk (PT) generates flow *into* the anomalous left coronary artery (LCA), while the normally originating right coronary artery (RCA) is perfused from the aorta. Intercoronary anastomoses are not yet functional. *B,* A decrease in neonatal pulmonary arterial pressure is accompanied by a parallel fall in flow into the anomalous left coronary. Intercoronary anastomoses are still not functional. *C,* When the pressure in the pulmonary trunk and anomalous left coronary artery falls *below* the pressure in the right coronary artery, flow proceeds from the right coronary artery into the *left* coronary artery through intercoronary anastomoses. The left coronary artery then drains *into* the pulmonary trunk and does not receive blood from it.

The Arterial Pulse, Jugular Venous Pulse, Precordial Movement, and Palpation

Pulsus alternans results from left ventricular failure.[21] The diastolic pressure is occasionally low because of aortic runoff through the fistulous communication.[30,40,100] The jugular venous pulse is elevated in the presence of congestive heart

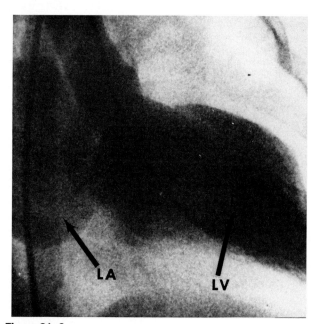

Figure 21–6

Left ventriculogram (right oblique projection) from a 5-year-old girl with anomalous origin of the left coronary artery from the pulmonary trunk. Mitral regurgitation was responsible for dilatation of the left atrium (LA) and left ventricle (LV).

failure but cannot be assessed in symptomatic infants. A left parasternal impulse is the result of an enlarged left atrium that expands in systole in response to mitral regurgitation.

Auscultation

Anomalous origin of the left coronary artery from the pulmonary trunk is accompanied by systolic, diastolic, or continuous murmurs or by no murmur at all. The holosystolic murmur of mitral regurgitation (Fig. 21–7) is the result of ischemic papillary muscle dysfunction.[8,15-17,23,31,70,86,91,117] Short mid-diastolic murmurs are analogous to mid-diastolic murmurs heard in other forms of mitral regurgitation.[70,91]

Continuous murmurs are generated by flow through intercoronary anastomoses (Figs. 21–7 and 21–8).[8,30,71,72,82,100] The configuration and location of these continuous murmur are only occasionally similar to patent ductus arteriosus,[30,32,71] which rarely coexists.[4,58,83] The continuous murmur of intercoronary anastomoses does not peak around the second heart sound but is softer in systole and louder in diastole (see Figs. 21–7 and 21–8) because transmural pressure generated by ventricular systole reduces intercoronary systolic flow. The occasional occurrence of an *isolated diastolic* murmur has been attributed to a reduction in systolic intercoronary flow caused by elevated pulmonary artery pressure provoked by left ventricular failure or mitral regurgitation.[70,100]

The continuous murmurs are located at the base of the heart or somewhat lower, to the left or right of the sternum but usually along the left sternal border (see Figs. 21–7 and

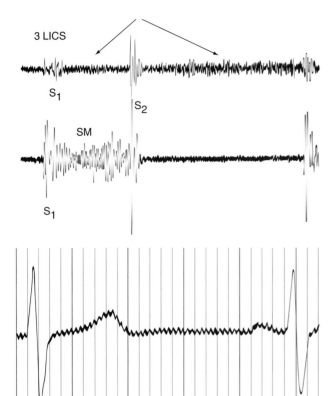

Figure 21–7

Phonocardiogram from a 13-year-old boy with anomalous origin of the left coronary artery from the pulmonary trunk. The continuous murmur in the third left intercostal space (3 LICS, *arrows*) is louder in diastole. A holosystolic murmur of mitral regurgitation (SM) was recorded at the apex. Lead 2 of the electrocardiogram reflects left axis deviation.

21–8).[30,70,71] An isolated diastolic murmur along the left or right sternal border is occasionally mistaken for semilunar valve regurgitation.[70] Third heart sounds coincide with left ventricular failure and mitral regurgitation.

The Electrocardiogram

There are three electrocardiographic features of anomalous origin of the left coronary artery from the pulmonary trunk: 1) deep but narrow q waves, 2) left ventricular hypertrophy, and 3) left axis deviation. In normal infants and children, q waves are consistently absent in leads 1 and aVL. Deep narrow q waves in leads 1 and aVL characterize anomalous origin of the left coronary artery from the pulmonary trunk[8,30,39,62,70,71,86,93,122] (Figs. 21–9A and 21–10) and are in striking contrast to the shallow broad q waves of adult ischemic heart disease. The depth of the q wave in lead aVL can equal or exceed the height of the R wave (Figs. 21–9A and 21–11). The q waves in infants can be small or absent[70,111] but become progressively more prominent with age. An abnormal tracing may improve with age[62,86,94] or may become more abnormal (see Fig. 21–9A, B). Q waves are rarely present in right precordial leads (Fig. 21–9B).[39,93]

Left ventricular hypertrophy, the second electrocardiographic characteristic of the coronary anomaly,[15,21,62] was featured in the title of the original Bland, White, and Garland publication, "Report of an unusual case associated with cardiac hypertrophy."[12] Although heart weights are increased,[8,122] it is the *posterobasal* region of the left ventricle that especially increases its mass.[15,90] From the gross morphologic point of view, this regional increase in mass is *hypertrophy*, but from the cell biologic point of view the posterobasal increase in mass is *hyperplasia* or *replication* of cardiomyocytes.[90] The basis for this cellular response is the capacity of immature cardiomyocytes to replicate in response to hypoxemia that is a feature of the hypoperfused but viable posterobasal left ventricular wall.[90]

Left ventricular hypertrophy is represented in the electrocardiogram by typical voltage and repolarization criteria (Figs. 21–11 and 21–12).[30,62,94,111,119] Deep narrow q waves in leads aVL and V_6 may reflect the initial force deformity of the coronary artery anomaly rather than left ventricular hypertrophy (Fig. 21–13). Electrocardiograms recorded during angina pectoris or exercise stress testing disclose ischemic ST segment depressions and T wave inversions.[119]

Left axis deviation is the third electrocardiographic characteristic of anomalous origin of the left coronary artery from the pulmonary trunk (see Fig. 21–9B).[8,71,92] The mechanism of left axis deviation has been attributed to the disproportionate increase in posterobasal left ventricular muscle mass that attracts the major depolarization vector in a left superior direction.[15,92]

Left atrial P wave abnormalities occur because of mitral regurgitation[16] (see Fig. 21–9B), which is occasionally responsible for atrial fibrillation.[16,64,117]

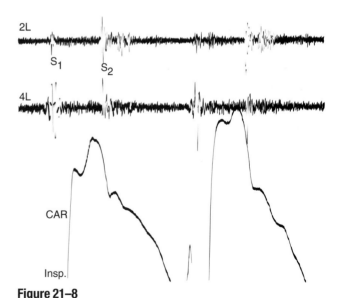

Figure 21–8

Phonocardiogram from a 33-year-old woman with anomalous origin of the left coronary artery from the pulmonary trunk misdiagnosed in childhood as patent ductus arteriosus. A continuous murmur appears in the second (2L) and fourth (4L) left intercostal spaces. Maximum intensity of the continuous murmur is *after* the second heart sound (S_2). Car, carotid; S_1, first heart sound.

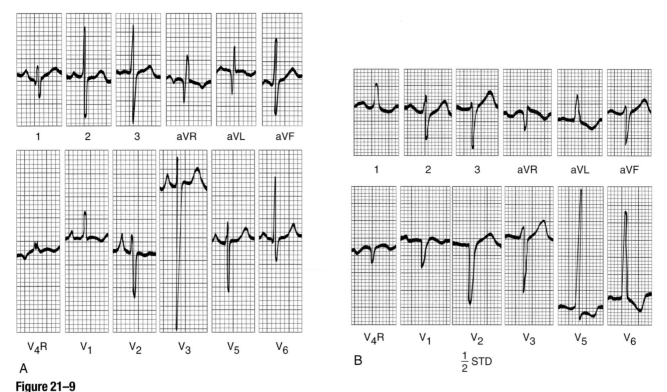

Figure 21–9

A, Electrocardiogram from a symptomatic 4-month-old girl with anomalous origin of the left coronary artery from the pulmonary trunk. The QRS axis is indeterminate (equidiphasic complexes in all six limb leads). A small but abnormal q wave is present in lead 1, and a deep narrow q wave is present in lead aVL. Left ventricular hypertrophy is reflected in the deep S wave in lead V_3 and the prominent R wave in lead V_6. *B,* Same patient at age 5 years. There is a left atrial P terminal force in lead V_4R. Left axis deviation is now present, and infarct q waves have developed in leads V_4R through V_2. Left ventricular hypertrophy is represented by voltage and repolarization criteria in leads V_{5-6}. All precordial leads are half standardized.

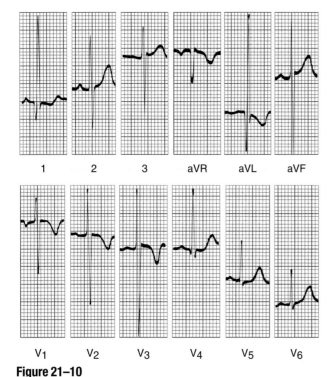

Figure 21–10

Electrocardiogram from a 9-year-old boy with anomalous origin of the left coronary artery from the pulmonary trunk. The QRS axis is leftward (minus 15 degrees). A deep narrow q wave is present in lead 1 but is especially evident in lead aVL.

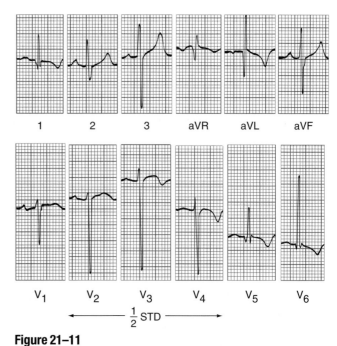

Figure 21–11

Electrocardiogram from a 15-year-old boy with anomalous origin of the left coronary artery from the pulmonary trunk. The small narrow but abnormal q wave in lead 1 is especially evident in lead aVL. The QRS axis is leftward (minus 10 degrees). Voltage and repolarization criteria for left ventricular hypertrophy are present in the precordial leads. Leads V_{2-4} are half standardized.

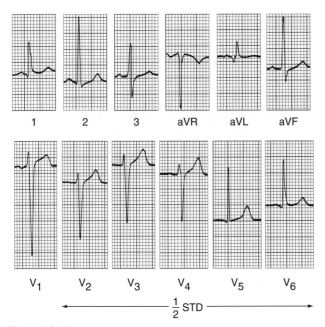

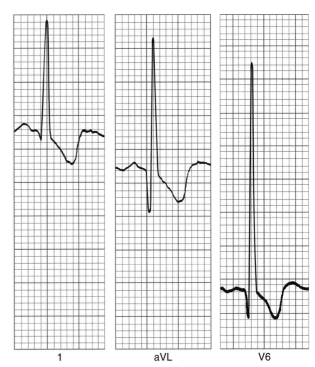

Figure 21–12

Electrocardiogram from a 19-year-old woman with anomalous origin of the left coronary artery from the pulmonary trunk. An unusual broad notched q wave is present in lead aVL. Left ventricular hypertrophy is reflected in the deep S wave in lead V_1 and the tall R waves in leads V_{5-6}. Leads V_{2-6} are half standardized.

Figure 21–13

Leads 1, aVL, and aV_6 from a 3-year-old asymptomatic girl with anomalous origin of the left coronary artery from the pulmonary trunk. The small but abnormal q wave in lead 1 and the deep narrow q waves in leads aVL and V_6 reflect initial force deformities of the coronary anomaly rather than left ventricular hypertrophy, which is represented by the tall R waves and inverted T waves.

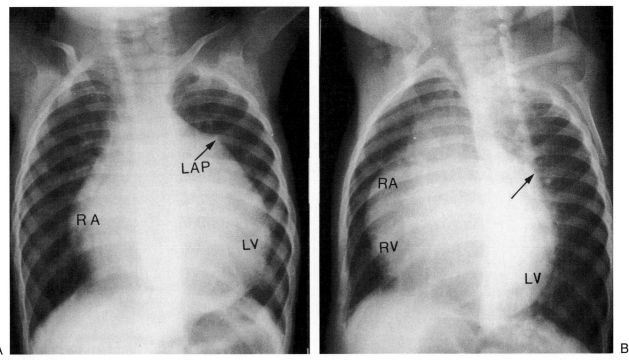

Figure 21–14

X-rays from a 10-month-old girl with anomalous origin of the left coronary artery from the pulmonary trunk. *A*, The left atrial appendage (LAP) is conspicuous, a dilated left ventricle (LV) occupies the apex, and an enlarged right atrium (RA) occupies the right cardiac border. *B*, In the left anterior oblique projection, the anterior border of the heart is formed by the right atrium and right ventricle (RV), the posterior border is formed by the dilated left ventricle, and a large left atrium lies beneath the left bronchus (*arrow*).

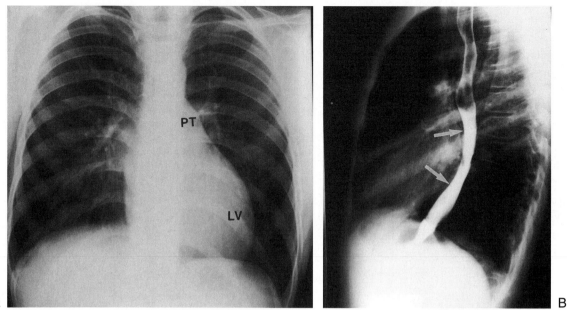

Figure 21–15

A, X-rays from the 13-year-old boy whose phonocardiogram is shown in Figure 21–7. A convex left ventricle occupies the apex, and there is slight prominence of the pulmonary trunk. *B*, The lateral view shows displacement of the barium-filled esophagus by a moderately large left atrium (*arrow*).

The X-Ray

The cardiac silhouette varies from massive cardiomegaly in symptomatic infants[62,70,110] (Fig. 12–14) to normal or nearly so in an occasional older child or adult (Fig. 21–15).[71] The most consistent radiologic feature is enlargement of the left ventricle (see Fig. 21–14).[13,62,101,102,110,123] Left atrial enlargement results from mitral regurgitation (see Figs. 21–6, 21–14, and 21–15).[16,62,86,101,102,117] Increased vascularity represents the pulmonary venous congestion of left ventricular failure (see Fig. 21–14). Dystrophic calcifica-

tion of the left ventricle has been described[8,61] but is not visible in the x-ray.[13]

The Echocardiogram

Echocardiography establishes the aortic origins of the left and right coronary arteries (Fig. 21–16) and identifies the origin of an anomalous left coronary artery from the pulmonary trunk (Fig. 21–17). Color flow imaging establishes the presence of continuous or diastolic flow entering the pul-

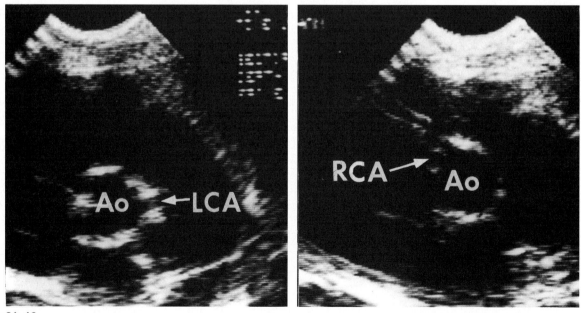

Figure 21–16

Echocardiograms in the short axis show normal origin of the left coronary artery (LCA) and normal origin of the right coronary artery (RCA). Ao, aorta.

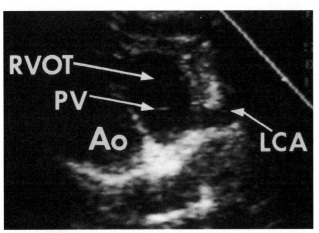

Figure 21–17
Echocardiogram in the short axis from a 4-year-old boy with anomalous origin of the left coronary artery (LCA) from the pulmonary trunk. The left coronary artery originates from the pulmonary trunk just above the pulmonary valve (PV). Ao, aorta; RVOT, right ventricular outflow tract.

monary trunk just distal to the pulmonary valve and adhering to the medial wall of the pulmonary trunk (Fig. 21–18).[17,49,57,60,104,105,113] A coronary arterial fistula into the pulmonary artery may exhibit similar flow patterns (see Chapter 22), but two coronary arteries are identified in their normal respective aortic sinuses.[50,113] Patent ductus arteriosus is characterized by color flow that enters near the *left* pulmonary artery, adheres to the *lateral* wall of the pulmonary trunk, and is directed *toward* the pulmonary valve (see Chapter 20). Echocardiography determines left ventricular size, wall motion, and ejection fraction, and color flow imag-

ing quantifies mitral regurgitation. Echogenic left ventricular papillary muscles indicate ischemic scarring (Fig. 21–19).

Summary

Infants with anomalous origin of the left coronary artery from the pulmonary trunk are normal at birth and may remain so as neonates, but irritability, pallor, fatigue, cough, weak cry, dyspnea, and diaphoresis subsequently develop due to ischemic pain and cardiac failure precipitated or aggravated by feeding, crying, or a bowel movement. Severity ranges from death in infancy (the dominant theme) to relatively asymptomatic adult survival. Precordial palpation detects a left ventricular impulse and occasionally anterior movement at the left sternal border due to systolic expansion of an enlarged left atrium. Auscultation reveals the murmur of mitral regurgitation, and flow through intercoronary anastomoses is responsible for a continuous murmur that tends to be softer in systole. The three electrocardiographic features include deep but narrow q waves in leads 1 and aVL, left ventricular hypertrophy, and left axis deviation. The x-ray varies from massive cardiomegaly due to left ventricular and left atrial enlargement in symptomatic infants and children to a normal or nearly normal x-ray in an occasional older child or young adult. Color flow imaging and Doppler interrogation identify the origin of the left coronary artery from the pulmonary trunk with retrograde flow. Left ventricular regional wall motion and ejection fraction can be established, and mitral regurgitation can be quantified.

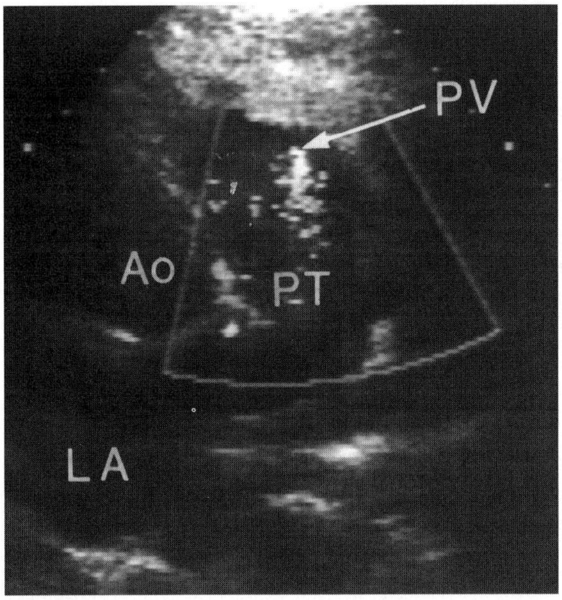

Figure 21–18
Black-and-white rendition of a color flow image in the short axis from a 22-year-old woman with anomalous origin of the left coronary artery from the pulmonary trunk. Flow from the anomalous left coronary artery enters the pulmonary trunk (PT) just above the pulmonary valve (PV). Ao, aorta; LA, left atrium.

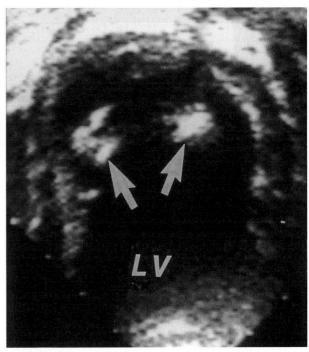

Figure 21–19
Echocardiogram from a 9-year-old girl with anomalous origin of the left coronary artery from the pulmonary trunk. *Arrows* point to left ventricular (LV) papillary muscles that are echogenic because of ischemic scarring.

REFERENCES

1. Abbott ME: Congenital cardiac disease. In Osler W: Modern Medicine. Philadelphia, Lea & Febiger, 1908.

2. Agusstson MH, Gasul BM, Lundquist R: Anomalous origin of the left coronary artery from the pulmonary artery (adult type). A case report. Pediatrics 29:274, 1962.

3. Agusstson MH, Gasul BM, Fell EH, et al: Anomalous origin of the left coronary artery from pulmonary artery. Diagnosis and treatment of infantile and adult type. JAMA 180:15, 1962.

4. Alexander RW, Griffith GC: Anomalies of the coronary artery and their clinical significance. Circulation 14:800, 1956.

5. Alexi-Meskishvili V, Berger F, Weng Y, et al: Anomalous origin of the left coronary artery from the pulmonary artery in adults. J. Card. Surg. 10:309, 1995.

6. Armer RM, Shumacker HB, Lurie PR, Fisch C: Origin of the left coronary artery from the pulmonary artery without collateral circulation. Pediatrics 32:588, 1963.

7. Arsan S, Naseri N, Keser N: An adult case of Bland White Garland syndrome with huge right coronary aneurysm. Ann. Thorac. Surg. 68:1832, 1999.

8. Askenazi J, Nadas AS: Anomalous left coronary artery originating from the pulmonary artery: Report on 15 cases. Circulation 51:976, 1975.

9. Baue AE, Baum S, Blakemore WS, Zinsser HF: A later stage of anomalous coronary circulation with origin of the left coronary artery from the pulmonary artery. Coronary artery steal. Circulation 36:878, 1967.

10. Bharati S, Chandra N, Stephenson LW, et al: Origin of the left coronary artery from the right pulmonary artery. J. Am. Coll. Cardiol. 3:1565, 1984.

11. Bharati S, Szarnicki RJ, Popper R, et al: Origin of both coronary arteries from the pulmonary trunk associated with hypoplasia of the aortic tract complex. J. Am. Coll. Cardiol. 3:437, 1984.

12. Bland EF, White PD, Garland J: Congenital anomalies of coronary arteries: Report of unusual case associated with cardiac hypertrophy. Am. Heart. J. 8:787, 1933.

13. Boostein, J. J.: Aberrant left coronary artery. Am. J. Roentgenol. 91:515, 1964.

14. Brooks, H. St. J.: Two cases of an abnormal coronary artery arising from the pulmonary artery. J. Anat. Physiol. 20:26, 1886.

15. Burch, G. E., and DePasquale, N. P.: The anomalous left coronary artery. An experiment of nature. (Editorial.) Am. J. Med. 37:159, 1964.

16. Burchell, H. B., and Brown, A. L., Jr.: Anomalous origin of coronary artery from pulmonary artery masquerading as mitral insufficiency. Am. Heart J. 63:388, 1962.

17. Canter, C. E., Gutierrez, F. R., Spray, T. L., and Martin, T. C.: Diagnosis of anomalous left coronary artery from the pulmonary trunk by color Doppler echocardiography. Am. Heart J. 116:885, 1988.

18. Cardo, M., Fernandez, B., Duran, A. C., Fernandez, M. C., Arque, J. M., Sans-Coma, V.: Anomalous origin of the left coronary from the dorsal aortic sinus and its relationship with aortic valve morphology in Syrian hamsters. J. Comp. Pathol. 112:373, 1995.

19. Cardo, M., Fernandez, B., Duran, A. C., Arque, J. M., Franco, D., Sans-Coma, V.: Anomalous origin of the left coronary artery from the pulmonary trunk and its relationship with the morphology of the cardiac semilunar valves in Syrian hamsters. Basic Res. Cardiol. 89:94, 1994.

20. Carvalho, J. S., Redington, A. N., Oldershaw, P. J., Shinebourne, E. A., Lincoln, C. R., and Gibson, D. G.: Analysis of left ventricular wall movement before and after reimplantation of anomalous left coronary artery in infancy. Br. Heart J. 65:218, 1991.

21. Case, R. B., Morrow, A. G., Stainsby, W., and Nestor, J. O.: Anomalous origin of the left coronary artery. Circulation 17:1062, 1958.

22. Castaneda, A. R., Indeglia, R. A., and Varco, R. L.: Anomalous origin of the left coronary artery from the pulmonary artery. Certain therapeutic considerations. Circulation 33 (Suppl. I):52, 1966.

23. Cayler, G. G., Smelloff, E. A., and Miller, G. E.: A new clinical sign of anomalous coronary artery. Dis. Chest 55:163, 1969.

24. Celermajer, D. S., Sholler, G. F., Howman-Giles, R., Celermajer, J. M.: Myocardial infarction in childhood: Clinical analysis of 17 cases and medium term followup of survivors. Br. Heart J. 65:332, 1991.

25. Chaitman, B. R., Bourassa, M. G., Lesperance, J., Dominguez, J. L. D., and Saltiel, J.: Aberrant course of the left anterior coronary artery

26. Chaitman, B. R., Bourassa, M. G., Lesperance, J., and Grondin, P.: Anomalous left coronary artery from pulmonary artery. Circulation 51:552, 1975.

27. Christensen, E. D., Johansen, J. B., Thayssen, P., Anderson, P. E., Alstrup, P.: Treatment of anomalous origin of the left coronary artery from the pulmonary artery in adulthood. Cardiology 87:260, 1996.

28. Colmers, R. A., and Siderides, C. I.: Anomalous origin of both coronary arteries from the pulmonary trunk. Am. J. Cardiol. 12:263, 1963.

29. Cronk, E. S., Sinclair, J. G., and Rigdon, R. H.: An anomalous coronary artery arising from the pulmonary artery. Am. Heart J. 42:906, 1951.

30. Cumming, G. R., and Ferguson, C. C.: Anomalous origin of the left coronary artery from the pulmonary artery functioning as a coronary arteriovenous fistula. Am. Heart J. 64:690, 1962.

31. Davachi, F., Moller, J. H., and Edwards, J. E.: Disease of the mitral valve in infancy. Circulation 43:565, 1971.

32. Davis, C., Jr., Dillon, R. F., Fell, E. H., and Gasul, B. M.: Anomalous coronary artery simulating patent ductus arteriosus. J.A.M.A. 160:1047, 1956.

33. Dent, E. D., Jr., and Fisher, R. S.: Single coronary artery: Report of two cases. Ann. Intern. Med. 44:1024, 1956.

34. Derrick, M. J., and Moreno-Cabral, R. J.: Anomalous origin of the left anterior descending artery from the pulmonary artery. J. Cardiac Surg. 6:24, 1991.

35. Edwards, J. E.: The direction of blood flow in coronary arteries arising from the pulmonary trunk. (Editorial.) Circulation 29:163, 1964.

36. El Habbal, M. M., De Leval, M., and Somerville, J.: Anomalous origin of the left anterior descending coronary artery from the pulmonary trunk: Recognition in life and successful surgical treatment. Br. Heart J. 60:90, 1988.

37. Evans, J. J., and Phillips, J. F.: Origin of the left anterior descending coronary artery from the pulmonary artery. J. Am. Coll. Cardiol. 3:219, 1984.

38. Fierens, C., Budts, W., Denef, B., Van De, W. F.: A 72 year old woman with ALCAPA. Heart. 83:E2, 2000.

39. Flaherty, J. T., Spach, M. S., Boineau, J. P., Canent, R. V., Barr, R. C., and Sabiston, D. C.: Cardiac potentials on body surface in infants with anomalous left coronary artery (myocardial infarction). Circulation 36:345, 1967.

40. Flamm, M. D., Stinson, E. B., Hultgren, H. N., Shumway, N. E., and Hancock, E. W.: Anomalous origin of the left coronary artery from the pulmonary artery. Circulation 38:113, 1968.

41. Frapier, J. M., Leclercq, F., Bodino, M., Chartal, P. A.: Malignant ventricular arrhythmias revealing anomalous origin of the left coronary from the pulmonary artery in two adults. Eur. J. Cardiothorac. Surg. 15:539, 1999.

42. Garcia, C. M., Chandler, J., and Russell, R.: Anomalous left circumflex coronary artery from the right pulmonary artery: First adult case report. Am. Heart J. 123:526, 1992.

43. Gasior, R. M., Winters, W. L., Glick, H., Sandiford, F., Chapman, D. W., and Morris, G. C.: Anomalous origin of left coronary artery from pulmonary artery. Am. J. Cardiol. 27:215, 1971.

44. Gasul, B. M., and Loeffler, E.: Anomalous origin of the left coronary artery from the pulmonary artery (Bland-White-Garland syndrome). Pediatrics 4:498, 1949.

45. George, J. M., and Knowlan, D. M.: Anomalous origin of the left coronary artery from the pulmonary artery in an adult. N. Engl. J. Med. 261:993, 1959.

46. Harthorne, J. S., Scannell, J. A., and Dinsmore, R. E.: Anomalous origin of the left coronary artery: Remediable cause of sudden death in adults. N. Engl. J. Med. 275:660, 1966.

47. Heidenreigh, F. P., Leon, D. F., and Shaver, J. A.: A case of anomalous right coronary artery to right atrial fistula presenting as atypical aortic insufficiency. Am. J. Cardiol. 23:453, 1969.

48. Heifetz, S. A., Robinowitz, M., Muller, K. H., and Virmanti, R.: Total anomalous origin of the coronary arteries from the pulmonary artery. Pediatr. Cardiol. 7:11, 1986.

49. Houston, A. B., Pollock, J. C. S., Doig, W. B., Gnanapragasam, J., Jamieson, M. P. G., Lilley, S., and Murtagh, E. P.: Anomalous origin of the left coronary artery from the pulmonary trunk: Elucidation with colour Doppler flow mapping. Br. Heart J. 63:50, 1990.

50. Hsu, S. Y., Lin, F. C., Chang, H. J., Yeh, S. J., Wu, D.: Multiplane transesophageal echocardiography in diagnosis of anomalous origin of the

left coronary artery from the pulmonary artery. J. Am. Soc. Echocardiogr. 11:668, 1998.

51. Huang, T., Hsueh, Y., and Tsung, S. H.: Endocardial fibroelastosis and myocardial calcification secondary to an anomalous right coronary artery arising from the pulmonary trunk. Hum. Pathol. 16:959, 1985.

52. Huritz, R. A., Caldwell, R. L., Girod, D. A., Brown, J., and King, H.: Clinical and hemodynamic course of infants and children with anomalous left coronary artery. Am. Heart J. 118:1176, 1989.

53. Hutchins, G., and Bannayan, G. A.: Development of endocardial fibroelastosis following myocardial infarction. Arch. Pathol. 91:113, 1971.

54. Iga, K., Hori, K., Matsumura, T., Gen, H.: Anomalous origin of left coronary from pulmonary artery in a 54 year old woman presenting with ventricular tachycardia from an anteroseptal scar. Jpn. Circ. J. 57:837, 1993.

55. Ihenacho, H. N. C., Singh, S. P., Astley, R., and Parsons, C. G.: Anomalous left coronary artery. Report of an unusual case with spontaneous remission of symptoms. Br. Heart J. 35:562, 1973.

56. Jameson, A. G., Ellis, K., and Levine, O. R.: Anomalous left coronary artery arising from the pulmonary artery. Br. Heart J. 25:251, 1963.

57. Jureidini, S. B., Nouri, S., Crawford, C. J., Chen, S., Pennington, G., and Fiore, A.: Reliability of echocardiography in the diagnosis of anomalous origin of the left coronary artery from the pulmonary trunk. Am. Heart J. 122:61, 1991.

58. Jurishica, A. J.: Anomalous left coronary artery: Adult type. Am. Heart J. 54:429, 1957.

59. Kafkas, P., and Miller, G. A. H.: Unusual left ventricular aneurysm in a patient with anomalous origin of left coronary artery from pulmonary artery. Br. Heart J. 33:409, 1971.

60. Karr, S. S., Parness, I. A., Spevak, P. J., van der Velde, M. E., Colan, S. D., and Sanders, S. P.: Diagnosis of anomalous left coronary artery by Doppler color flow mapping: Distinction from other causes of dilated cardiomyopathy. J. Am. Coll. Cardiol. 19:1271, 1992.

61. Kaunitz, P. E.: Origin of left coronary artery from pulmonary artery: Review of the literature and report of two cases. Am. Heart J. 33:182, 1947.

62. Keith, J. D.: Anomalous origin of left coronary artery from pulmonary artery. Br. Heart J. 21:149, 1959.

63. Kerwin, R. W., Westaby, S., Davies, G. J., and Blackwood, R. A.: Anomalous left coronary artery from the pulmonary artery presenting with infective endocarditis in an adult. Eur. Heart J. 6:545, 1985.

64. Kobayashi, J., Kosakai, Y., Kawashima, Y.: Maze procedure and anomalous coronary repair. Ann. Thorac. Surg. 61:1008, 1996.

65. Kutsche, L. M., and Van Mierop, L. H. S.: Anatomy and pathogenesis of aorticopulmonary septal defect. Am. J. Cardiol. 59:443, 1987.

66. Lampe, C. F. J., and Verheugt, A. P. M.: Anomalous left coronary artery. Adult type. Am. Heart J. 59:769, 1960.

67. Lerberg, D. B., Ogden, J. A., Zuberbuchler, J. R., and Bahnson, H. T.: Anomalous origin of the right coronary artery from the pulmonary artery. Ann. Thorac. Surg. 27:87, 1979.

68. Letcher, J. R., McCormick, D., Tendler, S., Ross, J., Chandrasekaran, K., and Brockman, S.: Left main coronary artery arising from the pulmonary trunk in a 56-year-old patient presenting with acute myocardial infarction. Am. J. Cardiol. 68:1257, 1991.

69. Levin, D. C., Fellows, K. E., and Abrams, H. L.: Hemodynamically significant primary anomalies of the coronary arteries. Circulation 58:25, 1978.

70. Liebman, J., Hellerstein, H. K., Ankeney, J. L., and Tucker, A.: The problem of the anomalous left coronary artery arising from the pulmonary artery in older children. Report of three cases. N. Engl. J. Med. 269:486, 1963.

71. Likar, I., Criley, J. M., and Lewis, K. B.: Anomalous left coronary artery arising from the pulmonary artery in an adult. A review of the therapeutic problem. Circulation 33:727, 1966.

72. Losekoot, G., Renaud, E. J., Meyne, N. G., and Van Dam, R. T.: Anomalous left coronary artery arising from the pulmonary artery. Br. Heart J. 28:646, 1966.

73. Mahdyoon, H., Brymer, J. F., Alam, M., and Khaja, F.: Anomalous right coronary artery from the pulmonary artery presenting with angina and aneurysmal left ventricular dilatation. Am. Heart J. 118:182, 1989.

74. Maurer, I., and Zierz, S.: Myocardial respiratory chain enzyme activities in anomalous origin of the left main coronary artery from the pulmonary trunk (Bland-White-Garland syndrome) and comparison with atherosclerotic coronary artery disease. Am. J. Cardiol. 70:1228, 1992.

75. Menahem, S., and Venables, A. W.: Anomalous left coronary artery from the pulmonary artery: A 15 year sample. Br. Heart J. 58:378, 1987.

76. Menke, J. A., Shaher, R. M., and Wolff, G. S.: Ejection fraction in anomalous origin of the left coronary artery from the pulmonary artery. Am. Heart J. 84:325, 1972.

77. Mesurolle, B., Qanadli, S. D., Merad, M., Mignon, F., Lacombe, P., Dubourg, O.: Anomalous origin of the left coronary artery arising from the pulmonary trunk. Eur. Radiol. 9:1570, 1999.

78. Midgley, F. M., Watson, D. C., Scott, L. P., Kuehl, K. S., Perry, L. W., Galioto, F. M., Ruckman, R. N., and Shapiro, S. R.: Repair of anomalous origin of the left coronary artery in the infant and small child. J. Am. Coll. Cardiol. 4:1231, 1984.

79. Moodie, D. S., Fyfe, D., Gill, C. C., Cook, S. A., Lytle, B. W., Taylor, P. C., Fitzgerald, R., and Sheldon, W. C.: Anomalous origin of the left coronary artery from the pulmonary artery (Bland-White-Garland syndrome in adult patients: Long-term follow-up after surgery). Am. Heart J. 106:381, 1983.

80. Murphy, M. L.: Single coronary artery. Am. Heart J. 74:557, 1967.

81. Nadas, A. S., Gamboa, R., and Hugenholtz, P. G.: Anomalous left coronary artery originating from the pulmonary artery. Circulation 29:167, 1964.

82. Neches, W. H., Mathews, R. A., Park, S. C., Lenox, C. C., Zuberbuhler, J. R., Siewers, R. D., and Bahnson, H. T.: Anomalous origin of the left coronary artery from the pulmonary artery. Circulation 50:582, 1974.

83. Nehgme, R. A., Dewar, M. L., Lutin, W. A., Talner, N. S., and Hellenbrand, W. E.: Anomalous left coronary artery from the main pulmonary trunk: Physiologic and clinical importance of its association with persistent ductus arteriosus. Pediatr. Cardiol. 13:97, 1992.

84. Newton, M. C., and Burwett, L. R.: Single coronary artery with myocardial infarction and mitral regurgitation. Am. Heart J. 95:126, 1978.

85. Nielsen, H. B., Perko, M., Aldershvile, J., Saunamaki, K.: Cardiac arrest during exercise: Anomalous left coronary artery from the pulmonary trunk. Scan. Cardiovasc. J. 33:369, 1999.

86. Noren, G. R., Raghib, G., Moller, J. H., Amplatz, K., Adams, P., Jr., and Edwards, J. E.: Anomalous origin of the left coronary artery from the pulmonary trunk with special reference to the occurrence of mitral insufficiency. Circulation 30:171, 1964.

87. Ogden, J. A.: Origin of a single coronary artery from the pulmonary artery. Am. Heart J. 78:251, 1969.

88. Ogden, J. A.: Congenital anomalies of the coronary arteries. Am. J. Cardiol. 25:474, 1970.

89. Pachinger, G. M., Van den Hoven, P., and Judkins, M. P.: Single coronary artery—a cause of angina pectoris. Am. J. Cardiol. 2:161, 1974.

90. Perloff, J. K. Normal myocardial growth and the development and regression of increased ventricular mass. In Perloff, J. K., and Child, J. S. (eds): Congenital Heart Disease in Adults, 2nd ed. Philadelphia, W. B. Saunders Company, 1998.

91. Perloff, J. K., and Roberts, W. C.: The mitral apparatus. Circulation 46:227, 1972.

92. Perloff, J. K., Roberts, N. K., and Cabeen, W. R.: Left axis deviation. Circulation 60:12, 1979.

93. Perry, L. W., and Scott, L. P.: Anomalous left coronary artery from pulmonary artery. Circulation 41:1043, 1970.

94. Puri, P. S., Rowe, R. D., and Neill, C. A.: Varying vectorcardiographic patterns in anomalous left coronary artery arising from the pulmonary artery. Am. Heart J. 71:616, 1966.

95. Purut, C. M., and Sabiston, D. C.: Origin of the left coronary artery from the pulmonary artery in older adults. J. Thorac. Cardiovasc. Surg. 102:566, 1991.

96. Rein, A. J. J. T., Colan, S. D., Parness, I. A., and Sanders, S. P.: Regional and global left ventricular function in infants with anomalous origin of the left coronary artery from the pulmonary trunk: Preoperative and postoperative assessment. Circulation 75:115, 1987.

97. Roche, A. H. G.: Anomalous origin of left coronary artery from the pulmonary artery in the adult. A report of uneventful ligation in two cases. Am. J. Cardiol. 20:561, 1967.

98. Rowe, G. G.: Inequalities of myocardial perfusion in coronary artery disease. Circulation 42:193, 1970.

99. Rudolph, A. M.: Effects of postnatal circulatory adjustments in congenital heart disease. Pediatrics 63:763, 1965.

100. Rudolph, A. M., Gootman, N. L., Kaplan, N., and Rohman, M.: Anomalous left coronary artery arising from the pulmonary

artery with large left-to-right shunt in infancy. J. Pediatr. 63:543, 1963.

101. Sabiston, D. C., Jr., Neill, C. A., and Taussig, H. B.: The direction of blood flow in anomalous left coronary artery arising from the pulmonary artery. Circulation 22:591, 1960.

102. Sabiston, D. C., Jr., Pelargonio, S., and Taussig, H. B.: Myocardial infarction in infancy. J. Thorac. Cardiovasc. Surg. 40:321, 1960.

103. Saenz, C. B., Taylor, J. L., Soto, B., Nanda, N. C., and Kirklin, J. K.: Acute myocardial infarction in a patient with anomalous right coronary artery. Am. Heart J. 112:1092, 1986.

104. Sanders, S. P., Parness, I. A., and Colan, S. D.: Recognition of abnormal connections of coronary arteries with the use of Doppler color flow mapping. J. Am. Coll. Cardiol. 13:922, 1989.

105. Schmidt, K. G., Cooper, M. J., Silverman, N. H., and Stanger, P.: Pulmonary artery origin of the left coronary artery: Diagnosis by two-dimensional echocardiography, pulsed Doppler ultrasound and color flow mapping. J. Am. Coll. Cardiol. 11:396, 1988.

106. Shah, R. M., Nanda, N. C., Hsiung, M. C., Moos, S., and Roitman, D.: Identification of anomalous origin of the right coronary artery from pulmonary trunk by Doppler color flow mapping. Am. J. Cardiol. 57:366, 1986.

107. Singh, A., Katkov, H., Zavoral, J. H., Sane, S. M., and McLeod, J. D.: Congenital aneurysms of the left ventricle. Am. Heart J. 99:25, 1980.

108. Smith, J. C.: Review of single coronary artery with report of two cases. Circulation 1:1168, 1950.

109. Soloff, L. A.: Anomalous coronary arteries arising from the pulmonary artery. Am. Heart J. 24:118, 1942.

110. Stein, H. L., Hagstrom, J. W. C., Ehlers, K. H., and Steinberg, I.: Anomalous origin of the left coronary artery from the pulmonary artery. Angiographic and pathologic study of a case. Am. J. Roentgenol. 93:320, 1965.

111. Summer, G. L., and Hendrix, G. H.: Surgical ligation of an anomalous left coronary artery arising from the pulmonary artery in an adult. Am. Heart J. 76:812, 1968.

112. Suzuki, Y., Murakami, T., and Kawai, C.: Detection of anomalous origin of left coronary from pulmonary artery by real-time Doppler color flow mapping in a 53-year-old asymptomatic female. Int. J. Cardiol. 34:339, 1992.

113. Swensson, R. E., Murillo-Olivas, A., Elias, W., Bender, R., Daily, P. O., and Sahn, D. J.: Noninvasive Doppler color flow mapping for detection of anomalous origin of the left coronary artery from the pulmonary artery and for evaluation of surgical repair. J. Am. Coll. Cardiol. 11:659, 1988.

114. Talner, N. S., Halloran, K. H., Mahdavy, M., Gardner, T. H., and Hipona, F.: Anomalous origin of left coronary artery from the pulmonary artery. A clinical spectrum. Am J. Cardiol. 15:689, 1965.

115. Tamer, D. F., Mallon, S. M., Garcia, O. L, and Wolff, G. S.: Anomalous origin of the left anterior descending coronary artery from the pulmonary artery. Am. Heart J. 108:341, 1984.

116. Tingelstad, J. B., Lower, R. R., and Eldredge, W. J.: Anomalous origin of the right coronary artery from the main pulmonary artery. Am. J. Cardiol. 30:670, 1972.

117. Usman, A., Fernandez, B., Uricchio, J. F., and Nichols, H. T.: Aberrant origin of left coronary artery combined with mitral regurgitation in an adult. Am. J. Cardiol. 8:130, 1961.

118. Van der Hauwaert, L. G., Stalpaert, G. L., and Verhaeghe, L.: Anomalous origin of the left coronary artery from the pulmonary artery. A therapeutic problem. Am. Heart J. 64:538, 1965.

119. Vesterlund, T., Thomsen, P. E. B., and Hansen, O. K.: Anomalous origin of the left coronary artery from the pulmonary artery in an adult. Br. Heart J. 54:110, 1985.

120. Vestermark, S.: Anomalous origin of left coronary artery from the pulmonary artery. Acta Paediatr. Scand. 54:387, 1965.

121. Wald, S., Stonecipher, K., Baldwin, B. J., and Nutter, D. O.: Anomalous origin of the right coronary artery from the pulmonary artery. Am. J. Cardiol. 27:677, 1971.

122. Wesselhoeft, H., Fawcett, J. S., and Johnson, A. L.: Anomalous origin of the left coronary artery from the pulmonary trunk. Circulation 38:403, 1968.

123. Wilder, R. J., and Perlman, A.: Roentgenographic demonstration of anomalous left coronary artery arising from the pulmonary artery. Am. J. Roentgenol. 91:511, 1964.

124. Wilson, C. L. Dlabal, P. W., and McGuire, S. A.: Surgical treatment of anomalous left coronary artery from the pulmonary artery: Follow-up in teenagers and adults. Am. Heart J. 98:440, 1979.

125. Wright, N. L., Baue, A. E., Baum, S., Blakemore, W. S., and Zinsser, H. F.: Coronary artery steal owing to anomalous left coronary artery originating from pulmonary artery. J. Thorac. Cardiovasc. Surg. 59:461, 1970.

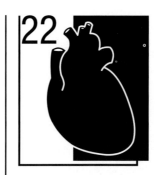

Congenital Coronary Arterial Fistula

Coronary arterial fistulas are the most frequent hemodynamically significant congenital malformations of the coronary circulation,[6,68,69,75,99,132,141] comprising 14% of congenital coronary artery anomalies (see Chapter 32).[141] In this anomaly, the right and left coronary arteries arise from their appropriate aortic sinuses, but a fistulous branch of one or more than one of the two coronary arteries drains into a cardiac chamber or into the pulmonary trunk, coronary sinus, vena cava, or a pulmonary vein. When the communication drains into a right cardiac chamber or into the pulmonary trunk, the fistula is *arteriovenous*,[94] an appropriate term because the fistulous communication allows arterialized systemic blood (*arterio*) to mix with unoxygenated blood in the right side of the heart (*venous*). When the fistula drains into the left atrium or left ventricle, the term coronary *arterial* fistula is correct, but the term *arteriovenous* is not correct.[94]

Congenital coronary arterial fistulas were described by Krause in 1865,[67] by Abbott in 1908,[1] and by Trevor in 1912.[126] Approximately half of these fistulas arise from the *right* coronary artery,[37,41,43,59,68] somewhat less than half from the *left* coronary artery,[16,29,68,108,128] and a distinct minority of 5% from *both* coronary arteries.[7,38,61,68,75,76,83,86,91,114,144] Even more rarely, all three coronary arteries are involved[13,26,89,93,100,104,135] or multiple fistulas arise from one coronary artery[110] or a congenitally single coronary artery gives rise to the fistula.[51] A fistula has been reported from the conus artery to the right atrium[70] and from the coronary sinus to left ventricle.[46] In approximately 3% of cases, the contralateral coronary artery is absent.[68]

The *drainage site* of a coronary arterial fistula is more important than the site of origin and consists of either single or multiple vascular channels or a maze of fine channels that form a diffuse network or plexus, a pattern especially likely when the left ventricle receives the fistula (see Fig. 22–4, 22–6).[13,26] Over 90% of congenital coronary arterial fistulas drain into the *right* side of the heart[33,59,75,104,128] and are therefore *arteriovenous*.[16,68,91,108,128] The substantial majority in approximate order of frequency enter the right ventricle (40%) or right atrium (25%) (see Fig. 22–3A),[44,68,85,94,108, 111,133,134] less commonly the pulmonary trunk (15%)* (Figs. 22–1 and 22–2) or coronary sinus (7%)[64,68,73,88,132] (Fig. 22–3B), and most rarely the superior vena cava.[33,42,58,69, 74,91,118] A recipient coronary sinus may be aneurysmal,[44,55] especially when it receives fistulas from *two* coronary arteries (see Fig. 22–20).[144] *Bilateral* coronary arterial fistulas usually drain into the pulmonary trunk.[7,76,86] The relatively few fistulas that do not communicate with the right side of the heart drain into the left atrium (5%)[5,21,29,41,68] (Fig. 22–5) or into the left ventricle (3%) (Figs. 22–4 and 22–6).† Coronary arterial fistulas are also known to drain into *both* ventricles[29,104] and into pulmonary veins.[37] A *coronary artery to left ventricular fistula* differs from an *aortic to left ventricular tunnel* (see Chapter 7).[117,121,123]

Small coronary arterial fistulas that exist without clinical evidence of their presence are often discovered incidentally during routine diagnostic coronary angiography[62,96] (see Fig. 22–2B) or during routine echocardiography (see Fig. 22–19). Coronary arterial fistulas are incidental findings in approximately 0.1% to 0.26% of patients undergoing coronary angiography.[30,140,141] In a series of 14,708 coronary arteriograms, 19 congenital coronary arterial fistulas were identified,[45] and in a series of 11,000 coronary angiograms, 13 fistulas were identified.[107] These unanticipated fistulas are characterized by one or more relatively small channels

---

*See references 6, 33, 38, 45, 47, 62, 68, 76, 86, 99, 107.
†See references 3, 5, 18, 22, 31, 37, 43, 68, 104, 108, 123, 128.

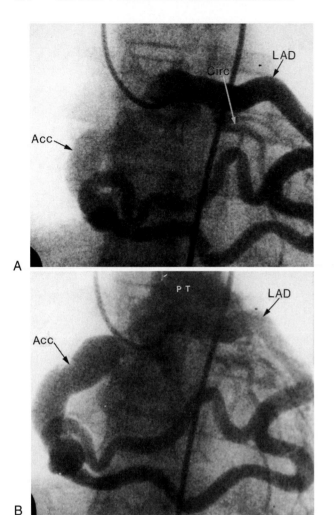

Figure 22–1

A, Selective left coronary arteriogram from a 10-year-old girl with a coronary arterial fistula from the left anterior descending coronary artery (LAD) to an accessory coronary artery (Acc). The vascular channels that form the fistula are large, dilated, and tortuous. Uninvolved branches of the circumflex system (Circ) are small. *B*, This later frame shows the large accessory coronary artery draining into the pulmonary trunk (PT).

that originate from the left anterior descending coronary artery and form a network that communicates with the pulmonary trunk at one or more sites (see Fig. 22–2B).[45] Importantly, a significant proportion of coronary arterial fistulas are *acquired* because of the prevalence of intravascular and interventional procedures.[122,141,145]

The coronary artery that gives rise to the fistula is characteristically dilated, elongated, and tortuous (see Fig. 22–1),[44,80,85,120] but the coronary arteries distal to the fistula are of normal caliber (see Fig. 22–2A).[68] The fistulous coronary artery often contains saccular aneurysms[69] that may reach an astonishing size[2,12,34,35,71,143] and may rupture.[17]

An estimated 1% to 2% of coronary arterial fistulas close spontaneously in infants, children, or adults,[*] and *spontaneous* closure occurred in a 44-year-old woman because of occlusion of an atherosclerotic coronary artery proximal to

the fistula.[63] Occasional fistulas harbor calcification of the wall[85] and thrombi with distal embolization.[106]

The *embryogenesis* of coronary arterial fistulas is uncertain. Fistulas entering the *right ventricle* have been related to the persistence of primitive intramyocardial sinusoids[34,131] or to the development of a rectiform vascular network in the distal branches of the involved coronary artery.[88] Fistulas entering the left ventricle are thought to result from direct flow through thebesian venous channels.[3,13,20] Interestingly, the veins of Thebesius were cited as evidence of direct passage of blood from one side of the heart to the other before William Harvey discovered the circulation (see Chapter 32).

There are six coronary anlagen in the embryo, three in the developing aorta and three in the developing pulmonary artery[56] (see Chapter 21). These anlagen normally involute except the two from the right and left aortic sinuses. A *coronary arterial to pulmonary artery fistula* may result from persistence of one or more of the pulmonary arterial anlagen, hence the term *accessory* coronary artery (see Fig. 22–1).[34,47] The relatively high incidence of *bilateral* coronary arterial fistulas to the pulmonary artery is in accord with this theory.[6,76,86] An accessory coronary artery consists of either a single large channel (see Fig. 22–1), one or more smaller channels, multiple tortuous channels, or a plexiform arrangement.[6,12,45,62,76,86,89,107]

The *physiologic responses to* coronary arterial fistulas are related to the volume of blood flowing through the fistula, the chamber or vascular bed into which the fistula drains, and the myocardial ischemia that results from a *coronary steal* caused by low-resistance vascular channels. About 10% of blood from the aortic root normally enters the coronary circulation, but the volume is considerably greater in the presence of a coronary arterial fistula. A *left-to-right* shunt is established when the fistula drains into the right atrium, right ventricle, or coronary sinus.[85] If drainage is into the right ventricular outflow tract, pulmonary trunk (see Figs. 22–1 and 22–2), left atrium (see Fig. 22–5), or left ventricle (see Figs. 22–4 and 22–6), the hemodynamic burden is borne by the left ventricle alone. When the fistula drains into the left ventricle, the hemodynamic result is analogous to aortic regurgitation because aortic-to-left ventricular flow through the fistula occurs during diastole,[*] although a fistulous coronary artery *receives* blood during *systole* when the stoma of the fistula is large.[37] If the fistula drains into the inflow tract of the right ventricle, volume overload of the right ventricle coexists. If drainage is either *directly* into the right atrium or *indirectly* into the right atrium through the coronary sinus (see Fig. 22–3), volume overload of right ventricle exists in addition to volume overload of the left side of the heart. If the fistula drains into the left atrium (see Fig. 22–5), the left ventricle is volume overloaded.[5,18,21,22,29,41]

The pulmonary-to-systemic flow ratios are typically small, even negligible, regardless of patient age.[44,63,69,94,132]

---

[*]See references 44, 48, 53, 72, 78, 82, 83, 92, 116, 124, 138, 139.

[*]See references 5, 13, 18, 22, 26, 34, 37, 43, 89, 93, 108, 119, 135.

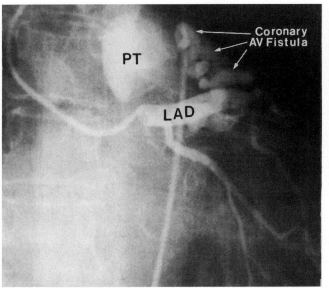
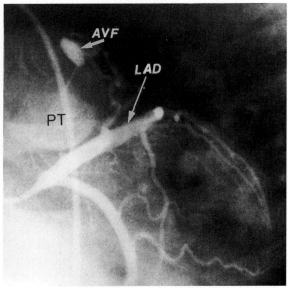

Figure 22-2

A, Left coronary arteriogram from a 62-year-old woman. A dilated left anterior descending artery (LAD) gave rise to a coronary arteriovenous fistula (coronary AV fistula) that drained into the pulmonary trunk (PT). Coronary arterial branches distal to the fistula are of normal caliber. *B*, Left coronary arteriogram from a 58-year-old man in whom a small coronary arterial fistula (AVF) from the left anterior descending artery (LAD) to the pulmonary trunk PT) was an incidental finding during routine coronary angiography.

Massive flow through a very large fistula is rare.[119] Shunts in excess of 2:1 are unusual,[44,63,69,133] but an occasional neonate experiences congestive heart failure because of an exceptionally large coronary arterial fistula that drains either into the left side of the heart[119] or into the right side of the heart (see Fig. 22–16).[131]

Myocardial ischemia occurs when a coronary arterial fistula functions as a low-resistance pathway that constitutes a *coronary steal*.[*] The coronary artery that gives rise to the fistula then assumes an important role, because steal from a major branch of the *left* coronary artery is more significant than steal from a smaller right coronary artery.[48] Acquired coronary artery stenosis *distal* to a congenital coronary arterial fistula aggravates the perfusion deficit because the fistula acts as a low-resistance alternative to the acquired obstruction.[62]

The History

The initial suspicion of a congenital coronary arterial fistula is likely to be a continuous murmur in an asymptomatic child or young adult[39,49,79] or in an older adult who comes to attention because of nonspecific symptoms.[143] A small acoustically silent coronary arterial fistula comes to light during coronary angiography or echocardiography done for other reasons. A continuous murmur exists from birth when a coronary arterial fistula drains into the low pressure right or left atrium because the pressure gradient responsible for the murmur is present in utero. Coronary

arterial fistulas that drain into the right ventricle or pulmonary trunk generate continuous murmurs after the neonatal fall in pulmonary vascular resistance. The continuous murmur is overlooked when it is soft and localized to an atypical site, and an isolated *diastolic* murmur may be heard but misinterpreted.[135] Clinically occult coronary artery to pulmonary artery fistulas are found in a small but consistent percentage of patients undergoing routine coronary angiography or echocardiography (see earlier). Coronary arterial fistulas are sometimes mistaken for patent ductus arteriosus[33,99,108] (Fig. 22–7), which occasionally coexists.[14,108,113,128]

The male-to-female ratio is about 1:1.[29,85,108,111,120] Survival into adulthood is expected, although life span is not normal.[41,47,63,64,69,85,88,120,132] Longevity has been reported from the sixth to ninth decade (see Fig. 22–15),[*] and the diagnosis has awaited the seventh to ninth decade.[142,140] A 68-year-old professional athlete was undiagnosed until acquired atherosclerotic coronary artery disease prompted coronary angiography, which disclosed bilateral coronary arterial fistulas.[7] Death may be from acquired coronary artery disease or from noncardiac causes.[62,64,69]

The majority of patients, especially those younger than 20 years ago, are asymptomatic when the coronary arterial fistula is first diagnosed.[†] An uncommon if not rare exception is the infant with an exceptionally large fistula (see Fig. 22–16).[119,131] Symptoms and complications in approximate order of frequency include dyspnea, fatigue, myocardial ischemia,[18,22,50,69] congestive heart failure,[65,68,109] sudden death,[137] infective

---

[*]See references 3, 7, 18, 22, 32, 33, 35, 36, 38, 44, 50, 66, 69, 85, 93, 105, 129.

[*]See references 10, 15, 18, 24, 29, 41, 55, 64, 69, 95, 134.
[†]See references 2, 9, 12, 25, 34, 44, 69, 88, 104, 106, 108, 132.

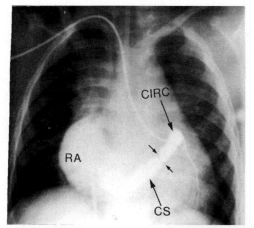

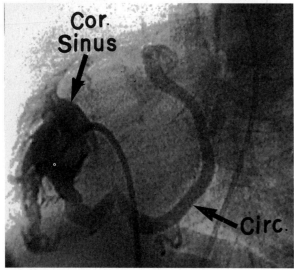

Figure 22–3

A, Left coronary arteriogram in an 8-year-old boy The dilated circumflex coronary artery (CIRC) narrows (*unlabeled paired arrows*) as it joins the coronary sinus (CS), which drains into a dilated right atrium (RA). *B,* Left coronary arteriogram in an 18-year-old woman with a coronary arterial fistula from a dilated circumflex artery (Circ.) to a dilated coronary sinus (Cor Sinus).

endocarditis,[*] and rupture.[52,68,104] Rarely, obstruction of the superior vena cava is caused by a large fistulous saccular aneurysm,[12,101] one of which ruptured at age 82 years.[17] Atrial fibrillation may herald congestive heart failure when a fistula drains into the right or left atrium or into the coronary sinus (see Fig. 22–15B).[5,69,108] A coronary steal may result in myocardial ischemia and angina pectoris without atherosclerotic coronary artery disease, and the ischemia has an undesirable effect on left ventricular function.[3,18,22,29,38,47,69] Spontaneous closure of a coronary arterial fistula is uncommon but not rare (see earlier).[†]

Physical Appearance

Growth and development are unaffected because the left-to-right shunts are relatively small. Catabolic effects of congestive heart failure are reserved for the rare occurrence of large fistulas in infants.

The Arterial Pulse

The arterial pulse and pulse pressure are normal because flow through the fistula is usually small. However, when the right ventricle, right atrium, or left atrium receives a large fistula, the arterial pulse is brisk and the pulse pressure is wide because the decrease in aortic *diastolic* pressure caused by flow into low pressure drainage sites is accompanied by an increase in *systolic* pressure in response to an increase in left ventricular stroke volume (see Fig. 22–8).[*] When a large fistula drains into the left ventricle, the hemodynamic results are analogous to aortic regurgitation.[34,37,43]

The Jugular Venous Pulse

The jugular venous pulse is normal even when the fistula drains into the right atrium. With the advent of congestive heart failure (see Fig. 22–15B), the mean jugular venous pressure rises.[35] Obstruction of the superior vena cava by a saccular aneurysm of a fistula that drained into the right atrium elevated the mean jugular venous pressure and damped the A and V waves.[12,101] A giant left atrium caused by a large coronary arterial-to-left atrial fistula in a 64-year-old man contributed to *inferior* vena caval obstruction.[41]

Precordial Movement and Palpation

A large fistula results in a hyperdynamic left ventricular impulse because left ventricular volume overload accompanies *all* drainage sites. If the fistula drains into the left atrium or left ventricle or into the pulmonary artery, an *isolated* left ventricular impulse is palpated. If the fistula drains into the right atrium or into the right ventricular inflow tract, volume overload is imposed on *both* ventricles, so both right *and* left ventricular impulses are palpated.

Auscultation

A continuous murmur is an auscultatory hallmark of coronary arterial fistulas[10,11,23,27,39,40,87] (see Figs. 22–7 through 22–11) and may be mistaken for the continuous murmur of patent ductus arteriosus.[14,108,113,128] The distinction is based on the configuration of the murmur[108,120] (see Fig. 22–7–22–11) and on its precordial location that is determined by the drainage site of the fistula, not by the coronary

---

[*]See references 9, 18, 32, 34, 58, 69, 101, 102, 118, 127.
[†]See references 48, 53, 72, 78, 82, 83, 92, 101, 124, 138, 139, 141.

---

[*]See references 5, 12, 16, 25, 29, 32, 60, 64, 65, 84, 108, 120.

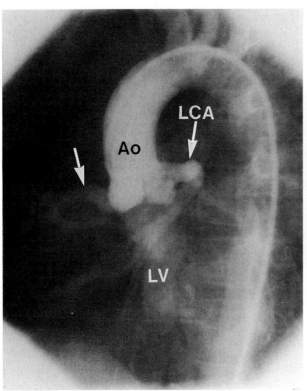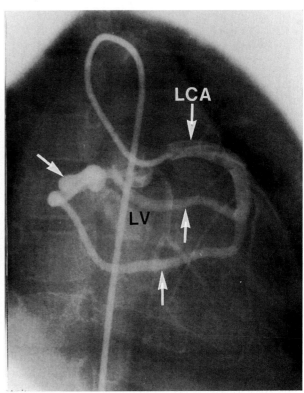

Figure 22–4

A, Aortogram (Ao) from a 5-year-old girl with a coronary arterial fistula that originated from the proximal left coronary artery (LCA) and drained into the left ventricle (LV). The proximal left coronary is dilated because it fed the tortuous fistula (*unmarked left arrow*). *B*, The left coronary arteriogram (LCA) visualized the dilated tortuous fistula (*unmarked white arrows*) that drained into the left ventricle (LV).

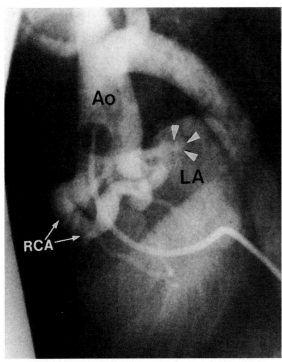

Figure 22–5

Aortogram (Ao) from an 11-month-old boy with a coronary arterial fistula that arose from the right coronary artery (RCA) and drained into the left atrium (LA).

artery of origin (Fig. 22–12).[16,85,108] When the fistula drains into the right atrium *directly* or drains into the right atrium *indirectly* through the coronary sinus (see Fig. 22–3A), intracardiac phonocardiography records the murmur within the right atrial cavity (see Fig. 22–9), and the thoracic wall site is topographically appropriate at the *right* upper or lower sternal border or over the sternum (see Fig. 22–12).[9,14,33,48,79,92] When a left circumflex coronary arterial fistula drains into the coronary sinus (see Fig. 22–3A), the continuous murmur is heard in the back between the spine and left scapula. When the fistula drains into the inflow tract of the right ventricle, the murmur sites are along the mid to lower *left* sternal border, over the *lower sternum* or subxiphoid (see Fig. 22–12).[106,108] When the fistula drains into the outflow tract of the right ventricle, the murmur is maximum along the upper to mid left sternal border (see Figs. 22–7 and 22–12).[8,16,27] When the fistula drains into the pulmonary trunk, the continuous murmur is prominent at the upper left sternal border (see Fig. 22–12).[4,10,11,29,39] A pulmonary arterial fistula discovered incidentally at coronary angiography is a small or plexiform communication (see Fig.22–2B) that is not accompanied by a murmur.[45,62,107] When the fistula drains into the left atrium, the murmur is maximum along the upper left sternal border (see Fig. 22–12) and may radiate toward the left anterior auxiliary line.[21,79,108] A fistula that drains into a left superior vena cava is accompanied by a continuous murmur at the upper to mid left sternal edge.[58,74,118]

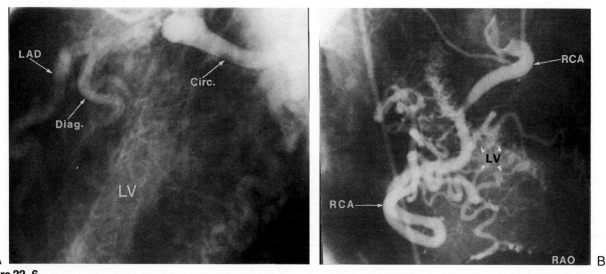

Figure 22–6

Coronary arteriograms from a 70-year-old asymptomatic woman who came to medical attention because of a diastolic murmur at the left sternal border. Left ventricular ejection fraction was 58%. *A,* The left anterior descending (LAD), diagonal (Diag), circumflex (Circ), and right coronary artery coronary artery (RCA; see panel *B*) were all dilated. *B,* The three dilated coronary arteries gave rise to a maze of tortuous fistulae that drained into the left ventricle (LV) through a fine intramural plexus.

Coronary arterial fistulas that are likely to be mistaken for a patent ductus arteriosus are those that drain into the pulmonary trunk, left atrium, or right ventricular outflow tract. Because the majority of coronary arterial fistulas drain into the body of the right ventricle or into the right atrium, the accompanying continuous murmurs are heard at sites *remote* from the ductus location. Spontaneous closure of a coronary arterial fistula is accompanied by diminution or disappearance of the murmur.[48,53,72,78]

Coronary arterial fistulas that drain into the right atrium, left atrium, or right ventricle generate continuous murmurs because pressure differences between the aortic root and the low pressure receiving chambers are continuous without interruption from systole into diastole. The *configuration* of continuous murmurs from these different fistulous sources differ from each other and differ from the continuous murmur of patent ductus arteriosus. When the fistula drains into the right atrium, coronary sinus, or left atrium, pressure gradients between aortic root and receiving chamber are much larger during systole than during diastole, so the murmur is louder in systole (see Fig. 22–9 22–10).[16,95,109] When the fistula communicates with the pulmonary trunk, the continuous murmur may increase around the second heart sound as in patent ductus but does not contain eddy sounds.[40,87] Flow patterns are more complex when the fistula drains into the right ventricle because right ventricular contraction compresses the fistula during its transmural course (see Fig. 22–7).[44] Compression reduces systolic flow, so the systolic portion of the continuous murmur softens (see Fig. 22–7C). If the fistula is only moderately compressed by right ventricular contraction, the intramural systolic gradient increases, so the systolic portion of the continuous murmur increases during systole (see Fig. 22–8).[60,84,94,98,128] A wide aortic pulse pressure (high systolic, low diastolic) reinforces the systolic portion of the continuous murmur (see Fig. 22–8). When congestive heart failure elevates right ventricular diastolic pressure, a continuous murmur may be confined to systole because elevated diastolic pressure decreases diastolic flow through the fistula.[24,55,57,134]

An early diastolic murmur is generated when a fistula drains into the left ventricle.[31,37,43,85] If a large fistulous stoma remains widely patent during left ventricular contraction, blood flow *into* the fistula during systole may generate a systolic murmur.[37] A coronary arterial to left ventricular

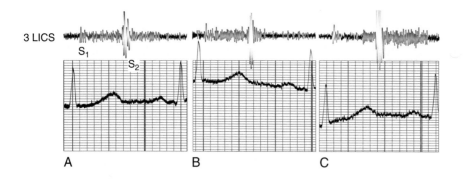

Figure 22–7

Phonocardiograms from a 37-year-old woman with a coronary arterial fistula between the right coronary artery and the outflow tract of the right ventricle. A continuous murmur peaked before and after the second heart sound (S₂) and was misdiagnosed as a patent ductus murmur even though the maximum location was the third left intercostal space (3 LICS) and even though the murmur changed configuration from beat to beat (*A, B, C*).

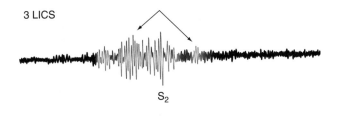

3 LICS

S₂

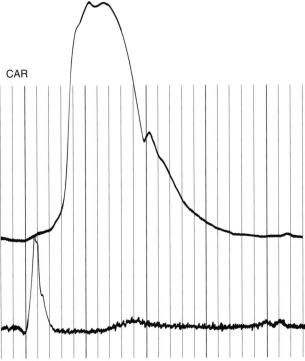

CAR

Figure 22–8
Phonocardiogram and carotid arterial pulse (CAR) from a 47-year-old man with a coronary arterial fistula between the right coronary artery and the outflow tract of the right ventricle. The continuous murmur was much louder in systole (*paired arrows*) and was maximum in the third left intercostal space (3 LICS). S₂, second heart sound. The wide systemic arterial pulse pressure was 170/68 mm Hg. Pulmonary to systemic flow ratio was 1.7:1.

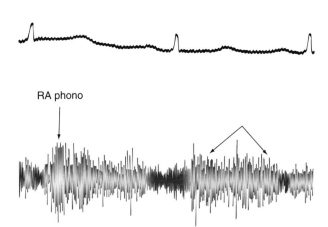

RA phono

Figure 22–9
Phonocardiogram recorded within the right atrium (RA PHONO) of a 27-year-old man with a coronary arterial fistula between the right coronary artery and right atrium. In the first cycle, the continuous murmur is louder in systole (*vertical arrow*). In the second cycle, the murmur is equal in systole and diastole (*paired arrows*).

fistula is silent when drainage is through thebesian venous channels.[3,20]

Coronary arterial fistulas usually deliver relatively small blood volumes through narrow pathways, so the accompanying continuous murmur is relatively localized, medium to moderately high frequency, and grade 3 or less.[19,44,81,120] Large fistulas generate coarse harsh rough murmurs that radiate and are accompanied by thrills.[39,44,106,128] The Valsalva maneuver may cause a coronary arterial to right ventricular fistulous murmur to soften as systolic pressure in the right ventricle increases.[39,128] Occasionally, a coronary arterial to right atrial fistulous continuous murmur diminishes appreciably during held inspiration and becomes tumultuous during exhalation.[39]

The second heart sound splits normally during respiration even when the right atrium receives the fistula. This is so for two reasons. *First*, the shunt volume is shared equally by the right and left sides of the heart because shunted blood must flow through *both* ventricles on its way back to the aorta. *Second*, inspiration results in an *increase* in right ventricular stroke volume and a *decrease* in left ventricular stroke volume because the shunt into the right atrium occurs with an intact atrial septum (see Chapter 15).

The Electrocardiogram

Electrocardiographic abnormalities are chiefly related to the chamber receiving the shunt and to the volume of

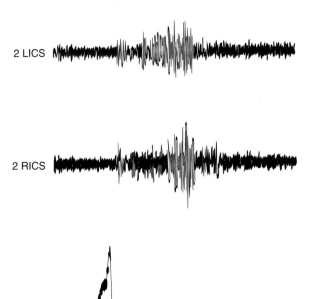

2 LICS

2 RICS

Figure 22–10
Phonocardiograms from an 8-year-old boy with a coronary arterial fistula from the circumflex coronary artery to the coronary sinus (see angiogram, Fig. 22–3A). The continuous murmur was louder in systole, and maximum in the second and third *right* intercostal spaces (2 RICS), topographically appropriate for the coronary sinus drainage site. 2 LICS, second left intercostal space. The electrocardiogram shows an incidental delta wave.

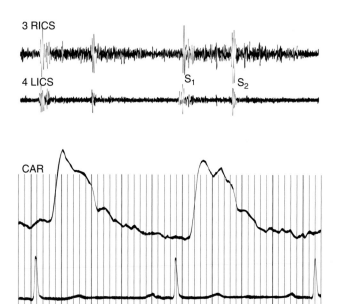

Figure 22–11

Phonocardiograms from a 23-year-old woman with a right coronary arterial fistula to the right atrium. A continuous murmur was loudest in the third *right* intercostal space (3 RICS). S_1 and S_2, first and second heart sounds; 4 LICS, fourth left intercostal space; CAR, carotid pulse.

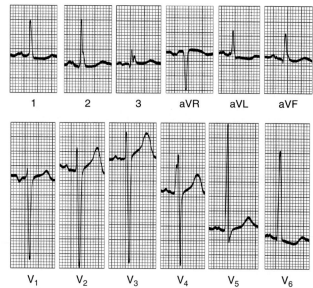

Figure 22–13

Electrocardiogram from the 47-year-old man with a right coronary arterial fistula that entered the right ventricular outflow tract. The phonocardiogram and carotid pulse are shown in Figure 22–8. The P waves are slightly bifid in leads 1, 2, and aVR, and the P terminal force is abnormal in lead V_1. Voltage and repolarization criteria for left ventricular hypertrophy are present in leads V_{5-6}.

blood flowing through the fistula.[29,69,85,94,108,120] Fistulas that drain into the right atrium or coronary sinus result in biatrial P wave abnormalities, drainage into the right ventricle, pulmonary trunk, or left atrium results in left atrial P wave abnormalities (Fig. 22–13), and drainage into the right atrium or coronary sinus results in right atrial P wave abnormalities.[5,44] Atrial fibrillation occasionally occurs in older patients with fistulas that drain into the right atrium, left atrium, or coronary sinus (see Fig. 22–15B).[5,69,108,144] Fistulas that drain into the right ventricular outflow tract, pulmonary trunk, left atrium, or left ventricle may cause left ventricular hypertrophy (see Fig. 22–13).[37,43,69,85] Biventricular hypertrophy may occur when the fistula drains into the right atrium or into the body of the right ventricle because shunted blood circulates through *both* ventricles.[8,13,34] A *coronary steal* may induce ischemic ST segment and T wave changes at rest or during exercise stress testing.[50,69,93,108] An ischemic pattern is more likely

if the coronary steal involves a major branch of the *left* coronary artery.[48] Myocardial infarction is rarely a feature of the electrocardiogram,[29,69] although a fistula may aggravate the perfusion deficit of coexisting acquired coronary artery disease.[62,69]

The X-Ray

The radiologic features of coronary arterial fistulas reflect the volume and duration of flow and the site of drainage. Young patients with small fistulas have normal x-rays,[44,63] whereas infants with large fistulas and congestive heart failure have appreciable cardiomegaly.[119,131] A large fistula that drains into the right atrium or coronary sinus is accompanied by increased pulmonary vascularity, a convex pulmonary trunk, and biventricular and biatrial enlargement

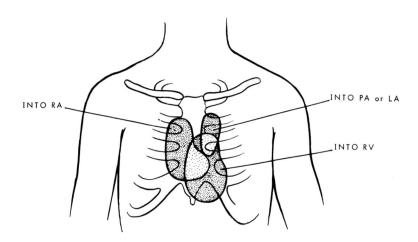

Figure 22–12

Schematic illustration of precordial murmur locations as determined by the site of coronary arterial fistula drainage. (Adapted from Sakakibara S, et al: Coronary arteriovenous fistula. Am Heart J 72:307, 1966.)

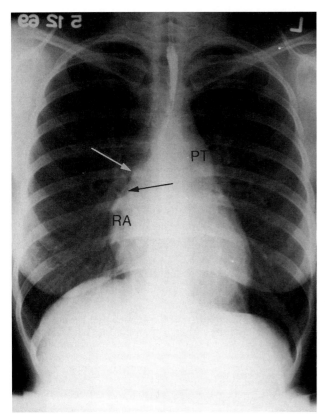

Figure 22–14

X-ray from a 23-year-old woman with a right coronary arterial fistula that drained into the right atrium (RA). The fistula reveals itself as a shadow to the right of the vertebral column (*arrows*). The pulmonary trunk (PT) is moderately dilated. The phonocardiogram is shown in Figure 22–11.

(Figs. 22–14 and 22–15).[2,8,35,44,65,85,88,133] Drainage into the right ventricle results in a similar picture but without dilation of the right atrium.[8] When a coronary arterial fistula drains into the pulmonary trunk or left atrium, chamber enlargement is confined to the left ventricle and left atrium (Fig. 22–14).[5,21] A giant left atrium was reported in a 64-year-old man with a right coronary arterial to left atrial fistula.[41]

Multiple saccular aneurysms of an enlarged tortuous coronary arterial fistula are occasionally recognized as an irregular silhouette along the right or left cardiac border (see Fig. 22–14).[2,21,37,44,108] A giant aneurysm of a left coronary artery to pulmonary artery fistula presented as a calcified mediastinal mass.[90] Calcification in the wall of a fistula is exceptional.[24]

The Echocardiogram

Transthoracic and transesophageal echocardiography with color flow imaging and Doppler interrogation identify the origin and drainage site of coronary arterial fistulas and assess their functional consequences.* The origin or stoma of a fistulous coronary artery considerably exceeds in size the origin of a normal coronary artery (Figs. 22–16 and 22–17).[130] The *drainage site* can be identified by color flow imaging[114,125] (Figs. 22–18 through 22–19) while Doppler interrogation establishes systolic and diastolic flow patterns[23,77,97,130] that shed light on the configuration of accompanying murmurs.

Coronary arterial fistulas drain into the pulmonary trunk immediately distal to the pulmonary valve, and flow proceeds upward along the medial wall (see Fig 22–18). Alternatively, a small fistula may drain into the pulmonary artery at a site more distal to the pulmonary valve and may exhibit exclusive diastolic flow (see Fig. 22–19).

---

*See references 23,77,97,102,114,125,130, 136,142,143.

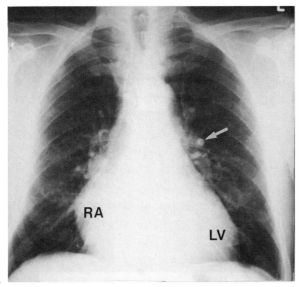

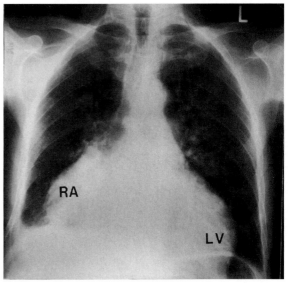

Figure 22–15

A, X-ray from a 64-year-old man with a large right coronary arterial to right atrial fistula. Pulmonary vascularity is increased. The *unmarked white arrow* identifies the cross section of an enlarged intrapulmonary artery reflecting increased flow. A dilated right atrium (RA) occupies the lower right cardiac border, and a moderately dilated left ventricle (LV) occupies the apex. *B*, X-ray from the same patient at age 75 years after the onset of atrial fibrillation. The size of the right atrium (RA) has increased dramatically. The left ventricle (LV) is much larger and extends below the left hemidiaphragm. There is a small right pleural effusion.

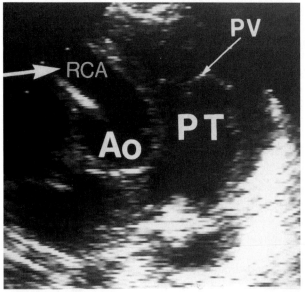

Figure 22–16

Echocardiogram (short axis) from a female neonate with congestive heart failure caused by a large right coronary arterial fistula that drained into outflow tract of the right ventricle. The proximal right coronary artery (RCA) is markedly dilated. Ao, aorta; PT, pulmonary trunk; PV, pulmonary valve.

Color flow imaging distinguishes a coronary arterial fistula that drains into the right atrium or right ventricle from a ruptured sinus of Valsalva aneurysm (see Chapter 23). A coronary arterial fistula that drains into the pulmonary trunk can be distinguished from a patent ductus arteriosus (see Chapter 20) and from anomalous origin of the left coronary artery from the pulmonary trunk (see Chapter 21), and a fistula that drains into the left ventricle can be distinguished from an aortic to left ventricular tunnel (see Chapter 7).

Echocardiography characterizes the hemodynamic response to flow delivered through a coronary arterial fistula and characterizes the response of the left ventricle to potential ischemic effects of a coronary steal. The coronary sinus is dilated when it receives one or more fistulas (see Figs. 22–3B and 22–20). Left ventricular ejection fraction reflects overload volume delivered through the fistula, and global and regional wall motion reflect potentially adverse ischemic effects of a coronary steal.

Summary

Physical appearance, the arterial pulse, and the jugular venous pulse are usually normal. Precordial palpation detects the impulses of either or both ventricles depending on the drainage site of the coronary arterial fistula. A precordial continuous murmur that is located inappropriately for a patent ductus arteriosus is often the first index of suspicion of a congenital coronary arterial fistula in an asymptomatic child or young adult. Suspicion is heightened if the murmur peaks in systole or diastole and not around the second heart sound. The electrocardiogram

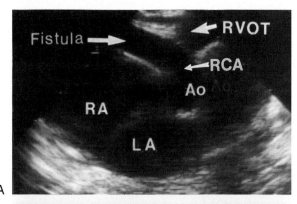

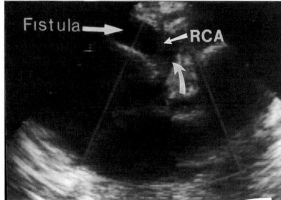

Figure 22–17

A, Echocardiogram (short axis) from a 3-week-old girl with a large coronary arterial fistula that drained into the right ventricular outflow tract (RVOT). The proximal right coronary artery (RCA) is markedly dilated. Ao, aorta; RA/LA, right and left atrium. *B*, Black-and-white print of a color flow image showing flow from aorta into the large right coronary artery from which the fistula originated.

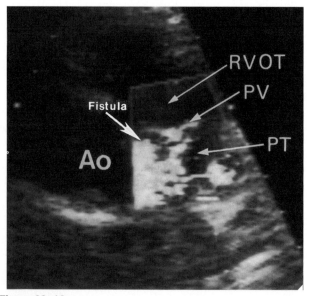

Figure 22–18

Black-and-white print of a color flow image from a 49-year-old woman with a coronary arterial fistula that drained into the pulmonary trunk (PT). The flow disturbance originates immediately distal to the pulmonary valve (PV) and then moves away from the valve along the medial wall of the pulmonary trunk. Ao, aorta; RVOT, right ventricular outflow tract.

Figure 22–19

Black-and-white prints of color flow images (short axis) from a 33-year-old woman with a tiny acoustically silent coronary arterial to pulmonary arterial fistula found incidentally. *A*, Flow through the tiny fistula was confined to diastole as timed with the low-pressure pulmonary regurgitation (PR). *B*, Entry site of the fistula was in the lateral wall of the pulmonary trunk relatively distal to the pulmonary valve (PV). Ao, aorta.

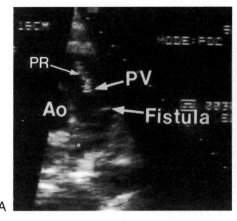
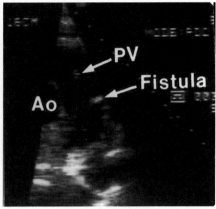

Figure 22–20

A, Anterior view of a three-dimensional magnetic resonance image data set obtained by using sequential acquisitions in transaxial planes in a 44-year-old man with coronary arterial fistulas from the right coronary artery (RCA) and the circumflex coronary artery (Circ) both of which entered an aneurysmal coronary sinus (CS). Ao, aorta; LAD, left anterior descending artery. *B*, Posterior view showing the aneurysmal coronary sinus to better advantage. LV, left ventricle.

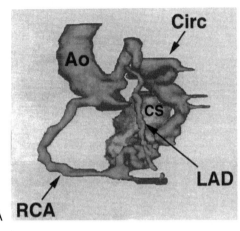
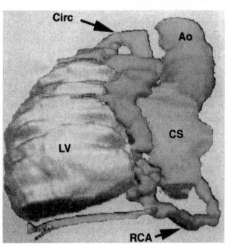

reflects the blood volume delivered through the fistula to the individual recipient chambers. More distinctive in young patients is left ventricular ischemia due to a coronary steal. The x-ray reflects the response of individual chambers to the size of the left-to-right shunt. Distinctive but rarely seen in the x-ray are the shadows of saccular aneurysms of a coronary arterial fistula as it courses along the right or left cardiac border. Echocardiography identifies the origin and drainage site of the fistula and establishes the physiologic consequences of the left-to-right shunt and the potential ischemic effects of a coronary steal.

REFERENCES

1. Abbott ME: Anomalies of the coronary arteries. In Osler W: Modern Medicine. Philadelphia, Lea & Febiger, 1908.
2. Abbott OA, Rivarola CH, Logue RB: Surgical correction of coronary arteriovenous fistula. J. Thorac. Cardiovasc. Surg. 42:660, 1961.
3. Ahmed SS, Haider B, Regan TJ: Silent left coronary artery-cameral fistula: Probable cause of myocardial ischemia. Am. Heart J. 104:869, 1982.
4. Amplatz K, Aguirre J, Lillehei CW: Coronary arteriovenous fistula into main pulmonary artery. JAMA 172:1384, 1960.
5. Arani DT, Greene DG, Klocke FJ: Coronary artery fistulas emptying into left heart chambers. Am. Heart J. 96:438, 1978.
6. Azcuna JI, Cabrera A, Arruza F, Iriar TEM: Fistulae between the coronary arteries and the right cavities of the heart. Br. Heart J. 33:451, 1971.
7. Baim DS, Kline H, Silverman JF: Bilateral coronary fistulas emptying into the left heart chambers. Circulation 65:810, 1982.
8. Barcia A, Kincaid OW, Swan HJC, et al: Coronary artery-to-right ventricle communication: Report of 2 cases studied by selective angiocardiography. Mayo Clin. Proc. 37:623, 1962.
9. Barnes RJ, Cheung ACS, Wu RWY: Coronary artery fistula. Br. Heart J. 31:299, 1969.
10. Baylis JH, Campbell M: An unusual cause for a continuous murmur. Guy's Hosp. Rep. 101:174, 1952.
11. Björk VD, Crafoord C: Arteriovenous aneurysm of the pulmonary artery simulating patent ductus arteriosus Botalli. Thorax 2:65, 1947.
12. Björk VO, Björk L: Coronary artery fistula. J Thorac Cardiovasc Surg 49:921, 1965.
13. Black IW, Loo CKC, Allan RM: Multiple coronary artery-left ventricular fistulae: Clinical, angiographic, and pathologic findings. Cathet. Cardiovasc. Diagn. 23:133, 1991.
14. Bosher, L. H., Jr., Vasli, S., McCue, C. M., and Belter, L. F.: Congenital coronary arteriovenous fistula associated with large patent ductus. Circulation 20:254, 1959.
15. Brack, M. J., Hubner, P. J. B., and Firmin, R. K.: Successful operation on a coronary arteriovenous fistula in a 74 year old woman. Br. Heart J. 65:107, 1991.
16. Braudo, J. L., Javett, S. N., Zion, M. M., and Adler, D. I.: Congenital coronary arteriovenous fistula. Br. Med. J. 1:601, 1962.
17. Bauer HH, Allmendinger PD, Flaherty J, Ovila D, Rossi MA, Chen C. Congenital coronary arteriovenous fistula: Spontaneous rupture with cardiac tamponade. Ann. Thorac. Surg. 62:1521, 1996.
18. Brooks, C. H., and Bates, P. D.: Coronary artery-left ventricular fistula with angina pectoris. Am. Heart J. 106:404, 1983.
19. Carmichael, D. B., and Davidson, D. G.: Congenital coronary arteriovenous fistula. Am. J. Cardiol. 8:846, 1961.
20. Cha, S. E., Singer, E., Maranhao, V., and Boldberg, H.: Silent coronary artery-left ventricular fistula: A disorder of the Thebesian system. Angiology 29:169, 1978.
21. Char, F., and Hara, M.: Congenital coronary artery fistula communication of the left coronary artery with the left atrium. J. Lancet 86:93, 1966.

22. Cheng, T. O.: Left coronary artery-to-left ventricular fistula: Demonstration of coronary steal phenomenon. Am. Heart J. 104:870, 1982.

23. Chia, B. L., Ee, G., Tan, A., Choo, M., and Tan, L.: Two-dimensional and pulsed Doppler echocardiographic abnormalities in coronary artery-pulmonary artery fistula. Chest 86:901, 1984.

24. Colbeck, J. C., and Shaw, J. M.: Coronary aneurysm with arteriovenous fistula. Am. Heart J. 49:270, 1954.

25. Cooley, D. A., and Ellis, P. R., Jr.: Surgical considerations of coronary arterial fistula. Am. J. Cardiol. 10:467, 1962.

26. Cottier, C., Kiowski, W., von Bertrab, R., Pfisterer, M., and Burkart, F.: Multiple coronary arteriocameral fistulas as a cause of myocardial ischemia. Am. Heart J. 115:181, 1988.

27. Davis, C., Jr., Dillon, R. F., Fell, E. H., and Gasul, B. M.: Anomalous coronary artery simulating patent ductus arteriosus. J.A.M.A. 160:1047, 1956.

28. Davis, C., Jr., Fell, E. H., and Dillon, R.: Congenital vascular lesions imitating the patent ductus. A.M.A. Arch. Surg. 72:838, 1956.

29. de Nef, J. J. E., Varghese, P. J., and Losekoot, G.: Congenital coronary artery fistula. Analysis of 17 cases. Br. Heart J. 33:857, 1971.

30. Vavuranakis M, Bush CA, Boudoulas H. Coronary artery fistulas in adults: Incidence, angiographic characteristics, natural history. Cath Cardiovasc Diagn. 35: 116, 1995.

31. Dobell, A. R. C., and Long, R. W.: Right coronary-left ventricular fistula mimicking aortic valve insufficiency in infancy. J. Thorac. Cardiovasc. Surg. 82:785, 1981.

32. Dubost C., Chevrier, J. L., and Metianu, C.: Congenital communication between the right coronary artery and the right atrium. A case report of successful repair. J. Cardiovasc. Surg. 2:60, 1961.

33. Edis, A. J., Schattenberg, T. T., Feldt, R. H., and Danielson, G. K.: Congenital coronary artery fistula. Mayo Clin. Proc. 47:567, 1972.

34. Edwards, J. E.: Anomalous coronary arteries with special reference to arteriovenous-like communications. Circulation 17:1001, 1958.

35. Edwards, J. E., Gladding, T. C., and Weir, A. B.: Congenital communication between the right coronary artery and the right atrium. J. Thorac. Cardiovasc. Surg. 35:662, 1958.

36. Effler, D. B., Sheldon, W. C, and Turner, J. C.: Coronary arteriovenous fistula. Surgery 41:41, 1967.

37. Eguchi, S., Nitta, H., Asano, K., Tanaka, M., and Hoshino, K.: Congenital fistula of the right coronary artery to the left ventricle. Am. Heart J. 80:242, 1970.

38. Eie, H., and Hillestad, L.: Arteriovenous fistulas of coronary arteries. Scand. J. Thorac. Cardiovasc. Surg. 5:34, 1971.

39. Engle, M. A., Goldsmith, E. I., Holswade, G. R., Goldberg, H. P., and Glenn, F.: Congenital coronary arteriovenous fistula. Diagnostic evaluation and surgical correction. N. Engl. J. Med. 264:856, 1961.

40. Ernst, C. B., Klassen, K. P., and Ryan, J. M.: Vascular malformation overlying the pulmonary artery simulating a patent ductus arteriosus. Circulation 23:759, 1961.

41. Floyd, W. L., Young, W. G., and Johnsrude, I. S.: Coronary arterial-left atrial fistula. Am. J. Cardiol. 25:716, 1970.

42. Galbraith, A. J., Werner, D., and Cutforth, R. H.: Fistula between left coronary artery and superior vena cava. Br. Heart J. 46:99, 1981.

43. Galioto, F. M., Raitman, M. J., Slovia, A. J., and Sarot, I. A.: Right coronary artery to left ventricle fistula. Am. Heart J. 82:93, 1971.

44. Gasul, B. M., Arcilla, R. A., Fell, E. H., Lynfield, J., Bicoff, J. P., and Luan, L. I.: Congenital coronary arteriovenous fistula. Pediatrics 25:531, 1960.

45. Gillebert, C., Van Hoof, R., Van de Werf, F., Piessens, J., and De Geest, H.: Coronary artery fistulas in an adult population. Eur. Heart J. 7:437, 1986.

46. Gnanapragasam, J. P., Houston, A. B., and Lilley, S.: Congenital fistula between the left ventricle and coronary sinus: Elucidation by colour Doppler flow mapping. Br. Heart J. 62:406, 1989.

47. Gobel, F. L., Anderson, C. F., Baltaxe, H. A., Amplatz, K., and Wang, Y.: Shunts between the coronary and pulmonary arteries with normal origin of the coronary arteries. Am. J. Cardiol. 25:655, 1970.

48. Griffiths, S. P., Ellis, K., Hordof, A. J., Martin, E., Levine, O. R., and Gersony, W. M.: Spontaneous complete closure of a congenital coronary artery fistula. J. Am. Coll. Cardiol. 2:1169, 1983.

49. Grob, M., and Kolb, E.: Congenital aneurysm of the coronary artery. Arch. Dis. Child. 34:8, 1959.

50. Gupta, N. C., and Beauvais, J.: Physiologic assessment of coronary artery fistula. Clin. Nucl. Med. 16:40, 1991.

51. Gupta, P. D., Rahimtoola, S. H., and Miller, R. A.: Single coronary artery-right ventricle fistula. Br. Heart J. 34:755, 1972.

52. Haberman, J. H., Howard, M. L., and Johnson, E. S.: Rupture of the coronary sinus with hemopericardium: A rare complication of coronary arteriovenous fistula. Circulation 28:1143, 1963.

53. Hackett, D., and Hallidie-Smith, K. A.: Spontaneous closure of coronary artery fistula. Br. Heart J. 52:477, 1984.

54. Haller, J. A., Jr., and Little, J. A.: Diagnosis and surgical correction of congenital coronary artery-coronary sinus fistula. Circulation 27:939, 1963.

55. Harris, A., Jefferson, K., and Chatterjee, K.: Coronary arteriovenous fistula with aneurysm of coronary sinus. Br. Heart J. 31:400, 1969.

56. Heifetz, S. A., Robinowitz, M., Mueller, K. H., and Virmani, R.: Total anomalous origin of the coronary arteries from the pulmonary artery. Pediatr. Cardiol. 7:11, 1986.

57. Heindenreich, F. P., Leon, D. F., and Shaver, J. A.: A case of anomalous right coronary artery to right atrial fistula presenting as atypical aortic insufficiency. Am. J. Cardiol. 23:453, 1969.

58. Hipona, F. A.: Congenital coronary arterial fistula to a persistent left superior vena cava. Am. J. Roentgenol. 97:355, 1966.

59. Hobbs, R. E., Millit, H. D., Raghavan, P. V., Moodie, D. S., and Sheldon, W. C.: Coronary artery fistulae: A 10 year review. Cleve. Clin. Q. 49:191, 1982.

60. Honey, M.: Coronary arterial fistula. Br. Heart J. 26:719, 1964.

61. Humblet, L., Delvigne, J., Kulbertus, H., Collignon, P., and Joris, H.: Arteriovenous fistula involving both coronary arteries and main pulmonary artery. Br. Heart J. 31:136, 1969.

62. Iskandrian, A. S., Kimbiris, D., Bemis, C. E., and Segal, B. L.: Coronary artery to pulmonary artery fistulas. Am. Heart J. 96:605, 1978.

63. Jaffe, R. B., Glancy, D. L., Epstein, S. E., Brown, B. G., and Morrow, A. G.: Coronary arterial-right heart fistulae. Circulation 47:133, 1973.

64. Kimbiris, D., Kasparian, H., Knibbe, P., and Brest, A. N.: Coronary artery-coronary sinus fistula. Am. J. Cardiol. 26:532, 1970.

65. Kitiyakara, K., Jumbala, B., and Sukrojana, K.: Congenital fistula between a coronary artery and the right atrium; report of a case successfully treated by open heart surgery. Acta Chir. Scand. 129:663, 1965.

66. Knoblich, R., and Rawson, A. J.: Arteriovenous fistula of heart. Am. Heart J. 52:474, 1956.

67. Krause, W.: Uber den Ursprung einer akzessorichen a. coronaria cordis aus der a. pulmonis. Z. Rationelle Med. 24:225, 1865.

68. Levin, D. C., Fellows, K. E., and Abrams, H. L.: Hemodynamically significant primary anomalies of the coronary arteries. Circulation 58:25, 1978.

69. Liberthson, R. R., Sagar, K., Berkoben, J. P., Weintraub, R. M., and Levine, F. H.: Congenital coronary arteriovenous fistula. Circulation 59:849, 1979.

70. Lipoff, J. I.: Anomalous origin of the left main coronary artery from the right sinus of Valsalva with coronary AV fistula of the conus artery. Chest 92:203, 1988.

71. Lim, C. H., Tan, N. C., Tan, L., Seah, C. S., and Tan, D.: Giant congenital aneurysm of the right coronary artery. Am. J. Cardiol. 39:751, 1977.

72. Mahoney, L. T., Schieken, R. M., and Lauer, R. M.: Spontaneous closure of a coronary artery fistula in childhood. Pediatr. Cardiol. 2:311, 1982.

73. Mantini, E., Grondin, C. M., Lillehei, C. W., and Edwards, J. E.: Congenital anomalies involving the coronary sinus. Circulation 33:317, 1966.

74. Marcus, B., Sivazlian, K., and Gordon, L. S.: Echocardiographic detection of left circumflex coronary artery to left superior vena cava fistula by use of Doppler color flow mapping. J. Am. Soc. Echocardiogr. 4:405, 1991.

75. McNamara, J. J., and Gross, R. E.: Congenital coronary fistula. Surgery 65:59, 1969.

76. Mehta, D., Redwood, D., and Ward, D. E.: Multiple bilateral coronary arterial to pulmonary artery fistulae in an asymptomatic patient. Int. J. Cardiol. 16:96, 1987.

77. Miyatake, K., Okamoto, M., Kinoshita, N., Fusejima, K., Sakakibara, H., and Nimura, Y.: Doppler echocardiographic features of coronary arteriovenous fistula. Complementary roles of cross sectional echocardiography and the Doppler technique Br. Heart J. 51:508, 1984.

78. Morgan, R. B., Forker, A. D., O'Sullivan, M. J., and Fosburg, R. D.: Coronary arterial fistulas. Seven cases with unusual features. Am. J. Cardiol. 30:432, 1972.

79. Mozen, H. E.: Congenital circoid aneurysm of a coronary artery with associated arterio-atrial fistula, treated by operation: A case report. Ann. Surg. 144:215, 1956.
80. Muir, C. S.: Coronary arterio-cameral fistula. Br. Heart J. 2:374, 1960.
81. Munkner, T., Petersen, O., and Vesterdal, J.: Congenital aneurysm of the coronary artery with an arteriovenous fistula. Acta Radiol. 50:333, 1958.
82. Muthusamy, R., Gupta, G., Ahmed, R. A. S., de Giovanni, J., and Singh, S. P.: Fistula between a branch of left anterior descending coronary artery and pulmonary artery with spontaneous closure. Eur. Heart J. 11:954, 1990.
83. Nakatani, S., Nanto, S., Nasuyama, T., Tamai, J., and Kodama, K.: Spontaneous near disappearance of bilateral coronary artery-pulmonary artery fistulas. Chest 99:1288, 1991.
84. Neill, C., and Mounsey, P.: Auscultation in patent ductus arteriosus with a description of two fistulae simulating patent ductus. Br. Heart J. 20:61, 1958.
85. Neufeld, H. N., Lester, R. G., Adams, P., Jr., Anderson, R. C., Lillehei, C. W., and Edwards, J. E.: Congenital communication of a coronary artery with a cardiac chamber or the pulmonary trunk ("coronary artery fistula"). Circulation 24:171, 1961.
86. Nishiguchi, T., Matsuoka, Y., Sennari, E., Okishima, T., Suzumiya, H., Akimoto, K., Takamura, K., Kawaguchi, K., Tashiro, S. Yamasaki, S., and Hayakawa, K.: Congenital coronary artery fistula: Diagnosis by two-dimensional Doppler echocardiography. Am. Heart J. 120:1244, 1990.
87. Nunn, D. B., Thrower, W. B., Boone, J. A., and Lipton, M.: Coronary arteriovenous fistula simulating patent ductus arteriosus. Am. Surg. 28:476, 1962.
88. Ogden, J. A.: Congenital anomalies of the coronary arteries. Am. J. Cardiol. 25:474, 1970.
89. Ogino, K., Hisatome, I., Kotake, H., Furuse, T., Mashiba, H., Kuroda, H., and Mori, T.: A case of four coronary artery fistulae originating from three vessels associated with aneurysm. Eur. Heart J. 8:1260, 1987.
90. Okita, Y., Miki, S., Jufuhara, K., Ueda, Y., Tahata, T., Sakai, T., Tatsumi, A., and Kitamo, M.: Aneurysm of coronary arteriovenous fistula presenting as a calcified mediastinal mass. Ann. Thorac. Surg. 54:771, 1992.
91. Oldham, H. N., Ebert, P. A., Young, W. G., and Sabiston, D. C.: Surgical management of congenital coronary artery fistula. Ann. Thorac. Surg. 12:503, 1971.
92. Farooki ZQ, Nowlen T, Hakimi M, Pinsky WW. Congenital coronary artery fistulae: A review of 18 cases with an emphasis on spontaneous closure. Pediatr Cardiol. 14: 208, 1993.
93. Oshiro, K., Shimabukuro, M., Nakada, Y., Chibana, T., Yoshida, H., Nagamine, F., Sunagawa, R., Gushiken, M., Murakami, K., and Mimura, G.: Multiple coronary LV fistulas: Demonstration of coronary steal phenomenon by stress thallium scintigraphy and exercise hemodynamics. Am. Heart J. 120:217, 1990.
94. Papaioannou, A., Agorogiannis, S., Nihoyanopoulos, J., and Lazzaridis, D.: Congenital coronary artery fistula. Am. J. Cardiol. 10:588, 1962.
95. Paul, O., Sweet, R. H., and White, P. D.: Coronary arteriovenous fistula. Case report. Am. Heart J. 37:441, 1949.
96. Phillips, P. A., and Libanoff, A. J.: Arteriovenous communication associated with obstructive arteriosclerotic coronary artery disease and myocardial infarction. Chest 65:106, 1974.
97. Pickoff, A. S., Wolff, G. S., Bennett, V. L., Kaiser, G., and Ferrer, P. L.: Pulsed Doppler echocardiographic detection of coronary artery to right ventricular fistula. Pediatr. Cardiol. 2:145, 1982.
98. Puyau, F. A., and Collins, H. A.: Congenital coronary arterio-venous fistula. Am. J. Dis. Child. 106:65, 1963.
99. Querimit, A. S., and Rowe, G. G.: Localization of coronary arteriovenous fistula by indicator-dilution curves. Am. J. Cardiol. 27:114, 1971.
100. Reddy, K., Gupta, M., and Hamby, R. I.: Multiple coronary arteriosystemic fistulas. Am. J. Cardiol. 33:304, 1974.
101. Rein, A. J. J. T., Yatsiv, I., and Simcha, A.: An unusual presentation of right coronary artery fistula. Br. Heart J. 59:598, 1988.
102. Ren. J. Y., and Goh, T. H.: Congenital coronary artery fistula to the right atrium. J. Cardiovasc. Ultrasonog. 4:21, 1985.
103. Rodgers, D. M., Wolf, N. M., Barrett, M. J., Zuckerman, G. L., and Meister, S. G.: Two-dimensional echocardiographic features of coronary arteriovenous fistula. Am. Heart J. 104:872, 1982.
104. Rose, A. G.: Multiple coronary arterioventricular fistulae. Circulation 58:178, 1978.
105. Rowe, G. G.: Inequalities of myocardial perfusion in coronary artery disease. Circulation 42:193, 1970.
106. Sabiston, D. C., Jr., Ross, R. S., Criley, J. M., Gaertner, R. A., Neill, C. A., and Taussig, H. B.: Surgical management of congenital lesions of the coronary circulation. Ann. Surg. 157:908, 1963.
107. Said, S. A. M., and Landman, G. H. M.: Coronary-pulmonary fistula: Long-term follow-up in operated and non-operated patients. Int. J. Cardiol. 27:203, 1990.
108. Sakakibara, S., Yokoyama, M., Takao, A., Nogi, M., and Gomi, H.: Coronary arteriovenous fistula; nine operated cases. Am. Heart J. 72:307, 1966.
109. Sanger, P. W., Taylor, F. H., Robicsek, F., and Cobey, W. G.: Coronary arterio-venous fistula. Ann. Surg. 149:572, 1959.
110. Schamroth, C. L., Sareli, P., Curcio, A., and Barlow, J. B.: Multiple coronary artery-right ventricle fistulas. Am. Heart J. 109:1388, 1985.
111. Schultz, J.: Coronary arteriovenous aneurysm. Review of the literature. Am. Heart J. 56:431, 1958.
112. Scott, D. H.: Aneurysm of coronary arteries. Am. Heart J. 36:403, 1948.
113. Shaffer, A. B., St. Ville, J., and Meckler, S. A.: Coronary arteriovenous fistula with patent ductus arteriosus. Am. Heart J. 65:758, 1963.
114. Shakudo, M., Yoshikawa, J., Yoshida, K., and Yamaura, Y.: Noninvasive diagnosis of coronary artery fistula by Doppler color flow mapping. J. Am. Coll. Cardiol. 13:1572, 1989.
115. Shizukuda, Y., Yonekura, S., Tsuchihashi, K., Tanaka, S., Komatsu, S., and Iimura, O.: A case of right coronary artery to left ventricle fistula observed over 20 years. Jpn. J. Med. 28:510, 1989.
116. Shubrooks, S. J., and Naggar, C. Z.: Spontaneous near closure of coronary artery fistula. Circulation 57:197, 1978.
117. Somerville, J., English, T., Ross, D. N.: Aorto-left ventricular tunnel. Br. Heart J. 36:321, 1974.
118. Stansel, H. C., Jr., and Fenn, J. E.: Coronary arteriovenous fistula between the left coronary artery and persistent left superior vena cava complicated by bacterial endocarditis. Ann. Surg. 160:292, 1964.
119. Starc, T. J., Bowman, F. O., and Hordof, A. J.: Congestive heart failure in a newborn secondary to coronary artery-left ventricular fistula. Am. J. Cardiol. 58:366, 1986.
120. Steinberg, I., Baldwin, J. S., and Dotter, C. T.: Coronary arteriovenous fistula. Circulation 17:372, 1958.
121. Sung, C., Leachman, R. D., Zerpa, F., Angelini, P., and Lufschanowski, R.: Aortico-left ventricular tunnel. Am. Heart J. 98:87, 1979.
122. Tabrah, F., Aintablian, A., and Hamby, R. I.: Coronary arteriovenous fistula complicating aorto-coronary bypass surgery. Am. Heart J. 85:534, 1973.
123. Takeda, K., Okuda, Y., Matsumura, K., Sakuma, H., Tagami, T., and Nakagawa, T.: Giant fistula between the right coronary artery and the left ventricle. Am. J. Radiol. 159:1087, 1992.
124. Tomita, H., Sawada, Y., Nagata, N., and Chiba, S.: Spontaneous near closure of coronary artery fistula: Doppler echocardiographic findings. Acta. Paediatr. Jpn. 33:389, 1991.
125. Trask, J. L., Bell, A., and Usher, B. W.: Doppler color flow imaging in detection and mapping of left coronary artery fistula to right ventricle and atrium. J. Am. Soc. Echocardiogr. 3:131, 1990.
126. Trevor, R. S.: Aneurysm of the descending branch of the right coronary artery, situated in the wall of the right ventricle and opening into the cavity of the ventricle, associated with great dilatation of the right coronary artery and non-valvular infective endocarditis. Proc. R. Soc. Med. 5:20, 1911–1912.
127. Tsagaris, T. J., and Hecht, H. H.: Coronary artery aneurysm and subacute bacterial endocarditis. Ann. Intern. Med. 57:116, 1962.
128. Upshaw, C. B., Jr.: Congenital coronary arteriovenous fistula. Report of a case with an analysis of 73 reported cases. Am. Heart J. 63:399, 1962.
129. Valdivia, E., Rowe, G. G., and Angevine, D. M.: Large congenital aneurysm of the right coronary artery. A.M.A. Arch. Pathol. 63:168, 1957.
130. Velvis, H., Schmidt, K. G., Silverman, N. H., and Turley, K.: Diagnosis of coronary artery fistula by two-dimensional echocardiography, pulsed Doppler ultrasound and color flow imaging. J. Am. Coll. Cardiol. 14:968, 1989.
131. Verani, M. S., and Lauer, R. M.: Echocardiographic findings in right coronary arterial-right ventricular fistulas. Report of a neonate with fatal congestive heart failure. Am. J. Cardiol. 35:444, 1975.

132. Vlodaver, Z., Johnson, T., Karnegis, J. N., Edwards, J. E., and Castaneda, A. R.: Clinical Pathologic Conference: Congenital communication of right coronary artery with coronary sinus. Am. Heart J. 85:689, 1973.

133. Walther, R. J., Starkey, G. W. B., Zervopoulos, E., and Gibbons, G. A.: Coronary arteriovenous fistula. Clinical and physiologic report of two patients, with review of the literature. Am. J. Med. 22:213, 1957.

134. Yenel, F.: Coronary arteriovenous communication. Report of a case and review of the literature. N. Engl. J. Med. 265:577, 1961.

135. Yokawa, S., Watanabe, H., and Kurosaki, M.: Asymptomatic left and right coronary artery-left ventricular fistula in an elderly patient with a diastolic murmur only. Int. J. Cardiol. 25:244, 1989.

136. Zahn, E. M., Smallhorn, J. F., Egger, G., Burrows, P. E., Rebecca, I. M., and Freedom, R. M.: Echocardiographic diagnosis of fistula between the left circumflex coronary artery and the left atrium. Pediatr. Cardiol. 13:178, 1992.

137. Lau G.: Sudden death arising from a congenital coronary fistula. Forensic Sci Int. 22:73, 1995.

138. Carrel T, Tkebuchava T, Jenni R, Arbenz U, Turina M.: Congenital coronary fistulas in children and adults. Cardiology 87: 325, 1996.

139. Sherwood MC, Rockenmacher S, Colon SD, Geva T.: Prognostic significance of clinically silent coronary artery fistulas. Am J Cardiol. 83: 407, 1999.

140. Ben-Gal T, Herz I, Solodky A, Snir E, Birnbaum Y.: Coronary artery-main pulmonary artery fistula. Clin Cardiol. 22: 310, 1999.

141. Said SAM, El Gamal MIH, van der Werf T.: Coronary arteriovenous fistulas: Collective review and management of six new cases. Clin Cardiol. 20: 748, 1997.

142. Tousoulis T, Brilli S, Aggelli K, Tentolouris C, Stefanadis C, Toutouzas K, Frogoudaki A, Toutouzas P.: Left main coronary to left atrial fistula causing mild pulmonary hypertension. Circulation. 103: 2028, 2001.

143. Zuppiroli A, Mori F, Santoro G, Dolara A.: Coronary arteriovenous aneurysmatic fistula draining into the right atrium. Circulation. 98: 1946, 1998.

144. Duerinckx AJ, Perloff JK, Currier JW.: Arteriovenous fistulas of the circumflex and right coronary arteries with drainage into an aneurysmal coronary sinus. Circulation. 99: 2827, 1999.

145. Wexberg et al. An introgenic coronary arteriovenous fistula, etc. Clin Cardiol 24:630, 2001.

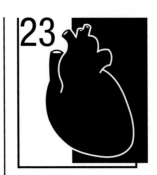

23

Congenital Aneurysms of the Sinuses of Valsalva

The sinuses of Valsalva are three small outpouchings in the wall of the aorta immediately above the attachments of each aortic cusp (Fig. 23–1). In 1839 Hope reported "a case of aneurysmal pouch of the aorta bursting into the right ventricle," the first account of a ruptured congenital aneurysm of a sinus of Valsalva.[53] A year later, Thurnam described Hope's case in greater detail and added five cases of *unruptured* aortic sinus aneurysms.[111] Thurnam named the sinuses according to their relationship to the coronary arteries as the *right* coronary sinus, the *left* coronary sinus, and the *noncoronary* sinus (Fig. 23–1),[111] designations that were accepted by Walmsley in 1929[114] and that remain in current use.[95]

Aneurysms of the sinuses of Valsalva account for 1% of congenital anomalies of the heart and circulation.[116] The aneurysms tend to be single, although exceptionally more than one sinus is involved.[14,41,71,88] There are reports of an aneurysm arising from each sinus of a *bicuspid* aortic valve[14] and from each sinus of a *trileaflet* aortic valve.[71,88]

The aortic sinuses are almost entirely intracardiac. Their anatomic relationship to adjacent structures determines the site into which a given congenital aneurysm ruptures.[60,95,110] Ninety percent to 95% originate in the *right* or *noncoronary* sinus and project into the *right ventricle* or *right atrium*, leaving less than 5% that originate in the left coronary sinus (Fig. 23–2).[31,38,46,51,90,95] Those arising in the *noncoronary* sinus almost all rupture into the *right atrium* (see Fig. 23–2). Those arising in the *right coronary* sinus rupture into the *right ventricle* or occasionally into the *right atrium* (see Fig. 23–2).[95] Rarely, rupture is into the pulmonary artery,[9,46,99] left ventricle,[32,74,95,108,115] left atrium,[47,57,95] or pericardial cavity.[31,63,74,95,103] Also rarely, a sinus aneurysm dissects into the interventricular septum and either remains unruptured or perforates into the left or right ventricle.[16, 32,41,63,70,81,89,116]

An aneurysm occasionally enters the right atrium and then crosses the tricuspid valve and ruptures into the right ventricle.[109] A large unruptured aneurysm may compress the superior vena cava, right atrium, right ventricle,[42,80] or a coronary artery[38,59] or may cause aortic regurgitation by interfering with coaptation of aortic leaflets.[44,93] It is sometimes difficult to distinguish a congenital aortic sinus aneurysm that is the site of infective endocarditis from aortic valve infective endocarditis causing perforation of an aortic sinus into the right side of the heart.[4,20,25,54,63,95] The congenital etiology of an aortic sinus aneurysm is debatable if it originates in the *left* coronary sinus and ruptures into the *left* side of heart.[47,74,95]

A congenital sinus of Valsalva aneurysm begins as a blind pouch or diverticulum that originates from a localized site in one aortic sinus and protrudes as a finger-like or nipple-like projection that perforates at its tip (Fig. 23–3).[68,85,95] The developmental fault is at the junction of the aortic media and the anulus fibrosis and sets the stage for avulsion and aneurysm formation.[30] The fault is present at birth, but with rare exception the aneurysm is not.[2,7,47,86,119]

The *physiologic consequences* of rupture depend on three factors: 1) the amount of blood flowing through the rupture, 2) the rapidity with which the rupture develops, and 3) the chamber that receives the rupture. Irrespective of the right-sided receiving site, shunted blood must flow through the pulmonary circulation, the left atrium, and the left ventricle before returning to the aorta, so volume overload of both sides of the heart is obligatory. When the right atrium receives the rupture, all four cardiac chambers are volume overloaded. A sudden large rupture provokes congestive heart failure because the heart cannot rapidly adapt to the hemodynamic burden. Small insidious perforations initially go unnoticed (Fig. 23–4).

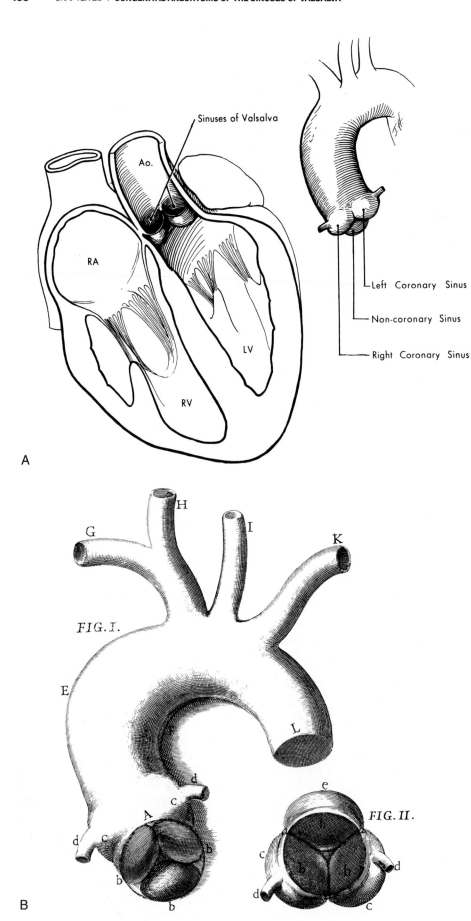

Figure 23–1

A, Illustration of the normal aortic root with the locations of the sinuses of Valsalva. RA, right atrium; Ao, aorta; LV, left ventricle; RV, right ventricle. *B,* Illustration of the aortic sinuses from Antonio Maria Valsalva's *Opera* published in 1740.

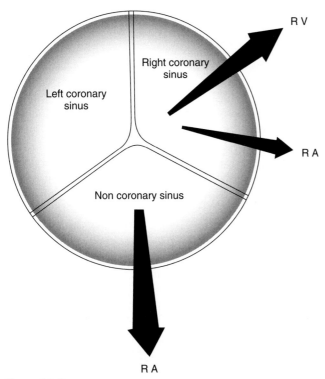

Figure 23–2

Ninety percent to 95% of congenital sinus of Valsalva aneurysms originate in the right or noncoronary sinus and rupture into the right ventricle or right atrium. This figure shows the relative distribution of the sinus of origin and the recipient chamber. RV, right ventricle; RA, right atrium.

across the aortic valve (Fig. 23–5),[50,66,68,70,92,93] while rupture of a sinus aneurysm into the left ventricle causes regurgitation through the rupture rather than across the aortic valve.[32] Aortic sinus aneurysms that rupture into the right ventricle or right atrium may be associated with a ventricular septal defect, especially subpulmonary,[12,23,40,47,49,95,97,106,119] an association that is not fortuitous (see Fig. 23–5).

Unruptured congenital sinus of Valsalva aneurysms were recognized by Thurnam in 1840 (see earlier).[111] Before echocardiography, approximately 20% of unruptured aneurysms were chance findings at necropsy or cardiac surgery.[6,10,36,51,58,63,70,92] Unruptured occult congenital aortic sinus aneurysms are now diagnosed with increasing frequency even in older adults (see Fig. 23–17).[15,27,28,38,59,91,93] An unruptured right coronary sinus aneurysm that projects into the right ventricle below the pulmonary valve can cause obstruction to right ventricular outflow (see earlier).[10,27,58,59] An unruptured aneurysm that protrudes into the right atrium at the level of the tricuspid valve can cause tricuspid regurgitation.[10] An unruptured aneurysm can compress a proximal coronary artery[10,31,38,51,59] or can dissect into the ventricular septum and cause complete heart block.[10,28,70,101] Protrusion into the left ventricle is occasionally responsible for aortic regurgitation,[6,66,70,93] less commonly for obstruction to left ventricular outflow.[92]

The History

Ruptured congenital sinus of Valsalva aneurysms occur chiefly in males, with a sex ratio as high as 4:1.[3,47,61,85,96,117]

A large ruptured or unruptured aneurysm in the outflow tract of the right ventricle can act as an obstructing mass.[10,12,40,42,52,59,64,69] Deformity of aortic cusps by a ruptured or unruptured aneurysm causes regurgitation

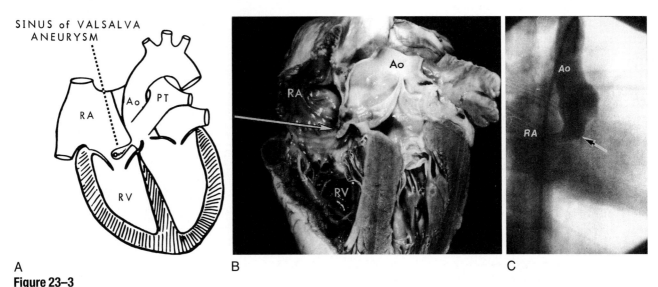

Figure 23–3

A, Illustration of a sinus of Valsalva aneurysm projecting into the right atrium (RA). The sinus itself is not dilated, but instead the aneurysm appears as a finger-like or nipple-like projection with a perforation at its tip. Ao, aorta; PT, pulmonary trunk; RV, right ventricle. *B,* Specimen from a 27-year-old woman whose heart was sectioned to correspond with the anatomic features in the schematic illustration. The ruptured aortic sinus aneurysm (*arrow*) extends as a finger-like projection into the right atrium (RA). *C,* Aortogram from a 20-year-old woman with rupture of a congenital aneurysm (*arrow*) of the right aortic sinus into the right atrium (RA).

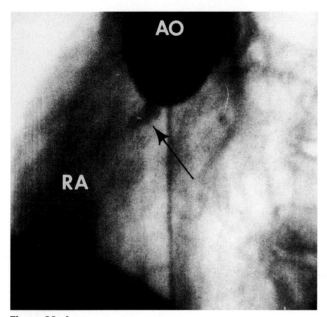

Figure 23–4
Left anterior oblique aortogram (Ao) from a 35-year-old man with an asymptomatic continuous murmur and a small noncoronary sinus aneurysm (*arrow*) that insidiously ruptured into the right atrium (RA).

Rupture during pregnancy is rare.[22] Attention has been called to an increased incidence in Asians.[43,67,97] There is a report of two brothers with aortic sinus aneurysms that perforated into the right atrium.[55]

Ruptured aortic sinus aneurysms typically express themselves in young men after puberty but before age 30 years.[3,117] Rupture rarely occurs in infancy or early childhood[2,7,11,19,37,42,47,86] and rarely as late as the seventh decade.[82,96,104] The average age of rupture was 34 years in one large series with a range of 11 to 67 years.[96] An occult *unruptured* congenital aneurysm of the right coronary sinus was an incidental necropsy finding in a 82-year-old man,[36] and an 85-year-old man came to attention because a previously unrecognized unruptured aortic sinus aneurysm in the right ventricular outflow tract caused a to-and-fro murmur (see Fig. 23–17).

Death from congestive heart failure usually occurs within a year after rupture.[3,35,96,110] *Sudden* death follows perforation into the pericardium,[6,41,98] and syncope or sudden death is an occasional sequel of complete heart block caused by a ruptured[62,81] or unruptured[10,15,28,101] aneurysm that dissects into the base of the ventricular septum. Conversely, long survival sometimes follows small slow perforations (see Fig. 23–4). One such individual lived for 30 years,[77] another lived for 17 years,[56] a 65-year-old man died of gastric carcinoma 10 years after rupture,[104] and rupture in infancy was followed by surgical repair 15 years later.[19] Small perforations come to attention because of an asymptomatic continuous murmur (see Fig. 23–4),[87] because of a systolic murmur caused by subpulmonary obstruction, because of a diastolic murmur caused by aortic regurgitation,[67,93] because of infective endocardi-

tis,[20,25,54,95] or because of diagnostic investigation or operation for ventricular septal defect.[43,67] A large unruptured saccular aneurysm filled with laminated thrombus came to attention because of a prominent paracardiac density on a routine chest x-ray,[91] and an unruptured aneurysm announced itself by cerebral and retinal emboli.[118] Compression of a coronary artery by an unruptured aneurysm is a rare cause of angina pectoris or myocardial infarction.[10,31,51] The 27-year-old man who represented the first successful surgical repair of a large acute rupture with a golf tee–shaped polyvinyl prosthesis[76] experienced a dramatic recurrent rupture three decades later (see second case history below).[48]

Congenital sinus of Valsalva aneurysms come to attention because of the *acute* development of a *large* perforation, *gradual* development of a *small* perforation, or because of an asymptomatic or symptomatic *unruptured* aneurysm. An *acute large rupture* is heralded by the dramatic onset of severe retrosternal or upper abdominal pain and intractable dyspnea.[60,65,73,76,78,96,106,110] The rupture often but not necessarily follows physical stress. The acute symptoms last for hours or days, sometimes subsiding gradually and leaving the patient temporarily improved,[60] but congestive heart failure reappears and relentlessly progresses.[60,110] Three case histories are illustrative.

The first history describes a 45-year-old man whose strenuous work included lifting 50- to 100-lb sacks of plaster.[106] He was in good health until 3 weeks previously, when he had an alarming experience. While carrying a 100-lb sack into a room, he suddenly became "out of

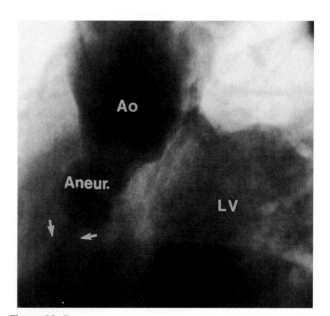

Figure 23–5
Aortogram (Ao) from a 31-year-old woman with an asymptomatic restrictive perimembranous ventricular septal defect, and moderate aortic regurgitation. Dyspnea, orthopnea, peripheral edema, and a coarse continuous murmur suddenly developed because of rupture of a right aortic sinus aneurysm (Aneur) into the right ventricle. The echocardiogram is shown in Figure 23–14. The holosystolic/early diastolic murmurs of ventricular septal defect and aortic regurgitation were obscured by superimposition of the continuous murmur. The left ventricle (LV) visualizes from the aorta because of aortic regurgitation.

breath" and fell to the floor. An extremely uncomfortable, raw feeling radiated from the epigastrium to the base of the neck. Despite severe weakness and shortness of breath, he finished carrying 20 more sacks and then sought his doctor. When seen by us he was relatively asymptomatic.

The second history is from the 27-year-old man (see earlier) whose health had been excellent and whose physical examinations in the military had been normal.[76] While sitting at his desk, the patient experienced the sudden onset of chest pain, shortness of breath, and epigastric discomfort. These symptoms persisted and he was admitted to an army hospital where his acute symptoms subsided following administration of digitalis and sodium restriction. Despite these measures, evidence of heart failure persisted.

The third history is from a 21-year-old woman who had previously been perfectly well[65]: About 24 hours after her usual weekend hike in the woods and hills and shortly after eating pizza, she had an episode of nausea and retching. The next morning she noticed gradually increasing dyspnea and severe substernal pressure radiating to the back followed by orthopnea and palpitation during the night. These symptoms remained severe for 1 week and then gradually subsided, leaving mild residual retrosternal pain and dyspnea.

Pain is presumably related to the rupture itself. Occasionally the aneurysm compresses a coronary artery so symptoms of myocardial ischemia or infarction coexist.[10,18,31,50] Rupture may be announced by acute dyspnea rather than pain,[41,60,110] or mild chest pain may occur for weeks before the onset of dyspnea and tightness in the upper abdomen.[33] When chest pain, dyspnea, and a continuous murmur suddenly develop in a patient with a *ventricular septal defect*, the reason is likely to be rupture of a coexisting aortic sinus aneurysm (see Fig. 23–5).

Small insidious perforations progress gradually and initially go unnoticed (see Figs. 23–4 and 23–16).[3,5,24,52,60,73,110] Mild dyspnea without pain sometimes precedes congestive heart failure by months or years.[3,52,109] Patients who present during a relatively asymptomatic interval have a continuous murmur that can be mistaken for a patent ductus arteriosus.[77]

Congenital aortic sinus aneurysms usually go unrecognized until they rupture.[6,36] However, unruptured aneurysms announce themselves by a to-and-fro murmur due to flow in and out of the intact aneurysmal pouch (see Fig. 23–17),[34] by a murmur of tricuspid regurgitation,[10] by a midsystolic murmur caused by obstruction to right ventricular outflow,[10,27,42,59] by myocardial ischemia due to coronary artery compression,[10,31,38,51,59] by aortic regurgitation caused by malapposition of aortic cusps,[66,67,92,93] by superior vena caval obstruction,[80] by a paracardiac mass in the chest x-ray,[91] by systemic emboli,[118] by complete heart block,[10,15,28,70,71,81,101] or by syncope or sudden death.[32,102]

Physical Appearance

Because rupture rarely occurs before puberty, growth and development are seldom affected by the catabolic effects of congestive heart failure.[60,76]

The Arterial Pulse

The arterial pulse shows all gradations of a rapid aortic runoff irrespective of which chamber or which side of the heart receives the rupture (Fig. 23–6).[13,32,34,41,72,73,76,110] Immediately after rupture, the pulse pressure may not be wide because the left ventricle has not adapted to the augmented volume and so the systolic pressure is not increased while left ventricular end diastolic pressure is elevated, analogous to acute severe aortic regurgitation.[75] If survival permits, the arterial pulse becomes bounding with a rapid rise, a rapid fall, a wide pulse pressure, and a bisferiens configuration. Carotid pulses become visible, Quincke pulses appear in the fingertips, and pistol shot sounds and Duroziez's murmur are detected over the femoral arteries.[73] The arterial pulse rate is slow when an aneurysm penetrates the base of the ventricular septum and causes complete heart block.[16,28,70]

The Jugular Venous Pulse

The height and wave form of the jugular venous pulse depend on the size and rapidity of the rupture and on

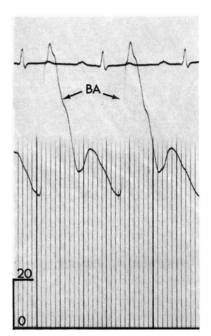

Figure 23–6
Brachial arterial pulse (BA) from a 17-year-old boy with a noncoronary sinus of Valsalva aneurysm that ruptured into the right atrium. Pulmonary blood flow was twice systemic. The upstroke of the brachial pulse is brisk, and the diastolic pressure is lower than normal.

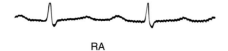

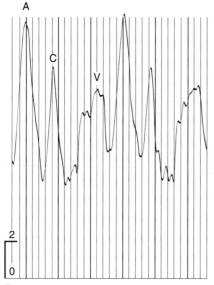

Figure 23–7
Right atrial (RA) pressure pulse from the 17-year-old boy referred to in Figure 23–6 with rupture of a noncoronary aortic sinus aneurysm into the right atrium. The A and V waves are elevated with a dominant A wave and a prominent C wave.

the presence and degree of right ventricular failure.[5,13,24,33,60,72,102,110] A small insidious rupture leaves the jugular venous pulse normal irrespective of which chamber receives the rupture. A large sudden rupture into the right atrium or right ventricle is accompanied by congestive heart failure, an elevated mean jugular venous pressure, and tall A and V waves (Fig. 23–7). The V wave is selectively elevated when an aortic sinus aneurysm projects into the right atrium at the level of the tricuspid valve and causes tricuspid regurgitation.[10] When an aneurysm causes obstruction of the superior vena cava, the mean jugular venous pressure is elevated, and the waveforms disappear. When an aneurysm results in obstruction to right ventricular outflow, the A wave selectively increases. Complete heart block is accompanied by the distinctive jugular pulse described in Chapter 4.

Precordial Movement and Palpation

Precordial impulses depend on the size, rapidity, and duration of the rupture rather than on the recipient chamber,[24,33,41,102] except when the rupture is directly into the left ventricle. The right and left ventricles are both hyperdynamic when rupture is into the right atrium or right ventricle because blood from the rupture circulates through all four chambers before reaching the aorta. A sinus aneurysm that ruptures into the left ventricle or that causes aortic regurgitation by compromising aortic cusp coaptation produces an isolated hyperdynamic left ventricular impulse.[93] An unruptured aneurysm that results in obstruction to right ventricular outflow is accompanied by an isolated *right* ventricular impulse and a systolic thrill generated across the obstruction.[45] A continuous thrill that is more prominent in either systole or diastole mirrors the loud coarse murmur associated with an acute large rupture. The maximum location of thrills varies with murmur site as described in the next section.

Auscultation

Auscultatory signs of rupture into the right side of the heart originate from the continuous murmur that is an essential part of the rupture and from additional murmurs that are not essential to the ruptured aneurysm but that often coexist. A hallmark of acute rupture of an aortic sinus aneurysm into the right side of the heart is the sudden appearance of a continuous murmur in a previously healthy individual, usually a young man.[96] The sudden appearance of a continuous murmur in a patient known to have a ventricular septal defect is a feature of rupture of a coexisting aortic sinus aneurysm (see Fig. 23–5).[96,97]

When the right atrium receives the rupture, the continuous murmur is maximum along the right or left sternal border or over the lower sternum (Fig. 23–8). When the rupture enters the body of the right ventricle, the continuous murmur is maximum at the mid to lower left sternal border (Fig.

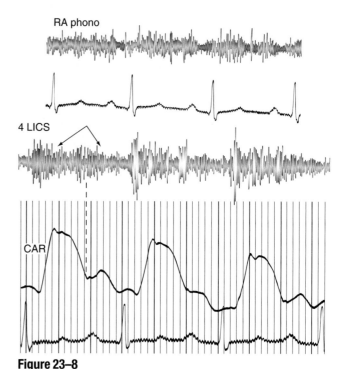

Figure 23–8
Intracardiac phonocardiogram from within the right atrial cavity (RA phono) and a simultaneous thoracic wall phonocardiogram from the fourth left intercostal space (4LICS) of the 17-year-old boy referred to in Figure 23–7 with rupture of a noncoronary sinus of Valsalva aneurysm into the right atrium. The intra-atrial continuous murmur does not peak around the second heart sound. The thoracic wall continuous murmur exhibits either systolic or diastolic accentuation from beat to beat (*paired arrows*). CAR, carotid pulse.

4 LICS

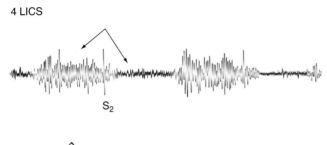

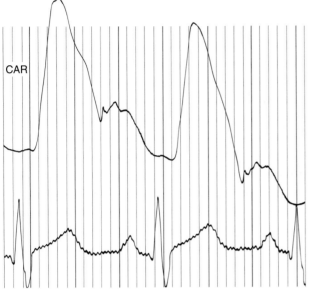

Figure 23–9

Phonocardiogram from the fourth left intercostal space (4 LICS) of a 28-year-old man with a right coronary sinus of Valsalva aneurysm that ruptured into the body of the right ventricle. Pulmonary blood flow was twice systemic. The continuous murmur is much louder in systole (*larger arrow*). CAR, carotid pulse; S₂, second heart sound.

23–9). Rupture into the outflow tract of the right ventricle results in a continuous murmur at the upper left sternal border. The *systolic* component of continuous murmurs tends to be louder at *higher* thoracic sites, and the *diastolic* component tends to be louder at *lower* thoracic sites.[33,65,68,72]

The quality, loudness, and configuration of the continuous murmur accompanying a sudden large rupture were stated in early reports. Hope described "a very loud, superficial sawing murmur prolonged continuously over the first and second heart sounds (probably weaker during the period of repose)."[53] Thurnam described "a superficial, harsh murmur and a peculiarly intense sawing or blowing sound, accompanied by an equally marked or purring tremor, heard over the varicose orifice and in the current circulation beyond it; this sound is continuous but is loudest during systole, less loud during diastole."[111] These descriptions carry an important message, namely, that the continuous murmur of a ruptured aortic sinus aneurysm does not peak around the second heart sound, in contrast to the continuous murmur of patent ductus arteriosus (Fig. 23–9).[60,77] Either the systolic or the diastolic portion of the murmur may be louder. Intensity may diminish around the second heart sound only to increase again in diastole, creating a to-and-fro cadence.[5,24,33,60,77,82,102]

From time to time, the continuous murmur exhibits either systolic or diastolic accentuation (see Figs. 23–8 and 23–9).[37] An aneurysm may be compressed by right ventricular systole, impeding systolic flow and accounting for diastolic accentuation of the continuous murmur.[13,33,39] Rupture directly into the left ventricle results in an early diastolic murmur of aortic regurgitation and a midsystolic murmur due to augmented flow into the aorta (see Fig. 23–10).[32,68] An unruptured aneurysm may cause an isolated diastolic murmur of aortic regurgitation by compromising aortic cusp apposition.[63,66,70,93]

Variations in murmur patterns are better understood by examining intracardiac phonocardiograms recorded at sites in and around the rupture (see Fig. 23–8).[72,102] Continuous murmurs are recovered from within the aneurysm itself. The systolic component may be more prominent in the proximal aortic portion of the aneurysm, and the diastolic component may be more prominent in the distal right atrial or right ventricular portion.[72]

In addition to continuous murmurs that originate within the aneurysm, other systolic and diastolic murmurs may coexist but tend to be obscured because the continuous murmur is louder. Tricuspid regurgitation,[109] mitral regurgitation,[32] or ventricular septal defect[3,97] results in holosystolic murmurs.[102] Midsystolic murmurs are caused by rapid ejection across the aortic and pulmonary valves.[72,102] An aneurysm may protrude into the right ventricular outflow tract and cause a midsystolic murmur,[45,59] or may compromise aortic cusp coaptation and cause the murmur of aortic regurgitation.

Prominent murmurs may accompany *unperforated* aortic sinus aneurysms. Murmurs in both phases of the cardiac

2 LICS

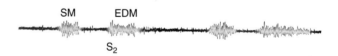

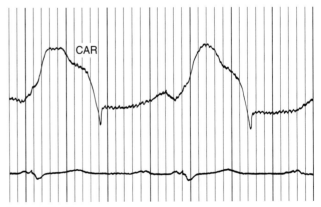

Figure 23–10

Phonocardiogram from the second left intercostal space (2 LICS) of a 24-year-old man with a right aortic sinus aneurysm that ruptured into the left ventricle. A soft early diastolic murmur of aortic regurgitation (EDM) was preceded by a short early systolic flow murmur (SM). CAR, carotid pulse.

cycle are generated as blood flows into and out of an unruptured aneurysmal pouch.[36] These to-and-fro murmurs are auscultatory counterparts of the phasic expansion and relaxation of unruptured aneurysms imaged on two-dimensional echocardiography (see Fig. 23–17) and are reflected in the to-and-fro signals recorded by pulsed Doppler echocardiography.[28] An unperforated aneurysm that obstructs the right ventricular outflow tract results in a midsystolic murmur across the obstruction,[10,45,59] and an unperforated aneurysm projecting into the right atrium can result in the murmur of tricuspid regurgitation.[10] An unruptured aneurysm that protrudes into the left ventricular outflow tract or into the base of the ventricular septum can cause murmurs of aortic regurgitation[66] and aortic stenosis.[44,92]

Third heart sounds originate in the right or left ventricle because of ventricular failure and increased atrioventricular flow. The second heart sound splits normally, and the pulmonary component is loud because pulmonary artery pressure is usually increased.

The Electrocardiogram

Small, slowly developing aortic sinus ruptures are accompanied by normal electrocardiograms. The rhythm is normal sinus even when a large rupture is into the right atrium. The PR interval tends to be prolonged (Fig. 23–11).[72,77] Atrioventricular conduction defects including complete heart block[*] and right or left bundle branch block or bifascicular block[15,32,41,60,63,115] result when a ruptured or unruptured aneurysm penetrates the base of the ventricular septum

---

[*]See references 1, 10, 15, 28, 29, 60, 62, 70, 71, 81, 101.

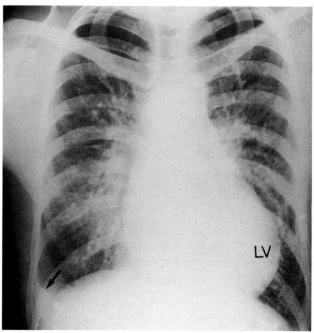

Figure 23–12
X-ray from a 21-year-old man with a right aortic sinus of Valsalva aneurysm that ruptured into the right ventricle. Pulmonary blood flow was 2.5 times systemic. The lung fields show marked pulmonary venous congestion and a small right pleural effusion (*arrow*). A moderately dilated left ventricle (LV) occupies the apex.

and injures the atrioventricular node or His bundle. The QRS axis is normal or rightward, occasionally leftward.[31,41,76,102]

A right atrial P wave abnormality is generated when the right atrium receives the rupture or when an aortic sinus aneurysm causes tricuspid regurgitation. Increased flow through the left atrium accounts for dilatation and for a left atrial or biatrial P wave abnormality.[72,102]

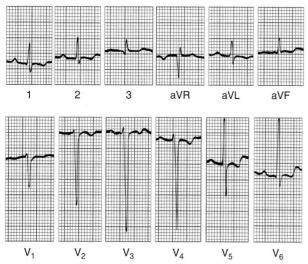

Figure 23–11
Electrocardiogram from the 17-year-old boy referred to in Figure 23–8 with a noncoronary aortic sinus aneurysm that ruptured into the right atrium. The PR interval is prolonged. The QRS axis is normal. Left ventricular hypertrophy is reflected in the deep S waves in leads V_{2-4} and in the prominent R waves and ST segment/T wave abnormalities in leads V_{5-6}.

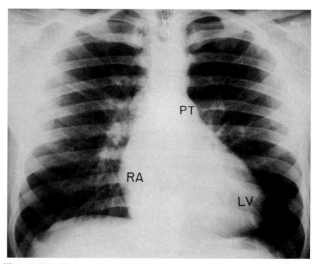

Figure 23–13
X-ray from the 17-year-old boy with a noncoronary aortic sinus aneurysm that ruptured into the right atrium. The right atrial pressure pulse is shown in Figure 23–7. Venous vascularity is manifested in the inner third of the lung fields. The pulmonary trunk (PT) is moderately dilated. An enlarged right atrium (RA) occupies the right lower cardiac border, and a dilated left ventricle (LV) occupies the apex.

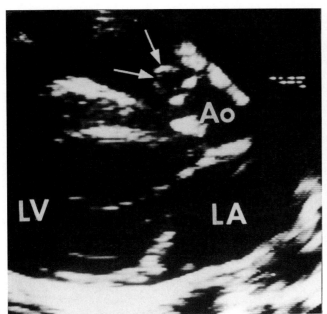
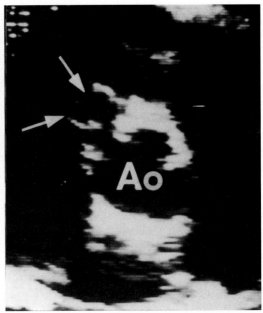

Figure 23–14

Parasternal long-axis (*left*) and short-axis (*right*) echocardiogram from a 31-year-old woman who had a restrictive perimembranous ventricular septal defect with mild aortic regurgitation. An aneurysm (*paired arrows*) from the right aortic sinus ruptured into the right ventricle near the attachment of the septal tricuspid leaflet. The aortogram is shown in Figure 23–5. Ao, aorta; LA, left atrium; LV, left ventricle.

Rupture into the right atrium or right ventricle results in volume overload of both ventricles, but the electrocardiogram usually shows *left* ventricular hypertrophy by voltage criteria and ST segment and T wave abnormalities (see Fig. 23–11).[60,96] Right ventricular hypertrophy may coexist but does not occur alone[8,13,60,96,102] and is usually reserved for aneurysms that cause right ventricular outflow obstruction.[45] An aneurysm that compresses a proximal coronary artery results in electrocardiographic changes of myocardial ischemia or infarction.[18,31,38,51,59,60,113]

The X-Ray

Because the majority of patients with ruptured congenital aortic sinus aneurysms were previously healthy adults, older routine chest x-rays are often available for comparison. Small insidious perforations leave the x-ray unchanged. Large acute ruptures are followed by pulmonary venous congestion that initially dominates because of the steep increase in end diastolic pressure in the unprepared left ventricle (Fig. 23–12),[75] and increased pulmonary arterial blood flow results in enlargement of the pulmonary trunk (Fig. 23–13).[8,13,26,43,60] Moderate left atrial enlargement is seen in the lateral projection, a right atrial convexity appears at the right lower cardiac border, and a moderately dilated left ventricle occupies the apex (see Fig. 23–13).[8,13,26,43,73,102] Volume overload of both ventricles with congestive heart failure accounts for the radiologic picture when an aortic sinus aneurysm ruptures into the right side of the heart (see Fig. 23–12).[43,60,73,102]

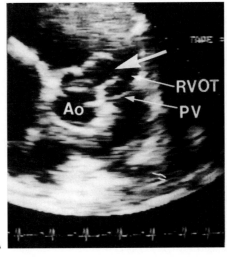
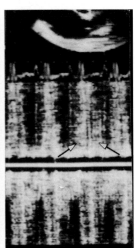

Figure 23–15

A, Parasternal short-axis echocardiogram of an aneurysm of the right sinus of Valsalva (*large unmarked arrow*) that ruptured into the right ventricular outflow tract (RVOT) in a 22-year-old man. PV, pulmonary valve. *B*, Pulsed Doppler with the sample volume in the aneurysm shows a continuous systolic and diastolic flow disturbance (*upper arrows*).

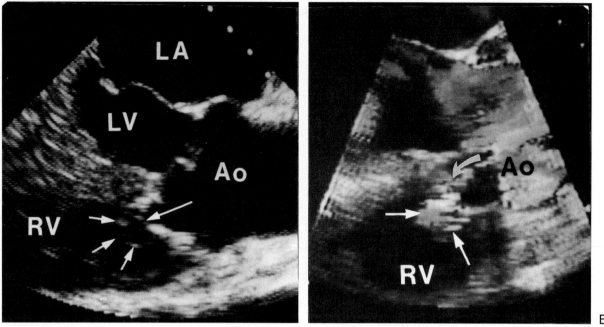

Figure 23–16
Transesophageal echocardiogram from a 32-year-old man with an asymptomatic continuous murmur. *A,* The three *unmarked oblique arrows* identify a sinus of Valsalva aneurysm that originated in the right aortic sinus (Ao) and projected into the right ventricular outflow tract (RV). LV, left ventricle; LA, left atrium. *B,* Black-and-white print of a color flow image shows high-velocity flow from the right aortic sinus (*curved arrow*) into the right ventricular outflow tract (RV) through a small rupture. (Courtesy of Dr. Ronald Van den Belt, Ann Arbor, Michigan.)

Rupture into the left ventricle causes pulmonary venous congestion without increased pulmonary arterial blood flow and with a selective increase in left ventricular size. Rarely, calcium is deposited in the aortic sinus aneurysm.[70,91] Also rarely an aneurysm of the *left* aortic sinus presents as a localized convex radiologic prominence immediately below the pulmonary trunk, or a large saccular aneurysm of the *right* aortic sinus presents as a prominent right paracardiac density.[31,51,57,91]

The Echocardiogram

Echocardiography with color flow imaging and Doppler interrogation establishes the diagnosis of a ruptured or unruptured sinus of Valsalva aneurysm (Figs. 23–14 through 23–18) and establishes the presence of associated abnormalities that are intrinsic features of the aneurysm or that are in addition to the aneurysm.[16,17,27,32,63,79,94,100,112] Echocardiography identifies small insidious asymptomatic ruptures suspected only by a continuous murmur (see Figs. 23–4 and 23–16). Two-dimensional imaging identifies the aneurysmal sac (see Figs. 23–14, 23–15, and 23–18A, B), the aortic sinus of origin (see Figs. 23–14, 23–15, and 23–18B), two normal sinuses, and a normal aorta above the aneurysm. Color flow imaging identifies flow into the recipient chamber (see Figs. 23–16B and 23–18A). Pulsed Doppler (see Fig. 23–15) and continuous-wave Doppler (see Fig. 23–18C) define the flow patterns in the ruptured aneurysm. A large, unruptured aortic sinus aneurysm (see Fig. 23–17) is character-

ized by phasic expansion and relaxation and to-and-fro pulsed Doppler signals at the site of origin from the aorta, but no color flow evidence of rupture.[28] Doppler interroga-

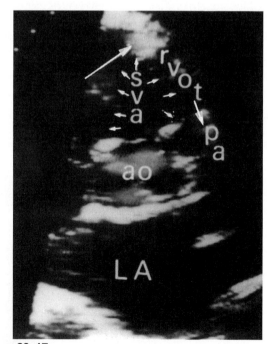

Figure 23–17
Black-and-white print of a color flow image from 85-year-old man with an unruptured sinus of Valsalva aneurysm (sva) that came to light because of an asymptomatic to-and-fro murmur. *Multiple small arrows* identify the unruptured aneurysm that projected into the right ventricular outflow tract (rvot, *long arrow*). Color flow imaging showed no rupture. pa, pulmonary artery; ao, aorta; LA, left atrium.

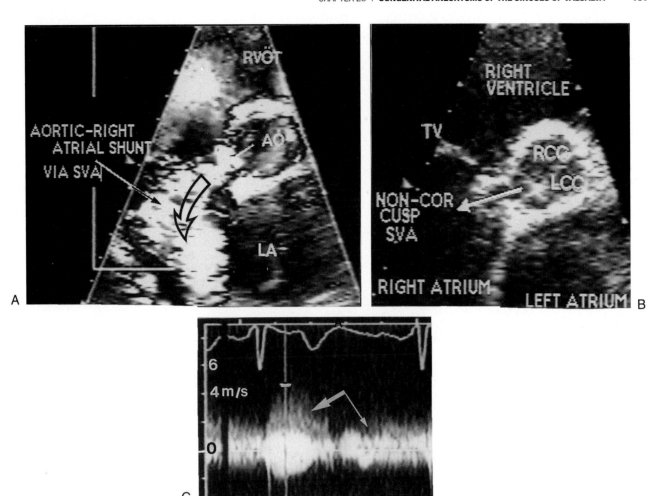

Figure 23–18

Echocardiograms with color flow imaging and Doppler interrogation from a 28-year-old man with an initially small asymptomatic rupture of a noncoronary sinus of Valsalva aneurysm (SVA) into the right atrium. The rupture gradual increased in size. *A,* Black-and-white print of a color flow image showing the aortic-to-right atrial rupture (*large curved arrow*). RVOT, right ventricular outflow tract; Ao, aorta; LA, left atrium. *B,* Short axis showing origin of the aneurysm from the noncoronary cusp (*arrow*). The right coronary cusp (RCC) and left coronary cusp (LCC) were normal. TV, tricuspid valve. *C,* Continuous wave Doppler within the rupture shows continuous flow that was distinctly greater during systole (*larger arrow*).

tion determines the presence and degree of subpulmonary obstruction when an aneurysm protrudes into the right ventricular outflow tract (see Fig. 23–16). The presence and degree of aortic regurgitation are established, a coexisting ventricular septal defect is identified, and the physiologic consequences of rupture into the right atrium, right ventricle, or left ventricle are determined. Real-time imaging identifies ischemic regional left ventricular wall motion abnormalities that result from compression of a coronary artery by an aortic sinus aneurysm.

Summary

Acute rupture of a large sinus of Valsalva aneurysm is clinically dramatic. Sudden chest pain and dyspnea develop in a previously healthy, young adult, usually male; a loud continuous murmur and relentless cardiac failure may follow a period of temporary improvement. The arterial pulse then resembles aortic regurgitation, the jugular venous pulse is ele-

vated, and dynamic biventricular impulses are palpable. A continuous murmur is maximum below the third intercostal space along the right or left sternal border or over the lower sternum. The murmur is louder in either systole or diastole and does not peak around the second heart sound. The electrocardiogram shows biatrial P wave abnormalities and left ventricular or combined ventricular hypertrophy. The x-ray initially exhibits pulmonary venous congestion followed by increased pulmonary arterial blood flow with dilatation of both ventricles and enlargement of the right atrium and left atrium. Echocardiography with color flow imaging and Doppler interrogation establishes the diagnosis of a ruptured or unruptured congenital aortic sinus aneurysm, identifies the chamber that receives the rupture, establishes coexisting abnormalities that are intrinsic to or in addition to the aneurysm, and assesses the physiologic consequences.

Small ruptures progress slowly and initially go unrecognized, ultimately coming to light because of a continuous murmur. An *unperforated* aneurysm may generate a to-and-fro murmur due to flow into and out of the intact aneurysm and can cause obstruction to right ventricular outflow and aortic regurgitation. Ruptured or unruptured aneurysms that penetrate the base of the ventricular septum cause atrioventricular conduction disturbances, complete heart block, syncope, or sudden death.

REFERENCES

1. Ahmad RAS, Sturman S, Watson RDS: Unruptured aneurysm of the sinus of Valsalva presenting with isolated heart block: Echocardiographic diagnosis and successful surgical repair. Br Heart J 61:375, 1989.
2. Ainger LE, Pate JW: Rupture of a sinus of Valsalva aneurysm in an infant. Surgical correction. Am J Cardiol 11:547, 1963.
3. Aletras H, Bjork VO, Cullhed I, Intonti F: Ruptured congenital aneurysm of the sinus of Valsalva with ventricular septal defect. Thorax 18:127, 1963.
4. Bardy GH, Valenstein P, Stack RS, et al: Two-dimensional echocardiographic identification of sinus of Valsalva-right heart fistula due to infective endocarditis. Am Heart J 103:1068, 1982.
5. Besterman EMM, Goldberg MJ, Sellors TH: Surgical repair of ruptured sinus of Valsalva. BMJ 2:410, 1963.
6. Boutefeu JM, Moret PR, Hahn C, Hauf E: Aneurysms of the sinus of Valsalva. Report of seven cases and review of the literature. Am J Med 65:18, 1978.
7. Breviere GM, Vaksmann G, Francart C: Rupture of a sinus of Valsalva aneurysm in a neonate. Eur J Pediatr 149:603, 1990.
8. Brofman BL, Elder JC: Cardio-aortic fistula; temporary circulatory occlusion as an aid in diagnosis. Circulation 16:77, 1957.
9. Brown JW, Health D, Whitaker W: Cardioaortic fistula. Circulation 12:819, 1955.
10. Bulkley BH, Hutchins GM, Ross RS: Aortic sinus of Valsalva aneurysms simulating primary right-sided valvular heart disease. Circulation 52:696, 1975.
11. Burakovsky, V. I., Podsolkov, V. P., Sabirow, B. N., Nasedkina, M. A., Alekian, B. G., and Dvinyaninova, N. B.: Ruptured congenital aneurysm of the sinus of Valsalva. J. Thorac. Cardiovasc. Surg. 95:836, 1988.
12. Burchell, H. B., and Edwards, J. E.: Aortic sinus aneurysm with communication into the right ventricle with associated ventricular septal defect. Proc. Staff Meet. Mayo Clin. 26:336, 1951.
13. Buzzi, A.: Evaluation of a precordial continuous murmur. Rupture of aneurysm of sinus of Valsalva into the right ventricle. Am. J. Cardiol. 4:551, 1959.
14. Chamsi-Pasha, H., Musgrove, C., and Lorton, R.: Echocardiographic diagnosis of multiple congenital aneurysms of the sinus of Valsalva. Br. Heart J. 59:724, 1988.
15. Channer, K. S., Hutter, J. A., and George, M.: Unruptured aneurysm of the sinus of Valsalva presenting with ventricular tachycardia. Eur. Heart J. 9:186, 1988.
16. Chen, W. W., and Tai, Y. T.: Dissection of interventricular septum by aneurysm of sinus of Valsalva. A rare complication diagnosed by echocardiography. Br. Heart J. 50:293, 1983.
17. Chiang, C., Lin, F., Fang, B., Kuo, C., Lee, Y., and Chang, C.: Doppler and two-dimensional echocardiographic features of sinus of Valsalva aneurysm. Am. Heart J. 116:1283, 1988.
18. Chipps, H. D.: Aneurysm of the sinus of Valsalva causing coronary occlusion. Arch. Pathol. 31:627, 1941.
19. Chojnacki, B.: Ruptured aneurysm of a sinus of Valsalva. J.A.M.A. 186:1176, 1963.
20. Conde, C. A., Meller, J., Donoso, E., and Dack, S.: Bacterial endocarditis with ruptured sinus of Valsalva and aorticocardiac fistula. Am. J. Cardiol. 35:912, 1975.
21. Cooperberg, P., Mercer, E. N., Mulder, D. S., and Winsberg, F.: Rupture of a sinus of Valsalva aneurysm. A report diagnosed preoperatively by echocardiography. Radiology 113:171, 1974.
22. Cripps, T., Pumphrey, C. W., and Parker, D. J.: Rupture of the sinus of Valsalva during pregnancy. Br. Heart J. 57:490, 1987.
23. Cullen, S., Sullivan, I. D.: Ruptured sinus of Valsalva with aorta-to right atrial fistula. Circulation 98:2503, 1998.
24. Datlow, D. W., and Massumi, R. A.: Asymptomatic rupture of aortic sinus (of Valsalva) into the right atrium. Report of a case. Med. Ann. D.C. 33:327, 1964.
25. Datta, D. N., Berry, J. N., and Khattri, H. N.: Infected aneurysm of sinus of Valsalva. Br. Heart J. 33:323, 1971.
26. Davidsen, H. G., Petersen, O., and Thompsen, G.: Roentgenologic findings in 5 cases of congenital aneurysm of the aortic sinuses (sinuses of Valsalva). Acta Radiol. 49:205, 1958.
27. Desai, A. G., Sharma, S., Kumar, A., Hansoti, R. C., and Kalke, B. R.: Echocardiographic diagnosis of unruptured aneurysm of right sinus of Valsalva. Am. Heart J. 109:363, 1985.
28. Dev, V., and Shrivaspava, S.: Echocardiographic diagnosis of unruptured aneurysm of the sinus of Valsalva dissecting into the ventricular septum. Am. J. Cardiol. 66:502, 1990.
29. Duras, P. F.: Heart block with aneurysm of the aortic sinus. Br. Heart J. 6:61, 1944.
30. Edwards, J. E., and Burchell, H. B.: Specimen exhibiting the essential lesion in aneurysm of the aortic sinus. Proc. Staff Meet. Mayo Clin. 31:407, 1956.
31. Eliot, R. S., Wollbrink, A., and Edwards, J. E.: Congenital aneurysm of the left aortic sinus. A rare lesion and a rare cause of coronary insufficiency. Circulation 28:951, 1963.
32. Engel, P. J., Held, J. S., Bel-Kahn, J. V., and Spitz, H.: Echocardiographic diagnosis of congenital sinus of Valsalva aneurysm with dissection of the interventricular septum. Circulation 63:705, 1981.
33. Evans, J. W., Harris, T. R., and Brody, D. A.: Ruptured aortic sinus aneurysm. Case report with review of clinical features. Am. Heart J. 61:408, 1961.
34. Falholt, W., and Thomsen, G.: Congenital aneurysm of the right sinus of Valsalva, diagnosed by aortography. Circulation 8:549, 1953.
35. Feldman, L., Friedlander, J., Dillon, R., and Wallyn, R.: Aneurysm of right sinus of Valsalva with rupture into right atrium and into right ventricle. Am. Heart J. 51:314, 1956.
36. Fishbein, M. C., Obma, R., and Roberts, W. C.: Unruptured sinus of Valsalva aneurysm. Am. J. Cardiol. 35:918, 1975.
37. Fowler, R. E. L., and Bevil, H. H.: Aneurysms of the sinuses of Valsalva. With report of a case. Pediatrics 8:340, 1951.
38. Gallet, B., Combe, E., Saudemont, J. P., Tetard, C., Barret, F., Gandjbakhch, I., and Hiltgen, M.: Aneurysm of the left aortic sinus causing coronary compression and unstable angina: Successful repair by isolated closure of the aneurysm. Am. Heart J. 115:1308, 1988.
39. Gerbode, F., Osborn, J. J., Johnston, J. B., and Kerth, W. J.: Ruptured aneurysms of the aortic sinuses of Valsalva. Am. J. Surg. 102:268, 1961.
40. Gialloreto, O. P., and Loiselle, G.: Aneurysm of aortic sinus of Valsalva associated with high ventricular septal defect. Am. J. Cardiol. 11:537, 1963.
41. Gibbs, N. M., and Harris, E. L.: Aortic sinus aneurysms. Br. Heart J. 23:131, 1961.
42. Gleason, M. M., Hardy, C., Chin, A. J., and Pigott, J. D.: Ruptured sinus of Valsalva aneurysm in childhood. Am. Heart J. 114:1235, 1987.
43. Guo, D. W., Cheng, T. O., Lin, M. L., and Gu, Z. Q.: Aneurysm of the sinus of Valsalva: A roentgenologic study of 105 Chinese patients. Am. Heart J. 114:1169, 1987.
44. Hands, M. E., Lloyd, B. L., and Hung, J.: Cross-sectional echocardiographic diagnosis of unruptured right sinus of Valsalva aneurysm dissecting into the interventricular septum. Int. J. Cardiol. 9:380, 1985.
45. Haraphongse, M., Ayudhya, R. K. N., Jugdutt, B., and Rossall, R. E.: Isolated unruptured sinus of Valsalva aneurysm producing right ventricular outflow obstruction. Cath. Cardiovasc. Diag. 19:98, 1990.
46. Heilman III, K. J., Groves, B. M., Campbell, D., and Blount, S. G.: Rupture of left sinus of Valsalva aneurysm into the pulmonary artery. J. Am. Coll. Cardiol. 5:1005, 1985.
47. Heiner, D. C., Hara, M., and White, H. J.: Cardioaortic fistulas and aneurysms of sinus of Valsalva in infancy. Pediatrics 27:415, 1961.
48. Hemp, J. R., Young, J. N., Harrell, J. E., and Woodworth, G. R.: Late recurrent rupture of a sinus of Valsalva aneurysm. Am. J. Cardiol. 63:761, 1989.
49. Henze, A., Huttunen, H., and Bjork, V. O.: Ruptured sinus of Valsalva aneurysms. Scand. J. Thorac. Cardiovasc. Surg. 17:249, 1983.
50. Heydorn, W. H., Nelson, W. P., Fitterer, J. D., Floyd, G. D., and Strevey, T. E.: Congenital aneurysm of the sinus of Valsalva protruding into the left ventricle. J. Thorac. Cardiovasc. Surg. 71:839, 1976.
51. Hiyamuta, K., Ohtsuki, T., Shimamatsu, M., Ohkita, Y., and Terasawa, M.: Aneurysm of the left aortic sinus causing acute myocardial infarction. Circulation 67:1151, 1983.

52. Hong, P. W., Lee, S. S., Kim, S. W., and Cha, H. D.: Unusual manifestation of ruptured aneurysm of the aortic sinus. Report of 2 cases. J. Thorac. Cardiovasc. Surg. 51:507, 1966.

53. Hope, J.: A Treatise on the Diseases of the Heart and Great Vessels, 3rd ed. London, J. Churchill & Sons, 1839.

54. Jick, H., Kasarjian, P. J., and Barsky, M.: Rupture of aneurysm of aortic sinus of Valsalva associated with acute bacterial endocarditis. Circulation 19:745, 1959.

55. Johnson, J.: Discussion from Sawyers, J. L., Adams, J. E., and Scott, H. W., Jr.: Surgical treatment for aneurysms of the aortic sinuses with aorticoatrial fistula. Surgery 41:26, 1957.

56. Jones, A. M., and Langley, F. A.: Aortic sinus aneurysms. Br. Heart J. 11:325, 1949.

57. Kay, J. H., Anderson, R. M., Lewis, R. R., and Reinberg, M.: Successful repair of sinus of Valsalva-left atrial fistula. Circulation 20:427, 1959.

58. Kerber, R. E., Ridges, J. D., and Kriss, J. P.: Unruptured aneurysm of the sinus of Valsalva producing right ventricular outflow obstruction. Am. J. Med. 53:775, 1972.

59. Kiefaber, R. W., Tabakin, B. S., Coffin, L. H., and Gibson, T. C.: Unruptured sinus of Valsalva aneurysm with right ventricular outflow obstruction diagnosed by two-dimensional and Doppler echocardiography. J. Am. Coll. Cardiol. 7:438, 1986.

60. Kieffer, S. A., and Winchell, P.: Congenital aneurysms of the aortic sinuses with cardioaortic fistula. Dis. Chest 38:79, 1960.

61. Kwittken, J., Christopoulos, P., Dua, N. K., and Bruno, M. S.: Congenital and acquired aortic sinus aneurysm. Arch. Intern. Med. 115:684, 1965.

62. Lee, E. B., Krieger, O. J., and Lee, N. K.: Congenital aneurysm of noncoronary sinus of Valsalva leading to complete heart block: Case report. Ann. Intern. Med. 45:525, 1956.

63. Lewis, B. S., and Agathangelou, N. E.: Echocardiographic diagnosis of unruptured sinus of Valsalva aneurysm. Am. Heart J. 107:1025, 1984.

64. Lin, T. K., Crockett, J. E., and Dimond, E. G.: Ruptured congenital aneurysm of sinus of Valsalva. Am. Heart J. 51:445, 1956.

65. Lippschutz, E. J., and Wood, L. W.: Rupture of an aneurysm of the sinus of Valsalva. Am. J. Med. 28:859, 1960.

66. London, S. B., and London, R. E.: Production of aortic regurgitation by unperforated aneurysm of the sinus of Valsalva. Circulation 24:1403, 1961.

67. Lukacs, L., Bartek, I., Haan, A., Hankoczy, J., and Arvay, A.: Ruptured aneurysms of the sinus of Valsalva. Eur. J. Cardiothorac Surg. 6:15, 1992.

68. Magidson, O., and Kay, J. H.: Ruptured aortic sinus aneurysms; clinical and surgical aspects of 7 cases. Am. Heart J. 65:597, 1963.

69. McGoon, D. C., Edwards, J. E., and Kirklin, J. W.: Surgical treatment of ruptured aneurysm of aortic sinus. Ann. Surg. 147:387, 1958.

70. Metras, D., Coulibaly, A. O., and Ouattara, K.: Calcified unruptured aneurysm of sinus of Valsalva with complete heart block and aortic regurgitation. Br. Heart J. 48:507, 1982.

71. Micks, R. H.: Congenital aneurysms of all three sinuses of Valsalva. Br. Heart J. 2:63, 1940.

72. Minkoff, S. M., Fort, M. L., and Sharp, J. T.: Rupture of an aneurysm of the sinus of Valsalva into the right atrium. Observations using a catheter-tip micromanometer microphone. Am. J. Cardiol. 19:278, 1967.

73. Morch, J. E., and Greenwood, W. F.: Rupture of the sinus of Valsalva. Am. J. Cardiol. 18:827, 1966.

74. Morgan, R. I., and Mazur, J. H.: Congenital aneurysm of aortic root with fistula to left ventricle. A case report and autopsy findings. Circulation 28:589, 1963.

75. Morganroth, J., Perloff, J. K., Zeldis, S. M., and Dunkman, W. B.: Acute severe aortic regurgitation. Ann. Intern. Med. 87:223, 1977.

76. Morrow, A. G., Baker, R. R., Hanson, H. E., and Mattingly, T. W.: Successful surgical repair of a ruptured aneurysm of the sinus of Valsalva. Circulation 16:533, 1957.

77. Neill, C., and Mounsey, P.: Auscultation of patent ductus arteriosus with a description of 2 fistulae simulating patent ductus. Br. Heart J. 20:61, 1958.

78. Nicholson, R. E.: Syndrome of rupture of aortic aneurysm into the pulmonary artery; review of the literature with report of 2 cases. Ann. Intern. Med. 19:286, 1943.

79. Nishimura, K., Hibi, N., Kato, T., Fukui, Y., Arakawa, T., Tatematsu, H., Miwa, A., Tada, H., Kambe, T., and Sakamoto, N.: Real time observation of ruptured right sinus of Valsalva aneurysm by high speed ultrasonocardiotomography. Circulation 53:732, 1976.

80. Okita, Y., Miki, S., Kusuhara, K., Ueda, Y., Tahata, T., Komeda, M., Yamanaka, K., Ishii, K., and Kawamua, K.: A giant aneurysm of the non-coronary sinus of Valsalva. Thorac. Cardiovasc. Surg. 35:316, 1987.

81. Onat, A., Ersanli, O., Kanuni, A., and Aykan, T. B.: Congenital aortic sinus aneurysms with particular reference to dissection of the interventricular septum. Am. Heart J. 72:158, 1966.

82. Oram, S., and East, T.: Rupture of aneurysm of aortic sinus (of Valsalva) into the right side of the heart. Br. Heart J. 17:541, 1955.

83. Pate, J. W.: Aneurysms of the sinus of Valsalva. Am. J. Surg. 102:502, 1961.

84. Paul, A. T., Somasunderam, K., and Jayewardene, F. L.: Two cases of aortico-ventricular fistulae. Br. Heart J. 23:203, 1961.

85. Perloff, J. K.: Sinus of Valsalva-right heart communications due to congenital aortic sinus defects. Am. Heart J. 59:318, 1960.

86. Perry, L. W., Martin, G. R., Galioto, F. M., and Midgley, F. M.: Rupture of congenital sinus of Valsalva aneurysm in a newborn. Am. J. Cardiol. 68:1255, 1991.

87. Peters, P., Juziuk, E., and Gunther, S.: Doppler color flow mapping detection of ruptured sinus of Valsalva aneurysm. J. Am. Soc. Echocardiogr. 2:195, 1989.

88. Pomerance, A., and Davis, M. J.: Congenital aneurysms of all three sinuses of Valsalva. J. Pathol. Bacteriol. 89:607, 1965.

89. Raffa, H., Mosieri, J., Sorefan, A. A., and Kayali, M. T.: Sinus of Valsalva aneurysm eroding into the interventricular septum. Ann. Thorac. Surg. 51:996, 1991.

90. Ramsey, T. L., and Mosquera, V. T.: Ruptured congenital aneurysm of the sinus of Valsalva with superimposed endocarditis with rupture of aortic cusp producing sudden death. Ohio Med. J. 42:843, 1946.

91. Reid, P. G., Goudevenos, J. A., and Hilton, C. J.: Thrombosed saccular aneurysm of a sinus of Valsalva: Unusual cause of a mediastinal mass. Br. Heart J. 63:183, 1990.

92. Rothbaum, D. A., Dillon, J. C., Chang, S., and Feigenbaum, H.: Echocardiographic manifestations of right sinus of Valsalva aneurysm. Circulation 49:768, 1974.

93. Rubin, D. C., Carliner, N. H., Salter, D. R., Plotnick, G. D., and Hawke, M. W.: Unruptured sinus of Valsalva aneurysm diagnosed by transesophageal echocardiography. Am. Heart J. 124:225, 1992.

94. Sahasakul, Y., Panchavinn, P., Chaithiraphan, S., and Sakiyal, A. K.: Echocardiographic diagnosis of a ruptured aneurysm of the sinus of Valsalva: Operation without catheterization in 7 patients. Br. Heart J. 64:195, 1990.

95. Sakakibara, S., and Konno, S.: Congenital aneurysm of the sinus of Valsalva; anatomy and classification. Am. Heart J. 63:405, 1962.

96. Sakakibara, S., and Konno, S.: Congenital aneurysm of the sinus of Valsalva: A clinical study. Am. Heart J. 63:708, 1962.

97. Sakakibara, S., and Konno, S.: Congenital aneurysm of the sinus of Valsalva associated with ventricular septal defect. Am. Heart J. 75:595, 1968.

98. Sawyers, J. L., Adams, J. E., and Scott, H. W., Jr.: Surgical treatment for aneurysms of the aortic sinuses with aorticoatrial fistula. Surgery 41:26, 1957.

99. Scagliotti, D., Fisher, E. A., Deal, B. J., Gordon, D., Chomaka, E. V., and Brundage, B. H.: Congenital aneurysm of the left sinus of Valsalva with an aortopulmonary tunnel. J. Am. Coll. Cardiol. 7:443, 1986.

100. Schatz, R. A., Schiller, N. B., Tri, T. B., Bowen, T. E., Ports, T. A., and Silverman, N. H.: Two-dimensional echocardiographic diagnosis of a ruptured right sinus of Valsalva aneurysm. Chest 79:584, 1981.

101. Segab, C., Davy, J. M., Scheuble, C., Bouchareine, F., Dussart, G., Aigueperse, J., and Motte, G.: Atrioventricular block disclosing an isolated congenital aneurysm of the sinus of Valsalva, extending into the septum and not ruptured. Arch. Mal. Coeur 74:1233, 1981.

102. Segal, B. L., Likeoff, W., and Novack, P.: Rupture of a sinus of Valsalva aneurysm. Am. J. Cardiol. 12:544, 1963.

103. Shumacker, H. B., Jr., and Judson, W. E.: Rupture of aneurysm of Valsalva into left ventricle and its operative repair. J. Thorac. Cardiovasc. Surg. 45:650, 1963.

104. Sorensen, E. W., and Kolsaker, L.: Ruptured aneurysm of sinus of Valsalva. Report of 2 cases. Acta Med. Scand. 172:369, 1962.

105. Steinberg, I., and Finby, N.: Clinical manifestations of the unperforated aortic sinus aneurysm. Circulation 14:115, 1956.

106. Szweda, J. A., and Drake, E. H.: Ruptured congenital aneurysms of the sinuses of Valsalva. Circulation 25:559, 1962.

107. Taguchi, K., Sasaki, N., Matsuura, Y., and Uemura, R.: Surgical correction of aneurysm of the sinus of Valsalva. Am. J. Cardiol. 23:180, 1969.

108. Tasaka, S., Yoshitoshi, Y., Seki, K., Koide, K., Ogata, E., and Nakamura, K.: Congenital aneurysm of the right coronary sinus of Valsalva with rupture into the left ventricle. Jpn. Heart J. 1:106, 1960.

109. Taylor, F. H., Sanger, P. W., Robicsek, F., and Ibrahim, K.: Herniation of ruptured sinus of Valsalva aneurysm through the tricuspid orifice. Case report. Am. Surg. 31:171, 1965.

110. Therkelsen, F., Fabricius, J., and Davidsen, H. G.: Aneurysm of the aortic sinus of Valsalva. Acta Chir. Scand. 283(Suppl):129, 1961.

111. Thurnam, J.: On aneurysms, and especially spontaneous varicose aneurysms of the ascending aorta. Trans. R. Med. Chir. Soc. (Glasgow) 23:323, 1840.

112. Vargas-Barron, J., Keirns, C., Attie, F., Gil-Moreno, M., and Aracil, C.: Congenital aneurysm of sinus of Valsalva detected by pulsed Doppler echocardiography. Am. Heart J. 111:181, 1986.

113. Venning, G. R.: Aneurysms of the sinuses of Valsalva. Am. Heart J. 42:57, 1951.

114. Walmsley, T.: The heart. In Quain's Elements of Anatomy, Vol. 4, Part 3. New York, Longmans, Green & Company, 1929.

115. Warthen, R.: Congenital aneurysm of the right anterior sinus of Valsalva with rupture into the left ventricle. Am. Heart J. 37:975, 1949.

116. Wells, T., Byrd, B., Nierste, D., Fleurelus, C.: Sinus of Valsalva aneurysm with rupture into the interventricular septum and left ventricular cavity. Circulation. 100:1843, 1999.

117. Winfield, M. E.: Rupture of an aneurysm of the posterior sinus of Valsalva into the right atrium. Am. J. Cardiol. 3:688, 1969.

118. Wortham, D. C., Gorman, P. D., Hull, R. W., Vernalis, M. N., and Gaither, N. S.: Unruptured sinus of Valsalva aneurysm presenting with embolization. Am. Heart J. 125:896, 1993.

119. Yacoub, M. H., Lise, M., and Muir, J.: Aneurysms of two sinuses of Valsalva with a ventricular septal defect and aortic regurgitation. Br. Heart J. 31:661, 1969.

120. Yoshida, S., Togashi, M., Chida, A., and Miyahara, M.: Ruptured sinus of Valsalva aneurysm into the left ventricle. Jpn. Heart J. 19:954, 1978.

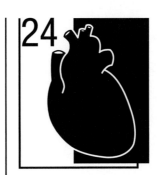

Pulmonary Atresia with Intact Ventricular Septum

In his first edition of *Malformations of the Human Heart*,[50] Thomas Peacock wrote: ". . . the orifice or trunk of the pulmonary artery is entirely impervious. A case of this description was described by John Hunter in 1783.[38] The child was born at the eighth month, was very livid . . . and died in convulsions on the thirteenth day. The pulmonary artery was found entirely impervious. The septum of the ventricles was entire, and the right ventricle had scarcely any cavity left, while the left ventricle was large and powerful. The foramen ovale continued open, and the pulmonary branches received their supply of blood from the aorta, through the medium of the arterial duct."

Peacock's description refers to the malformation now called *pulmonary atresia with intact ventricular septum*, which is characterized by complete anatomic obstruction to forward flow from the right ventricle to the pulmonary trunk because of an imperforate pulmonary valve and an intact ventricular septum (Fig. 24–1). The reported incidence of the malformation varies from 1 per 22,000 live births[42] to 4.2 per 100,00 live births.[3] An interatrial communication that is usually a restrictive foramen ovale is the only exit from the right atrium. The imperforate pulmonary valve consists of three fused but well-formed cusps with triradiate commissural ridges that converge at the center of the sealed orifice.[5,11] The valve is structurally similar to if not identical with critical pulmonary valve stenosis in which a triradiate valve has a pinpoint opening at its apex.[13,22,29,45,53] Less commonly commissural ridges are confined to the periphery of the valve, which has a smooth imperforate dimple at the center.[11] A well-developed pulmonary trunk (see Fig. 24–1) implies that there was forward flow across a pulmonary valve, that was stenotic but patent during much if not most of fetal life.[53] A normally formed ductus arteriosus also implies that

intrauterine blood flow was from the right ventricle into the pulmonary trunk through the ductus and into the aorta (see Fig. 24–5). This is in contrast to pulmonary atresia with Fallot's tetralogy in which an abnormally formed long tortuous ductus functions as a systemic artery that carries blood flow from the aorta into the pulmonary artery in the fetus rather than vice versa (see Chapter 18).

The *normal right ventricle* consists of an *inlet portion* that is part of the diastolic filling mechanism and a trabecular and an infundibular portion that are part of the systolic pump mechanism.[13] Over three quarters of cases of pulmonary atresia with intact ventricular septum are characterized by a small right ventricle (see Figs. 24–1A and 24–2A, B) in which these three portions are represented.[13,22,35,45,57,63] A small right ventricle is associated with small trabecular and infundibular cavities (see Figs. 24–1A and 24–2A, B), a thick wall, myocardial fiber disarray, and endocardial fibroelastosis.[8,12,13,33] Capillary disorganization coincides with myocardial fiber disarray.[16] Pinpoint neonatal pulmonary valve stenosis occasionally exists with a diminutive right ventricular cavity analogous to pulmonary atresia with intact ventricular septum.[29]

The morphology and function of the tricuspid valve vary with right ventricular size. When the right ventricle is small and thick-walled, the tricuspid anulus is small, the tricuspid valve is small and thickened, the chordal attachments are poorly delineated, and the papillary muscles are hypoplastic.[49] When the right ventricle is dilated and thin-walled, the tricuspid valve is incompetent and resembles Ebstein's malformation.[8,49] *Functional* pulmonary atresia exists when a dilated mechanically inadequate right ventricle with tricuspid regurgitation cannot generate sufficient systolic pressure to open a stenotic but nonarteritic pulmonary valve.[60] Functional pulmonary atresia

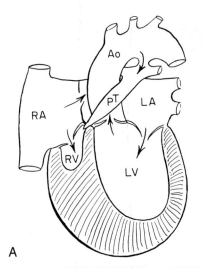

A

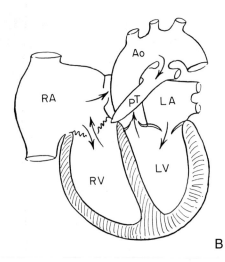

B

Figure 24–1

Illustrations of two varieties of pulmonary atresia with intact ventricular septum. In both varieties the pulmonary valve is by definition imperforate. The pulmonary trunk (PT) is well-formed. A restrictive foramen ovale is the only exit from the right atrium (RA). Pulmonary blood flow depends on tenuous patency of a ductus arteriosus. *A,* In this more common variety, the right ventricle (RV) is small and thick-walled, the tricuspid valve is small but competent, and the right atrium is moderately enlarged. Ao, aorta; LA, left atrium; LV, left ventricle. *B,* In this less common variety, the right ventricle is thin-walled and normal-sized or enlarged. The tricuspid valve is incompetent because of an Ebstein-like malformation, so the right atrium is dilated.

also occurs during transient neonatal tricuspid regurgitation.[32]

The coronary circulation in pulmonary atresia with intact ventricular septum and small right ventricle is a focus of lively interest.[9,16,23,24,28,33,40,48] *Intramyocardial sinusoids* were described in 1926[34] and play important roles in the pathogenesis of right ventricular to coronary artery communications (see Fig. 24–2).[4,5,13,14,33,40,49] Morphogenetic studies of the coronary circulation have shed new light on the abnormalities of the coronary vascular bed in pulmonary atresia with intact ventricular septum and small right ventricle (see Chapter 32).[33,39,48] The coronary vascular bed evolves in an orderly chronology represented by the sequential development of blood islands, coronary venous connections, and coronary artery to aortic connections. The blood islands proliferate and coalesce and form networks of vascular channels that have no connections with other blood islands or with the ventricular cavity. Suprasystemic systolic pressure drives blood from the small isovolumetrically contracting right ventricle through primitive vascular channels that are composed of thickened intima and fibroelastic walls[48] and that connect the right ventricular cavity to epicardial coronary arteries (see Fig. 24–2A, B).[13,14,30,40,48,49] Abnormalities of the coronary vascular bed in pulmonary atresia with intact ventricular septum and small right ventricle are secondary to the hemodynamic derangements of the malformation.[13,40] Myocardial sinusoids as primary developmental faults are rare.[26] Epicardial veins may be prominent and thick-walled.[48] Ventriculo-coronary arterial connections are located chiefly in the region of the apex of the right ventricle, and communicate chiefly with the distal left anterior descending coronary arterial system (see Fig. 24–2A, B).[30,48] Intramyocardial channels that end blindly punctuate the endocardium of the thick-walled right ventricle and create the appearance of a highly trabeculated muscular wall (Figs. 24–3 and 24–4).[48,49]

Ventriculo-coronary arterial communications have been described in the *inverted* left ventricle of congenitally corrected transposition of the great arteries with pulmonary atresia and intact ventricular septum.[58,61] Left ventricular to coronary arterial connections in *aortic* atresia with intact ventricular septum differ from right ventricular to coronary arterial connections in pulmonary atresia with intact ventricular septum (see Chapters 31 and 32).[6,48,51,54]

Myocardial ischemia is an important sequel of ventriculo-coronary arterial connections.[14,33,40,48] Large unobstructed connections (see Fig. 24–2A, C) function as a fistulous steal because blood from the aortic root flows freely into the right ventricular cavity during diastole.[49] More commonly and more importantly, ischemia results from obstructing luminal abnormalities that range from mild medial and intimal thickening to luminal obliteration that extend from the origins of the intramyocardial connections to the coronary artery ostia in the aortic sinuses.[13,33,40,48,49] Luminal obstructive lesions that originate in the fetus and neonate can evolve into severe stenoses or obliteration.[33,40,48] *Proximal* discontinuity of a coronary artery, which is the most egregious form of this prejudicial coronary circulation, results from acquired ostial obliteration or from congenital atresia of an aortic sinus ostium.[9] Proximal discontinuity and severe luminal obstruction set the stage for a *right ventricular-dependent coronary circulation* in which suprasystemic pressure is required to generate retrograde blood flow and myocardial perfusion.[7,9,14,33] Myocardial ischemia and infarction can result in left ventricular aneurysm[63] and in right ventricular rupture[7,37] and are largely responsible for the high mortality.[33,40]

The right atrium enlarges moderately when the right ventricle is diminutive,[22,25] but the right atrium can be aneurysmal when the right ventricle is dilated and tricuspid regurgitation is severe (see Fig. 24–4).[8,22] The left atrium enlarges because it receives venous return from both the systemic and pulmonary circulations.[25,53] The left

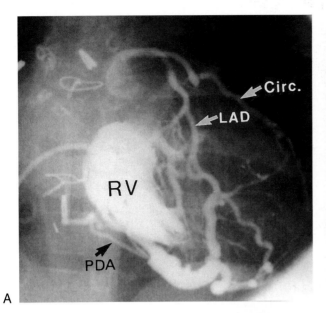

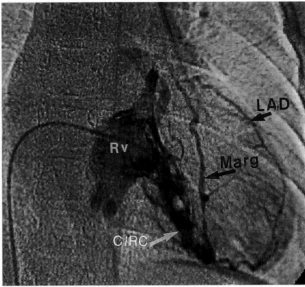

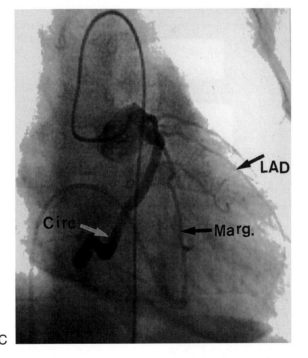

Figure 24–2

A, Right ventriculogram from a 3-year-old girl with pulmonary atresia, intact ventricular septum, and metal sutures from a bidirectional Glenn operation. The small right ventricle (RV) ends blindly. The left anterior descending (LAD), circumflex (Circ), and posterior descending (PDA) coronary arteries are visualized through ventriculo-coronary arterial communications. The luminal irregularities were nonobstructive. The circumflex coronary artery outlines an enlarged left ventricle. *B and C*, Angiograms from a 4-year-old boy with pulmonary atresia, an intact ventricular septum, and a small right ventricle (RV). *B*, A large circumflex coronary artery (Circ) and the left anterior descending (LAD) and marginal (Marg) coronary arteries were visualized through right ventricular sinusoids. *C*, Contrast material injected into the left aortic sinus visualized the large circumflex coronary artery and the left anterior descending and marginal coronary arteries.

ventricle is initially large and powerful as Peacock described (Fig. 24–5),[50] but its compliance and ejection fraction diminish because it pumps the entire output for both circulations.[22,25,53,55,56]

The *physiologic derangements* in pulmonary atresia with intact ventricular septum are implicit in the anatomic features of the malformation. Physiologic classification is based on the tripartite morphology of the right ventricle and on the degree of right ventricular hypoplasia as mild, moderate, or severe. Flow from the right ventricle into the pulmonary trunk is impossible by definition. Venous blood reaches the systemic circulation via an interatrial

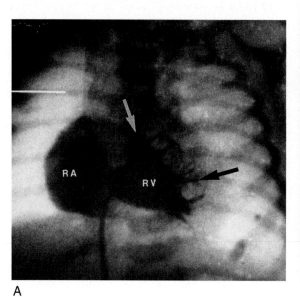
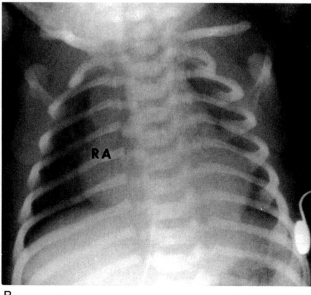

Figure 24–3

A, Right ventriculogram from a 1-day-old boy with pulmonary atresia (*upper arrow*), intact ventricular septum, and a moderate-sized right ventricle (RV) that contained an inlet portion, a trabecular portion, and a well-formed infundibulum. Intramyocardial sinusoids end blindly (*lower right arrow*). Tricuspid regurgitation filled a large right atrium (RA). *B,* X-ray from the same patient shows oligemic lung fields, a large right atrium (RA), and a well-formed left ventricle at the apex.

communication that is usually a restrictive patent foramen ovale and is the only exit for the right atrium (see Fig. 24–1).[25] Unoxygenated right atrial blood mixes with oxygenated left atrial blood. The mixture flows into the left ventricle and into the aorta, so systemic arterial oxygen saturation is reduced. Blood from the aorta reaches the pulmonary circulation through a tenuously patent ductus arteriosus upon which survival depends[62] (see Figs. 24–1 and 24–5). When the ductus closes, effective pulmonary blood flow ceases.[25,62] Systemic to pulmonary collateral vessels are inadequate for survival.[62]

These physiologic patterns from the right atrium to the left side of the heart are relatively constant from

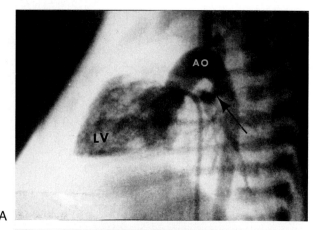

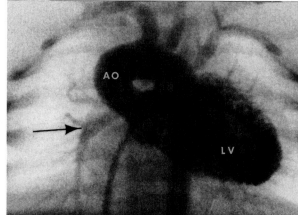

Figure 24–5

A, Lateral left ventriculogram from a 3-day-old girl with pulmonary atresia, intact ventricular septum, a diminutive right ventricle, and a large left ventricle (LV). The *oblique arrow* on the right points to a normally formed ductus arteriosus that narrowed at its pulmonary insertion. Ao, aorta. *B,* Left ventriculogram shows the large left ventricle (LV) and a prominent ascending aorta (Ao). Pulmonary arteries (*left arrow*) filled through the patent ductus arteriosus.

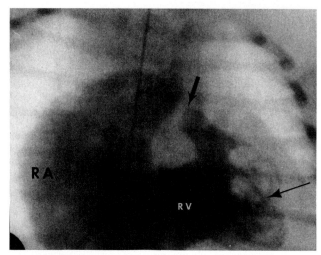

Figure 24–4

Right ventriculogram from a 1-day-old girl with pulmonary atresia, intact ventricular septum, and a normal-sized right ventricle (RV) that contained an inlet portion, a trabecular portion (*lower right arrow*), and a blind infundibular portion (*upper arrow*). Severe tricuspid regurgitation filled a huge right atrium (RA).

patient to patient, but the patterns in the *right* side of the heart vary considerably. When the right ventricle is small, little blood enters or leaves its cavity because the diminutive chamber and the diminutive tricuspid valve obstruct right atrial flow, which is further obstructed by the thick ventricular wall and endocardial fibroelastosis.[49] Whatever blood enters the right ventricle during diastole is trapped during systole except for the small portion that exits through ventriculo-coronary arterial connections. When the right ventricle is dilated and thin-walled and the tricuspid valve is incompetent, right atrial blood copiously enters the ventricular cavity during diastole only to be returned to the right atrium during the next systole. Systolic pressure is comparatively low when the right ventricle and right atrium communicate freely across an incompetent tricuspid valve.[22] Although right atrial blood readily flows *into* the right ventricle, no useful purpose is served because forward flow into the pulmonary trunk is impossible. Back-and-forth movement of blood across the tricuspid orifice results in progressive enlargement of the right side of the heart, which becomes massive.

The History

Pulmonary atresia with intact ventricular septum is equally represented in males and females.[43] There are reports of the malformation in siblings[19,27] and a report in first cousins,[20] but familial recurrence is rare. Over half of newborns die in the first month of life, a considerable majority die within the first three months, and very few live beyond the first year.[22,25] Survival hinges on tenuous patency of the ductus arteriosus and on the size of the interatrial communication, which is usually a restrictive patent foramen ovale.[25,55,62] Cyanosis begins immediately after birth, and the degree of cyanosis depends on patency of the ductus arteriosus.[22,25,55,62] Pulmonary blood flow diminishes as the ductus involutes, and when the ductus closes pulmonary blood flow ceases. Despite this ominous outlook, isolated examples of survival have been reported to age 3.5 years[41] and to age 14 years,[2] and four patients lived for 20 to 21 years.[1,10,21,52] The 21-year-old woman had a closed ductus arteriosus at necropsy, but instead had a sizable connection between the aortic root and pulmonary trunk and a large atrial septal defect.[52] Another 21-year-old woman survived without a patent ductus because the anterior descending branch of the left coronary artery originated from the pulmonary trunk and provided adequate pulmonary blood flow via intercoronary anastomoses.[64]

Physical Appearance

Birth weights are normal and neonatal physical appearance is normal except for cyanosis.[55] Survival beyond the newborn period is accompanied by increasing cyanosis, progressive dyspnea, right-sided heart failure, and physical underdevelopment. The exceptional 21-year-old woman mentioned previously was well-developed.[52]

The Arterial Pulse and Jugular Venous Pulse

The arterial pulse is normal or diminished.[25,55] Large A waves are generated by powerful right atrial contraction when the right ventricle and tricuspid valve are small.[49] Large systolic venous waves are generated when the right ventricle is enlarged and the Ebstein tricuspid valve is incompetent.

Precordial Movement and Palpation

A right ventricular impulse is necessarily absent when pulmonary atresia with intact ventricular septum occurs with a small right ventricle. The impulse of an enlarged left ventricle occupies the apex (see Fig. 24–5). A right ventricular impulse is readily palpated when the right ventricle is dilated and the tricuspid valve is incompetent. The thrill of tricuspid regurgitation may be present at the lower left sternal edge.[55] A very large right atrium with severe tricuspid regurgitation generates a visible and palpable systolic impulse at the right sternal border and over the liver.

Auscultation

When the right ventricle is small, the first heart sound consists of the single mitral component because the hypoplastic tricuspid valve mechanism generates no closure sound. When the right ventricle is dilated, audibility of the tricuspid component of the first heart sound depends on mobility of the anterior leaflet of the Ebstein-like valve (Fig. 24–6).

A transient soft systolic murmur has been ascribed to flow through the patent ductus prior to involution.[25] A soft midsystolic aorta flow murmur is occasionally caused by increased left ventricular stroke volume.[62] The murmur of tricuspid regurgitation is present on the first day of life when the right ventricle is dilated and the malformed tricuspid valve is incompetent (see Fig. 24–6).[55] The murmur is usually medium frequency and decrescendo because the right ventricular systolic pressure is relatively low. Maximum intensity is along the lower left sternal edge and toward the apex topographically coinciding with the displaced tricuspid valve, but the murmur may radiate to the right side of the chest and even to the right axilla when a very large right atrium receives tricuspid regurgitant flow (see Fig. 24–4).[55]

Continuous murmurs originating in the ductus arteriosus are rare because ductal patency is transient.[22] In the 21-year-old woman referred to earlier, a continuous murmur was generated by flow through intercoronary anastomoses between the right coronary artery and the anterior descending branch of the left coronary artery.[64] In the other 21-year-old woman referred to, a systolic/diastolic

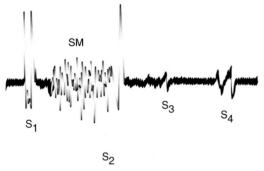

Figure 24–6
Phonocardiogram at the lower left sternal border of a 2-day-old boy with pulmonary atresia, intact ventricular septum, a normal-sized right ventricle, and tricuspid regurgitation. A long crescendo systolic murmur (SM) goes up to a prominent single second heart sound (S_2) that represented aortic valve closure. S_1, first heart sound; S_3, third heart sound; S_4, fourth heart sound.

murmur originated in a communication between the aortic root and the pulmonary trunk.[52] A 2-month-old girl with bidirectional ventriculo-coronary arterial flow had a murmur that was to and fro rather than continuous.[65]

The second heart sound is necessarily single because there is only one functional semilunar valve. Third and fourth heart sounds occur with tricuspid regurgitation because of rapid mid-diastolic filling and an increased force of right atrial contraction transmitted into an unobstructed right ventricle. (see Fig. 24–6).[55]

The Electrocardiogram

The electrocardiogram is a key to the clinical recognition of pulmonary atresia with intact ventricular septum and a small right ventricle because it calls attention to the combination of *cyanosis* with a dominant *left ventricle*. The electrocardio-

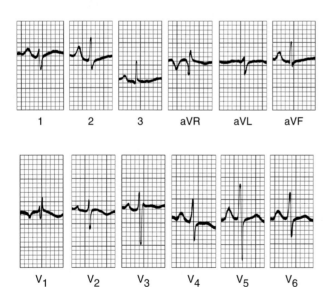

Figure 24–7
Electrocardiogram from a 15-hour-old boy with pulmonary atresia, intact ventricular septum, and a diminutive right ventricle. A tall peaked right atrial P wave is present in lead 2. The QRS axis is rightward, depolarization is clockwise, and there is adult QRS progression in the precordial leads.

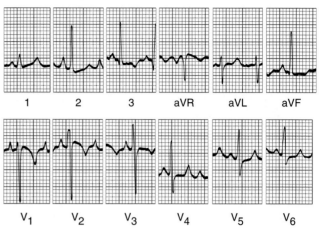

Figure 24–8
Electrocardiogram from a 2-week-old girl with pulmonary atresia, intact ventricular septum, and a small right ventricle. Tall peaked right atrial P waves are present in lead 2 and in leads V_{1-3}. The QRS axis is vertical, depolarization is clockwise, and there is adult QRS progression in the precordial leads.

gram also distinguishes this malformation from tricuspid atresia, which it physiologically resembles (see Chapter 25).

Peaked right atrial P waves appear in limb leads and in right precordial leads when the right ventricle is small (Figs. 24–7 and 24–8).[25,31,55] Biatrial P waves occasionally evolve because the left atrium receives systemic *and* pulmonary venous return.[25,31] The QRS shows *a normal or rightward mean axis and clockwise deplorization*[25,31] (see Figs. 24–7 and 24–8), which is a useful means of distinguishing pulmonary atresia with intact ventricular septum and small

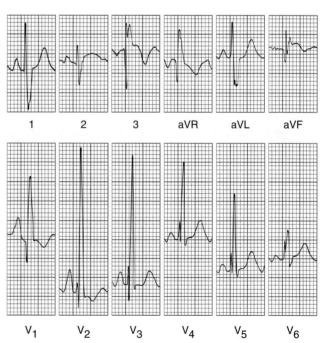

Figure 24–9
Electrocardiogram from a 1-day-old girl with pulmonary atresia, intact ventricular septum, a dilated right ventricle, severe tricuspid regurgitation, and a large right atrium. Exceptionally tall right atrial P waves appear in lead 1 and in right precordial leads. Right atrial enlargement is indicated by the qR pattern in lead V_1. Tall R waves in V_{1-3} reflect the enlarged right ventricle.

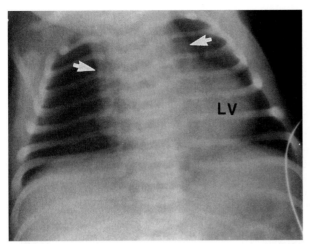

Figure 24–10
X-ray from a 2-day-old girl with pulmonary atresia, intact ventricular septum, and a diminutive right ventricle. The lung fields (*arrows*) are oligemic. An enlarged convex left ventricle occupies the apex. Thymus obscures the base of the heart.

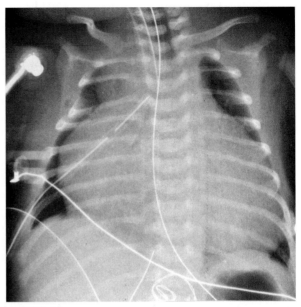

Figure 24–12
X-ray from a 5-month-old boy with pulmonary atresia, intact ventricular septum, a dilated right ventricle, and severe tricuspid regurgitation. The immense cardiac silhouette is the result of right atrial and right ventricular dilatation. The largely obscured lung fields are oligemic.

right ventricle from tricuspid atresia which is characterized by *left* axis deviation and *counterclockwise depolarization.*[22,25,31] Precordial leads display an adult QRS pattern (see Figs. 24–7 and 24–8).[31,57] Right ventricular hypertrophy is conspicuously absent. The small right ventricle does not generate large precordial QRS amplitudes despite its thick wall because its cavity contains little blood.[31] Similar electrocardiographic patterns may occur in neonates with pinpoint pulmonary stenosis and diminutive right ventricle (see Chapter 11).[29,45] Left ventricular hypertrophy is reflected by voltage criteria,[31] but ST segment abnormalities reflect left ventricular ischemia rather than hypertrophy.

In the first week of life, the electrocardiogram does not reliably distinguish pulmonary atresia with intact ventricular septum and *small* right ventricle from pulmonary atresia with intact ventricular septum and a *large* right ventricle.[45] Shortly thereafter, the electrocardiogram associated with a dilated right ventricle and tricuspid regurgitation reveals itself because of a rightward QRS axis and right ventricular hypertrophy in precordial leads (Fig. 24–9).[18,31,55,57] Right

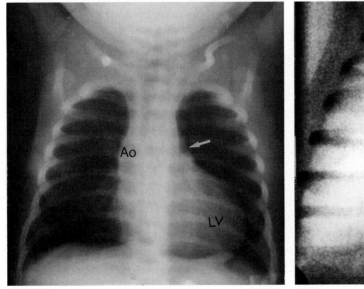
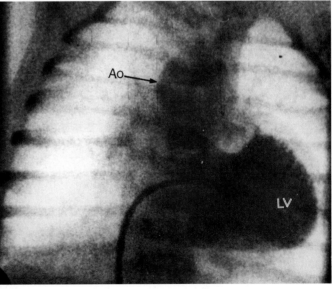

A B

Figure 24–11
A, X-ray from a 3-week-old girl with pulmonary atresia, intact ventricular septum, and a small right ventricle. The lung fields are oligemic. The ascending aorta (Ao) is enlarged, the main pulmonary artery segment (arrow) is normal, and an enlarged convex left ventricle (LV) occupies the apex. *B,* Angiogram showing the enlarged left ventricle (LV) and the dilated ascending aorta (Ao).

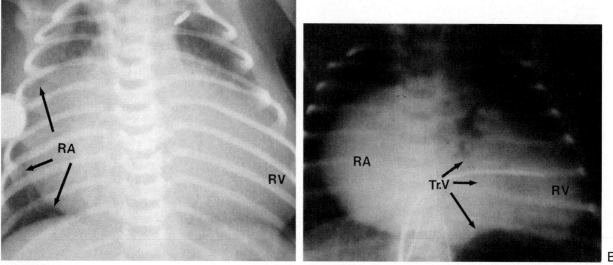

Figure 24–13

A, X-ray from a 7-day-old girl with pulmonary atresia, intact ventricular septum, a dilated right ventricle, and severe tricuspid regurgitation. The cardiac silhouette is immense because of striking enlargement of the right atrium (RA) and right ventricle (RV). *B,* Contrast injection into the dilated right ventricle (RV) identified the displaced tricuspid valve leaflets (TrV) and a huge right atrium (RA).

atrial enlargement is reflected in exceptionally tall P waves and a qR pattern in lead V_1 (see Fig. 24–9).

The X-Ray

When the right ventricle is small, the cardiac silhouette at birth may be normal or nearly so (Fig. 24–10).[18,35] The pulmonary artery segment is normal because the pulmonary trunk develops normally despite pulmonary valve atresia (Fig. 24–11). The ascending aorta is enlarged (see Figs. 24–5B and 24–11).[22,41] The right atrial shadow is moderately prominent (see Fig. 24–11). A well-formed convex left ventricle occupies the apex (see Figs. 24–5, 24–10, and 24–11).[41]

The x-ray differs appreciably when the right ventricle is dilated and the tricuspid valve is incompetent.[41,55] The cardiac silhouette virtually fills the chest because of remarkable enlargement of the right atrium and right ventricle (Figs. 24–12 and Fig. 24–13).[8,55]

The Echocardiogram

Echocardiography with color flow imaging and Doppler interrogation establishes the diagnosis of pulmonary atresia with intact ventricular septum, identifies the atretic pulmonary valve and the well-formed pulmonary trunk, and distinguishes a small right ventricle with a small tricuspid valve from a dilated right ventricle with tricuspid regurgitation.[32,43,60] The malformation can be recognized in utero.[17,23]

Hypoplasia of the right ventricle is judged as mild, moderate, or severe (Fig. 24–14), and the inlet, trabecular, and outlet portions can be identified.[43] Deep endocardial recesses represent blind penetrations of the

proximal segments of ventriculo-coronary arterial communications (see Fig. 24–14). Retrograde flow into the aorta can be detected with pulsed Doppler or can be suspected because of dilatation of a proximal coronary artery.[33] Color flow imaging with Doppler interrogation confirms the absence of flow across the atretic pul-

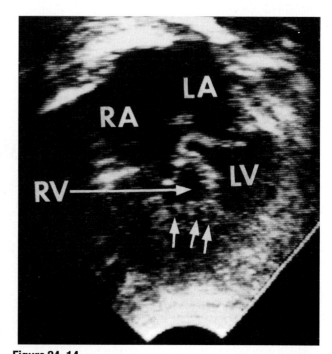

Figure 24–14

Echocardiogram (apical four-chamber view) from an 8-month-old boy with pulmonary atresia, intact ventricular septum, and a diminutive right ventricle (RV). Blind ventriculocoronary artery sinusoids (*three vertical arrows*) penetrate the right ventricular wall. The right atrium (RA) is enlarged. The size of the left atrium (LA) and left ventricle (LV) are normal.

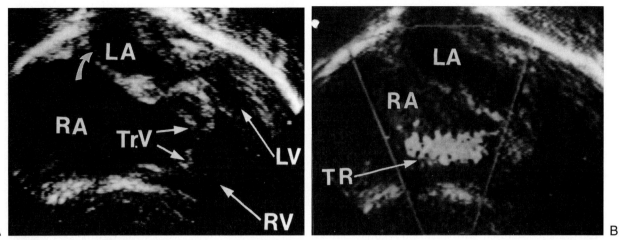

Figure 24–15

A, Echocardiogram from a 6-day-old boy with pulmonary atresia, intact ventricular septum, a dilated right ventricle, and severe tricuspid regurgitation. The Ebstein-like tricuspid valve (TrV) is apically displaced into the enlarged right ventricle (RV). The right atrium (RA) is huge. The size of the left atrium (LA) and left ventricle (LV) are normal. The *unmarked curved arrow* between the right and left atrium identifies a restrictive patent foramen ovale. *B,* Black-and-white print of a color flow image showing the jet of severe tricuspid regurgitation (Tr) into the huge right atrium (RA).

monary valve, which appears as an immobile dense line that moves but fails to open. Initial patency of the ductus is identified with color flow imaging, which also detects a right-to-left shunt across a restrictive interatrial communication.

When the right ventricle is dilated, echocardiography identifies the Ebstein-like malformation of the tricuspid valve with displacement and immobility of the septal and posterior leaflets (Figs. 24–15A and 24–16A). Color flow imaging establishes the degree of tricuspid regurgitation (see Figs. 24–15B and 24–16B). The right atrium can be immense (see Figs. 24–15A and 24–16A). Ebstein's anom-

aly with *functional* pulmonary atresia in which a patent but stenotic pulmonary valve fails to open can be distinguished from *anatomic* pulmonary atresia and a malformed Ebstein-like tricuspid valve.[60]

Summary

Pulmonary atresia with intact ventricular septum is suspected in neonates and infants with cyanosis, a dominant left ventricle, and reduced pulmonary blood flow. When the right ventricle *is* small, the physical examination

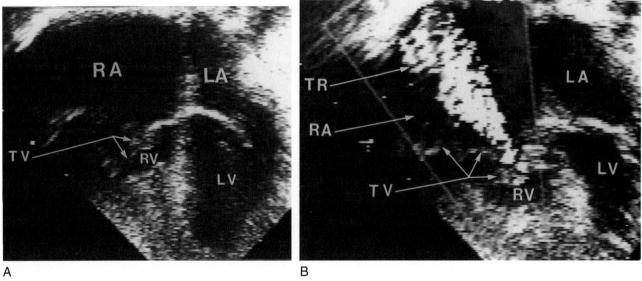

Figure 24–16

A, Echocardiogram (four chamber view) from a 2-day-old girl with pulmonary atresia, intact ventricular septum, a moderate sized right ventricle, and severe tricuspid regurgitation. The tricuspid valve (TV) is thickened and recessed into the right ventricle (RV) whose apex is filled with hypertrophied muscle. The right atrium (RA) is immense. The size of the left atrium (LA) is normal, and the left ventricle (LV) is moderately enlarged. *B,* Black-and-white print of a color flow image showing a huge right atrium (RA) and severe tricuspid regurgitation (TR) that originated within the right ventricle (RV) from a recessed tricuspid valve (TV).

reveals an isolated left ventricular impulse and either no murmur at all or a soft aortic midsystolic flow murmur. The electrocardiogram shows right atrial P waves, a vertical QRS axis with clockwise depolarization, and adult QRS progression in the precordial leads. An initially normal radiologic cardiac silhouette increases moderately because of moderate enlargement of the right atrium and left ventricle. The lung fields are oligemic, and the main pulmonary artery segment is normal. Echocardiography with color flow imaging and Doppler interrogation identifies an imperforate pulmonary valve, a well-formed pulmonary trunk, a small thick-walled right ventricle, a small tricuspid valve, and moderate enlargement of the right atrium and left ventricle.

A dilated right ventricle with tricuspid regurgitation is characterized on physical examination by a right ventricular impulse and a tricuspid regurgitation murmur that radiates to the right of the sternum. The electrocardiogram shows strikingly tall peaked right atrial P waves. The QRS axis is rightward with clockwise depolarization. Right ventricular hypertrophy is reflected in tall right precordial R waves. The x-ray reveals a cardiac silhouette that virtually fills the chest because of massive dilatation of the right atrium and right ventricle. The echocardiogram with color flow imaging and Doppler interrogation identifies a dilated right ventricle, an Ebstein-like malformation of the tricuspid valve, severe tricuspid regurgitation, and striking enlargement of the right atrium.

REFERENCES

1. Abbott, M.E.S.: Atlas of Congenital Cardiac Diseases. New York, American Heart Association, 1936.
2. Allanby K.D., Brinton, W.D., Campbell, M., and Gardner, F.: Pulmonary atresia and collateral circulation to lungs. Guy's Hosp. Rep. 99:110, 1950.
3. Ekman, J.B.M., Sunnegardh, J., and Hanseus, K., et al: Outcome of children born with pulmonary atresia and intact ventricular septum in Sweden from 1980 to 1999. Scand. Cardiovasc. J. 35:192, 2001.
4. L'Ecuyer, T.J., Poulik, J.M., and Vincent J.A.: Myocardial infarction due to coronary abnormalities in pulmonary atresia with intact ventricular septum. Pediatr. Cardiol. 22:68, 2001.
5. Arom, K.V., and Edwards J.E.: Relationship between right ventricular muscle bundles and pulmonary valve: Significance in pulmonary atresia with intact ventricular septum. Circulation 54:111, 1976.
6. Baffa, J.M., Chen, S., Guttenberger, M.E., et al: Coronary artery abnormalities and right ventricular histology in hypoplastic left heart syndrome. J. Am. Coll. Cardiol. 20:350, 1992.
7. Powell, A.J., Mayer, J.E., Lang, P., and Lock J.E.: Outcome in infants with pulmonary atresia, intact ventricular septum, and right ventricular-dependent coronary circulation. Am. J. Cardiol. 86:1272, 2000.
8. Bharati, S., McAllister, H.A., Chiemmongkoltip, P., and Lev, M.: Congenital pulmonary atresia with tricuspid insufficiency. Am. J. Cardiol. 40:70, 1977.
9. Freedom, R.M., Yoo, S.J., and Jovois, A.: A most peculiar coronary circulation in a patient with pulmonary atresia and intact ventricular septum. Cardiol. Young. 10:60, 2000.
10. Bostoen, H., Robiscek, S., and Sanger, P. W.: Atresia of the pulmonary valve with normal pulmonary artery and intact ventricular septum in a 21-year-old woman. Coll. Works Cardiopulm. Dis. 11:753, 1966.
11. Braulin, E. A., Formanek, A. G., Moller, J. H., and Edwards, J. E.: Angio-pathological appearances of pulmonary valve in pulmonary atresia with intact ventricular septum. Br. Heart J. 47:281, 1982.
12. Bulkley, B. H., D'Amico, B., and Taylor, A. L.: Extensive myocardial fibral disarray in aortic and pulmonary atresia—relevance to hypotrophic cardiomyopathy. Circulation 67:191, 1983.
13. Bull, C., de Leval, M. R., Mercanti, C., Macartney, F. J., and Anderson, R. H.: Pulmonary atresia and intact ventricular septum: A revised classification. Circulation 66:266, 1982.
14. Burrows, P. E., Freedom, R. M., Benson, L. N., and Moes, C. A. F.: Coronary angiography in pulmonary atresia with intact ventricular septum. Am. J. Roentgenol. 154:789, 1990.
15. Buzzi, A.: Description of congenital pulmonary atresia and tricuspid stenosis (Delmas 1826). Am. J. Cardiol. 4:691, 1959.
16. Oosthoek, P.W., Moorman, A.F., Sauer, U., and Gittengerger-de Groot, A.C.: Capillary distribution in the ventricles of hearts with pulmonary atresia and intact ventricular septum. Circulation 91:1790, 1995
17. Patel, C.R., Shah, D.M., Dahms, B.B.: Prenatal diagnosis of a coronary fistula in a fetus with pulmonary atresia with intact ventricular septum and trisomy 18. J. Ultrasound Med. 18:429, 1999.
18. Celermajer, J. M., Bowdler, J. D., Gengos, D. C., Cohen, D. H., and Stuckey, D. S.: Pulmonary valve fusion with intact ventricular septum. Am. Heart J. 76:452, 1968.
19. Chitayat, D., McIntosh, N., and Fouron, J.: Pulmonary atresia with intact ventricular septum and hypoplastic right heart in sibs: A single gene disorder? Am. J. Med. Genet. 42:304, 1992.
20. Grossfeld, P.D., Lucas, V.W., Sklansky, M.S., Kashani, I.A., Rothman, A.: Familial occurrence of pulmonary atresia and intact ventricular septum. Am J Med Genet. 72:294, 1997
21. Costa, A.: Atresia congenita del'ostio della pulmonare, consetto interventriculare chiuso e dotto di Botallo persistente in nomo de 20 anni. Clin. Med. Ital. 61:567, 1930.
22. Davignon, A. L., Greenwold, W. E., DuShane, J. W., and Edwards, J. E.: Congenital pulmonary atresia with intact ventricular septum. Clinicopathologic correlation of two anatomic types. Am. Heart J. 62:591, 1961.
23. Patel, C. R., Dahms, B. B., and Sallee, D.: Pulmonary atresia with intact ventricular septum, right-sided aortic arch and ventriculocoronary connection-prenatal echocardiographic diagnosis. Cardiol Young. 11:352, 2001
24. Garcia, J.A., Zellers, T.M., Weinstein, E.M., Mahony, L.: Usefulness of Doppler echocardiography in diagnosing right ventricular coronary arterial communications in patients with pulmonary atresia and intact ventricular septum and comparison with angiography. Am J. Cardio 81:103, 1998.
25. Elliott, L. P., Adams, P., Jr., and Edwards, J. E.: Pulmonary atresia with intact ventricular septum. Br. Heart J. 25:489, 1963.
26. Engberding, R., and Bender, F.: Identification of a rare congenital anomaly of the myocardium by two-dimensional echocardiography: Persistence of isolated myocardial sinusoids. Am. J. Cardiol. 53:1733, 1984.
27. Eriksen, N. L., Buttino, L., and Juberg, R. C.: Congenital pulmonary atresia with intact ventricular septum, tricuspid insufficiency, and patent ductus arteriosus in two sibs. Am J. Med. Genet. 32:187, 1989.
28. Satou, G. M., Perry, S. B., Gauvreau, K., and Geva, T.: Echocardiographic predictors of coronary artery pathology in pulmonary atresia with intact ventricular septum. Am. J. Cardiol. 85:1319, 2000.
29. Freed, M. D., Rosenthal, A., Bernhard, W. F., Litwin, S. B., and Nadas, A. S.: Critical pulmonary stenosis with a diminutive right ventricle in neonates. Circulation 48:875, 1973.
30. Freedom, R. M., and Harrington, D. P.: Contributions of intramyocardial sinusoids in pulmonary atresia and intact ventricular septum to a right-sided circular shunt. Br. Heart J. 36:1061, 1974.
31. Gamboa, R., Gersong, W. M., and Nadas, A. S.: The electrocardiogram in tricuspid atresia and pulmonary atresia with intact ventricular septum. Circulation 34:24, 1966.
32. Gewillig, M., Dumoulin, M., and Van der Hauwaert, L.: Transient neonatal tricuspid regurgitation: A Doppler echocardiographic study of three cases. Br. Heart J. 60:446, 1988.
33. Gittenberger-de Groot, A. C., Sauer, U., Bindl, L., Babic, R., Essed, C. E., and Buhlmeyer, K.: Competition of coronary arteries and ventriculo-coronary arterial communications in pulmonary atresia with intact ventricular septum. Int. J. Cardiol. 18:243, 1988.
34. Grant, R. T.: Unusual anomaly of coronary vessels in malformed heart of child. Heart 13:273, 1926.

35. Greenwald, W. E., and Edwards, J. E.: Congenital pulmonary atresia with intact ventricular septum: Two anatomic types. Circulation 14:945, 1956.

36. Horne, M. K., and Rowlands, D. T.: Hypoplastic right heart complex in a 46 year old woman. Br. Heart J. 33:167, 1971.

37. Hubbard, J. F., Girod, D. A., Caldwell, R. L., Hurwitz, R. A., Mahony, L. A., and Waller, B. F.: Right ventricular infarction with cardiac rupture in an infant with pulmonary valve atresia with intact ventricular septum. J. Am. Coll. Cardiol. 2:363, 1983.

38. Hunter, J.: Medical Observations and Inquiries. 6:291, 1783 (see reference 50, Peacock, T.B.).

39. Hutchins, G. M., Kessler-Hanna, A., and Moore, G. W.: Development of the coronary arteries in the embryonic human heart. Circulation 77:1250, 1988.

40. Kasznica, J., Ursell, P. C., Blanc, W. A., and Gersony, W. M.: Abnormalities of the coronary circulation in pulmonary atresia and intact ventricular septum. Am. Heart J. 114:1415, 1987.

41. Kieffer, S. A., and Carey, L. S.: Radiological aspects of pulmonary atresia with intact ventricular septum. Br. Heart J. 25:655, 1963.

42. Daubeney, P. E., Sharland, G. K., Cook, A. C., Keeton, B.R., Anderson, R. H., and Webber, S. A.: Pulmonary atresia with intact ventricular septum: Impact of fetal echocardiography on incidence at birth and postnatal outcome. Circulation 98:562, 1998.

43. Leung, M. P., Mok, C., and Hui, P.: Echocardiographic assessment of neonates with pulmonary atresia and intact ventricular septum. J. Am. Coll. Cardiol. 12:719, 1988.

44. Mahoney, L. T., Knoedel, D. L., Wagman, A. J., and Marvin, W. J.: Pulsed-Doppler demonstration of retrograde coronary artery flow in pulmonary atresia with intact ventricular septum. J. Cardiovasc. Ultrasonogr. 6:101, 1987.

45. Miller, G. A. H., Restifo, M., Shinebourne, E. A., Paneth, M., Joseph, M. C., Lennox, S. C., and Kerr, I. H.: Pulmonary atresia with intact ventricular septum and critical pulmonary stenosis presenting in first month of life. Br. Heart J. 35:9, 1973.

46. Newfeld, E. A., Cole, R. B., and Paul, M. H.: Ebstein's malformation of the tricuspid valve in the neonate. Functional and anatomic pulmonary outflow tract obstruction. Am. J. Cardiol. 19:727, 1967.

47. O'Connor, W. N., Cottrill, C. M., Johnson, G. L., Noonan, J. A., and Todd, E. P.: Pulmonary atresia with intact ventricular septum and ventriculocoronary communications. Circulation 61:805, 1982.

48. O'Connor, W. N., Stahr, B. J., Cottrill, C. M., Todd, E. P., and Noonan, J. A.: Ventriculocoronary connections in hypoplastic right heart syndrome: Autopsy serial section study of six cases. J. Am. Coll. Cardiol. 11:1061, 1988.

49. Patel, R. G., Freedom, R. M., Moes, C. A. F., Bloom, K. R., Olley, P. M., Williams, W. G., Trusler, G. A., and Rowe, R. D.: Right ventricular volume determinations in 18 patients with pulmonary atresia and intact ventricular septum. Circulation 61:428, 1980.

50. Peacock, T. B.: On Malformations of the Human Heart. London, J. Churchill & Sons, 1858.

51. Raghib, G., Bloemendaal, R., Kanjuh, V., and Edwards, J. E.: Aortic atresia and premature closure of foramen ovale. Myocardial sinusoids and coronary arteriovenous fistula serving as outflow channel. Am. Heart J. 70:476, 1965.

52. Robicsek, F., Bostoen, H., and Sanger, P. W.: Atresia of the pulmonary valve with normal pulmonary artery and intact ventricular septum in a 21-year old woman. Angiology 17:896, 1966.

53. Santos, M. A., Moll, J. N., Drummond, C., Araujo, W. B., Romao, N., and Reis, N. B.: Development of the ductus arteriosus in right ventricular outflow tract obstruction. Circulation 62:818, 1980.

54. Sauer, U., Gittenberger-de Groot, A. C., Geishauser, M., Babic, R., and Buhlmeyer, K.: Coronary arteries in the hypoplastic left heart syndrome: Histopathologic and histometrical studies and implications for surgery. Circulation 80(Suppl. I): I-186, 1989.

55. Schrire, V., Sutin, G. J., and Barnard, C. N.: Organic and functional pulmonary atresia with intact ventricular septum. Am. J. Cardiol. 8:100, 1961.

56. Scognamiglio, R., Daliento, L., Razzolini, R., Boffa, G. M., Pellegrino, P. A., Chioin, R., and Volta, S. D.: Pulmonary atresia with intact ventricular septum: A quantitative cineventriculographic study of the right and left ventricular function. Pediatr. Cardiol. 7:183, 1986.

57. Shams, A., Fowler, R. S., Trusler, G. A., Keith, J. D., and Mustard, W. T.: Pulmonary atresia with intact ventricular septum: Report of 50 cases. Pediatrics 74:370, 1971.

58. Shimizu, T., Ando, M., and Takao, A.: Pulmonary atresia with intact ventricular septum and corrected transposition of the great arteries. Br. Heart J. 45:471, 1981.

59. Sideris, E. B., Olley, P. M., Spooner, E., Farina, M., Foster, E., Trusler, G., and Shaher, R.: Left ventricular function and compliance in pulmonary atresia with intact ventricular septum. J. Thorac. Cardiovasc. Surg. 84:192, 1982.

60. Smallhorn, J. F., Izukawa, T., Benson, L., and Freedom, R. M.: Noninvasive recognition of functional pulmonary atresia by echocardiography. Am. J. Cardiol. 54:925, 1984.

61. Steeg, C. N., Ellis, K., Bransilver, B., and Gersony, W. M.: Pulmonary atresia and intact ventricular septum complicating corrected transposition of the great vessels. Am. Heart J. 82:382, 1971.

62. Venables, A. W.: The patterns of pulmonary circulation in pulmonary atresia. Br. Heart J. 26:760, 1964.

63. Zuberbuhler, J. R., and Anderson, R. H.: Morphological variations in pulmonary atresia with intact ventricular septum. Br. Heart J. 41:281, 1979.

64. McArthur JD, Munsi SC, Sukumar IP, Cherian G. Pulmonary atresia with intact ventricular septum.Circulation 44:740, 1971

65. Ogden JA. Secondary coronary arterial fistulas. J Pediatr. 78:78, 1971.

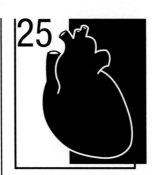

Tricuspid Atresia

Tricuspid atresia was described in 1817.[55] Because of the morphologic heterogeneity of the malformation and because "manifold anatomic combinations can result in this haemodynamic arrangement,"[2] almost a century elapsed before the great arterial relationships were defined.[38] Incidence has been estimated at 0.06 per 1000 live births with a prevalence of 1% to 3% of congenital heart disease.[57,64] This chapter is concerned with hearts in *situs solitus* without ventricular inversion in which no physiologic or anatomic connection exists between the morphologic right atrium and the morphologic right ventricle. Systemic venous return cannot directly reach the ventricular portion of the heart but instead traverses the atrial septum from a morphologic right atrium into a morphologic left atrium where it mixes with pulmonary venous return before crossing a solitary atrioventricular valve into a morphologic left ventricle, which is the only pumping chamber for the pulmonary and systemic circulations (Fig. 25–1).[2] Atresia of the tricuspid valve with Ebstein's anomaly and atresia of the right atrioventricular valve with single ventricle are dealt with in Chapters 13 and 26.

Tricuspid atresia as just defined has certain anatomic features that consistently recur from case to case and certain features that are variable.[19,51,64] Consistent features include: 1) physiologic and anatomic absence of a connection between the morphologic right atrium and the morphologic right ventricle, 2) hypoplasia of the morphologic right ventricle, 3) an interatrial communication, and 4) a morphologic left ventricle that is equipped with a morphologic mitral valve. Variable features provide the rationale for a clinical classification based on two morphologic features[19,51,64,71]: 1) whether or not the great arteries are transposed, and 2) whether or not pulmonary stenosis coexists (Figs. 25–2 and 25–3). An embryologic classification is based on two

microscopic characteristics: 1) the rudiments of an atretic tricuspid apparatus that form a dimple on the floor of the right atrium that can be localized with transillumination by a light source placed within the hypoplastic right ventricle,[18,51,52,59,61,69] and 2) a fibrous atrioventricular remnant that forms a microscopic tract from the right atrium to a tiny inlet component of the subjacent right ventricle.[77] Failure of expansion of the exceedingly small inlet component during early embryogenesis is believed to be the pathogenetic

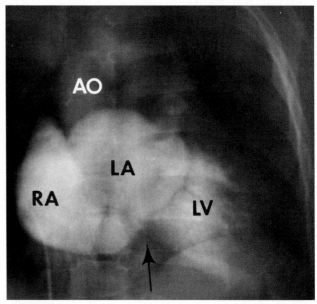

Figure 25–1
Angiocardiogram from an 8-year-old boy with tricuspid atresia, normally related great arteries, and a restrictive ventricular septal defect that closed spontaneously. Contrast material injected into the right atrium (RA) sequentially fills the left atrium (LA), left ventricle (LV), and aorta (Ao). The right ventricle (*unmarked arrow*) remains unopacified as a wedge-shaped area of negative contrast.

TRICUSPID ATRESIA WITHOUT TRANSPOSITION

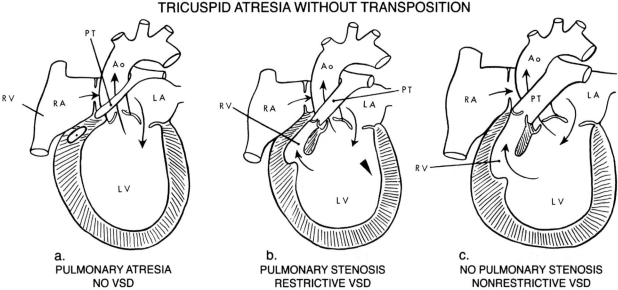

a.
PULMONARY ATRESIA
NO VSD

b.
PULMONARY STENOSIS
RESTRICTIVE VSD

c.
NO PULMONARY STENOSIS
NONRESTRICTIVE VSD

Figure 25–2

Illustrations of three principal varieties of tricuspid atresia without transposition of the great arteries. Anatomic arrangements proximal to the mitral valve are similar. An interatrial communication provides the right atrium (RA) with its only exit. Anatomic arrangements distal to the mitral valve vary. *A, Pulmonary atresia* is represented by an intact ventricular septum. All left ventricular blood enters the aorta (Ao). The pulmonary trunk (PT) is hypoplastic. Pulmonary blood flow depends on patency of the ductus arteriosus or on systemic arterial collaterals. The left atrium (LA) and left ventricle (LV) are normal-sized. *B, Subpulmonary stenosis* is represented by a restrictive ventricular septal defect between the normal-sized left ventricle (LV) and the small right ventricle (RV). The pulmonary trunk is normal or small. *C,* A nonrestrictive ventricular septal defect permits unobstructed blood flow into the pulmonary trunk. When pulmonary vascular resistance is low, pulmonary blood flow is increased, so the left atrium and left ventricle are dilated.

mechanism responsible for approximately two thirds of cases of tricuspid atresia.[77] *Congenital tricuspid stenosis* is a less severe form of the malformation in which a transilluminated dimple separates the right atrium from the right ventricle but a well-formed tricuspid valve joins a small inlet portion of the right ventricle (Fig. 25–4).[18,59,69]

An *interatrial communication* in the form of a restrictive patent foramen ovale is present in approximately three fourths of cases.[17] The valve of the foramen ovale occasionally protrudes aneurysmally as the obstructed right atrium vainly seeks an exit,[24,56] and the aneurysmal protrusion can obstruct left atrial flow.[56] An atrial septal defect is a

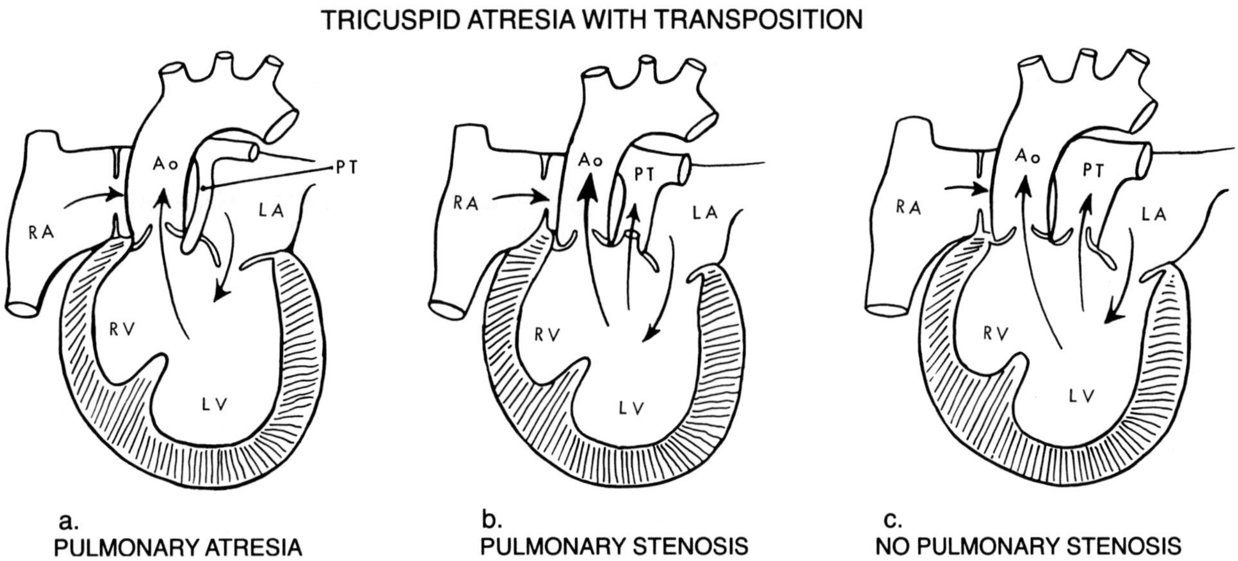

TRICUSPID ATRESIA WITH TRANSPOSITION

a.
PULMONARY ATRESIA

b.
PULMONARY STENOSIS

c.
NO PULMONARY STENOSIS

Figure 25–3

Illustration of three principal varieties of tricuspid atresia with complete transposition of the great arteries. The anatomic arrangements proximal to the mitral valve are similar. An interatrial communication provides the right atrium (RA) with its only exit. A nonrestrictive ventricular septal defect permits unobstructed blood flow from the left ventricle (LV) to the transposed aorta (Ao). Anatomic arrangements distal to the mitral valve vary. *A,* With *atresia of the pulmonary valve,* all left ventricular blood enters the aorta (Ao) through the nonrestrictive ventricular septal defect. The right ventricle (RV) is well-formed. The pulmonary trunk (PT) is hypoplastic. Pulmonary blood flow depends on patency of the ductus arteriosus or on systemic arterial collaterals. The left atrium (LA) and left ventricle (LV) are normal-sized. *B,* Valvular or subvalvular pulmonary stenosis regulates pulmonary blood flow. The pulmonary trunk is well-developed. The left atrium and left ventricle remain normal-sized. *C,* With no pulmonary stenosis and low pulmonary vascular resistance, pulmonary blood flow is increased, so the left atrium and left ventricle are enlarged.

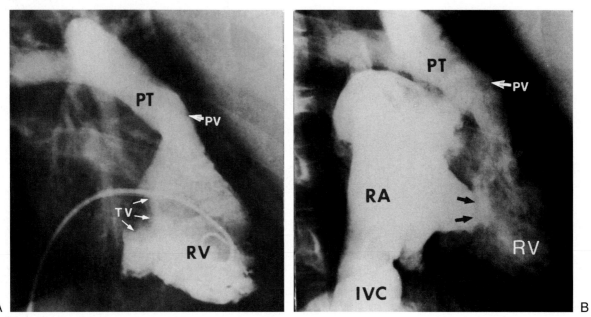

Figure 25–4

A, Right ventriculogram (RV) from a 50-year-old woman with congenital tricuspid stenosis, a well-formed right ventricles, and no obstruction to right ventricular outflow. The stenotic tricuspid valve (TV) domes in diastole. PV, pulmonary valve; PT, pulmonary trunk. *B*, Contrast material injected into the right atrium (RA) identifies diastolic doming of the stenotic tricuspid valve (*unmarked paired arrows*). Negative contrast faintly visualizes a normal pulmonary valve (PV). The inferior vena cava (IVC) visualized because right atrial (RA) pressure was elevated.

much less common form of interatrial communication that is almost always an ostium secundum defect.[17,19]

The great arteries are nontransposed in approximately 90% of cases.[17,71] Pulmonary blood flow depends on the condition of the ventricular septum (see Fig. 25–2). The usual arrangement at birth is a restrictive ventricular septal defect (see Figs. 25–2*B*) that constitutes physiologically advantageous subpulmonary stenosis when the result is adequate but not excessive pulmonary blood flow. That advantage is lost in about 40% of cases because the defect decreases in size or closes spontaneously—*acquired pulmonary atresia* (see Figs. 25–2*A* and 25–6).[17,50,52,54,60,64] The time course of spontaneous closure is similar to that of isolated perimembranous ventricular septal defects (see Chapter 17) with the majority that are destined to close doing so in the first year of life[17,50,54,60,70] Rarely, the ventricular septum is congenitally intact and the pulmonary valve is atretic, completely denying the left ventricle access to the pulmonary circulation (see Fig. 25–2*A*). Also rarely, the pulmonary valve is bicuspid and stenotic, and obstruction is exclusively at valve level.[37] A nonrestrictive ventricular septal defect (see Figs. 25–2*C* and 25–5) permits unobstructed flow from left ventricle to main pulmonary artery and coincides with a well-developed right ventricle and a normally formed pulmonary valve. Pulmonary blood flow is regulated by pulmonary vascular resistance.[40,64]

Tricuspid atresia with *complete transposition of the great arteries* typically occurs with a nonrestrictive ventricular septal defect and no pulmonary stenosis (see Fig. 25–3).[17,40,71] Left ventricular blood has unobstructed access to the transposed aorta through a well-developed right ventricle. Pulmonary blood flow is regulated by pulmonary vascular resistance because the transposed

pulmonary trunk originates from the left ventricle (see Fig. 25–3). Pulmonary vascular disease usually develops in the first year of life (Figs. 25–7 and 25–8).[17] A decrease in size or spontaneous closure of the ventricular septal defect is uncommon,[50] but constitutes *subaortic stenosis* because the transposed aorta arises from the right ventricle.[37,40,44,52] Pulmonary stenosis is infrequent and pulmonary atresia is rare (see Fig. 25–3).[34,71]

The *coronary artery distribution* in tricuspid atresia is analogous to if not identical with that of univentricular hearts with a single morphologic left ventricle and an outlet chamber (see Chapters 26 and 32).[14] The rudimentary right ventricle of tricuspid atresia and the right ventricular remnant of the single ventricle are both delimited by coronary arteries.[14]

Additional anatomic variables associated with tricuspid atresia involve the mitral valve,[43] the ductus arteriosus, the ascending aorta and aortic isthmus, the atrial appendages, and the pulmonary valve.[78] *Abnormalities of the mitral valve* are represented by myxomatous, redundant, or prolapsing leaflets,[43] a cleft anterior leaflet, and direct attachment of leaflets to papillary muscles.[43] When the great arteries are nontransposed and the ventricular septum is congenitally intact—physiologic pulmonary atresia—the fetal ductus arteriosus functions as an aortic tributary and is small and malformed.[63] The ascending aorta and isthmus are large because the aorta receives the entire cardiac output. When the great arteries are transposed and the ventricular septal defect is restrictive, left ventricular blood is diverted into the pulmonary trunk, so the ductus arteriosus enlarges and the ascending aorta and isthmus are underfilled and hypoplastic.[17,29] Very rarely, the pulmonary valve is absent.[78] Juxtaposition of the atrial

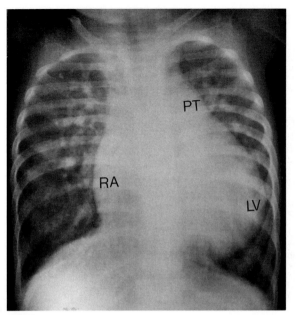
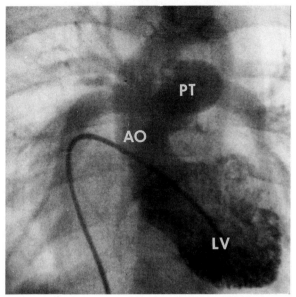

Figure 25–5

A, X-ray from a 6-year-old girl with tricuspid atresia, normally related great arteries, a nonrestrictive ventricular septal defect with low pulmonary vascular resistance, and a large ostium secundum atrial septal defect (see Fig. 25–2C). Pulmonary blood flow is markedly increased, the pulmonary trunk (PT) is prominent, the right atrium (RA) is enlarged, and a dilated left ventricle (LV) occupies the apex. B, Left ventriculogram (LV) from a 4-year-old girl with tricuspid atresia, normally related great arteries, a nonrestrictive ventricular septal defect, and low pulmonary vascular resistance. The pulmonary trunk (PT) and its branches are dilated, and the left ventricle is enlarged. Compare with Figure 25–2C.

appendages, a condition in which both appendages lie on one side of the great arteries,[7,11,15,17] almost always means that the great arteries are transposed (see Chapter 27). Juxtaposition is present in about 50% of patients with tricuspid atresia and complete transposition.

The *physiologic consequences* of tricuspid atresia begin with the obligatory right-to-left shunt at the atrial level. The left atrium indirectly receives the entire systemic venous return across the interatrial communication and directly receives the entire return from the pulmonary veins.[53] The left atrial mixture flows across a morphologic mitral valve into a morphologic left ventricle, which is the sole pumping chamber for the systemic and pulmonary circulations. Pulmonary blood flow is reduced when the great arteries are not transposed because a restrictive ventricular septal defect constitutes a zone of subpulmonary stenosis (see Figs. 25–2 and 25–6), an arrangement that accounts for about 90% of cases. Left ventricular volume overload is curtailed at the price of increased cyanosis. When the ventricular septal defect is nonrestrictive and pulmonary vascular resistance is low, pulmonary blood flow and left ventricular volume overload are excessive and cyanosis is mild (see Fig. 25–5). When the great arteries are transposed, the ventricular septal defect is usually nonrestrictive, pulmonary stenosis is usually absent (see Fig. 25–3), low pulmonary vascular resistance results in increased pulmonary blood flow and left ventricular volume overload, and cyanosis is mild.[39,42] Regulation of pulmonary vascular resistance that achieves adequate but not excessive pulmonary blood flow is a delicate balance that is seldom realized (see Figs. 25–7 and 25–8).[17,40]

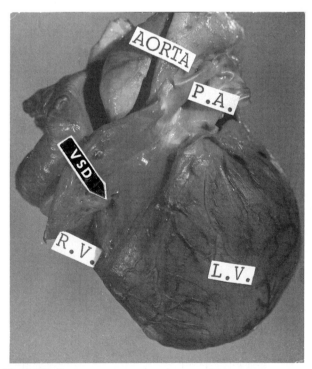

Figure 25–6

Necropsy specimen from a 2-year-old boy with tricuspid atresia, normally related great arteries, and a slitlike ventricular septal defect (VSD) seen from the cavity of the small right ventricle (RV). The pulmonary valve and main pulmonary artery (PA) were normally formed, implying that a previously advantageous ventricular septal defect decreased in size. The left ventricle (LV) is moderately enlarged.

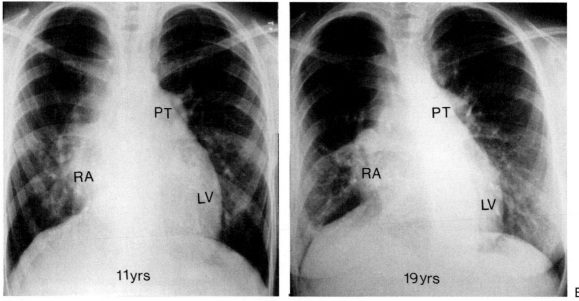

Figure 25–7

X-rays from a girl with tricuspid atresia, normally related great arteries, a nonrestrictive ventricular septal defect, and a large ostium secundum atrial septal defect. At age 11 years, pulmonary vascular resistance was below systemic, pulmonary vascularity was increased, the left ventricle (LV) was enlarged, and the pulmonary trunk (PT) and right atrium (RA) were dilated. At age 19 years, the pulmonary vascular resistance was suprasystemic, pulmonary vascularity was normal, the pulmonary trunk and right atrium remained dilated, but the left ventricle was no longer enlarged. Overlying breast tissue accounts for prominent lower lung field radiodensities.

The History

The defect occurs with equal frequency in male and female when tricuspid atresia occurs with normally related great arteries,[17] but males predominate when the great arteries are transposed[17] unless there is juxtaposition of the atrial appendages.[15] There are reports of tricuspid atresia in siblings,[31,62,76] in families,[22] and in experimental animals.[4] Birth is premature in about 6% of infants with tricuspid atresia.[57]

Survival depends on two variables, namely, an adequate interatrial communication and an adequate regulation of pulmonary blood flow.[17,34] Increased longevity incurs the

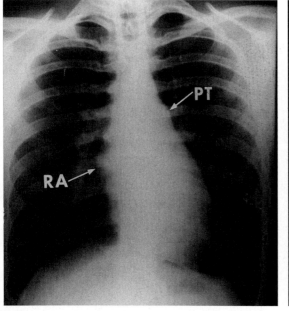
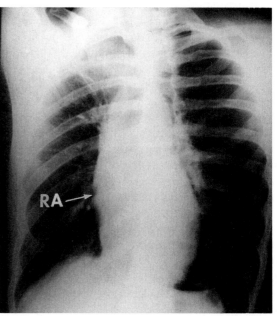

Figure 25–8

X-rays from an 18-year-old man with tricuspid atresia, complete transposition of the great arteries, a nonrestrictive ventricular septal defect, and suprasystemic pulmonary vascular resistance. *A*, Pulmonary vascularity is diminished, and the dilated hypertensive posterior pulmonary trunk is border-forming (PT). The right cardiac silhouette is *hump-shaped* because of a prominent superior border caused by an enlarged right atrium (RA) and a receding inferior border caused by a hypoplastic right ventricle. *B*, Left anterior oblique projection highlights the hump-shaped configuration.

risk of infective endocarditis, paradoxical emboli, and brain abcess.[17,44,46] Actuarial survival has been reported at 72% at 1 year, 52% at 5 years, and 46% at 10 years. Life span is less than 6 months when tricuspid atresia occurs with normally related great arteries and pulmonary atresia (see Fig. 25–2A) but exceptional survivals have been recorded to age 21 years[9] and 22 years.[74] Acquired pulmonary atresia takes the form of delayed spontaneous closure of the ventricular septal defect, an eventuality that usually occurs in the first year of life.[17,52,54] Survival depends on patency of the ductus arteriosus, which is seldom realized.[50] Exceptional survival has nevertheless been reported at age 8 years (see Fig. 25–1), 18 years,[17] and 27 years,[60] in addition to a 21-year-old woman who survived because adequate pulmonary blood flow was achieved by an anomalous artery connecting the ascending aorta to the pulmonary trunk.[2] The most exceptional survival was a 65-year-old man with tricuspid atresia, pulmonary atresia, an ostium secundum atrial septal defect, and large aortic-to-pulmonary arterial collaterals.[6]

The majority of patients with tricuspid atresia and normally related great arteries die in their first year because a restrictive ventricular septal defect decreases in size or spontaneously closes.[17] When the ventricular septal defect adequately regulates pulmonary blood flow, survivals have been realized from the second decade into the fifth decade.[10,12] Two patients lived to 57 years of age,[34] and a 30-year-old woman had a relatively uneventful pregnancy and a dysmature but otherwise normal offspring.[79] If the ventricular septal defect is nonrestrictive (see Fig. 25–2C), increased pulmonary blood flow results in excessive volume overload of the left ventricle and congestive heart failure.[40] However, one such patient was alive at age 6 years (see Fig. 25–5), and survivals have been reported to age 32 years and 45 years[27,30,46] with an exceptional survival to age 57 years.[45]

The same longevity patterns occur with tricuspid atresia, complete transposition of the great arteries, and a nonrestrictive ventricular septal defect (see Fig. 25–3C). Regulation of pulmonary blood flow depends on pulmonary vascular resistance (see Fig. 25–8). Exceptional survivals have been reported to the mid and late teens.[17,66] Satisfactory regulation of pulmonary blood flow is more likely to be achieved by pulmonary stenosis (see Fig. 25–3B).[17] Isolated patients have lived into the second, third, and fourth decades[21,34,46] with one patient dying at age 56 years.[80]

Survival in *congenital tricuspid stenosis* depends on the degree of obstruction and on the presence of an adequate interatrial communication.[35,69] A 20-year-old woman was acyanotic (see Fig. 25–11),[69] a woman with cyanosis underwent surgical repair at age 50 years (see Fig. 25–4), and a man with cyanosis survived to age 57 years.[35]

Hypoxic spells are precipitated by a reduction in size or spontaneous closure of a restrictive ventricular septal defect[52] and are characterized by sudden deepening of cyanosis followed by paroxysmal dyspnea, lethargy, and syncope.[17,64] Older children may squat for relief of dyspnea.[10,34] Syncope has been attributed to intermittent occlusion of the interatrial communication by a large spinnaker-like valve of the sinus venosus.[33]

Physical Appearance

Physical appearance in tricuspid atresia reflects the cyanosis of venoarterial mixing and decreased pulmonary blood flow, and the catabolic effects of congestive heart failure and excessive pulmonary blood flow. A left precordial bulge seldom occurs because the right ventricle is underdeveloped. The *cat-eye syndrome* is a distinctive although uncommon physical appearance characterized by fissures of the iris (congenital coloboma) that result in an oblong pupillary shape.[23]

The Arterial Pulse

The arterial pulse is normal (see Fig. 25–9B) unless pulmonary blood flow is excessive and the left ventricle has

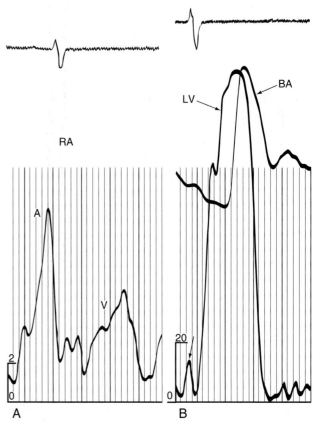

Figure 25–9
Tracings from the 18-year-old man with tricuspid atresia, complete transposition of the great arteries, and pulmonary vascular disease whose x-rays are shown in Figure 25–8. A, Right atrial pressure pulse (RA) showing a prominent A wave. B, Presystolic distention of the *left* ventricle (*unmarked lower left arrow*) reflected the prominent right atrial A wave that was transmitted into the left ventricle (LV) through a nonrestrictive atrial septal defect. BA, brachial artery pulse.

failed. Arterial pulses are feeble if not undetectable when the aorta is hypoperfused because of tricuspid atresia with transposition of the great arteries and a restrictive ventricular septal defect.[20]

The Jugular Venous Pulse

The *A wave* is increased when a restrictive interatrial communication obstructs egress from the right atrium (Fig. 25–10), and large A waves are features of congenital tricuspid stenosis (Fig. 25–11). The Y descent is slow when a restrictive interatrial communication impedes right atrial flow during the passive filling phase. The A wave increases when a thick-walled left ventricle resists right atrial contraction (see Fig. 25–9A). A and V waves are both increased when left ventricular failure causes a rise in mean pressure in the left atrium that is in continuity with the right atrium. Large V waves of mitral regurgitation are transmitted from the left atrium into the right atrium when the interatrial communication is nonrestrictive.[10]

Precordial Movement and Palpation

A key to the clinical recognition of tricuspid atresia is the combination of a *left* ventricular impulse in a *cyanotic* patient in whom a *right* ventricular impulse is conspicuously absent. The left ventricle remains palpable even when pulmonary blood flow is reduced because it handles the entire output of the systemic and pulmonary circulations. When pulmonary blood flow is increased, the

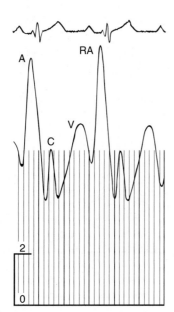

Figure 25–10
Right atrial pressure pulse (RA) from a 9-month-old girl with tricuspid atresia, normally related great arteries, a restrictive ventricular septal defect, and a patent foramen ovale. The A wave is prominent. The C and V waves are normal.

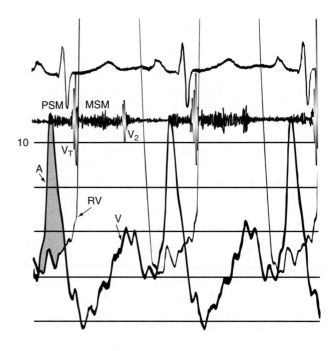

Figure 25–11
Right ventricular (RV) and right atrial pressure pulses with phonocardiogram at the lower left sternal border of a 20-year-old woman with congenital tricuspid stenosis and pulmonary valve stenosis. The large right atrial A wave exceeded right ventricular end-diastolic pressure (*shaded area*) and generated a presystolic murmur (PSM). A midsystolic murmur (MSM) was generated across the stenotic pulmonary valve. The height of the V wave was normal. A₂, aortic component of the second heart sound.

impulse of the volume overload left ventricle is increased.[39] A gentle right ventricular impulse is reserved for the patient with a nonrestrictive ventricular septal defect and a relatively well- developed right ventricle.

Auscultation

Auscultatory signs are determined by the anatomic variations beyond the mitral valve. The single first heart sound is necessarily the mitral component because the tricuspid valve is atretic.[48] When the *great arteries are not transposed*, a holosystolic systolic murmur is generated across the restrictive ventricular septal defect (Figs. 25–12, 25–13, and 25–14). The murmur is maximum at the mid to lower left sternal edge but radiates to the second left intercostal space when the left ventricle ejects through the ventricular septal defect into the pulmonary trunk (see Fig. 25–13). When the ventricular septal defect decreases in size or closes spontaneously, the holosystolic murmur becomes early systolic before vanishing altogether.[50,52,70] The second heart sound is represented by the aortic component, although a soft delayed pulmonary component is occasionally detected because the restrictive ventricular septal defect is functionally subpulmonary stenosis (see

3 LICS

4 LICS

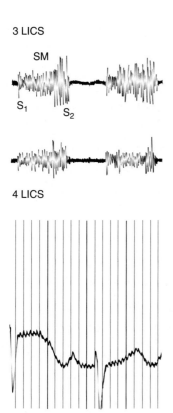

Figure 25–12
Phonocardiogram from a 20-month-old boy with tricuspid atresia and normally related great arteries. A holosystolic murmur (SM) in the third and fourth left intercostal spaces (3 LICS/4 LICS) originated at a slitlike ventricular septal defect that constituted a zone of subpulmonary stenosis. S_1, single first heart sound; S_2, second heart sound.

2 LICS

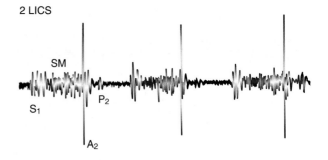

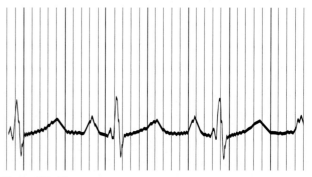

Figure 25–13
Phonocardiogram from a 9-month-old girl with tricuspid atresia, normally related great arteries, and a restrictive ventricular septal defect. A holosystolic murmur (SM) radiated to the second left interspace (2 LICS) because the left ventricle ejected across the ventricular septal defect into the pulmonary trunk. The pulmonary closure sound (P_2) is soft and delayed. The first heart sound (S_1) is single. A_2, aortic component of the second heart sound.

Fig. 25–13). When the ventricular septum is intact from birth (functional congenital pulmonary atresia, see Fig. 25–2A), there is either no murmur at all or a short midsystolic murmur into a dilated aortic root. *Continuous murmurs* through aortopulmonary collaterals are exceptional (Fig. 25–15).[60]

When tricuspid atresia occurs with *transposition of the great arteries* (see Fig. 25–3C), a holosystolic murmur is generated across the ventricular septal defect, which is usually nonrestrictive (Fig. 25–16). The single second heart sound is the aortic component and is loud because the transposed aorta is anterior (see Fig. 25–16). A third heart sound introduces a middiastolic murmur generated by increased flow across the mitral valve (see Fig. 25–16). When elevated pulmonary vascular resistance reduces pulmonary blood flow, left ventricular stroke volume falls, the ventricular septal defect murmur softens or disappears (Fig. 25–17), and a soft midsystolic murmur is generated into the anterior aortic root. The second heart sound is audibly split because the hypertensive dilated posterior pulmonary trunk generates a loud pulmonary component (see Fig. 25–17). *Pulmonary or subpulmonary stenosis generates*

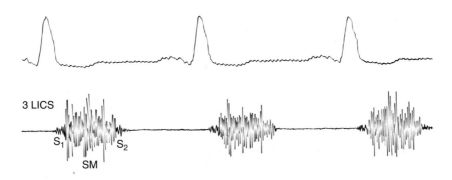

3 LICS

Figure 25–14
Phonocardiogram from the third left intercostal space (3 LICS) of a 28-year-old man with tricuspid atresia, normally related great arteries, a restrictive ventricular septal defect, and stenosis of the pulmonary valve and infundibulum. The variation in configuration of the systolic murmur (SM) was caused by the combined effects of a holosystolic ventricular septal defect murmur and a midsystolic pulmonary stenotic murmur. S_1, first heart sound; S_2, second heart sound.

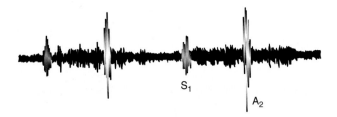

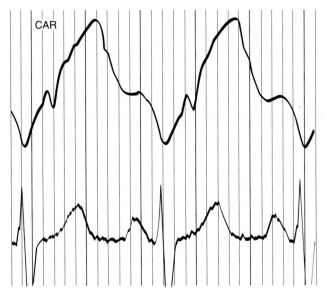

Figure 25–15

Phonocardiogram from the right anterior chest of a 7-year-old boy with tricuspid atresia, pulmonary atresia, normally related great arteries, and a continuous murmur due to systemic to pulmonary arterial collaterals. S_1, first heart sound; A_2, aortic component of the second heart sound; CAR, carotid pulse.

a midsystolic murmur, the loudness and length of which vary inversely with the degree of obstruction because the more severe the stenosis, the more left ventricular blood is diverted into the aorta via the ventricular septal defect (see Fig. 25–3B). Flow across the stenotic sites falls reciprocally, so the pulmonary stenotic murmur softens and shortens (Fig. 25–18). The posterior position of the pulmonary trunk softens the murmur still further.

Left ventricular fourth heart sounds occur when the interatrial communication is nonrestrictive and the increased force of right atrial contraction is transmitted into the left ventricle. Presystolic murmurs are expected in congenital tricuspid stenosis[69] (Fig. 25–19) and are possible in tricus-

pid atresia when powerful right atrial contraction is exerted against a restrictive interatrial communication.

The Electrocardiogram

Tall peaked right atrial P waves are typical (Figs. 25–20 and 25–21),[13,17,27,68] and the P terminal force may be negative in lead V_1 (see Fig. 25–21). The left atrium is seldom represented in the P wave despite the fact that it receives the entire return from the systemic and pulmonary veins.[13,27] There is no necessary relationship between P wave morphology and the size of the interatrial communication.[13,17]

The diagnosis of tricuspid atresia without transposition of the great arteries and with a restrictive ventricular septal defect can be entertained when *left axis deviation and left ventricular hypertrophy occur in the presence of cyanosis* (see Figs. 25–20 and 25–21).[13,17,25,27,28,68] Left axis deviation was commented on in 1929,[58] and its diagnostic value was emphasized in 1936 by Helen Taussig.[72] The cause of left axis deviation has not been firmly established,[8,13,28,49,65] but left anterior fascicular block is not the mechanism.[8,65] The central fibrous body in tricuspid atresia is abnormally formed whether or not the great arteries are transposed.[8] A fibrous strand has been traced through the central fibrous body to the cavity of the rudimentary right ventricle,[77] and the atrioventricular node pierces the central fibrous body to form the His bundle.[8] The left bundle branches originate close to the AV node/His bundle junction and undergo early arborization, whereas the right bundle branch is elongated.[27,28] It is doubtful that early arborization of the left bundle accounts for left axis deviation.[27,28] The QRS axis appears to depend in large part on the relative mass of the right and left ventricles[13,27,28] because arborization patterns of the bundle branches are the same in all varieties of tricuspid atresia.[27,28] Left axis deviation occurs with adult progression of the precordial QRS pattern (see Figs. 25–20 and 25–21).[27,28,68] Left ventricular hypertrophy is represented by deep S waves in right precordial leads and tall R waves with repolarization abnormalities in leads aVL and V_{5-6} (see Figs. 25–20 and 25–21).

Tricuspid atresia with complete transposition of the great arteries typically occurs with a nonrestrictive ventric-

Near apex

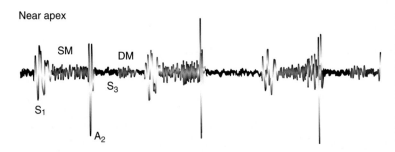

Figure 25–16

Phonocardiogram from a 13-month-old boy with tricuspid atresia, transposition of the great arteries, a nonrestrictive ventricular septal defect, and low pulmonary vascular resistance. The holosystolic murmur (SM) originated at the ventricular septal defect. The mid-diastolic murmur (DM) and the third heart sound (S_3) were caused by increased flow across the mitral valve. The aortic component of the second heart sound (A_2) was prominent because the transposed aorta was anterior. S_1, single first heart sound.

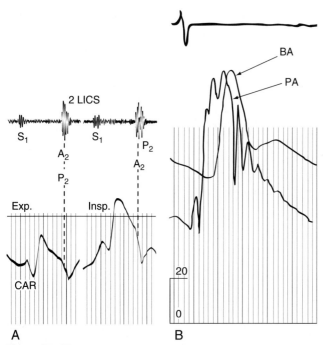

Figure 25–17

Tracings from the 18-year-old man with tricuspid atresia, complete transposition of the great arteries, and pulmonary vascular disease whose x-rays are shown in Figure 25–8. *A*, Phonocardiogram from the second left intercostal space (2 LICS) recorded a single first heart sound (S_1) and no murmur. There was close inspiratory splitting of the second heart sound (A_2/P_2) because pulmonary vascular resistance was lower than systemic vascular resistance (see diastolic pressures in panel *B*). The pulmonary component of the second sound was prominent because the posterior pulmonary trunk was dilated and hypertensive. CAR, carotid. *B*, Brachial arterial (BA) and pulmonary arterial (PA) pressures were equal during systole but diverged during diastole.

ular septal defect and a well-developed right ventricle. Increased pulmonary blood flow adds materially to left atrial volume, so left atrial enlargement and right atrial enlargement coexist and P waves are broad and bifid as well as peaked (Fig. 25–22).[13,17,25,27] The well-developed right ventricle contributes to the normal QRS axis, and may influence the QRS pattern in the precordial leads (see Fig. 23–22).[1,17,27,28,40,68]

The X-Ray

The cardiac silhouette may be distinctive in tricuspid atresia without transposition of the great arteries with a restrictive ventricular septal defect (Figs. 25–23 and 25–24).[10,36,37] The right cardiac contour exhibits a prominent superior border caused by enlargement of the right atrium and its appendage and a flat receding inferior border caused by absence of the right ventricle (Figs. 25–23B, 25–24, and 25–25B). A convex left ventricle occupies the apex (see Figs. 25–23A and 25–25A), but left atrial enlargement is seldom evident. Pulmonary vascularity is reduced, the main pulmonary artery segment is

inconspicuous, and the ascending aorta is relatively prominent (see Figs. 25–23 and 25–25). When a congenitally intact ventricular septum causes functional pulmonary atresia (see Fig. 25–2A), the ascending aorta is more conspicuous, and the lung fields exhibit the lacy vascular pattern of systemic arterial collateral vessels (Fig. 25–26).[10,36] When the ventricular septal defect is nonrestrictive and pulmonary vascular resistance is low (see Fig. 25–2C), there is increased pulmonary vascularity, an enlarged pulmonary trunk, enlargement of the left and right atria, and a prominent apex-forming left ventricle (see Figs. 25–5A and 25–7).

The x-ray in tricuspid atresia with *complete transposition of the great arteries*, a nonrestrictive ventricular septal defect, and low pulmonary vascular resistance (see Fig. 25–3C) is characterized by increased pulmonary vascularity, enlargement of the left and right atria, and a prominent apex-forming left ventricle. The vascular pedicle is narrow because the great arteries are transposed. The x-ray resembles complete transposition of the great arteries with similar pulmonary vascular resistance (see Chapter 27).[40] The left cardiac border is straight if left-sided juxtaposition of the atrial appendages coexists. When pulmonary vascular resistance is increased, the lungs are oligemic and the heart size is normal or nearly so, but the right cardiac border may retain its hump-shaped contour even though the right ventricle is not rudimentary (see Fig. 25–8).[17]

3 LICS

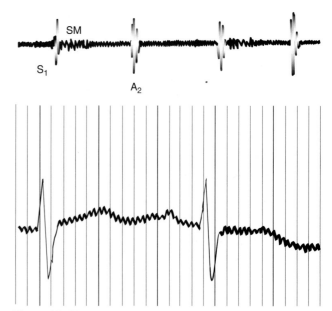

Figure 25–18

Phonocardiogram from the third left intercostal space (3 LICS) of an 18-month-old boy with tricuspid atresia, transposition of the great arteries and severe pulmonary stenosis. The pulmonary stenotic murmur (SM) was trivial because left ventricular blood was diverted away from the pulmonary trunk and across a nonrestrictive ventricular septal defect into the transposed aorta (see Fig. 25–3B). The aortic component of the second heart sound was prominent (A_2) because the transposed aorta was anterior.

3 LICS

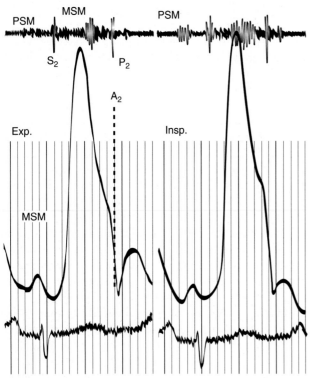

Figure 25–19

Phonocardiogram from the third left intercostal space (3 LICS) of the 20-year-old woman with tricuspid stenosis and pulmonary stenosis whose right atrial and right ventricular pressure pulses are shown in Figure 25–11. The presystolic murmur of tricuspid stenosis (PSM) increased during inspiration (INSP). The midsystolic murmur (MSM) was across the stenotic pulmonary valve. CAR, carotid pulse; Exp., expiration.

The x-ray in tricuspid atresia with transposition of the great arteries and pulmonary stenosis (see Figs. 25–3B and 25–27) shows normal or reduced pulmonary vascularity, a prominent right atrium, and a convex left ventricle, but a narrow vascular pedicle because the great arteries are transposed.

The Echocardiogram

Echocardiography with color flow imaging and Doppler interrogation establishes the diagnosis of tricuspid atresia and establishes the positions of the great arteries, the condition of the ventricular septum, and the nature of the interatrial communication (Figs. 25–28 and 25–29).[21] An echodense band produced by fibrofatty tissue in the right atrioventricular groove represents absence of the right AV connection that characterizes tricuspid atresia (see Figs. 25–28 and 25–29). When the great arteries are not transposed, the right ventricular cavity is small, the ventricular septal defect is restrictive, and the left ventricle is moderately enlarged (see Fig. 25–28). When the interatrial communication is restrictive, the right atrium is enlarged and the atrial septum is concave to the left. When

the great arteries are transposed and pulmonary resistance is low, echocardiography identifies a nonrestrictive ventricular septal defect, a well-formed right ventricle, enlarged right and left atria and a dilated volume-overloaded left ventricle (see Fig. 25–29). The echocardiogram characterizes the structural abnormalities of the mitral valve.[43] Color flow mapping with Doppler interrogation establishes the size of the interatrial communication and the condition of the ventricular septum. When the great arteries are transposed, continuous-wave Doppler interrogates the left ventricular outflow tract for the presence and degree of pulmonary stenosis.

Summary

Tricuspid atresia without transposition of the great arteries and with a restrictive ventricular septal defect presents with cyanosis from birth and a clinical picture dominated by hypoxemia. A right ventricular impulse is conspicuously absent. A left parasternal holosystolic systolic murmur is generated through the restrictive ventricular septal defect that is functionally subpulmonary stenosis. The electrocardiogram exhibits tall, peaked, right atrial P waves, left axis deviation, counterclockwise depolarization, and adult progression of the precordial QRS pattern. The x-ray discloses a distinctive hump-shaped appearance of the right cardiac border. Echocardiography with color

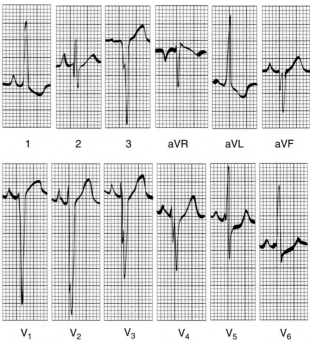

Figure 25–20

Electrocardiogram from a 9-month-old girl with tricuspid atresia, normally related great arteries, and a slit-like ventricular septal defect. Tall peaked right atrial P waves appear in lead 2 and in right precordial leads. There is left axis deviation with adult progression of the precordial QRS. Left ventricular hypertrophy is manifested by the tall R wave and inverted T wave in lead aVL and the deep S waves in right precordial leads.

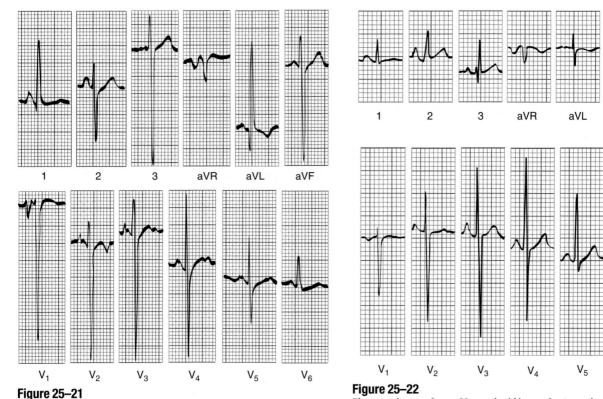

Figure 25–21

Electrocardiogram from a 7-year-old boy with tricuspid atresia, normally related great arteries, and pulmonary atresia due to spontaneous closure of a restrictive ventricular septal defect. Biatrial abnormalities are manifested by tall right atrial P waves in leads 1 and 2 and bifid left atrial P waves in mid and left precordial leads. There is left axis deviation with adult progression of the precordial QRS. Left ventricular hypertrophy is manifested by the tall R wave and inverted T wave in lead aVL and the deep S waves in right precordial leads.

Figure 25–22

Electrocardiogram from a 32-month-old boy with tricuspid atresia, transposition of the great arteries, a nonrestrictive ventricular septal defect, and low pulmonary vascular resistance. Biatrial P wave abnormalities are manifested by tall peaked right atrial P waves in leads 2, aVF, and V_3 and a bifid left atrial P wave in lead aVL. The QRS axis is normal. Precordial leads show adult progression with large biphasic RS complexes of biventricular hypertrophy in leads V_{3-4}.

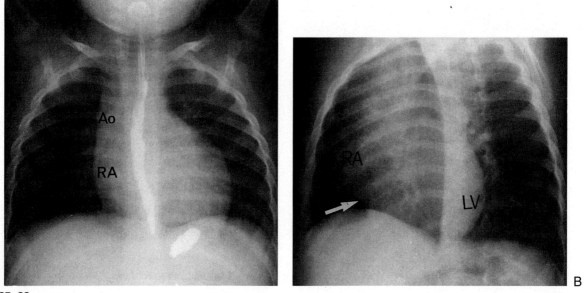

Figure 25–23

A, X-ray from a 10-month-old boy with tricuspid atresia, normally related great arteries and a restrictive ventricular septal defect (see Fig. 25–2*B*). Pulmonary vascularity is reduced, the ascending aorta (Ao) is prominent, the main pulmonary artery segment is inconspicuous, the dilated right atrium (RA) recedes acutely because of absence of the right ventricle, and a large left ventricle occupies the apex. *B*, Shallow left anterior oblique projection highlights the hump-shaped appearance caused by right atrial enlargement (RA) in the absence of a right ventricle (*arrow*). LV, left ventricle.

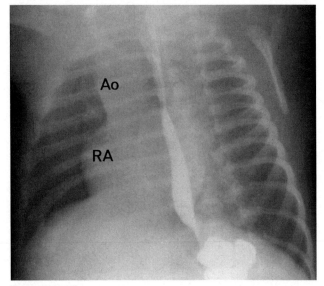

Figure 25–24

Left anterior oblique x-ray from a 4-month-old boy with tricuspid atresia, normally related great arteries, and a restrictive ventricular septal defect. The right atrium (RA) creates a distinctive *hump-shaped* appearance highlighted by the prominent ascending aorta (Ao). (Also see Fig. 25–23.)

flow imaging and Doppler interrogation identifies an echo-dense band in the location of the atretic tricuspid valve, a restrictive ventricular septal defect, a small right ventricle, normally related great arteries, and an interatrial communication that is usually restrictive.

Tricuspid atresia with complete transposition of the great arteries, a nonrestrictive ventricular septal defect, and low pulmonary vascular resistance presents with mild cyanosis and a clinical picture dominated by congestive heart failure and its catabolic effects. A left ventricular impulse is prominent, and a right ventricular impulse is present but less conspicuous. A systolic murmur is generated through the ventricular septal defect, and an apical mid-diastolic murmur is generated by increased flow across the mitral valve. The electrocardiogram shows biatrial P wave abnormalities and a normal or vertical axis with adult progression of the precordial QRS. The x-ray is characterized by increased pulmonary blood flow, a narrow vascular pedicle, enlargement of the right and left atria, and enlargement of the left ventricle. Echocardiography with color flow imaging and Doppler interrogation identifies the atretic tricuspid valve, a nonrestrictive ventricular septal defect, a well-formed right ventricle, and enlargement of the left atrium, right atrium, and left ventricle. When pulmonary stenosis coexists, cyanosis ranges from mild to severe, the left ventricle is palpable but not dynamic, and the length and loudness of the pulmonary stenotic murmur vary inversely with severity. The electrocardiogram shows right atrial P waves, a normal or vertical QRS axis, and adult progression of the precordial QRS pattern. The x-ray shows the narrow vascular pedicle, normal or decreased pulmonary vascularity, a prominent right atrium, and a convex left ventricle. The echocardiogram identifies the atretic tri-

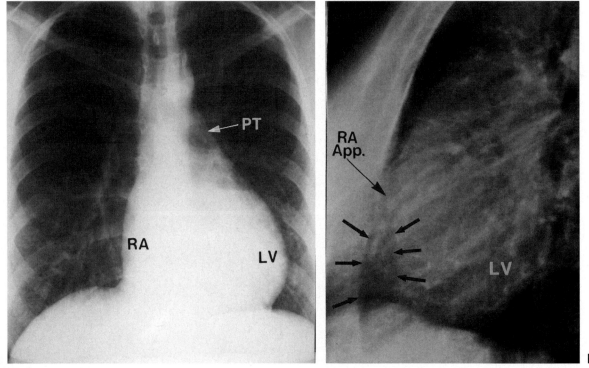

Figure 25–25

A, X-ray from a 25-year-old woman with tricuspid atresia, normally related great arteries, and a moderately restrictive ventricular septal defect. Congestive heart failure in infancy improved as the ventricular septal defect decreased in size. Pulmonary vascularity and the pulmonary trunk (PT) are normal, the right atrium (RA) is moderately dilated, and an enlarged convex left ventricle (LV) occupies the apex. *B,* Lateral projection shows the right atrial appendage (RA App) against the sternum and a receding inferior border because the right ventricle is absent (*unmarked arrows*). Left ventricular enlargement is confirmed.

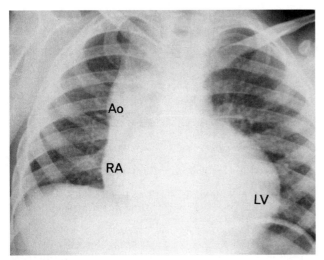

Figure 25–26

A, X-ray from a 7-year-old boy with tricuspid atresia, normally related great arteries, and pulmonary atresia due to a congenitally intact ventricular septum. The lung fields exhibit the lacy appearance of collateral arterial circulation. The main pulmonary artery segment is concave, the ascending aorta is conspicuously dilated (Ao), an enlarged convex left ventricle (LV) extends below the left hemidiaphragm, and a dilated right atrium (RA) occupies the lower right cardiac border.

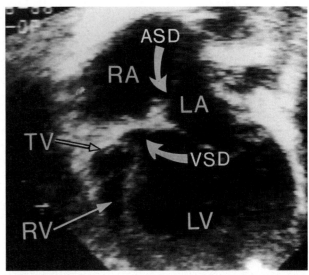

Figure 25–28

Echocardiogram (four-chamber view) from a 4-year-old boy with tricuspid atresia, normally related great arteries, and a restrictive ventricular septal defect. The atretic tricuspid valve (TV) is represented by a dense band of bright echoes. The right ventricle (RV) is small, and the left ventricle (LV) is dilated. There was a left-to-right shunt (*lower curved arrow*) across the ventricular septal defect (VSD) and a right-to-left shunt (*upper arrow*) across an ostium secundum atrial septal defect (ASD). RA, right atrium; LA, left atrium.

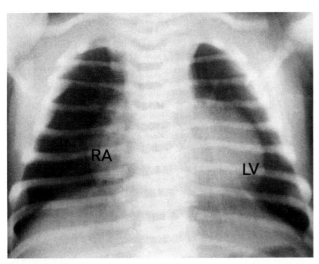

Figure 25–27

X-ray from a 10-month-old girl with tricuspid atresia, transposition of the great arteries, and severe pulmonary stenosis. Pulmonary vascularity is decreased, the main pulmonary artery segment is not seen, a prominent right atrium (RA) occupies the lower right cardiac border, and an enlarged convex left ventricle (LV) occupies the apex.

cuspid valve, transposed great arteries and a nonrestrictive ventricular septal defect. Continuous-wave Doppler establishes the presence and degree of pulmonary stenosis.

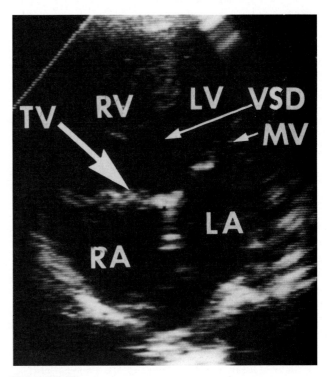

Figure 25–29

Echocardiogram (four chamber view) from an 18-month-old boy with tricuspid atresia, transposition of the great arteries, a nonrestrictive ventricular septal defect (VSD), and low pulmonary vascular resistance. The atretic tricuspid valve (TV) is represented by a dense band of echoes (*large arrow*). The right ventricular cavity (RV) is well-developed, the right atrium (RA) is enlarged, and a normal mitral valve (MV) lies between the left ventricle (LV) and the left atrium (LA).

REFERENCES

1. Abrams, R., Saldana, M., Kastor, J.A., Shelburne, J.C.: Tricuspid and pulmonary valve atresia with aortopulmonary fistula: Survival of a patient to 21 years of age. Chest 68:263, 1975.
2. Anderson, R.H., Rigby, M.L.: The morphologic heterogeneity of "tricuspid atresia." Int. J. Cardiol. 16:67, 1987.
3. Rydberg, A., BarAm, S., Teien, D.E., et al: The abnormal contralateral atrioventricular valve in mitral and tricuspid atresia in neonates: An echocardiographic study. Pediatr. Cardiol. 20:200, 1999.

4. Svensson, E.C., Huggins, G.S., Lin, H., et al: A syndrome of tricuspid atresia in mice with a targeted mutation of the gene encoding Fog-2. Nat. Genet. 25:353, 2000.
5. Baron, M.G.: Hypoplasia of the inflow portion of the right ventricle: An angiocardiographic sign of tricuspid atresia. Circulation 44:746, 1971.
6. Beaver, T.R., Shroyer, K.R., Muro-Cacho, C.A., et al: Survival to age 65 years with tricuspid atresia and pulmonic valve atresia. Am. J. Cardiol. 62:165, 1988.
7. Becker, A.E., Becker, M.J.: Juxtaposition of atrial appendages associated with normally oriented ventricles and great arteries. Circulation 41:685, 1970.
8. Bharati, S., Lev, M.: The conduction system in tricuspid atresia with and without regular (d-) transposition. Circulation .:423, 1977.
9. Breisch, E.A., Wilson, D.B., Laurenson, R.D., et al: Tricuspid atresia (type 1a): Survival to 21 years of age. Am. Heart. J. 106:149, 1983.
10. Brown, J.W., Heath, D., Morris, T.L., Whitaker, W.: Tricuspid atresia. Br. Heart J. 18:499, 1956.
11. Charuzi, Y., Spanos, P.K., Amplatz, K., Edwards, J.E.: Juxtaposition of the atrial appendages. Circulation 47:620, 1973.
12. Cooley, R.N., Sloan, R.D., Hanlon, C.R., Bahnson, H.T.: Angiocardiography in congenital heart disease of cyanotic type. II. Observation on tricuspid stenosis or atresia with hypoplasia of the right ventricle. Radiology 54:848, 1950.
13. Davachi, F., Lucas, R.V., Moller, J.H.: The electrocardiogram and vectorcardiogram in tricuspid atresia. Correlation with pathologic anatomy. Am. J. Cardiol. 25:18, 1970.
14. Deanfield J.E., Tommasini G., Anderson R.H., Macartney F.J.: Tricuspid atresia: Analysis of coronary artery distributions and ventricular morphology. Br. Heart J. 48:485, 1982.
15. Deutsch, V., Shem-Tov, A., Yahini, J.H., Neufeld, H.N.: Juxtaposition of atrial appendages: Angiographic observations. Am. J. Cardiol. 34:240, 1974.
16. Dick, M., Behrendt, D.M., Byrum, C.J., et al: Tricuspid atresia and the Wolff-Parkinson-White syndrome. Am. Heart J. 101:496, 1981.
17. Dick, M., Fyler, D.C., Nadas, A.S.: Tricuspid atresia: Clinical course in 101 patients. Am. J. Cardiol. 36:327, 1975.
18. Dimich, I., Goldfinger, P, Steinfeld, L., Lukban, S.B.: Congenital tricuspid stenosis. Am. J. Cardiol. 31:89, 1973.
19. Edwards, J.E., Burchell, H.B.: Congenital tricuspid atresia; classification. Med. Clin. North Am. 33:1177, 1949.
20. Folger, G. M.: Systemic hypoperfusion in a neonate with tricuspid atresia and transposition of the great arteries. Angiology 31:721, 1980.
21. Orie, J.D., Anderson C., Ettedgui, J.A, Zuberbuhler, J.R., Anderson, R.H.: Echocardiographic-morphologic correlations in tricuspid atresia. J. Am. Coll. Cardiol. 26:750, 1995.
22. Bonnet D., Fermont L., Kachaner J., Sidi D., Amiel J., Lyonnet S.: Tricuspid atresia and conotruncal malformations in five families. J. Med. Genet. 36:349, 1999.
23. Freedom, R. M., and Gerald, P. S.: Congenital cardiovascular disease and the "cat-eye" syndrome. Am. J. Dis. Child. 126:16, 1973.
24. Freedom, R. M., and Rowe, R. D.: Aneurysm of the atrial septum in tricuspid atresia. Am. J. Cardiol. 38:265, 1976.
25. Gambea, R., Gersony, W. M., and Nadas, A. S.: The electrocardiogram in tricuspid atresia and pulmonary atresia with intact ventricular septum. Circulation 34:24, 1966.
26. Gasul, B. M., Fell, E. H., Marvelis, W., and Casas, R.: Diagnosis of tricuspid atresia or stenosis in infants. Pediatrics 6:862, 1950.
27. Guller, B., Titus, J. L., and Du Shane, J. W.: Electrocardiographic diagnosis of malformations associated with tricuspid atresia: Correlation with morphologic features. Am. Heart J. 78:180, 1969.
28. Guller, B., Du Shane, J. W., and Titus, J. L.: The atrioventricular conduction system in two cases of tricuspid atresia. Circulation 40:217, 1969.
29. Gyepes, M. T., Marcano, B. A., and Desilets, D. T.: Tricuspid atresia, transposition, and coarctation of aorta. Radiology 97:633, 1970.
30. Hart, A. S., and Vacek, J. L.: Prolonged survival in tricuspid atresia with Eisenmenger's physiology. Clin. Cardiol. 7:555, 1984.
31. Lin, A. E., Rosti, L.: Tricuspid atresia in sibs. J. Med. Genet. 35:1055, 1998.
32. Holmes, W. F.: Case of malformation of the heart. Trans. Med. Chir. Soc. Edinburgh 1:252, 1824.
33. Jones, R. N., and Niles, N. R.: Spinnaker formation of sinus venosus valve. Case report of a fatal anomaly in a ten-year-old boy. Circulation 38:468, 1968.
34. Jordon, J. C., and Sanders, C. A.: Tricuspid atresia with prolonged survival. A report of two cases with a review of the world literature. Am. J. Cardiol. 18:112, 1966.
35. Karalis, D. G., Chandrasekaran, K., Victor, M. F., and Mintz, G. S.: Prolonged survival despite severe cyanosis in an adult with right ventricular hypoplasia and atrial septal defect. Am. Heart J. 120:701, 1990.
36. Kieffer, S. A., and Carey, L. S.: Tricuspid atresia with normal aortic root. Roentgen-anatomic correlation. Radiology 80:605, 1963.
37. Kroop, I. G.: Congenital tricuspid atresia. Am. Heart J. 41:549, 1951.
38. Kuhne, M.: Uber zwei falle kongenitaler atresia des ostium venosum dextrum. Jahresb. Kinderheilk. 63:225, 1906.
39. La Corte, M. A., Dick, M., Scheer, G., La Farge, C. G., and Fyler, D. C.: Left ventricular function in tricuspid atresia. Circulation 52:996, 1975.
40. Marcano, B. A., Reimenschneider, T. A., Ruttenberg, H. D., Goldberg, S. J., and Gyepes, M.: Tricuspid atresia with increased pulmonary blood flow. Circulation 40:399, 1969.
41. McDermid, H. E., Duncan, A. M. V., Brasch, K. R., Holden, J. J. A., Magenis, E., Sheehy, R., Burn, J., Kardon, N., Noel, B., Schinzel, A., Teshima, I., and White, B. N.: Characterization of the supernumerary chromosomes in cateye syndrome. Science 232:646, 1986.
42. Nishioka, K., Kamiya, T., Ueda, T., Hayashidera, T., Mori, C., Konishi, Y., Tatsuta, N., and Jarmakani, J. M.: Left ventricular volume characteristics in children with tricuspid atresia before and after surgery. Am. J. Cardiol. 47:1105, 1981.
43. Ottenkamp, J., and Wenink, A. C. G.: Anomalies of the mitral valve and of the left ventricular architecture in tricuspid valve atresia. Am. J. Cardiol. 48:880, 1981.
44. Patel, R., Fox, K., Taylor, J. F. H., and Graham, G. R.: Tricuspid atresia: Clinical course in 62 patients. Br. Heart J. 40:1408, 1978.
45. Patel, M. M., Overy, D. C., Kozonis, M. C., and Hadley-Fowlkes, L. L.: Long-term survival in tricuspid atresia. J. Am. Coll. Cardiol. 9:338, 1987.
46. Patterson, W., Baxley, W. A., Karp, R. B., Soto, B., and Bargerson, L. L.: Tricuspid atresia in adults. Am. J. Cardiol. 49:141, 1982.
47. Perloff, J. K.: Auscultatory and phonocardiographic manifestations of pulmonary hypertension. Prog. Cardiovasc. Dis. 9:303, 1967.
48. Perloff, J. K.: Physical Examination of the Heart and Circulation, 3rd ed., Philadelphia, W. B. Saunders Company, 2000.
49. Perloff, J. K., Roberts, N. K., and Cabeen, W. R.: Left axis deviation. Circulation 60:12, 1979.
50. Rao, P. S.: Natural history of the ventricular septal defect in tricuspid atresia and its surgical implications. Br. Heart J. 39:276, 1977.
51. Rao, P. S.: A unified classification for tricuspid atresia. Am. Heart J. 99:799, 1980.
52. Rao, P. S.: Further observations on the spontaneous closure of physiologically advantageous ventricular septal defects in tricuspid atresia. Ann. Thorac. Surg. 35:121, 1983.
53. Rao, P. S.: Left to right atrial shunting in tricuspid atresia. Br. Heart J. 49:345, 1983.
54. Rao, P. S., and Sissman, N. J.: Spontaneous closure of physiologically advantageous ventricular septal defects. Circulation 43:83, 1971.
55. Rashkind, W. J.: Tricuspid atresia: A historical review. Pediatr. Cardiol. 2:85, 1982.
56. Reder, R. F., Yeh, H., and Steinfeld, L.: Aneurysm of the interatrial septum causing pulmonary venous obstruction in an infant with tricuspid atresia. Am. Heart J. 102:786, 1981.
57. Report of the New England Regional Infant Cardiac Program. Pediatrics 65 (Suppl. 2):392, 1980.
58. Rihl, J., Terplan, K., and Weiss, F.: Uber einen fall von agenesie der tricuspidalklappe. Med. Klin. 25:1543, 1929.
59. Riker, W. L., Potts, W. J., Grana, L., Miller, R. A., and Lev, M.: Tricuspid stenosis or atresia complexes. A surgical and pathologic analysis. J. Thorac. Cardiovasc. Surg. 45:423, 1963.
60. Roberts, W. C., Morrow, A. G., Mason, D. T., and Braunwald, E.: Spontaneous closure of ventricular septal defect. Anatomic proof in an adult with tricuspid atresia. Circulation 27:90, 1963.
61. Rosenquist, G. C., Levy, R. J., and Rowe, R. D.: Right atrial-left ventricular relationships in tricuspid atresia: Position of the presumed site of atretic valve as determined by transillumination. Am. Heart J. 80:493, 1970.
62. Kumar, A., Victoria, B. E., Gessner, I. H., Alexander, J. A.: Tricuspid atresia and annular hypoplasia: report of a familial occurrence. Pediatr. Cardiol. 15:201, 1994.

63. Rudolph, A. M., Heymann, M. A., and Spitznas, V.: Hemodynamic considerations in the development of narrowing of the aorta. Am. J. Cardiol. 30:514, 1972.

64. Sade, R. M., and Fyfe, D. A.: Tricuspid atresia: Current concepts in diagnosis and treatment. Pediatr. Clin. North Am. 37:151, 1990.

65. Schatz, J., Kongrad, E., and Malm, J. R.: Left anterior and left posterior hemiblock in tricuspid atresia and transposition of the great vessels: Observations on electrocardiographic nomenclature and electrophysiologic mechanisms. Circulation 54:1010, 1976.

66. Shariatzadeh, A. N., King, H., Girod, D., and Shumacker, H. B.: Tricuspid atresia: A review of 68 cases. Chest 71:538, 1977.

67. Sieveking, E. H.: Congenital malformation of the heart. Absence of the right auricular-ventricular orifice, patulous foramen ovale, defective interventricular septum. Trans. Pathol. Soc. Lond. 5:97, 1854.

68. Somlyo, A. P., and Halloran, K. H.: Tricuspid atresia. An electrocardiographic study. Am. Heart J. 63:171, 1962.

69. Steelman, R. B., Perloff, J. K., Cochran, P. T., and Ronan, J. A.: Congenital stenosis of the pulmonic and tricuspid valves. Am. J. Med. 54:788, 1973.

70. Syamasundar, R. P.: Natural history of the ventricular septal defect in tricuspid atresia and its surgical implications. Br. Heart J. 39:276, 1977.

71. Tandon, R., and Edwards, J. E.: Tricuspid atresia. A re-evaluation and classification. J. Thorac. Cardiovasc. Surg. 67:530, 1974.

72. Taussig, H. B.: Clinical and pathological findings in congenital malformations of heart due to defective development of right ventricle associated with tricuspid atresia or hypoplasia. Bull. Johns Hopkins Hosp. 59:435, 1936.

73. Van Praagh, S., Vangi, V., Sul, J. H., Metras, D., Parness, I., Casteneda, A. R., and Van Praagh, R.: Tricuspid atresia or severe stenosis with partial common atrioventricular canal: Anatomic data, clinical profile and surgical considerations. J. Am. Coll. Cardiol. 17:932, 1991.

74. Voci, G., Diego, J. N., Shafia, H., Alavi, M., Ghusson, M., and Banka, V. S.: Type Ia tricuspid atresia with extensive coronary artery anomalies in a living 22 year old woman. J. Am. Coll. Cardiol. 10:1100, 1987.

75. Warnes, C. A., and Sommerville, J.: Tricuspid atresia with transposition of the great arteries in adolescents and adults. Br. Heart J. 57:543, 1987.

76. Weigel, T. J., Driscoll, D. J., and Michels, V. V.: Occurrence of congenital heart defects in siblings of patients with univentricular heart and tricupid atresia. Am. J. Cardiol. 64:768, 1989.

77. Wenink, A. C. G., and Ottenkamp, J.: Tricuspid atresia. Microscopic findings in relation to "absence" of the atrioventricular connexion. Int. J. Cardiol. 16:57, 1987.

78. Litovsky, S., Choy, M., Park, J., Parrish, M., Waters, B., and Nagashima, M.: Absent pulmonary valve with tricuspid atresia or severe tricuspid stenosis. Pediatr. Dev. Pathol. 3:353, 2000.

79. Hatjis, C. G., Gibson, M., Capless, E. L., Auletta, F. J., and Anderson, G. G.: Pregnancy in a patient with tricuspid atresia. Am. J. Obstet. Gynecol. 145:114, 1983.

80. Fontana, R. S. and Edwards, J. E.: Congenital Cardiac Disease. Philadelphia. W. B. Saunders, 1962.

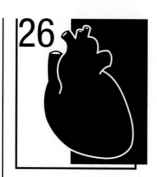

The Univentricular Heart

"The auricular sinuses are separated by a more or less complete septum, and there are generally two auriculo-ventricular apertures; while the ventricle is either wholly undivided or presents only a very rudimentary septum. Two arteries are usually given off—an aorta and pulmonary artery. A case that appears to have been of this description was described by Chemineau in 1699. The cases which have just been quoted corresponded so far as that the heart consisted of two auricles and only one ventricle."[55] Nearly a century and a half after Thomas Peacock's description, there is no consensus regarding the terminology for hearts with only *one ventricle (sic)*.[8,55,74] *Single* and *univentricular* are synonymous (*single* = *uni* = *one*), so these terms are interchangeable and are appropriate when two atria are related entirely or almost entirely to one ventricular compartment that qualifies on purely morphologic grounds as a left, right, or indeterminate ventricle.[3,8,74] Univentricular atrioventricular connection or double inlet ventricle is characterized according to gross morphologic characteristics of the ventricular mass[7,43,48,67,79] and according to the *atrioventricular connections* to that mass.[3,8,67,69,74,75] Clinically undetectable and clinically irrelevant developmental considerations are important but should not determine clinical terminology. Inherently contradictory terms should be avoided such as ventricular septal defect[13] and interventricular communication[68] that imply the presence of two morphologically distinct ventricles and an authentic septum between them. To say that a ventricular septal defect exists in a heart with a single ventricle and "not a trace of an inter-ventricular septum" (Peacock[55]) is a contradiction in terms irrespective of theoretical arguments to the contrary. In this chapter, the terms *univentricular* and *single ventricle* are applied to hearts in which one ventricular chamber receives the entire flow from the right atrium and the left atrium, both of which, with the entire atrioventricular junction, are related to the univentricular or single ventricle heart.

Single ventricle as just defined accounts for about 1% of congenital malformations of the heart at birth.[42] In 80% to 90% of cases, the ventricular chamber that receives the atrioventricular connections has *left ventricular* morphologic features and incorporates at its base an *outlet chamber* that is an infundibular remnant devoid of a sinus or inlet component and that is remote from the crux of the heart (Figs. 26–1, 26–2, 26–3, and 26–4).[39,48,67,75] In 10% to 25% of cases, the ventricular chamber that receives the atrioventricular connections has *right ventricular* morphologic features and incorporates within its mass a rudimentary compartment that represents a left ventricular remnant or *trabecular pouch* that is related to the crux and varies in size from well-formed to microscopic (see Figs. 26–31 and 26–32).[67,69,73] The trabecular pouch occupies a posterior, inferior, or lateral position within the ventricular mass and may or may not communicate with the cavity.[37,67,69,74,75] In less than 10% of cases, the single ventricle has *indeterminate* morphologic features and incorporates neither an outlet chamber nor a trabecular pouch.[48] Because the indeterminate ventricle contains remnants of neither a rudimentary morphologic right ventricle nor a rudimentary morphologic left ventricle, the term *univentricular heart* or *single ventricle* is unassailable on morphologic grounds.[44,48]

The *atrioventricular connections* that guard the inlet of a univentricular heart consist of either two separate valves, one patent valve with atresia of the other valve or a common atrioventricular valve.[8,29,37,58,68,70] It is customary to refer to *right* atrioventricular or *left* atrioventricular valves rather than *tricuspid* and *mitral* valves because tricuspid and mitral valve morphologic features cannot always be

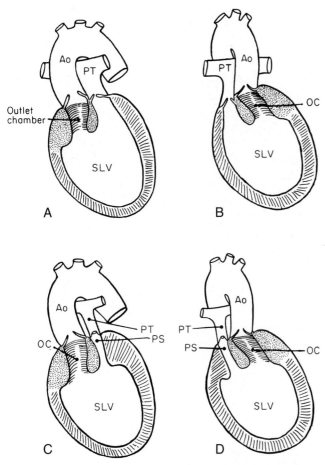

Figure 26–1

Illustrations of the most frequent types of univentricular heart represented by a single morphologic left ventricle (SLV). The anterosuperior outlet chamber (OC) is located at the base of the single ventricle and is either right-sided (noninverted) (*A* and *C*) or left-sided (inverted) (*B* and *D*). Pulmonary stenosis (PS) is absent (*A* and *B*) or present (*C* and *D*). PT, pulmonary trunk; Ao, aorta.

recognized.[13] An atrioventricular valve is likely to be abnormal when it is *concordant* with the ventricular loop (*right* AV valve with *noninverted* outlet chamber, *left* AV valve with *inverted* outlet chamber).[13,29,71] When the outlet chamber is *inverted*, the *left* AV valve tends to be stenotic, and when the outlet chamber is *noninverted*, the *right* atrioventricular valve tends to be incompetent.[13] A *common atrioventricular valve* is usually four-leaflet,[70] and isomerism is the usual pattern of the right atrial appendages.[68,70] Straddling of a right or a left AV valve or a common AV valve refers to attachments of tensor apparatus to both sides of an outlet foramen or to both sides of a trabecular pouch.[8,13,29,61,67,71,74]

In univentricular hearts that are morphologically *left ventricular*, the outlet chamber is anterosuperior and lies to the right or left of midline.[28,37,38] *Noninverted* is applied to a *right anterosuperior position* of the outlet chamber, and *inverted* is applied to a *left anterosuperior position* (see Figs. 26–1 through 26–4).[44,48,52] The outlet chamber is either smooth-walled and devoid of trabeculations[48,74,79] (see Fig. 26–4) or contains scanty trabeculations that are not clinically identified and are therefore not clinically relevant.[38,74] The aorta arises discordantly from the outlet

chamber, and the pulmonary trunk arises discordantly from the single morphologic left ventricle[44,48,75] (see Figs. 26–1 through 26–4) so *transposition of the great arteries* appropriately applies (see Chapter 27). In the uncommon Holmes heart, the aorta arises concordantly from the single morphologic left ventricle and the pulmonary trunk arises concordantly from the outlet chamber (see Fig. 26–23). Andrew Fernando Holmes was Canadian, but his 1824 publication on single ventricle was in a Scottish journal[36] because his medical training was at the University of Edinburgh. Rarely, the outlet chamber gives rise to both great arteries, to neither great artery, or to a common arterial trunk.[28] In univentricular hearts characterized by *a single morphologic right ventricle*, both great arteries originate from the right ventricle,[67,69] an arrangement that is a form of *double outlet right ventricle* (see Chapter 19). Occasionally, the pulmonary trunk originates concordantly from the single right ventricle, and the aorta originates concordantly from the trabecular pouch, which is a left ventricular remnant.[67,69] A *morphologically indeterminate* single ventricle incorporates neither an outlet chamber nor a trabecular pouch, so both great arteries necessarily arise from the indeterminate single ventricle.

The orifice that joins a single left ventricle to an outlet chamber has been variously referred to as a *bulboventricular foramen*,[28] a *ventricular septal defect*,[13] and an *interventricular communication*.[68] *Bulboventricular foramen* assumes that the embryologic bulboventricular foramen is the same communication that exists in the univentricular heart, which is not necessarily the case. *Ventricular septal defect* and *interventricular communication* are discouraged as inherently contradictory terms in univentricular hearts. *Outlet foramen* is a simple descriptive term that will be used herein to refer to the orifice between the single left ventricle and the outlet chamber. A restrictive outlet foramen is a form of subaortic stenosis which may be present at birth[10,28,30,44,48,56,68,75] or may be acquired subsequently,[13,28,30,68] and is often accompanied by coarctation of the aorta.[10,28,30,44,48,56,75]

Pulmonary stenosis is either subpulmonary or in a bicuspid pulmonary valve when the pulmonary trunk originates from a single morphologic left ventricle (see Figs. 26–1, 26–2C, and 26–3).[28,48,75] The degree of stenosis varies from mild to severe (see Figs. 26–2 and 26–3) to pulmonary atresia (Fig. 26–5), which was recognized by Thomas Peacock:

"The case of Fleischmann differed in some degree from these, as though the heart consisted of three cavities, the ventricle only gave rise to one vessel, the orifice of the pulmonary artery being impervious. The child had lived twenty one weeks."[55]

Pulmonary stenosis is a feature of the Holmes heart[36] (Fig. 26–23) and usually results from obstruction of the outlet foramen of the concordant subpulmonary outlet chamber.[41,47]

Coronary artery origins in univentricular hearts of left ventricular morphology depend on the location of the

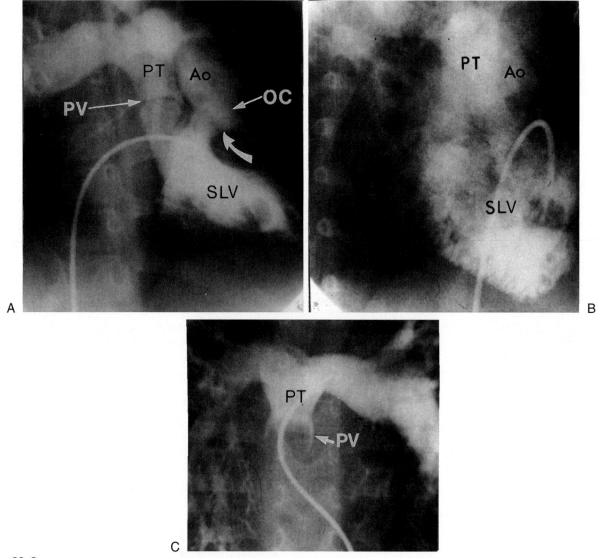

Figure 26–2
Angiocardiograms from a 7-year-old boy with univentricular heart of left ventricular morphology. *A,* The aorta (Ao) originates from an inverted outlet chamber (OC) that joins the single left ventricle (SLV) through a nonrestrictive outlet foramen (unmarked curved arrow). The pulmonary trunk (PT) originates from the single ventricle. Pulmonary stenosis was caused by a mobile stenotic pulmonary valve (PV) shown in C. *B,* Lateral ventriculogram showing the fine trabecular pattern of a morphologic left ventricle. The great arteries are side by side. *C,* Pulmonary arteriogram showing the mobile dome stenotic pulmonary valve (PV).

outlet chamber (see Chapters 6 and 32).[39,44] A major branch of each coronary artery usually outlines or *delimits* the surface boundaries of the outlet chamber.

The *morphogenesis* of univentricular hearts is believed to reside in an abnormality of the ventricular trabecular components of the developing heart.[7,21,38,75] Normally, the *left ventricular* trabecular component is derived from the inlet portion of the embryonic heart tube, and the *right ventricular* trabecular component is derived from the outlet portion. As the ventricular mass develops, the atrioventricular junction is shared between the left ventricular trabecular component and the right ventricular trabecular component. When the atrioventricular junction retains its connection to the *left* ventricular trabecular component, the result is double inlet to a morphologic *left* ventricle.

When the atrioventricular junction retains its connection to the *right* ventricular trabecular component, the result is double inlet to a morphologic *right* ventricle. When right and left ventricular trabecular components fail to develop, the result is double inlet to an *indeterminate* ventricle.

The *physiologic derangements* associated with univentricular hearts are related to: 1) the inherent mechanics of a single ventricle,[6,12,19,27,32] 2) the mechanics of a morphologic right ventricle versus a morphologic left ventricle,[81] 3) the morphology and functional state of the atrioventricular valve(s) that guard the inlet to a single ventricle, 4) the degree of mixing within the single ventricle, 5) the pulmonary vascular resistance, and 6) the presence and degree of pulmonary stenosis or subaortic stenosis.[45,47,48,52]

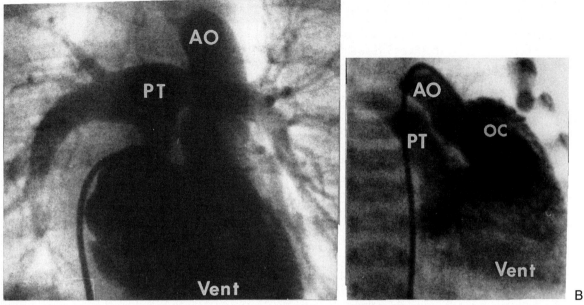

Figure 26–3

A, Ventriculogram from a 3-year-old girl with single morphologic left ventricle (Vent) and pulmonary stenosis (gradient 60 mm Hg). An inverted outlet chamber gives rise to the aorta (AO), which is convex to the left. The posteromedial pulmonary trunk (PT) is not border forming. *B,* Ventriculogram from a 5-week-old female with single morphologic left ventricle and mild pulmonary stenosis (gradient 25 mm Hg). The inverted outlet chamber (OC) forms a striking leftward convexity and gives rise to the aorta (AO). The morphologic left ventricle (Vent) is finely trabeculated.

In hearts with two ventricles, the mechanics of each ventricle augment the function of the other ventricle.[12,19] *Ventricular-ventricular interaction* is an integral part of cardiac mechanics and results from mechanical coupling of two ventricles through the interventricular septum and through an anatomic continuum that joins the mural myocardium of the two ventricles.[12,19] Ventricular interdependence cannot occur unless a right ventricle contributes to left ventricular function and a left ventricle contributes to right ventricular function. Accordingly, ventricular interdependence does not exist in univentricular hearts, resulting in abnormal systolic and diastolic function irrespective of the morphology of the single ventricle.[2,54] Because a single ventricle is the only pump for the systemic and pulmonary circulations, the

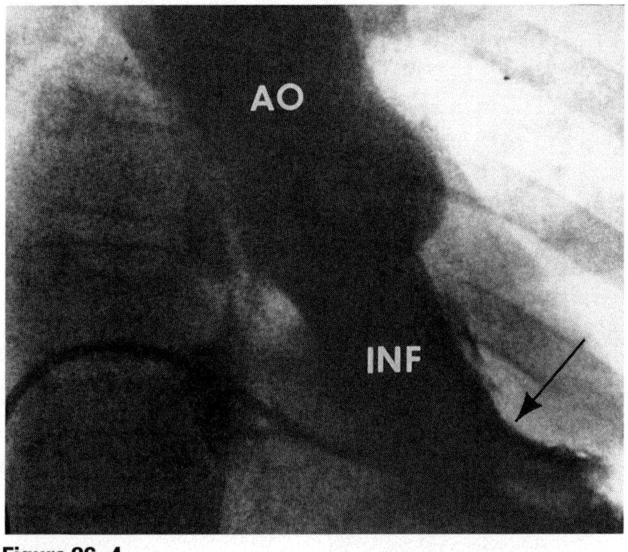

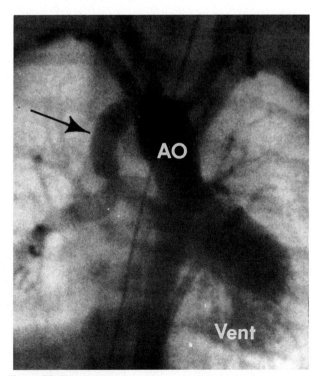

Figure 26–4

Ventriculogram from a 9-year-old boy with a univentricular heart of the left ventricular type and an inverted outlet chamber (INF) that is devoid of trabeculations and that gives rise to the aorta (AO). The outlet foramen (unmarked arrow) is nonrestrictive.

Figure 26–5

Ventriculogram from a 1-day-old girl with single ventricle (Vent) of the left ventricular type and pulmonary atresia. An enlarged aorta (AO) originates from an inverted outlet chamber. A large anomalous systemic arterial collateral (unmarked arrow) communicated with the right pulmonary artery.

volume handled by a univentricular heart is increased and provokes an adaptive increase in ventricular mass.[2,54,64] In univentricular hearts of *right ventricular morphology*, the indices that reflect an adaptive increase in ventricular mass are significantly reduced including mass *per se*, wall thickness, ratio of wall thickness to transverse ventricular diameter and ratio of ventricular mass to end-diastolic volume.[64] Inadequate mass relative to chamber volume reflects poor adaptation of univentricular hearts of right ventricular morphology.[64,81]

The *physiology of the circulation* in univentricular hearts is materially influenced by atrioventricular valve structure and function. Incompetence, stenosis or atresia of an atrioventricular valve affects flow into the single ventricle and modifies its loading conditions. Atrioventricular valve regurgitation adds to the volume overload of the single ventricle. Atresia of the right or left atrioventricular valve results in a single inlet that does not disturb the circulation provided there is free access to the single ventricle via a nonrestrictive interatrial communication and across the contralateral atrioventricular valve. However, the right atrium is obstructed when the right atrioventricular valve is atretic and the interatrial communication is restrictive.[15,58] Similarly, the *left* atrium is obstructed when the left atrioventricular valve is atretic and the interatrial communication is restrictive.

The streams of right atrial venous blood and left atrial arterialized blood remain remarkably separated within the single ventricular chamber.[45,48] Separation of the streams is greater when pulmonary resistance is low and when the outlet chamber is inverted.[45,48] Unoxygenated blood from the systemic venous atrium selectively finds it way into the pulmonary trunk, and oxygenated blood from the pulmonary venous atrium selectively finds its way into the aorta. Subaortic stenosis diverts even more blood into the pulmonary circulation.[10,56] Cyanosis is mild and occasionally absent.[52] However, the benefits of increased pulmonary blood flow are achieved at the price of volume overload of the single ventricle.

Pulmonary vascular disease and *pulmonary stenosis* curtail pulmonary blood flow and adversely affect streaming within the single ventricle. When pulmonary stenosis or pulmonary

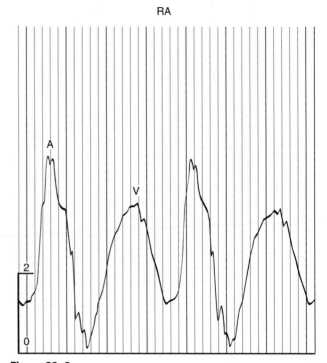

Figure 26–6
Right atrial pressure pulse (RA) from an 18-year-old boy with single morphologic left ventricle and pulmonary stenosis (gradient 50 mm Hg). The pressure pulse is normal in height and waveform.

vascular disease are severe, cyanosis is conspicuous because a smaller volume of oxygenated blood reaches the left atrium, and because there is greater mixing of unoxygenated and oxygenated blood within the single ventricle.[47,67]

Because 80% to 90% of univentricular hearts are characterized by a single morphologic left ventricle with an outlet chamber, the following sections deal principally with this more prevalent type of single ventricle.

The History

The male/female ratio is between 2 to 1 and 4 to 1.[35,48,52] Recurrence in siblings is rare.[66] Neonates or infants come

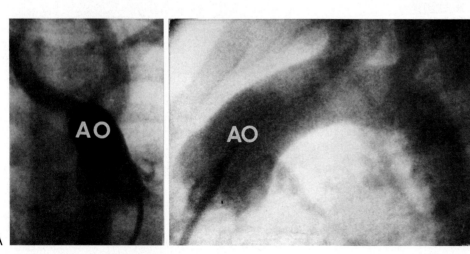

Figure 26–7
Aortograms from a 2-year-old boy with single morphologic left ventricle and pulmonary stenosis (gradient 55 mm Hg). An inverted outlet chamber gave rise to the aorta (AO) which is convex to the left (*A*) and anterior (*B*).

to attention because of congestive heart failure, cyanosis, or a murmur. The type of presentation and the survival patterns depend on the pulmonary vascular resistance, the presence and degree of pulmonary stenosis, the morphology of the single ventricle, and the presence and degree of subaortic stenosis. Fifty percent of patients with univentricular hearts of left ventricular morphology are dead within 14 years with an annual attrition rate of 4.8%.[51] Fifty percent of patients with univentricular hearts of right ventricular morphology are dead within 4 years.[51]

Infants with increased pulmonary blood flow present with congestive heart failure, mild cyanosis and poor growth and development.[47,48,67] Congestive heart failure is refractory when subaortic stenosis augments already excessive pulmonary blood flow.[56] Pulmonary vascular resistance seldom achieves satisfactory regulation of pulmonary flow. An exceptional case similar if not identical to the 24-year-old man referred to in Figure 26–18 was described by Peacock[55]:

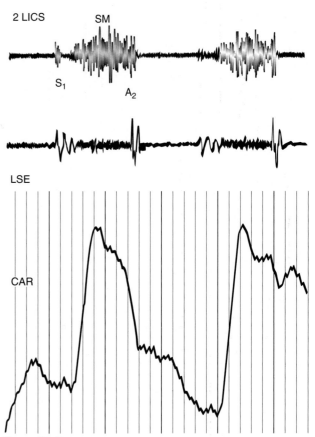

Figure 26–9
Phonocardiogram and carotid pulse (CAR) from a 6-year-old girl with single morphologic left ventricle, pulmonary stenosis (gradient 85 mm Hg), and an inverted outlet chamber. A prominent pulmonary stenotic murmur (SM) was maximum in the second left intercostal space (2 LICS). The single second heart sound (A₂) was aortic because the aorta was anterior to the pulmonary trunk. LSE, left sternal edge.

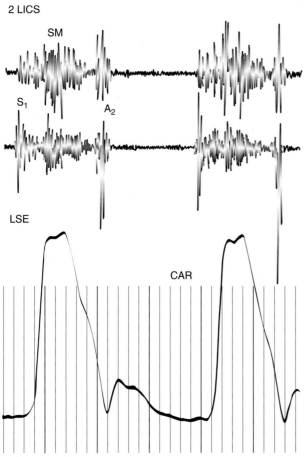

Figure 26–8
Phonocardiograms and carotid arterial pulse (CAR) from a 12-year-old boy with single morphologic left ventricle, pulmonary stenosis (gradient 60 mm Hg), and an inverted outlet chamber. The pulmonary stenotic murmur (SM) was louder in the second left intercostal space (2 LICS) compared to the mid left sternal edge (LSE). The single second heart sound (A₂, aortic component) was loud because the aorta was anterior to the pulmonary trunk.

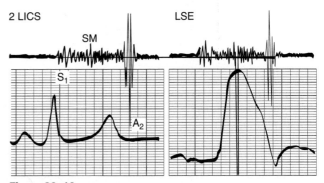

Figure 26–10
Tracings from an 8-year-old boy with single morphologic left ventricle and severe pulmonary stenosis (gradient 100 mm Hg). The pulmonary stenotic murmur (SM) in the second left intercostal space (2 LICS) and at the lower left sternal edge (LSE) is soft and short. The second heart sound (A₂, aortic component) was loud because an anterior aorta arose from an inverted outlet chamber. The pulmonary component was inaudible because the pulmonary valve was posterior to the aorta. Lower right tracing, carotid pulse.

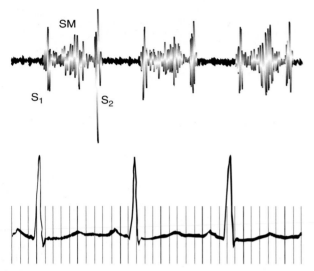

Figure 26–11

Phonocardiogram from a 2-month-old boy with single morphologic left ventricle and a restrictive outlet foramen (subaortic gradient 30 mm Hg). The mid systolic stenotic murmur (SM) radiated to the second *right* intercostal space (2 RICS) because the outlet chamber was noninverted and gave rise to an aorta with a rightward convexity. S_1, first heart sound, S_2, second heart sound.

"The heart was very greatly enlarged, and the walls of the ventricle fully three times their usual thickness: there was not a trace of inter-ventricular septum, but the positions of the vessels of the heart were natural, and the orifices were somewhat dilated."

The oldest reported survivor with a single morphologic left ventricle and pulmonary vascular disease was a 59-year-old man.[34]

Pulmonary stenosis is more effective than pulmonary vascular resistance in regulating pulmonary blood flow (see Figs. 26–2 and 26–3). Peacock described a patient with single ventricle and pulmonary stenosis who suffered from *morbus caeruleus* but lived to age 11 years: "The heart was found to have two auricles and one ventricle, and from the latter cavity the aorta and pulmonary artery arose."[55] Survival into adolescence and early adulthood is not rare. Longevity occasionally extends into the fourth or fifth decade[1,5,11,18,33,36,41,46,50,62,63,80] (see Figs. 26–12 and 26–24) with one patient reaching 56 years of age. Moderate pulmonary stenosis is physiologically desirable, but severe pulmonary stenosis or atresia results in deep, even profound cyanosis (see Fig. 26–5). Squatting may attenuate dyspnea.[67] Hypoxic spells seldom occur.[48]

Subaortic stenosis caused by a restrictive outlet foramen has an adverse effect on longevity by augmenting pulmonary blood flow and augmenting volume overload of the single ventricle. The outlet foramen can become progressively more restrictive.[13,68]

The multisystem systemic disorders associated with cyanotic congenital heart disease and Eisenmenger syndrome are important features in the history of patients with univentricular hearts (See Chapter 17).[5]

Physical Appearance

An underdeveloped, diaphoretic, mildly cyanotic tachypneic infant is the expected appearance associated with increased pulmonary blood flow and congestive heart failure. Profound cyanosis is the expected appearance with severe pulmonary stenosis or atresia and metabolic acidosis.

The Arterial Pulse

In neonates and infants with congestive heart failure, the arterial pulses are small and the rate is rapid. In single left ventricle with subaortic stenosis, the brachial and femoral pulses should be compared because of the incidence of coarctation of the aorta.[28,68]

The Jugular Venous Pulse

The height and waveform of the jugular pulse are normal when moderate pulmonary stenosis curtails excessive pulmonary blood flow (Fig. 26–6). Incompetence of the right atrioventricular valve increases the V wave. Atresia of the *right* atrioventricular valve increases the A wave when the interatrial communication is restrictive. Atresia of the *left* atrioventricular valve results in a large jugular venous A wave when an atrial septal defect is nonrestrictive.

Precordial Movement and Palpation

Single ventricle of left ventricular morphology generates precordial movement analogous to a morphologic left ventricle in a biventricular heart. When pulmonary blood flow is increased, the impulse of the volume overloaded single

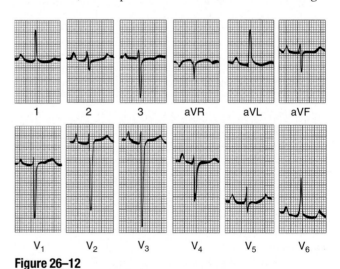

Figure 26–12

Electrocardiogram from a 45-year-old woman with single morphologic left ventricle, a noninverted outlet chamber, and pulmonary stenosis (gradient 80 mm Hg). The PR interval is prolonged. Tall peaked right atrial P waves appear in leads 2, aVF and V_{2-6}. There is left axis deviation with counterclockwise depolarization. The rS patterns in leads V_{1-4} are stereotyped.

left ventricle is hyperdynamic. A visible and palpable systolic impulse in the third left intercostal space is a result of the leftward and anterior position of an inverted outlet chamber (Fig. 26–2*A, B*). The second heart sound is loud and palpable because the aorta is anterior whether the outlet chamber is inverted or noninverted (Fig. 26–7*B*). A systolic thrill at the mid left sternal border is evidence of subaortic stenosis caused by a restrictive outlet foramen. Potential pulmonary stenotic thrills are attenuated by the posterior position of the pulmonary trunk. A *single morphologic right ventricle* imparts an impulse at the mid to lower left sternal border and subxiphoid area analogous to a morphologic right ventricular impulse of a biventricular heart. There is no impulse in the third left intercostal space because there is no underlying outlet chamber.

Auscultation

A potential pulmonary ejection sound that originates in a mobile stenotic pulmonary valve (see Fig. 26–2*C*) is attenuated because of the posterior position of the pulmonary trunk. Pulmonary ejection sounds do not occur with subpulmonary stenosis (see Fig. 26–3). An *aortic ejection sound* is generated in the dilated anterior ascending aorta in the presence of pulmonary atresia (see Figs. 26–5 and 26–25).

A prominent systolic murmur at the mid left sternal border originates in the outlet foramen when pulmonary blood flow is increased. The murmur begins early because flow into the outlet chamber commences before the aortic valve opens.[52] The murmur is decrescendo and ends before the aortic component of the second heart sound because forward flow decelerates and stops before the aortic valve closes.[52]

Pulmonary stenotic murmurs are most prominent at the mid or lower left sternal border when the stenosis is subpulmonary[48] and vary inversely in length and loudness according to the degree of stenosis (Figs. 26–8, 26-9, and 26–10). As the stenosis increases, more blood is diverted into the aorta and less blood enters the pulmonary trunk, so the stenotic murmur softens and shortens. The murmur is dampened further because of the posterior position of the pulmonary trunk.

The murmur of subaortic stenosis caused by a restrictive outlet foramen is midsystolic and radiates from the mid left sternal border to the left or right base depending on whether the outlet chamber is inverted or noninverted (Fig. 26–11). Ventricular failure decreases the gradient across the outlet foramen and decreases the subaortic murmur.[56] Because coarctation of the aorta tends to coexist with subaortic stenosis, auscultation should include the interscapular area over the spine in search of the systolic murmur of coarctation (see Chapter 8).

The *second heart sound* splits normally. A rise in pulmonary vascular resistance abolishes the split. The aortic component is loud because the aorta is anterior. The pulmonary component is transmitted when the posterior pulmonary trunk is hypertensive and dilated. In the pres-

ence of pulmonary stenosis, the loud and single second heart sound is aortic. In the presence of subaortic stenosis, the second heart sound tends to be single because the aortic component is attenuated and a prominent pulmonary component originates in the hypertensive posterior pulmonary trunk (see Fig. 26–11). The aortic component of the second sound is loud in single morphologic right ventricle because the aorta is anterior to the pulmonary trunk or side by side.[67]

Two types of diastolic murmurs occur with univentricular hearts. When pulmonary blood flow is increased, a large volume of blood enters the left atrium and flows across the left atrioventricular valve, generating a mid-diastolic murmur.[48,52] A rise in pulmonary vascular resistance attenuates the mid-diastolic flow murmur and results in a high frequency early diastolic Graham Steell murmur of pulmonary hypertensive pulmonary regurgitation.[46,48,52]

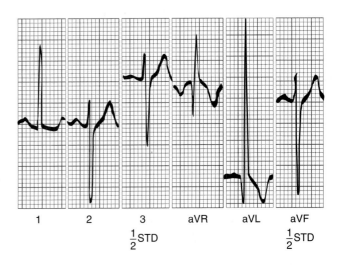

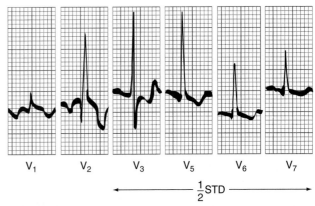

Figure 26–13

Electrocardiogram from a 6-year-old boy with single morphologic left ventricle, a noninverted outlet chamber, low pulmonary vascular resistance, and increased pulmonary blood flow. A left atrial P wave abnormality is represented by broad negative terminal forces in leads V_{1-2}. There is left axis deviation with counterclockwise depolarization. The QRS pattern is stereotyped in leads V_{2-7}, and QRS amplitude is strikingly increased in limb leads and in midprecordial leads. Leads 3, aVF and V_{3-7} are half standardized. Small Q waves appear in right and left precordial leads. In lead aVL, the tall R wave and inverted T wave are patterns of left ventricular hypertrophy.

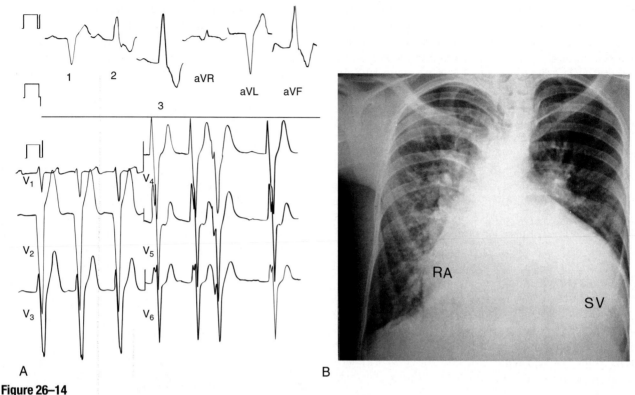

Figure 26–14

A, Electrocardiogram from a 7-year-old boy with single morphologic left ventricle, noninverted outlet chamber, and pulmonary vascular disease. The QRS axis is rightward despite noninversion of the outlet chamber. There is an intraventricular conduction defect with a QRS duration of 164 msec. The PR interval is 267 msec. The amplitude of QRS complexes is striking in limb and precordial leads, all of which are half standardized. Leads V_1 through V_6 are stereotyped. *B,* X-ray from the same patient showing pulmonary venous congestion and a narrow vascular pedicle caused by noninversion of the outlet chamber and a posterior non–border-forming pulmonary trunk. The single ventricle (SV) is strikingly dilated, and the right atrium (RA) is enlarged.

The Electrocardiogram

A ventricular septal structure is lacking at the inlet portion of the ventricular mass with single morphologic left ventricle, so the *posterior* AV node is hypoplastic and does not form a His bundle or establish a ventricular connection.[4,14,77,78] Instead, a well-developed *anterior accessory* AV node gives rise to the His bundle and establishes atrioventricular connections. When the outlet chamber is *noninverted*, a long nonbranching penetrating bundle runs

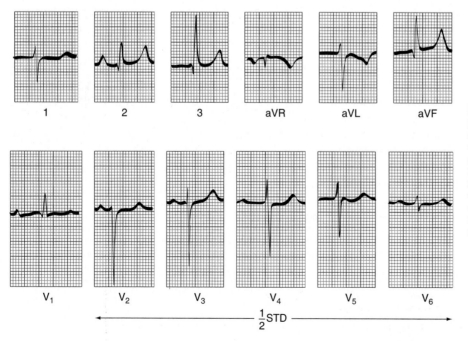

Figure 26–15

Electrocardiogram from a 30-year-old cyanotic woman with single morphologic left ventricle, inversion of the outlet chamber, and pulmonary stenosis (gradient 85 mm Hg). There is complete heart block with narrow QRS complexes. The QRS axis is rightward, appropriate for an inverted outlet chamber. The rS complexes in leads V_2 through V_5 are stereotyped and the amplitudes are increased (half standardized).

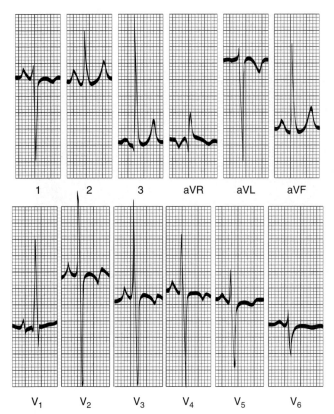

Figure 26–16
Electrocardiogram from an 18-year-old man with single morphologic left ventricle, inversion of the outlet chamber, and pulmonary stenosis (gradient 50 mm Hg). Tall peaked right atrial P waves are present in leads 2, aVF, and V_{1-5}. The QRS axis is rightward, appropriate for an inverted outlet chamber. The RS complexes are stereotyped in leads V_2 through V_5 with increased amplitude in leads V_{2-4}. There is a tall monophasic R wave in lead V_1 despite a morphologic left ventricle.

down the right parietal wall of the single ventricle toward the outlet foramen before bifurcating into right and left bundle branches.[4] When the outlet chamber is *inverted*, the penetrating bundle encircles the outflow tract of the single ventricle before branching at the outlet foramen. The left bundle branch is concordant with the left ventricular morphology of the single left ventricle, and the right bundle branch is concordant with the outlet chamber.[4,69]

An inlet septum is also lacking in univentricular hearts with a *morphologic right ventricle* and a rudimentary trabecular pouch. However, the ventricular segment between the morphologic right ventricle and the trabecular pouch extends to the crux of the heart, so a regular posterior AV node and His bundle are formed at the crux.[26] Distribution of the bundle branches apparently depends on the right/left orientation of the trabecular pouch.

When a univentricular heart is morphologically *indeterminate* (no outlet chamber, no trabecular pouch), neither the inlet septum nor trabecular septal tissue reaches the crux. Accordingly, the AV node is anterior or anterolateral, and the penetrating bundles descend as single fascicles among free-running trabeculae.

Diversity in the electrocardiogram reflects diversity of the anatomic variations of univentricular hearts.[25,31,52,53,60,65,67] Electrocardiographic interpretations become clearer when related to specific morphologic types of single ventricles and their associated physiologic derangements.

In a single morphologic left ventricle with a *noninverted outlet chamber*, the PR interval is usually normal because atrioventricular conduction is normal despite an elongated

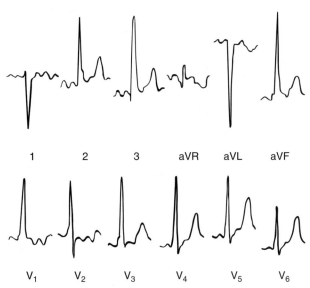

Figure 26–17
Electrocardiogram from a 19-year-old man with single morphologic right ventricle and pulmonary stenosis (gradient 50 mm Hg). There is coarse atrial fibrillation. The QRS axis is rightward, appropriate for an inverted outlet chamber. The amplitude of QRS complexes is increased in the limb leads. The Rs pattern is stereotyped in leads V_1 through V_6.

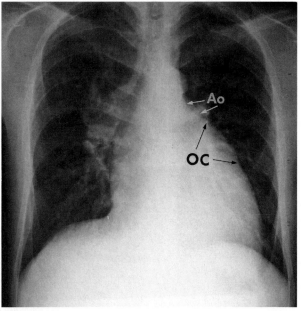

Figure 26–18
X-ray from a 24-year-old man with single morphologic left ventricle and pulmonary vascular disease. Pulmonary vascularity was not increased because pulmonary resistance was elevated. An inverted outlet chamber (OC) forms a convex bulge at the left upper cardiac border and gives rise to the aorta (Ao). The large right pulmonary artery is tilted upward creating a *waterfall* appearance. The single ventricle and right atrium are dilated.

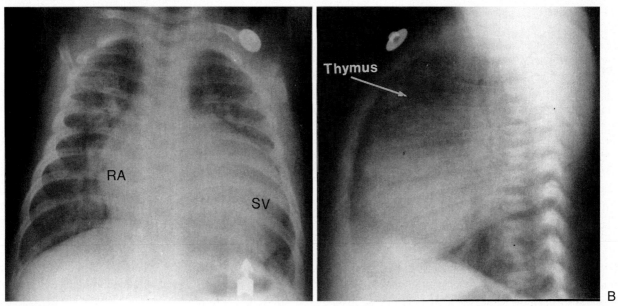

Figure 26–19

X-rays from a 3-week-old neonate with a single morphologic left ventricle and a noninverted outlet chamber. *A,* The posteroanterior projection shows a narrow vascular pedicle appropriate for complete transposition of the great arteries. Pulmonary venous congestion is marked, and the single ventricle (SV) and right atrium (RA) are strikingly dilated. *B,* The lateral projection shows a thymic shadow, which implies that complete transposition is occurring with single ventricle and not an isolated malformation.

nonbranching penetrating bundle (see Fig. 26–14). The P waves show left atrial or biatrial abnormalities when pulmonary blood flow is increased (see Fig. 26–13) and right atrial abnormalities when pulmonary blood flow is reduced (Fig. 26–12).

The QRS axis is directed away from the noninverted outlet chamber toward the main ventricular mass and is leftward and inferior or leftward and superior (left axis deviation) (see Figs. 26–12 and 26–13).[20,60] Initial depolarization forces are anterior and leftward, so small Q

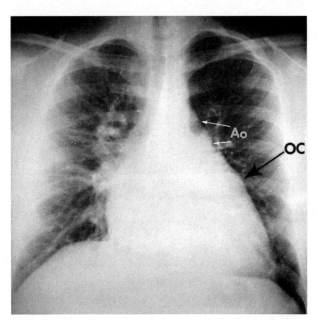

Figure 26–20

X-ray from a 19-year-old man with single morphologic left ventricle, pulmonary stenosis (gradient 50 mm Hg), and increased pulmonary blood flow. The inverted outlet chamber (OC) forms a convex bulge at the upper left cardiac border and gives rise to the aorta (Ao). The single ventricle and right atrium are dilated.

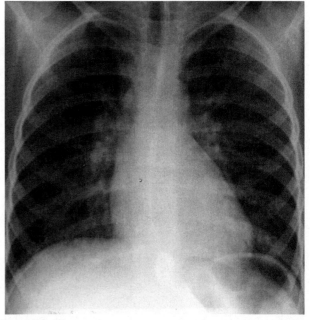

Figure 26–21

X-ray from a 7-year-old girl with single morphologic left ventricle and severe pulmonary stenosis (gradient 105 mm Hg). Pulmonary arterial vascularity is reduced. The vascular pedicle is narrow because a noninverted outlet chamber gave rise to an anterior aorta that ascended vertically, and the posterior pulmonary trunk was not border forming. The size and shape of the heart are virtually normal.

waves occasionally appear in left precordial leads (Fig. 26–13).[20] Left ventricular hypertrophy is the prevailing pattern and is especially striking when pulmonary blood flow is increased and the single ventricle is volume overload (see Fig. 26–13). Precordial QRS complexes exhibit stereotyped patterns (see Figs. 26–13 and 26–14).[20,25,60] QRS voltages of remarkably great amplitude in one or more limb leads and precordial leads are noteworthy features (see Figs. 26–13 and 26–14).[65]

When the outlet chamber is *inverted,* atrioventricular conduction is often abnormal and PR interval prolongation occasionally culminates in complete heart block.[4,48] The P wave axis shifts to the left in the horizontal plane, so tall peaked right atrial P waves appear in mid and left precordial leads (see Fig. 26–16),[65] a pattern that also occurs with noninversion of the outlet chamber (see Fig. 26–12).[65] The QRS axis is inferior and to the right, directed away from the inverted outlet chamber toward the main ventricular mass (Figs. 26–15 and 26–16).[20,60] Ventricular depolarization is clockwise so Q waves appear in leads 2, 3 and aVF. Because initial forces of ventricular depolarization are posterior and *leftward,* Q waves may be present in right precordial leads but do not appear in left precordial leads (see Figs. 26–15 and 26–16).[20,25] Even though the univentricular heart is morphologically a left ventricle, precordial leads may show a dominant R wave in

lead V_1 and large equidiphasic RS complexes in midprecordial leads (Fig. 26–16).

In univentricular hearts with a *morphologic right ventricle* and a trabecular pouch, atriventricular conduction is normal because a regular posterior AV node and His bundle are formed at the crux.[26,67] Right axis deviation and tall stereotyped precordial R waves are features of a single morphologic right ventricle (Fig. 26–17).[67] The QRS axis is usually rightward (Fig. 26–17) but is occasionally leftward and superior.[67]

The X-Ray

The location of the outlet chamber is an important feature of the x-ray. An *inverted* outlet chamber forms a localized convexity at the left upper cardiac border and gives rise to an aorta that is convex to the left or that rises vertically[16,24,52] (Figs. 26–2A, 26–3, 26–18 ; see Fig. 26–20) as in congenitally corrected transposition of the great arteries (see Chapter 6).[24,48] In the Holmes heart, the inverted outlet chamber is distinctively convex but gives rise to a concordant pulmonary trunk (see Fig. 26–23).[47] A *noninverted* outlet chamber is not border forming on the left (Figs. 26–19A and 26–21) and gives rise to an aorta that is convex to the right (see Fig. 26–1A) as in complete

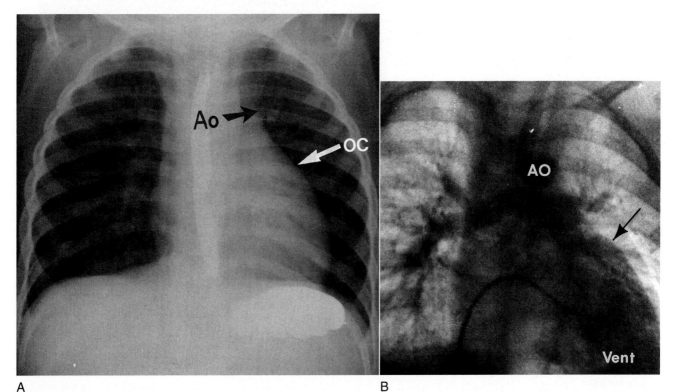

A   **B**

Figure 26–22

A, X-ray from a 1-year-old boy with single morphologic left ventricle, an inverted outlet chamber, and pulmonary stenosis (gradient 65 mm Hg). The straight left upper cardiac border is caused by the inverted outlet chamber (OC) and ascending aorta (Ao). The size and shape of the heart are otherwise virtually normal. *B,* Ventriculogram in the same patient showing the fine trabecular pattern of a morphologic left ventricle (Vent). The aorta (Ao) arises from an inverted outlet chamber (*arrow*).

transposition of the great arteries (see Chapter 27).[24] With the exception of the Holmes heart (see Fig. 26–23),[20,24,36,47] the great arteries are transposed, with the aorta originating discordantly from the outlet chamber and the pulmonary trunk originating discordantly from the morphologic left ventricle (see Fig. 26–1). A transposed posteromedial pulmonary trunk may lift its dilated right branch and create a *waterfall* appearance

(see Fig. 26–18).[16,24,52] *Absence of a thymic* shadow is an important radiologic feature of complete transposition of the great arteries in biventricular hearts (see Chapter 27), but is not a feature of complete transposition in a univentricular heart (Fig. 26–19B).

The cardiac silhouette increases in response to excessive pulmonary blood flow and volume overload of the single ventricle (Figs 26–14B and 26–19A).[16,29,35] Left

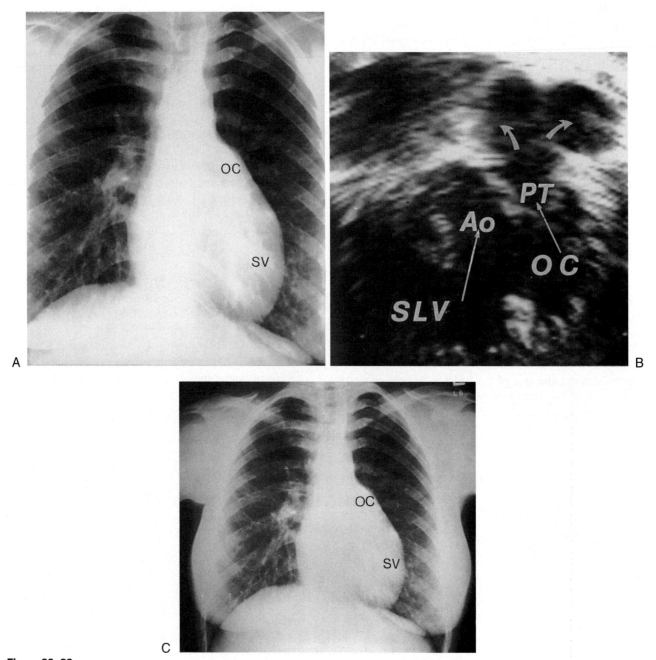

Figure 26–23

A, X-ray from a 20-month-old boy with the Holmes heart characterized by a single morphologic left ventricle (SV) that gave rise to a concordant aorta and an inverted outlet chamber (OC) that gave rise to a concordant pulmonary trunk. Subpulmonary stenosis was caused by a restrictive ostium of the outlet chamber. *B*, Echocardiogram from the same patient showing the aorta (Ao) arising concordantly from the single left ventricle (SLV) and the pulmonary trunk (PT) arising concordantly from the inverted outlet chamber (OC). *C*, X-ray from a 20-year-old woman with the Holmes heart and a cardiac silhouette that is virtually identical with that of the 20-month-old boy shown in *A*.

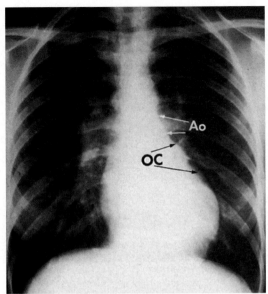

Figure 26–24

X-ray from a 30-year-old woman with single morphologic left ventricle, pulmonary stenosis (gradient 85 mm Hg), inversion of the outlet chamber, and a normal heart size. Pulmonary vascularity is reduced. The vascular pedicle is narrow because the pulmonary trunk was posterior and the inverted outlet chamber (OC) gives rise to an aorta (Ao) that was anterior and ascended vertically.

atrial enlargement is best identified in lateral films or by barium esophagram[16] because what appears to be a left atrial appendage in the posteroanterior projection is likely to represent an inverted outlet chamber (Figs. 26–18 and 26–20). Right atrial dilatation accompanies congestive heart failure, which is reinforced by subaortic stenosis (Figs. 26–14*B* and 26–19*A*).

In *single morphologic left ventricle* with *severe pulmonary stenosis*, the size of the heart is normal or nearly normal, but an inverted outlet chamber reveals itself as a bulge at the left upper cardiac border (Figs. 26–21, 26–22 ; see Fig. 26–24). Also distinctive is a dilated aorta that

arises from an inverted outlet chamber and presents as a convexity to the left (see Figs. 26–18, 26–20, and 26–23) or that ascends vertically and is not border-forming on either side (Fig. 26–24). Pulmonary *atresia* with an inverted outlet chamber has a box-like cardiac silhouette with the dilated ascending aorta forming the left upper border that merges with a small underfilled ventricle below, and the vertebral column forming the straight right border (Fig. 26–25).

In univentricular hearts of *right ventricular* morphology, both great arteries arise from the single right ventricle.[67] The vascular pedicle is narrow because the aorta is anterior and the pulmonary trunk is posterior to the aorta or side by side.[67] Pulmonary stenosis is common, so pulmonary vascularity is normal or reduced and the heart size is not significantly increased.[67]

The Echocardiogram

Echocardiography with color flow imaging and Doppler interrogation identifies a single morphologic left ventricle that incorporates an outlet chamber at its base.[13,22,29,37,57,68] The internal architecture of the single ventricle is characterized (see Figs. 26–27 and 26–28), and two separate patent atrioventricular valves are usually present (Fig. 26–26). Right and left AV valve morphology is concordant with inversion or noninversion of the outlet chamber.[13] An atrioventricular valve can be incompetent, stenotic, or imperforate, and part of the tensor apparatus can straddle the outlet foramen.[13,37,61,68] Color flow imaging establishes the presence and degree of incompetence of the right or left AV valve. A common atrioventricular valve is a feature of atrial isomerism with a univentricular heart (see Chapter 3).

Echocardiography identifies an inverted or noninverted outlet chamber (Figs. 26–27, 26–28, 26–29, and 26–30). from which the aorta arises discordantly, and identifies a single left ventricle from which the

Figure 26–25

X-rays from a 22-year-old man with single morphologic left ventricle and pulmonary atresia. *A,* Pulmonary vascularity markedly is reduced. The cardiac silhouette has a box-like configuration with the left upper border of the box formed by a dilated aorta that ascends vertically from the inverted outlet chamber, and the straight right border of the box formed by the vertebral column above and a barely visible right atrium below. *B,* The aortogram shows the dilated convex ascending aorta (AO) and a nonfunctional right Blalock-Taussig shunt (*arrow*).

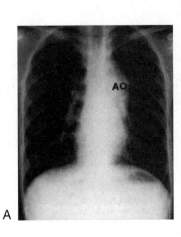

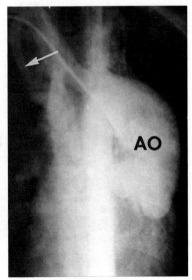

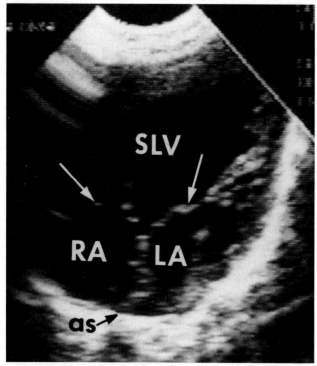

Figure 26–26
Echocardiogram (apical view) from a 1-month-old boy with single morphologic left ventricle (SLV) and separate right and left atrioventricular valves (oblique arrows). The atrial septum (as) is intact. RA, right atrium; LA, left atrium.

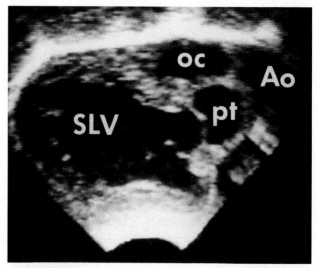

Figure 26–28
Echocardiogram (subcostal) from a 10-month-old boy with a finely trabeculated single morphologic left ventricle (SLV) from which the pulmonary trunk (pt) originates, and an outlet chamber (OC) from which the aorta (Ao) originates.

pulmonary trunk arises discordantly (see Figs. 26–28 to 26–30). In the Holmes heart, the outlet chamber is concordant with the pulmonary trunk, and the aorta is concordant with the single morphologic left ventricle (Fig. 26–23B). Color flow imaging with continuous-wave

Doppler establishes the presence and degree of pulmonary stenosis or subaortic stenosis caused by a restrictive outlet foramen. When subaortic stenosis exists from infancy, the aortic arch should be interrogated with two-dimensional imaging, and color flow with continuous-wave Doppler because of the increased incidence of arch hypoplasia and coarctation of the aorta.

A univentricular heart of *right ventricular* morphology is recognized by the morphologic characteristics of the ventricular endocardium and a trabecular pouch (Figs.

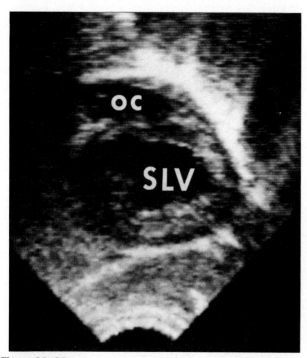

Figure 26–27
Echocardiogram (short axis) from a 16-month-old boy with a finely trabeculated single morphologic left ventricle (SLV). OC, outlet chamber.

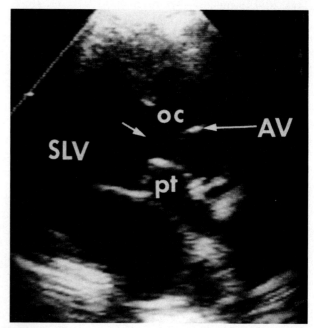

Figure 26–29
Echocardiogram (parasternal long axis) from a 13-year-old boy with a single morphologic left ventricle (SLV) from which the pulmonary trunk (pt) originates, and a noninverted outlet chamber (OC) from which the aorta originates. AV, aortic valve.

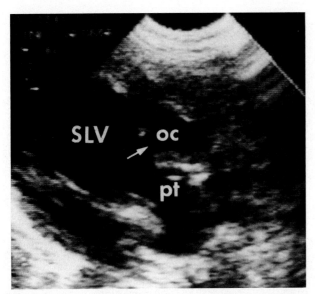

Figure 26–30
Echocardiogram (parasternal long axis) from a 1-month-old boy with single morphologic left ventricle (SLV) from which the pulmonary trunk (pt) originates, and an inverted outlet chamber (OC) from which the aorta originates. The outlet foramen (*arrow*) was restrictive by continuous wave Doppler.

26–31 and 26–32*A*) that may be straddled by elements of the atrioventricular valve tensor apparatus. Two-dimensional echocardiography with color flow imaging shows two side-by-side great arteries arising from the single right ventricle (Figs. 26–32*B, C*). Continuous-wave Doppler identifies the presence and degree of pulmonary stenosis.

A univentricular heart of *indeterminate* morphology can be suspected based on endocardial morphology and on the absence of either an outlet chamber or a trabecular pouch.

Summary

Single ventricular or *univentricular* refers to hearts with atrioventricular connections that are exclusively or primarily assigned one main ventricular chamber that is morphologically a left, right, or indeterminate ventricle. This chapter is concerned with three major types of univentricular hearts: 1) a single morphologic *left* ventricle with an anterobasal outlet chamber that is either inverted or noninverted, 2) a single morphologic *right* ventricle with a rudimentary trabecular pouch (left ventricular remnant) that is directly posterior or posteroinferior and left-sided or right-sided, and 3) a single ventricle that is morphologically *indeterminate* and is devoid of either an outlet chamber or a trabecular pouch. The physiologic derangements and clinical manifestations depend on the absence, presence, and degree of pulmonary vascular disease, pulmonary stenosis or subaortic stenosis, and on the morphology and functional state of the atrioventricular connections. Because

univentricular atrioventricular connections to a single morphologic *left* ventricle with an outlet chamber represent 80% to 90% of cases, this chapter and summary deal chiefly with that arrangement.

Single morphologic left ventricle with increased pulmonary blood flow presents in infancy with mild cyanosis and congestive heart failure. Physical appearance reflects the poor growth and development caused by the catabolic effects of congestive heart failure. Arterial pulses are sometimes diagnostically useful because subaortic stenosis (restrictive outlet foramen) is associated with coarctation of the aorta. Precordial palpation identifies a ventricular impulse with left ventricular characteristics together with a visible and palpable left basal impulse of an inverted outlet chamber. Auscultation detects a prominent long decrescendo systolic murmur at the mid left sternal border due to flow through the outlet foramen. Electrocardiographic features associated with a noninverted outlet chamber include left axis deviation, left ventricular hypertrophy, QRS complexes of great amplitude, and stereotyped precordial QRS patterns. Electrocardiographic features associated with an inverted outlet chamber include PR interval prolongation, an inferior or rightward QRS axis, absent left precordial Q waves, QRS complexes of great amplitude, and stereotyped precordial QRS patterns. The chest x-ray shows increased pulmonary vascularity and an inverted convex outlet chamber that gives rise to an aorta that is convex to the left. Echocardiography with color flow imaging and Doppler interrogation identifies two atrioventricular valves that enter a single ventricle with left ventricular morphology that incorporates at its base an inverted or noninverted outlet chamber from which the aorta arises discordantly.

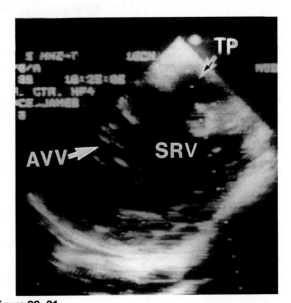

Figure 26–31
Transesophageal echocardiogram from a 36-year-old man with a coarsely trabeculated single morphologic right ventricle (SRV). A trabecular pouch (TP) arises from the posteroinferior wall of the single ventricle. The atrioventricular valve (AVV) tensor apparatus did not straddle the trabecular pouch.

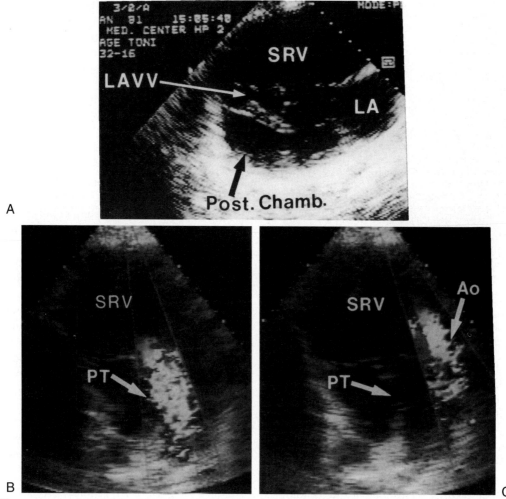

Figure 26–32

Echocardiogram (parasternal long axis) from a 29-year-old woman with a single morphologic right ventricle (SRV) and pulmonary stenosis (gradient 65 mm Hg). *A,* A trabecular pouch (Post Chamb) arises from the posterior wall of the single ventricle. Tensor apparatus from the left atrioventricular valve (LAVV) did not straddle the trabecular pouch. *B,* Black-and-white print of a color flow image showing flow from the single right ventricle (SRV) into the pulmonary trunk (PT). *C,* Black-and-white print of a color flow image showing flow from the single right ventricle into the aorta (Ao). The aorta (Ao) and pulmonary trunk (PT) are side by side.

A *single morphologic left ventricle* with *pulmonary stenosis* presents with cyanosis rather than congestive heart failure. The ventricular impulse is modest compared to the dynamic impulse of a volume-overloaded single ventricle. Auscultation detects a pulmonary stenotic murmur whose loudness and length vary inversely with severity. A loud single second heart sound is aortic. The electrocardiogram does not reflect either the presence or degree of pulmonary stenosis. The chest x-ray discloses normal or decreased pulmonary blood flow, a heart size that is normal or nearly normal, and a left basal convexity of the inverted outlet chamber. Color flow imaging and continuous wave Doppler interrogation establish the degree of pulmonary stenosis. In the presence of pulmonary atresia, a dilated ascending aorta is dramatically border forming, and the cardiac silhouette is box-like.

Univentricular hearts of right ventricular morphology are more likely to present with cyanosis than with congestive heart failure because of coexisting pulmonary stenosis.

The length and intensity of the pulmonary stenotic murmur vary inversely with the degree of stenosis. Precordial QRS complexes are stereotyped and show right ventricular hypertrophy patterns with increased amplitude. The chest x-ray discloses a narrow vascular pedicle because the aorta is side by side or anterior to the pulmonary trunk. An outlet chamber is conspicuously absent. Pulmonary vascularity and heart size vary inversely with the severity of pulmonary stenosis and the degree of pulmonary vascular disease.

REFERENCES

1. Abbott, M.E.: Atlas of Congenital Cardiac Disease. New York, The American Heart Association, 1936.
2. Akagi, T., Benson, L.N., Green, M., et al: Ventricular performance before and after Fontan repair for univentricular atrioventricular connection: angiographic and radionuclide assessment. J. Am. Coll. Cardiol. 20:920, 1992.
3. Anderson, R.H.: Weasel words in paediatric cardiology. Single ventricle. Int. J. Cardiol. 2:425, 1983.

4. Anderson, R.H., Arnold, R., Thapar, M.K., et al: Cardiac specialized tissue in hearts with an apparently single ventricular chamber (double inlet left ventricle). Am. J. Cardiol. 33:95, 1974.

5. Niwa, K., Perloff, J.K., Child, J.S., Miner, P.D.: Eisenmenger syndrome in adults: Ventricular septal defect, truncus arteriosus, univentricular heart. J. Am. Coll. Cardiol. 34:223, 1999.

6. Santamore, W.P., Lynch, P.R., Meier, G., et al: Myocardial interaction between the ventricles. J. App. Physiol. 4:362, 1976.

7. Anderson, R.H., Becker, A.E., Wilkinson, J.L., Gerlis, L.M.: Morphogenesis of univentricular hearts. Br. Heart J. 38:558, 1976.

8. Anderson, R.H., Macartney, F.J., Tynan, M., et al: Univentricular atrioventricular connection: The single ventricle trap unsprung. Pediatr. Cardiol. 4:273, 1983.

9. Anderson, R.H., Penkoske, P.A., Zuberbuhler, J.R.: Variable morphology of ventricular septal defect in double inlet left ventricle. Am. J. Cardiol. 55:1561, 1985.

10. Barber, G., Hagler, D.J., Edwards, W.D., et al: Surgical repair of univentricular heart (double inlet left ventricle) with obstructed anterior subaortic outlet chamber. J. Am. Coll. Cardiol. 4:771, 1984.

11. Barry, D.R., Isaac, D.H.: Case of cor triloculare biatriatum and survival to adult life. BMJ 2:921, 1953.

12. Fogel, M.A., Weinberg, P.M., Fellows, K.E., Hoffman, E.A.: A study in ventricular-ventricular interaction: single right ventricles compared with systemic right ventricles in a dual-chambered circulation. Circulation 92:219, 1995.

13. Bevilacqua, M., Sanders, S.P., Van Praagh, S., et al: Double-inlet single left ventricle: Echocardiographic anatomy with emphasis on the morphology of the atrioventricular valves and ventricular septal defect. J. Am. Coll. Cardiol. 18:559, 1991.

14. Bharati, S., Lev, M.: The course of the conduction system in single ventricle and inverted (l) loop and inverted (l) transposition. Circulation 51:723, 1975.

15. Cabrera A., Azcuna, J.I., Bilbao, F.: Single primitive ventricle with d-transposition of the great vessels and atresia of the left AV valve. Am. Heart J. 88:225, 1974.

16. Carey, L.S., Ruttenberg, H.D.: Roentgenographic features of common ventricle with inversion of the infundibulum. Corrected transposition with rudimentary left ventricle. AJR 92:652, 1964.

17. Carns, M.L., Ritchie, G., Musser, M.J.: Unusual case of congenital heart disease in a woman who lived for 44 years and 6 months. Am. Heart J. 21:522, 1941.

18. Chambers, W. N., Criscitello, M. G., and Goodale, F.: Cor triloculare biatriatum. Survival to adult life. Circulation 23:91, 1961.

19. Fogel, M.A., Weinberg, P.M., Gupta, K.B., Rychik J., Hubbard, A., Hoffman, E.A., Haselgrove J.: Mechanics of the single ventricle. A study in ventricular-ventricular interaction II. Circulation 98:330, 1998

20. Davachi, F., and Moller, J. H.: Electrocardiogram and vectorcardiogram in single ventricle. Am. J. Cardiol. 23:19, 1969.

21. De la Cruz, M. V., and Miller, B. L.: Double inlet left ventricle: Two pathologic specimens with comments on the embryology and on the relation to single ventricle. Circulation 37:249, 1968.

22. DiSessa, T. G., Isabel-Jones, J. B., Heins, H., Hernandez, J. G., Bloor, C., and Friedman, W. F.: Two-dimensional echocardiographic features of the univentricular heart. J. Cardiovasc. Ultrasonog. 3:89, 1984.

23. Driscoll, D. J., Staats, B. A., Heise, C. T., Rice, M. J., Puga, F. J., Danielson, G. K., and Ritter, D. G.: Functional single ventricle: Cardiorespiratory response to exercise. J. Am. Coll. Cardiol. 4:337, 1984.

24. Elliott, L. P., and Gedgaudas, E.: The roentgenologic findings in common ventricle with transposition of the great vessels. Radiology 82:850, 1964.

25. Elliott, L. P., Ruttenberg, H. D., Eliot, R. S., and Anderson, R. C.: Vectorial analysis of the electrocardiogram in common ventricle. Br. Heart J. 26:302, 1964.

26. Essed, C. E., Ho, S. Y., Hunter, S., and Anderson, R. H.: Atrioventricular conduction system in univentricular heart of right ventricular type with right-sided rudimentary chamber. Thorax 35:123, 1980.

27. Damiano RJ, La Follette P, Cox JL, Lowe JE, Santamore WP.: Significant left ventricular contribution to right ventricular systolic function. Am J Physiol. 261:H1514, 1991.

28. Freedom, R. M., and Rowe, R. D.: Morphological and topographical variations of the outlet chamber in complex congenital heart disease. Cathet. Cardiovasc. Diagn. 4:345, 1978.

29. Freedom, R. M., Picchio, F., Duncan, W. J., Harder, J. R., Moes, C. A. F., and Rowe, R. D.: The atrioventricular junction in the univentricular heart: A two-dimensional echocardiographic analysis. Pediatr. Cardiol. 3:105, 1982.

30. Freedom, R. M., Sondheimer, H., Dische, R., and Rowe, R. D.: Development of "subaortic stenosis" after pulmonary arterial banding for common ventricle. Am. J. Cardiol. 39:78, 1977.

31. Freireich, A. W., and Nicolson, G. B.: A rare electrocardiographic finding occasionally seen in single ventricle hearts. Am. Heart J. 43:526, 1952.

32. Williams RV, Ritter S, Tani LY, Pogotto LT, Minich LL.: Quantitative assessment of ventricular function in children with single ventricles using the Doppler myocardial performance index. Am J Cardiol. 86:1106, 2000.

33. Ammash NM, Warnes CA.: Survival into adulthood of patients with unoperated single ventricle. Am J Cardiol. 77:543, 1996.

34. Habeck, J., Reinhardt, G., and Findeisen, V.: A case of double inlet left ventricle in a 59-year-old man. Int. J. Cardiol. 30:119, 1991.

35. Hallerman, F. J., Davis, G. D., Ritter, D. G., and Kincaid, O. W.: Roentgenographic features of common ventricle. Radiology 87:409, 1966.

36. Holmes, A. F.: Case of malformation of the heart. Trans. Med. Chir. Soc. Edinburgh 1:252, 1824.

37. Huhta, M. D., Seward, J. B., Tajik, A. J., Hagler, D. J., and Edwards, W. D.: Two-dimensional echocardiographic spectrum of univentricular atrioventricular connection. J. Am. Coll. Cardiol. 5:149, 1985.

38. Hutchins, G. M., Meredith, M. A., and Moore, G. W.: The cardiac malformations. Hum. Pathol. 12:242, 1981.

39. Keeton, B. R., Lie, J. T., McGoon, D. C., Danielson, G. K., Ritter, D. G., and Wallace, R. B.: Anatomy of coronary arteries in univentricular hearts and its surgical implications. Am. J. Cardiol. 43:569, 1979.

40. Kitamura, S., Kawashima, Y., Shimazaki, Y., Mori, T., Nakano, S., Beppu, S., and Kozuka, T.: Characteristics of ventricular function in single ventricle. Circulation 60:849, 1979.

41. Klaus, A. P., Smith, R. M., Schneider, A. B., and Parker, B. M.: Single ventricle with normal relationship of the great vessels and pulmonic stenosis. A case report of an adult with the "Holmes heart." Am. Heart J. 78:530, 1969.

42. Steinberg EH, Danzker DR. Single ventricle with severe pulmonary hypertension: survival into the third decade of life. Am Heart J. 125:1451, 1993.

43. Lev, M.: Pathologic variations of positional variations in cardiac chambers in congenital heart disease. Lab. Invest. 3:71, 1954.

44. Lev, M., Liberthson, R. R., Kirkpatrick, J. R., Eckner, F. A. O., and Arcilla, R. A.: Single (primitive) ventricle. Circulation 39:577, 1969.

45. Macartney, F. J., Partridge, J. B., Scott, O., and Deverall, P. B.: Common or single ventricle: An angiocardiographic and hemodynamic study of 42 patients. Circulation 53:543, 1976.

46. Mandel, A., and Hirsch, V.: Cor triloculare biatriatum. Report of a case with survival to the age of 29 years. Am. Heart J. 66:104, 1963.

47. Marin-Garcia, J., Tandon, R., Moller, J. H., and Edwards, J. E.: Common (single) ventricle with normally related great vessels. Circulation 49:565, 1974.

48. Marin-Garcia, J., Tandon, R., Moller, J. H., and Edwards, J. E.: Single ventricle with transposition. Circulation 49:994, 1974.

49. Mann, J. D.: Cor triloculare biatriatum. Br. Med. J. 1:614, 1907.

50. Mehta, J. B., and Hewlett, R. F. L.: Cor triloculare; unusual adult heart. Br. Heart J. 7:41, 1945.

51. Moodie, D. S., Ritter, D. G., Tajik, A. J., and O'Fallon, W. M.: Longterm follow-up in the unoperated univentricular heart. Am. J. Cardiol. 53:1124, 1984.

52. Morgan, A. D., Krovetz, J., Bartley, T. D., Green, J. R., Jr., Shanklin, D. R., Wheat, M. W., Jr., and Schiebler, G. L.: Clinical features of single ventricle with congenitally corrected transposition. Am. J. Cardiol. 17:379, 1966.

53. Neill, C. A., and Brink, A. J.: Left axis deviation in tricuspid atresia and single ventricle. The electrocardiogram in 36 autopsied cases. Circulation 12:612, 1955.

54. Parikh, S. R., Huritz, R. A., Caldwell, R. L., and Girod, D. A.: Ventricular function in the single ventricle before and after Fontan surgery. Am. J. Cardiol. 67:1390, 1991.

55. Peacock, T. B.: On Malformations of the Human Heart. London, John Churchill, 1858.

56. Penkoske, P. A., Freedom, R. M., Williams, W. G., Trusler, G. A., and Rowe, R. D.: Surgical palliation of subaortic stenosis in the univentricular heart. J. Thorac. Cardiovasc. Surg. 87:767, 1984.

57. Child JS: Transthoracic and transesophageal echocardiographic imaging: Anatomic and hemodynamic assessment. In Perloff JK and

Child JS.: Congenital Heart Disease in Adults, 2nd edition, W B Saunders, Co. Philadelphia, 1998, p 91.

58. Quero, M.: Atresia of the left atrioventricular orifice associated with a Holmes heart. Circulation 42:739, 1970.

59. Quero, M.: Coexistence of single ventricle with atresia of one atrioventricular orifice. Circulation 46:794, 1972.

60. Quero-Jimenez, M., Casanova-Gomez, M., Castro-Gussoni, C., Moreno-Granado, F., Perez-Martinez, V., and Merino-Batres, G.: Electrocardiographic findings in single ventricle and related conditions. Am. Heart J. 86:449, 1973.

61. Rice, M. J., Seward, J. B., Edwards, W. D., Hagler, D. J., Danielson, G. K., Puga, F. J., and Tajik, A. J.: Straddling atrioventricular valve. Am. J. Cardiol. 55:505, 1985.

62. Rogers, H. M., and Edwards, J. E.: Cor triloculare biatriatum: An analysis of the clinical and pathologic features of nine cases. Am. Heart J. 41:299, 1951.

63. Sagar, K. B., and Mauck, H. P.: Univentricular heart in adults: Report of nine cases with review of the literature. Am. Heart J. 110:1059, 1985.

64. Sano, T., Ogawa, M., Yabuuchi, H., Matsuda, H., Nakano, S., Shimazaki, Y., Taniguchi, K., Arisawa, J., Hirose, H., and Kawashima, Y.: Quantitative cineangiographic analysis of ventricular volume and mass in patients with single ventricle: Relation to ventricular morphologies. Circulation 77:62, 1988.

65. Shaher, R. M.: The electrocardiogram in single ventricle. Br. Heart J. 25:465, 1963.

66. Shapiro, S. R., Ruckman, R. N., Kapur, S., Chandra, R., Galioto, F. M., Perry, L. W., and Scott, L. P.: Single ventricle with truncus arteriosus in siblings. Am. Heart J. 102:456, 1981.

67. Shinebourne, E. A., Lan, K., Calcaterra, G., and Anderson, R. H.: Univentricular heart of right ventricular type. Am. J. Cardiol. 46:439, 1980.

68. Shiraishi, H., and Silverman, N. H.: Echocardiographic spectrum of double inlet left ventricle: Evaluation of interventricular communication. J. Am. Coll. Cardiol. 15:1401, 1990.

69. Soto, B., Bertranou, E. G., Bream, P. R., Souza, A., and Bargeron, L. M.: Angiographic study of univentricular heart of right ventricular type. Circulation 60:1325, 1979.

70. Stein, J. I., Smallhorn, J. F., Coles, J. G., Williams, W. G., Trusler, G. A., and Freedom, R. M.: Common atrioventricular valve guarding double inlet atrioventricular connexion: Natural history and surgical results in 76 cases. Int. J. Cardiol. 28:7, 1990.

71. Tandon, R., Becker, A. E., Moller, J. H., and Edwards, J. E.: Double inlet left ventricle. Straddling tricuspid valve. Br. Heart J. 36:747, 1974.

72. Thiene, G., Daliento, L., Frescura, C., De Tommasi, M., Macartney, F. J., and Anderson, R. H.: Atresia of the left atrioventricular orifice. Br. Heart J. 45:393, 1981.

73. Thies, W. R., Soto, B., Diethelm, E., Bargeron, L. M., and Pacifico, A. D.: Angiographic anatomy of hearts with one ventricular chamber: The true single ventricle. Am. J. Cardiol. 55:1363, 1985.

74. Van Praagh, R., David, I., and Van Praagh, S.: What is a ventricle? The single ventricle trap. Pediatr. Cardiol. 2:79, 1982.

75. Van Praagh, R., Ongley, P. A., and Swan, H. J. C.: Anatomic types of single or common ventricle in man. Morphologic and geometric aspects of 60 necropsied cases. Am. J. Cardiol. 13:367, 1964.

76. Weigel, T. J., Driscoll, D. J., and Michels, V. V.: Occurrence of congenital heart defects in siblings of patients with univentricular heart and tricuspid atresia. Am. J. Cardiol. 64:768, 1989.

77. Wenink, A. C. G.: Development of the human cardiac conduction system. J. Anat. 121:617, 1976.

78. Wenink, A. C. G.: The conduction tissues in primitive ventricle with outlet chamber. J. Thorac. Cardiovasc. Surg. 75:747, 1978.

79. Wilkinson, J. L., Anderson, R. H., Arnold, R., Hamilton, D. I., and Smith, A.: The conduction tissues in primitive ventricular hearts with an outlet chamber. Circulation 53:930, 1976.

80. Young, A. H.: Rare anomaly of the human heart—a three chambered heart in an adult aged 35 years. J. Anat. Physiol. Lond. 41:190, 1907.

81. Piran S, Veldtman G, Siu S, Webb GD, Liu PP. Heart failure and ventricular dysfunction in patients with single or systemic right ventricles. Circulation 105:1189, 2002.

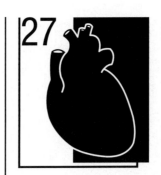

Complete Transposition of the Great Arteries

In 1797, Matthew Baillie described "a singular malformation in which the pulmonary artery arises from the left ventricle and the aorta from the right ventricle."[9] Seventeen years later, John Farre used the term *transposition* to characterize Baillie's singular malformation.[31] Each great artery is placed across the ventricular septum: *positio* means "placed," and *trans* means "cross." The term *transposition of the great arteries* is used herein in its original sense to signify that the aorta arises from the morphologic right ventricle and the pulmonary trunk arises from the morphologic left ventricle—ventriculoarterial discordance (Figs. 27–1 through 27–4).[24–26,30,56] The designation *complete* indicates that ventriculoarterial discordance is associated with atrioventricular concordance. The single discordance between ventricles and great arteries makes the transposition physiologically complete. The alignments result in a unique extrauterine circulation in which two independent circulations function in parallel (Fig. 27–5). *Congenitally corrected transposition* (see Chapter 6) refers to atrioventricular *and* ventriculoarterial discordance. The double discordance physiologically corrects the transposition, which is therefore not complete, so there is one circulation in series, as in the normal heart. The term *malposition of the great arteries* refers to abnormal spatial relations but concordant ventricular alignments.[3,22,108]

The term D-*transposition* is synonymous with *complete transposition*. Because D- refers to a dextro (rightward) bend in the bulboventricular loop, the designation is appropriate because virtually all examples of complete transposition of the great arteries are accompanied by a D-ventricular loop (see Figs. 27–2A and 27–4A). Segmental analysis identifies situs solitus (S), a dextro-ventricular loop (D) and a rightward (D) and anterior aorta (see Figs. 27–2A, 27–3, and 27–4). In about one third of cases, the aorta is anterior and to the left, directly anterior or, rarely,

posterior to the pulmonary trunk.[24,30,109,113,119] The great arteries rise in parallel and do not cross, as in the normal heart (see Figs. 27–1, 27–34, and 27–35).[70,102]

The origin and course of the coronary arteries are physiologically unimportant but anatomically pivotal because of the arterial switch operation for complete transposition (see Chapter 32).[2,28,36,75,86,95,99] The morphologic right coronary artery is concordant with the morphologic right ventricle, and the morphologic left coronary artery is concordant with the morphologic left ventricle. Two aortic

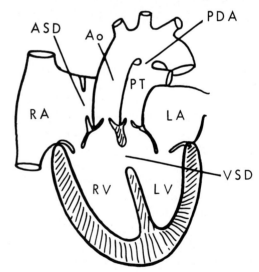

Figure 27–1

Illustration of complete transposition of the great arteries. The aorta (Ao) arises from the morphologic right ventricle (RV), is convex to the right, and is positioned to the right of and anterior to the pulmonary trunk (PT), which arises from the morphologic left ventricle (LV). The great arteries are parallel to each other and do not cross. The systemic and pulmonary circulations are joined by three types of communications: atrial septal defect (ASD), ventricular septal defect (VSD), and patent ductus arteriosus (PDA). LA, left atrium; RA, right atrium.

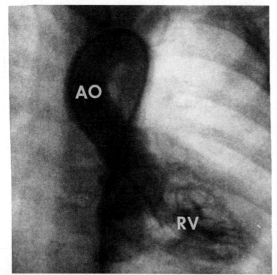

A

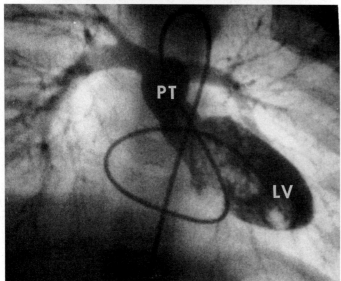

B

Figure 27–2

Ventriculograms from an 8-month-old boy with complete transposition of the great arteries, a patent foramen ovale, an intact ventricular septum, and a closed ductus arteriosus. A balloon atrial septostomy was performed at 6 days of age. *A,* The right ventricle (RV) gives rise to the ascending aorta (AO), which is convex to the right. *B,* The left ventricle (LV) gives rise to a centrally placed pulmonary trunk (PT) with a rightward inclination. The great arteries are parallel to each other and do not cross. Blood flow in the left pulmonary artery is less than jblood flow in the right pulmonary artery.

sinuses face the right ventricular outflow tract (Fig. 27–6) irrespective of the spatial relations between the ascending aorta and the pulmonary artery.[36,75,86,99] The two facing sinuses are the left sinus (#1) and the posterior sinus (#2).[36,86,99] The right aortic sinus does not face the right ventricular outflow tract (see Fig. 27–6).

Dual sinus origin indicates that a coronary artery arises from each of the two facing sinuses (see Fig. 27–6).[99] Dual sinus origin accounts for about 90% of cases,[12,75,99] in the majority of which the left main coronary artery arises from the left aortic sinus and gives rise to the anterior descending and circumflex coronary arteries, and the right coronary artery arises by a single ostium from the posterior aortic sinus (see Fig. 27–6A).[99] In the less common type of dual sinus origin, the left anterior descending coronary artery originates from the left aortic sinus, and the circumflex and right coronary arteries originate by a single ostium in the posterior aortic sinus (see Fig. 27–6B).[99] *Single sinus origin* indicates that both coronary arteries arise from one of the two but not both of the facing sinuses by a single

ostium or by multiple ostia.[99] In a small minority of cases of single sinus origin, the left anterior descending, circumflex, and right coronary arteries arise by ostia in the posterior aortic sinus.[75,99] The sinus node artery originates from the proximal right coronary artery and courses upward and to the right, partially imbedded in the limbus of the atrial septum. An aberrant anterior descending coronary artery may pass intramurally between the aortic root and pulmonary trunk.[37,63]

The incidence of complete transposition of the great arteries is estimated at 1 in 2300 to 1 in 5100 live births.[41,57] The malformation represents approximately 5% to 8% of congenital cardiac malformations but accounts for 25% of deaths from congenital heart disease in the first year of life.[58] The morphogenesis of the ventriculoarterial discordance that characterizes complete transposition focuses on the conus as the crucial connection between the ventricles and the great arteries.[20] The segmental components of the heart—the atria, the ventricles, and the great arteries—appear at different developmental stages.[24] The straight

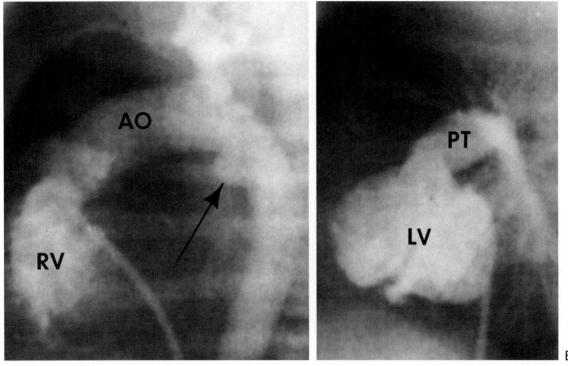

Figure 27–3

Lateral ventriculograms from a 4-day-old boy with complete transposition of the great arteries, a patent foramen ovale, and an intact ventricular septum. A balloon atrial septostomy was performed at 4 days of age. *A*, The aortic root (AO) curves anteriorly as it arises from the morphologic right ventricle (RV), so the plane of the aortic valve is tilted upward. *Arrow* points to a dimple at the aortic insertion of the closed ductus. *B*, The posterior pulmonary trunk (PT) arises from the morphologic left ventricle (LV).

heart tube is formed from primordia of the trabeculated portions of both ventricles. During looping, the atria are at the caudal end of the embryonic tube and the conus is at the cephalic end of the tube. When the truncus appears, the developing heart has three segments—atrial, ventricular, and arterial.[24] The ventral end of the arterial segment is continuous with the conus, and the dorsal end is continuous with the aortic arches. The spiral division that develops within the truncus progresses from the aortic arches toward the truncal ridges. Conal development is then pivotal.[20] The subaortic portion of the conus persists in complete transposition of the great arteries, while the

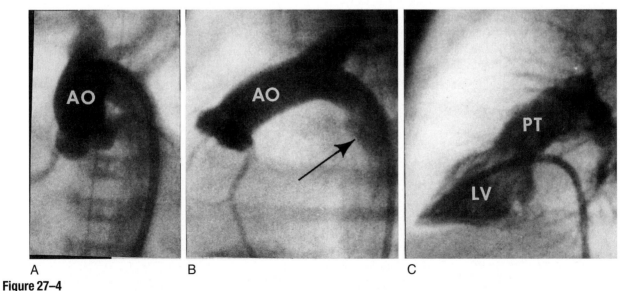

Figure 27–4

Angiocardiograms from a 3-day-old boy with complete transposition of the great arteries, a patent foramen ovale, an intact ventricular septum, and a closed ductus arteriosus. *A*, Aortogram (anteroposterior) showing a midline ascending aorta (AO) with slight rightward convexity. *B*, Lateral aortogram showing the anterior position of the aortic root with the plane of the aortic valve tilted upward. *Arrow* points to a dimple at the aortic end of the closed ductus. *C*, Lateral left ventriculogram showing the posterior pulmonary trunk (PT) arising from the morphologic left ventricle (LV).

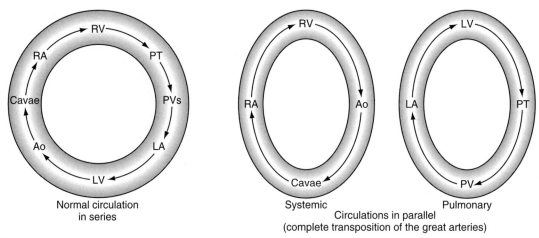

Figure 27–5

Illustrations of the normal circulation and the distinctive circulation in transposition of the great arteries. In the normal heart, there is a single circulation in series with flow from the right ventricle (RV) into the pulmonary trunk (PT), pulmonary veins (PV), left atrium (LA), left ventricle (LV), aorta (Ao), systemic venous bed, venae cavae, right atrium (RA), and back to the right ventricle. In complete transposition of the great arteries, there are two circulations in parallel. The systemic circulation is characterized by flow from the right ventricle into the aorta, systemic venous bed, venae cavae, right atrium, and back to the right ventricle. The pulmonary circulation is characterized by flow from left ventricle into pulmonary trunk, pulmonary veins, left atrium, and back to the left ventricle.

subpulmonary conus is absorbed (conal inversion). The aortic valve moves anteriorly and the pulmonary valve moves inferoposteriorly into fibrous continuity with the mitral valve. The maldeveloped conus is inappropriate for the ventricular loop, so the great arteries are discordant relative to their ventricles of origin. There is pulmonary/mitral continuity because a left-sided subpulmonary conus is absent, and there is aortic/tricuspid discontinuity because a right-sided subaortic conus is present. Aortic/tricuspid discontinuity causes the aortic valve to lie superior to the pulmonary valve and causes the ascending aorta to lie parallel to the pulmonary trunk.

The ductus arteriosus in complete transposition is usually closed or insignificantly patent (Fig. 27–7, and see Figs. 27–3 and 27–4) and is only occasionally widely patent (Fig. 27–8).[116] Interatrial communications take the form of a patent foramen ovale or an ostium secundum atrial septal defect.[13,30,34,56] Ventricular septal defects are inlet, muscular, perimembranous, or infundibular.[52,65,67,68,77] Inlet defects caused by malalignment with the atrial septum

result in a straddling tricuspid valve.[8] Perimembranous ventricular septal defects extend into the inlet septum and into the muscular septum. Infundibular septal defects result from malalignment of the infundibular septum, which can be shifted leftward and posterior or rightward and anterior, and the malalignment defect can be subaortic, subpulmonary, or doubly committed.[52,65,67,68,77]

Pulmonary stenosis is represented by obstruction to left ventricular outflow and occurs in approximately 15% of cases of complete transposition.[30,87,96,97,103,104,111] Fixed subpulmonary stenosis is characterized by a circumferential fibrous membrane or diaphragm (Fig. 27–9A), a fibromuscular ridge, herniating tricuspid leaflet tissue, anomalous septal attachments of the mitral valve, accessory mitral leaflet tissue, tissue tags from the membranous septum, and hypertrophy of the anterolateral muscle bundle.[30,87,96,97,104,111] Leftward and posterior deviation of the infundibular septum causes tunnel or tubular subpulmonary stenosis.[51,65,67,68,77,87,97] Pulmonary valve stenosis is uncommon.[87,96]

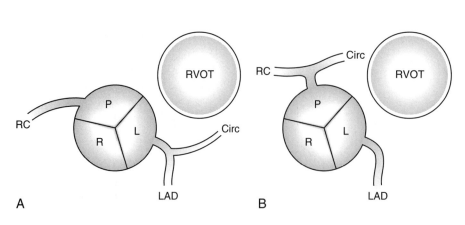

Figure 27–6

Illustrations of the coronary artery origins in complete transposition of the great arteries. The two coronary sinuses that face the right ventricular outflow tract (RVOT) are the left sinus (L) (sinus #1) and the posterior sinus (P) (sinus #2). The right (R) sinus does not face the right ventricular outflow tract. *A*, The left main coronary artery arises from left sinus and branches into the circumflex (Circ) and left anterior descending (LAD) arteries. The right coronary artery (RC) arises from the posterior sinus (P). *B*, The left main coronary artery arises from the posterior sinus (P) and branches into the right coronary artery (RC) and the circumflex coronary artery (Circ). The left anterior descending coronary artery arises from the left sinus (L).

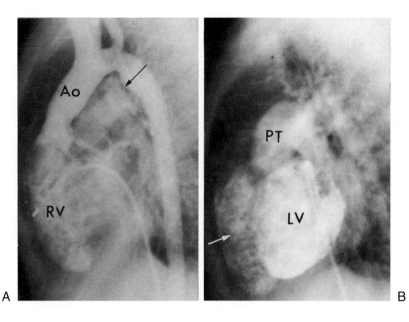

Figure 27–7

Lateral angiocardiograms from an 18-month-old girl with complete transposition of the great arteries, an atrial septal defect, a nonrestrictive ventricular septal defect, and a restrictive ductus arteriosus. *A*, The right ventricle (RV) gives rise to an anterior aorta (Ao) whose valve is in a horizontal plane. *Arrow* points to a small patent ductus. *B*, The left ventricle (LV) gives rise to a posterior pulmonary trunk (PT). The right ventricle (*arrow*) is opacified through the ventricular septal defect. This unoperated patient is alive and functional with pulmonary vascular disease at the age of 43 years.

Dynamic subpulmonary stenosis is not present at birth but develops during the first few weeks of life and is associated with systolic anterior motion of the anterior mitral leaflet (see Figs. 27–9B and 27–36).[7,87,103,104] The obstruction is *dynamic* because the degree varies spontaneously and is augmented by isoproterenol and reduced by beta blockade.[7] The development of dynamic subpulmonary stenosis coincides with a fall in pulmonary vascular resistance and a fall in left ventricular systolic pressure in the face of persistent systemic systolic pressure in the adjacent right ventricle. Systemic right ventricular pressure results in systolic movement of the base of the ventricular septum into the outflow tract of the adjacent low-pressure left ventricle. Systolic anterior motion of the anterior mitral leaflet is then caused by the Venturi effect that is generated by hyperkinetic ejection of a volume-overloaded left ventricle into a low-resistance pulmonary vascular bed (see Fig. 27–9B).

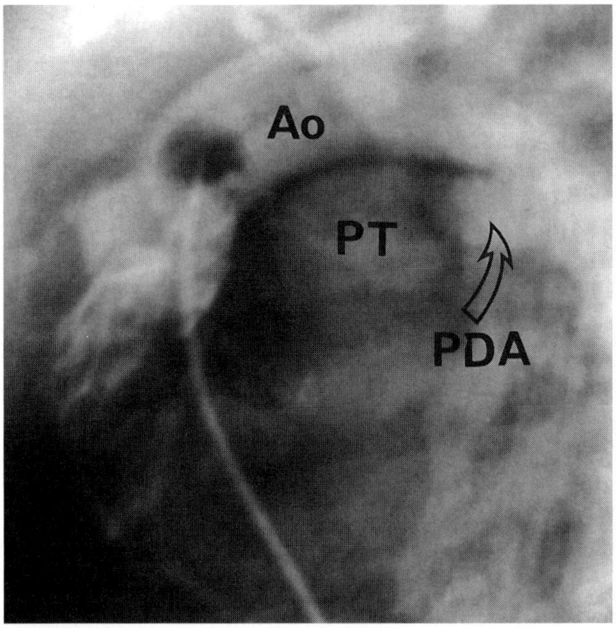

Subaortic stenosis is caused by rightward and anterior deviation of a malaligned infundibular septum.[52,55,65,67,68,77,91,117] Aortic arch anomalies are represented by hypoplasia, coarctation, and interruption and have been attributed to reduced flow during morphogenesis.[51,64,67,68,77]

Juxtaposition of the atrial appendages refers to an anomaly in which both atrial appendages or the left appendage and part of the right appendage are adjacent to each other (juxtaposed) on the same side of the heart. Juxtaposition is a rare congenital anomaly that is strongly associated with complete transposition of the great arteries[11,19,26,105,106] and occurs in 2% to 6% of cases of anatomically corrected malpositions.[11,22] Juxtaposition reduces the size and volume of the right atrium. Left-sided juxtaposition is six times as frequent as right-sided juxtaposition. There is female preponderance with juxtaposition of the atrial appendages, in contrast to marked male preponderance with complete transposition of the great arteries without juxtaposition (see The History).[26]

Tricuspid valve abnormalities occur in about 30% of patients with complete transposition and inlet ventricular septal defects.[8,43,67] The abnormalities include straddling or overriding of chordae, overriding of the tricuspid annulus, abnormal chordal attachments, and, less commonly, tricuspid valve dysplasia, accessory tricuspid tissue, and double orifice tricuspid valve. Mitral valve abnormalities occur in 20% to 30% of necropsy specimens of complete transposition. Mitral abnormalities include a cleft anterior leaflet, straddling of the mitral valve, abnormal size or position,

Figure 27–8

Lateral aortogram from a 3-day-old girl with complete transposition of the great arteries and a large patent ductus arteriosus (PDA, *arrow*) that was the only communication between the two circulations. Shunting was essentially unidirectional from the anterior aorta (AO) through the ductus into the posterior pulmonary trunk (PT).

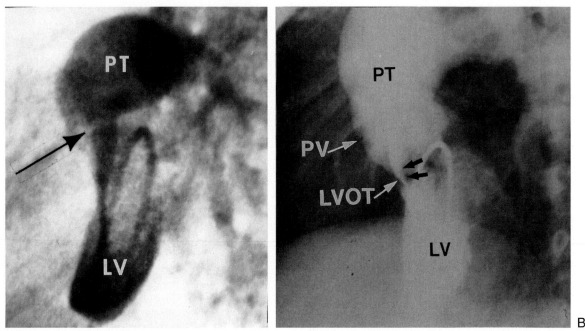

Figure 27–9
A, Lateral left ventriculogram (LV) from a 9-month-old girl with complete transposition of the great arteries and intact ventricular septum. *Arrow* points to a subpulmonary membrane or diaphragm. Left ventricular systolic pressure was 60 mm Hg and pulmonary artery systolic pressure was 18 mm Hg. The pulmonary trunk (PT) is dilated. *B,* Left ventriculogram from a 3-week-old male neonate with complete transposition of the great arteries, intact ventricular septum, and dynamic subpulmonary stenosis. Systolic anterior motion of the anterior mitral leaflet (*paired unmarked black arrows*) caused obstruction of the left ventricular outflow tract (LVOT). PT, pulmonary trunk; PV, pulmonary valve.

anomalous mitral tissue strands, redundant mitral valve tissue, and abnormal papillary muscles.[66,67,84]

Matthew Baillie described the anatomic features of the singular malformation of complete transposition of the great arteries.[9] The malformation is even more singular in physiologic terms. The normal heart is associated with a single circulation in series (see Fig. 27–5) with flow from right ventricle into pulmonary artery, pulmonary veins, left atrium, left ventricle, aorta, systemic venous bed, venae cavae, right atrium, and back to the right ventricle. Blood at any given location must traverse both sides of the circulation before returning to that location (see Fig. 27–5). In complete transposition of the great arteries, there are two circulations in parallel (see Fig. 27–5). The systemic circulation is characterized by flow from right ventricle into aorta, systemic venous bed, venae cavae, right atrium, and back to the right ventricle. The pulmonary circulation is characterized by flow from the left ventricle into the pulmonary artery, pulmonary capillary bed, pulmonary veins, left atrium, and back to the left ventricle. Blood within the systemic circulation recirculates within the systemic circulation, and blood within the pulmonary circulation recirculates within the pulmonary circulation. The two circulations do not cross unless they are joined by communications at the atrial, ventricular, or great arterial level, upon which survival depends. These communications permit blood from the systemic circulation to enter the pulmonary circulation for oxygenation and permit oxygenated blood from the pulmonary circulation to enter the systemic circulation.

The net volume of blood exchanged between the systemic and pulmonary circulations must be isovolumetric over short periods of time or the donor circulation would be rapidly depleted and the recipient circulation would be rapidly overloaded. The amount of blood exchanged between the two parallel circulations is small relative to the volume recirculating within each circulation. The volume of effective bidirectional mixing depends on the location and size of the communication that joins the two circulations and on the magnitude of pulmonary blood flow.[39,59,74,104] Survival is tightly coupled to the delicate interplay between the intercirculatory communications and pulmonary blood flow. The circulation in a neonate with complete transposition, a restrictive foramen ovale, and a nonpatent ductus arteriosus is represented by the circulations in parallel illustrated in Figure 27–5. The tendency for neonatal pulmonary vascular resistance to fall prompts an increase in pulmonary blood flow, but that advantage is lost because the oxygenated blood cannot enter the systemic vascular bed. The value of an adequate interatrial communication is dramatized by the immediate response to balloon atrial septostomy.[78,80] An adequate interatrial communication permits quantitatively equal bidirectional shunting that is right-to-left during ventricular diastole and left-to-right during ventricular systole.[59,60,88]

An adequately sized ventricular septal defect permits bidirectional shunting that is determined by instantaneous pressure differences between the two ventricles. When pulmonary vascular resistance is low, there is a preferential right-to-left systolic shunting into the low resistance pulmonary circulation and a preferential left-to-right diastolic shunting away from the volume-loaded left ventricle. A large patent ductus arteriosus (Fig. 27–8) is initially accompanied by bidirectional flow that is replaced by virtually exclusive systemic to pulmonary flow as pulmonary vascular resistance falls.[116] The temporary value of ductal patency is witnessed by the response to prostaglandin-induced ductal dilatation as a pharmacologic bridge to balloon septostomy.[54] Because ductal flow is essentially unidirectional, the pulmonary circulation becomes volume overloaded with no egress except a restrictive foramen ovale.

Low pulmonary vascular resistance with an increase in pulmonary blood flow provides a large volume of oxygenated blood for intercirculatory mixing.[59] Elevated pulmonary vascular resistance and pulmonary stenosis decrease pulmonary blood flow and result in a smaller volume of oxygenated blood for intercirculatory mixing. The increase in left ventricular afterload incurred by pulmonary vascular disease or pulmonary stenosis results in a reduction in left ventricular compliance that adversely affects intracardiac mixing.[59,60,104] Hypoxemia provokes a fall in systemic vascular resistance and an increase in the volume of unsaturated blood recirculating in the systemic vascular bed.[59,60]

The geometry of the left ventricle in complete transposition is governed by volume overload imposed by increased pulmonary blood flow and pressure overload imposed by increased pulmonary vascular resistance or pulmonary stenosis. Right ventricular free wall thickness exceeds normal in the neonate and outstrips left ventricular wall thickness. Septal thickness and right ventricular free wall thickness then increase in parallel, so the septum becomes disproportionately thick relative to the left ventricular wall.[38,39,44,46,49,53,61,98] When the ventricular septum bows into a low-pressure left ventricle, the right ventricle becomes spherical and the left ventricle resembles a prolate ellipsoid.[107]

When left ventricular pressure is elevated, the septum flattens or bows into the right ventricle, resulting in a more normal septal position and better left ventricular function.[38,46] During the first few weeks of life, left ventricular function is normal, but mass does not increase in proportion to volume,[23] a discrepancy that is responsible for decreased left ventricular function. The right ventricle functions normally at birth, but contractility and ejection fraction then decline.[23,45] Mass, geometry, and the coronary circulation conspire to make a morphologic subaortic right ventricle ill equipped to support the systemic circulation (see Chapter 6).

Pulmonary vascular disease is prevalent in patients with complete transposition of the great arteries, especially in the presence of a nonrestrictive ventricular septal defect[21,53,71,102,104,115,120] or a large patent ductus arteriosus.[16,116] Grade 3 or 4 Heath-Edwards changes of pulmonary vascular disease are found in 20% of infants before 2 months of age and in about 80% after 1 year.[21,42] A reduction in the number of intra-acinar pulmonary arteries has been identified by quantitative morphometric studies.[27,79] Vasoconstriction of pulmonary arterioles is induced by hypoxemic blood carried in systemic arterial collaterals, accelerating the pulmonary vascular disease.[6] Early pulmonary vascular disease is more prevalent with a nonrestrictive ventricular septal defect and complete transposition than with an equivalent isolated ventricular septal defect.[6,42,112] Even with an isolated atrial septal defect, the incidence of pulmonary vascular disease is about 6%, although progression is slower.[21,53,71,72]

The History

Males outnumber females by a ratio as high as 4:1,[30,33,58] unless there is juxtaposition of the atrial appendages.[26] Complete transposition of the great arteries seldom occurs in first-born infants, but a twofold increase in incidence has been reported in offspring of mothers who have had three or more pregnancies.[58,74] Familial recurrence of concordant cardiac defects within affected family members supports monogenic or oligogenic inheritance in selected pedigrees.[14] Complete transposition and congenitally corrected transposition sometimes segregate in the same family, probably because of monogenic transmission, supporting a pathogenetic link between complete transposition and looping disorders.[14]

Cyanosis begins as early as the first day of life in more than 90% of infants with an intact ventricular septum.[57,74] Severe pulmonary stenosis or atresia results in intense neonatal cyanosis. Mild cyanosis with delayed onset is a feature of complete transposition with a nonrestrictive ventricular septal defect[46,58,74,94] or patent ductus arteriosus.[116] A large isolated ductus (see Fig. 27–8) is associated with severe congestive heart failure in the first few days of life. Spontaneous closure results in a sudden fall in systemic arterial oxygen saturation, rapid clinical deterioration, and death.[116] Dynamic subpulmonary stenosis or a rise in pulmonary vascular resistance curtails pulmonary blood flow and alleviates congestive heart failure at the expense of increasing hypoxemia. Pulmonary stenosis is occasionally responsible for hypercyanotic spells characterized by intense cyanosis, tachypnea, extreme irritability, and hypothermia but seldom by loss of consciousness.[7,74] Squatting is rare.[74]

Survival is tightly coupled to the delicate interplay between intercirculatory communications and pulmonary blood flow.[10] The neonate with complete transposition depends for survival on connections between the systemic and pulmonary circulations (see earlier). The older infant depends for survival on adequate pulmonary blood flow. Outcome is bleak, with an overall death rate of 30% in the first week, 50% in the first month, and 90% in the first year.[13,58,89,101] Survival is poorest when the foramen ovale is restrictive, the ventricular septum is intact, and the ductus is closed. The salutary effect of an adequately sized interatrial communication is underscored by the immediate response to balloon septostomy (see earlier),[80] after which 75% of patients survive for 6 months, 65% survive for 1 year, and many survive into their teens.[78] A nonrestrictive ventricular septal defect with pulmonary vascular disease carries a 6-month survival rate of about 30% and a 1-year survival rate of about 20%. Moderate pulmonary stenosis improves longevity by regulating pulmonary blood flow, with three quarters of patients surviving for a year or more. The majority of patients who reach their teens have a nonrestrictive ventricular septal defect with pulmonary vascular disease or pulmonary stenosis.[51] Sporadic examples of unusual longevity have been recorded in the third, fourth, and fifth decades (see Fig. 27–7),[1,47,64,73,92] and complete transposition of the great arteries was confirmed at necropsy in a 56-year-old patient.[122] Brain abscess is rare in patients younger than 2 years of age but reportedly has a predilection for complete transposition of the great arteries or Fallot's tetralogy.[32]

Physical Appearance

Birth weights in infants with complete transposition are on average greater than normal, with a substantial proportion above 8 pounds,[5,85] in contrast to newborns with other forms of congenital heart disease, who average less than normal birth weights for gestational age.[58] The illusion of robust health is soon dispelled by the catabolic effects of congestive heart failure (Fig. 27–10).[58,74] Increased anteroposterior chest dimensions are associated with hyperinflation of the lungs (see The X-Ray). Intense early cyanosis reflects poor intercirculatory mixing and low pulmonary blood flow. Mild delayed cyanosis reflects good intercirculatory mixing and increased pulmonary blood flow. Complete transposition with a large patent ductus, pulmonary vascular disease, and an intact ventricular septum is associated with reversed differential cyanosis—feet less cyanotic than hands—because oxygenated blood from the pulmonary artery enters the aorta distal to the left subclavian artery and flows selectively to the lower extremities (see Chapter 19).[16,74,116] Deeply cyanotic patients with pulmonary vascular disease or severe pulmonary stenosis have varicosities of the scalp and arms because of the large volume of highly unsaturated blood in the systemic circulation.[74]

The Arterial Pulse

In 1957, Cleland described peripheral arterial pulses that were of remarkably full volume (Fig. 27–11) with visible pulsations of the dorsalis pedis and posterior tibial arteries.[123] Shaher attributed the bounding pulses, the scalp varices, and the warm extremities to the large volume of highly unsaturated blood recirculating in the hyperkinetic low-resistance systemic vascular bed. Bounding pulses are not associated with patent ductus arteriosus because ductal flow is essentially systolic from aorta into pulmonary trunk and does not enter the right ventricle from which the aorta and systemic arteries arise.[116] Diminished femoral pulses call attention to complete transposition with coarctation of the aorta and anterior and rightward deviation of the infundibular septum (subaortic stenosis).

The Jugular Venous Pulse

The jugular venous pulse is elevated under two widely divergent physiologic circumstances. The first and most

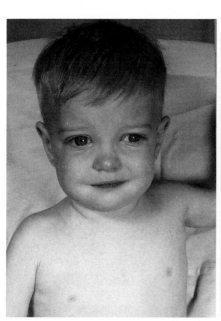
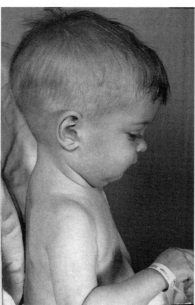

A   B

Figure 27–10
Physical appearance of a 15-month-old boy with complete transposition of the great arteries. Birth weight was 9 pounds 2 ounces. The child's head is large, although his body and arms have lost the robust appearance with which he was born.

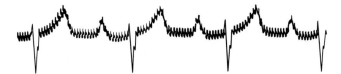

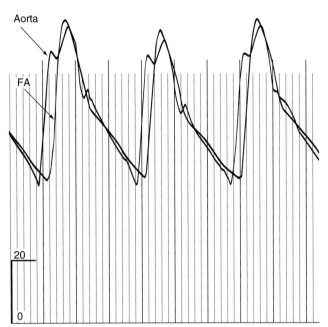

Figure 27–11
Aortic and femoral artery pulses (FA) from a deeply cyanosed 15-month-old boy with complete transposition of the great arteries, a ventricular septal defect, and severe pulmonary stenosis. The pulse pressure is wide because the diastolic pressure is low. The rate of the rise is brisk, and the aortic pulse (*upper arrow*) is bisferiens (twin peaked).

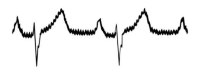

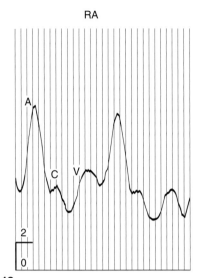

Figure 27–12
Right atrial pressure pulse (RA) from the deeply cyanotic 15-month-old boy referred to in Figure 27–11. The A wave is dominant, and the mean right atrial pressure is elevated.

common is congestive heart failure that accompanies a nonrestrictive ventricular septal defect with low pulmonary vascular resistance. The second circumstance is right ventricular failure in deeply cyanotic patients with a large volume of unsaturated blood recirculating through the right ventricle and right atrium (Fig. 27–12).

Precordial Movement and Palpation

The right ventricular impulse is transiently normal or nearly normal in neonates with complete transposition of the great arteries. The impulse becomes prominent in response to congestive heart failure that accompanies a nonrestrictive ventricular septal defect and is especially prominent when the right ventricle is overloaded by the large volume of unoxygenated blood that recirculates in a hypervolemic hyperdynamic systemic vascular bed.

A loud palpable second heart sound at the left base originates in the aortic valve (Fig. 27–13) because the transposed aorta is anterior. A dilated hypertensive posterior pulmonary trunk does not transmit its impulse. A right aortic arch occurs in about 8% of patients with complete transposition

and occasionally reveals itself as a right sternoclavicular impulse, especially when the aortic root is pulsatile and hyperkinetic in deeply cyanotic patients.[62] A left ventricular impulse is not identified in neonates and is overshadowed by

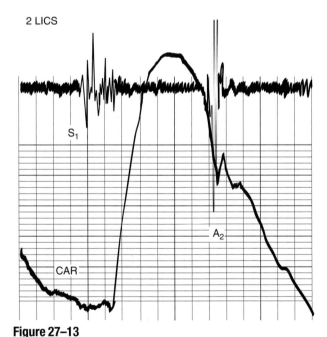

Figure 27–13
Phonocardiogram and carotid pulse (CAR) from a 2-year-old boy with complete transposition of the great arteries, a nonrestrictive atrial defect, low pulmonary vascular resistance, and increased pulmonary blood flow. The aortic component of the second heart sound (A₂) was loud because the aortic root was anterior. There were no murmurs. 2 LICS, second left intercostal space; S₁, first heart sound.

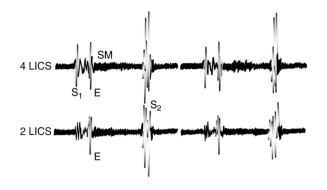

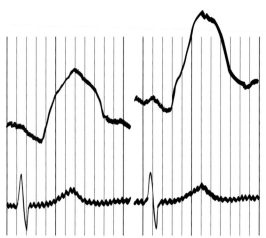

Figure 27–14

Tracings from a 5-year-old girl with complete transposition of the great arteries, a nonrestrictive ventricular septal defect, and pulmonary vascular disease. The soft decrescendo systolic murmur (SM) at the fourth left intercostal space (4 LICS) was caused by systolic shunting across the ventricular septal defect. The pulmonary ejection sound (E) originated in a dilated hypertensive posterior pulmonary trunk. 2 LICS, second left intercostal space. The second heart sound (S_2) was single because of synchronous closure of the aortic and pulmonary valves. The second sound was loud because of amplification caused by the anterior aortic root in conjunction with amplification caused by the dilated hypertensive posterior pulmonary trunk. Carotid pulse is shown below.

the right ventricular impulse in older patients. The left ventricle is palpable when a nonrestrictive ventricular septal defect exists with low pulmonary vascular resistance because the left ventricle is both volume overloaded and pressure overloaded. The left ventricle is seldom palpable despite volume overload when there is a nonrestrictive atrial septal defect and an intact ventricular septum (see Fig. 27–28) because ejection is at a low systolic pressure.

Auscultation

A pulmonary ejection sound (Fig. 27–14) originates in a dilated hypertensive posterior pulmonary trunk (Fig. 27–15).[74,118] The ejection sound does not selectively decrease during inspiration because the transposed pulmonary trunk arises from the left ventricle. Aortic ejection sounds occasionally occur when complete transposition is accompanied by a dilated aortic root associated with leftward and posterior malalignment of the infundibular septum (subaortic stenosis).

Midsystolic flow murmurs originate in the transposed anterior aorta, especially when the systemic circulation is hypervolemic and hyperkinetic. Midsystolic flow murmurs potentially originate in a dilated posterior pulmonary trunk (see Fig. 27–15), but these inherently soft murmurs are likely to be rendered inaudible by the anterior aorta (Fig. 27–16, and see Fig. 27–13).

A holosystolic murmur of ventricular septal defect awaits the neonatal fall in pulmonary vascular resistance to express itself (Fig. 27–17; see Chapter 17).[74,118] A subsequent rise in pulmonary resistance shortens and ultimately abolishes the murmur,[76] as in patients with Eisenmenger syndrome (see Fig. 27–14). A restrictive ventricular septal defect generates a holosystolic murmur or a soft early systolic murmur that disappears when the defect spontaneously closes.

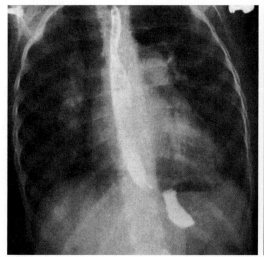

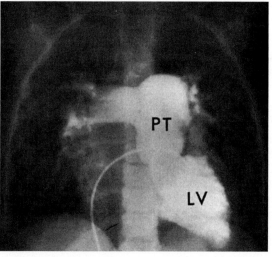

Figure 27–15

X-ray and angiocardiogram from a 7-year-old boy with complete transposition of the great arteries, a nonrestrictive atrial septal defect, an intact ventricular septum, and pulmonary vascular disease. *A,* The hypertensive posterior pulmonary trunk is sufficiently dilated to be border forming to the left. *B,* Angiocardiogram shows the dilated hypertensive pulmonary trunk (PT) arising from the morphologic left ventricle (LV).

2 LICS

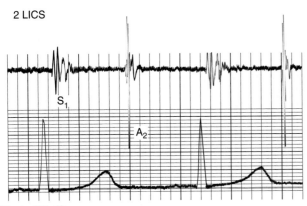

Figure 27–16

Phonocardiogram from the second left intercostal space (2 LICS) of an 18-month-old girl with complete transposition of the great arteries, a nonrestrictive atrial septal defect, low pulmonary vascular resistance, and increased pulmonary blood flow. There were no murmurs. The second heart sound was loud because the aortic component (A_2) originated in an anterior aortic root.

The midsystolic murmur of fixed pulmonary stenosis is present at birth. The midsystolic murmur of dynamic obstruction to left ventricular outflow appears after the first few weeks of life and progressively increases in length and loudness. Pulmonary stenotic murmurs are heard best in the third left intercostal space at the left sternal border because stenosis is usually subvalvular. The murmur radiates upward and to the right because of the rightward course of the transposed pulmonary trunk (see Fig. 27–2B). The midsystolic murmur of pulmonary stenosis with a nonrestrictive ventricular septal defect varies inversely in length and loudness with the degree of stenosis, as in Fallot's tetralogy (see Chapter 18). A soft pulmonary stenotic murmur is rendered inaudible by the anterior aortic root (Fig. 27–18).

The murmur of nonrestrictive patent ductus arteriosus is systolic rather than continuous because flow from the aorta into the pulmonary trunk is almost exclusively systolic.[116] High neonatal pulmonary vascular resistance curtails diastolic flow and curtails the diastolic portion of the continuous murmur (see Chapter 20).[76] A continuous murmur potentially originates in a restrictive patent ductus but is damped by the anterior aorta. Continuous murmurs seldom originate in the large systemic arterial collaterals that occasionally accompany complete transposition (see earlier).

Mid-diastolic murmurs are generated across the mitral valve when pulmonary blood flow is increased (see Fig. 27–17).[118] Mid-diastolic murmurs across the tricuspid valve are generated in deeply cyanotic patients because the systemic circulation is hypervolemic and hyperkinetic.[118] A high-frequency early diastolic Graham Steell murmur of pulmonary hypertensive pulmonary regurgitation is difficult to hear because of the posterior position of the pulmonary trunk.

A loud and single second heart sound is the aortic component because the aorta is anterior (see Figs. 27–13,

27–14, 27–16, and 27–17). The sequence of semilunar valve closure is normal because the aortic component precedes the pulmonary component despite ventriculoarterial discordance because low pulmonary vascular resistance and increased pulmonary capacitance result in normal timing or only a slight delay of the pulmonary arterial dicrotic notch.[35] Right bundle branch block causes paradoxical splitting of the second sound because the aortic component is delayed, occurring after the pulmonary component.[121] Pulmonary hypertension increases the audibility of the pulmonary component, provided that pulmonary vascular resistance remains sufficiently low to permit inspiratory splitting. When pulmonary and systemic resistances equalize, the semilunar valves close simultaneously, the second sound is single, and its intensity is reinforced, as in Eisenmenger syndrome with a ventricular septal defect (see Fig. 27–14; see Chapter 17). With pulmonary stenosis, splitting is not audible because the inherently soft pulmonary component is further attenuated by the posterior position of the pulmonary trunk.

A left ventricular third heart sound is generated when increased pulmonary blood flow causes volume overload of the left ventricle in mildly cyanosed patients, especially when the left ventricle fails (see Fig. 27–17). A right ventricular third heart sound is generated when increased systemic blood

LSE

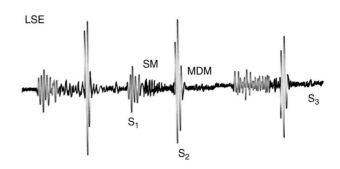

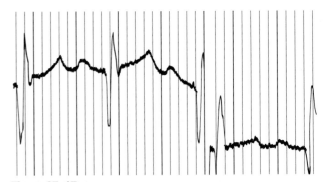

Figure 27–17

Phonocardiogram at the lower left sternal edge (LSE) of a 10-month-old boy with complete transposition of the great arteries, a nonrestrictive ventricular septal defect, low pulmonary vascular resistance, and increased pulmonary blood flow. The decrescendo holosystolic murmur (SM) originated across the ventricular septal defect. The second heart sound (S_2) was the aortic component that was loud because the aortic root was anterior. A mid-diastolic murmur (MDM) and a third heart sound (S_3) resulted from augmented mitral valve flow.

2 LICS

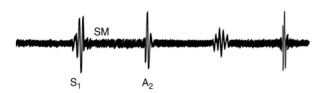

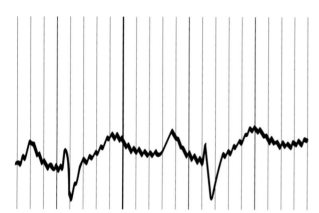

Figure 27–18

Phonocardiogram from a deeply cyanotic 13-month-old boy with complete transposition of the great arteries, a nonrestrictive ventricular septal defect, and severe fixed subpulmonary stenosis. The pulmonary stenotic murmur (SM) was virtually absent because flow was reduced and the pulmonary trunk was posterior. 2 LICS, second left intercostal space; S_1, first heart sound; A_2, aortic component of the second heart sound.

flow causes volume overload of the right ventricle in deeply cyanosed patients, especially when the right ventricle fails.

The Electrocardiogram

The electrocardiogram may be normal in the first few days of life (Fig. 27–19).[17,81,93] Tall peaked right atrial P waves soon emerge because mean right atrial pressure is increased (congestive heart failure) or because right atrial volume is increased (hypervolemic systemic circulation) (Figs 27–20 and 27–21).[29,50,100] Left atrial P wave abnormalities are reserved for patients with a large atrial septal defect and increased pulmonary blood flow (Fig. 27–22).

Right axis deviation is moderate or absent when the left ventricle is volume-overloaded in the presence of a nonrestrictive ventricular septal defect and increased pulmonary blood flow. Right axis deviation occurs when left ventricular volume overload is curtailed by pulmonary vascular disease or pulmonary stenosis (Fig. 27–23, and see Fig. 27–21).

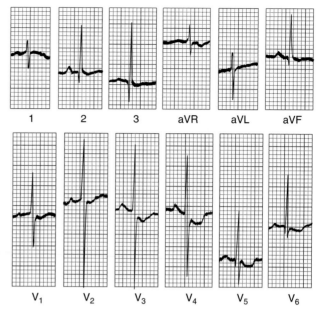

Figure 27–19

Electrocardiogram from a 7-day-old girl with complete transposition of the great arteries and a nonrestrictive ventricular septal defect. For the first few days of life, the electrocardiogram was normal and is virtually normal here except for nonspecific ST segment and T waves changes in leads V_{5-6}. The QRS axis is +90 degrees. Compare with Figure 27–20, which is the electrocardiogram from the same patient at 4 years of age.

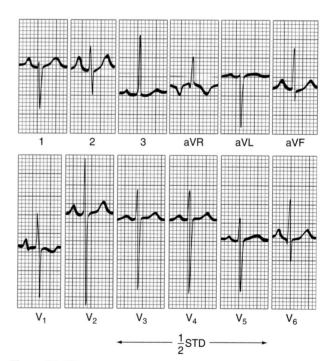

$\frac{1}{2}$STD

Figure 27–20

Electrocardiogram at 4 years of age from the patient whose normal neonatal electrocardiogram is shown in Figure 27–19. Tall peaked right atrial P waves are present in lead 2 and in leads V_{1-2}. Precordial leads exhibit combined ventricular hypertrophy reflected in the large R/S complexes in leads V_{2-5}, which are half standardized. Left ventricular volume overload is manifested by the Q wave and the well-developed R wave in lead V_6. Right ventricular pressure overload is manifested by right axis deviation, a monophasic R wave in lead aVR, and a prominent S wave in lead V_6.

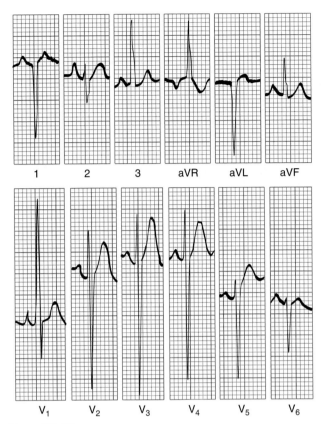

Figure 27–21

Electrocardiogram from a deeply cyanotic 15-month-old boy with complete transposition of the great arteries, a nonrestrictive ventricular septal defect, and severe fixed subpulmonary stenosis. Peaked right atrial P waves appear in lead 2 and aVF and in lead V_1. Pure right ventricular hypertrophy is reflected in marked right axis deviation, tall monophasic R waves in lead aVR and in V_1, and deep S waves in left precordial leads. T waves are taller in right precordial leads than in left precordial leads.

Right axis deviation is most striking when an atrial septal defect occurs with increased pulmonary blood flow, normal pulmonary artery pressure, and pure right ventricular hypertrophy (see Fig. 27–22). Left precordial R waves are small and Q waves are absent despite left ventricular volume overload (see Fig. 27–22). Pure right ventricular hypertrophy also occurs when pulmonary stenosis or a nonrestrictive ventricular septal defect with pulmonary vascular disease reduces left ventricular volume, and when a hypervolemic systemic circulation increases right ventricular volume (see Figs. 27–21 and 27–23). Biventricular hypertrophy is evidence of a nonrestrictive ventricular septal defect with low pulmonary vascular resistance and both volume and pressure overload of the left ventricle (see Fig. 27–20).[93] Right precordial T waves are seldom deeply inverted, even when the systemic right ventricle is volume overloaded. Right precordial T waves are often not only positive but tend to be distinctly taller than left precordial T waves (see Figs. 27–21 and 27–22).

The X-Ray

An initially normal neonatal x-ray assumes typical features of complete transposition as pulmonary vascular resistance

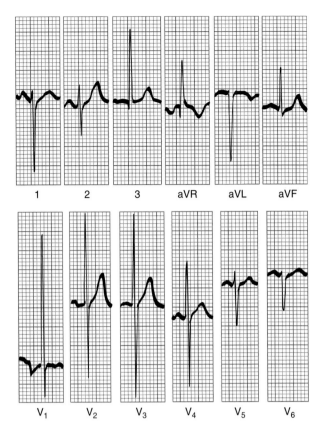

Figure 27–22

Electrocardiogram from a 2-year-old girl with complete transposition of the great arteries, a nonrestrictive atrial septal defect, low pulmonary vascular resistance, and increased pulmonary blood flow. The broad deep P terminal force in lead V_1 indicates a left atrial abnormality. Except for large equidiphasic RS complexes in leads V_{2-3}, there is pure right ventricular hypertrophy manifested by marked right axis deviation, a tall monophasic R wave in lead V_1, and rS complexes in leads V_{5-6}. The T wave amplitude is much greater in lead V_2 than in lead V_6.

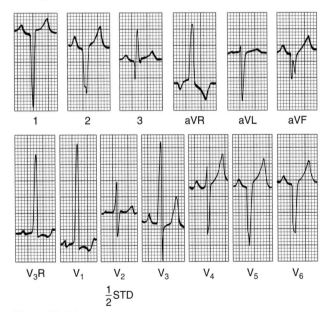

$\frac{1}{2}$STD

Figure 27–23

Electrocardiogram from a 16-month-old boy with complete transposition of the great arteries, a nonrestrictive ventricular septal defect, and suprasystemic pulmonary vascular resistance. Tall peaked right atrial P waves are present in leads 1, 2, and aVF. Pure right ventricular hypertrophy is manifested by marked right axis deviation, tall monophasic R waves in leads V_3R and V_1, and the deep S waves in leads V_{4-6}.

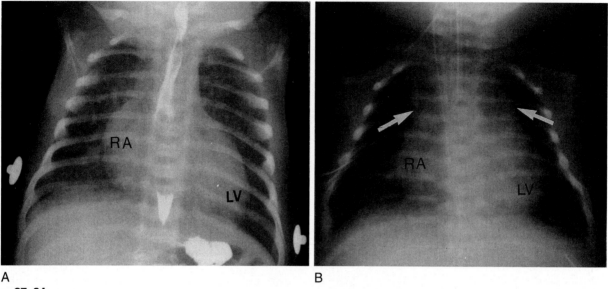

Figure 27–24

A, X-ray from a 4-day-old boy with complete transposition of the great arteries and a nonrestrictive ventricular septal defect. The thymus is characteristically absent, disclosing a narrow vascular pedicle. The right atrium (RA) is prominent, and a convex left ventricle (LV) occupies the apex. Pulmonary vascularity is increased in this overpenetrated film. B, X-ray from an identical 4-day-old boy with complete transposition of the great arteries and an uncharacteristically present thymus (*paired arrows*) that obscures the vascular pedicle.

falls and pulmonary blood flow increases.[57,74] Increased pulmonary vascularity is sometimes evident within the first few days of life (Figs. 27–24 and 27–25). The distribution of pulmonary blood flow favors the right lung because of the rightward direction of the pulmonary trunk (see Figs. 27–2B and 27–25B).[70,110] A progressive increase in flow to the right lung may culminate in a substantial decrease in flow to the left lung.[70] The crural portions of the hemidiaphragms are low when the lungs are hyperinflated.

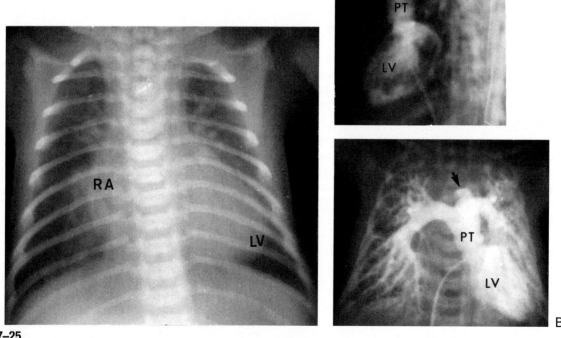

Figure 27–25

X-ray and angiocardiograms from a 5-day-old boy with complete transposition of the great arteries, a patent foramen ovale, an intact ventricular septum, and a large patent ductus arteriosus. A, Increased pulmonary blood flow is evident at this young age. Absence of thymic shadow discloses a narrow vascular pedicle. The right atrium (RA) is prominent, and a dilated left ventricle (LV) occupies the apex. B, Contrast material injected into the left ventricle (LV). The lateral projection (*top*) shows the pulmonary trunk (PT) arising from the left ventricle. The frontal projection (*bottom*) shows the pulmonary trunk arising from the left ventricle and proceeding rightward with disproportionate flow into the right pulmonary artery. Relatively little contrast material enters the ductus (*small upper arrow*).

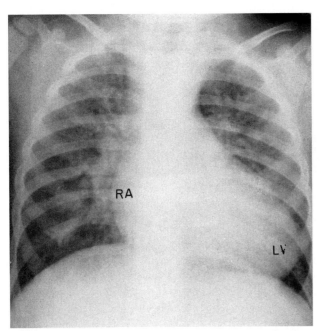

Figure 27–26

X-ray from a 1-year-old boy with complete transposition of the great arteries, a nonrestrictive ventricular septal defect, and increased pulmonary vascularity. The vascular pedicle is narrow, and a distinctive egg-shaped cardiac silhouette results from an enlarged right atrium (RA) at the right cardiac border and an enlarged left ventricle (LV) at the apex.

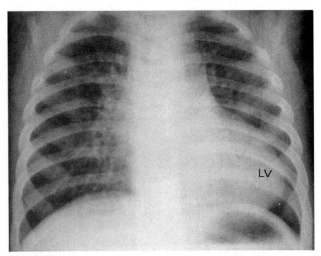

Figure 27–27

X-ray from a 9-month-old boy with complete transposition of the great arteries, a patent foramen ovale, and an intact ventricular septum. An atrial septostomy was performed at 2 days of age. Pulmonary vascularity is increased, the vascular pedicle is narrow, and an enlarged convex left ventricle (LV) occupies the apex.

Thymic shadow is almost always absent after the first 12 hours of life (see Fig. 27–24A) and therefore seldom obscures the distinctive radiologic appearance of the vascular pedicle, which is characteristically narrow (Figs. 27–26 and 27–27, and see Figs. 27–24 and 27–25) because the pulmonary trunk is posterior and medial (see Figs. 27–2B, 27–3B, and 27–25B).[18,102] The pedicle is narrowest when the ascending aorta courses vertically upward directly anterior to the pulmonary trunk (Fig. 27–28). The aortic root is seldom sufficiently rightward to be border forming (see Figs. 27–2A and 27–4), except when the ascending aorta enlarges in the presence of leftward and posterior malalignment of the infundibular septum (Fig. 27–29). The vascular pedicle is also wide when a dilated hypertensive posterior pulmonary trunk is convex to the left (Fig. 27–30).[5] A right aortic arch is present in 11% to 16% cases of complete transposition when pulmonary stenosis and ventricular septal defect coexist.[18,30,40,48,62,90]

The size and shape of the heart are determined chiefly by the magnitude of pulmonary blood flow. When pulmonary vascular resistance is low and pulmonary blood flow is increased, the cardiac silhouette often has the distinctive appearance of a tilted egg lying on its side pointing downward and to the left (see Figs. 27–26 and 27–27).[18,102] The blunter right border of the egg consists of the right atrium, and the convex left border consists of the left ventricle.[39] In the lateral projection, the heart assumes a circular appearance because an enlarged right ventricle merges with the anterior aorta and an enlarged

left ventricle merges with the dilated posterior left atrium (see Fig. 27–3). Juxtaposition of the atrial appendages is recognized by a localized bulge along the mid-left cardiac border that represents the contiguous mass of the two appendages together.[15]

As pulmonary vascular resistance increases, lung vascularity decreases, the size of the left ventricle and left atrium decrease, and a dilated hypertensive posterior pulmonary trunk emerges at the left base (Fig. 27–31, and see Figs. 27–15 and 27–30). Severe fixed pulmonary stenosis is associated with decreased pulmonary vascularity, a small left ventricle, a small left atrium, and enlargement of the right ventricle and right atrium because of the hypervolemic systemic circulation (see Fig. 27–29).[39,56]

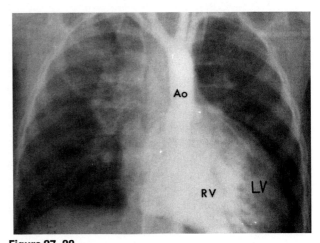

Figure 27–28

Angiocardiogram from a 29-month-old boy with complete transposition of the great arteries and a nonrestrictive atrial septal defect. The aorta (Ao) originates from the right ventricle (RV) and arises vertically. An enlarged unopacified left ventricle occupies the apex.

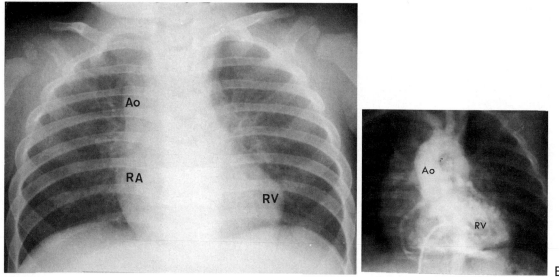

Figure 27–29

A, X-ray from a 15-month-old boy with complete transposition of the great arteries, a nonrestrictive ventricular septal defect, and severe fixed subpulmonary stenosis caused by posterior and leftward deviation of the infundibular septum. Pulmonary vascularity is reduced, and the vascular pedicle is uncharacteristically wide because of a dilated ascending aorta (Ao). The right atrium (RA) is moderately enlarged, but the apex-forming right ventricle (RV) is not dilated. B, The right ventriculogram discloses a dilated ascending aorta (Ao) with a rightward convexity, accounting for the wide vascular pedicle in the x-ray.

The Echocardiogram

Echocardiography with color flow imaging and Doppler interrogation establishes the ventricular origins of the great arteries (ventriculoarterial discordance), their spatial relationships, the presence of a ventricular septal defect or an atrial septal defect, and the presence and degree of obstruction to ventricular outflow.[4,69,114] The spiral relationship of the aorta and main pulmonary artery segment in the normal heart is represented in the short axis by an anterior "sausage" caused by the right ventricular outflow tract and main pulmonary artery segment transected tangentially and a posterior circle, which is the aorta. In complete transposition, the great arteries appear as double circles with the aorta anterior and to the right or side-by-side and to the right of the main pulmonary artery (Fig. 27–32A). Identification of each great artery rests more securely on imaging the right and left branches of the main pulmonary

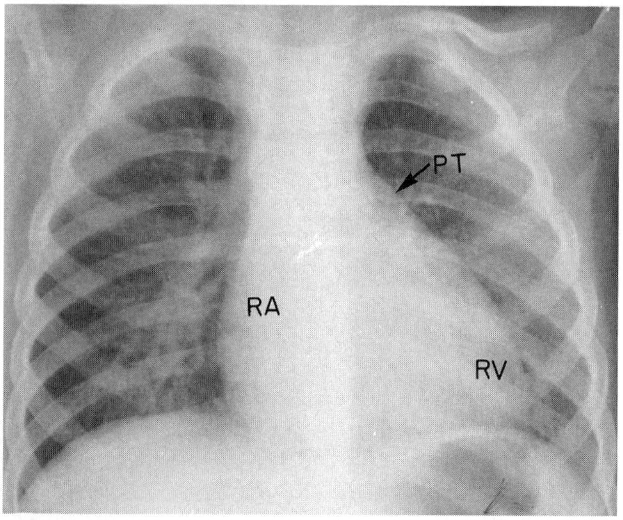

Figure 27–30

X-ray from a 16-month-old boy with complete transposition of the great arteries, a nonrestrictive ventricular septal defect, and pulmonary vascular disease. A dilated hypertensive posterior pulmonary trunk (PT) emerges to the left (*arrow*). The right ventricle (RV) occupies the apex, and the right atrium (RA) occupies the right lower cardiac border.

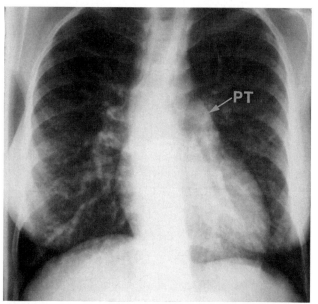

Figure 27–31

X-ray from a 30-year-old woman with complete transposition of the great arteries, a nonrestrictive ventricular septal defect, and pulmonary vascular disease. The lung fields have the lacy pattern of neovascularity. A dilated hypertensive posterior pulmonary trunk (PT) reveals itself at the left base. The left branch is obscured, but the dilated right branch is well seen. The right atrium is slightly convex, and a moderately enlarged right ventricle occupies the apex.

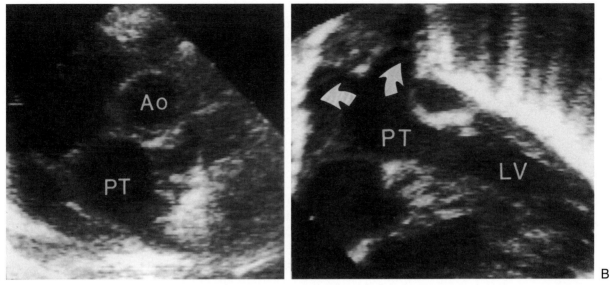

Figure 27–32

Echocardiograms from a 3-month-old boy with complete transposition of the great arteries, a patent foramen ovale, and an intact ventricular septum. An atrial septostomy was performed at 4 days of age. *A*, The great arteries are represented in the short axis by two circles, with the aorta (Ao) anterior and rightward and the pulmonary trunk (PT) posterior and leftward. *B*, The subxiphoid image shows alignment of the morphologic left ventricle (LV) with the pulmonary trunk (PT), which is identified by its bifurcation into right and left branches (*curved arrows*).

artery (Fig. 27–33, and see Fig. 27–32*B*) and imaging the brachiocephalic branches of the aortic arch with continuation as the descending thoracic aorta (Fig. 27–34). The anterior aortic root and posterior pulmonary trunk run parallel to each other (see Fig. 27–34) and do not cross as in the normal heart. The ventricle of origin of each discordant great artery can be properly assigned (see Figs. 27–32, 27–33, and 27–34). An important role of echocardiography is in determining the origin and course of the coronary arteries.[2,75]

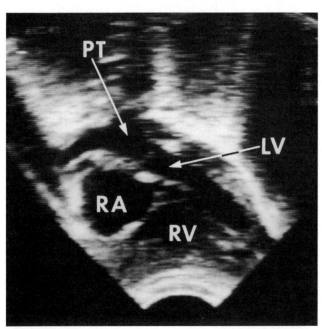

Figure 27–33

Echocardiogram (subcostal) from a male neonate with complete transposition of the great arteries, a patent foramen ovale, and an intact ventricular septum. The left ventricle (LV) gives rise to the pulmonary trunk (PT), which is directed upward and rightward and is identified by right and left branches. A normal left ventricular outflow tract is delineated beneath delicate pulmonary valve echoes. Compare to the angiocardiogram in Figure 27–2*B*. RA, right atrium; RV, right ventricle.

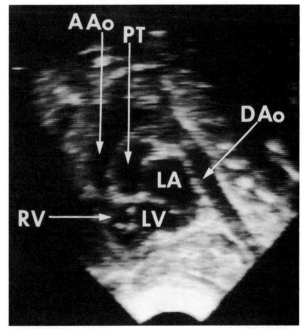

Figure 27–34

Echocardiogram (subcostal) from a male neonate with complete transposition of the great arteries, a patent foramen ovale, and an intact ventricular septum. The ascending aorta (AAo) is anterior, rises vertically from the right ventricle (RV), and gives off the brachiocephalic arteries before continuing as the descending aorta (DAo). Compare with the angiocardiogram in Figure 27–2*A*. The left ventricle (LV) gives rise to the pulmonary trunk (PT), which is posterior and parallel to the ascending aorta. LA, left atrium.

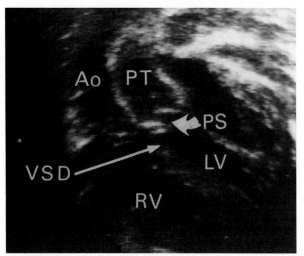

Figure 27–35

Echocardiogram (subcostal) from a 2-month-old boy with complete transposition of the great arteries, a moderately restrictive ventricular septal defect (VSD), and pulmonary valve stenosis (PS). The two great arteries are parallel and do not cross. The mildly dilated pulmonary trunk (PT) originates from the left ventricle (LV), and the aorta (Ao) originates from the right ventricle (RV).

Echocardiography with color flow imaging and Doppler interrogation establishes the presence of a ventricular septal defect or an atrial septal defect. Visualization of the left ventricular outflow tract determines the absence (see Figs. 27–32 and 27–33), presence, and degree of obstruction as well as its morphologic type (Figs. 27–35 and 27–36),[69,83,114] and continuous-wave Doppler interrogation establishes the magnitude of the gradient. Fixed obstruction to left ventricular outflow is characterized by pulmonary valve stenosis (see Fig. 27–35) or posterior and leftward malalignment of the infundibular septum.[83,114] Dynamic obstruction to left ventricular outflow is characterized by systolic anterior movement of the anterior mitral leaflet that can be recognized with two-dimensional real time imaging (see Fig. 27–36A).[69] The combination of systolic anterior movement of the anterior mitral leaflet, abnormal systolic movement of the base of the ventricular septum, and a hyperkinetic left ventricular free wall conspire to produce the left ventricular outflow gradient of dynamic subpulmonary stenosis (Fig. 27–36B).[69,114]

Juxtaposition of the atrial appendages is recognized in the two-dimensional echocardiogram as malposition of the right atrial appendage with an abnormal plane of the atrial septum.[82] Tricuspid valve anomalies can be identified, especially straddling or overriding.

Summary

The clinical recognition of complete transposition of the great arteries is based on the following features: (1) male child, (2) large birth weight, (3) cyanosis in the neonatal period or shortly thereafter, (4) radiologic evidence of increased pulmonary blood flow in the presence of cyanosis

and an egg-shaped cardiac silhouette with a narrow vascular pedicle and absent thymic shadow, and (5) echocardiographic identification of aortic alignment with the morphologic right ventricle, pulmonary trunk alignment with the morphologic left ventricle (ventricular/arterial discordance), and right atrial alignment with right ventricle and left atrial alignment with left ventricle (atrioventricular concordance).

Complete transposition with a restrictive foramen ovale presents with rapidly progressive cyanosis beginning on the first day of life. The electrocardiogram and x-ray can be transiently normal, and apart from conspicuous cyanosis, the physical signs are disarmingly unimpressive, with a normal arterial pulse, a moderate right ventricular impulse, and no cardiac murmur.

Complete transposition with nonrestrictive ventricular septal defect presents with congestive heart failure and relatively mild cyanosis that coincide with the neonatal fall in pulmonary vascular resistance. A right ventricular impulse is accompanied by a palpable left ventricle, there is a loud holosystolic left parasternal murmur, the electrocardiogram shows moderate right axis deviation and biventricular hypertrophy, and the x-ray shows increased pulmonary blood flow and an egg-shaped cardiac silhouette with a narrow vascular pedicle. Pulmonary vascular disease causes a decrease in pulmonary blood flow, progressive cyanosis, a decrease in size of the left ventricle

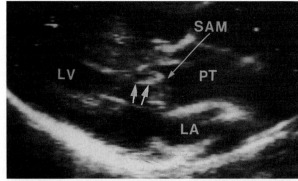

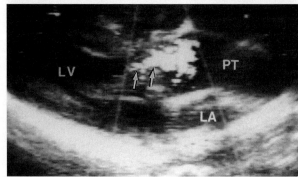

Figure 27–36

A, Echocardiogram (parasternal long axis) from an 8-week-old boy with dynamic subpulmonary stenosis caused by systolic anterior motion (SAM) of the anterior mitral leaflet (*unmarked paired arrows*). B, Black and white print of a color flow image showing accelerated flow across the narrow left ventricular outflow tract (*paired unmarked arrows*). Compare to Figure 27–9B. LA, left atrium; LV, left ventricle; PT, pulmonary trunk.

and left atrium, loss of the left ventricular impulse, a pulmonary ejection sound, an inconspicuous or absent midsystolic murmur, a loud single second sound, and a Graham Steell murmur. The electrocardiogram shows pure right ventricular hypertrophy. The vascular pedicle in the x-ray is narrow, but a dilated posterior pulmonary trunk may emerge at the left base.

Dynamic subpulmonary stenosis reveals itself several weeks after birth. The midsystolic murmur increases in length and loudness as the dynamic obstruction to left ventricular outflow progresses. Neonates with fixed subpulmonary stenosis caused by leftward and posterior malalignment of the infundibular septum and a nonrestrictive ventricular septal defect present with conspicuous cyanosis and a pulmonary stenotic murmur that varies inversely in loudness length with the degree of obstruction. The pulmonary stenotic murmur radiates upward and to the right because of the rightward direction taken by the pulmonary trunk. The second heart sound is loud because the aorta is anterior and is single because the pulmonary component is inaudible, owing to the posterior position of the pulmonary trunk. The right ventricle is palpable but not the left ventricle. Arterial pulses are bounding because the systemic circulation is hypervolemic and hyperkinetic. The vascular pedicle may widen because of rightward convexity of a dilated aortic root. The electrocardiogram shows pure right ventricular hypertrophy and marked right axis deviation.

When complete transposition is associated with a nonrestrictive atrial septal defect, cyanosis is mild, the right ventricular impulse is conspicuous, but the left ventricle is not palpable. The pulmonary midsystolic flow murmur is damped by the anterior aorta and is followed by the loud second sound of aortic valve closure. The electrocardiogram shows marked right axis deviation with pure right ventricular hypertrophy. The x-ray is similar to complete transposition with a nonrestrictive ventricular septal defect and increased pulmonary blood flow, but the left ventricle is less dilated.

Complete transposition with a nonrestrictive patent ductus arteriosus presents in neonates with mild to moderate cyanosis and tachypnea but without bounding pulses and without a continuous murmur.

REFERENCES

1. Allwork SP, Urban AE, Anderson RH: Left juxtaposition of the auricles with L-position of the aorta: Report of 6 cases. Br Heart J 39:299, 1977.
2. Sim EK, van Son JA, Edwards WD, et al: Coronary artery anatomy in complete transposition of the great arteries. Ann Thorac Surg 57:890, 1994.
3. Anderson RH, Becker AE, Losekoot TG, Gerlis LM: Anatomically corrected malposition of great arteries. Br Heart J 37:993, 1975.
4. Pasquini L, Sanders SP, Parness IA, et al: Conal anatomy in 119 patients with D-loop transposition of the great arteries and ventricular septal defect: An echocardiographic and pathologic study. J Am Coll Cardiol 21:1712, 1993.
5. Aziz KU, Nanton MA, Kidd L, et al: Variations in the size and distensibility of the pulmonary arteries in D- transposition of the great arteries. Am J Cardiol 38:452, 1976.
6. Aziz KU, Paul MH, Rowe RD: Bronchopulmonary circulation in D-transposition of the great arteries: Possible role in genesis of accelerated pulmonary vascular disease. Am J Cardiol 39:432, 1977.
7. Aziz KU, Paul MH, Idriss FS, et al: Clinical manifestations of dynamic left ventricular outflow tract stenosis with D-transposition of the great arteries with intact ventricular septum. Am J Cardiol 44:290, 1979.
8. Aziz KU, Paul MH, Muster AJ, Idriss FS: Positional abnormalities of the atrioventricular valves in transposition of the great arteries including double outlet right ventricle, atrioventricular valve straddling and malattachment. Am J Cardiol 44:1135, 1979.
9. Baillie M: Morbid Anatomy of Some of the Most Important Parts of the Human Body, 2nd ed. London, Johnson and Nicol, 1797.
10. Maeno YV, Kamenir SA, Sinclair B, et al: Prenatal features of ductus arteriosus constriction and restrictive foramen ovale in D-transposition of the great arteries. Circulation 99:1209, 1999.
11. Becker AE, Becker MJ: Juxtaposition of atrial appendages associated with normally oriented ventricles and great arteries. Circulation 41:685, 1970.
12. Yoo S, Burrows P, Moes F, et al: Evaluation of coronary artery patterns in complete transposition by laid-back aortography. Cardiol Young. 6:149, 1996.
13. Boessen I: Complete transposition of the great vessels: Importance of septal defects and patent ductus arteriosus. Analysis of 132 patients dying before age 4. Circulation 28:885, 1963.
14. Digilio MC, Casey B, Toscano A, et al: Complete transposition of the great arteries: Patterns of congenital heart disease in familial precurrence. Circulation 104:2809, 2001.
15. Bream PR, Elliott LP, Bargeron LM: Plain film findings of anatomically corrected malposition: Its association with juxtaposition of the atrial appendages and right aortic arch. Radiology 126:589, 1978.
16. Buckley MJ, Mason DT, Ross J Jr, Braunwald E: Reversed differential cyanosis with equal desaturation of the upper limbs: Syndrome of complete transposition of the great vessels with complete interruption of the aortic arch. Am J Cardiol 15:111, 1965.
17. Calleja HB, Hosier DM, Grajo MZ: The electrocardiogram in complete transposition of the great vessels. Am Heart J 69:31, 1965.
18. Carey LS, Elliott LP: Complete transposition of the great vessels: Roentgenographic findings. Am J Roentgenol 91:529, 1964.
19. Charuzi Y, Spanos PK, Amplatz K, Edwards JE: Juxtaposition of the atrial appendages. Circulation 47:620, 1973.
20. Chuaqui B: Doerr's theory of morphogenesis of arterial transposition in light of recent research. Br Heart J 41:481, 1979.
21. Clarkson PM, Neutze JM, Wardill JC, Barratt-Boyes BG: The pulmonary vascular bed in patients with complete transposition of the great arteries. Circulation 53:539, 1976.
22. Colli AM, de Leval M, Somerville J: Anatomically corrected malposition of the great arteries. Am J Cardiol 55:1367, 1985.
23. Daliento L, Cuman G, Isabella G, et al: Ventricular development and function in complete transposition: Angiocardiographic evaluation. Int J Cardiol 12:341, 1986.
24 De la Cruz MV, Arteaga M, Espino-Vela J, et al: Complete transposition of the great arteries: Types and morphogenesis of ventriculoarterial discordance. Am Heart J 102:271, 1981.
25. De la Cruz MV, Berrazueta JR, Arteaga M, et al: Rules for diagnosis of atrioventricular discordances and spatial identification of ventricles: Crossed great arteries and transposition of the great arteries. Br Heart J 38:341, 1976.
26. Deutsch V, Shem-Tov A, Yahini JH, Neufeld HN: Juxtaposition of atrial appendages: Angiographic observations. Am J Cardiol 34:240, 1974.
27. Dick M, Heidelberger K, Crowley D, et al: Quantitative morphometric analysis of the pulmonary arteries in two patients with D-transposition of the great arteries and persistence of the fetal circulation. Pediatr Res 15:1397, 1981.
28. Elliott LP, Amplatz K, Edwards JE: Coronary arterial patterns in transposition complexes: Anatomic and angiocardiographic studies. Am J Cardiol 17:362, 1966.
29. Elliott LP, Anderson RC, Tuna N, et al: Complete transposition of the great vessels. II. An electrocardiographic analysis. Circulation 27:1118, 1963.
30. Elliott LP, Neufeld HN, Anderson RC, et al: Complete transposition of the great vessels. I. An anatomic study of sixty cases. Circulation 27:1105, 1963.
31. Farre JR: On Malformations of the Human Heart. London, Longman, Hurst, Rees, Orme and Brown, 1814.

32. Fischbein CA, Rosenthal A, Fischer EG, et al: Risk factors for brain abscess in patients with congenital heart disease. Am J Cardiol 34:97, 1974.

33. Flyer DC: Report of the New England Regional Infant Cardiac Program. Pediatrics 65(Suppl):377, 1980.

34. Folse R, Roberts WC, Cornell WP: Increased bronchial collateral circulation in a patient with transposition of the great vessels and pulmonary hypertension. Am J Cardiol 8:282, 1961.

35. Fouron JC, Douste-Blazy MY, Ducharme G, et al: Hang-out time of pulmonary valve in d-transposition of great arteries. Br Heart J 47:277, 1982.

36. Gittenberger-de Groot AC, Saucer U, Oppenheimer-Dekker A, Quaegebeur J: Coronary arterial anatomy in transposition of the great arteries: A morphological study. Pediatr Cardiol 4(Suppl 1):15, 1983.

37. Grittenberger-de Groot AC, Sauer U, Quaegebeur J: Aortic intramural coronary artery in three hearts with transposition of the great arteries. J Thoracic Cardiovasc Surg 91:566, 1986.

38. Graham TP, Atwood GF, Boucek RJ, et al: Right heart volume characteristics in transposition of the great arteries. Circulation 51:881, 1975.

39. Graham TP, Jarmakani JM, Canent RV, Jewett PH: Quantification of left heart volume and systolic output in transposition of the great arteries. Circulation 44:899, 1971.

40. Guerin R, Soto B, Karp RB, et al: Transposition of the great arteries: Determination of the position of the great arteries in conventional chest roentgenograms. Am J Roentgenol Radium Ther Nuclear Med 110:747, 1970.

41. Gutgesell HP, Garson A, McNamara DG: Prognosis for the newborn with transposition of the great arteries. Am J Cardiol 44:96, 1979.

42. Haworth SG, Radley-Smith R, Yacoub M: Lung biopsy findings in transposition of the great arteries with ventricular septal defect: Potentially reversible pulmonary vascular disease is not always synonymous with operability. J Am Coll Cardiol 9:327, 1987.

43. Huhta JC, Edwards JE, Danielson GK, Feldt RH: Abnormalities of the tricuspid valve in complete transposition of the great arteries with ventricular septal defect. J Thorac Cardiovasc Surg 83:569, 1982.

44. Huhta JC, Edwards WD, Feldt RH, Puga FJ: Left ventricular wall thickness in complete transposition of the great arteries. J Thorac Cardiovasc Surg 84:97, 1982.

45. Hurwitz RA, Caldwell RL, Girod DA, et al: Ventricular function in transposition of the great arteries: Evaluation by radionuclide angiocardiography. Am Heart J 110:600, 1985.

46. Jarmakani JMM, Canent RV: Preoperative and postoperative right ventricular function in children with transposition of the great vessels. Circulation 50:II-39, 1974.

47. Johnson CD: Longevity in transposition of the great arteries. Bol Asoc Med P R 73:344, 1981.

48. Jue KL, Adams P Jr, Pryor R, et al: Complete transposition of the great vessels in total situs inversus: Anatomic, electrocardiographic and radiologic observations. Am J Cardiol 17:389, 1966.

49. Keane JF, Ellison RC, Rudd M, Nadas AS: Pulmonary blood flow and left ventricular volumes in transposition of the great arteries and intact ventricular septum. Br Heart J 35:521, 1973.

50. Khoury GH, Shaher RM, Fowler RS, Keith JD: Preoperative and postoperative electrocardiogram in complete transposition of the great vessels. Am Heart J 72:199, 1966.

51. Kidd L, Humphries JO: Transposition of the great arteries in the adult. Cardiovasc Clin 10:365, 1979.

52. Kurosawa H, Van Mierop LHS: Surgical anatomy of the infundibular septum in transposition of the great arteries with ventricular septal defect. J Thorac Cardiovasc Surg 91:123, 1986.

53. Lakier JB, Stanger P, Heymann MA, et al: Early onset of pulmonary vascular obstruction in patients with aortopulmonary transposition and intact ventricular septum. Circulation 51:875, 1975.

54. Lang P, Freed MD, Norwood WI, Nadas AS: Use of prostaglandin E1 in infants with D-transposition of the great arteries and intact ventricular septum. Am J Cardiol 44:76, 1979.

55. Layman TE, Edwards JE: Anomalies of the cardiac valves associated with complete transposition of the great vessels. Am J Cardiol 19:247, 1967.

56. Lev M, Rimoldi HJA, Paiva R, Arcilla RA: The quantitative anatomy of simple complete transposition. Am J Cardiol 23:409, 1969.

57. Levin DL, Paul MH, Muster AJ, et al: The clinical diagnosis of d-transposition of the great vessels in the neonate. Arch Intern Med 137:1421, 1977.

58. Liebman J, Cullum L, Belloe NB: Natural history of transposition of the great arteries. Circulation 40:237, 1969.

59. Mair DD, Ritter DG: Factors influencing intercirculatory mixing in patients with complete transposition of the great arteries. Am J Cardiol 30:653, 1972.

60. Mair DD, Ritter DG: Factors influencing systemic arterial oxygen saturation in complete transposition of the great arteries. Am J Cardiol 31:742, 1973.

61. Maroto E, Fouron J, Douste-Blazy M, et al: Influence of age on wall thickness, cavity dimensions and myocardial contractility of the left ventricle in simple transposition of the great arteries. Circulation 67:1311, 1983.

62. Mathew R, Rosenthal A, Fellows K: The significance of right aortic arch in D-transposition of the great arteries. Am Heart J 87:314, 1974.

63. Mayer JE, Sanders SP, Jonas RA, et al: Coronary artery pattern and outcome of arterial switch operation for transposition of the great arteries. Circulation 82(Suppl IV):IV-139, 1990.

64. Messeloff CR, Weaver JC: A case of transposition of the large vessels in an adult who lived to the age of 38 years. Am Heart J 42:467, 1951.

65. Milanesi O, Ho SY, Thiene G, et al: The ventricular septal defect in complete transposition of the great arteries: Pathologic anatomy in 57 cases with emphasis on subaortic, subpulmonary, and aortic arch obstruction. Hum Pathol 18:392, 1987.

66. Moene RJ, Oppenheimer-Dekker A: Congenital mitral valve anomalies in transposition of the great arteries. Am J Cardiol 49:1972, 1982.

67. Moene RJ, Oppenheimer-Dekker A, Wenink ACG, et al: Morphology of ventricular septal defect in complete transposition of the great arteries. Am J Cardiol 55:1566, 1985.

68. Moene RJ, Ottenkamp J, Oppenheimer-Dekker A, Bartelings MM: Transposition of the great arteries and narrowing of the aortic arch. Br Heart J 53:58, 1985.

69. Moro E, ten Cate FJ, Tirtaman C, et al: Doppler and two-dimensional echocardiographic observations of systolic anterior motion of the mitral valve in d-transposition of the great arteries: An explanation of the left ventricular outflow tract gradient. J Am Coll Cardiol 7:889, 1986.

70. Muster AJ, Paul MH, van Grondelle A, Conway JJ: Asymmetric distribution of the pulmonary blood flow between the right and left lungs in D-transposition of the great arteries. Am J Cardiol 38:352, 1976.

71. Newfeld EA, Paul MH, Muster AJ, Idriss FS: Pulmonary vascular disease in complete transposition of the great arteries: A study of 200 patients. Am J Cardiol 34:75, 1974.

72. Newfeld EA, Paul MH, Muster AJ, Idriss FS: Pulmonary vascular disease in transposition of the great vessels and intact ventricular septum. Circulation 59:525, 1979.

73. Nichol AD, Segal AJ: Complete transposition of the main arterial stems: Report of a case. JAMA 147:645, 1951.

74. Noonan JA, Nadas AS, Rudolph AM, Harris GBC: Transposition of the great arteries: A correlation of clinical, physiological and autopsy data. N Engl J Med 263:592, 637, 739, 1960.

75. Pasquini L, Sanders SP, Parness IA, Colan SD: Diagnosis of coronary artery anatomy by two-dimensional echocardiography in patients with transposition of the great arteries. Circulation 75:557, 1987.

76. Perloff JK: Auscultatory and phonocardiographic manifestations of pulmonary hypertension. Prog Cardiovasc Dis 9:303, 1967.

77. Pigott JD, Chin AJ, Weinberg PM, et al: Transposition of the great arteries with aortic arch obstruction: Anatomical review and report of surgical management. J Thorac Cardiovasc Surg 94:82, 1987.

78. Powell TG, Dewey M, West CR, Arnold R: Fate of infants with transposition of the great arteries in relation to balloon atrial septostomy. Br Heart J 51:371, 1984.

79. Rabinovitch M, Haworth SG, Casteneda AR, et al: Lung biopsy in congenital heart disease: A morphometric approach to pulmonary vascular disease. Circulation 58:107, 1978.

80. Rashkind WJ, Miller WW: Creation of an atrial septal defect without thoracotomy. JAMA 196:991, 1966.

81. Rastieaux NJ, Ellison C, Albers WH, Nadas AS: The Frank electrocardiogram in complete transposition of the great arteries. Am Heart J 83:219, 1972.

82. Rice MJ, Seward JB, Hagler DJ, et al: Left juxtaposed atrial appendages: Diagnosis by two-dimensional echocardiographic features. J Am Coll Cardiol 5:1330, 1983.

83. Riggs TW, Muster AJ, Aziz KV, et al: Two-dimensional subpulmonary stenosis due to tricuspid valve pouch in complete transposition of the great arteries. J Am Coll Cardiol 2:484, 1984.

84. Rosenquist GC, Stark J, Taylor JFN: Congenital mitral valve disease in transposition of the great arteries. Circulation 51:731, 1975.

85. Rosenthal G, Wilson PD, Permutt T, et al: Birth weight and cardiovascular malformations: A population-based study. Am J Epidemiol 133:1273, 1991

86. Rossi MB, Ho SY, Anderson RH, et al: Coronary arteries in complete transposition: The significance of the sinus node artery. Ann Thorac Surg 42:574, 1986.

87. Sansa M, Tonkin IL, Bargeron LM, Elliott LP: Left ventricular outflow tract obstruction in transposition of the great arteries. Am J Cardiol. 44:88, 1979.

88. Satomi G, Nakazawa M, Takao A, et al: Blood flow patterns of the interatrial communication in patients with complete transposition of the great arteries: A pulsed Doppler echocardiographic study. Circulation 73:95, 1986.

89. Schmaltz AA, Knab I, Seybold-Epting W, Apitz J: Prognosis of children with transposition of the great arteries, treated in a regional heart centre between 1967 and 1979. Eur Heart J 5:570, 1982.

90. Schneeweiss A, Blieden LC, Shem-Tov A, et al: Wide vascular pedicle on the thoracic roentgenogram in complete transposition of the great arteries. Clin Cardiol 5:75, 1982.

91. Schneeweiss A, Motro M, Shem-Tov A, Neufeld HN: Subaortic stenosis: An unrecognized problem in transposition of the great arteries. Am J Cardiol 48:336, 1981.

92. Shaher RM: Prognosis of transposition of the great vessels with or without atrial septal defect. Br Heart J 25:211, 1963.

93. Shaher RM, Deuchar DC: The electrocardiogram in complete transposition of the great vessels. Br Heart J 28:265, 1966.

94. Shaher RM, Kidd L: Acid-base balance in complete transposition of the great vessels. Br Heart J 29:207, 1967.

95. Shaher RM, Puddu GC: Coronary arterial anatomy in complete transposition of the great vessels. Am J Cardiol 17:355, 1966.

96. Shirvastava S, Tadavarthy SM, Fukuda T, Edwards JE: Anatomic causes of pulmonary stenosis in complete transposition. Circulation 54:154, 1976.

97. Silberbach M, Castro WL, Goldstein MA, et al: Comparison of types of pulmonary stenosis with the state of the ventricular septum in complete transposition of the great arteries. Pediatr Cardiol 10:11, 1989.

98. Smith A, Wilkinson JL, Arnold R, et al: Growth and development of ventricular walls in complete transposition of the great arteries with intact septum. Am J Cardiol 49:362, 1982.

99. Smith A, Arnold R, Wilkinson JL, et al: An anatomical study of the patterns of the coronary arteries and sinus nodal artery in complete transposition. Int J Cardiol 12:295, 1986.

100. Southall DP, Keeton BR, Leanage R, et al: Cardiac rhythm and conduction before and after Mustard's operation for complete transposition of the great arteries. Br Heart J 43:21, 1980.

101. Sterns LP, Baker RM, Edwards JE: Complete transposition of the great vessels: Unusual longevity in a case with subpulmonary stenosis. Circulation 29:610, 1964.

102. Tonkin IL, Kelley MJ, Bream PR, Elliot LP: The frontal chest film as a method of suspecting transposition complexes. Circulation 53:1016, 1976.

103. Tonkin IL, Sausa M, Elliot LP, Bargeron LM: Recognition of developing left ventricular outflow tract obstruction in complete transposition of the great arteries. Radiology 134:53, 1980.

104. Tynan M: Transposition of the great arteries: Changes in the circulation after birth. Circulation 46:809, 1972.

105. Tyrrell MJ, Moes CAF: Congenital levoposition of the right atrial appendage. Am J Dis Child 121:508, 1971.

106. Urquhart W, Farmer MB: Left-sided juxtaposition of the atrial appendages. Br Heart J 35:1184, 1973.

107. Van Doesburg NH, Bierman FZ, Williams RG: Left ventricular geometry in infants with D-transposition of the great arteries and intact ventricular septum. Circulation 68:733, 1983.

108. Van Praagh R, Durnin RE, Jockin H, et al: Anatomically corrected malposition of the great arteries. Circulation 51:20, 1975.

109. Van Praagh R, Perez-Trevino C, Lopez-Cuellar M, et al: Transposition of the great arteries with posterior aorta, anterior pulmonary artery, subpulmonary conus and fibrous continuity between aortic and atrioventricular valve. Am J Cardiol 28:621, 1971.

110. Vidne BA, Duszynski D, Subramanian S: Pulmonary blood flow distribution in transposition of the great arteries. Am J Cardiol 38:62, 1976.

111. Vidne BA, Subramanian S, Wagner HR: Aneurysm of the membranous ventricular septum in transposition of the great arteries. Circulation 53:157, 1976.

112. Viles PH, Ongley PA, Titus JL: The spectrum of pulmonary vascular disease in transposition of the great arteries. Circulation 40:31, 1969.

113. Virdi IS, Keeton BR, Monro JL: Complete transposition with posteriorly located aorta and multiple ventricular septal defects. Int J Cardiol 21:347, 1988.

114. Vitarelli A, D'Addio AP, Gentile R, Burattini M: Echocardiographic evaluation of left ventricular outflow tract obstruction in complete transposition of the great arteries. Am Heart J 108:531, 1984.

115. Wagenvoort CA, Nauta J, van der Schaar PJ, et al: The pulmonary vasculature in complete transposition of the great vessels as judged from lung biopsies. Circulation 38:746, 1968.

116. Waldman JD, Paul MH, Newfeld EA, et al: Transposition of the great arteries with intact ventricular septum and patent ductus arteriosus. Am J Cardiol 39:232, 1977.

117. Waldman JD, Schneeweiss A, Edwards WD, et al: The obstructive subaortic conus. Circulation 70:339, 1984.

118. Wells B: The sounds and murmurs in transposition of the great vessels. Br Heart J 25:748, 1963.

119. Wilkinson JL, Arnold R, Anderson RH, Acerete F: Posterior transposition reconsidered. Br Heart J 37:757, 1975.

120. Yamaki S, Tezuka F: Quantitative analysis of pulmonary vascular disease in complete transposition of the great arteries. Circulation 54:805, 1976.

121. Zuberbuhler JR, Bauersfeld SR, Pontius RG: Parodoxic splitting of the second sound with transposition of the great vessels. Am Heart J 74:816, 1967.

122. Kato K: Congenital transposition of cardiac vessels: Clinical and pathologic study. Am J Dis Child 39:363, 1930.

123. Cleland PM, Goodwin JF, Steiner RE, Zoob M: Transposition of the aorta and pulmonary artery with pulmonary stenosis. Am Heart J 54:10, 1957.

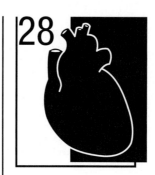

Truncus Arteriosus

Truncus arteriosus was recognized in 1798,[78] and the clinical and necropsy manifestations were described in 1864.[10] Humphreys summarized the cases reported up to 1932,[39] and Lev and Saphir critically reviewed published accounts during the following decade.[46] The malformation accounts for approximately 1% to 2% of cases of congenital heart disease at necropsy and approximately 0.7% to 1.2% of all congenital cardiac malformations.[13,54,69,79,87]

In truncus arteriosus, a single great artery with a single semilunar valve leaves the base of the heart and gives rise to the coronary, pulmonary, and systemic circulations.[3,13,16,17,66,69,73,74] A second semilunar valve is neither present nor implied. The single arterial trunk receives the output from both ventricles, so a ventricular septal defect is obligatory.[2,13,17,60,67] Type IV, or pseudotruncus with a biventricular aorta and an atretic pulmonary valve, is classified as pulmonary atresia with ventricular septal defect rather than truncus arteriosus (see Chapter 18).[39,72,86] Edwards, with disarming candor, stated, "Twenty-eight years after the introduction of the term, we doubt that the condition which Collett and Edwards had called truncus Type IV exists."[17,66] Similarly, a solitary pulmonary trunk referred to in 1814 by Farrell[24] is classified as a variety of aortic atresia.[1,61] *Hemitruncus*, a term no longer used, referred to a rare anomaly in which one pulmonary artery branch arose from the ascending aorta just above the aortic sinuses, and the main pulmonary artery with the other branch arose in their normal positions.[25,26]

A *right aortic arch* accompanies truncus arteriosus in about 30% of cases (Figs. 28–1 and 28–5).[13,31,34,35,69,74] The truncus is large because it accepts the entire output of the systemic and pulmonary circulations (see Figs. 28–1 and 28–2A), although inherent medial abnormalities contribute to the dilatation.[51a] Agenesis of the ductus arteriosus occurs in 50% to 75% of cases,[12,13,60,74] which is not surprising because a fetal ductus is not required to channel pulmonary arterial blood into the aorta.[60,82]

In 1949, Collett and Edwards classified truncus arteriosus into four types based on the origins of the pulmonary arteries.[17] Type 4 of Collett and Edwards is now considered pulmonary atresia with ventricular septal defect (see earlier and see Chapter 18). The first three types were reconsidered by van Praagh in 1965[74] and form the basis for current terminology (Fig. 28–3). The most common variety is type 1, which is characterized by a short main pulmonary artery that originates from the truncus and gives rise to the right and left pulmonary arteries (see Figs. 28–2A, 28–4, and 28–5).[74] Type 2 and type 3 of Collett and Edwards were originally defined by right and left pulmonary arteries that arose from separate ostia at either the side or the back of the truncus (see Fig. 28–3).[13,17] These two types are now considered as a single category[74] and are referred to herein as type 2 (see Figs. 28–1B and 28–3). In about 15% of cases, the right or left pulmonary artery is absent or hypoplastic (see Fig. 28–4B). An absent or hypoplastic pulmonary artery is usually concordant with the side of the aortic arch.[29]

The truncal valve is quadricuspid in 40% to 50% of cases (see Figs. 28–10 and 28–22), bicuspid in a distinct minority, and very rarely pentacuspid or hexacuspid.[*] A normal trileaflet aortic valve differs from a trileaflet truncal valve because of the presence of truncal raphes and cuspal inequality,[44] and because trileaflet truncal valves tend to be thickened and focally or diffusely dysplastic.[12,28,84] A trileaflet truncal valve with raphes and cusps in excess of three represents a morphogenetic combination of aortic and pulmonary valves.[72,74] The truncal valves are poorly supported and are frequently incompetent.[13,19,28,30] Stenotic

---

[*]See references 12, 13, 16, 17, 28, 30, 39, 60, 63, 69, 74.

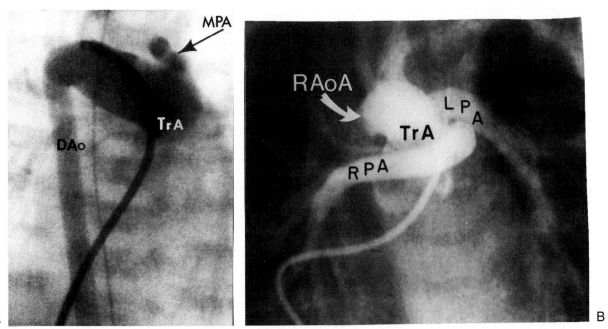

Figure 28–1

A, Angiogram from a 1-week-old girl with truncus arteriosus type 1 (TrA). A main pulmonary artery (MPA) arose from the truncus that continued as a right aortic arch and a right descending aorta (DAo). *B*, Angiogram from a 4-month-old girl with truncus arteriosus type 2. Separate right and left pulmonary arteries (RPA, LPA) arose by separate ostia from the truncus, which continued as a right aortic arch (RAoA).

truncal valves are less common[11,13,44,45,53] but can calcify in older adults.[48]

The coronary arteries in truncus arteriosus are defined by their relationships to the truncal sinuses and by their epicardial courses (see Fig. 32–32).[2,8,20,63,68,74] During normal morphogenesis, the coronary arterial ostia appear after division of the embryonic truncus is complete.[36] There are initially six coronary artery anlagen, three from the aorta and three from the pulmonary artery.[33] Anlagen in the three pulmonary sinuses and in one of the three aortic sinus normally undergo involution, leaving two coronary arteries that arise from two persistent anlagen in the right and left aortic sinuses. In truncus arteriosus, the sinus substrates to which coronary arteries are assigned are disturbed by failure of septation of the embryonic truncus and by developmental abnormalities of the truncal valve.[20,68] The left coronary

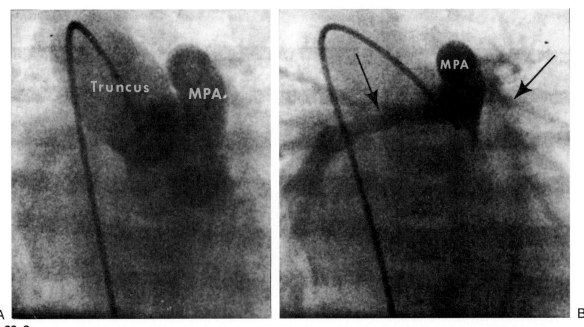

Figure 28–2

Angiograms from a 14-week-old boy with truncus arteriosus type 1. *A*, The main pulmonary artery (MPA) arose directly from the truncus. *B*, The right and left branches (*two unmarked arrows*) arose from the main pulmonary artery.

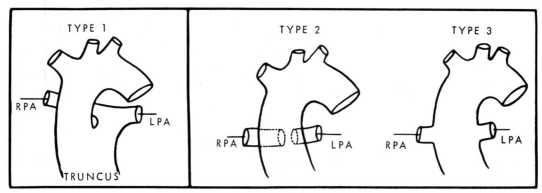

Figure 28–3

Illustrations of three anatomic types of truncus arteriosus. Type 1: A short main pulmonary artery originates from the truncus and gives rise to right and left pulmonary arteries (RPA, LPA). Type 2 and type 3: Right and left pulmonary arteries arise by separate ostia directly from the posterior or lateral wall of the truncus. Type 2 and type 3 are now considered as one category.

artery tends to arise from the left posterior aspect of the truncus, and the right coronary artery tends to arise from the right anterior aspect of the truncus whether the truncal valve is bicuspid, tricuspid, or quadricuspid (see Fig. 32–32).[2] When the truncal valve is quadricuspid, which is usually the case, coronary artery orifices originate in opposite sinuses rather than in adjacent sinuses, and high ostial origins are frequent.[2,68] The right coronary artery is dominant in about 85% of cases, and the conus branch of the right coronary artery is large and the left anterior descending artery is small.[2,8] The incidence of single coronary artery is increased (see Chapter 32).[20,68] An ostial membrane of the left coronary artery has been reported.[38]

A ventricular septal defect that results from absence or deficiency of the infundibular septum is almost always nonrestrictive and is roofed by the truncal valve, setting the stage for inadequate support and truncal valve regurgitation.[16,59] The biventricular truncal valve is either assigned equally to the two ventricles or predominantly to the right ventricle but infrequently to the left ventricle.[12,13,16,60,73]

Cardiovascular anomalies associated with truncus arteriosus include a right aortic arch (see Figs. 28–1 and 28–5), truncal valve abnormalities (see Figs. 28–10 and 28–22), anomalies of origin and distribution of the coronary arteries (see Fig. 32–12), absence of the right or left pulmonary artery (see Fig. 28–4B), and atresia of the ductus arteriosus.

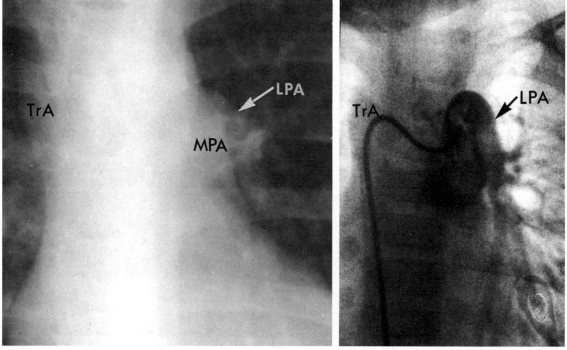

Figure 28–4

X-rays from a 7-year-old boy with truncus arteriosus type 1. *A*, The truncus (TrA) formed a right aortic arch. A main pulmonary artery (MPA) arose directly from the truncus and bifurcated into a left pulmonary artery (LPA) and a right pulmonary artery (not shown). The left pulmonary artery formed a hilar comma, delineated in the accompanying angiogram. *B*, Angiogram from a 16-month-old boy with truncus arteriosus type 1 and a right aortic arch. The left pulmonary artery (LPA) formed a distinctive hilar comma. The right pulmonary artery was absent.

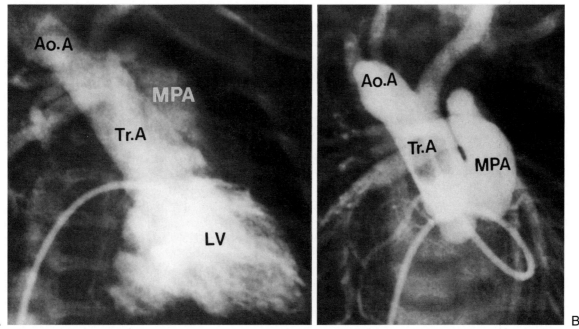

Figure 28–5

Angiocardiograms from a male neonate with truncus arteriosus type 1 and DiGeorge syndrome (see Fig. 28–6). *A*, The left ventriculogram (LV) visualized the truncus (TrA) that continued as a right aortic arch (AoA). The main pulmonary artery (MPA) originated directly from the truncus. *B*, Contrast material into the truncus delineated a main pulmonary artery originating directly from the truncus, which continued as a right aortic arch (AoA).

Abnormalities that occur sporadically include single ventricle, aberrant subclavian artery, left superior vena cava, and total anomalous pulmonary venous connection.[4,51,57,86] When truncus arteriosus occurs with complete interruption of the aortic arch, the interruption is distal to the origin of the left carotid artery.[12] The left subclavian artery arises from the descending aorta, and a patent ductus provides continuity from truncus to descending aorta.[12]

Importantly, a truncus arteriosus is a feature of normal early embryogenesis, an understanding of which sheds light on the morphogenesis of persistent truncus arteriosus.[42,52,60,72,85] Septation of the arterial pole of the normal heart begins with the appearance of two opposing truncal cushions that rapidly enlarge and fuse to form the truncal septum.[42] The proximal truncal septum normally fuses with the distal infundibular septum, a process that completes the spiral division of the truncus arteriosus and establishes left ventricular origin of the aorta and right ventricular origin of the pulmonary trunk. The aortic and pulmonary valves and their sinuses develop from truncal tissue at the line of fusion of the truncal and infundibular septa. In persistent truncus arteriosus, the truncal septum fails to develop and the infundibular septum is deficient or absent. The deficient or absent infundibular septum is responsible for the nonrestrictive ventricular septal defect that is roofed by the truncal valve. Vestigial development of the distal truncal septum is responsible for the short main pulmonary artery that arises from the truncus. When the truncal septum is absent altogether with no vestigial remnant, the main pulmonary artery is absent, so the right and left pulmonary arteries arise directly from the truncus by separate ostia.

Physiologic consequences of truncus arteriosus depend on the size of the pulmonary arteries and on the pulmonary vascular resistance. Right ventricular pressure is identical with systemic because both ventricles communicate directly with the biventricular truncus via the nonrestrictive ventricular septal defect. When a main pulmonary artery arises directly from the truncus, blood flow from the left and right ventricles tends to cross, so oxygen content is higher in the aorta than in the pulmonary artery.[69] Systemic arterial oxygen saturation is high when pulmonary resistance is low and pulmonary blood flow is increased, an advantage purchased at the price of volume overload of the left ventricle and congestive heart failure. Truncal valve regurgitation or truncal valve stenosis adds to the hemodynamic burden of the volume-overloaded left ventricle,[11,13,28,30,50,53] and the hemodynamic derangements are imposed on the right ventricle because the truncus is biventricular. As pulmonary vascular resistance rises, pulmonary blood flow falls. Volume overload of the left ventricle is curtailed at the price of increased cyanosis. Occasionally, mild to moderate hypoplasia of both pulmonary arteries adequately regulates pulmonary blood flow. In patients with truncus arteriosus and an absent right or left pulmonary artery, vascular disease develops early in the contralateral pulmonary artery (see Fig. 28–16A).[29]

The History

Truncus arteriosus occurs with equal frequency in males and females.[12,69] Isolated examples have been reported in siblings[9,12,32,62] and in twins,[6,43,58] and there is a relatively high incidence of congenital cardiac malformations in siblings of children with truncus arteriosus.[54] Familial recurrence of nonsyndromic truncus arteriosis with interrupted aortic arch has been described.[22] Truncus arteriosis has been reported with chromosome 22q11 deletion,[65] trisomy 18,[80] and trisomy 21.[79]

Truncus arteriosus comes to attention in the first few weeks of life because of tachypnea, diaphoresis, poor feeding, and failure to thrive.[50,69] As pulmonary resistance falls, pulmonary blood flow increases and neonatal cyanosis diminishes or may virtually vanish.[50,69] Truncal valve regurgitation is responsible for biventricular failure because regurgitant flow is received by both ventricles.[30,50] Appearance of the systolic murmur awaits the fall in neonatal pulmonary vascular resistance analogous to the time course with ventricular septal defect (see Chapter 17).

Infants with truncus arteriosus seldom reach their first birthday.[12,17,30,50,69] The majority die with congestive heart failure in the first few months of life. In van Praagh's necropsy series, mean age at death was 5 weeks.[74] A rise in pulmonary vascular resistance occasionally regulates pulmonary blood flow and relieves the volume-overloaded left ventricle. Symptoms of congestive heart failure improve while cyanosis deepens, and a small but not insignificant number of patients reach their third, fourth, or fifth decade[14,17,37,50,64] (see Figs. 28–15 through 28–18) with an occasional survival into the sixth decade.[15,18] Patients with truncus arteriosus and Eisenmenger syndrome experience the multisystem systemic disorders described in Chapter 17. Morbidity and mortality are also influenced by a host of noncardiac abnormalities that coexist with truncus arteriosus,[4] as described later.

Physical Appearance

Infants with increased pulmonary blood flow and congestive heart failure are frail and poorly developed, with cyanosis that is inconspicuous or absent. When truncus arteriosus occurs with hypoplasia of a pulmonary artery, the ipsilateral hemithorax tends to be small (see Fig. 28–16A).[13] DiGeorge syndrome is an important aspect of truncus arteriosus.[27,56,71,83] Typical appearance includes hypertelorism, low-set ears, micrognathia, a small fishlike mouth, a short philtrum, short down-slanting palpebral fissures, deformed or absent pinnae, cleft lip, a high-arched or cleft palate, a malformed nose, and bilateral cataracts (Fig. 28–6). Extracardiac congenital abnormalities involve the limbs, kidneys, and intestines.[56] Infants experience hypocalcemic seizures and severe infections due to deficient cell-mediated immunity and absence of the thymus and parathyroid glands.[56] The CHARGE association includes coloboma, heart disease, choanal atresia, retardation of growth and mental development, genital hypoplasia, and ear anomalies.[47] Conotruncal anomalies, especially truncus arteriosus, have been reported in 42% of patients with CHARGE association.[47]

The Arterial Pulse

The pulse pressure is wide because low pulmonary vascular resistance permits a diastolic runoff from the truncus into the pulmonary bed (Fig. 28–7). The rate of rise of the arterial pulse is brisk because a large left ventricular stroke volume is rapidly ejected. A brisk arterial pulse is especially conspicuous in the context of left ventricular failure and pulsus alternans (see Fig. 28–7). Truncal valve regurgitation inde-

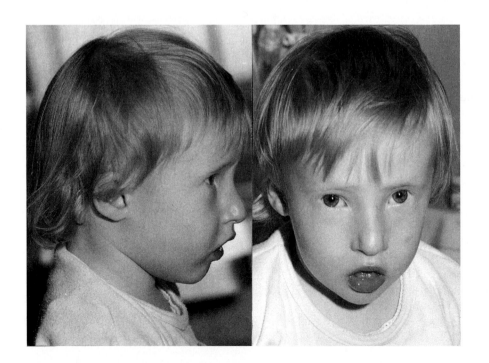

Figure 28–6
A 2-year-old girl with DiGeorge syndrome and truncus arteriosus. Facial dysmorphism included hypertelorism, low-set ears, micrognathia, a small fishlike mouth, short philtrum, down-slanting palpebral fissures, and a malformed nose. (From Radford DJ, Perkins L, Lachman R, Thong YH: Pediatr Cardiol 9:95, 1988.)

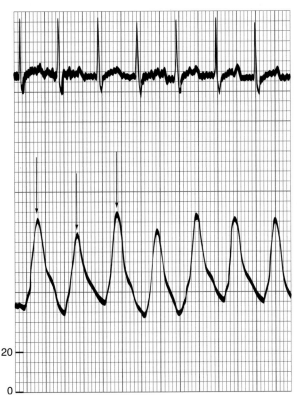

Figure 28–7
Aortic pressure pulse from an 18-day-old girl with a truncus arteriosus type 1. A short main pulmonary artery arose directly from the truncus and bifurcated into large right and left branches. The pulse pressure is wide, with a brisk rate of rise despite depressed left ventricular function reflected in the pulsus alternans (*arrows*).

pendently causes a bounding arterial pulse analogous to the waterhammer pulse of aortic regurgitation.[13,19,30,50]

The Jugular Venous Pulse

In infants with congestive heart failure, the jugular veins are distended, the liver is enlarged, and neither waveform nor a liver pulse can be identified. In adults with truncus arteriosus and Eisenmenger syndrome, the jugular venous pulse is normal or nearly so, analogous to the jugular pulse in patients with Eisenmenger syndrome and nonrestrictive ventricular septal defect (see Chapter 17).

Precordial Movement and Palpation

The impulse of a volume-overloaded hyperdynamic left ventricle is accompanied by a parasternal and subxiphoid impulse of a systemic right ventricle. Both impulses are augmented by regurgitant flow across an incompetent biventricular truncal valve. The main pulmonary artery of type 1 truncus arteriosus can be palpated in the second left intercostal space. The second heart sound is palpable because the truncal valve closes at systemic pressure and because truncal dilatation brings the valve closer to the

chest wall. A systolic thrill appears at the midleft sternal edge as neonatal pulmonary vascular resistance falls and as the left ventricle ejects a large stroke volume through the ventricular septal defect. A right sternoclavicular impulse indicates a right aortic arch.

In adults with truncus arteriosus and pulmonary vascular disease, the left ventricle is not volume overloaded and right ventricular pressure remains at systemic level, so the precordial impulse is from the right ventricle alone. Biventricular regurgitation across the truncal valve makes both ventricles palpable irrespective of pulmonary vascular resistance.

Auscultation

A normal first heart sound is followed by a high-pitched ejection sound generated within the dilated truncus (Figs. 28–8 and 28–9).[69,76] The systolic murmur through the ventricular septal defect and into the truncus is decrescendo, beginning with the ejection sound and ending before the second heart sound (see Figs. 28–8 and 28–9).[69,76] The murmur is harsh and blowing and usually grade 3/6 to 4/6 with maximum intensity in the third or fourth left intercostal space. Radiation is upward and to the right because the truncus takes the course of an ascending aorta (see Fig. 28–5).[69] The murmur is more prominent when the biventricular truncus arises chiefly above the right ventricle and is less prominent and often midsystolic when the truncus arises chiefly above the left ventricle or when pulmonary vascular disease minimizes the shunt. Flow is then across the truncal valve rather than across the ventricular septal defect. When the truncal valve is

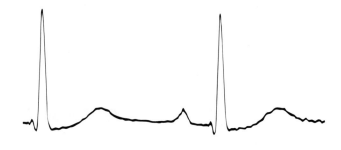

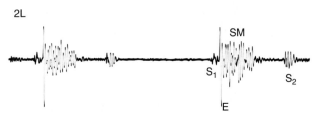

Figure 28–8
Phonocardiogram in the second left intercostal space (2L) of a 3-week-old male with truncus arteriosus type 2. The first heart sound (S_1) is followed by an ejection sound (E) and an early systolic decrescendo murmur (SM) that ended well before the second heart sound (S_2).

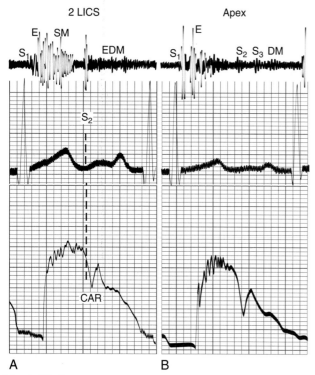

Figure 28–9

Phonocardiograms from an 11-year-old boy with truncus arteriosus type 2 from which right and left pulmonary arteries arose directly. *A*, In the second left intercostal space (2 LICS), there is an ejection sound (E) and a prominent decrescendo systolic murmur (SM) that ends before a loud single second sound (S_2). A decrescendo early diastolic murmur (EDM) of truncal valve regurgitation issued from the single truncal second heart sound. CAR, carotid; S_1, first heart sound. *B*, A third heart sound (S_3) and a short mid-diastolic murmur (DM) were recorded at the apex, together with the transmitted ejection sound and systolic murmur.

thickened, dysplastic, or stenotic, the murmur is midsystolic, as in aortic stenosis (see Chapter 7).

Systolic or continuous murmurs that are louder in systole are generated at the origins of hypoplastic pulmonary arteries as they emerge from the truncus. Continuous murmurs are seldom generated by the systemic arterial collaterals that supply the ipsilateral lung when a pulmonary artery is absent.

The truncal valve closure sound is prominent because the enlarged truncus is closer to the chest wall and because the truncal valve closes at systemic pressure (see Fig. 28–9). Splitting should not be possible because the truncus is equipped with only one valve. However, the second heart sound of a truncal valve equipped with three or more well-formed cusps may be impure or reduplicated on auscultation, but phonocardiograms show that the vibrations merge and do not represent two sounds separated by a distinct interval. On the other hand, the phonocardiogram occasionally records two components that have been assigned to cuspal inequality with asynchronous closure of tricuspid or quadricuspid truncal valves.[76]

A high-frequency blowing early diastolic murmur is caused by truncal valve regurgitation (Fig. 28–10, and see Fig. 28–9A).[13,19,30] An apical mid-diastolic murmur intro-

duced by a third heart sound (see Fig. 28–9B) results from increased mitral valve flow in response to low pulmonary vascular resistance and increased pulmonary blood flow. Mid-diastolic or presystolic Austin Flint murmurs are believed to result from severe truncal valve regurgitation.

The Electrocardiogram

Tall peaked right atrial P waves appear in limb leads and in precordial leads (Figs. 28–11 and 28–12) and are often accompanied by notched bifid left atrial P waves.[55,69] Infants may exhibit isolated left atrial P waves in response to increased pulmonary blood flow.

The conduction system is related to the location of the ventricular septal defect.[7] When pulmonary blood flow is reduced, the QRS axis is rightward and depolarization is clockwise because an underfilled left ventricle is coupled with a systemic right ventricle (Fig. 28–13, and see Fig. 28–12). The axis is normal or leftward when increased pulmonary blood flow overloads the left ventricle (see Fig. 28–11).[13,69] Precordial leads exhibit biventricular hypertrophy (see Figs. 28–11 and 28–12) with pure right ventricular hypertrophy reserved for adults with pulmonary vascular disease (see Fig. 28–13).[13,18,69] When pulmonary blood flow is increased, left precordial leads exhibit the deep Q waves, tall R waves, and inverted T waves of left ventricular hypertrophy, while right precordial leads continue to exhibit the tall R waves of right ventricular

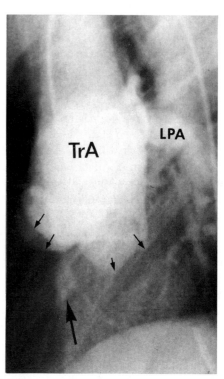

Figure 28–10

Lateral angiocardiogram from a 6-year-old boy with type 2 truncus arteriosus (TrA) and a quadricuspid truncal valve (*four small arrows*) that was incompetent (*large arrow*). LPA, left pulmonary artery.

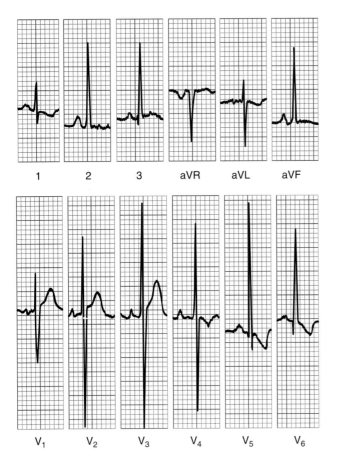

Figure 28–11
Electrocardiogram from a 3-week-old boy with truncus arteriosus type 1. Peaked right atrial P waves appear in leads 2 and aVF and in mid-precordial leads. The QRS axis is normal. Left ventricular hypertrophy is manifested by tall R waves and inverted T waves in leads V_{5-6}. Biventricular hypertrophy is manifested by large equidiphasic RS complexes in leads V_{2-4}.

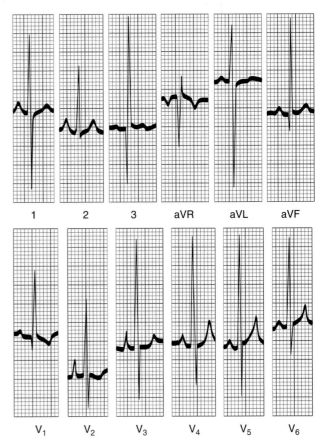

Figure 28–12
Electrocardiogram from a 2-year-old girl with truncus arteriosus type 1 and absent left pulmonary artery. Tall peaked right atrial P waves appear in lead 2 and in leads V_{2-4}. The Q wave in lead V_1 reflects right atrial enlargement. The QRS axis is +90 degrees. Right ventricular hypertrophy is manifested by the tall monophasic R wave in lead V_1 and by the prominent S waves in leads V_{4-6}. Left ventricular hypertrophy is manifested by the tall R waves and peaked T waves in leads V_{4-6} and by tall R waves in leads 3 and aVF.

hypertrophy (see Figs. 28–11 and 28–12). Large equidiphasic QRS complexes in central chest leads indicate combined ventricular hypertrophy (see Fig. 28–11).

The X-Ray

Increased pulmonary vascularity reflects both pulmonary blood flow and pulmonary venous congestion (Fig. 28–14).[69] A main pulmonary artery segment is absent when right and left pulmonary arteries arise directly from the truncus (see Fig. 28–14B).[69] The concave profile stands out in the right anterior oblique projection (see Fig. 28–17B). A dilated left pulmonary artery may occupy the concavity, but its shadow is usually recognized as such (see Fig. 28–17A). A prominent left pulmonary artery may reveal itself as a high shadow that curves upward to form a left hilar comma (see Fig. 28–4) that is especially evident when the aortic arch is right-sided.[13,34] The convex main pulmonary artery segment of truncus type 1 tends to arise at a higher level (see Fig. 28–18) compared with other forms of pulmonary artery dilatation. In older adults with pulmonary vascular disease, the dilated hypertensive main

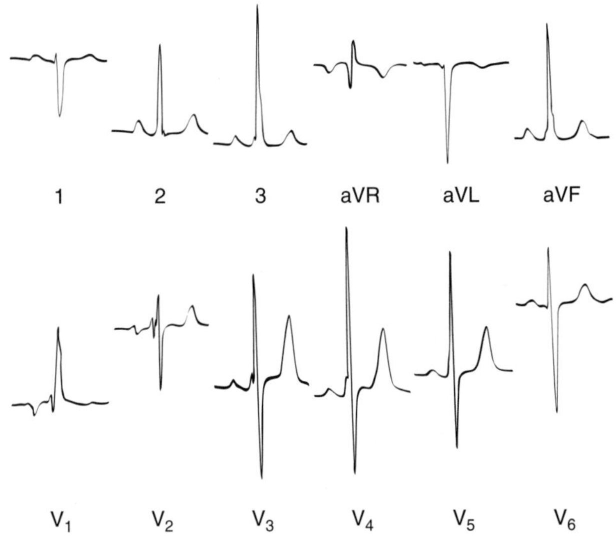

Figure 28–13
Electrocardiogram from a 42-year-old man with truncus arteriosus type 1 and pulmonary vascular disease whose x-rays are shown in Figure 28–18. The P wave in lead 2 is slightly peaked, and the negative P terminal force in lead V_1 is a right atrial abnormality. There is right axis deviation. Right ventricular hypertrophy is manifested by a tall monophasic R wave in lead V_1, by deep S waves in left precordial leads, and by increased amplitude of the R waves in leads 3 and aVF. The R waves in leads V_{4-5} indicate a well-developed left ventricle.

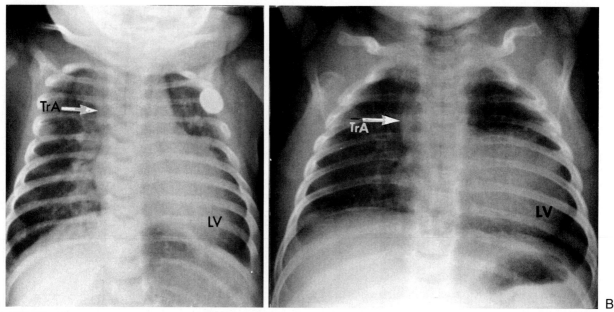

Figure 28–14

A, X-ray from a 3-week-old boy with truncus arteriosus type 1 that reveals itself at the right base (TrA, *arrow*). Pulmonary vascularity is increased, and the left ventricle (LV) is markedly dilated. *B,* X-ray from a 2-month-old boy with a truncus arteriosus type 2 that is prominent at the right base (TrA, *arrow*). A main pulmonary artery is conspicuously absent. Pulmonary vascularity is increased, and the left ventricle (LV) is strikingly dilated.

pulmonary artery segment is especially prominent (see Fig. 28–18). A large truncus arteriosis resembles a large ascending aorta (see Fig. 28–14) that may continue as a right aortic arch (see Fig. 28–5) and a high transverse aorta (Fig. 28–15).

The left ventricle dilates in response to volume overload associated with low pulmonary vascular resistance and increased pulmonary blood flow (see Figs. 28–14 and 28–15A). Enlargement of the right ventricle and right atrium is evident with congestive heart failure and when the right ventricle receives regurgitant flow across an incompetent biventricular truncal valve. Hypoplasia or absence of a pulmonary artery is accompanied by reduced vascularity and a smaller ipsilateral hemithorax (Fig.

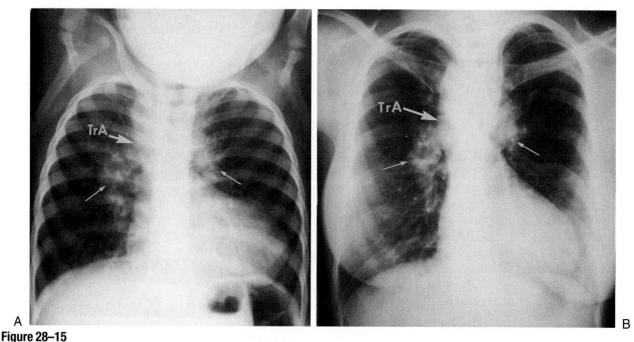

Figure 28–15

X-rays at 18 months and at 21 years of age from the same female patient with truncus arteriosus type 2. *A,* The truncus (TrA) continued as a right aortic arch and a high transverse aorta. Two separate pulmonary arteries (*small unmarked arrows*) originated by separate ostia directly from the truncus. Pulmonary vascularity is increased. The volume-overloaded left ventricle is dilated. *B,* Twenty years later, pulmonary vascular resistance was suprasystemic. Large right and left pulmonary arteries (*arrows*) stand out in bold relief against the clear lung fields of reduced pulmonary blood flow. The left ventricle remained enlarged because of truncal valve regurgitation.

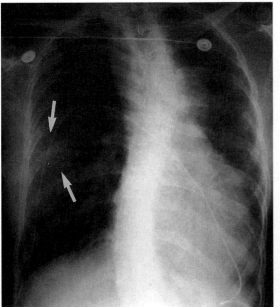 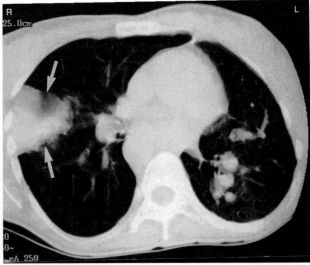

Figure 28–16

X-ray (*A*) and magnetic resonance image (*B*) from a 32-year-old woman with truncus arteriosus type 2. Scoliosis rotated the heart into a partial right anterior oblique position. The left pulmonary artery was hypoplastic, the left lung is hypoperfused, and the left hemithorax is small. The right pulmonary artery was normally formed, and there was pulmonary vascular disease in the right lung. *Arrows* bracket a density that the magnetic resonance image identified as an intrapulmonary hemorrhage.

28–16*A*). Absence of a pulmonary artery is usually on the same side as the aortic arch[49] (see Fig. 28–4*B*) in contrast to Fallot's tetralogy (see Chapter 18).

The x-ray in adults with high pulmonary vascular resistance shows decreased pulmonary vascularity, increased prominence of the main pulmonary artery and its right and left branches, and a relatively normal left ventricle (Figs. 28–17 and 28–18).

The Echocardiogram

Echocardiography with color flow imaging and Doppler interrogation establishes the type of truncus arteriosus, the relationship of the truncus to the left and right ventricles, the morphology and functional derangements of the truncal valve, and the physiologic consequences of the

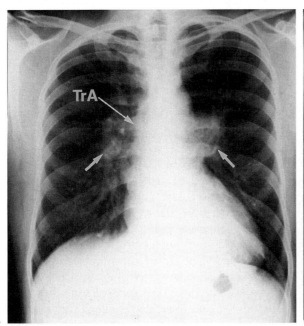 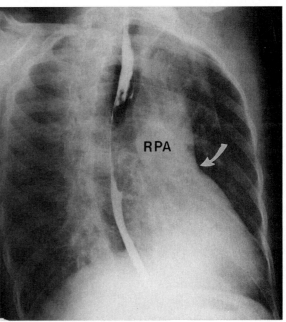

Figure 28–17

A, X-rays from a 30-year-old man with truncus arteriosus type 2 (TrA). Pulmonary vascularity is reduced because of pulmonary vascular disease. The hypertensive right and left pulmonary arteries are huge (*two unmarked arrows*). *B*, The right anterior oblique projection highlights the absence of a main pulmonary artery segment (*unmarked curved arrow*) in contrast to enlargement of the pulmonary artery branches. RPA, right pulmonary artery.

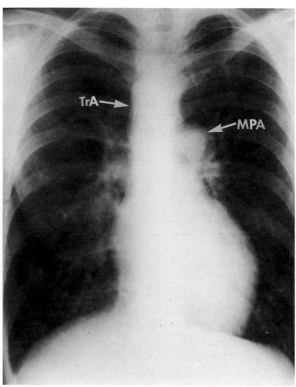

Figure 28–18

X-rays at 10 years (*A*) and at 42 years (*B*) of age from the same man with truncus arteriosus type 1 and pulmonary vascular disease. The electrocardiogram is shown in Figure 28–13. The two films are virtually identical except for body size. A dilated main pulmonary artery (MPA) originated from the truncus (TrA), which gave rise to enlarged hypertensive right and left branches. The truncus continued as a right aortic arch, a high transverse aorta, and a right descending aorta. Pulmonary vascularity was reduced because of pulmonary vascular disease. The convex left ventricle is of normal size.

malformation.[5,88] A single great arterial trunk overrides a nonrestrictive ventricular septal defect in the infundibular septum (Figs. 28–19 and 20–20*A*). The truncal valve forms the roof of the defect (see Fig. 28–20*A*). Right and left pulmonary arteries either arise from a short main pulmonary artery (see Figs. 28–19 and 28–20*A*) or arise directly from the truncus by separate ostia. Color flow imaging delin-

eates the truncus and the pulmonary arterial arrangements (Fig. 28–21, and see Fig. 28–20*B*). Unbalanced biventricular right or left ventricular origin of the truncus can be determined (see Figs. 28–20*A* and 28–21), and the morphology of the truncal valve can be established (Fig. 28–22). Color flow imaging determines the presence and degree of truncal valve regurgitation, and continuous-wave Doppler determines the presence and degree of truncal valve stenosis.

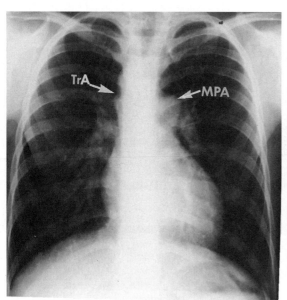

Figure 28–19

Echocardiogram (subcostal) showing truncus arteriosus type 1 (TrA) communicating with a main pulmonary artery (MPA) that gave rise to right and left branches. AAo, ascending aorta; RA, right atrium; LV, left ventricle.

Summary

Truncus arteriosus typically comes to attention in early infancy because increased pulmonary blood flow results in congestive heart failure. Cyanosis is mild or absent. A systolic murmur across the ventricular septal defect becomes evident as neonatal pulmonary vascular resistance falls. The arterial pulse is bounding despite congestive heart failure. Left and right ventricular impulses are conspicuous, and a main pulmonary artery impulse is palpable in truncus type 1. Auscultation reveals an ejection sound and a relatively long decrescendo systolic murmur maximum in the third left intercostal space with radiation upward and to the right. A mid-diastolic murmur is caused by augmented flow across the mitral valve. When the shunt across the ventricular septal defect is reduced by increased

Figure 28–20

A, Echocardiogram (subcostal) from a 3-year-old boy with truncus arteriosus type 1. The biventricular truncus (Tr) arises above a nonrestrictive ventricular septal defect (VSD) that is roofed by the truncal valve (*short unmarked arrow*). The main pulmonary artery (MPA) arises directly from the truncus. *B,* Black and white print of a color flow image showing the truncus arteriosus and the main pulmonary artery originating from it.

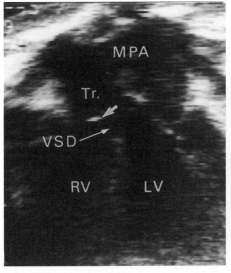
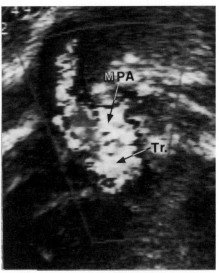

pulmonary vascular resistance, a soft midsystolic murmur emerges across the truncal valve. The midsystolic truncal murmur is louder and longer when the valve is dysplastic or stenotic. The second heart sound is loud, single, and reduplicated. An early diastolic murmur is caused by truncal valve regurgitation.

The electrocardiogram shows right atrial or biatrial P waves, and the QRS pattern exhibits varying degrees of combined ventricular hypertrophy. Pure right ventricular hypertrophy is reserved for adults with elevated pulmonary vascular resistance. The x-ray shows increased vascularity because of pulmonary arterial blood flow and because of pulmonary venous congestion. The truncus often continues as a right aortic arch and a high transverse arch. The main pulmonary artery segment is prominent in truncus type 1 but is concave when the right and left pulmonary arteries arise directly from the truncus by separate ostia. The left pulmonary artery may form a distinctive hilar comma. The left and right ventricles dilate in response to congestive heart failure and in response to biventricular truncal valve regurgitation. In adults with pulmonary vascular disease, the lungs are oligemic, the main pulmonary artery segment and the left and right branches are prominent, but the heart size is normal or nearly so unless the truncal valve is regurgitant or stenotic. Echocardiography with color flow imaging and Doppler interrogation establishes the type of truncus arteriosus, the relationship of the truncus to the right and left ventricles, the morphology and functional derangements of the truncal valve, and the physiologic consequences of the malformation.

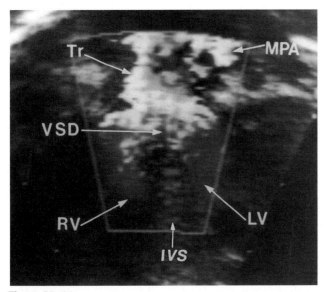

Figure 28–21

Black and white print of a color flow image from a 3-week-old boy with truncus arteriosus type 1. The biventricular truncus (Tr) arises above a nonrestrictive ventricular septal defect (VSD). A main pulmonary artery (MPA) arose directly from the truncus. IVS, interventricular septum; RV/LV, right and left ventricle.

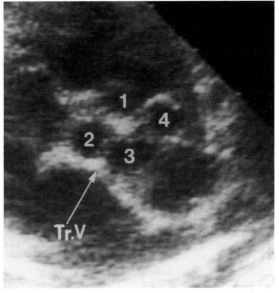

Figure 28–22

A quadricuspid truncal valve (Tr.V) in the short axis.

REFERENCES

1. Allwork SP, Bentall RHC: Truncus solitarius pulmonalis. Br Heart J 35:977, 1973.
2. Anderson KR, McGoon DC, Lie JT: Surgical significance of the coronary arterial anatomy in truncus arteriosus communis. Am J Cardiol 41:76, 1978.
3. Anderson RH, Wilkinson JL, Arnold R, Lubkiewicz K: Morphogenesis of bulboventricular malformations. 1: Considerations of embryogenesis in the normal heart. Br Heart J 36:242, 1974.
4. Williams JM, de Leeuw M, Black MD, et al: Factors associated with outcome of persistent truncus arteriosus. J Am Coll Cardiol 34:545, 1999.
5. Duke C, Sharland GK, Jones AMR, Simpson JM: Echocardiographic features and outcome of truncus arteriosus diagnosed during fetal life. Am J Cardiol 88:1379, 2001.
6. Benesova D, Sikl H: Rare concordant malformation in monochoriate twins: Persistent common arterial trunk. J Pathol Bacteriol 67:367, 1954.
7. Bharati S, Karp R, Lev M: The conduction system in truncus arteriosus and its surgical significance. J Thorac Cardiovasc Surg 104;954, 1992.
8. Bharati S, McAllister HA, Rosenquist GC, et al: The surgical anatomy of truncus arteriosus communis. J Thorac Cardiovasc Surg 67:501, 1974.
9. Brunson SC, Nudel DB, Grootman N, Aftalion B: Truncus arteriosus in a family. Am Heart J 96:419, 1978.
10. Buchanan A: Malformation of the heart: Undivided truncus arteriosus. Heart otherwise double. Trans. Pathol Soc Lond 15:89, 1864.
11. Burnell RH, McEnery G, Miller GAH: Truncal valve stenosis. Br Heart J 33:423, 1971.
12. Butto F, Lucas RV, Edwards JE: Persistent truncus arteriosus: Pathologic anatomy in 54 cases. Pediatr Cardiol 7:95, 1986.
13. Calder L, Van Praagh R, Van Praagh S, et al: Truncus arteriosus communis: Clinical, angiographic, and pathologic findings in 100 patients. Am Heart J 92:23, 1976.
14. Carr FB, Goodale RH, Rockwell AEP: Persistent truncus arteriosus in man aged 36 years. Arch Pathol 19:833, 1935.
15. Carter JB, Blieden LC, Edwards JE: Persistent truncus arteriosus: Report of survival to age 52 years. Minn Med 56:280, 1973.
16. Ceballos R, Soto B, Kirklin JW, Bargeron LM: Truncus arteriosus: An anatomical-angiographic study. Br Heart J 49:589, 1983.
17. Collett RW, Edwards JE: Persistent truncus arteriosus: Classification according to anatomic types. Surg Clin North Am 29:1245, 1949.
18. Niwa K, Perloff JK, Kaplan S, et al: Eisenmenger syndrome in adults: Ventricular septal defect, truncus arteriosus, univentricular heart. J Am Coll Cardiol 34:223, 1999.
19. Deely WJ, Hagstrom JWC, Engle MA: Truncus insufficiency: Common truncus arteriosus with regurgitant truncus valve. Am Heart J 65:542, 1963.
20. de la Cruz MV, Cayre R, Angelini P, et al: Coronary arteries in truncus arteriosus. Am J Cardiol 66:1482, 1990.
21. Di George AM: Congenital absence of the thymus and its immunologic consequences: Occurrence with congenital hypoparathyroidism. Birth Defects 4:116, 1986.
22. Digilio MC, Marino B, Musolino Am, et al: Familial recurrence of nonsyndromic interrupted aortic arch and truncus arteriosus with atrioventricular canal. Teratology 61:329, 2000.
23. Edwards JE, McGoon DC: Absence of anatomic origin from heart of pulmonary arterial supply. Circulation 47:393, 1973.
24. Farre JR: Pathological researches: Essay I: On malformation of the human heart. London, Longman, 1814.
25. Fong LV, Anderson RH, Siewers RD, et al: Anomalous origin of one pulmonary artery from the ascending aorta: A review of echocardiographic, catheter, and morphological features. Br Heart J 62:389, 1989.
26. Fontana GP, Spach MS, Effmann EL, Sabiston DC: Origin of the right pulmonary artery from the ascending aorta. Ann Surg 206:102, 1987.
27. Freedom RM, Rosen FS, Nadas AS: Congenital cardiovascular disease and anomalies of the third and fourth pharyngeal pouch. Circulation 46:165, 1972.
28. Fuglestad SJ, Puga FJ, Danielson GK, Edwards WD: Surgical pathology of the truncal valve: A study of 12 cases. Am J Cardiovasc Pathol 2:39, 1988.
29. Fyfe DA, Driscoll DJ, DiDonato RM, et al: Truncus arteriosus with single pulmonary artery. J Am Coll Cardiol 5:1168, 1985.
30. Gelband H, Van Meter S, Gersony WM: Truncal valve abnormalities in infants with persistent truncus arteriosus. Circulation 45:397, 1972.
31. Glew D, Hartnell GG: The right aortic arch revisited. Clin Radiol 43:305, 1991.
32. Goodyear JE: Persistent truncus arteriosus in two siblings. Br Heart J 23:194, 1961.
33. Hackensellner HA: Ueber akessorische, von der Arteria Pulmonalis abgehende Herzgefaesse und ihre bei den Tung fuer das Verstaendis der formalen Genese des Ursprunges einer oder beider Coronararterien von der Lungenschlagader. Frankf Z Path 66:263, 1955.
34. Hallerman FJ, Kincaid OW, Tsakiris AG, et al: Persistent truncus arteriosus: Radiographic and angiographic study. Am J Roentgenol 107:827, 1969.
35. Hastreiter AR, D'Cruz IA, Cantez T: Right-sided aorta. Br Heart J 28:722, 1966.
36. Heifetz SA, Robinowitz M, Muller KH, Virmani R: Total anomalous origin of the coronary arteries from the pulmonary artery. Pediatr Cardiol 7:11, 1986.
37. Hicken P, Evans D, Heath D: Persistent truncus arteriosus with survival to the age of 38 years. Br Heart J 28:284, 1966.
38. Van Son JA, Autschbach R, Hambsch J: Congenital ostial membrane of left coronary artery in truncus arteriosus. J Thorac Cardiovasc Surg 118:1132, 1999.
39. Humphreys EM: Truncus arteriosus communis persistens; criteria for identification of common arterial trunk, with report of case with 4 semilunar cusps. Arch Pathol 14:671, 1932.
40. Hunter OB Jr: Truncus arteriosus communis persistens. Arch Pathol 37:328, 1944.
41. Johnson JL, Turner AF: Persistent truncus arteriosus with interruption of the aortic arch. Vasc Dis 4:244, 1967.
42. Kutsche LM, Van Mierop LHS: Anatomy and pathogenesis of aorticopulmonary septal defect. Am J Cardiol 59:443, 1987.
43. Lang MJ, Aughton DJ, Riggs TW, et al: Dizygotic twins concordant for truncus arteriosus. Clin Genet 39:75, 1991.
44. Ledbetter MK, Tandon R, Titus JL, Edwards JE: Stenotic semilunar valve in persistent truncus arteriosus. Chest 69:182, 1976.
45. Lee MH, Bellon EM, Liebman J, Perrin EV: Truncal valve stenosis. Am Heart J 85:397, 1973.
46. Lev M, Saphir O: Truncus arteriosus communis persistens. J Pediatr 20:74, 1942.
47. Lin AE, Chin AJ, Devine W, et al: The pattern of cardiovascular malformation in the CHARGE association. Am J Dis Child 141:110, 1987.
48. MacGilpin HH Jr: Truncus arteriosus communis persistens. Am Heart J 39:615, 1950.
49. Mair DD, Ritter DG, Danielson GK, et al: Truncus arteriosus with unilateral absence of a pulmonary artery. Circulation 55:641, 1977.
50. Marcelletti C, McGoon DC, Mair DD: The natural history of truncus arteriosus. Circulation 54:108, 1976.
51. Litovsky SH, Ostfeld I, Bjornstad PG, et al: Truncus arteriosus with anomalous pulmonary venous connection. Am J Cardiol 83:801, 1999.
51a. Niwa K, Perloff JK, Bhuta S, Laks H: Structural abnormalities of great arterial walls in congential heart disease. Circulation 103:393, 2001.
52. Orts-Llorca F, Fonolla JP, Sobrado J: The formation, septation and fate of the truncus arteriosus in man. J Anat 134:41, 1982.
53. Patel RG, Freedom RM, Bloom KR, Rowe RD: Truncal or aortic valve stenosis in functionally single arterial trunk. Am J Cardiol 42:800, 1978.
54. Pierpont MEA, Gobel JW, Moller JH, Edwards JE: Cardiac malformations in relatives of children with truncus arteriosus or interruption of the aortic arch. Am J Cardiol 61:423, 1988.
55. Portillo B, Perez-Martin R: Truncus arteriosus communis: Electrocardiographic study in 17 cases. Arch Inst Cardiol Mex 30:609, 1960.
56. Radford DJ, Perkins L, Lachman R, Thong YH: Spectrum of DiGeorge syndrome in patients with truncus arteriosus. Pediatr Cardiol 9:95, 1988.
57. Paris YM, Bhan I, Marx GR, Rhodes J: Truncus arteriosus with a single left ventricle. Am Heart J 133:377, 1997.

58. Mas C, Delatycki MB, Weintraub RG: Persistent truncus arteriosus in monozygotic twins. Am J Genet 82:146, 1999.

59. Rosenquist CG, Bharati S, McAllister HA, Lev M: Truncus arteriosus communis. Am J Cardiol 37:410, 1976.

60. Rothko K, Moore GW, Hutchins GM: Truncus arteriosus malformation. Am Heart J 99:17, 1980.

61. Sennari E, Nishiguchi T, Okishima T, et al: Truncus solitarius pulmonalis. Pediatr Cardiol 11:50, 1990.

62. Shapiro SR, Ruckman RN, Kapur S, et al: Single ventricle with truncus arteriosus in siblings. Am Heart J 102:456, 1981.

63. Shrivastava S, Edwards JE: Coronary arterial origin in persistent truncus arteriosus. Circulation 55:551, 1977.

64. Silverman JJ, Scheinesson GP: Persistent truncus arteriosus in a 43 year old man. Am J Cardiol 17:94, 1966.

65. Momma K, Ando M, Matsuoka R: Truncus arteriosus communis associated with chromosome 22q11 deletion. J Am Coll Cardiol 30:1067, 1997.

66. Sotomora RF, Edwards JE: Anatomic identification of so-called absent pulmonary artery. Circulation 57:624, 1978.

67. Stone FM, Amplatz K, Lucas RV, et al: Ventricular septal defect, solitary aortic trunk, and ductal origins of pulmonary arteries. Am Heart J 92:506, 1976.

68. Suzuki A, Ho SY, Anderson RH, Deanfield JE: Coronary arterial and sinus anatomy in hearts with a common arterial trunk. Ann Thorac Surg 48:792, 1989.

69. Tandon R, Hauck AJ, Nadas AS: Persistent truncus arteriosus: A clinical, hemodynamic, and autopsy study of nineteen cases. Circulation 28:1050, 1963.

70. Todd EP, Lindsay WG, Edwards JE: Bilateral ductal origin of the pulmonary arteries. Circulation 54:834, 1976.

71. Van Mierop LHS, Kutsche LM: Cardiovascular anomalies in DiGeorge syndrome and importance of neural crest as a possible pathogenetic factor. Am J Cardiol 58:133, 1986.

72. Van Mierop LHS, Patterson DF, Schnarr WR: Pathogenesis of persistent truncus arteriosus in light of observations made in a dog embryo with the anomaly. Am J Cardiol 41:755, 1978.

73. Van Praagh R: Classification of truncus arteriosus communis (TAC). Am Heart J 92:129, 1976.

74. Van Praagh R, Van Praagh S: The anatomy of common aorticopulmonary trunk (truncus arteriosus communis) and its embryologic implications: A study of 57 necropsy cases. Am J Cardiol 16:406, 1965.

75. Victorica BE, Elliott LP: Roentgenologic findings and approach to persistent truncus arteriosus in infancy. Am J Roentgenol 104:440, 1968.

76. Victorica BE, Gessner IH, Schiebler GL: Phonocardiographic findings in persistent truncus arteriosus. Br Heart J 30:812, 1968.

77. Webb AC: Truncus arteriosus communis persistens. Arch Pathol 42:427, 1946.

78. Wilson J: Description of a very unusual malformation of the human heart. Philos Trans R Soc Lond 18:346, 1798.

79. Francalanci P, Gallo P, Dallapiccola B, et al: A genetic assessment of trisomy 21 in a patient with persistent truncus arteriosus who died 38 years ago. Am J Cardiol 79:245, 1997.

80. Moore JW, Wight NE, Jones MC, Krous HF: Truncus arteriosus associated with trisomy 18. Pediatr Cardiol 15:154, 1994.

81. Alboliras ET, Lombardo S, Antillon J: Truncus arteriosus with double aortic arch: Two dimensional and color flow Doppler echocardiographic diagnosis. Am Heart J 129:415, 1995.

82. Mello DM, McElhinney DB, Parry AJ, et al: Truncus arteriosus with patent ductus and normal aortic arch. Ann Thorac Surg 64:1808, 1997.

83. Farrell MJ, Stadt H, Wallis KT, et al: HIRA, a DiGeorge syndrome candidate gene, is required for cardiac outflow tract septation. Circ Res 84:127, 1999.

84. Marino B, Digilio MC, Dallapiccola B: Severe truncal valve dysplasia: Association with DiGeorge syndrome? Ann Thorac Surg 66:980, 1998.

85. Yu IT, Hutchins GM: Truncus arteriosus malformation: A developmental arrest at Carnegie stage 14. Teratology 53:31, 1996.

86. Berdjis F, Wells WJ, Starnes VA: Truncus arteriosus with total anomalous pulmonary venous return and interrupted aortic arch. Ann Thorac Surg 61:220, 1996.

87. Slavik Z, Keeton BR, Salmon AP, et al: Persistent truncus arteriosus operated during infancy. Ped Cardiol 15:112, 1994.

88. Child JS: Transthoracic and transesophageal echocardiographic imaging: Anatomic and hemodynamic assessment. In Perloff JK, Child JS (eds): Congenital Heart Disease in Adults, 2nd ed. Philadelphia, WB Saunders, 1998, p. 91.

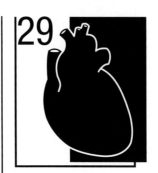

Congenital Anomalies of Vena Caval Connection

Anomalous vena caval connections represent a wide range of malformations that vary from minor to major and that occur either in isolation or with coexisting congenital heart disease. This chapter focuses on isolated anomalous vena caval connections in situs solitus hearts (Table 29–1). Anomalies of vena caval connection with cardiac malpositions and with atrial isomerism are dealt with in Chapter 3.

In early embryonic development, the common cardinal veins are bilaterally symmetric and are potentially responsible for bilateral superior venae cavae.[61] The left common cardinal vein initially drains into the left portion of the sinus venosus, which becomes the coronary sinus.[61] Failure of obliteration of the left common cardinal vein results in persistent connection of a left superior vena cava to the coronary sinus (Fig. 29–1),[55,61] a relatively common anomaly estimated at 0.3% to 0.5% in the general population and 1.5% to 10% of patients with congenital heart disease.[11,28,54,55,71] An isolated left superior vena cava in itself produces no physiologic derangements when it drains harmlessly into the right atrium via the coronary sinus (see Fig. 29–1).[26,54,55] However, the coronary sinus dilates sometimes appreciably,[2,71] especially if there is atresia of its right atrial orifice[39] or absence of the right superior vena cava.[14,84] When the right superior vena cava is absent, the sinus node pacemaker is absent, because the pacemaker is normally located at the junction of the right superior vena cava and the morphologic right atrium.[18,19,36,40,47,49,59,85] A persistent left superior vena cava is a significant anomaly when it connects directly to the left atrium (Figs. 29–2 and 29–3).* The coronary sinus is usually absent,[55,83] with absence including partial or complete unroofing of its anterosuperior wall. Unroofing results in a connection

between the left atrium and the right atrium—a coronary sinus type of atrial septal defect (see Chapter 15).[15,55,67] A right-to-left shunt coexists through the left superior vena caval-to-left atrial connection.[20,26,55,56,62,77] An absent coronary sinus with bilateral superior venae cavae (right superior cava connected to the right atrium,[26,34] left superior cava connected to the left atrium) is believed to represent a developmental complex.[25,34,67] If the right superior vena cava is absent or atretic (see Fig. 29–3), the innominate vein crosses the midline and terminates in the left superior vena cava.[21,78] The left atrium occasionally receives the azygos vein, the hepatic vein, or the coronary sinus,[10,21,44,77] variations that are not considered in this chapter.

Direct connections between venae cavae and left atrium are uncommon.* Rarely, a right superior vena cava con-

---

*13,21,26,52,53,67,68,72,73,81,84

Table 29–1   Congenital Anomalies of Vena Caval Connection

Left superior vena cava
   connected to coronary sinus
   connected to left atrium
Right superior vena cava
   absent
   connected to left atrium
Bilateral superior venae cavae
Inferior vena cava
   connected to left atrium
   interruption with azygous continuation
Superior and inferior venae cavae both connected to left atrium (total anomalous systemic venous connection)

---

*See references 1, 27, 32, 34, 41, 44, 55, 67, 73, 74, 77, 79.

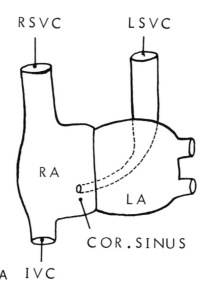
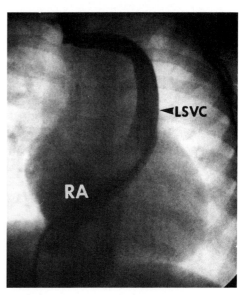

Figure 29–1

A, Persistent left superior vena cava (LSVC) drains into the right atrium (RA) via the coronary sinus. The right superior vena cava (RSVC) and the inferior vena cava (IVC) drain normally into the right atrium. B, Left superior vena cava draining into the coronary sinus in a 3-year-old child.

nects to the left atrium.[4,8,23,42,43,45,64,76] Still more rarely, a right superior vena cava connects to the left atrium, and a left superior vena cava connects to the right atrium.[51] Connection of a right superior vena cava to the left atrium must be distinguished from drainage of a right superior vena cava into both atria caused by a contiguous superior vena caval sinus venosus atrial septal defect (see Chapter 15).[55,72] When a right superior vena cava is congenitally absent (see Fig. 29–3), brachiocephalic veins join a left superior vena cava that connects to the coronary sinus.[3,14,17,55,85]

Bilateral superior venae cavae[11] are illustrated in Figure 29–2. The innominate bridge that connects the two superior cavae may be widely patent, narrow, or atretic (see Fig. 29–2), and the size of the left superior vena cava ranges from large to rudimentary.[11] Bilateral superior venae cavae with atrial isomerism are dealt with in Chapter 3.

Anomalous connection of the inferior vena cava to the left atrium consists of a morphogenetic spectrum represented by combinations of persistence of the valve of the right sinus venosus, fusion of the valve with the septum secundum, and incomplete development of the atrial septum.[58] The inferior vena cava penetrates the diaphragm at its expected site.[5,29,55] An enlarged azygos vein may arise from the anomalous inferior cava and convey inferior caval blood into the right atrium (see Fig. 29–5).[12,29,30,75,81] An isolated left-sided abdominal inferior vena cava usually crosses to the right after receiving the renal veins, then penetrates the diaphragm and enters the right atrium at the normal site.[9] A distinction must be made between connection of the inferior vena cava to the left atrium and anomalous inferior vena caval drainage into the left atrium due to persistence of a large eustachian valve (right valve of the sinus venosus) that directs flow toward a patent foramen

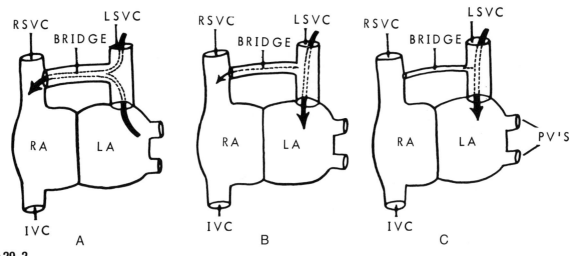

Figure 29–2

A, Persistent left superior vena cava (LSVC) communicating directly with the left atrium (LA). The right superior vena cava (RSVC) and the inferior vena cava (IVC) drain normally into the right atrium (RA). The bilateral superior venae cavae communicate through a large innominate bridge. The direction of blood flow is from the left atrium into the anomalous left superior vena cava and then across the innominate bridge into the right superior vena cava. These pathways constitute a left-to-right shunt. B, A restrictive innominate bridge offers resistance so that left superior vena caval blood is diverted into the left atrium with only a small portion flowing across the bridge. C, An atretic innominate bridge diverts left superior vena caval blood entirely into the left atrium. PV'S, pulmonary veins.

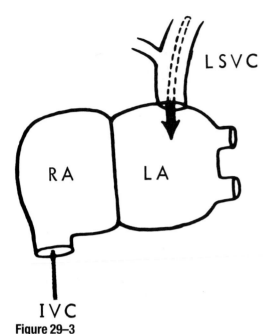

Figure 29–3

A persistent left superior vena cava (LSVC) connects directly to the left atrium (LA). The right superior vena cava is absent, but the inferior vena cava (IVC) drains normally into the right atrium (RA).

ovale or across an ostium secundum atrial septal defect (see Chapter 15).[28,58]

Inferior vena caval interruption with azygous continuation is rare as an isolated malformation and is of no physiologic significance[55] but can be mistaken for the descending thoracic aorta (Fig. 29–4).[6] Interruption is immediately proximal to the renal veins and continues into a dilated azygos vein that enters the thorax to the right of the aorta,

runs in the posterior mediastinum, and connects to a right superior vena cava (see Fig. 29–4). There is an association with congenital absence of the portal vein.[48] Inferior vena caval interruption with azygos continuation and left isomerism is dealt with in Chapter 3.

Anomalous connection of either vena cava to the left atrium is rare enough, but connection of the right superior vena cava *and* the inferior vena cava to the left atrium—total anomalous systemic venous connection—is even rarer (see Figs. 29–7 and 29–9).[33,55,66,69,72,82] Survival depends on adequate mixing through an interatrial communication.

The physiologic consequences of anomalous vena caval connections to the left atrium take into account two variables: (1) the direction and volume of blood flow through the connection, and (2) the effect of the connection on the amount of blood flow entering the right and left sides of the heart. Flow patterns are complex when a persistent left superior vena cava communicates with the left atrium (see Fig. 29–2).[56,62,77] The left superior vena cava may be the only superior cava (see Fig. 29–3) or bilateral superior cavae may fail to communicate with each other because of stenosis or atresia of the innominate bridge (see Fig. 29–2B,C). All or nearly all of left superior vena caval blood is then channeled into the left atrium (see Fig. 29–2B,C), so cyanosis is obligatory. Alternatively, when bilateral superior venae cavae communicate freely through a nonrestrictive innominate bridge, the direction of blood flow is from the left atrium into the anomalous left superior vena cava, across the innominate bridge and into the right superior vena cava (see Fig. 29–2A).[46,56,62] The pathway constitutes a left-to-right shunt, so cyanosis is absent.[56,77] With this exception, communications between venae cavae and

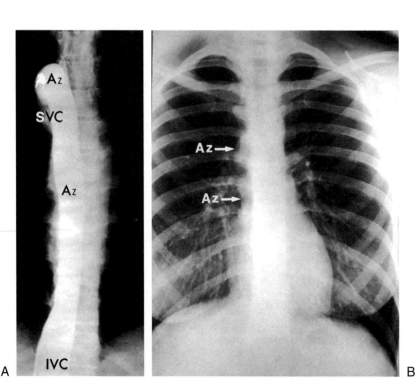

Figure 29–4

A, Inferior vena cavagram from a 28-year-old woman with isolated inferior vena caval interruption (IVC) and azygous (Az) continuation to a right superior vena cava (SVC). *B,* The x-ray shows the azygos vein ascending along the right side of the vertebral column (lower Az), forming a knuckle as it joins the right superior cava (upper Az).

left atrium result in right-to-left shunts and in a decrease in systemic arterial oxygen saturation. When a right superior vena cava connects to the left atrium, caval blood flow is into the left atrium, so cyanosis is obligatory. When the inferior vena cava connects to the left atrium, unoxygenated blood is directed into the left atrium despite a large azygos vein, so cyanosis is also obligatory (Fig. 29–5).

Consider now the relative amounts of blood flowing through the two sides of the heart in the presence of vena caval-to-left atrial connections. Normally, the entire systemic venous return from the superior and inferior venae cavae enters the right side of the heart, while the entire pulmonary venous return from the pulmonary veins enters the left side of the heart. If one vena cava connects to the left atrium, the right side of the heart is effectively bypassed, so right ventricular output and pulmonary blood flow fall reciprocally.[38,56] Left ventricular output theoretically remains unchanged,[56] because the increment in anomalous caval flow into the left atrium is matched by the reciprocal decrement in pulmonary venous flow. Accordingly, as systemic venous return to the left atrium increases, pulmonary venous return to the left atrium decreases by the same amount, so total blood flow to the left side of the heart remains unchanged. In the absence of compensatory mechanisms, anomalous caval connections to the left atrium should be associated with reduced pulmonary flow and normal systemic flow,[38,56] patterns that should pertain irrespective of whether the superior or inferior vena cava connects anomalously. Do these circulatory patterns really exist? Clinical and experimental observations indicate that right atrial and right ventricular pressures are normal or low[20,38,43,57] and pulmonary blood flow is usually[5,20,38,56] but not always reduced.[78] Necropsy descriptions of a small right atrium and a small right ventricle are relevant.[5,29,43,80] However, left ventricular output tends to be moderately increased.[5,20,38,57,78] The mechanisms responsible for these deviations from theoretical blood flow patterns are not known.

When the superior vena cava and inferior vena cava *both* connect to the left atrium—total anomalous systemic venous connection—flow patterns are modified by obligatory mixing at atrial level. The left atrium receives blood from both cavae *and* from the pulmonary veins. Part of this mixture reaches the left ventricle directly across the mitral valve, and the remainder enters the right side of the heart across an atrial septal defect. Pulmonary blood flow is not increased even in the presence of a nonrestrictive atrial septal defect and normal pulmonary vascular resistance (see Fig. 29–9).

The inferior vena cava normally carries about twice the volume of systemic venous return compared with the superior vena cava. Accordingly, an anomalously connecting inferior cava delivers a larger proportion of blood to the left atrium than an anomalously connecting superior vena cava. However, the magnitude of systemic blood flow (cardiac output) does not depend on which vena cava delivers its return to the left atrium, provided that pulmonary venous return falls by an equivalent amount.

The History

Isolated anomalous vena caval connection to the left atrium has an equal sex distribution.[56] Cyanosis dates from birth or infancy,[5,20,29,43,58,72,78] unless bilateral superior cavae are connected by a nonrestrictive innominate bridge (see Fig. 29–2A). There is a paucity of symptoms despite conspicuous cyanosis[5,20,29,54,57,58,64,81]—the syndrome of cyanosis and clubbing with a "normal" heart.[57] Adult survival is expected, with longevities recorded in the sixth, seventh, and eighth decades.[1,7,9,23,44,56,72] Mild effort intolerance, dyspnea, and light-headedness develop late if at all.[20,23,57,70,72,81] One man tolerated training in the armed forces.[58] Brain abscess and paradoxical embolus have been reported.[42,64,65,72,79]

The cause of death is usually unrelated to isolated congenital anomalies of vena caval connection.[5,29,78] However, unexplained sudden death has been reported with isolated left superior vena caval connection to the coronary sinus, especially if the right superior vena cava is absent (see The Electrocardiogram).[40,49]

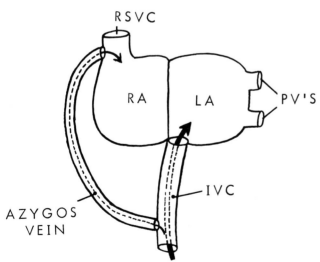

Figure 29–5
The inferior vena cava (IVC) connects directly to the left atrium (LA). The anomalous inferior vena cava gives rise to an enlarged azygos vein that joins a normal right superior vena cava (RSVC). A small portion of inferior vena caval blood is diverted through the azygos vein into the right superior vena cava and into the right atrium (RA). PV'S, pulmonary veins.

Physical Appearance

Cyanosis and clubbing are the only abnormalities of physical appearance.[5,8,20,29,43,72] Cyanosis increases with effort because caval venous return increases, and cyanosis is greater when the inferior vena cava connects to the left atrium because approximately twice as much blood is delivered to the heart via the inferior vena cava (see earlier).[38,50,78] Because a large azygos venous system allows substantial inferior vena caval flow into the right atrium and proportionately less flow into the left atrium (see Fig. 29–5), cyanosis is relatively mild.[81] A superior vena cava that connects to the left atrium (see Fig. 29–3) results in conspicuous cyanosis.[20,43] Cyanosis is absent when a nonrestrictive innominate bridge joins bilateral superior venae cavae because the direction of flow is from the left atrium into the anomalous left superior vena cava (see Fig. 29–2A).[56,62]

The Arterial Pulse and Jugular Venous Pulse

The arterial pulse is normal because left ventricular stroke volume increases little, if at all.

Attention has been called to a new physical sign, namely, relative prominence of the left internal jugular venous pulse because of persistence of the left superior vena cava.[18] The jugular venous pulse is confined to the left side of the neck when there is congenital absence of the right superior vena cava.

Precordial Movement and Palpation

The left ventricular impulse is normal or only moderately increased, reflecting the normal or only moderate increase in systemic output. A right ventricular impulse is absent. These physical signs indicate that cyanosis is occurring with a dominant left ventricle—an important observation in the clinical recognition of cyanotic congenital heart disease (see Table 1–1).

Auscultation

Left ventricular stroke volume is seldom sufficient to generate a flow murmur into the aorta.[23,29,57,72,78,81] The second heart sound is single because decreased right ventricular stroke volume and decreased pulmonary capacitance result in early pulmonary valve closure and synchrony or near synchrony of the two components.[23,57,72] The intensity of the pulmonary component is normal or reduced because pulmonary arterial pressure is normal or low.[20,38,57,78]

The Electrocardiogram

When a left superior vena cava connects to the coronary sinus (see Fig. 29–1), the atrial rhythm is likely to be ectopic, and abnormalities of atrioventricular conduction may coexist.[17,18,40,49,55,60,61] When a right superior vena cava is absent or connects to the left atrium, the sinus node is absent, so the atrial focus is ectopic and the P wave axis is

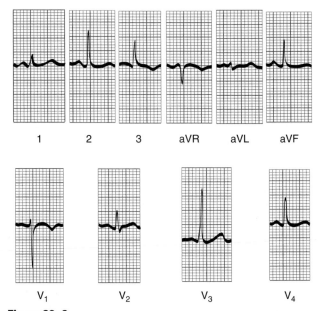

Figure 29–6

Normal electrocardiogram from a 9-year-old girl with isolated connection of the inferior vena cava to the left atrium. (From Venables AW: Isolated drainage of the inferior vena cava to the left atrium. Br Heart J 25:545, 1963).

abnormal (see Fig. 29–7).[47] Atresia or absence of the segment of superior vena cava adjacent to the right atrium is accompanied by developmental abnormalities of the sinus node and an ectopic atrial focus.[49]

The QRS pattern is normal with vena caval-to-left atrial connections (see Figs. 29–6 and 29–8). Adult survival anticipates age-related electrocardiographic abnormalities.[1,9,43,56,64,72,81] Right ventricular hypertrophy is absent because flow into the right side of the heart is normal or

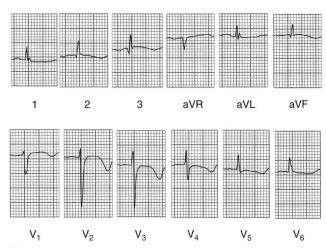

Figure 29–7

Electrocardiogram from a 28-year-old woman in whom both the superior and inferior vena cava joined the left atrium—total anomalous systemic venous connection. A large ostium secundum atrial septal defect permitted interatrial mixing upon which survival depended. The sinus node was absent because there was no junction between the superior vena cava and right atrium, so the P wave axis is directed upward and to the left, indicating an ectopic atrial focus. Broad notched P waves in leads 1, 3, and aVL reflect total caval drainage into the left atrium. The T wave abnormalities are nonspecific.

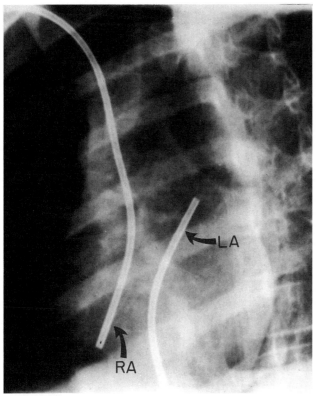

Figure 29–8

Left anterior oblique projection from a 9-year-old girl with isolated inferior vena caval connection to the left atrium. One catheter entered the right atrium (RA) from the superior vena cava, and a second catheter entered the left atrium (LA) from the inferior vena cava (see Fig. 29–6 for electrocardiogram). (From Venables AW: Isolated drainage of the inferior vena cava to the left atrium. Br Heart J 25:545, 1963.)

reduced. Left ventricular electrical forces retain their normal adult dominance (Figs. 29–6 and 29–7), but the modest increment in left ventricular volume is seldom sufficient to cause hypertrophy.[56,57,78]

The X-Ray

The size and configuration of the heart are normal (Fig. 29–8),[20,29,43,57,72,78,80,81] even when both superior and inferior venae cavae connect to the left atrium (Fig. 29–9). A left superior vena cava may form a concave or crescentic shadow as it emerges from beneath the middle third of the left clavicle.[22,26,31,55,62,77] When the inferior vena cava communicates with the left atrium, the inferior vena caval shadow is absent from its expected location at the angle formed by the posterior cardiac silhouette and the diaphragm (see Fig. 29–9B).[29] An inferior vena caval shadow is also absent when there is inferior caval interruption with azygos continuation (see Fig. 29–4). The azygos vein ascends along the right edge of the vertebral column, forming a knuckle as it courses anteriorly to join the right superior vena cava (see Fig. 29–4).

The Echocardiogram

Echocardiography with color flow and contrast imaging establishes the diagnoses of most if not all of the

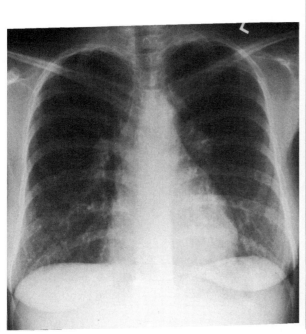

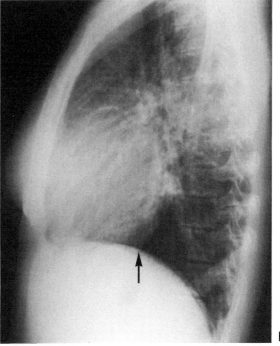

Figure 29–9

X-rays from the 28-year-old woman with total anomalous systemic venous connection whose electrocardiogram is shown in Figure 29–7. *A,* The size and configuration of the heart are normal. Pulmonary vascularity is not reduced. Markings in the left lower lung field are the result of superimposed breast tissue. *B,* In the lateral projection, the inferior vena caval shadow is absent (*arrow*).

varieties of vena caval connection described in this chapter,[15,16,24,35,37,63,64] including the intrauterine diagnoses.[71] A dilated coronary sinus in the parasternal long-axis view arouses suspicion of a hitherto unsuspected connection of a left superior vena cava to the coronary sinus (Fig. 29–10). The coronary sinus is absent when a left superior vena cava connects directly to the left atrium (see Fig. 29–2). Color flow imaging confirms the course of a persistent left superior vena cava (Fig. 29–11), which can sometimes be visualized together with the innominate bridge associated with bilateral cavae (see Fig. 29–2). When the right superior vena cava is absent, a persistent left superior vena cava is imaged along the left side of the aorta.

Contrast echocardiography identifies specific vena caval-to-left atrial connections.[24,63,64] When a left superior vena cava connects directly to the left atrium, injection of echo-contrast into the left antecubital vein is followed by immediate opacification of the left atrium.[24] Conversely, when a right superior vena cava connects directly to the left atrium, injection of contrast material into the right antecubital vein promptly opacifies the left atrium.[24] Contrast echocardiography is more complex when the inferior vena cava connects to the left atrium because material injected into the femoral vein may appear in the right as well as the left atrium, depending on the size of the azygos vein that leaves the inferior vena cava and joins the right atrium via a right superior vena cava (see Fig. 29–5). When a right superior vena cava and an inferior vena cava both connect to the left atrium (see Fig. 29–9), injection of contrast material into the right antecubital vein and into the femoral vein results in a combination of the patterns just described.

Summary

A left superior vena cava can connect anomalously to the coronary sinus or left atrium. A right superior vena cava can connect anomalously to the left atrium or can be absent altogether. Bilateral superior venae cavae can be connected by an innominate bridge that is either widely patent, narrow, or atretic. An inferior vena cava can connect to the left atrium or can be interrupted with azygous continuation. Superior and inferior venae cavae can both connect to the left atrium—total anomalous systemic venous connection.

Persistent left superior vena cava is suspected in the x-ray by a shadow that emerges from beneath the middle third of the left clavicle and passes downward toward the left upper border of the aortic arch. Echocardiography with color flow imaging and echo-contrast confirms the diagnosis and determine whether the caval connection is to the coronary sinus or to the left atrium. A left superior vena cava-to-coronary sinus connection is often first suspected on routine echocardiography because of dilatation of the coronary sinus. Isolated superior vena caval connection to the left atrium is a form of cyanotic congenital heart disease with a dominant left ventricle, which is palpable at the apex without a palpable right ventricle. Cyanosis dates from birth or early life, but cardiac symptoms are absent or mild even when cyanosis is conspicuous. The electrocardiogram shows normal adult left ventricular dominance. Echocardiography with color flow and echo-contrast identifies the left superior vena cava entering the left atrium. A dilated coronary sinus effectively excludes direct connection of a left superior vena cava to the left atrium. Bilateral superior venae cavae and an innominate bridge can be imaged.

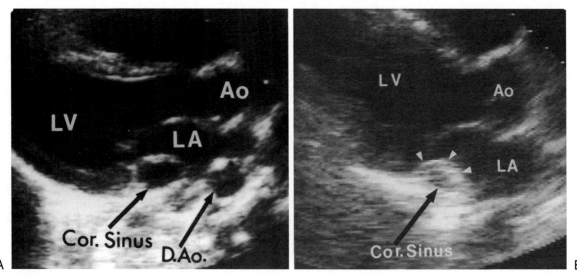

Figure 29–10

A, Echocardiogram (parasternal long axis) from a normal 9-month-old boy whose coronary sinus (Cor Sinus) was dilated because of connection to a persistent left superior vena cava. The large size of the coronary sinus is evident when it is compared to the cross-sectional area of the descending aorta (DAo). LA, left atrium; LV, left ventricle. *B*, Echocardiogram from a normal 12-month-old girl showing a normal-sized coronary sinus.

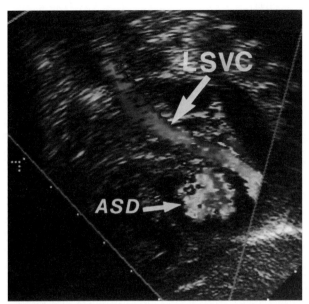

Figure 29-11
Black and white print of a color flow image showing the course of a persistent left superior vena cava (LSVC) that communicated with a dilated coronary sinus in a 3-day-old boy with an ostium secundum atrial septal defect (ASD).

Inferior vena caval connection to the left atrium is accompanied by conspicuous cyanosis unless a large azygos vein preferentially channels inferior caval return into the right atrium. The inferior vena caval shadow is absent from its expected location in the lateral chest x-ray. Contrast echocardiography with injection into the femoral vein opacifies the left atrium.

REFERENCES

1. Arsenian MA, Anderson RA: Anomalous venous connection of the superior vena cava to the left atrium. Am J Cardiol 62:989, 1988.
2. Ascuitto RJ, Ross-Ascuitto NT, Kopf GS, et al: Persistent left superior vena cava causing subdivided left atrium. Ann Thorac Surg 44:546, 1987.
3. Bartram U, Van Praagh S, Levine JC, et al: Absent right superior vena cava in visceroatrial situs solitus. Am J Cardiol 80:175, 1997.
4. Bharati S, Lev M: Direct entry of the right superior vena cava into the left atrium with aneurysmal dilatation and stenosis of its entry into the right atrium with stenosis of pulmonary veins. Pediatr Cardiol 5:123, 1984.
5. Black H, Smith GT, Goodale WT: Anomalous inferior vena cava draining into the left atrium associated with intact interatrial septum and multiple pulmonary arteriovenous fistulae. Circulation 29:258, 1964.
6. Blanchard DG, Sobek JL, Hope J, et al: Infrahepatic interruption of the inferior vena cava with azygous continuation. J Am Soc Echocardiogr 11:1078, 1998.
7. Bourdillon PD, Foale RA, Sommerville J: Persistent left superior vena cava with coronary sinus and left atrial connection. Eur J Cardiol 11:227, 1979.
8. Braudo M, Beanlands DS, Trusler G: Anomalous drainage of the right superior vena cava into the left atrium. Can Med Assoc J 99:715, 1968.
9. Brickner ME, Eichhorn EJ, Netto D, et al: Left-sided inferior vena cava draining into the coronary sinus via persistent left superior vena cava. Catheterization Cardiovasc Diag 20:189, 1990.
10. Brochard P, Lejonc JL, Loisance DY, Nitenberg A: A rare cause of cyanosis and polycythemia. Eur Heart J 2:227, 1981.
11. Buirski G, Jordan SC, Joffe HS, Wilde P: Superior vena caval abnormalities: Their occurrence rate, associated cardiac abnormalities and angiographic classification in a paediatric population with congenital heart disease. Clin Radiol 37:131, 1986.
12. Cabrera A, Arriola J, Llorente A: Anomalous connection of inferior vena cava to the left atrium. Int J Cardiol 46:79, 1994.
13. Campbell M, Deuchar DC: The left-sided superior vena cava. Br Heart J 16:423, 1954.
14. Chan KL, Abdulla A: Images in cardiology: Giant coronary sinus and absent right superior vena cava. Heart 83:704, 2000.
15. Chen MC, Hung JS, Chang KC, et al: Partially unroofed coronary sinus and persistent left superior vena cava: Intracardiac echocardiographic observation. J Ultrasound Med 15:857, 1996.
16. Chin AJ: Subcostal two-dimensional echocardiographic identification of right superior vena cava connecting to the left atrium. Am Heart J 127:939, 1994.
17. Choi JY, Anderson RH, Macartney FJ: Absent right superior caval vein (vena cava) with normal atrial arrangement. Br Heart J 57:474, 1987.
18. Colman AL: Diagnosis of left superior vena cava by clinical inspection, a new physical sign. Am Heart J 73:115, 1967.
19. Davis D, Pritchett ELC, Klein GJ, et al: Persistent left superior vena cava in patients with congenital atrioventricular preexcitation conduction abnormalities. Am Heart J 101:677, 1981.
20. Davis WH, Jordaan FR, Snyman HW: Persistent left superior vena cava draining into the left atrium as an isolated anomaly. Br Heart J 57:616, 1959.
21. DeLeval MR, Ritter DG, McGoon DC, Danielson GK: Anomalous systemic venous connection. Mayo Clin Proc 50:599, 1975.
22. Elliott LP, Jue KL, Amplatz K: A roentgen classification of cardiac malpositions. Invest Radiol 1:17, 1966.
23. Ezekowitz MD, Alderson PO, Bulkley BH, et al: Isolated drainage of the superior vena cava into the left atrium in a 52 year old man. Circulation 58:751, 1978.
24. Foale R, Bourdillon PD, Sommerville J, Rickards A: Anomalous venous return: Recognition by two-dimensional echocardiography. Eur Heart J 4:186, 1983.
25. Foster ED, Baeza OR, Farina MF, Shaher RM: Atrial septal defect associated with drainage of left superior vena cava to left atrium and absence of the coronary sinus. J Thorac Cardiovasc Surg 76:718, 1978.
26. Fraser RS, Dvorkin J, Rossall RW, Eidem J: Left superior vena cava. Am J Med 31:711, 1961.
27. Freed MD, Rosenthal A, Bernhard WF: Balloon occlusion of a persistent left superior vena cava in the preoperative evaluation of systemic venous return. J Thorac Cardiovasc Surg 65:835, 1973.
28. Gallaher ME, Sperling DR, Gwinn JL, et al: Functional drainage of the inferior vena cava into the left atrium. Am J Cardiol 12:561, 1963.
29. Gardner DL, Cole L: Long survival with inferior vena cava draining into left atrium. Br Heart J 17:93, 1955.
30. Genoni M, Jenni R, Vogt PR, et al: Drainage of the inferior vena cava to the left atrium. Ann Thorac Surg 67:543, 1999.
31. Gensini GG, Caldini P, Casaccio F, Blount SG Jr: Persistent superior vena cava. Am J Cardiol 4:677, 1959.
32. Gerlis LM, Partridge JB, Fiddler GI: Anomalous connection of left atrial appendage with persistent left superior vena cava. Br Heart J 48:73, 1982.
33. Gueron M, Hirsh M, Borman J: Total anomalous systemic venous drainage into the left atrium. J Thorac Cardiovasc Surg 58:570, 1969.
34. Helseth HK, Peterson CR: Atrial septal defect with termination of left superior vena cava in the left atrium and absence of the coronary sinus. Ann Thorac Surg 17:186, 1974.
35. Hibi N, Fukui Y, Nishimura K, et al: Cross-sectional echocardiographic study on persistent left superior vena cava. Am Heart J 100:69, 1980.
36. Huang SK: Persistent left superior vena cava in a man with ventricular fibrillation. Chest 89:155, 1986.
37. Huhta JC, Smallhorn JF, Macartney FJ, et al: Cross-sectional echocardiographic diagnosis of systemous venous return. Br Heart J 48:388, 1982.
38. Hultgren HN, Gerbode F: A physiological study of experimental left atrium-inferior vena caval anastomoses. Am J Physiol 177:164, 1954.
39. Imai S, Matsubara T, Yamazoe M, et al: Atresia of the right atrial orifice of the coronary sinus with persistent left superior vena cava. J Cardiol 34:341, 1999.
40. James TN, Marshall TK, Edwards JE: Cardiac electrical instability in the presence of a left superior vena cava. Circulation 54:689, 1976.
41. Kabbani SS, Feldman M, Angelini P: Single (left) superior vena cava draining into the left atrium. Ann Thorac Surg 16:518, 1973.

42. King RE, Plotnick GD: Isolated right superior vena cava into the left atrium detected by contrast echocardiography. Am Heart J 122:583, 1991.

43. Kirsch WM, Carlsson E, Hartmann AF: A case of anomalous drainage of the superior vena cava into the left atrium. J Thorac Cardiovasc Surg 41:550, 1961.

44. Konstam MA, Levine BM, Strauss HW, McKusick VA: Left superior vena cava to left atrial communication diagnosed with radionuclide angiography and with differential right to left shunting. Am J Cardiol 43:149, 1979.

45. Kothari SS, Sharma R, Taneja K: Anomalous drainage of right superior vena cava into the left atrium. Indian Heart J 50:332, 1998.

46. Lam W, Danoviz J, Witham D, et al: Left-to-right shunt via left superior vena cava communication with left atrium. Chest 79:700, 1981.

47. Langford EJ, Sulke AN, Curry PV: Atrial permanent pacing for sinus node dysfunction with absent right superior vena cava. Int J Cardiol 40:177, 1993.

48. LeBorgne J, Paineau J, Hamy A, et al: Interruption of the inferior vena cava with azygous termination associated with congenital absence of the portal vein. Surg Radiol Anat 22:197, 2000.

49. Lenox CC, Hashida Y, Anderson RH, Hubbard JD: Conduction tissue anomalies in absence of the right superior caval vein. Int J Cardiol 8:251, 1985.

50. Levy SE, Blalock A: Fractionation of output of heart and of oxygen consumption of normal unanesthetized dogs. Am J Physiol 118:368, 1937.

51. Leys D, Manouvrier J, Dupard T, et al: Right superior vena cava draining into the left atrium with left superior vena cava draining into the right atrium. Br Med J 293:855, 1986.

52. Maillis MS, Cheng TO, Meyer JF, et al: Cyanosis in patients with atrial septal defect due to systemic venous drainage into the left atrium. Am J Cardiol 33:674, 1974.

53. Mankin HT, Burchell HB: Clinical considerations in partial anomalous pulmonary venous connection: Report of 2 unusual cases. Proc Staff Meet Mayo Clin 28:463, 1953.

54. Mantini E, Grondin CM, Lillehei CW, Edwards JE: Congenital anomalies involving the coronary sinus. Circulation 33:317, 1966.

55. Mazzucco A, Bortolotti U, Stellin G, Gallucci V: Anomalies of systemic venous return: A review. J Cardiac Surg 5:122, 1990.

56. Meadows WR, Sharp JT: Persistent left superior vena cava draining into the left atrium without arterial oxygen unsaturation. Am J Cardiol 16:273, 1965.

57. Meadows WR, Bergstrand I, Sharp JT: Isolated anomalous connection of a great vein to the left atrium: The syndrome of cyanosis and clubbing, "normal" heart, and left ventricular hypertrophy on electrocardiogram. Circulation 24:669, 1961.

58. Meyers DG, Latson LA, McManus BM, Fleming WH: Anomalous drainage of the inferior vena cava into a left atrial connection. Cathet Cardiovasc Diag 16:239, 1989.

59. Momma K, Linde LM: Abnormal rhythms associated with persistent left superior vena cava. Pediatr Res 3:210, 1969.

60. Naik AM, Doshi R, Peter CT, Chen PS: Electrical potentials from a persistent left superior vena cava draining into the coronary sinus. J Cardiovasc Electrophysiol 10:1559, 1999.

61. Nsah EN, Moore W, Hutchins GM: Pathogenesis of persistent left superior vena cava with a coronary sinus connection. Pediatr Pathol 11:261, 1991.

62. Odman P: A persistent left superior vena cava communicating with the left atrium and pulmonary vein. Acta Radiol 40:554, 1953.

63. Pan CW, Chen CC, Wang SP, et al: Echocardiographic evidence for drainage of a persistent left superior vena cava into the left atrium. J Cardiovasc Ultrasonog 3:329, 1984.

64. Park H, Summerer MH, Preuss K, et al: Anomalous drainage of the right superior vena cava into the left atrium. J Am Coll Cardiol 2:358, 1983.

65. Potter EL: Diffuse angiectasis of the cerebral meninges of the newborn infant. Arch Pathol 46:87, 1948.

66. Pugliese P, Murzi B, Redaelli S, Eufrate S: Total anomalous systemic venous drainage into the left atrium. G Ital Cardiol 13:62, 1983.

67. Raghib G, Ruttenberg HD, Anderson RC, et al: Termination of left superior vena cava in left atrium, atrial septal defect, and absence of coronary sinus: A developmental complex. Circulation 31:906, 1965.

68. Rastelli GC, Ongley PA, Kirklin JW: Surgical correction of common atrium with anomalously connected persistent left superior vena cava: Report of a case. Proc Mayo Clin 40:528, 1965.

69. Roberts KD, Edwards JM, Astley R: Surgical correction of total anomalous systemic venous drainage. J Thorac Cardiovasc Surg 64:803, 1972.

70. Rosenkranz S, Stablein A, Deutsch HJ, et al: Anomalous drainage of the right superior vena cava into the left atrium. Int J Cardiol 64:285, 1998.

71. Salazar J, Garcia MD, Romo A, et al: Left superior vena cava drainage to the coronary sinus: Fetal cardiac Doppler. Rev Esp Cardiol 50:529, 1997.

72. Shapiro EP, Al-Sadir J, Campbell NPS, et al: Drainage of right superior vena cava into both atria. Circulation 63:712, 1981.

73. Shumacker HB Jr, King H, Waldhausen JA: The persistent left superior vena cava: Surgical implications with special reference to caval drainage into the left atrium. Ann Surg 165:797, 1967.

74. Sibley YDL, Roberts KD, Silove ED: Surgical correction of isolated persistent left superior vena cava draining to left atrium in a neonate. Br Heart J 55:605, 1986.

75. Singh A, Doyle EF, Danilowicz D, Spencer FC: Masked abnormal drainage of the inferior vena cava into the left atrium. Am J Cardiol 38:261, 1976.

76. Tandon R: Anomalous drainage of right superior vena cava into the left atrium. Indian Heart J 51:345, 1999.

77. Taybi H, Kurlander GJ, Lurie PR, Campbell JA: Anomalous systemic venous connection to the left atrium or to a pulmonary vein. Am J Roentgenol 94:62, 1965.

78. Tuchman H, Brown JF, Huston JH, et al: Superior vena cava draining into left atrium. Am J Med 21:481, 1956.

79. Tuma S, Samanek M, Voriskova M, et al: Anomalies of the systemic venous return. Pediatr Radiol 5:193, 1977.

80. Vazquez-Perez J, Frontera-Izquierdo P: Anomalous drainage of the right superior vena cava into the left atrium as an isolated anomaly. Am Heart J 97:89, 1979.

81. Venables AW: Isolated drainage of the inferior vena cava to the left atrium. Br Heart J 25:545, 1963.

82. Viart P, Le Clerc JL, Primo G: Total anomalous systemic venous drainage. Am J Dis Child 131:195, 1977.

83. Wiles HB: Two cases of left superior vena cava draining directly to a left atrium with a normal coronary sinus. Br Heart J 65:158, 1991.

84. Winter SF: Persistent left superior vena cava. Survey of world literature and report of 30 additional cases. Angiology 5:90, 1954.

85. Yilmaz AT, Arisan M, Demirkilic U, et al: Partially unroofed coronary sinus syndrome with persistent left superior vena cava, absent right superior vena cava and right-sided pericardial defect. Eur J Cardiothorac Surg 10:1027, 1996.

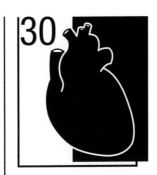

Congenital Pulmonary Arteriovenous Fistula

In 1897, Churton described the necropsy findings of congenital pulmonary arteriovenous fistulae in a 12-year-old boy.[31] Four decades later, the anomaly was recognized in a living subject.[113] Pulmonary arteriovenous fistulae are the result of a developmental fault in the vascular complex that is responsible for pulmonary arteries and veins.[6,84] The fistulae can be solitary or multiple, unilateral or bilateral, or minute and diffuse throughout both lungs.* Approximately 75% of congenital pulmonary arteriovenous fistulae involve the lower lobes or right middle lobe (Figs. 30–1 through 30–4, Fig. 30–6).[9,18,36,73,84,102] Congenital pulmonary arteriovenous fistulae usually occur without coexisting congenital heart disease, but isolated exceptions have been reported with left isomerism[4,63] (see Chapter 3) and with atrial septal defect (see Chapter 15).[69,103]

A fistula consists of one or more relatively large vascular trunks, a thin aneurysmal sac, or a tangle of distended tortuous vascular channels (Figs. 30–5 and 30–7, and see Figs. 30–1 through 30–4, Fig. 30–6).[53,84] The arterial supply is through enlarged tortuous branches of a pulmonary artery, and drainage is through dilated pulmonary veins (see Figs. 30–1 through 30–4 and 30–5).[6,73] Fistulous rupture results in hemorrhage into the pulmonary parenchyma or into the pleural space.[33,45,84] Exceptionally, the arterial supply is from a bronchial, intercostal, anomalous systemic artery or a coronary artery (see Chapter 22), so the fistula is then systemic arteriovenous rather than pulmonary arteriovenous.[5,14,20,53,62,67,73] A rare anatomic variation consists of a congenital connection between a pulmonary artery and the left atrium, an anomaly in which an initial connection exists between a pulmonary artery and a pulmonary vein, but during vascular development the pulmonary vein becomes incorporated into the left atrium.[61,70,76,84,106,126,127] Extralobar arteriovenous fistulae are represented by pulmonary sequestrations, but the arterial supply and venous drainage are systemic rather than pulmonary.[46]

The physiologic consequences of pulmonary arteriovenous fistulae depend on the amount of unoxygenated blood delivered through the malformation and on the size of the malformation, which tends to increase with age.[121,124] The volume of blood delivered through the fistula is sufficient to cause cyanosis[36,54,62,84] but is only rarely sufficient to incur a hemodynamic burden (see Fig. 30–7).[50] Pulmonary artery pressure is normal, with rare exception.[104] In experimental pulmonary arteriovenous fistulae, cardiac output and left ventricular stroke volume are increased,[129] but in a congenital pulmonary arteriovenous fistula, blood flow through the malformation increases while blood flow through the uninvolved lung decreases by a comparable amount.[54,84] Accordingly, the net volume of blood reaching the left side of the heart is little if at all affected, so left ventricular stroke volume and cardiac output remain normal or nearly so.[54,84] Rarely, a large pulmonary arteriovenous malformation imposes an excess volume load on the left side of the heart and induces congestive heart failure (see Fig. 30–7).[50,84]

Blood flow through pulmonary arteriovenous fistulae is affected by certain mechanical factors.[52] Flow through lower lobe fistulae is augmented in the upright position because of increased perfusion of dependent portions of the lungs. A decubitus position compresses the dependent lung and reduces blood flow through an ipsilateral pulmonary arteriovenous fistula. An example was the large pulmonary arteriovenous fistula in an infant in whom ipsilateral chest wall compression was therapeutic, immediately decreasing the cyanosis and relieving the dyspnea (see Fig. 30–7).[50] Elevation of the diaphragm during

---

*See reference 18, 21, 36, 43, 47, 49, 62, 84, 105, 115, 125.

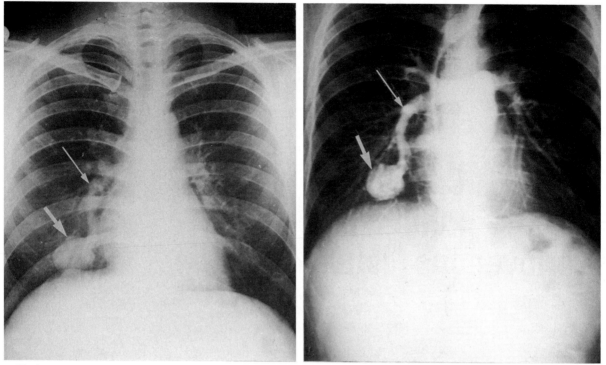

Figure 30–1

A, X-ray of a 21-year-old man with a congenital right lower lobe pulmonary arteriovenous fistula (*thick arrow*). The lobulated density is connected to the hilus (*thin arrow*) by dilated vessels that enter and leave the fistula. The x-ray is otherwise normal. *B,* Angiocardiogram showing the fistula (*thick arrow*) with its pulmonary arterial connection (*thin arrow*).

pregnancy compressed a lower lobe fistula and abolished the accompanying murmur, which reappeared after delivery.[52]

Acquired pulmonary arteriovenous fistulae are occasional sequelae of cavopulmonary shunts, especially Glenn shunts.[12,92] Acquired pulmonary arteriovenous fistulae occur in children with liver cirrhosis and portal hypertension, especially with biliary atresia and right isomerism[10,39,101] (see Chapter 3) and regress after liver transplantation.[10] Large hepatic arteriovenous fistulae sometimes occur with Rendu-

Osler-Weber disease without pulmonary arteriovenous fistulae.[26,34,96,97] Hepatic, cerebral, and pulmonary arteriovenous fistulae may coexist.[15,29,79] Isolated congenital varicose pulmonary veins are rare and are not the result of arteriovenous malformations.[87]

In 1865, Babington called attention to familial epistaxis,[7] and in 1876 Legg described recurrent epistaxes and cutaneous telangiectasia in three generations.[72] Twenty years later, Rendu published his classic description of familial epistaxes and telangiectasia (cutaneous angiomatas) of the

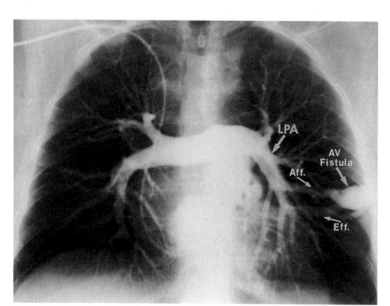

Figure 30–2

Pulmonary arteriogram from a 35-year-old woman with a solitary left lower lobe congenital pulmonary arteriovenous fistula (AV Fistula). An afferent (Aff.) channel enters the fistula, and an efferent (Eff.) channel leaves the fistula. LPA, left pulmonary artery.

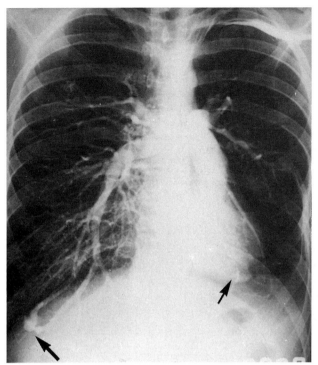

Figure 30–3

Angiocardiogram from a 32-year-old man with congenital bilateral pulmonary arteriovenous fistulae of the right and left lower lobes (*arrows*). The afferent and efferent vascular channels that join and leave the fistula are readily seen on the right. The left lower lobe fistula (*upper arrow*) was behind the cardiac apex, inviting a mistaken diagnosis of intracardiac origin. The heart size is normal.

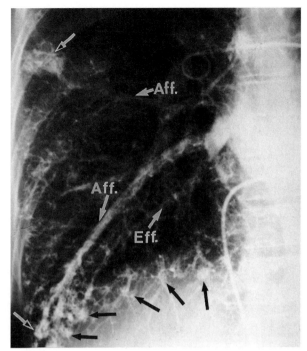

Figure 30–4

Right pulmonary arteriogram from a 50-year-old woman with hereditary hemorrhagic telangiectasia and multiple pulmonary arteriovenous fistulae. Afferent (Aff.) and efferent (Eff.) vascular channels enter and leave the fistulae. *Unmarked arrows* identify multiple fistulae in the right lower lobe and right middle lobe.

nose, cheeks, and upper lip.[99] In 1901, Osler reported "On a family form of recurring epistaxis associated with multiple telangiectases of the skin and mucous membranes,"[32,88] and in 1907, Weber reported on "Multiple hereditary developmental angiomata (telangiectases) of the skin and mucous membranes associated with recurring haemorrhages."[131] In 1909, Hanes referred to the disorder as hereditary hemorrhagic telangiectasia,[51,53] but the eponym *Rendu-Osler-Weber* remains in use with no consensus on the most appropriate sequence of names[45,59,91,107,118] and with no inclusion of Legg.[72]

In 1917, Wilkins reported telangiectasia and epistaxes in a patient who died of massive hemothorax and at necropsy had three pulmonary arteriovenous fistulae.[133] The association of hemorrhagic telangiectasia and pulmonary arteriovenous fistula has been amply confirmed.* Clinical diagnostic criteria have changed remarkably little over the last century.[107]

---

*See references 14, 18, 21, 29, 36, 38, 53, 59, 84, 91, 107, 116.

Figure 30–5

A, Selective injection of contrast material into the right pulmonary artery (RPA) of a 73-year-old woman with multiple small bilateral congenital pulmonary arteriovenous fistulae but no telangiectasia. *Arrows* point to at least four fistulae in the right lower lobe. B, Contrast material injected into the left pulmonary artery (LPA) of the patient's 71-year-old brother who also had multiple small bilateral pulmonary arteriovenous fistulae and no telangiectasia. *Arrows* identify at least five left lower lobe fistulae. These siblings represent the rare occurrence of familial congenital pulmonary arteriovenous fistulae without telangiectasia.

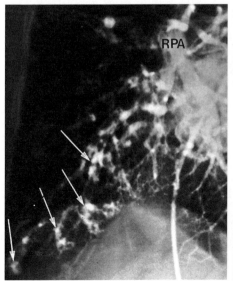
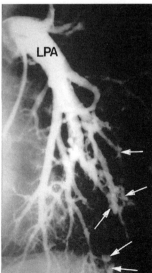

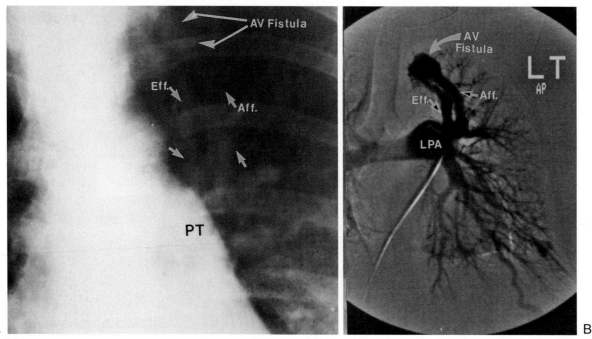

Figure 30–6

A, Close-up of the chest x-ray of a 26-year-old woman with a single large left upper lobe pulmonary arteriovenous fistula (AV Fistula). She had endured two brain abscesses. The solitary fistula and its afferent (Aff.) and efferent (Eff.) vascular channels are faintly seen. PT, pulmonary trunk. *B*, Contrast material selectively injected into the left pulmonary artery (LPA) visualized the afferent channel that entered the fistula and the efferent channel that left the fistula.

Pulmonary arteriovenous fistulae occur in 5% to 30% of patients with telangiectasia, and 30% to 60% of patients with pulmonary arteriovenous fistulae have telangiectasia.[14,16,29,35,36,38,84,116,122] The incidence is 1 in 50,000, with autosomal dominant transmission and a 20% mutation rate. The mucocutaneous lesions are tiny localized arteriovenous fistulae composed of thin dilated vascular membranes with a layer of endothelium and no muscular or elastic coat.[53,81] The fragile lesions easily rupture.[53,84] Telangiectasia are found on the skin and lips (Fig. 30–9), on nasal, oral, and vaginal mucous membranes, beneath the nails, and in the gastrointestinal tract, liver, central nervous system, kidney, and retina.[17,29,48,53,55,84,93,98,134]

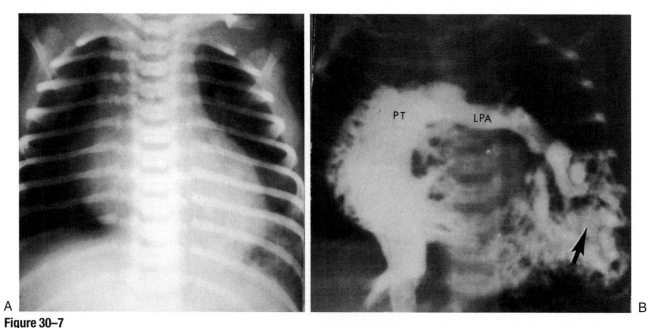

Figure 30–7

X-ray and angiocardiogram from a 4-day-old cyanotic infant with a massive left lower lobe congenital pulmonary arteriovenous fistula. *A*, The fistulous mass is seen in the x-ray as a hazy density above the left hemidiaphragm. The cardiac silhouette is enlarged because of congestive heart failure. *B*, Angiocardiogram with contrast material injected into the inferior vena cava visualized the pulmonary trunk (PT) and an elongated left pulmonary artery (LPA) that entered a large left lower lobe vascular malformation (*arrow*) that displaced the heart to the right. (From Hall RJ, et al: Massive pulmonary arteriovenous fistula in the newborn. Circulation 31:762, 1965.)

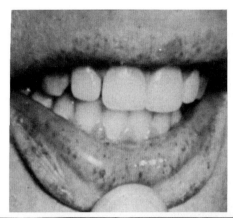

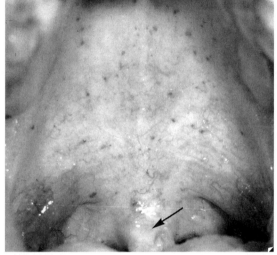

Figure 30–8

A, Typical hemorrhagic telangiectasia on the lips of a 25-year-old woman. *B*, Telangiectasia on the palate and uvula (*arrow*) of a 30-year-old man. Both patients had pulmonary arteriovenous fistulae.

The History

Pulmonary arteriovenous fistulae and autosomal dominant hereditary hemorrhagic telangiectasia afflict males and females with equal frequency.[*] The fistulae tend to increase in size and number with the passage of time[60,84,121,124] and are seldom recognized until adulthood.[80,84,114,120] Symptoms are the same whether malformations are multiple or single (see Figs. 30–1 through 30–3), except for minute diffuse fistulous channels (see Figs. 30–4 and 30–6).[36] Mean patient age in a large series was 39 years (range, 3 to 73 years), with a distinct majority older than 20 years.[36] However, the first description of a pulmonary arteriovenous fistula was at necropsy in a 12-year-old boy,[31] and, despite adult prevalence, cyanosis is occasionally present shortly after birth[50,57,100] and the malformation is occasionally manifest in childhood (Fig. 30–8).[36,57,60,62,69,85,109]

Asymptomatic acyanotic pulmonary arteriovenous fistulae usually come to light because of abnormal shadows on a chest x-ray.[73,74,84,117] Symptoms and complications are

related to the pulmonary malformation per se and to coexisting hereditary hemorrhagic telangiectasia.[129] Congestive heart failure is reserved for the rare large fistula in an infant (see Fig. 30–7).[50] The right-to-left shunt inherent in the fistulous communication results in cyanosis that seldom causes significant symptoms.[36,43,57,73] Dyspnea and fatigue coincide with anemia provoked by bleeding telangiectasia.[14,60] Rupture of fistulae into a contiguous bronchus causes hemoptysis that varies from mild and occasional to recurrent and massive.[8,14,15,22,24,30,73,77] Chest pain accompanies pleural involvement,[123] and hemothorax results from rupture of a subpleural fistula.[24,33,45,53,73,75] Intrapulmonary hemorrhage can be massive and fatal.[42] Pregnancy exerts a number of adverse effects, including hemothorax,[44] hemoptysis,[19,40] enlargement of existing fistulae with increasing cyanosis,[40,44] and expansion of occult fistulae that resolve after delivery.[132] However, pregnancy also exerts favorable effects because elevation of the diaphragm compresses fistulae in the lower lobes, which is where they are usually located.[52] Fistulae are rarely substrates for infective endocarditis.[73]

Hemorrhagic telangiectases, as the name implies, are announced by bleeding. An annotation in *The Lancet* vividly described the classic pattern[38]:

Every large general hospital is certain to have on its list of frequent attenders a small group of unfortunate adults who come to the casualty department complaining of recurrent bleeding from the nose, lips, or mouth. The blood is seen to stem from an insignificant leak in the center of a small ruby patch, many of which are usually to be found scattered here and there on the mucous membrane [see Fig. 30–9]. Although the flow of blood is seldom vigorous it may eventually, by its persistence, cause some concern. Its arrest can be infuriatingly difficult. Each ruby patch marks the position of a tiny arteriovenous communication at the capillary level. Presumably these vessels are very close to the surface or else they are abnormally fragile. Whatever the cause, they can be induced to bleed by the most trivial of injuries.

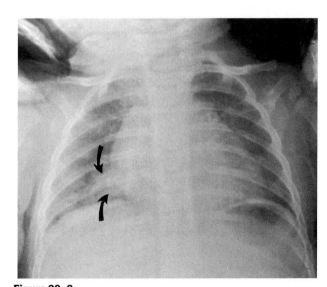

Figure 30–9

X-ray of a 6-month-old cyanotic girl with a congenital right lower lobe pulmonary arteriovenous fistula that faintly revealed itself (*arrows*). Mucocutaneous telangiectasia were not identified. Cyanosis disappeared after coil embolization.

[*]See references 2, 35, 36, 38, 53, 74, 80, 90, 105, 116.

Epistaxis is the most frequent and usually the first overt hemorrhagic event.[53,84] Cutaneous lesions bleed easily, especially when exposed to sunlight.[53,84] Tracheobronchial telangiectases set the stage for hemoptysis,[53,84] and appropriately placed lesions elsewhere cause melena, hematuria, intraocular hemorrhage, vaginal bleeding, and cerebrovascular accidents.[22,43,46,53,55,81,84,96,98]

Cerebral events deserve special comment with reference to a peculiar constellation of symptoms including dizziness, vertigo, paresthesias, tinnitus, faintness, visual disturbances, speech defects, headache, weakness of the limbs, hemiplegia, mental confusion, and convulsions.* Cerebral episodes may be brief or prolonged, isolated or recurrent and may manifest similar patterns with recurrent attacks.[53] Pathogenesis has not been established, but occurrence in acyanotic patients without pulmonary arteriovenous fistulae incriminates telangiectases,[53,78,111] which have been described with a cerebral arteriovenous malformation characterized by a plexiform nidus with an arterial feeding pedicle and a draining vein.[95]

Pulmonary arteriovenous fistulae set the stage for paradoxical emboli, stroke, and brain abscess (see Fig. 30–6).† Intracranial malformations have induced fatal grand mal siezures.[27] Sudden death can result from massive intrapulmonary hemorrhage and massive hemothorax.[1,23,33,42,43,53,58,85] The 41-year-old woman described by Brown Kelly in 1906 died of intractable epistaxes.[65]

Physical Appearance

Cyanosis and clubbing are intense when the fistulous shunt is large,[41,53] but anemia caused by bleeding telangiectasia can virtually abolish the cyanosis, although clubbing persists.[41,43,53] Cyanosis is absent when systemic arteries rather than pulmonary arteries feed the fistulae.[53,62]

The distinctive physical feature of patients with pulmonary arteriovenous fistulae is the coexisting mucocutaneous telangiectases—clusters of tiny ruby lesions on the nasal and oral mucous membranes (see Fig. 30–9) and on the face, tongue, skin, retina, and nail beds.[14,36,38,53,84,118] The lesions blanch with the slightest pressure and bleed with the slightest provocation. Unlike spider angioma, blanching with pressure is usually incomplete.[38] Telangiectases, which are rarely evident in infants and young children, may be the first clue of a pulmonary arteriovenous fistula.

The Arterial Pulse and Jugular Venous Pulse

The arterial pulse and the jugular venous pulse are normal because left ventricular stroke volume is normal or only modestly increased, and congestive heart failure is rare.[50] Isolated examples of an increased arterial pulse occur with a massive pulmonary arteriovenous fistula[50] (see Fig. 30–7) and when coexisting intrahepatic arteriovenous fistulae cause a hyperdynamic circulatory state.[26,96,97]

Precordial Movement and Palpation

The extra amount of blood pumped by the right or left ventricle is relatively small (see Physiologic Consequences), so the ventricular impulses are normal. Precordial impulses are hyperdynamic in the rare event of a massive pulmonary arteriovenous fistula (see Fig. 30–7),[50] and hepatic arteriovenous fistulae are accompanied by hyperdynamic ventricular impulses, hepatomegaly, and a hepatic thrill.[26,96,97]

Auscultation

Pulmonary arteriovenous fistulae transmit murmurs to overlying chest wall sites because the fistulae are close to the periphery of the lungs (see Figs. 30–1 through 30–3).[43,57,119] Murmurs are absent when fistulae lie deeply within the lungs or when they are small and diffuse (see Figs. 30–4 and 30–6).[53,103,116] Murmurs are missed when they are faint and assigned to non-precordial sites,[57,120] and the clinical diagnosis is untenable in acyanotic patients with no murmur and no telangiectases.[36] If arteriovenous fistulae are hepatic, the abdominal location of the murmur is responsible for oversight.[26,34,96,98]

Murmurs are typically less than grade 3 and therefore rarely cause thrills.[11,69,73] Loud harsh murmurs are exceptional.[50] Auscultation should be carried out in a quiet room with the patient comfortable and the thorax relaxed to avoid the interference of muscle tremor. The entire chest should be examined in addition to the liver and the cranium. Respiration should be shallow and quiet and should include gentle held exhalation. Because 75% of pulmonary arteriovenous fistulae are in the lower lobes and right middle lobe, these overlying chest wall sites warrant special auscultatory attention.[62,74,84,102] Murmurs overlying the lingula of the left lung can be mistaken for intracardiac murmurs (see Fig. 30–3).[43,60,84]

Pulmonary arteriovenous fistulae generate murmurs that are either systolic or continuous (Figs. 30–10 and 30–11).* In the first clinically diagnosed case, the murmur was continuous.[113] The major pressure gradient across the fistula is systolic.[73,84,135] Diastolic gradients are negligible or absent, so the diastolic portion of the murmur is negligible or absent, accounting for the high incidence of murmurs that are confined to systole (see Fig. 30–10). Isolated diastolic murmurs are rare.[84,135] Fistulae are downstream from the right ventricle, so an interval elapses from the onset of right ventricular ejection to arrival of blood flow

*See references 14, 15, 52, 53, 73, 78, 83, 84, 96, 111, 119.
†See references 25, 28, 38, 53, 56, 60, 68, 82, 91, 93, 94, 124, 128.

*See references 8, 11, 14, 43, 53, 60, 69, 73, 86, 116, 135.

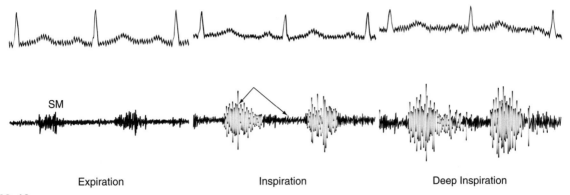

Expiration   Inspiration   Deep Inspiration

Figure 30–10

Phonocardiogram from the left mid-axillary line of the 35-year-old woman whose solitary left lower lobe pulmonary arteriovenous fistula is shown in Figure 30–2. The systolic murmur (sm) that was recorded during expiration becomes continuous and increases appreciably during deep inspiration.

through the fistula. This interval is responsible for the delayed onset and late crescendo exhibited by the murmurs, which begin late and finish after the second heart sound (see Fig. 30–11).[14,86]

The normal inspiratory increase in right ventricular volume is available for forward flow through the fistulae, and simultaneous inspiratory depression of the diaphragm reduces compression of lower lobe fistulae. Accordingly, the murmur decreases during expiration and increases during inspiration, especially during deep held inspiration (see Fig. 30–10).[36,52,53,60,73,84,135] The murmur may be heard only at the end of an exaggerated inspiratory effort, so unless this maneuver is performed, the response of the murmur will be missed. Inspiration may also cause a systolic murmur to become continuous (see Fig. 30–10). To detect these respiratory effects, auscultation should be carried out at the end of normal expiration and at the height of deep, momentarily held inspiration. Two purposes are served by these maneuvers, namely, respiratory interference is minimized, and held inspiration provides time for right ventricular blood to reach the fistula. The Valsalva and Müller maneuvers exaggerate these effects.[73,116] Flow through the fistula diminishes during the Valsalva maneuver, so the murmur softens or vanishes. When straining is released, flow abruptly accelerates and the murmur intensifies. The Müller maneuver (forced inspiration against a closed glottis) increases flow through the fistula and increases the intensity of the fistulous murmur. Standing increases perfusion of the dependent portions of the lungs and increases audibility of lower lobe murmurs.[52] A lateral decubitus position on the side of a fistula compresses the ipsilateral lung and decreases the murmur.[52] Pregnancy elevates the diaphragm, compresses lower lobe fistulae, and decreases or abolishes the murmur (see earlier).[52]

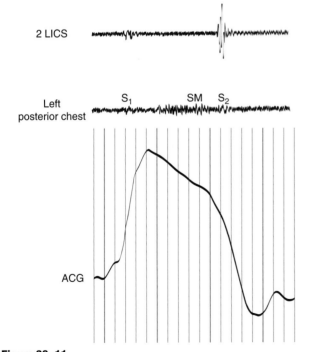

2 LICS

Left posterior chest

S_1 SM S_2

ACG

Figure 30–11

Phonocardiograms from a 38-year-old woman with a congenital pulmonary arteriovenous fistula of the left lower lobe. Recordings from the second left intercostal space (2 LICS) disclosed no murmur, but recordings from the left posterior chest disclosed a soft delayed systolic murmur (SM). ACG, apex cardiogram; S_1/S_2, first and second heart sounds.

The Electrocardiogram

The electrocardiogram is usually normal because the hemodynamic burden is modest.[36,60,84] Flow through the fistula is associated with a reciprocal decrease in flow through the uninvolved lung, so right ventricular output is normal and the volume entering the left side of the heart is normal. The increment of blood shunted through the fistula seldom imposes volume load on either ventricle. These circulatory adjustments are less effective when fistulae are large (see Fig. 30–7), which may account for the occasional presence of either right or left axis deviation.[11,73,135] When a large pulmonary arteriovenous fistula or a large pulmonary arterial-to-left atrial fistula exists in utero,[50,84] right ventricular blood preferentially flows through the low-resistance fistula and imposes volume overload on the left side of the heart.[50] This mechanism is held responsible for left ventricular hypertrophy and left atrial P wave abnormalities in the electrocardiogram.[50,84]

The X-Ray

The rare large fistula is associated with an increase in heart size (see Fig. 30–7),[50,73,105] but the size and shape of the heart are otherwise normal (see Figs. 30–1 and 30–2). The most important feature of the x-ray is the abnormal density cast by the fistula itself (see Figs. 30–1A, 30–3, 30–5A, 30–7A, and 30–9). Lateral views should be examined because the density may be hidden by the heart or diaphragm (see Fig. 30–3).[18,60,153,235] Multiple small fistulae are difficult to identify on the x-ray and impart hazy radiodensities rather than circumscribed lesions.[6,29,36,49,53,73] Fistulae in infants are usually poorly defined on the x-ray (see Fig. 30–9) but tend to increase in size and radiodensity.[60,84,121,124] Large fistulae are exceptional (see Fig. 30–7).

Pulmonary arteriovenous fistulae can be single or multiple, unilateral or bilateral and typically involve the lower lobes and right middle lobe (see Figs. 30–1 through 30–4).[36,62,74,84] Upper lobe fistulae are uncommon (see Fig. 30–6). The densities vary in size and shape from small focal opacities (see Figs. 30–4 and 30–6) to large homogeneous densities that have been mistaken for coin lesions or metastatic carcinoma (see Figs. 30–1 and 30–2).[36,116] The densities are round or lobulated with well-demarcated edges[73,74,84] (Figs. 30–1 and 30–2) or hazy and ill-defined borders (see Figs. 30–7A and 30–9).[29,53,73,74,117,118] Lateral projections confirm that the opacities are within the lung parenchyma.[36,53,74] Calcification is exceptional.[112,116] Hemorrhage may obscure the lesion,[84,105] and intrapleural rupture causes painful hemothorax.[33,38,45,53,84,105]

Vascular shadows connecting the parenchymal density to the hilus establish the lung lesion as a pulmonary arteriovenous fistula (see Figs. 30–1 through 30–4 and 30–6).[29,53,73,74,78,84,105,110,116] The linear vascular shadows correspond to dilated afferent pulmonary arterial channels that join the fistula and efferent channels that leave the fistula (see Figs. 30–1 through 30–4 and 30–6). Rarely, localized notching of ribs is caused by dilated tortuous intercostal arteries that enter the fistula.[73,96,119] Subtle variations in the size of a fistula can be induced by changes in intrathoracic pressure.[29,73,74,84,116] The Valsalva maneuver diminishes the fistula by decreasing flow. The Müller maneuver enlarges the fistula by increasing flow.[84]

The Echocardiogram

Pulmonary arteriovenous fistulae are seldom imaged because the lesions are within the lung parenchyma. An exception is a solitary large paracardiac fistula.[61] Pulsed Doppler echocardiography has recorded bidirectional flow into and out of the fistula,[64] and the diagnosis has been made by color Doppler and amplitude ultrasound angiography and by transcranial echocardiography.[66,130] Contrast echocardiography can detect relatively small right-to-left fistulous shunts and can establish the shunts as extracardiac.[36,61,71,89,108] Agitated saline injected into a peripheral vein, vena cava, or pulmonary artery is promptly detected in pulmonary veins or in the left atrium by transthoracic and transesophageal echocardiograpy.[36,37,61,89,108,124]

Summary

Pulmonary arteriovenous fistulae are usually discovered in young adults because of abnormal densities on routine chest x-rays or because of cyanosis or mucocutaneous telangiectasia. Dyspnea and fatigue do not correspond to the degree of cyanosis but are related to anemia caused by familial hemorrhagic telangiectasia. The history is characterized by recurrent epistaxis, hemoptysis, and bleeding from mouth, lips, and gastrointestinal tract. Cerebral, intrapulmonary, and intrapleural hemorrhage can be lethal. Peculiar cerebral symptoms include dizziness, tinnitus, vertigo, paresthesias, faintness, visual aberrations, speech disturbances, headache, extremity weakness, mental confusion, and seizures. Pulmonary arteriovenous malformations set the stage for paradoxical embolism, stroke, and brain abscess. Physical appearance is characterized by cyanosis and clubbing but especially by clusters of small ruby patches (telangiectases) on the face, nasal and oral mucous membranes, tongue, lips, and skin. The arterial pulse, the jugular venous pulse, and the precordial movements are usually normal. Auscultation detects systolic or continuous murmurs at non-precordial sites corresponding to the lower lobe or right middle lobe locations of the majority of pulmonary arteriovenous fistulae. Systolic murmurs increase in intensity and become continuous during inspiration, during the Müller maneuver, or with standing, and decrease in intensity during exhalation, during the Valsalva maneuver, or in an ipsilateral decubitus position. The electrocardiogram is normal, and the size and shape of the heart on x-ray are normal. However, the lung fields show distinctive fistulous densities that are single or multiple, unilateral or bilateral, small or large and are typically located in the lower lobes or right middle lobe. The densities are round or lobulated, are well demarcated, and are attached to the hilus by shadows that represent dilated afferent and efferent vessels entering and leaving the fistula. The radiologic size of a fistula decreases with the Valsalva maneuver and increases with the Müller maneuver. Contrast echocardiography confirms small right-to-left fistulous shunts and identifies the shunts as extracardiac.

REFERENCES

1. Adegboyega PA, Youh G, Adesokan A: Recurrent massive hemothorax in Rendu-Weber-Osler syndrome. South Med J 89:1193, 1996.
2. Alexander LL, Harrington LA: Multiple arteriovenous fistulas of the lung. N Y J Med 55:2807, 1955.
3. Allen SW, Whitfield JM, Clarke DR, et al: Pulmonary arteriovenous malformation in the newborn: A familial case. Pediat Cardiol 14:58, 1993.
4. Amodeo A, Marino B: Pulmonary arteriovenous fistulas in patients with left isomerism and cardiac malformations. Cardiol Young 8:283, 1998.

5. Anabtawi IN, Ellison RG: Maldevelopment of the pulmonary veins and pulmonary arteriovenous aneurysms. Am Surg 30:770, 1964.

6. Anabtawi IN, Ellison RG, Ellison LT: Pulmonary arteriovenous aneurysms and fistulas: Anatomical variations, embryology, and classification. Ann Thorac Surg 1:277, 1965.

7. Babington BG: Hereditary epistaxis. Lancet 2:362, 1865.

8. Baer S, Behrend A, Goldburgh HL: Arteriovenous fistulas of the lungs. Circulation 1:602, 1950.

9. Baker C, Trounce JR: Arteriovenous aneurysm of lung. Br Heart J 11:109, 1949.

10. Barbe T, Losay J, Grimon G, et al: Pulmonary arteriovenous shunting in children with liver disease. J Pediatr 126:571, 1995.

11. Batinica S, Gagro A, Bradic I, Marinovic B: Congenital pulmonary arteriovenous fistula: A rare cause of cyanosis in childhood. Thorac Cardiovasc Surg 39:105, 1991.

12. Bernstein HS, Brook MM, Silverman NH, Bristow J: Development of pulmonary arteriovenous fistulae in children after cavopulmonary shunt. Circulation 92(Suppl 9):II309, 1995.

13. Berthezene Y, Howarth NR, Revel D: Pulmonary arteriovenous fistula: Detection with magnetic resonance angiography. Eur Radiol 8:1403, 1998.

14. Björk VO, Intonti F, Aletras H, Madsen R: Varieties of pulmonary arteriovenous aneurysms. Acta Chir Scand 125:69, 1963.

15. Blatchford JW, Bolman RM, Hunter DW, Amplatz K: Concomitant pulmonary and cerebral arteriovenous fistulae. Chest 88:782, 1985.

16. Bosher LH Jr, Blake A, Byrd BR: An analysis of the pathologic anatomy of pulmonary arteriovenous aneurysms with particular reference to the applicability of local excision. Surgery 45:91, 1959.

17. Boston LN: Gastric hemorrhage due to familial telangiectasis. Am J Med Sci 180:798, 1930.

18. Boczko ML: Pulmonary arteriovenous fistulas. Mayo Clin Proc 74:1305, 1999.

19. Bradshaw DA, Murray KM, Mull NH: Massive hemoptysis in pregnancy due to a solitary pulmonary arteriovenous malformation. West J Med 161:600, 1994.

20. Brain R, Kauntze R: Systemic-pulmonary arteriovenous aneurysm of chest wall and lung. Guy's Hosp Rep 109:110, 1960.

21. Brian CA, Payne RM, Link KM, et al: Pulmonary arteriovenous malformation. Circulation 100:e29, 1999.

22. Brink AJ: Telangiectasis of lungs; with 2 case reports of hereditary haemorrhagic telangiectasia with cyanosis. Q J Med 19:239, 1950.

23. Britt CI, Andrews NC, Klassen KP: Pulmonary arteriovenous fistula. Am J Surg 101:727, 1961.

24. Brummelkamp WH: Unusual complication of pulmonary arteriovenous aneurysm: Intrapleural rupture. Dis Chest 39:218, 1961.

25. Brydon HL, Akinwunmi J, Selway R, Ul-Haq I: Brain abscesses associated with pulmonary arteriovenous malformations. Br J Neurosurg 13:265, 1999.

26. Burckhardt D, Stalder GA, Ludin H, Bianchi L: Hyperdynamic circulatory state due to Osler-Weber-Rendu disease with intrahepatic arteriovenous fistulas. Am Heart J 85:797, 1973.

27. Byard RW, Schliebs J, Koszyca BA: Osler-Weber-Rendu syndrome: Pathological manifestations and autopsy considerations. J Forensic Sci 46:698, 2001.

28. Chambers WR.: Brain abscess associated with pulmonary arteriovenous fistula. Ann Surg 141:276, 1955.

29. Chandler D: Pulmonary and cerebral arteriovenous fistula with Osler's disease. Arch Intern Med 116:277, 1965.

30. Chung Y, Ahrens WR, Singh J: Massive hemoptysis in a child due to pulmonary arteriovenous malformation. J Emerg Med 15:317, 1997.

31. Churton T: Multiple aneurysms of pulmonary artery. Br Med J 1:1223, 1897.

32. Cooper B: William Osler on telangiectatic syndromes. BUMC Proceedings 12:238, 1999.

33. Dalton ML, Goodwin FC, Bronwell AW, Rutledge R: Intrapleural rupture of pulmonary arteriovenous aneurysm. Diseases Chest 52:97, 1967.

34. Danchin N, Thisse JY, Neimann JL, Faivre G: Osler-Weber-Rendu disease with multiple intrahepatic arteriovenous fistulas. Am Heart J 105:856, 1983.

35. Dines DE, Clagett OT, Bonebrake RA: Hereditary telangiectasia and pulmonary fistula. Arch Intern Med 119:195, 1967.

36. Dines DE, Seward JB, Bernatz PE: Pulmonary arteriovenous fistula. Mayo Clin Proc 58:176, 1983.

37. Duch PM, Chandrasekaran K, Mulhern CB, et al: Transesophageal echocardiographic diagnosis of pulmonary arteriovenous malformation. Chest 105:1694, 1994.

38. Editorial: Pulmonary arteriovenous fistula in hereditary haemorrhagic telangiectasia. Lancet 1:158, 1960.

39. El Gamal M, Stoker JB, Spiers EM, Whitaker W: Cyanosis complicating hepatic cirrhosis: Report of a case due to multiple pulmonary arteriovenous fistulas. Am J Cardiol 25:490, 1970.

40. Esplin MS, Varner MW: Progression of pulmonary arteriovenous malformation during pregnancy: Case report and review of the literature. Obstet Gynecol Surv 52:248, 1997.

41. Fawcett AW, Dhillon BS: Pulmonary arterio-venous fistula; review of world literature and report on 2 additional cases. Postgrad Med J 32:353, 1956.

42. Ference BA, Shannon TM, White RI, et al: Life-threatening pulmonary hemorrhage with pulmonary arteriovenous malformations and hereditary hemorrhagic telangiectasia. Chest 106:1387, 1994.

43. Foley RE, Boyd DP: Pulmonary arteriovenous aneurysm. Surg Clin North Am 41:801, 1961.

44. Freixinet J, Sanchez-Palacios M, Guerrero D, et al: Pulmonary arteriovenous fistula ruptured to pleural cavity in pregnancy. Scand J Thorac Cardiovasc Surg 29:39, 1995.

45. Gammon RB, Miksa AK, Keller FS: Osler-Weber-Rendu disease and pulmonary arterial venous fistulas. Chest 98:1522, 1990.

46. Goldblatt E, Vimpani G, Brown JH: Extralobar pulmonary sequestration. Am J Cardiol 29:100, 1972.

47. Gossage JR, Kanj G: Pulmonary arteriovenous malformations: A state of the art review. Am J Resp Crit Care Med 158:643, 1998.

48. Grung P: Telangiectasia haemorrhagica hereditaria Osler with arteriovenous aneurysms of lung and with hepatosplenomegaly. Case report. Acta Med Scand 150:95, 1954.

49. Hales MR: Multiple small arteriovenous fistulae of lungs. Am J Pathol 32:927, 1956.

50. Hall RJ, Nelson WP, Blake HA, Geiger JP: Massive pulmonary arteriovenous fistula in the newborn; a correctable form of "cyanotic heart disease"; an additional cause of cyanosis with left axis deviation. Circulation 31:762, 1965.

51. Hanes FM: Multiple hereditary telangiectases causing hemorrhagic (hereditary hemorrhagic) telangiectasia. Bull Johns Hopkins Hosp 20:63, 1909.

52. Hazlett DR, Medina J: Postural effects on the bruit and right to left shunt of pulmonary arteriovenous fistula. Chest 60:89, 1971.

53. Hodgson CH, Burchell HB, Good CA, Clagett OT: Hereditary hemorrhagic telangiectasia and pulmonary arteriovenous fistula; survey of a large family. N Engl J Med 261:625, 1959.

54. Hultgren HN, Gerbode F: Physiologic studies in a patient with a pulmonary arteriovenous fistula. Am J Med 17:126, 1954.

55. Humphries JE, Frierson HF, Underwood PB: Vaginal telangiectasias: Unusual presentation of the Osler-Weber-Rendu syndrome. Obstet Gynecol 81:865, 1993.

56. Hunter DD: Pulmonary arteriovenous malformation: An unusual cause of cerebral embolism. Can Med Assoc J 93:662, 1965.

57. Husson GS: Pulmonary arteriovenous aneurysms in childhood. Pediatrics 18:871, 1956.

58. Israel HL, Gosfield E Jr: Fatal hemoptysis from pulmonary arteriovenous fistula: Report of case in patient with hereditary haemorrhagic telangiectasia. JAMA 152:40, 1953.

59. Iqbal M, Rossoff LJ, Steingerg HN, et al: Pulmonary arteriovenous malformations: A clinical review. Postgrad Med J 76:390, 2000.

60. Jeresaty RM, Knight HF, Hart WE: Pulmonary arteriovenous fistulas in children: Report of two cases and review of literature. Am J Dis Child 111:256, 1966.

61. Jimenez M, Fournier A, Choussat A: Pulmonary artery to left atrium fistula as an unusual cause of cyanosis in the newborn. Pediatr Cardiol 10:216, 1989.

62. Kafka V, Padovcova H, Kabelka M, Kleint Z: A congenital arteriovenous pulmonary aneurysm in a 2 1/2 year old boy: Case report and review of the literature. J Cardiovasc Surg 2:396, 1961.

63. Kapur S, Rome J, Chandra RS: Diffuse pulmonary arteriovenous malformation in a child with polysplenia syndrome. Pediatr Pathol Lab Med 15:462, 1995.

64. Kataoka H, Matsuno O: Rendu-Osler-Weber disease: Transthoracic Doppler ultrasonographic findings. Circulation 103:e36, 2001.

65. Kelly AB: Multiple telangiectases of the skin and mucous membranes of the nose and mouth. Glas Med J 65:411, 1906.

66. Kimura K, Minematsu K, Wada K, et al: Transcranial Doppler of a paradoxical brain embolism associated with a pulmonary arteriovenous fistula. Am J Neuroradiol 20:1881, 1999.

67. Kiphart RJ, MacKenzie JW, Templeton AW, Martin RA: Systemic pulmonary arteriovenous fistula of the chest wall and lung. J Thorac Cardiovasc Surg 54:113, 1967.

68. Kjeldssen AD, Oxhoj H, Anderson PE, et al: Prevalence of pulmonary arteriovenous malformations and occurrence of neurologic symptoms in patients with hereditary hemorrhagic telangiectasia. J Intern Med 248:255, 2000.

69. Knight WB, Bush A, Busst CM, et al: Multiple pulmonary arteriovenous fistulas in childhood. Int J Cardiol 23:105, 1989.

70. Kroeker EJ, Adams HD, Leon AS, Pouget JM: Congenital communication between a pulmonary artery and the left atrium. Am J Med 34:721, 1963.

71. Kuramochi T, Izumi S, Nakayama K, et al: Contrast echocardiographic detection of pulmonary arteriovenous shunt in a hypoxic patient with liver cirrhosis. J Cardiol 24:155, 1994.

72. Legg JW: Case of haemophilia complicated with multiple naevi. Lancet 2:856, 1876.

73. LeRoux BT: Pulmonary arteriovenous fistulae. Q J Med 28:1, 1959.

74. LeRoux BT: Pulmonary hamartomata. Thorax 19:236, 1964.

75. Livingston SO, Carr RE: Hereditary hemorrhagic telangiectasia; report of case with hemothorax. J Thorac Cardiovasc Surg 31:497, 1956.

76. Lucas RV Jr, Lund GW, Edwards JE: Direct communication of a pulmonary artery with the left atrium: An unusual variant of the pulmonary arteriovenous fistula. Circulation 24:1409, 1961.

77. Lyons HA, Mannix EP Jr: Successful resections for bilateral pulmonary arteriovenous fistulas. N Engl J Med 254:969, 1956.

78. Mallin SR, Brest AN, Moyer JH: The differential diagnosis of pulmonary arteriovenous fistula. Dis Chest 40:322, 1961.

79. Maryuama J, Watanabe M, Onodera S, et al: A case of Rendu-Osler-Weber disease with cerebral hemangioma, multiple pulmonary arteriovenous fistulas and hepatic arteriovenous fistula. Jpn Med J 28:651, 1989.

80. McKusick VA: A genetical view of cardiovascular disease. Circulation 30:326, 1964.

81. Mestre JR, Andres JM: Hereditary hemorrhagic telangiectasia causing hematemesis in an infant. J Pediatr 101:577, 1982.

82. Momma F, Ohara S, Ohyama T, et al: Brain abscess associated with congenital pulmonary arteriovenous fistula. Surg Neurol 34:439, 1990.

83. Moussouttas M, Fayad P, Rosenblatt M, et al: Pulmonary arteriovenous malformations: Cerebral ischemia and neurologic manifestations. Neurology 55:959, 2000.

84. Moyer JH, Glantz G, Brest AN: Pulmonary arteriovenous fistulas. Am J Med 32:417, 1962.

85. Muri JW: Arteriovenous aneurysm of lung. Am J Surg 89:265, 1955.

86. Neill C, Mounsey P: Auscultation in patent ductus arteriosus with a description of 2 fistulae simulating patent ductus. Br Heart J 20:61, 1958.

87. Nelson WP, Hall RJ, Garcia E: Varicosities of the pulmonary veins simulating arteriovenous fistulas. JAMA 195:13, 1966.

88. Osler W: On family form of recurring epistaxis, associated with multiple telangiectases of skin and mucous membranes. Bull Johns Hopkins Hosp 12:333, 1901.

89. Ozkutlu S, Saraclar M: Two-dimensional contrast echocardiography in pulmonary arteriovenous fistula. Jpn Heart J 30:425, 1989.

90. Perry WH: Clinical spectrum of hereditary hemorrhagic telangiectasia (Osler-Weber-Rendu Disease). Am J Med 82:989, 1987.

91. Pick A, Deschamps C, Stanson AW: Pulmonary arteriovenous fistula: Presentation, diagnosis, and treatment. World J Surg 23:1118, 1999.

92. Premsekar R, Monro JL, Salmon AP: Diagnosis, management and pathophysiology of post-Fontan hypoxaemia secondary to Glenn shunt related pulmonary arteriovenous malformation. Heart 82:528, 1999.

93. Press OW, Ramsey PG: Central nervous system infections associated with hereditary hemorrhagic telangiectasia. Am J Med 77:86, 1984.

94. Preston DC, Shapiro BE: Pulmonary arteriovenous fistula and brain abscess. Neurology 56:418, 2001.

95. Putman CM, Chaloupka JC, Fulbright RK, et al: Exceptional multiplicity of cerebral arteriovenous malformations associated with hereditary hemorrhagic telangiectasia (Osler-Weber-Rendu syndrome). Am J Neuroradiol 17:1733, 1996.

96. Radtke WE, Smith HC, Fulton RE, Adson MA: Misdiagnosis of atrial septal defect in patients with hereditary telangiectasia (Osler-Weber-Rendu disease) and hepatic arteriovenous fistula. Am Heart J 95:235, 1978.

97. Razi B, Beller BM, Ghidoni J, et al: Hyperdynamic circulatory state due to intrahepatic fistula in Osler-Weber-Rendu disease. Am J Med 50:809, 1971.

98. Reilly PJ, Nostrant TT: Clinical manifestations of hereditary hemorrhagic telangiectasia. Am J Gastroenterol 79:363, 1984.

99. Rendu H: Epistaxis répetée chez un sujet porteur de petits angiomes cutanés et muqueaux. Bull Mém Soc Méd d'Hôp Paris 13:731, 1896.

100. Ronald J: Pulmonary arterio-venous fistula. Br Heart J 16:34, 1954.

101. Rydell R, Hoffbauer FW: Multiple pulmonary arteriovenous fistulas in juvenile cirrhosis. Am J Med 21:450, 1956.

102. Sahn SH, Bluth I, Schub H: Pulmonary arteriovenous fistula. Dis Chest 44:542, 1963.

103. Sanders JS, Martt JM: Multiple small pulmonary arteriovenous fistulas: Diagnosis by cardiac catheterization. Circulation 25:383, 1962.

104. Sapru RP, Hutchinson DCS, Hall JI: Pulmonary hypertension in patients with pulmonary arteriovenous fistulae. Br Heart J 31:559, 1969.

105. Seaman WB, Goldman A: Roentgen aspects of pulmonary arteriovenous fistula. Arch Intern Med 89:70, 1952.

106. Sheikhzadeh A, Hakim H, Ghabusi P, et al: Right pulmonary artery-to-left atrial communication. Am Heart J 107:396, 1984.

107. Shovlin CL, Guttmacher AE, Buscarini E, et al: Diagnostic criteria for hereditary hemorrhagic telangiectasia. Am J Genet 91:66, 2000.

108. Shub C, Tajik AJ, Seward JB, Dines DE: Detecting intrapulmonary right to left shunt with contrast echocardiography: Observations in a patient with diffuse pulmonary arteriovenous fistulas. Mayo Clin Proc 51:81, 1976.

109. Shumacker HB Jr, Waldhausen JA: Pulmonary arteriovenous fistulas in children. Ann Surg 158:713, 1963.

110. Singleton EB, Leachman RD, Rosenberg HS: Congenital abnormalities of the pulmonary arteries. Am J Roentgenol 91:487, 1964.

111. Sisel RJ, Parker BM, Bahl OP: Cerebral symptoms in pulmonary arteriovenous fistula. Circulation 41:123, 1970.

112. Sloan RD, Cooley RN: Congenital pulmonary arteriovenous aneurysm. Am J Roentgenol 70:183, 1953.

113. Smith HL, Horton BT: Arteriovenous fistula of lung associated with polycythemia vera: Report of a case in which diagnosis was made clinically. Am Heart J 18:589, 1939.

114. Standefer JE, Tabakin BS, Hanson JS: Pulmonary arteriovenous fistulas: Case report with cine-angiographic studies. Am Rev Respir Dis 89:95, 1964.

115. Steinberg I: Diagnosis and surgical treatment of pulmonary arteriovenous fistula: Report of three new and review of 19 consecutive cases. Surg Clin North Am 41:523, 1961.

116. Steinberg I, Finby N: Roentgen manifestations of pulmonary arteriovenous fistula. Am J Roentgenol 78:234, 1957.

117. Steinberg I, Maisel B, Vogel FS: Pulmonary arteriovenous fistula associated with capillary telangiectasia (Rendu-Osler-Weber disease): Report of a case illustrating use of metal casting for demonstrating the lesion. J Thorac Cardiovasc Surg 35:517, 1958.

118. Steinberg I, McClenahan JL: Pulmonary arteriovenous fistula; angiocardiographic observations in 9 cases. Am J Med 19:549, 1955.

119. Stork WJ: Pulmonary arteriovenous fistula. Am J Roentgenol 74:44, 1955.

120. Stringer CJ, Stanley AL, Bates RC, Summers JE: Pulmonary arteriovenous fistula. Am J Surg 89:1054, 1955.

121. Swanson KL, Prakash UB, Stanton AW: Pulmonary arteriovenous fistulas: Mayo Clinic experience. Mayo Clin Proc 74:671, 1999.

122. Taber RE, Ehrenhaft JL: Arteriovenous fistulae and arterial aneurysms of pulmonary arterial tree. AMA Arch Surg 73:567, 1956.

123. Taiana JA, Schieppati E, Pini A: Arteriovenous fistula of lung: Surgical treatment of 2 cases. Ann Surg 141:417, 1955.

124. Teragaki M, Akioka K, Yasuda M, et al: Case report: Hereditary hemorrhagic telangiectasia with growing pulmonary arteriovenous fistulas followed for 24 years. Am J Med Sciences 295:545, 1988.

125. Terry TB, Barth KH, Kaufman SL, White RI: Balloon embolism for treatment of pulmonary arteriovenous fistulas. N Engl J Med 302:1189, 1980.

126. Trilomis T, Busch T, Aleksic I, et al: Pulmonary arteriovenous fistula drainage into the left atrium. Thor Cardiovasc Surg 48:37, 2000.

127. Tuncali T, Aytac A: Direct communication between right pulmonary artery and left atrium. J Pediatr 71:384, 1967.

128. Walder LA, Anastasia LF, Spodick DH: Pulmonary arteriovenous malformations with brain abscess. Am Heart J 127:227, 1994.

129. Waldhausen JA, Abel FL: The circulatory effects of pulmonary arteriovenous fistula. Surgery 59:76, 1966.

130. Wang HC, Kuo PH, Liaw YS, et al: Diagnosis of pulmonary arteriovenous malformations by color Doppler ultrasound and amplitude ultrasound angiography. Thorax 53:372, 1998.

131. Weber FP: Multiple hereditary developmental angiomata (telangiectases) of the skin and mucous membranes associated with recurring hemorrhages. Lancet 2:160, 1907.

132. Wilmshurst P, Jackson P: Arterial hypoxemia during pregnancy caused by pulmonary arteriovenous microfistulas. Chest 110:1368, 1996.

133. Wilkins GD: Ein Fall von multiplen Pulmonalis Aneurysmen. Beitr Klin Tuberk 38:1, 1917.

134. Wollstein M: Malignant hemangioma of lung with multiple visceral foci: report of a case. Arch Pathol 12:562, 1931.

135. Yater WM, Finnegan J, Giffin HM: Pulmonary arteriovenous fistula (varix): Review of the literature and report of two cases. JAMA 141:581, 1949.

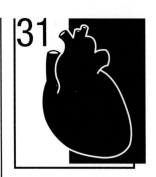

Hypoplastic
Left Heart

In 1952, Lev called attention to congenital hypoplasia of major components of the left side of the heart.[31] In 1958, Noonan and Nadas referred to these malformations as the *hypoplastic left heart syndrome,*[47] which includes aortic atresia with a hypoplastic but perforate mitral valve (Fig. 31–1) and aortic atresia with an atretic mitral valve (Fig. 31–2).[2,32,56,86,87] Aortic atresia in both settings is accompanied by a hypoplastic ascending aorta that serves as a common coronary artery (see Figs. 31–1 and 31–2). This differs fundamentally from absence of the aortic arch (Steidele's complex,[33] see Chapter 8). A hypoplastic but patent mitral valve is accompanied by a hypoplastic but patent left ventricle (see Fig. 31–1). Mitral atresia is accompanied by a blind, slitlike left ventricular cavity imbedded in ventricular muscle (see Fig. 31–2). An experimental model in chick embryos is represented by atresia or hypoplasia of the mitral valve, left ventricle, aortic valve, and thoracic aorta.[24] Hypoplasia or atresia of the mitral valve leaves the left atrium with no exit except a restrictive patent foramen ovale (see Figs. 31–1 and 31–2), which is further compromised by hypoplasia of the limbus of the foramen that is rotated and deviated close to the orifice of the superior vena cava.[57] An intact atrial septum is accompanied by either a thick muscular septal wall and a small left atrium, or by a thick septum secundum, a thin septum primum, and an enlarged left atrium.[8] Alternative decompression pathways for the obstructed left atrium consist of vascular channels from a levoatrial cardinal vein to the innominate vein, an accessory vein from left atrium to the superior vena cava, a venous connection from left atrium to hepatic veins, a coronary venous connection from left atrium to coronary sinus, and a coronary sinoseptal defect.[8] Vasoconstriction during early embryogenesis leads to decreased growth and development of pulmonary veins and to alveolar capillary dysplasia, forcing arterial

blood to bypass the deficient capillary bed and to drain through anomalous bronchial veins.[83] Lymphatics are strikingly enlarged, and dilated pulmonary veins are thick and arterialized with multiple elastic laminae.[8,63]

Aortic atresia with a hypoplastic but perforate mitral valve is the subject of the first section of this chapter (see Fig. 31–1). The second section deals with aortic atresia and mitral atresia (see Fig. 31–2). Hypoplastic left heart, as herein

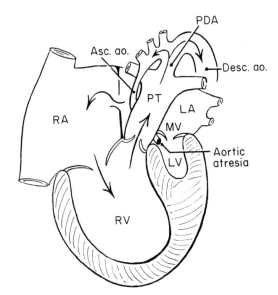

Figure 31–1

Illustration of the essential anatomic and physiologic derangements in a hypoplastic left heart with aortic atresia, a hypoplastic but perforate mitral valve (MV), and a hypoplastic left ventricle (LV). There is retrograde filling of a hypoplastic ascending aorta (Asc ao) that functions as a common coronary artery. The right ventricle (RV) serves the pulmonary circulation through the pulmonary trunk (PT) and serves the systemic circulation through pulmonary trunk–ductus–descending aortic continuity. A patent foramen ovale is the only exit for the left atrium (LA). Des ao, descending aorta; PDA, patent ductus arteriosus; RA, right atrium.

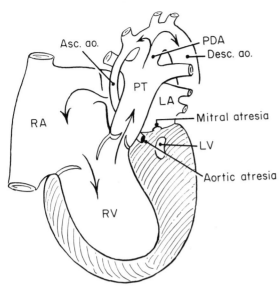

Figure 31–2

Illustration of the essential anatomic and physiologic derangements in a hypoplastic left heart with aortic atresia and mitral atresia. The left ventricular cavity (LV) is a rudimentary blind slit. The physiologic derangements are as described in Figure 31–1.

defined, occurs in 0.04 to 0.16 per 1000 live births[37,43] and accounts for 7.5% of infants with congenital heart disease.[5,19]

Aortic Atresia with Hypoplastic but Perforate Mitral Valve

The pathway to the systemic circulation is a single arterial trunk represented by pulmonary artery–ductus–descending aortic continuity (see Fig. 31–1). A hypoplastic ascending aorta serves as a common coronary artery,[18,26,35,53,56,71] and in 50% to 75% of cases is accompanied by moderate coarctation[2,18] that is located either proximal to the ductus (preductal) or distal to the junction of the ductus and the aortic arch (paraductal) (Fig. 31–3).[2,18] The right ventricle is hypertrophied because it is the sole pumping chamber for the systemic and pulmonary circulations[25,26,56,71] and harbors histologic changes of ischemia and infarction.[34] The blind hypoplastic left ventricle is thick-walled and lined with endocardial fibroelastosis.[47,48,56,60] Isovolumetric contraction causes myofiber disarray but does not cause direct ventricular–coronary artery communications.[13,48] Pinpoint neonatal aortic stenosis with small left ventricular cavity (see Chapter 7) is associated with intramyocardial sinusoids but not with direct ventricular-coronary communications.[39,40,48,59,61] The left ventricle is adequately formed in the presence of a ventricular septal defect and a patent or absent aortic valve.[2,20,32,42,49,50,52,56,67]

The coronary circulation is a matter of lively interest.[5,34,47,48,54,56,61] The hypoplastic ascending aorta functions as a common coronary artery that receives retrograde systolic and diastolic flow from the patent ductus (see Figs. 31–1 and 31–3).[34,47,56] The small tubular ascending aorta is not an impediment to retrograde flow, and the

preductal coarctation (see Fig. 31–3) is a seldom realized impediment to flow into the common coronary artery.[34] Intramyocardial coronary abnormalities analogous to those of pulmonary atresia with intact ventricular septum might be anticipated (see Chapter 24) because isovolumetric contraction generates excessive systolic pressure that could act as a driving force for direct ventricular–coronary arterial communications.[5,61] However, the differences between pulmonary atresia with intact ventricular septum and aortic atresia with a hypoplastic but patent mitral valve are as pronounced as the similarities.[5,61]

Myocardial sinusoids are restrictive vascular networks that spare the coronary arteries from the impact of high ventricular systolic pressure that is delivered through direct ventricular–coronary arterial communications.[5,61] In aortic atresia with a hypoplastic but patent mitral valve (see Fig. 31–1), the intramyocardial communications are sinusoidal.[5,61] Accordingly, epicardial and subepicardial coronary arteries do not receive the impact of high isovolumetric systolic pressure and are spared the luminal obliterative features of pulmonary atresia with an intact ventricular septum (see Chapter 24).[5,61]

The physiologic consequences of hypoplastic left heart with aortic atresia and a hypoplastic but perforate mitral valve are determined by the size of the ductus arteriosus, the pulmonary vascular resistance, and the condition of the atrial septum. Constriction of the ductus compromises flow into the systemic circulation and into the hypoplastic ascending aorta, which functions as a common coronary artery (see earlier). Right ventricular function suffers

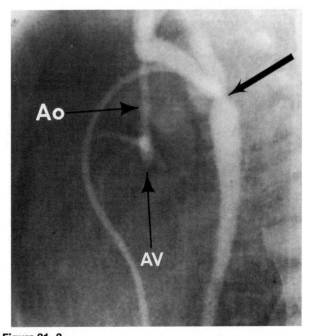

Figure 31–3

Lateral aortogram with catheter across a patent ductus arteriosus in a male neonate with aortic valve atresia (AV) and a hypoplastic but perforate mitral valve (see Fig. 31–1). A hypoplastic ascending aorta functioned as a common coronary artery. The *large unmarked arrow* at the upper right identifies coarctation of the aorta.

because of the ischemic effects of inadequate coronary blood flow,[15,26,34,48,70,71] because of obligatory pulmonary hypertension caused by the high pressure in the obstructed left atrium,[29] and because a large left ventricular mass has disadvantageous effects on right ventricular end-diastolic volume and right ventricular wall motion.[3,4,87] Competence of the tricuspid valve is important for survival, yet tricuspid dysplasia with multiple papillary muscles is common.[85] Low pulmonary vascular resistance permits increased pulmonary arterial blood flow that is received by the obstructed left atrium from which the only effective egress is a restrictive patent foramen ovale (see Fig. 31–1).[25,71] In the presence of an adequate interatrial communication,[29,64] increased pulmonary blood flow makes a large volume of oxygenated left atrial blood available for mixing in the right atrium, so systemic arterial oxygen saturation is relatively high.[29] However, preferential blood flow through the ductus into the lungs is accompanied by a reciprocal fall in systemic blood flow and a shocklike state.[60] When pulmonary vascular resistance is high, systemic blood flow is maintained at the price of increasing cyanosis.[60]

THE HISTORY

Hypoplastic left heart represents 7% to 8% of symptomatic heart disease in the first year of life[6] and is responsible for 25% of cardiac deaths in the first week of life.[19,74] The malformation has been called the most malignant form of congenital heart disease,[25] a conclusion underscored by an average lifespan of only 5 to 14 days.[19,56,75] Precarious survival depends on three tenuous variables: patency of the ductus arteriosus, pulmonary vascular resistance, and an adequate interatrial communication.[7] Risk is greatest during the time of normal ductal closure when systemic blood flow and coronary blood flow decrease or cease altogether.[11] Tachypnea, tachycardia, and cyanosis are present during the brief interval of ductal patency.[6] A fall in pulmonary vascular resistance diverts blood from the systemic circulation into the pulmonary circulation and augments flow into the obstructed left atrium. A rise in pulmonary vascular resistance improves systemic blood flow at the price of hypoxemia. Ninety-five percent of afflicted infants die within the first month of life.[19,41] Two cases of extraordinary survival include a 22-year-old woman with a large patent ductus arteriosus and an adequately sized atrial septal defect[72] and a 24-year-old man with a patent ductus arteriosus and a ventricular septal defect.[38]

There is male prevalence of 55% to 70% in aortic atresia with a hypoplastic but perforate mitral valve.[10,25,43,47,56,60] Maternal age tends to be above average, with a mean of 31 years.[2] First-degree relatives of probands have an increased prevalence of congenital heart disease.[6,12,43] The malformation is occasionally familial[28,55,60] and has been reported in siblings as an autosomal recessive inheritance.[88] A mosaic chromosomal 22q11 deletion is associated with hypoplastic left heart,[58,68] and genetic disorders include Turner syndrome, trisomy 13, trisomy 18, and trisomy 21.[44,45,69]

Hypoxemia and hypotension are associated with hypoxic-ischemic cerebral injury and intracranial hemorrhage.[22] Major and minor congenital central nervous system abnormalities include microcephaly, micrencephaly, abnormal cortical mantle, agenesis of the corpus callosum, and holoprosencephaly.[23] The overall frequency of extracardiac anomalies, including central nervous system abnormalities, is 12% to 37%.[44]

PHYSICAL APPEARANCE

Tachypnea and cyanosis are present even during the brief period of ductal patency. Cyanosis is mildest when an adequate interatrial communication and a patent ductus are accompanied by low pulmonary vascular resistance and increased pulmonary blood flow. A fall in pulmonary resistance is accompanied by systemic hypoperfusion and a shocklike state. Cyanosis is profound when pulmonary resistance is high and the ductus is restrictive.

Turner syndrome (see Chapter 8) is associated with a hypoplastic left heart.[44,45,69,77] Another association is Rubenstein-Taybi syndrome, a mendelian dominant disorder characterized by mental retardation, typical facies, broad thumbs, and short stature.[79]

THE ARTERIAL PULSE, THE JUGULAR VENOUS PULSE, AND PRECORDIAL PALPATION

Brachial and carotid artery pulses remain palpable because the ascending aortic tubular hypoplasia does not include the arch (see Figs. 31–1 and 31–2).[47] Femoral artery pulses are palpable because of pulmonary trunk–ductal–descending aortic continuity (see Figs. 31–1 and 31–2) and because coarctation is usually mild and preductal or paraductal (see Fig. 31–3). When low pulmonary vascular resistance diverts blood from the systemic circulation, all of the arterial pulses diminish if not vanish.[60]

High right atrial A and V waves are not amenable to clinical assessment. Precordial palpation is dominated by a striking right ventricular impulse and a palpable pulmonary closure sound.

AUSCULTATION

Unimpressive auscultatory signs are in contrast to the dramatic clinical picture. Murmurs are usually absent (Fig. 31–4),[6,47] or a soft midsystolic murmur is generated by ejection into the dilated hypertensive pulmonary trunk.[51] A systolic murmur is more likely to be caused by tricuspid regurgitation.[85] The second heart sound is loud because of pulmonary hypertension and is single because the aortic valve is atretic (see Fig. 31–4). A diastolic triple rhythm is caused by summation of right ventricular third and fourth heart sounds (see Fig. 31–4).

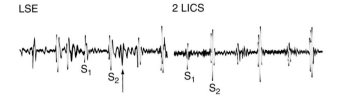

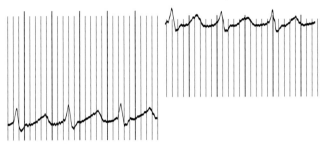

Figure 31–4

Phonocardiograms from a 9-day-old boy with aortic atresia and a hypoplastic but perforate mitral valve. Necropsy findings were as illustrated in Figure 31–1. A loud filling sound (*unmarked arrow*) with after-vibrations at the lower left sternal edge (LSE) was caused by summation of right ventricular third and fourth heart sounds. The second heart sound (S_2) in the second left intercostal space (2 LICS) was loud because of pulmonary hypertension and was single because of aortic valve atresia. S_1, first heart sound.

THE ELECTROCARDIOGRAM

Tall peaked right atrial P waves are common (Figs. 31–5 and 31–6) but not invariable (Fig. 31–7). The PR interval is occasionally prolonged (see Fig. 31–5). Despite

abnormalities of the left bundle branch, left axis deviation is uncommon and left bundle branch block is virtually unknown.[47,66] Changes in the branching portion of the bundle of His and the left bundle branch depend on the size of the left ventricular cavity, with major changes reserved for absence or virtual absence of a cavity.[9] When the left ventricular cavity is small but not slitlike, the left bundle branch has a peripheral Purkinje network, and the right bundle branch is normal in size.[9] Wolff-Parkinson-White bypass tracks are rare even though there are persistent connections of the left bundle branch to ventricular septal musculature with abundant Mahaim fibers.[9]

The QRS complex reflects pure right ventricular hypertrophy (see Figs. 31–5 and 31–6).[60] Left ventricular hypertrophy is not a feature despite an increase in mass, because end-diastolic volume affects the magnitude of the QRS waveform.[73] Left ventricular forces are absent when the cavity is small but may be present when the cavity is adequately developed (see Fig. 31–7).[20]

THE X-RAY

Dilatation of the right atrium and right ventricle are responsible for cardiac enlargement (Fig. 31–8).[82] The shadow of the hypoplastic ascending artery is necessarily absent, and the hypertensive pulmonary trunk is dilated (see Fig. 31–8). Pulmonary venous congestion is obligatory,[82] but the amount of lung available for assessment may be limited by remarkable cardiomegaly, even in the first 24 to 48 hours of life.

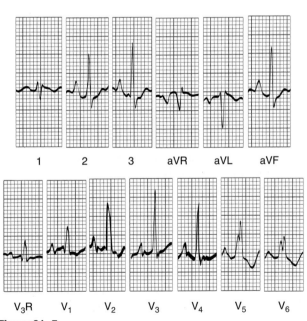

Figure 31–5

Electrocardiogram from the 9-day-old boy with aortic atresia and a hypoplastic but perforate mitral valve whose phonocardiogram is shown in Figure 31–4. Tall peaked right atrial P waves are present in leads 2, 3, aVF, and V_{2-4}, and right atrial enlargement is indicated by qR complexes in leads V_3R and V_1. The PR interval is prolonged. Right ventricular hypertrophy is reflected in the vertical QRS axis and the tall monophasic R waves in right and mid-precordial leads. The splintered QRS in leads V_{5-6} is due to a right ventricular conduction defect. The left ventricle is not represented.

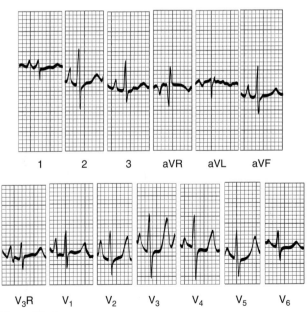

Figure 31–6

Electrocardiogram from a 3-week-old boy with aortic atresia and a hypoplastic but perforate mitral valve. Necropsy findings were as illustrated in Figure 31–1. Tall peaked right atrial P waves are present in leads 2, 3, aVF, and V_{1-3}. Right ventricular dominance is indicated by the rightward QRS axis, prominent R waves in leads V_{2-4}, and upright right precordial T waves.

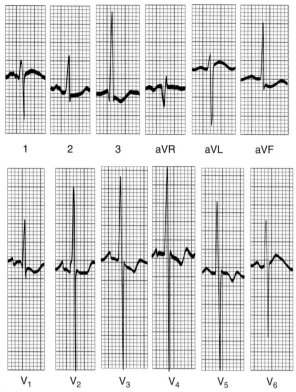

Figure 31–7

Electrocardiogram from a 4-week-old boy with aortic atresia and a hypoplastic but perforate mitral valve. The P waves are normal despite an enlarged right atrium and a high-pressure left atrium. Right ventricular hypertrophy is indicated by right axis deviation, a tall R wave in lead V_1, and a deep S wave in lead V_6. Large RS complexes in leads V_{2-5} suggest biventricular hypertrophy. The left ventricle at necropsy was thick-walled, and the small cavity was lined with endocardial fibroelastosis.

THE ECHOCARDIOGRAM

Echocardiography with color flow imaging and Doppler interrogation establishes the diagnosis of hypoplastic left heart with aortic atresia and a hypoplastic but perforate mitral valve.[36,59] Fetal echocardiography permits the diagnosis as early as the 24th week of gestation.[4,11,39,59,67,76,78,81,84] Flow patterns in the fetal ductus can be monitored,[30] and the condition of the atrial septum can be determined.[65] A hypoplastic but perforate mitral valve communicates with a small left ventricle that gives rise to an atretic aortic valve and a hypoplastic tubular ascending aorta (Fig. 31–9). The ventricular septum and the free wall of the hypoplastic left ventricle are thick and immobile, and the cavity is lined with endocardial fibroelastosis (see Fig. 31–9). Coarctation is identified as a thin discrete posterior ledge extending across the lumen of the aorta at the level of the ductus arteriosus or as kinking and narrowing at the site of ductal insertion. The left atrium is small and thick-walled (see Fig. 31–9). Function of the enlarged hypertrophied right ventricle and competence of the tricuspid valve can be established (see Fig. 31–9).[14,80,85] Ductus–pulmonary trunk–descending aortic continuity is confirmed by color flow imaging. Doppler interrogation establishes retrograde flow into the hypoplastic ascending aorta and occasionally identifies biphasic flow in the proximal coronary arteries.[72] Direct ventricular–coronary artery communications can be identified.[46]

SUMMARY

A patient with hypoplastic left heart represented by aortic atresia and a hypoplastic but perforate mitral valve presents as a tachypneic, listless, often moribund male neonate with cyanosis that varies from mild to profound. Brachiocephalic and femoral arterial pulses are palpable. A right ventricular impulse is conspicuous. Auscultation occasionally detects a tricuspid regurgitant murmur, a

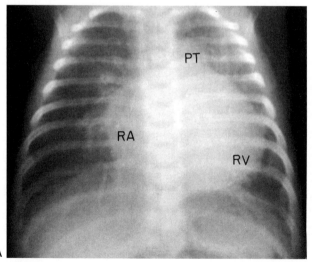

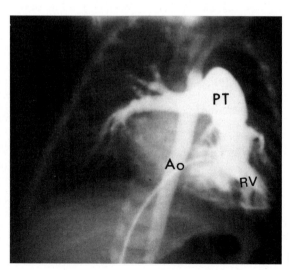

Figure 31–8

X-ray and angiocardiogram from a 2-day-old boy with aortic atresia and a hypoplastic but perforate mitral valve. Necropsy findings were as illustrated in Figure 31–1. *A*, The lungs exhibit pulmonary venous congestion. The right atrium (RA) and right ventricle (RV) are enlarged, the pulmonary trunk (PT) is dilated, but the ascending aorta is conspicuously absent. *B*, The right ventricular angiocardiogram visualizes the large pulmonary trunk (PT) with pulmonary artery–ductus–descending aortic continuity. Ao, descending aorta.

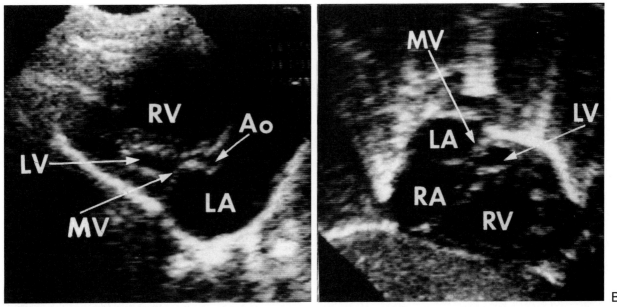

Figure 31–9

A, Echocardiogram (parasternal long axis) from a male neonate with aortic atresia and a hypoplastic but perforate mitral valve (MV). The hypoplastic left ventricle is lined with endocardial fibroelastosis. The ascending aorta (Ao) is hypoplastic, the left atrium (LA) is thick-walled but not enlarged, and the right ventricle (RV) is dilated. *B*, Subcostal four-chamber view shows a hypoplastic but patent mitral valve (MV), a hypoplastic left ventricular cavity with endocardial fibroelastosis, a nondilated left atrium, and dilatation of the right ventricle (RV) and right atrium (RA).

pulmonary midsystolic murmur, or, more often than not, no murmur at all. The electrocardiogram displays right atrial P waves and right ventricular hypertrophy. The x-ray discloses pulmonary venous congestion and dilatation of the right atrium, right ventricle, and pulmonary trunk but conspicuous absence of the ascending aorta. Echocardiography with color flow imaging and Doppler interrogation identifies a hypoplastic perforate mitral valve, a hypoplastic left ventricle lined with endocardial fibroelastosis, a hypoplastic tubular ascending aorta guarded by an atretic aortic valve, and a single arterial trunk that consists of pulmonary artery–ductus–descending aortic continuity.

Hypoplastic Left Heart with Aortic Atresia and Mitral Atresia

The major physiologic derangements of hypoplastic left heart with aortic atresia and mitral atresia are similar to those of aortic atresia with a hypoplastic but perforate mitral valve, but there are anatomic differences and subtle clinical differences. The attachment of the valve of the fossa ovalis may be malaligned relative to the muscular rim of the fossa.[2] Mitral atresia is represented by an imperforate macroscopic membrane on the floor of the left atrium or a microscopic fibrous remnant between the floor of the left atrium and a putative left ventricular cavity represented by a minute blind slit devoid of endocardial fibroelastosis (see Fig. 31–2).[17,21,27,56] Myofiber disarray does not

occur because isovolumetric contraction does not occur.[5,17,27,48,56,61]

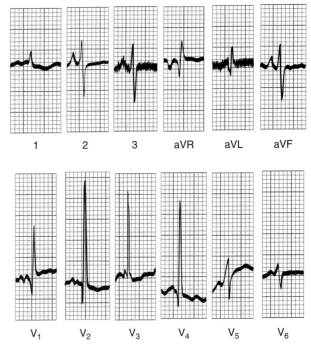

Figure 31–10

Electrocardiogram from a 3-week-old boy with aortic atresia and mitral atresia. Necropsy findings were as illustrated in Figure 31–2. Peaked right atrial P waves are present in leads 2 and 3, and right atrial enlargement is indicated by the qR pattern in lead V_1. Pure right ventricular hypertrophy is reflected in the vertical and superior QRS axis and the tall monophasic R waves in leads V_{2-4}.

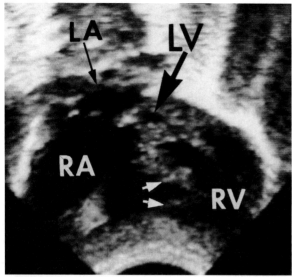

Figure 31–11

Echocardiogram (subcostal four-chamber view) from a 1-day-old boy with aortic atresia and mitral atresia. A blind slitlike cavity without endocardial fibroelastosis is imbedded in the left ventricular (LV) muscle mass. The left atrium (LA) is small and thick-walled. A dilated right atrium (RA) communicates (*arrows*) with a dilated right ventricle (RV).

There is no left ventricular cavity to develop excessive systolic pressure, so ventricular–coronary arterial connections do not develop and epicardial and subepicardial coronary arteries are neither thickened nor tortuous.[5,48,61] A ventricular septal defect or absence of the right ventricular sinus is associated with a well-formed left ventricle.[56,62,67] The physiologic consequences are the same and longevity patterns are similar[16] whether aortic atresia is accompanied by mitral atresia or by a hypoplastic but perforate mitral valve (see Figs. 31–1 and 31–2).

Female twins have been reported,[10] but male sex predominates.[17,64] Subtle clinical points favor hypoplastic left heart with mitral atresia. The electrocardiogram shows pure right ventricular hypertrophy[17] devoid of left ventricular potentials because a left ventricular cavity does not exist (Fig. 31–10).[73] The left bundle branch does not develop a Purkinje network because there is no left ventricular cavity in which to do so.[9] Mahaim fibers are the only extensions of the left bundle branch that maintain continuity with ventricular septal muscle.[9] The right bundle branch enlarges because it is responsible for conduction to virtually all of the ventricular muscle mass.[9]

These unusual pathways of atrioventricular conduction and ventricular activation are not represented in the electrocardiogram. The echocardiogram identifies atresia of both the aortic and mitral valves and occasionally identifies the blind rudimentary left ventricular cavity devoid of endocardial fibroelastosis (Fig. 31–11).

REFERENCES

1. Abbot M: Congenital cardiac disease. In Osler's Modern Medicine, 3rd ed. Philadelphia, Lea & Febiger, 1927.
2. Aiello VD, Ho SY, Thiene G: Morphologic features of the hypoplastic left heart syndrome: Reappraisal. Pediatr Pathol 10:931, 1990.
3. Alberman ED, Fedrick JM, Schutt WH: Hypoplastic left heart complex. J Med Genet 4:83, 1967.
4. Allan LD, Cook A, Sullivan I, Sharland GK: Hypoplastic left heart syndrome: Effects of fetal echocardiography on birth prevalence. Lancet 337:959, 1991.
5. Baffa JM, Chen S, Guttenberg ME, et al: Coronary artery abnormalities and right ventricular histology in hypoplastic left heart syndrome. J Am Coll Cardiol 20:350, 1992.
6. Bailey LL, Gundry SR: Hypoplastic left heart syndrome. Pediatr Clin North Am 37:137, 1990.
7. Hoshino K, Ogawa K, Hishitani T, et al: Hypoplastic left heart syndrome: Duration of survival without surgical intervention. Am Heart J 137:535, 1999.
8. Rychik J, Rome JJ, Collins MH, et al: Hypoplastic left heart syndrome with intact atrial septum: Atrial morphology, pulmonary vascular histopathology and outcome. J Am Coll Cardiol 34:554, 1999.
9. Bharati S, Lev M: The conduction system in hypoplasia of the aortic tract complex. Circulation 59:1324, 1979.
10. Bjornstad PG, Michalsen H: Coexistent mitral and aortic valve atresia with intact ventricular septum in sibs. Br Heart J 36:302, 1974.
11. Blake DM, Copel JA, Kleinman CS: Hypoplastic left heart syndrome: Prenatal diagnosis, clinical profile, and management. Am J Obstet Gynecol 165:529, 1991.
12. Boughman JA, Berg KA, Astemborski JA, et al: Familial risks of congenital heart defect assessed in a population-based epidemiologic study. Am J Med Genet 26:839, 1987.
13. Bulkley BH, Weisfelt ML, Hutchins GM: Isometric cardiac contraction. N Engl J Med 296:135, 1977.
14. Kimball TR, Witt SA, Khoury PR, Daniels SR: Automated echocardiographic analysis of systemic ventricular performance in hypoplastic left heart syndrome. J Am Soc Echocardiogr 9:629, 1996.
15. Deely WJ, Ehlers KH, Levin AR, Engle MA: Hypoplastic left heart syndrome: Anatomic, physiologic, and therapeutic considerations. Am J Dis Child 121:168, 1971.
16. Ehrlich M, Bierman FZ, Ellis K, Gersony WM: Hypoplastic left heart syndrome: Report of a unique survivor. J Am Coll Cardiol 7:361, 1986.
17. Eliot RS, Shone JD, Kanjuh VI, et al: Mitral atresia: A study of 32 cases. Am Heart J 70:6, 1965.
18. Elzenga NJ, Gittenberger-de Groot AC: Coarctation and related aortic arch anomalies in hypoplastic left heart syndrome. Int J Cardiol 8:379, 1985.
19. Fyler DC: Report of the regional infant cardiac program. Pediatrics 65:436, 1980.
20. Freedom RM, Dische MR, Rowe RD: Conal anatomy in aortic atresia, ventricular septal defect and normally developed left ventricle. Am Heart J 94:689, 1977.
21. Gittenberger-de Groot AC, Wenink ACG: Mitral atresia: Morphological details. Br Heart J 51:252, 1984.
22. Glauser TA, Rorke LB, Weinberg PM, Clancy RR: Acquired neuropathologic lesions associated with the hypoplastic left syndrome. Pediatrics 85:991, 1990.
23. Glauser TA, Rorke LB, Weinberg PM, Clancy RR: Congenital brain anomalies associated with the hypoplastic left heart syndrome. Pediatrics 85:984, 1990.
24. Harh JY, Paul MH, Gallen WJ, et al: Experimental production of hypoplastic left heart syndrome in the chick embryo. Am J Cardiol 31:51, 1973.
25. Hastreiter AR, van der Horst RL, Dubrow IR, Eckner FO: Quantitative angiographic and morphologic aspects of aortic valve atresia. Am J Cardiol 51:1705, 1983.
26. Hawkins JA, Doty DB: Aortic atresia: Morphologic characteristics affecting survival and operative palliation. J Thorac Cardiovasc Surg 88:620, 1984.
27. Kanjuh VI, Eliot RS, Edwards JE: Coexistent mitral and aortic valvular atresia. Am J Cardiol 15:611, 1965.
28. Kojima H, Ohgimi Y, Mizzutani K, Nishimura Y: Hypoplastic left heart syndrome in siblings. Lancet 2:701, 1969.
29. Krovetz LJ, Rowe RD, Scheibler GL: Hemodynamics of aortic valve atresia. Circulation 42:953, 1970.
30. Rychik J, Gullquist SD, Jacobs ML, Norwood WI: Doppler echocardiographic analysis of flow in the ductus arteriosus of infants with hypoplastic left heart syndrome. J Am Soc Echocardiogr 9:166, 1996.

31. Lev M: Pathologic anatomy and interrelationship of hypoplasia of the aortic tract complex. Lab Invest 1:61, 1952.
32. Lev M: Some newer concepts of the pathology of congenital heart disease. Med Clin North Am 50:3, 1966.
33. Lie JT: The malformation complex of the absence of the arch of the aorta-Steidele's complex. Am Heart J 73:615, 1967.
34. Lloyd TR, Marvin WJ: Age at death in the hypoplastic left heart syndrome: Multivariate analysis and importance of the coronary arteries. Am Heart J 117:1337, 1989.
35. Lopez W: Aortic atresia without significant hypoplasia of the ascending aorta. AJR 92:88, 1964.
36. Ludman P, Foale R, Alexander N, Nihoyannopoulos P: Cross sectional echocardiographic identification of hypoplastic left heart syndrome and differentiation from other causes of right ventricular volume overload. Br Heart J 63:355, 1990.
37. Grech V: Decreased prevalence of hypoplastic left heart syndrome in Malta. Pediatr Cardiol 20:355, 1999.
38. Maxwell P, Somerville J: Aortic atresia: Survival to adulthood without surgery. Br Heart J 64:336, 1990.
39. Satomi G, Yashukochi S, Shimizu T, et al: Has fetal echocardiography improved the prognosis of congenital heart disease? Comparison of patients with hypoplastic left heart syndrome with and without prenatal diagnosis. Pediatr Int 41:728, 1999.
40. Mocellin R, Sauer B, Simon M, et al: Reduced left ventricular cavity size and endocardial fibroelastosis as correlates of mortality in newborns and young infants with severe aortic valve stenosis. Pediatr Cardiol 4:265, 1983.
41. Moodie DS, Gallen WJ, Griedberg D: Congenital aortic atresia: Report of a long survival. J Thorac Cardiovasc Surg 63:726, 1972.
42. Moreno F, Quero M, Diaz LP: Mitral atresia with normal aortic valve: A study of 18 cases and a review of the literature. Circulation 53:1004, 1976.
43. Morris CD, Outcalt J, Menashe VD: Hypoplastic left-heart syndrome: Natural history in a geographically defined population. Pediatrics 85:977, 1990.
44. Natowicz M, Chatten J, Clancy R, et al: Genetic disorders and major extracardiac anomalies associated with hypoplastic left heart syndrome. Pediatrics 82:698, 1988.
45. Natowicz M, Kelley RI: Association of Turner syndrome with hypoplastic left-heart syndrome. Am J Dis Child 141:218, 1987.
46. Bensky AS, Covitz W: Echocardiographic demonstration of a ventriculocoronary artery communication in a neonate with hypoplastic left heart syndrome. J Am Soc Echocardiogr 7:324, 1994.
47. Noonan JA, Nadas AS: The hypoplastic left heart syndrome: An analysis of 101 cases. Pediatr Clin North Am 5:1029, 1958.
48. O'Connor WN, Cash JB, Cottril CM, et al: Ventriculocoronary connections in hypoplastic left hearts. Circulation 66:1078, 1982.
49. Parikh SR, Huritz RA, Caldwell RL, Waller B: Absent aortic valve in hypoplastic left heart syndrome. Am Heart J 119:977, 1990.
50. Pelligrino PA, Thiene G: Aortic valve atresia with a normally developed left ventricle. Chest 69:121, 1976.
51. Perloff JK: Auscultatory and phonocardiographic manifestations of pulmonary hypertension. Prog Cardiovasc Dis 9:303, 1967.
52. Perry LW, Scott LP, Shapiro SR, et al: Atresia of the aortic valve with ventricular septal defect. Chest 72:757, 1977.
53. Pillsbury RC, Lower RR, Shumway NE: Atresia of the aortic arch. Circulation 30:749, 1964.
54. Raghib G, Bloemendaal RD, Kanjuh VI, Edwards JE: Aortic atresia and premature closure of foramen ovale: Myocardial sinusoids and coronary arteriovenous fistula serving as outflow channel. Am Heart J 70:476, 1965.
55. Rao SS, Gootman N, Platt N: Familial aortic atresia. Am J Dis Child 118:919, 1969.
56. Roberts WC, Perry LW, Chandra RS, et al: Aortic valve atresia: A new classification based on necropsy study of 73 cases. Am J Cardiol 37:753, 1976.
57. Rammell-Dow DR, Bharati S, Avis JT, et al: Hypoplasia of the eustachian valve and abnormal orientation of the limbus of the foramen ovale in hypoplastic left heart syndrome. Am Heart J 130:148, 1995.
58. Grossfeld PD: The genetics of hypoplastic left heart syndrome. Cardiol Young 9:627, 1999.
59. Sahn DJ, Shenker L, Reed KL, et al: Prenatal ultrasound diagnosis of hypoplastic left heart syndrome in utero associated with hydrops fetalis. Am Heart J 104:1368, 1982.
60. Saied A, Folger GM: Hypoplastic left heart syndrome. Am J Cardiol 29:190, 1972.
61. Sauer U, Gittenberger-deGroot AC, Geishauser M, et al: Coronary arteries in hypoplastic left heart syndrome: Histopathologic and histometrical studies and implications for surgery. Circulation 80 (Suppl. I):I-168, 1989.
62. Shinpo H, Van Praagh S, Parness I, et al: Mitral atresia with a large left ventricle and an underdeveloped or absent right ventricular sinus. J Am Coll Cardiol 19:1561, 1992.
63. Shone JD, Edwards JE: Mitral atresia associated with pulmonary venous anomalies. Br Heart J 26:241, 1964.
64. Sinha SN, Rusnak SL, Sommers HM, et al: Hypoplastic left ventricle syndrome. Am J Cardiol 21:166, 1968.
65. Better DJ, Apfel HD, Zidere V, Allan LD: Pattern of pulmonary venous blood flow in hypoplastic left heart syndrome in the fetus. Heart 81:646, 1999.
66. Soloff LA: Congenital aortic atresia: Report of the first case with left axis deviation of the electrocardiogram. Am Heart J 37:123, 1949.
67. Thiene G, Gallucci V, Macartney FJ, et al: Anatomy of aortic atresia. Circulation 59:173, 1979.
68. Conaevage MW, Seip JR, Belchis DA, et al: Association of a mosaic chromosomal 22q11 deletion with hypoplastic left heart syndrome. Am J Cardiol 77:1023, 1996.
69. Van Egmond H, Orye E, Praet M, et al: Hypoplastic left heart syndrome and 45X karyotype. Br Heart J 60:69, 1988.
70. Van der Horst RL, Hastreiter AR: Ascending aortic obstruction of retrograde coronary blood flow in aortic atresia. Am Heart J 101:345, 1981.
71. Van der Horst RL, Hastreiter AR, DuBrow IW, Eckner FAO: Pathologic measurements in aortic atresia. Am Heart J 106:1411, 1983.
72. Vargas-Barron J, Rijlaarsdam M, Romero-Cardenas A, et al: Hypoplastic left heart syndrome: Report of a case of spontaneous survival to adulthood. Am Heart J 123:1713, 1992.
73. Voukydis PC: Effect of intracardiac blood on the electrocardiogram. N Engl J Med 291:612, 1974
74. Allen LD, Apfel HD, Printz BF: Outcome after prenatal diagnosis of the hypoplastic left heart syndrome. Curr Opin Cardiol 12:44, 1997.
75. Cohen DM, Allen HD: New developments in the treatment of hypoplastic left heart syndrome. Curr Opin Cardiol 12:44, 1997.
76. Kumar RK, Newberger JW, Gauvreau K, et al: Comparison of outcome when hypoplastic left heart syndrome and transposition of the great arteries are diagnosed prenatally versus when diagnosis of these two conditions is made only postnatally. Am J Cardiol 83:1649, 1999.
77. Reis PM, Punch MR, Bove EL, van de Ven CJ: Outcome of infants with hypoplastic left heart and Turner syndromes. Obstet Gynecol 93:532, 1999.
78. Simpson JM: Hypoplastic left heart syndrome. Ultrasound Obstet Gynecol 15:271, 2000.
79. Bartsch O, Wagner A, Hinkel, et al: FISH studies in 45 patients with Rubinstein-Taybi syndrome: Deletions associated with polysplenia, hypoplastic left heart and death in infancy. Eur J Hum Genet 7:748, 1999.
80. Altmann K, Printz BF, Soloiejczky DE, et al: Two-dimensional echocardiographic assessment of right ventricular function as a predictor of outcome in hypoplastic left heart syndrome. Am J Cardiol 86:964, 2000.
81. Brackley KJ, Kilby MD, Wright JG, et al: Outcome after prenatal diagnosis of hypoplastic left heart syndrome. Lancet 356:1143, 2000.
82. Bardo DM, Frankel DG, Applegate KE, et al: Hypoplastic left heart syndrome. Radiographics 21:705, 2001.
83. Rabah R, Poulik JM: Congenital alveolar capillary dysplasia with misalignment of pulmonary veins associated with hypoplastic left heart syndrome. Pediatr Dev Pathol 4:167, 2001.
84. Donner RM: Hypoplastic left heart syndrome. Curr Treat Options Cardiovasc Med 2:469, 2000.
85. Stamm C, Anderson RH, Ho SY: The morphologically tricuspid valve in hypoplastic left heart syndrome. Eur J Cardiothorac Surg 12:587, 1997.
86. Tchervenkov CI, Jacobs ML, Tahta SA: Congenital heart surgery nomenclature and database project: Hypoplastic left heart syndrome. Ann Thorac Surg 69:S170, 2000.
87. Sugiyama H, Yutani C, Iida K, et al: The relation between right ventricular function and left ventricular morphology in hypoplastic left heart syndrome: Angiographic and pathological studies. Pediatr Cardiol 20:422, 1999.
88. Grobman W, Pergament E: Isolated hypoplastic left heart syndrome in three siblings. Obstet Gynecol 88:673, 1996.

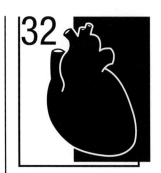

Congenital Anomalies of the Coronary Circulation

Coronary is a term derived from the Latin *coronarius* ("pertaining to a crown") translated from the Greek *stephanos* ("wreath") and referring to the crown-like or wreath-like arrangement of arteries that encircle the heart.[2] This chapter deals with the coronary circulation—arterial and venous—including the morphogenesis, the normal coronary arteries, and the congenital anomalies classified in Table 32–1.

Leonardo da Vinci made accurate anatomical drawings of the coronary arteries and the great cardiac vein (coronary sinus) and called attention to two vessels (coronary arteries) that arise from two external openings (aortic sinuses) (see Fig. 32–3A).[15] Two hundred years later, the dual coronary artery circulation was characterized,[162] and after another 200 years, congenital anomalies of the coronary arteries were recognized.[17] Andreas Vesalius of Brussels, the celebrated sixteenth century Flemish anatomist, had depicted an anomalous right coronary

artery originating from the left aortic sinus and passing anterior to the right ventricular outflow tract (*De Humani Corporis Fabrica*, Basel, 1543). Selective coronary angiography, introduced in 1962,[163] was a major step forward in imaging coronary artery anatomy in the living, beating human heart.[43,146,159] Imaging techniques continue to evolve and include transesophageal echocardiography, magnetic resonance imaging, computed tomography, electron beam tomography, and three-dimensional reconstruction.[169,173,175]

Myocardial morphogenesis is characterized by the early emergence of trabeculations in the luminal layers of the ventricle that permit an increased mass in the absence of a coronary circulation.[164] Cardiac jelly in the embryonic luminal layer is the primitive site of metabolic exchange between the cardiac mesenchyma and blood in the ventricular cavity.* The human heart begins to beat as early as the 22nd day after conception, and a few days later an ebb-and-flow circulation permits metabolic exchange.

The sequence of development of the coronary vascular bed consists of blood islands and coronary venous connections followed by coronary artery-to-aortic connections.[4,63,165] Blood islands, which are the first stage of development, are epicardial layers of endothelial cells distended by nucleated erythrocytes. The blood islands proliferate, coalesce, and form rudimentary networks of vascular channels with no discernible connections to other islands or to the cavity of the ventricle.[63] The second stage of development is a venous connection between the network of vascular channels and the coronary sinus, an arrangement that drains the blood islands, which become reduced in size. The distal coronary bed remains a loose intermingling vascular

Table 32–1 | A Classification of Congenital Anomalies of the Coronary Circulation

Congenital anomalies of coronary arteries unassociated with congenital heart disease

    Anomalous aortic origin

    Anomalous proximal course

    Anomalous distal connection

    Anomalous pulmonary arterial origin

    Anomalies of size—atretic, hypoplastic, ectatic, aneurysmal

Congenital anomalies of coronary arteries associated with congenital heart disease

Acquired anomalies of coronary arteries secondary to congenital heart disease

Congenital anomalies of the coronary venous circulation

---

*See references 4, 17, 30, 55, 59, 63, 90, 108, 115, 137, 138, 145, 155.

network until myocardial mass develops. In the third stage of development, the coronary arteries join the aorta through an arterial connection to the plexus of vascular channels. The third stage is established after aortopulmonary septation and after formation of the semilunar valves. Flow commences from the aorta into the proximal coronary arteries, then through myocardial capillaries, and then into coronary veins and into the coronary sinus.[165]

It is not known why the two coronary arteries originate from the right and left aortic sinuses that face the right ventricular outflow tract (Fig. 32–1A). The embryonic great arteries contain six sinuses, three in the aorta and three in the pulmonary trunk. The endothelial outgrowths, or anlagen (buds, sprouts), in the third aortic sinus and in all three pulmonary sinuses undergo rapid involution or do not develop.[55] Aortic-to-coronary artery connections

become evident before the appearance of precursor connections in the aortic sinuses.[63] What determines the aortic sinus sites of the two coronary ostia? It has been speculated that mural tension is increased by a catenoid configuration of the right and left aortic sinuses so that endothelium penetrates the aortic wall preferentially in the right and left sinus sites, establishing connections with the epicardial coronary plexus.[63]

The capillary bed, which is interposed between the coronary arterial and coronary venous circulations, plays a pivotal role in the transport of oxygen and nutrients to the myocardium. Capillary density, defined as the ratio of the number of capillaries to the number of cardiomyocytes, is basic to the metabolic exchange between blood and tissues. Capillary density depends on angiogenesis—the capacity of capillaries to replicate. Fetal capillaries replicate in response to the hypoxic intrauterine environment. Postnatal angiogenesis is a diminishing continuation of that response.[115,145]

The coronary circulation includes three separate systems of veins.[65] The largest system terminates in the coronary sinus and drains blood from most of the left ventricle. A second venous system drains most of the blood from the right ventricle. Adam Christian Thebesius (1686–1732) described the third venous system, which consists of small veins that drain portions of blood directly into the cavities of the right ventricle and the right atrium.[65]

Patterns of blood flow in the coronary circulation are unique and differ distinctively in the right and left ventricles. In the normal thin-walled right ventricle, coronary flow is continuous because pressure in the aorta continuously exceeds right ventricular intramural pressure.[6] In the normal relatively thick-walled left ventricle, a higher diastolic pressure in the aorta coincides with a diastolic fall in intramyocardial pressure that results in brisk diastolic flow into the epicardial coronary arteries. Isovolumetric left ventricular contraction exerts disproportionate pressure on the subendocardial third of the wall, expressing blood from the subendocardial perforating branches and arresting flow into extramural branches.[6] The pressure in the aorta during ventricular systole generates transient flow into the extramural coronary arteries and into the contiguous subepicardial myocardium because subepicardial pressure is appreciably lower than pressure in the subendocardium.[6]

The round or ovoid ostia of the two coronary arteries are located in the right and left anterior aortic sinuses, which are therefore called the *coronary sinuses*.[2] The posterior aortic sinus is devoid of a coronary ostium and is therefore called the *noncoronary sinus*.[2] Normal coronary artery ostia are located in the middle of an aortic sinus just below the sinotubular junction and just above the upper margin of the aortic cusps. Abnormally located ostia originate above the sinotubular junction or in the posterior aortic sinus or eccentrically near a commissure.[4,106] Two coronary ostia are the norm, but three or four ostia are considered normal variants.[4] A third ostium usually results from a separate conus branch in the right coronary sinus (see Fig. 32–1A).

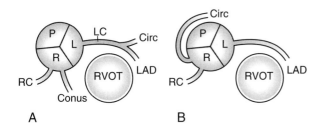

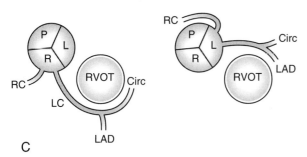

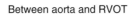

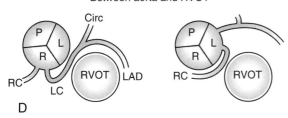

Figure 32–1

A, Illustration of the normal origin of the left coronary artery (LC) and the right coronary artery (RC). A conus artery arises by a separate ostium from the right aortic sinus. L, left aortic sinus; P, posterior aortic sinus; R, right aortic sinus. *B,* The left anterior descending coronary artery (LAD) arises normally from the left aortic sinus, and the circumflex coronary artery (Circ) arises aberrantly from the right aortic sinus. *C,* First illustration shows an aberrant left coronary artery (LC) passing anterior to the right ventricular outflow tract (RVOT), and second illustration shows an aberrant right coronary (RC) artery passing posterior to the right ventricular outflow tract. *D,* First illustration shows an aberrant left coronary artery (LC) passing between the aorta and the right ventricular outflow tract (RVOT), and the second illustration shows an aberrant right coronary artery passing between the aorta and the right ventricular outflow tract.

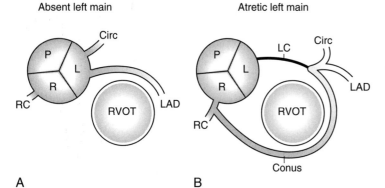

Absent left main   Atretic left main

A   B

Figure 32–2

A, Absent left main coronary artery as represented in the left aortic sinus (L) by separate origins of the ostia of the circumflex coronary artery (Circ) and the left anterior descending coronary artery (LAD). *B,* Atresia of the ostium and proximal segment of the left main coronary artery (LC). A large conus branch from the right coronary artery (RC) supplies the circumflex coronary artery (Circ) and the left anterior descending coronary artery (LAD).

Less commonly, three coronary ostia result from the origin of the left anterior descending and circumflex coronary arteries from the left aortic sinus together with the origin of the right coronary artery from the right aortic sinus, an arrangement that has been designated *absent left main coronary artery* (Fig. 32–2A).[4]

Coronary arteries that originate from normally located ostia arise at a right angle from the aortic wall. Coronary arteries that originate from ectopic ostia arise from the aortic wall at an acute angle and run tangential to the aortic wall. Normal proximal coronary arteries are epicardial, but in about a quarter of cases the proximal left anterior descending coronary artery is intramural and is recognized as such by angiographic narrowing of the intramural segment.

The relatively large left ventricular mass is served by both the left and right coronary arteries. One coronary artery can be dominant, with right or left dominance encompassing a wide range. Extreme dominance assumes that the dominant and nondominant coronary arteries arise from separate ostia in separate aortic sinuses, in contrast to dominance that results from a single coronary artery that originates from a single coronary ostium in a single aortic sinus.[119]

Congenital Anomalies of the Coronary Arteries Unassociated with Congenital Heart Disease

ANOMALIES OF AORTIC ORIGIN (TABLE 32–2)

Congenital anomalies of the coronary arteries are included in comprehensive clinical and necropsy reviews.[3,4,45,53,81,119] The widespread use of selective coronary angiography has helped establish the types and prevalence of many of these anomalies.[25,43,45,53,60,72,84] Among 13,010 adults who underwent coronary angiography, 0.61% had congenital anomalies,[43,146] and the incidence was 1.3% among 126,595 patients who underwent coronary arteriography at the Cleveland Clinic.[159] Transesophageal echocardiography provides accurate information on the origin and proximal course of anomalous coronary arteries.[47,58,69,73,92,110,129]

Anomalous aortic origins of coronary arteries unassociated with congenital heart disease are listed in Table 32–2. Origin of a coronary artery is considered anomalous when the ostium is located above the sinotubular junction, in the

Table 32–2	**Congenital Anomalies of Coronary Arteries Unassociated with Congenital Heart Disease**

Anomalous aortic origin

   Eccentric ostium within an aortic sinus

   Ectopic ostium above an aortic sinus

   Conus artery from the right aortic sinus

   Circumflex coronary artery from the right aortic sinus or from the right coronary artery

   Absence of the left main coronary artery—origin of left anterior descending and circumflex coronary artery from separate ostia in the left aortic sinus

   Atresia of the left main coronary artery

   Origin of the left anterior descending coronary artery from the right aortic sinus or from the right coronary artery

   Origin of the right coronary artery from the left aortic sinus, from posterior aortic sinus or from left coronary artery

   Origin of a single coronary artery from the right or left aortic sinus

   Anomalous origin from a noncardiac systemic artery

Anomalous aortic origin with anomalous proximal course

   Acute proximal angulation

   Ectopic right coronary artery passing between aorta and pulmonary trunk

   Ectopic left main coronary artery

      Between aorta and pulmonary trunk

      Anterior to the pulmonary trunk

      Posterior to the aorta

      Within the ventricular septum (intramyocardial)

   Ectopic left anterior descending coronary artery anterior, posterior or between the aorta and pulmonary trunk

Anomalous origin from the pulmonary trunk

   Left main coronary artery

   Left anterior descending coronary artery

   Right coronary artery

   Right and left coronary arteries

   Circumflex coronary artery

   Accessory coronary artery

posterior aortic sinus, or in close proximity to an aortic commissure rather than in the middle of the sinus (see earlier).[4,17,104,106,153,155]

In 30% to 50% of normal human hearts, a small conus artery arises separately from the right aortic sinus and is of no functional significance (see Fig. 32–1A).[4,41,43,60] The circumflex coronary artery may arise from a separate ostium in the right aortic sinus and pass behind the aorta (see Fig. 32–1B) or may arise from the proximal right coronary artery and enter the left atrioventricular groove as if it were a proximal branch of the left coronary artery.[25,72,84,103,111,146,159,160] Anomalous origin of the circumflex coronary artery is regarded as benign, but there is one report of myocardial ischemia in the absence of coronary atherosclerosis.[111] Also regarded as benign is the exceptional absence of the circumflex coronary artery with a dominant right coronary artery that perfuses the lateral and posterolateral left ventricular walls.[9,43,159]

The left anterior descending coronary artery can arise from the right aortic sinus or from the right coronary artery.[72,128,146,155] The anomalous left anterior descending artery usually passes anterior or posterior to the great arteries, but occasionally passes between the aorta and the right ventricular outflow tract, where it poses a potential risk.[146] Rarely, the left anterior descending coronary artery, the circumflex coronary artery, and right coronary arteries arise by separate ostia from the right aortic sinus.[112]

Origin of the left main coronary artery from the right aortic sinus is uncommon but clinically important.[10,25,43,60,64,71,72,119,146,159] The right coronary artery and the left main coronary artery can arise from separate ostia in the right aortic sinus (see Fig. 32–1C).[75] The left main coronary artery passes either anterior or posterior to the right ventricular outflow tract (see Fig. 32–1C) or between the right ventricular outflow tract and the aorta (see Fig. 32–1D) or is intramyocardial within the ventricular septum.[10,64,71,119,122,159] The risk associated with passage of the left main coronary artery between the aorta and right ventricular outflow tract has been convincingly established (see later).

Absence of a left main coronary artery refers to a rare anomaly in which the left anterior descending and circumflex coronary arteries originate from separate ostia in the left aortic sinus (see Fig. 32–2A).[4,40,60,72,119,155,159] Both arteries are then normally distributed, so the arrangement is functionally benign.[159]

Atresia of the left main coronary artery includes atresia of the ostium, which is represented by an imperforate dimple, and atresia of the proximal course of the coronary artery, which is represented by a fibrous strand (see Fig. 32–2B). A large conus branch originates from the right coronary artery and supplies the left anterior descending artery and the circumflex coronary artery (see Fig. 32–2B).

Origin of the right coronary artery from the left aortic sinus (Fig. 32–3B, and see Fig. 32–1C,D) represents about one quarter of ectopic coronary artery origins.[25,41,]

[60,72,75,119,121,146,167] Less common is origin of the right coronary artery from the posterior aortic sinus or from the left coronary artery.[98,146,155,159] The functional significance of these arrangements does not depend on the anomalous origin but on whether the ectopic right coronary artery passes between the aorta and the right ventricular outflow tract (see Figs. 32–1D and 32–3B,C).[75,119,121,146,159]

Single coronary artery, which is an anomaly that has been known since 1903,[7] originates from a single ostium in the left or right aortic sinus and gives rise to the entire coronary circulation (Figs. 32–4 and 32–5).[37,119,159] A second coronary ostium is neither present nor implied. An isolated single coronary artery unassociated with congenital heart disease divides into normally formed and normally distributed branches irrespective of the aortic sinus from which it originates (see Fig. 32–4C,D).[14,54,119,135,139,155,159] A single coronary artery associated with congenital heart disease is characterized by branching patterns that bear no resemblance to normal.[119] A single coronary artery functions normally unless a major branch is congenitally hypoplastic[101] or passes between the aorta and right ventricular outflow tract (Fig. 32–6).

Anomalous origin of a coronary artery from an extracardiac systemic artery is relatively rare (see Table 32–2).[4] The anomalous coronary can originate from the innominate, subclavian, internal mammary, carotid, or bronchial artery or from the descending aorta.[4,37,126]

The Coronary Artery Surgery Study (1989) posed the question as to whether a coronary artery that originated anomalously from an aortic sinus was predisposed to atherosclerosis.[28] It was concluded that atherosclerosis was more prevalent in subjects with anomalous circumflex coronary arteries than in matched control subjects with non-anomalous circumflex coronary arteries.

The courses taken by anomalous coronary arteries and their branches are far more important than their ectopic origins.[4,10,27,64,112,119,122,123] These courses include (1) passage anterior to the right ventricular outflow tract (see Fig. 32–1C), (2) passage posterior to the aorta (see Fig. 32–1C), (3) passage between the aorta and the right ventricular outflow tract (see Fig. 32–1D), and (4) intramyocardial passage (tunneling) that incurs little or no risk.[123] Angina pectoris, myocardial infarction, and sudden death are, with few exceptions, reserved for anomalous coronary arteries that pass between the aorta and the right ventricular outflow tract.*

Ischemic risk is determined by a number of variables in addition to the course of the anomalous coronary artery between the aorta and the right ventricular outflow tract, namely[10,29,50,75,119,142] (1) the coronary artery or branch that is involved, (2) the slitlike ostium and acute angulation of the origin of the ectopic coronary artery,[4,11,25,27,71,97,125,142] (3) coronary dominance,[75] and (4) the effect of

---

*See references 10, 11, 25, 27, 36, 71, 84, 93, 97, 99, 119, 122, 142, 144, 147, 155.

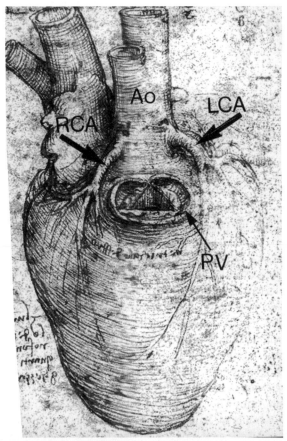

A

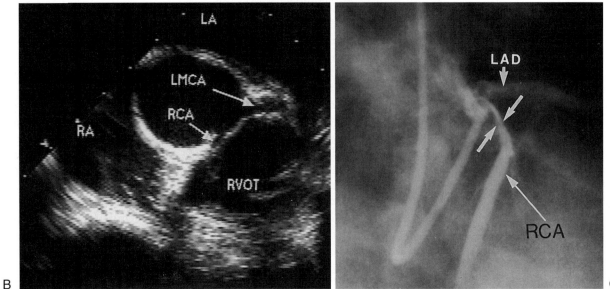

B   C

Figure 32–3

A, Drawing of a bullock's heart by Leonardo da Vinci, circa 1513, with labels by the author. "The heart from the right side. The pulmonary artery has been removed to expose the pulmonary orifice and the semilunar valves guarding it. From the aorta spring the right and left coronary arteries." Ao, aorta; LCA, left coronary artery; PV, pulmonary valve; RCA, right coronary artery. *B,* Echocardiogram (short axis) from an asymptomatic 23-year-old man in whom the right coronary artery (RCA) originated from the left aortic sinus and passed between the aorta and right ventricular outflow tract (RVOT). The left main coronary artery (LMCA) originated from the left aortic sinus by a separate ostium and divided into the left anterior descending and circumflex coronary arteries (compare to Fig. 32–1*D,* second illustration). *C,* Coronary arteriogram from a 29-year-old woman with angina pectoris. The right coronary artery (RCA) originated from the left aortic sinus and was compressed (*paired arrows*) as it passed between the aorta and the right ventricular outflow tract (compare to Fig. 32–1*D,* second illustration). The left coronary artery originated by a separate ostium from the left aortic sinus and divided into the left anterior descending (LAD) and circumflex coronary arteries.

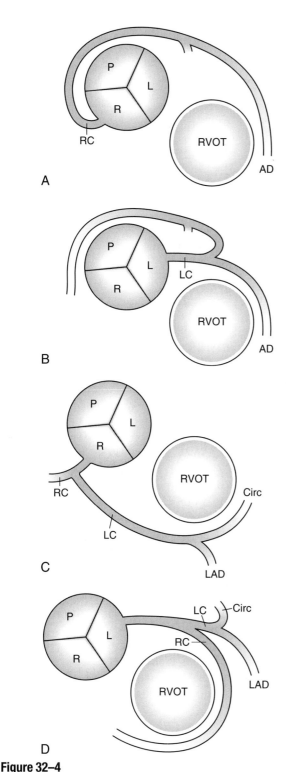

Figure 32–4

A, Illustration of a single coronary artery arising from a single ostium in the right aortic sinus (R) and then branching as a right coronary artery (RC). AD, anterior descending artery. *B,* A single coronary artery arising from a single ostium in the left aortic sinus (L) and then branching as a left coronary artery (LC). *C,* A single coronary artery arising from a single ostium in the right aortic sinus and then branching into the right coronary (RC) and left coronary (LC) artery. *D,* A single coronary artery arising from a single ostium in the left aortic sinus and then branching into right (RC) and left coronary (LC) arteries.

strenuous exercise.[10,27,64,71,83,99,125,144,170] Risk is greatest when the left main coronary artery arises from the right aortic sinus and courses between the aorta and the right ventricular outflow tract[10,27,64,71,122,144,147,171,172] (see Fig. 32–1D) or when the left branch of a single coronary artery courses between the aorta and the right ventricular outflow tract (see Fig. 32–6B).[142] Risk is less when the right coronary artery originates from the left aortic sinus and passes between the aorta and the right ventricular outflow tract (see Fig. 32–1D).[11,75,97,99,125,144,170] Sudden death typically occurs during or immediately following physical exercise.[10,27,64,71,83,84,122,147]

Fatal impairment of coronary blood flow appears to be a sporadic occurrence in light of the fact that highly trained competitive athletes with ectopic coronary arteries perform intense physical exercise repeatedly and for many years before experiencing sudden death.[178] It has been proposed that expansion of the aortic root and pulmonary trunk during exercise is responsible for increasing the already acute angulation of the ectopic coronary artery and for flaplike closure of its slit-shaped ostium.[10,119,178] An analogous risk potentially confronts the fetus during the hemodynamic stress of labor and delivery.[89] A stillborn term fetus died during labor, and at necropsy the right coronary artery originated from the left aortic sinus.[97] Exercise-induced dilatation of the aortic root compresses an ectopic coronary artery against the base of the pulmonary trunk to which the infundibular septum is firmly anchored.[10,119] This mechanism may account for sudden death in patients with an ectopic coronary artery that is not characterized by acute angulation or a slit-like ostium.[75,142]

Coronary arteries that originate normally from their respective aortic sinuses can have abnormal distal connections. A small coronary arterial fistula incidentally discovered during routine coronary arteriography was a case in point (see Chapter 22).[43,52,159] Another example is a functionally benign distal intercoronary communication in which contiguous peripheral coronary artery branches form an open-ended circulation with bidirectional flow.[159]

Anomalous pulmonary arterial origins of coronary arteries[57,119,141,159] are listed in Table 32–2. Anomalous origin of the left coronary artery from the pulmonary trunk is the most important of these abnormalities (see Chapter 21). Anomalous origin of the right coronary artery from the pulmonary trunk is a rare anomaly that was first reported in 1885[176] and may be discovered incidentally at necropsy.[166,168] Rarer still is anomalous origin of both coronary arteries from the pulmonary trunk.[117]

Anomalies of coronary arterial size include congenital hypoplasia or atresia or, conversely, congenital coronary artery ectasia or aneurysm[21] (see Tables 32–1 and 32–4). Atresia of the ostium of the left main coronary artery extends proximally as a fibrous chord opposite a blind

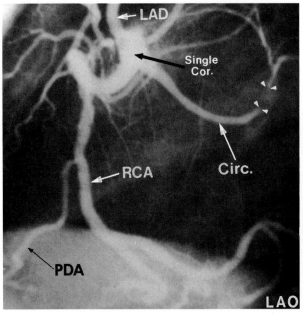

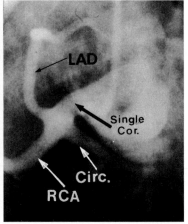

Figure 32–5
Coronary arteriograms from a 54-year-old woman. *A*, A single ostium in the right aortic sinus gave rise to a single coronary artery (Single Cor) from which originated the left anterior descending (LAD), the circumflex (Circ), and the right coronary (RCA) arteries. *B*, Injection into the right aortic sinus shows the single coronary artery from which the left anterior descending, circumflex, and right coronary arteries originate.

dimple in the left aortic sinus (see Fig. 32–2*B*).[12,13,20,46,60,74,96,119,143,150] Survival depends on the adequacy of connections between a normally arising right coronary artery and the distal nonhypoplastic portion of the left coronary artery (see Fig. 32–2*B*). Myocardial infarction and death have occurred from infancy[20] to the teens[150] to 60 years and 71 years of age.[46,96] The clinical presentation of infants with ostial atresia or left main coronary artery atresia is similar to the presentation of infants with anomalous origin of the left coronary artery from the pulmonary trunk (see Chapter 21).[20]

Hypoplasia of coronary arteries exists when the right coronary artery and the left circumflex coronary artery do not go beyond the lateral border of the heart.[24,142] Hypoplasia of the left main coronary artery is analogous to atresia, described earlier (see Fig. 32–2*B*).[24]

Coronary artery ectasia accompanies the erythrocytosis of cyanotic congenital heart disease (see Fig. 32–14). Hereditary hemorrhagic telangiectasia, or Rendu-Osler-Weber disease, is another cause of coronary ectasia (see Chapter 30).[76] Congenital aneurysms in the proximal right or left coronary artery are believed to result from an occult developmental fault that is present at birth.[32,56,133,155,157]

CONGENITAL CORONARY ARTERY ANOMALIES ASSOCIATED WITH CONGENITAL HEART DISEASE
(TABLE 32–3)

Fallot's tetralogy is associated with anomalies of origin, course, and distribution of coronary arteries, with an incidence of 10% to 36% (see Chapter 18).[35,44,62,86,95,116,155,174] The most common anomalies are origin of a conus artery from the right coronary artery or from the right aortic sinus (Fig. 32–7*A*), origin of a circumflex coronary artery from the right coronary artery or origin of a left anterior descending artery from the right aortic sinus (see Fig. 32–7*B*), and origin of a single coronary artery from the right aortic sinus (Fig. 32–8, and see Fig. 32–7*C*). Less common anomalies include origin of a coronary artery from the posterior aortic sinus,[155] anastomoses between coronary arteries and bronchial arteries,[34,161] fistulas between coronary arteries and pulmonary arteries or right atrium,[34] hypoplastic coronary arteries,[155] and pulmonary arterial origin of the left anterior descending coronary artery.[158] The physiologic consequences of these coronary anomalies are unimportant. What is important is the surgical risk incurred when anomalous coronary arteries cross the right ventricular outflow tract (see Fig. 32–7*B*,*C*).

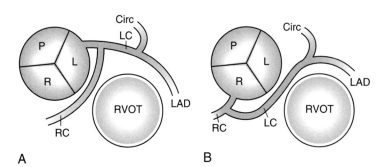

Figure 32–6
A, A single coronary artery originates from the left coronary sinus (L), and the right coronary artery branch (RC) passes between the aorta and the right ventricular outflow tract (RVOT). *B*, A single coronary artery originates from the right coronary sinus (R), and the left coronary artery branch (LC) passes between the aorta and the right ventricular outflow tract.

Table 32–3	Congenital Anomalies of the Coronary Arteries Associated with Congenital Heart Disease

Fallot's tetralogy

Complete transposition of the great arteries

Congenitally corrected transposition of the great arteries

Double-outlet ventricle

Univentricular heart

Tricuspid atresia

Truncus arteriosus

Isolated quadricuspid aortic valve

Isolated bicuspid aortic valve

Characterization of the origins of the coronary arteries in complete transposition of the great arteries (see Chapter 27) is relevant to arterial switch operations.[42,51,94,134,140] Coronary artery morphology and ventricular morphology are concordant, that is, the morphologic right coronary artery is assigned to the morphologic subaortic right ventricle, and the morphologic left coronary artery is assigned to the morphologic subpulmonary left ventricle. The two sinuses that face the right ventricular outflow tract are the left aortic sinus and the posterior aortic sinus (Fig. 32–9). The left sinus is rightward and is designated *sinus 1*.[51,127,140] The posterior sinus is leftward and is designated *sinus 2* (see Fig. 32–9).[51,127,140]

Dual sinus origin means that a main coronary artery branch arises from each of the two sinuses that face the right ventricular outflow tract, an arrangement that is present in 90% of these cases.[140] The majority of dual sinus origins are represented by the circumflex coronary artery and the left anterior descending artery arising from left aortic sinus and the right coronary artery arising from the posterior sinus[140] (see Fig. 32–9A). Less common is dual sinus origin represented by the circumflex coronary artery and the right coronary artery from the posterior sinus and origin of the left anterior descending artery from the left aortic sinus (see Fig. 32–9B).[140] *Single sinus origin* means that main coronary arterial branches arise from one of the two but not both of the sinuses that face the right ventricular outflow tract.[140] In single sinus origin, the anterior descending, circumflex, and right coronary arteries arise from the posterior sinus.[140] Rarely, an anomalous coronary artery is intramyocardial or passes between the aorta and the right ventricular outflow tract.[51]

In congenitally corrected transposition of the great arteries, morphologic right and morphologic left coronary arteries are concordant with morphologic right and morphologic left ventricles (see Chapter 6).[42,87,155] The two aortic sinuses that face the right ventricular outflow tract are designated right posterior and left posterior (Fig. 32–10). The nonfacing anterior sinus is noncoronary (see Fig. 32–10). The morphologic right coronary artery

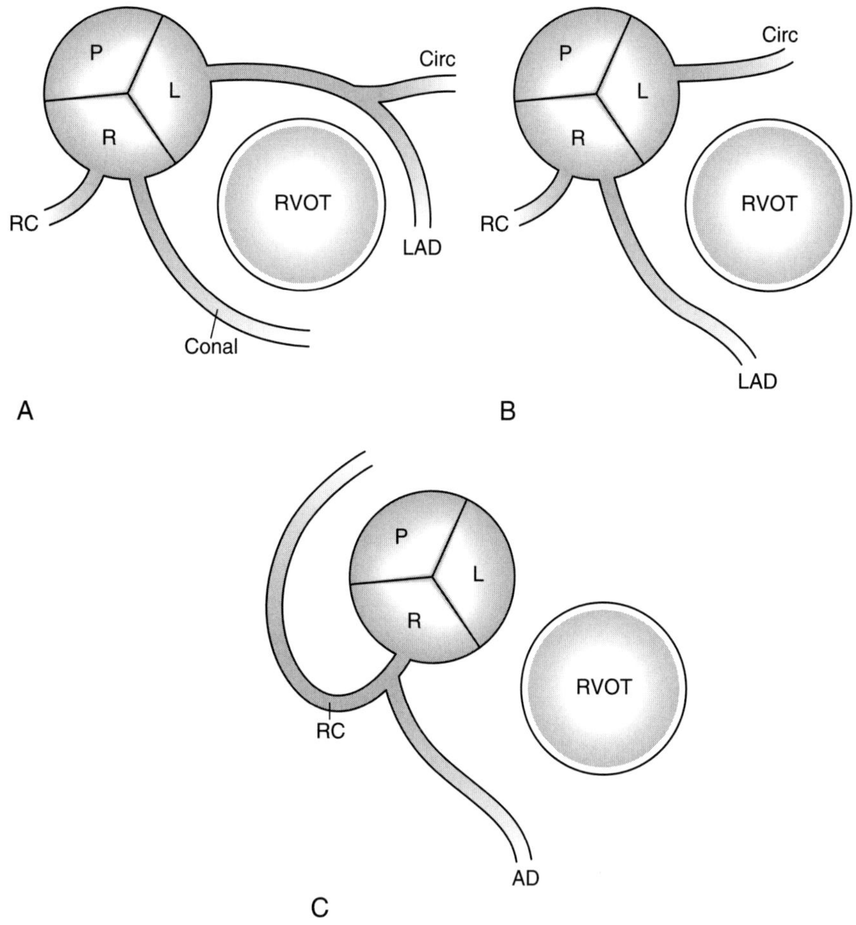

Figure 32–7

Illustrations of the coronary artery anomalies in Fallot's tetralogy. *A*, A conal artery arises by a separate ostium from the right aortic sinus (R) and passes anterior to the right ventricular outflow tract (RVOT). *B*, Left anterior descending coronary artery (LAD) arises by a separate ostium from the right aortic sinus and passes anterior to the right ventricular outflow tract (RVOT). *C*, The anterior descending branch (AD) of a single coronary artery passes anterior to the right ventricular outflow tract. RC, right coronary artery branch.

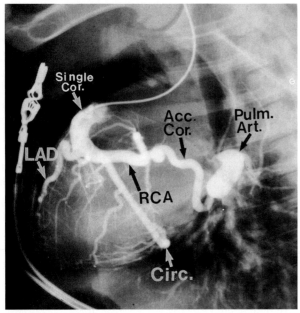

Figure 32–8

Coronary arteriogram from a 3-week-old Holstein calf with Fallot's tetralogy confirmed at necropsy. A single coronary artery (Single Cor) originated from the right aortic sinus and branched into the left anterior descending (LAD), circumflex (Circ), and right coronary (RCA) arteries. An accessory coronary artery (Acc Cor) connected the right coronary artery (RCA) to the pulmonary artery (Pulm Art). (Courtesy of Dr. Sidney Moise, New York College of Veterinary Medicine, Cornell University, Ithaca, New York.)

originates from the left posterior sinus, and the morphologic left coronary artery originates from the right posterior sinus, arrangements that are inverted (see Fig. 32–10). The course of the left anterior descending coronary artery delineates the position of the ventricular septum. Coronary anomalies are uncommon, but there are reports of hypoplasia of the circumflex and left anterior descending coronary arteries[33] and of a single coronary ostium arising from the right posterior sinus.[33,87]

The origin, course, and distribution of the coronary arteries in double outlet right ventricle are the same as in the normal heart (see Chapter 19).[42,152,155] The right coronary artery arises from the right aortic sinus, and the left coronary artery arises from the left aortic sinus (Fig. 32–11).[42,152,155]

Occasionally, both coronary arteries arise from the same aortic sinus, rarely, four coronary ostia arise from the right aortic sinus,[153] or a single coronary artery arises from a single coronary artery ostium.[155] Double outlet left ventricle is associated with a relatively high incidence of congenital anomalies of the origin and course of coronary arteries, including single coronary artery, right aortic sinus origin of the left anterior descending artery, and origin of both coronary arteries or all three coronary arteries from the right or left aortic sinus.[31]

In univentricular hearts of left ventricular morphology (see Chapter 26), the aortic sinus from which the right or left coronary artery originates is determined by inversion or noninversion of the outlet chamber.[155] When the outlet chamber is inverted, the aortic sinus from which each coronary artery originates is the same as in congenitally corrected transposition of the great arteries with biventricular hearts (see Fig. 32–10), but a major branch of each coronary artery delimits, or outlines, the surface boundaries of the outlet chamber.[80] When the outlet chamber is noninverted, the aortic sinus from which each coronary artery originates is the same as in complete transposition of the great arteries with biventricular hearts (see Fig. 32–9). Tricuspid atresia (see Chapter 25) is characterized by delimiting coronary arteries that meet at the apex of the rudimentary morphologic right ventricle.[38]

Coronary artery origins in truncus arteriosus (see Chapter 28) correspond to the number and spatial relationships of the quadricuspid, tricuspid, or bicuspid truncal valve (Fig. 32–12).[39,136,151] Truncal cusps that face the atrioventricular orifices lie posterior, and the cusp or cusps that do not face the atrioventricular orifices lie anterior.[39] When the truncal valve is tricuspid, the right coronary artery arises from the right anterior sinus, and the left coronary artery arises from the posterior sinus or the left anterior sinus (Fig. 32–12A). Bicuspid truncal valve cusps are oriented right/left or anterior/posterior (see Fig. 32–12B). When the cusps are anterior/posterior, the left coronary artery or a single coronary artery arises from the posterior sinus, and the right coronary artery arises from the anterior sinus (see Fig. 32–12B).[1,39] When bicuspid truncal valves are oriented right/left, the right coronary artery arises from the right sinus, and the left coronary artery arises from the left sinus.[39] Quadricuspid truncal valves are associated with two types of coronary artery arrangements. When two of the four truncal cusps are posterior and two are anterior, the left coronary artery arises from the left posterior sinus, and the right coronary

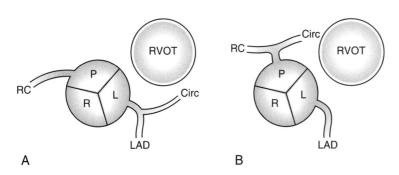

A   **B**

Figure 32–9

Illustrations of the coronary arteries in complete transposition of the great arteries. The two aortic sinuses facing the right ventricular outflow tract (RVOT) are designated the left sinus (L) and the posterior sinus (P). The right (R) sinus does not face the right ventricular outflow tract. A, The left coronary artery arises from the left sinus (L) and divides into the circumflex coronary artery (Circ) and the left anterior descending artery (LAD). The right coronary artery (RC) arises from the posterior sinus (P). B, The left anterior descending coronary artery arises from the left sinus (L), and a second coronary artery arises from the posterior sinus (P) and branches into the right coronary artery (RC) and the circumflex coronary artery (Circ).

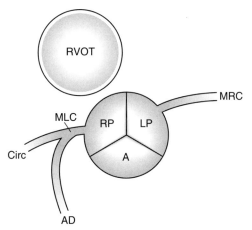

Figure 32–10

Illustration of the coronary arteries in congenitally corrected transposition of the great arteries. The left posterior sinus (LP) and the right posterior sinus (RP) face the right ventricular outflow tract (RVOT). The anterior sinus (A) is noncoronary. The morphologic right coronary artery (MRC) arises from the left posterior sinus. The morphologic left coronary artery (MLC) arises from the right posterior sinus and divides into the circumflex coronary artery (Circ) and the anterior descending artery (AD).

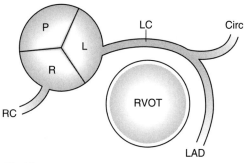

Figure 32–11

Illustration of the coronary arteries in double-outlet right ventricle. The right coronary artery (RC) arises from the right aortic sinus (R), and the left coronary artery (LC) arises from the left aortic sinus (LC) and branches into the left anterior descending coronary artery (LAD) and the circumflex artery (Circ), as in the normal heart.

artery arises from the right or left anterior sinus (see Fig. 32–12C).[1,39,155] In both of these arrangements, high origins of right and left coronary artery ostia are frequent.[1,155]

Isolated quadricuspid valves are rare (see Chapter 7).[77,78] In one such patient, a single coronary artery arose from the right anterior sinus.[70] Isolated bicuspid aortic valves are associated with two types of cusp relationships and coronary artery origins (Fig. 32–13). The two cusps may be oriented anterior/posterior with both coronary arteries arising from the anterior sinus (see Fig. 32–13A), or the cusps may be oriented right/left with the right coronary artery arising from the right sinus and the left coronary artery arising from the left sinus (see Fig. 32–13B). Bicuspid aortic valves tend to be associated with left coronary artery dominance and have a relatively high incidence of immediate bifurcation of the left coronary artery into circumflex and left anterior descending arteries.[66,85,118,132]

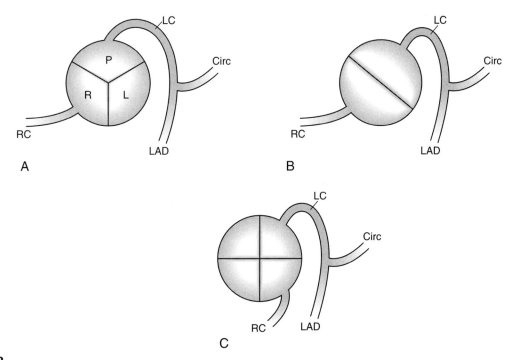

Figure 32–12

Illustrations of the coronary arteries in truncus arteriosus. A, When the truncal valve is trileaflet, the left coronary artery (LC) arises from the posterior sinus and divides into the circumflex coronary artery (Circ) and the left anterior descending artery (LAD). The right coronary artery (RC) arises from the right aortic sinus (R). B, When the truncal valve is bicuspid, the right coronary artery (RC) arises from the anterior sinus, and the left coronary artery (LC) arises from the posterior sinus and divides into the circumflex coronary artery (Circ) and the left anterior descending artery (LAD). C, When the truncal valve is quadricuspid, two of the aortic sinuses are posterior and two are anterior. The right coronary artery (RC) arises from the left anterior sinus. The left coronary artery (LC) arises from the left posterior sinus and divides into the circumflex coronary artery (Circ) and the left anterior descending artery (LAD).

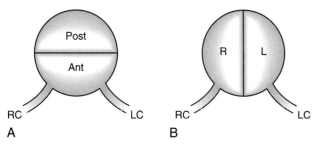

Figure 32–13
Illustrations of the coronary arteries when the aortic valve is bicuspid. *A*, When the two cusps are posteroanterior, the right coronary artery (RC) and the left coronary artery (LC) both originate in the sinus of the anterior cusp. *B*, When the two cusps are right/left, the right coronary artery (RC) and the left coronary artery (LC) each arise concordantly from the right coronary sinus (R) and the left coronary sinus (L).

ACQUIRED ANOMALIES OF CORONARY ARTERIES SECONDARY TO CONGENITAL HEART DISEASE
(TABLE 32–4)

Coarctation of the aorta is associated with extramural and intramural abnormalities of the coronary arteries (see Chapter 8). Systemic hypertension causes intimal proliferation and medial thickening and is a risk factor for premature coronary atherosclerosis.[131,154,155] Luminal size increases in proportion to medial thickness.[88,155] Intramural coronary arteries and arterioles have thick walls, a rich adventitia, and dense collagen and elastic fibers.[131]

Supravalvular aortic stenosis (see Chapter 7) is associated with extramural coronary artery abnormalities analogous to coarctation of the aorta[100,105,120,149,155] Ostial obstruction is caused by aortic medial proliferation or by adherence of an aortic cusp.[105] Because the extramural coronary arteries are exposed to systolic hypertension proximal to the supravalvular stenosis, they are thick-walled, dilated, tortuous, and prematurely atherosclerotic.

Severe chronic bicuspid aortic regurgitation is accompanied by large, smooth-walled extramural coronary arteries in response to the increase in left ventricular mass of a geometrically normal but magnified left ventricle. Coronary artery ectasia refers to elongation, tortuosity, and dilatation of extramural coronary arteries in adults with cyanotic congenital heart disease (Fig. 32–14).[16,109] High viscosity of the erythrocytic perfusate increases endothelial shear stress, with release of vasodilatory nitric oxide and prostaglandins.[177]

In pulmonary atresia with intact ventricular septum (see Chapter 24), suprasystemic pressure in the blind hypoplastic right ventricle generates flow through intramural intratrabecular channels with the development of ventricular-coronary artery connections.[18,19,22,68,107] These vascular abnormalities are not primary disorders of coronary artery development. Myocardial ischemia is caused by the fistulous steal associated with aortic diastolic runoff into the right ventricle through large unobstructed intramural channels.[107] Ischemia is also caused by epicardial, intramural, medial, and intimal thickening with luminal narrowing of the ventricular-coronary arterial channels that extend from their right ventricular origins to the coronary ostia.[19,22,61,68] The luminal narrowing ranges from mild to obliteration to coronary ostial discontinuity.[19,68,79,148]

The coronary circulation in aortic atresia with mitral atresia is not accompanied by ventricular-coronary artery channels because the sealed left ventricle cannot generate suprasystemic pressure.[5,102,114,124,130] When a hypoplastic mitral valve is perforate, the small left ventricle receives diastolic flow, contracts isovolumetrically, and generates suprasystemic pressure. Nevertheless, intramyocardial sinusoids with direct ventricular-coronary artery connections do not develop, so the suprasystemic left ventricular pressure is not transmitted into epicardial coronary arteries, which are spared the morphologic changes that characterize pulmonary atresia with intact ventricular septum. A sinusoidal-capillary network develops, but coronary arterial abnormalities, if present at all, consist of tortuosity and an increase in wall thickness, not luminal narrowing.[5,130]

Paradoxical emboli to the coronary arteries are rare secondary complications of cyanotic congenital heart disease.[48,67] A right-to-left intracardiac shunt potentially delivers paradoxical emboli from a peripheral thromboembolic source.

CONGENITAL ANOMALIES INVOLVING THE CORONARY SINUS (TABLE 32–5)

The coronary sinus is the site of a variety of congenital abnormalities.[8,91,137] Partial or complete absence results from absence of the roof, from absence of the entire coronary sinus, or from an atrial septal defect that occupies the site of the ostium of the coronary sinus (see Chapter 15). Hypoplasia of the coronary sinus is a response to diversion of blood from the sinus into dilated thebesian veins. Stenosis or atresia of the ostium is characterized by a coronary sinus that is hypoplastic or that ends blindly.[156] A left superior vena cava carries coronary sinus blood retrograde into the left innominate vein (see

---

Table 32–4 Acquired Anomalies of Coronary Arteries Secondary to Congenital Heart Disease

Coarctation of the aorta

Supravalvular aortic stenosis

Aortic regurgitation

Coronary ectasia with cyanotic congenital heart disease

Pulmonary atresia with intact ventricular septum and hypoplastic right ventricle

Aortic atresia with intact ventricular septum and hypoplastic left ventricle

Paradoxical coronary artery emboli

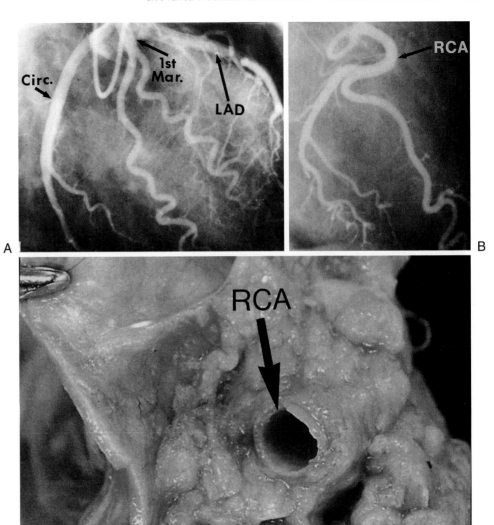

Figure 32-14
Coronary arteriograms from a 50-year-old cyanotic man with a nonrestrictive ventricular septal defect and Eisenmenger syndrome. *A*, The circumflex coronary artery (Circ) and the left anterior descending artery (LAD) are dilated, and the first marginal artery (1st Mar) is dilated and tortuous. *B*, The right coronary artery (RCA) is dilated and tortuous. *C*, Dilated right coronary artery (RCA) from a 40-year-old cyanotic woman with double-outlet right ventricle, a subpulmonary ventricular septal defect (Taussig Bing), and pulmonary vascular disease.

Table 32-5	Congenital Anomalies of the Coronary Sinus

Partial or complete absence:

   Coronary sinus atrial septal defect

   Unroofed coronary sinus

Hypoplasia of the coronary sinus

Stenosis or atresia of the ostium of the coronary sinus

Enlargement of the coronary sinus

   Without left-to-right shunt:

      Persistent left superior vena cava

      Anomalous inferior vena caval drainage

      Partial anomalous hepatic venous connection

   With left-to-right shunt:

      Total anomalous pulmonary venous connection

      Unroofed coronary sinus

      Coronary artery to coronary sinus fistula

Modified from Mantini E, Grondin CW, Lillehei CW, Edwards JE: Congenital anomalies involving the coronary sinus. Circulation 33:317, 1966.

Chapter 29).[49] The coronary sinus enlarges when it receives a left superior vena cava or a hepatic vein, when it is joined by a left superior vena cava that receives blood from the inferior vena cava via the hemiazygos vein (see Chapter 29), when it is the drainage site for total anomalous pulmonary venous connection (see Chapter 15), or when there is a coronary artery to coronary sinus fistula (see Chapter 22).

REFERENCES

1. Anderson KR, McGoon DC, Lie JT: Surgical significance of the coronary arterial anatomy in truncus arteriosus. Am J Cardiol 41:77, 1978.
2. Anderson RH, Becker AE: Cardiac Anatomy. London, Gower Medical Publishing, 1980.
3. Anderson RH, Becker AE, Lucchesse FE, et al: Morphology of Congenital Heart Disease. Baltimore, University Park Press, 1983.
4. Angelini P: Normal and anomalous coronary arteries: Definitions and classification. Am Heart J 117:418, 1989.
5. Baffa JM, Chen S, Guttenberg ME, et al: Coronary artery abnormalities and right ventricular histology in hypoplastic left heart syndrome. J Am Coll Cardiol 20:350, 1992.

6. Baird RJ, Manktelow RT, Shah PA, Ameli FM: Intramyocardial pressure. J Thorac Cardiovasc Surg 59:810, 1970.

7. Banchi A: Morfolgia della arteriae coronariae cordis. Arch Ital Anat Embriol 3:89, 1903.

8. Bankl H: Congenital Malformations of the Heart and Great Vessels. Baltimore, Urban & Schwarzenberg, 1977.

9. Barresi V, Susmano A, Colandrea MA, et al: Congenital absence of the circumflex coronary. Am Heart J 86:811, 1973.

10. Barth CW, Roberts WC: Left main coronary artery originating from the right sinus of Valsalva and coursing between the aorta and pulmonary trunk. J Am Coll Cardiol 7:366, 1986.

11. Barth CW, Bray M, Roberts WC: Sudden death in infancy associated with origin of both left main and right coronary arteries from a common ostium above the left sinus of Valsalva. Am J Cardiol 57:365, 1986.

12. Bedogni F, Castellani A, LaVecchia L, et al: Atresia of the left main coronary artery: Clinical recognition and surgical treatment. Cathet Cardiovasc Diagn 25:35, 1992.

13. Beretta L, Lemma M, Santoli C: Isolated atresia of the left main coronary artery in an adult. Eur J Cardiothorac Surg 4:169, 1990.

14. Biffani G, Lioy E, Loschiavo P, Parma A: Single coronary artery, anomalous origin of the right coronary artery from the left anterior descending artery. Eur Heart J 12:1326, 1991.

15. O'Malley CD, Saunders JB de CM: Translations, Text and Introduction. Leonardo Da Vinci On the Human Body. New York, Greenwich House, 1982.

16. Bjork L: Ectasia of the coronary arteries. Radiology 87:33, 1966.

17. Blake HA, Manion WC, Mattingly TW, Baroldi G: Coronary artery anomalies. Circulation 30:927, 1964.

18. Bull C, de Laval MR, Mercanti C, et al: Pulmonary atresia with intact ventricular septum. Circulation 66:266, 1982.

19. Burrows PE, Freedom RM, Benson LN, Moes CAF: Coronary angiography and pulmonary atresia with intact ventricular septum. Am J Roent 154:789, 1990.

20. Byrum CJ, Blackman MS, Schneider B, et al: Congenital atresia of the left coronary ostium and hypoplasia of the left main coronary artery. Am Heart J 99:354, 1980.

21. Caffersky EA, Crawford DW, Turner SF, et al: Congenital aneurysm of the coronary artery with myocardial infarction. Am J Med Sci 257:320, 1969.

22. Calder AL, Co EE, Shee MD: Coronary arterial abnormalities in pulmonary atresia with intact ventricular septum. Am J Cardiol 59:436, 1987.

23. Calder L, Van Praagh R, Van Praagh S, et al: Truncus arteriosus communus. Am Heart J 92:23, 1976.

24. Casta A: Hypoplasia of the left coronary artery complicated by reversible myocardial ischemia in a newborn. Am Heart J 114:1238, 1987.

25. Chaitman BR, Lesperance J, Saltiel J, Bourassa MJ: Clinical, angiographic, and hemodynamic findings in patients with anomalous origin of the coronary arteries. Circulation 53:122, 1976.

26. Cheatham JP, Ruyle NA, McManus BM, Bammel GE: Origin of the right coronary from the descending thoracic aorta. Cathet Cardiovasc Diagn 13:321, 1987.

27. Cheitlin MD, De Castro CM, McAllister HA: Sudden death as a complication of anomalous left coronary origin from the anterior sinus of Valsalva: A not-so-minor congenital anomaly. Circulation 50:780, 1974.

28. Click RL, Holms DR, Vlietstra RE, et al: Anomalous coronary arteries: Location, degree of atherosclerosis and effect on survival: A report from the coronary artery surgery study. J Am Coll Cardiol 13:531, 1989.

29. Cohen LS, Shaw LD: Fatal myocardial infarction in an 11 year old boy associated with a unique coronary artery anomaly. Am J Cardiol 19:420, 1967.

30. Conte G, Pellegrini A: On the development of the coronary arteries in human embryos, stages 14–19. Anat Embryol 169:209, 1984.

31. Coto EO, Jimenez MQ, Anderson RH, et al: Double outlet left ventricle. In Anderson RH, Macartney FJ, Shinebourne EA, Tynan M (eds): Paediatric Cardiology. Edinburgh, Churchill Livingstone, 1983.

32. Crocker DW, Sobin S, Thomas WC: Aneurysm of the coronary arteries. Am J Pathol 33:819, 1957.

33. Dabizzi RP, Barletta GA, Caprioli G, et al: Coronary artery anatomy in corrected transposition of the great arteries. J Am Coll Cardiol 12:486, 1988.

34. Dabizzi RP, Caprioli G, Aiazzi L, et al: Distribution and anomalies of coronary arteries in tetralogy of Fallot. Circulation 61:95, 1980.

35. Dabizzi RP, Teodori G, Barletta GA, et al: Associated coronary and cardiac anomalies in the tetralogy of Fallot: An angiographic study. Eur Heart J 11:692, 1990.

36. Davia JE, Green DC, Cheitlin MD, et al: Anomalous left coronary artery origin from the right coronary sinus. Am Heart J 108:165, 1984.

37. Davis JS, Lie JT: Anomalous origin of a single coronary artery from the innominate artery. Angiology 28:775, 1977.

38. Deanfield JE, Tommasini G, Anderson JH, Macartney FJ: Tricuspid atresia: Analysis of coronary artery distribution and ventricular morphology. Br Heart J 48:485, 1982.

39. de la Cruz MV, Cayre R, Angelini P, et al: Coronary arteries in truncus arteriosus. Am J Cardiol 66:1482, 1990.

40. Dicicco BS, McManus BM, Waller BF, Roberts WC: Separate aortic ostium of the left anterior descending and left circumflex coronary arteries from the left aortic sinus of Valsalva (absent left main coronary artery). Am Heart J 104:153, 1982.

41. Donaldson RM, Raphael MJ: Missing coronary artery: Review of technical problems in coronary arteriography resulting form anatomical variants. Br Heart J 47:62, 1982.

42. Elliott LP, Amplatz K, Edwards JE: Coronary arterial patterns in transposition complexes. Am J Cardiol 17:362, 1966.

43. Engle HJ, Torres C, Page H: Major variations in anatomical origin of the coronary arteries: Angiographic observations in 4,250 patients without associated congenital heart disease. Cathet Cardiovasc Diagn 1:157, 1975.

44. Fellows KE, Freed MD, Keane JF, et al: Results of routine preoperative coronary angiography in tetralogy of Fallot. Circulation 51:561, 1975.

45. Fernandes ED, Kadivar H, Hallman GL, et al: Congenital malformations of the coronary arteries: The Texas Heart Institute Experience. Ann Thorac Surg 54:732, 1992.

46. Fortuin NJ, Roberts WC: Congenital atresia of the left main coronary artery. Am J Med 50:385, 1971.

47. Gaither NS, Rogan KM, Stajduhar K, et al: Anomalous origin and course of coronary arteries in adults: Identification and improved imaging utilizing transesophageal echocardiography. Am Heart J 122:69, 1991.

48. Gerber RS, Sherman CT, Sack JB, Perloff JK: Isolated paradoxical embolus to the right coronary artery. Am J Cardiol 70:1634, 1992.

49. Gerlis LM, Gibbs JL, Williams GJ, Thomas GDH: Coronary sinus orifice atresia and persistent left superior vena cava. Br Heart J 52:648, 1984.

50. Gibson R, Nihill MR, Mullins CE, et al: Congenital coronary artery obstruction associated with aortic valve anomalies in children. Circulation 64:857, 1981.

51. Gittenberger-de Groot AC, Sauer U, Quaegebeur J: Aortic intramural coronary artery in three hearts with transposition of the great arteries. J Thorac Cardiovasc Surg 91:566, 1986.

52. Gobel FL, Anderson CF, Baltaxe HA, et al: Shunts between the coronary and pulmonary arteries with normal origin of the pulmonary arteries. Am J Cardiol 25:656, 1970.

53. Greenberg MA, Fish BG, Spindola-Franco H: Congenital anomalies of the coronary arteries: Classification and significance. Radiol Clin N Am 27:1127, 1989.

54. Habbab MA, Senft AG, Haft JI: Origin of the right coronary artery from the left anterior descending coronary artery: A very rare anomaly of coronary arterial origin. Am Heart J 114:169, 1987.

55. Hackensellner HA: Aksessorische Kranzgefassanlagen der Arteria pulmonalis unter 63 menschlichen Embryonenserien mit einer grossten Lange von 12 bis 36 mm. Mikroscopischanat Forsch 62:153, 1956.

56. Harris PN: Aneurysmal dilatation of the cardiac coronary arteries. Am J Pathol 13:89, 1937.

57. Heifetz SA, Robinowitz M, Mueller KH, Viramini R: Total anomalous origin of the coronary arteries from the pulmonary artery. Pediatr Cardiol 7:11, 1986.

58. Henson KD, Geiser EA, Billett J, et al: Use of transesophageal echocardiography to visualize an anomalous right coronary artery arising from the left main coronary artery (single coronary artery). Clin Cardiol 15:462, 1992.

59. Hirakow R: Development of the cardiac blood vessels in staged human embryos. Acta Anat 115:220, 1983.

60. Hobbs RE, Millit HD, Raghavan PV, et al: Congenital coronary artery anomalies. Cardiovasc Clin 12:43, 1982.

61. Hubbard JF, Girod DA, Caldwell RL, et al: Right ventricular infarction with cardiac rupture in an infant with pulmonary valve atresia with intact ventricular septum. J Am Coll Cardiol 2:363, 1983.

62. Hurwitz RA, Smith W, King H, et al: Tetralogy of Fallot with abnormal coronary artery: 1967 to 1977. J Thorac Cardiovasc Surg 80:129, 1980.
63. Hutchins GM, Kessler-Hanna A, Moore GW: Development of the coronary arteries in the embryonic human heart. Circulation 77:1250, 1988.
64. Ishikawa T, Brandt PWT: Anomalous origin of the left main coronary artery from the right anterior aortic sinus. Am J Cardiol 55:770, 1985.
65. James TN: Anatomy of the Coronary Arteries. New York, Paul B. Hoeber, 1961.
66. Johnson AD, Detwiler JH, Higgins CB: Left coronary arterial anatomy in patients with bicuspid aortic valves. Br Heart J 40:489, 1978.
67. Jungbluth A, Erbel R, Darius H, et al: Paradoxical coronary embolism: Case report and review of the literature. Am Heart J 116:879, 1988.
68. Kasznica J, Ursell PC, Blanc WA, Gersony WM: Abnormalities of the coronary circulation in pulmonary atresia with intact ventricular septum. Am Heart J 114:1415, 1987.
69. Kessler KM, Feldman T, Harding L, et al: Anomalous origin of the right coronary artery from the left sinus of Valsalva: Echocardiographic-angiographic correlations. Am Heart J 115:470, 1988.
70. Kim H, McBirde RA, Titus JL: Quadricuspid aortic valve and single coronary ostium. Arch Pathol Lab Med 112:842, 1988.
71. Kimbris D: Anomalous origin of the left main coronary artery from the right sinus of Valsalva. Am J Cardiol 55:765, 1985.
72. Kimbris D, Iskandrian AS, Segal BL, Bemis CE: Anomalous aortic origin of coronary arteries. Circulation 58:606, 1978.
73. Koh KK: Confirmation of anomalous origin of the right coronary artery from the left sinus of Valsalva by means of transesophageal echocardiography. Am Heart J 122:851, 1991.
74. Koh E, Nakagawa M, Hamaoka K, et al: Congenital atresia of the left coronary ostium: Diagnosis and surgical treatment. Pediatr Cardiol 10:159, 1989.
75. Kragel AH, Roberts WC: Anomalous origin of either the right or left main coronary artery from the aorta with subsequent coursing between aorta and pulmonary trunk: Analysis of 32 necropsy cases. Am J Cardiol 62:771, 1988.
76. Kurnik PB, Heymann WR: Coronary artery ectasia associated with hereditary hemorrhagic telangiectasia. Arch Intern Med 149:2357, 1989.
77. Kurosawa H, Wagenaar SS, Becker AE: Sudden death in a youth: A case of quadricuspid aortic valve with isolation of origin of left coronary artery. Br Heart J 46:211, 1981.
78. Lanzillo G, Breccia PA, Intoni F: Congenital quadricuspid aortic valve with displacement of the right coronary orifice. Scand J Thorac Cardiovasc Surg 15:149, 1981.
79. Lenox CC, Briner J: Absent proximal coronary arteries associated with pulmonic atresia. Am J Cardiol 30:666, 1972.
80. Lev M, Liberthson RR, Kirkpatrick JK, et al: Single (primitive) ventricle. Circulation 39:577, 1969.
81. Levin DC, Fellows KE, Abrams HL: Hemodynamically significant primary anomalies of the coronary arteries. Circulation 58:25, 1978.
82. Levin SE, Zarvos P, Milner S, Schmaman A: Arteriohepatic dysplasia. Pediatrics 66:876, 1980.
83. Liberthson RR: Congenital anomalies of the coronary arteries. Cardiovasc Med 9:857, 1984.
84. Liberthson RR, Dinsmore RE, Bharati S, et al: Aberrant coronary artery origin from the aorta: Diagnosis and clinical significance. Circulation 50:774, 1974.
85. Line DE, Babb JD, Pierce WS: Congenital aortic valve anomaly; aortic regurgitation with left coronary artery isolation. J Thorac Cardiovasc Surg 77:533, 1979.
86. Longenecker CG, Reemstma K, Creech O Jr: Anomalous coronary artery distribution associated with tetralogy of Fallot: A hazard in open cardiac repair. J Thorac Cardiovasc Surg 42:258, 1961.
87. Losekoot TG, Anderson RH, Becker AE, et al: Congenitally Corrected Transposition. Edinburgh, Churchill Livingstone, 1983.
88. MacAlpin RN, Abbasi AS, Grollman JH, Eber L: Human coronary artery size during life. Diagn Radiol 108:567, 1973.
89. MacMahon HE, Dickinson PCT: Occlusive fibroelastosis of coronary arteries in the newborn. Circulation 35:3, 1967.
90. Manasek FJ: Histogenesis of the embryonic myocardium. Am J Cardiol 25:149, 1970.
91. Mantini E, Grondin CW, Lillehei CW, Edwards JE: Congenital anomalies involving the coronary sinus. Circulation 33:317, 1966.
92. Maron BJ, Leon MB, Swain JA, et al: Prospective identification by two-dimensional echocardiography of anomalous origin of the left main coronary artery from the right sinus of Valsalva. Am J Cardiol 68:140, 1991.
93. Maron BJ, Roberts WC, McAllister HA, et al: Sudden death in young athletes. Circulation 62:218, 1980.
94. Mayer JE, Sanders SP, Jonas RA, Castaneda AR, Wernovsky G: Coronary artery pattern and outcome of arterial switch operation for transposition of the great arteries. Circulation 82(Suppl IV):IV-139, 1990.
95. Meng CC, Eckner FA, Lev M: Coronary artery distribution in tetralogy of Fallot. Arch Surg 90:363, 1965.
96. Murphy ML: Single coronary artery. Am Heart J 74:557, 1967.
97. Muus CJ, McManus BM: Common origin of right and left coronary arteries from the region of left sinus of Valsalva: Association with unexpected intrauterine fetal death. Am Heart J 107:1285, 1984.
98. Nath A, Kennett JD, Politte LL, et al: Anomalous right coronary artery arising from the midportion of the left anterior descending coronary artery. Angiology 38:142, 1987.
99. Nelson-Piercy C, Rickards AF, Yacoub MH: Aberrant origin of the right coronary artery as a potential cause of sudden death: Successful anatomical correction. Br Heart J 64:208, 1990.
100. Neufeld HN, Wagenvoort CA, Ongley PA, Edwards JE: Hypoplasia of the ascending aorta. Am J Cardiol 10:746, 1962.
101. Newton MC, Burwell LR: Single coronary artery with myocardial infarction and mitral regurgitation. Am Heart J 95:126, 1978.
102. O'Connor WN, Cash JB, Cottril CM, et al: Ventriculocoronary connections in hypoplastic left hearts. Circulation 66:1078, 1982.
103. Page HL, Siegel HJ, Campbell WB, Thomas CS: Anomalous origin of the left circumflex coronary artery. Circulation 50:768, 1974.
104. Palomo AR, Shrager BR, Chahine RA: Anomalous origin of the right coronary artery from the ascending aorta high above the left posterior sinus of Valsalva of a bicuspid aortic valve. Am Heart J 109:902, 1985.
105. Pansegrau DG, Kioshos JM, Durnin RE, Kroetz FW: Supravalvular aortic stenosis in adults. Am J Cardiol 31:635, 1973.
106. Partridge JB: High leftward origin of the right coronary artery. Int J Cardiol 13:83, 1986.
107. Patel RG, Freedom RM, Moes CAF, et al: Right ventricular volume determinations in 18 patients with pulmonary atresia and intact ventricular septum. Circulation 61:428, 1980.
108. Patten BM: The development of the heart. In Gould SE (ed): Pathology of the Heart. Springfield, Illinois, Charles C Thomas, 1968.
109. Perloff JK, Urschell CW, Roberts WC, Caulfield WH: Aneurysmal dilatation of the coronary arteries in cyanotic congenital heart disease. Am J Med 45:802, 1968.
110. Piovesana P, Corrado D, Contessotto F, et al: Echocardiographic identification of anomalous origin of the left circumflex coronary artery from the right sinus of Valsalva. Am Heart J 119:205, 1990.
111. Piovesana P, Corrado D, Verlato R, et al: Morbidity associated with anomalous origin of the left circumflex coronary artery from the right aortic sinus. Am J Cardiol 63:762, 1989.
112. Pollack BD, Belkin RN, Lazar S, et al: Origin of all three coronary arteries from separate ostia in the right sinus of Valsalva. Catheter Cardiovasc Diag 26:26, 1992.
113. Price AC, Lee DA, Kagen KE, Baker WP: Aortic dysplasia in infancy simulating anomalous origin of the left coronary artery. Circulation 48:434, 1973.
114. Raghib G, Bloemendaal RD, Kanjuh VI, Edwards JE: Aortic atresia and premature closure of foramen ovale: Myocardial sinusoids and coronary arteriovenous fistula serving as outflow channel. Am Heart J 70:746, 1965.
115. Rakusan K, Flanagan MF, Geva T, et al: Morphometry of human coronary capillaries during normal growth and the effect of age in left ventricular pressure-overload hypertrophy. Circulation 86:38, 1992.
116. Reemstma K, Longenecker CG, Creech O Jr: Surgical anatomy of the coronary artery distribution in congenital heart disease. Circulation 24:782, 1961.
117. Roberts WC: Anomalous origin of both coronary arteries from the pulmonary artery. Am J Cardiol 10:595, 1962.
118. Roberts WC: Congenitally bicuspid aortic valve: A study of 85 autopsy patients. Am J Cardiol 26:72, 1970.

119. Roberts WC: Major anomalies of coronary arterial origin seen in adulthood. Am Heart J 111:941, 1986.

120. Roberts WC: Valvular, subvalvular and supravalvular aortic stenosis. Cardiovasc Clin 5:104, 1973.

121. Roberts WC, Kragel AH: Anomalous origin of either the right or left main coronary artery from the aorta without coursing of the anomalistically arising artery between aorta and pulmonary trunk. Am J Cardiol 62:1263, 1988.

122. Roberts WC, Shirani J: The four subtypes of anomalous origin of the left main coronary artery from the right aortic sinus (or from the right coronary artery). Am J Cardiol 70:119, 1992.

123. Roberts WC, Dicicco BS, Waller BF, et al: Origin of the left main from the right coronary artery or from the right aortic sinus with intramyocardial tunneling to the left side of the heart via the ventricular septum. Am Heart J 104:303, 1982.

124. Roberts WC, Perry LW, Chandra RS, et al: Aortic valve atresia. Am J Cardiol 37:753, 1976.

125. Roberts WC, Siegel RJ, Zipes DM: Origin of the right coronary artery from the left sinus of Valsalva and its functional consequences. Am J Cardiol 49:863, 1982.

126. Robicsek F: Origin of the left anterior descending coronary artery from the left mammary artery. Am Heart J 108:1377, 1984.

127. Rossi MB, Ho SY, Anderson RH, et al: Coronary arteries in complete transposition: The significance of the sinus node artery. Ann Thorac Surg 42:573, 1986.

128. Russo G, Tamburino C, Licciardello G, et al: Isolated, anomalous origin of the left anterior descending coronary artery from the right coronary artery with angina pectoris. Eur Heart J 12:558, 1991.

129. Samdarshi TE, Hill DL, Nanda NC: Transesophageal color Doppler diagnosis of anomalous origin of left circumflex coronary artery. Am Heart J 122:571, 1991.

130. Sauer U, Gittenberger-de Groot AC, Geishauer M, et al: Coronary arteries in the hypoplastic left heart syndrome: Histopathologic and histometrical studies and implications for surgery. Circulation 80(Suppl. I):I-168, 1989.

131. Schneeweiss A, Sherf L, Lehrer E, et al: Segmental study of the terminal coronary vessels in coarctation of the aorta. Am J Cardiol 49:1996, 1982.

132. Scholz DG, Lynch JA, Willerscheidt AB, et al: Coronary arterial dominance associated with congenital bicuspid aortic valve. Arch Pathol Lab Med 104:417, 1980.

133. Scott DH: Aneurysms of the coronary arteries. Br Heart J 36:403, 1948.

134. Shaher RM, Pudder GC: The coronary arterial anatomy in complete transposition of the great vessels. Am J Cardiol 16:406, 1965.

135. Sharbaugh AH, White RS: Single coronary artery: Analysis of the anatomic variation, clinical importance, and report of five cases. JAMA 230:243, 1974.

136. Shrivastava S, Edwards JE: Coronary arterial origin in persistent truncus arteriosus. Circulation 55:551, 1977.

137. Silver MA, Rowley NE: The functional anatomy of the human coronary sinus. Am Heart J 115:1080, 1988.

138. Sissman N: Developmental landmarks in cardiac morphogenesis: Comparative chronology. Am J Cardiol 25:141, 1970.

139. Smith JC: Review of single coronary artery with report of two cases. Circulation 1:1168, 1950.

140. Smith A, Arnold R, Wilkinson JL, et al: An anatomical study of the patterns of the coronary arteries and sinus nodal artery in complete transposition. Int J Cardiol 12:295, 1986.

141. Sreenivasan VV, Jocobstein MD: Origin of the right coronary artery from the pulmonary trunk. Am J Cardiol 69:1513, 1992.

142. Taylor AJ, Rogan KM, Virmani R: Sudden cardiac death associated with isolated congenital coronary artery anomalies. J Am Coll Cardiol 20:640, 1992.

143. Teplitsky I, Wurzel M, Melamed R, Aygen M: Anomalous origin of the coronary arteries. Angiology 38:128, 1987.

144. Thomas D, Salloum J, Montalescout G, et al: Anomalous coronary arteries coursing between the aorta and pulmonary trunk: Clinical indications for coronary artery bypass. Eur Heart J 12:832, 1991.

145. Tomanek RJ: Age as a modulator of coronary capillary angiogenesis. Circulation 86:320, 1992.

146. Topaz O, DeMarchena EJ, Perin E, et al: Anomalous coronary arteries: Angiographic findings in 80 patients. Int J Cardiol 34:129, 1992.

147. Tsung SH, Huang TY, Chang HH: Sudden death in young athletes. Arch Pathol Lab Med 106:168, 1982.

148. Ueda K, Saito A, Nakano H, Hamazaki Y: Absence of proximal coronary arteries associated with pulmonary atresia. Am Heart J 106:596, 1983.

149. Underhill WL, Tredway JB, D'Angelo GL, Baay JEW: Familial supravalvular aortic stenosis: Comments on the mechanisms of angina pectoris. Am J Cardiol 27:560, 1971.

150. Van der Hauwaert LG, Dumoulin M, Moerman P: Congenital atresia of the left coronary ostium. Br Heart J 48:298, 1982.

151. Van Praagh R, Van Praagh S: The anatomy of common aortico-pulmonary trunk (truncus arteriosus communis) and its embryologic implications. Am J Cardiol 16:406, 1965.

152. Van Praagh R, Davidoff A, Chin A, et al: Double outlet right ventricle: Anatomic types and developmental implications based on a study of 101 autopsied cases. Coeur 8:389, 1982.

153. Virmani R, Chun PKC, Rogan K, Riddick L: Anomalous origin of four coronary ostia from the right sinus of Valsalva. Am J Cardiol 63:760, 1989.

154. Vlodaver Z, Neufeld HN: The coronary arteries in coarctation of the aorta. Circulation 37:449, 1968.

155. Vlodaver Z, Neufeld HN, Edwards JE: Coronary Arterial Variations in the Normal Heart and in Congenital Heart Disease. New York, Academic Press, 1975.

156. Watson GH: Atresia of the coronary sinus orifice. Pediatr Cardiol 6:99, 1985.

157. Wong CK, Cheng CH, Lau CP, Leung WH: Asymptomatic congenital coronary artery aneurysm in adulthood. Eur Heart J 10:947, 1989.

158. Yamaguchi M, Tsukube T, Yosokawa Y, et al: Pulmonary origin of left anterior descending coronary artery in tetralogy of Fallot. Ann Thorac Surg 52:310, 1991.

159. Yamanaka O, Hobbs RE: Coronary artery anomalies in 126,595 patients undergoing coronary arteriography. Cathet Cardiovasc Diagn 21:28, 1990.

160. Young-Hyman PJ, Tommaso CL, Singleton RT: A new double coronary artery anomaly: The right coronary artery originating above the coronary sinus giving off the circumflex artery. J Am Coll Cardiol 4:1329, 1984.

161. Zureikat HY: Collateral vessels between the coronary and bronchial arteries in patients with cyanotic congenital heart disease. Am J Cardiol 45:599, 1980.

162. Baroldi G, Scomazzoni G: Coronary Circulation in the Normal Heart and the Pathologic Heart. Washington, DC, United States Government Printing Office, 1967.

163. Sones FM, Shirey EK: Cine coronary arteriography. Mod Conc Cardiovasc Dis 31:735, 1962.

164. Sedmera D, Vuillemin M, Thompson RP, Anderson RH: Developmental patterning of the myocardium. Anat Rec 258:319, 2000.

165. Cortis BS, Serratto M: The collateral coronary circulation in the human fetus. Cardiologia 43:77, 1998.

166. Hekmat V, Rao SM, Chhabra M, et al: Anomalous origin of the right coronary artery from the main pulmonary artery. Clin Cardiol 21:773, 1998.

167. Poullis M: Anomalous origin of the right coronary artery. Clin Cardiol 22:815, 1999.

168. Albertal J, Lynch FG, Vaccarino G, Vrancic M: Anomalous origin of right coronary artery. Circulation 103:e73, 2001.

169. Ropers D, Moshage W, Daniel WG, Jessel J: Visualization of coronary artery anomalies and their anatomic course by contrast-enhanced electron beam tomography and three-dimensional reconstruction. Am J Cardiol 87:193, 2001.

170. Cox ID, Bunce N, Fluck DS: Failed sudden cardiac death in a patient with an anomalous origin of the right coronary artery. Circulation 102:1461, 2000.

171. Davis JA, Cecchin F, Jones TK, Portman MA: Major coronary artery anomalies in a pediatric population. J Am Coll Cardiol 37:593, 2001.

172. Pelliccia A: Congenital coronary anomalies in young patients. J Am Coll Cardiol 37:598, 2001.

173. Taylor AM, Thorne SA, Rubens MB, Jhooti P, Keegan J: Coronary artery imaging in grown up congenital heart disease. Complementary role of magnetic resonance and x-ray coronary angiography. Circulation 101:1670, 2000.

174. Weber HS, Zangwill SD, Zachary CH, Cyran SE: Transvenous approach to coronary angiography in infants with tetralogy of Fallot. Am J Cardiol 83:630, 1999.

175. Fernandez F, Alam M, Smith S: The role of transesophageal echocardiography in identifying anomalous coronary arteries. Circulation 88:2532, 1995.

176. Brooks H: Two cases of abnormal coronary artery of the heart arising from the pulmonary artery. J Anat 20:26, 1885.

177. Perloff JK, Rosove MH, Sietsema KE: Cyanotic congenital heart disease: A multisystem systemic disorder. In Perloff JK, Child JS (eds): Congenital Heart Disease in Adults, 2nd ed. Philadelphia, WB Saunders, 1998, p 199.

178. Basso C, Maron BJ, Corrado D, Thiene G: Clinical profile of congenital coronary artery anomalies with origin from the wrong aortic sinus leading to sudden death in young competitive athletes. J Am Coll Cardiol 35:1493, 2000.

Index

Note: Page numbers followed by the letter f refer to figures; those followed by the letter t refer to tables.